Pharmaceutical Inhalation Aerosol Technology

DRUGS AND THE PHARMACEUTICAL SCIENCES

A Series of Textbooks and Monographs

Series Executive Editor
James Swarbrick
Pharmaceutech, Inc.
Pinehurst, North Carolina

Recent Titles in Series

Good Manufacturing Practices for Pharmaceuticals, Seventh Edition, *Graham P. Bunn*

Pharmaceutical Extrusion Technology, Second Edition, *Isaac Ghèbre-Sellassie, Charles E. Martin, Feng Zhang, and James Dinunzio*

Biosimilar Drug Product Development, *Laszlo Endrenyi, Paul Declerck, and Shein-Chung Chow*

High Throughput Screening in Drug Discovery, *Amancio Carnero*

Generic Drug Product Development: International Regulatory Requirements for Bioequivalence, Second Edition, *Isadore Kanfer and Leon Shargel*

Aqueous Polymeric Coatings for Pharmaceutical Dosage Forms, Fourth Edition, *Linda A. Felton*

Good Design Practices for GMP Pharmaceutical Facilities, Second Edition, *Terry Jacobs and Andrew A. Signore*

Handbook of Bioequivalence Testing, Second Edition, *Sarfaraz K. Niazi*

Generic Drug Product Development: Solid Oral Dosage Forms, Second Edition, *edited by Leon Shargel and Isadore Kanfer*

Drug Stereochemistry: Analytical Methods and Pharmacology, Third Edition, *edited by Krzysztof Jozwiak, W. J. Lough, and Irving W. Wainer*

Pharmaceutical Powder Compaction Technology, Second Edition, *edited by Metin Çelik*

Pharmaceutical Stress Testing: Predicting Drug Degradation, Second Edition, *edited by Steven W. Baertschi, Karen M. Alsante, and Robert A. Reed*

Pharmaceutical Process Scale-Up, Third Edition, *edited by Michael Levin*

Sterile Drug Products: Formulation, Packaging, Manufacturing, and Quality, *Michael J. Akers*

Pharmaceutical Inhalation Aerosol Technology

Third Edition

Edited by

Anthony J. Hickey
Sandro R.P. da Rocha

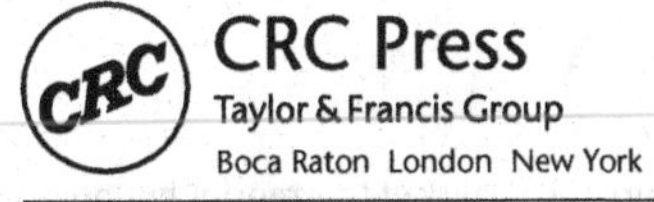

CRC Press is an imprint of the
Taylor & Francis Group, an **informa** business

CRC Press
Taylor & Francis Group
6000 Broken Sound Parkway NW, Suite 300
Boca Raton, FL 33487-2742

First issued in paperback 2021

ISBN 13: 978-1-03-209322-2 (pbk)
ISBN 13: 978-1-1380-6307-5 (hbk)

Library of Congress Cataloging-in-Publication Data

Names: Hickey, Anthony J., 1955- editor.
Title: Pharmaceutical inhalation aerosol technology
/ [edited by] Anthony J. Hickey, Sandro R.P. da Rocha.
implementing game mechanics, art, design and programming / Penny de Byl.
Description: Third edition. | Boca Raton, Florida : CRC Press, [2019] |
Drugs and the pharmaceutical sciences |
Includes bibliographical references and
index
Identifiers: 2018044344| ISBN 9781138063075 (hardback : alk.paper)
ISBN 9780429055201 (ebook)
Subjects: LCSH: Aerosol therapy.
Classification: LCC RM161 .P55 2019 | DDC 615/.6--dc23
LC record available at https://lccn.loc.gov/2018044344

Visit the Taylor & Francis Web site at
http://www.taylorandfrancis.com

and the CRC Press Web site at
http://www.crcpress.com

Publisher's Note
The publisher has gone to great lengths to ensure the quality of this reprint but points out that some imperfections in the original copies may be apparent.

Contents

Section IV Particle Engineering/Processing

Section V Drug Product Formulation

Section VI Devices

Section VII Drug Product Testing

Section VIII Regulatory Considerations

Section IX Preclinical Testing

Section X Clinical Testing

Preface

Two previous editions of the book *Pharmaceutical Inhalation Aerosol Technology* (PhIAT) were published in 1993 and 2004. The first edition appeared at a time when few books on aerosol technology were available, notably those of WC Hinds (*Aerosol Technology*, Wiley) and PC Reist (*Introduction to Aerosol Science*) that had only been available for a decade. There were few general texts on medical aerosols, and those were in specialized areas, notably several volumes by Stephen Newman. With this background, the original PhIAT book was intended to broadly cover all aspects of the field from lung biology (pharmacology, physiology, and anatomy) to drug product manufacturing, performance, and clinical applications. In the intervening decades many new volumes have appeared and much more has been published on aerosol physics, formulation and device development, and therapeutic strategies, supported by the commercialization of many new drug products.

This edition of PhIAT not only provides an update on many topics addressed in the 2nd edition, but also expands the "technology" focus of the original volumes to address the title more directly. Since the major purpose of any book should be its utility to the reader, it is logical to look at the topic from the perspective of clear unmet needs. The new text covers all aspects of product development and manufacturing encompassing the important areas of preformulation, formulation, device selection, and drug product evaluation. In order to expand the scope to consider previously unaddressed aspects of pharmaceutical inhalation aerosol technology, considerations of the patient interface have been restricted to those aspects of aerosol delivery, lung deposition, and clearance that are used as measures of effective dose delivery.

The introduction of Dr. Sandro da Rocha as co-editor of the new edition reflects the intention to bring engineering principles to bear on this important topic and to stress the importance of pharmaceutical engineering as a foundational element of all inhaler products and their application to pulmonary drug delivery.

We are grateful to the publishing staff, in particular, Hilary LaFoe and Jessica Poile for their assistance in navigating the manuscript through the process.

This book is dedicated in memory of Professor Paul Myrdal, outstanding scientist, educator, family man, and friend. He is missed by all.

Anthony J. Hickey
Chapel Hill, NC

Sandro R.P. da Rocha
Richmond, VA
September 2018

Editors

Anthony J. Hickey is Distinguished RTI Fellow at the Research Triangle Institute, Emeritus Professor of Molecular Pharmaceutics of the Eshelman School of Pharmacy (2010–present, Professor 1993–2010), and Adjunct Professor of Biomedical Engineering in the School of Medicine at the University of North Carolina at Chapel Hill. He obtained PhD (1984) and DSc (2003) degrees in Pharmaceutical Sciences from Aston University, Birmingham, United Kingdom. Following postdoctoral positions, at the University of Kentucky (1984–1988), Dr. Hickey joined the faculty at the University of Illinois at Chicago (1988–1993). In 1990 he received the AAPS Young Investigator Award in Pharmaceutics and Pharmaceutical Technology. He is a Fellow of the Royal Society of Biology (2000), the American Association of Pharmaceutical Scientists (2003), the American Association for the Advancement of Science (2005), and the Royal Society of Biology (2017). He received the Research Achievement Award of the Particulate Presentations and Design Division of the Powder Technology Society of Japan (2012), the Distinguished Scientist Award of the American Association of Indian Pharmaceutical Scientists (2013); the David W. Grant Award in Physical Pharmacy of the American Association of Pharmaceutical Scientists (2015); Thomas T. Mercer Joint Prize for Excellence in Inhaled Medicines and Pharmaceutical Aerosols of the American Association for Aerosol Research and the International Society for Aerosols in Medicine (2017). He has published numerous papers and chapters (over 250) in the pharmaceutical and biomedical literature, one of which received the AAPS Meritorious Manuscript Award in 2001. He has edited five texts on pharmaceutical inhalation aerosols and co-authored three others on "pharmaceutical process engineering," "pharmaceutical particulate science," and "pharmaco-complexity." He holds 25 United States patents on a variety of inhaler device technologies, pulmonary, and oral drug delivery formulation technologies. He is founder (1997, and formerly President and CEO, 1997–2013) of Cirrus Pharmaceuticals, Inc., which was acquired by Kemwell Pharma in 2013; founder (2001, and formerly CSO, 2002–2007) of Oriel Therapeutics, Inc, which was acquired by Sandoz in 2010; founder and CEO of Astartein, Inc. (2013–present); member of the Pharmaceutical Dosage Forms Expert Committee of the United States Pharmacopeia (USP, 2010–2015, Chair of the Sub-committee on Aerosols); and formerly Chair of the Aerosols Expert Committee of the USP (2005–2010). Dr. Hickey conducts a multidisciplinary research program in the field of pulmonary drug and vaccine delivery for treatment and prevention of a variety of diseases.

Sandro R.P. da Rocha is a full professor in the Department of Pharmaceutics in the School of Pharmacy and director for Pharmaceutical Engineering—School of Pharmacy at Virginia Commonwealth University (VCU). He also holds a joint appointment in Chemical and Life Science Engineering and is a full member of the Massey Cancer Center at VCU. He obtained his BSc and MSc in Chemical Engineering at USFM and UFSC, respectively, in Brazil, and a PhD in 2000 from the University of Texas at Austin in Chemical Engineering. After a postdoctoral position in Chemistry and Biochemistry also at the University of Texas at Austin, Dr. da Rocha joined the faculty at Wayne State University in Detroit, MI, where he worked until 2015. Professor da Rocha has contributed extensively to the area of pulmonary drug delivery, particularly through the development of novel pressurized metered dose inhaler formulations and of nanotherapeutics for pulmonary drug delivery, both areas having potential applications in the treatment of a variety of pulmonary disorders. Professor da Rocha has received numerous awards and recognition for his work, including visiting appointments at foreign institutions where he has developed collaborative efforts and taught in the area of nanomedicine and pulmonary drug delivery. Professor da Rocha has delivered a number of lectures nationally and internationally in the area of pulmonary nanotherapeutics and has written manuscripts and book chapters with his collaborators that include visiting faculty, postdoctoral fellows, PhD, undergraduate, graduate, and high-school students, who now hold key positions in the industry, academia, and government in various areas including pulmonary pharmaceutics.

Contributors

Ana Aguiar-Ricardo
LAQV-REQUIMTE
Department of Chemistry
Faculty of Science and Technology
NOVA University of Lisbon
Caparica, Portugal

Abeer M. Al-Ghananeem
Department of Pharmaceutical Sciences
Sullivan University
Louisville, Kentucky

Balaji Bharatwaj
Merck & Co., Inc.,
Rahway, New Jersey

Elizabeth R. Bielski
Department of Pharmaceutics School of Pharmacy
Virginia Commonwealth University
Richmond, Virginia

Robert J. Bischof
Hudson Institute of Medical Research
Melbourne, Victoria, Australia
and
Allergenix Pty Ltd.
Melbourne, Victoria, Australia

Jürgen B. Bulitta
Department of Pharmaceutics
University of Florida
Gainesville, Florida

Elise Burmeister Getz
Oriel Therapeutics, Inc., a Novartis Company
Clinical Department
Emeryville, California USA

Patrick Carius
Helmholtz Institute for Pharmaceutical Research Saarland (HIPS)
Helmholtz Center for Infection Research (HZI)
Saarland University
Saarbrücken, Germany
and
Department of Pharmacy
Saarland University
Saarbrücken, Germany

Nicholas Carrigy
Department of Mechanical Engineering
University of Alberta
Edmonton, Alberta, Canada

Hak-Kim Chan
Sydney Pharmacy School
Faculty of Medicine and Health
The University of Sydney
Camperdown, NSW, Australia

Lai Wah Chan
Department of Pharmacy
National University of Singapore
Singapore

Mong-Jen Chen
Department of Pharmaceutics
University of Florida
Gainesville, Florida

Jeremy Clarke
GlaxoSmithKline
Pharma Supply Chain
Ware, United Kingdom

Joon Chong Yee
Bristol-Myers Squibb, Co.
New York City, New York

David Cipolla
Aradigm
Hayward, California

Eunice Costa
Inhalation, R&D Drug Product Development
Hovione FarmaCiencia
Lisboa, Portugal

Gabriella Costabile
Department of Pharmacy
Ludwig-Maximilians-Universität München
Munich, Germany

Peter A. Crooks
University of Arkansas for Medical Sciences
Little Rock, Arkansas

Sandro R.P. da Rocha
Department of Pharmaceutics
Center for Pharmaceutical Engineering
Virginia Commonwealth University
Richmond, Virginia

Wilbur de Kruijf
Medspray
Enschede, the Netherlands

Anne H. de Boer
Department of Pharmaceutical Technology and Biopharmacy
University of Groningen
Groningen, the Netherlands

Myrna B. Dolovich
Faculty of Health Sciences
Department of Medicine
McMaster University
Hamilton, Ontario, Canada

Stefanie K. Drescher
Department of Pharmaceutics
University of Florida
Gainesville, Florida

Joachim Eicher
Boehringer Ingelheim Pharma GmbH and Co. KG
HP Supply Germany
Ingelheim am Rhein
Germany

Warren H. Finlay
Department of Mechanical Engineering
University of Alberta
Edmonton, Alberta

Laleh Golshahi
Department of Mechanical Engineering
Virginia Commonwealth University
Richmond, Virginia

Floris Grasmeijer
PureIMS
Roden, the Netherlands
University of Groningen
Groningen, the Netherlands

Ailin Guo
Pharmaceutical Sciences
South Dakota State University
Brookings, South Dakota

Jayne E. Hastedt
JDP Pharma Consulting, LLC
San Carlos, California

Ross H.M. Hatley
Respironics Respiratory Drug Delivery (UK) Ltd.
A business of Philips Electronics UK Limited
Chichester, West Sussex, United Kingdom

Rebecca L. Heise
Department of Biomedical Engineering
Virginia Commonwealth University
Richmond, Virginia

Paul Wan Sia Heng
Department of Pharmacy
National University of Singapore
Singapore

Rodrigo S. Heyder
Department of Pharmaceutics
Virginia Commonwealth University
Richmond, Virginia

Anthony J. Hickey
University of North Carolina
Chapel Hill, North Carolina
and
RTI International
Research Triangle Park, North Carolina

Günther Hochhaus
Department of Pharmaceutics
University of Florida
Gainesville, Florida

Susan Hoe
AstraZeneca Pharmaceuticals LP
South San Francisco, California
Cambridge, United Kingdom

Allen Horhota
Moderna Therapeutics
Greater Boston Area
Boston, Massachusetts

Stephen T. Horhota
BIND Therapeutics
Westford, Massachusetts

Justus C. Horstmann
Helmholtz Institute for Pharmaceutical Research Saarland (HIPS)
Helmholtz Center for Infection Research (HZI)
Saarland University
Saarbrücken, Germany
and
Department of Pharmacy
Saarland University
Saarbrücken, Germany

Jibriil P. Ibrahim
Monash Institute of Pharmaceutical Sciences
Parkville, Victoria, Australia

Mary E. Krause
Bristol-Myers Squibb, Co.
New York City, New York

Philip Chi Lip Kwok
Sydney Pharmacy School
Faculty of Medicine and Health
The University of Sydney
Camperdown, NSW, Australia

David Lechuga-Ballesteros
AstraZeneca Pharmaceuticals LP
South San Francisco, California

Claus-Michael Lehr
Helmholtz Institute for Pharmaceutical Research Saarland (HIPS)
Helmholtz Center for Infection Research (HZI)
Saarland University
Saarbrücken, Germany
and
Department of Pharmacy
Saarland University
Saarbrücken, Germany

Stefan Leiner
Boehringer Ingelheim Pharma GmbH and Co. KG
Quality & Records Management
Ingelheim am Rhein
Germany

Benjamin W. Maynor
Liquidia Technologies
Research Triangle Park, North Carolina, USA

Michelle P. McIntosh
Monash Institute of Pharmaceutical Sciences
Parkville, Victoria, Australia

Bernice Mei Jin Tan
Department of Pharmacy
National University of Singapore
Singapore

Olivia M. Merkel
Department of Pharmacy
Ludwig-Maximilians-Universität München
Munich, Germany

Jolyon Mitchell
Inhaler Consulting Services Inc.
London, Ontario, Canada
and
Affiliate Professor
University of Hawai'i, College of Pharmacy
Hilo, Hawai'i

Beth Morgan
AstraZeneca Pharmaceuticals
Research Triangle Park, North Carolina

Ajit S. Narang
Small Molecule Pharmaceutical Sciences
Genentech, Inc.
San Francisco, California

Steven C. Nichols
Director
OINDP Consultancy
Rugby, Warwichshire, UK

Narsimha R. Penthala
Department of Pharmaceutical Sciences
University of Arkansas for Medical Sciences
Little Rock, Arkansas

Shelly Pizarro
Genentech, Inc.
San Francisco, California

John N. Pritchard
Respironics Respiratory Drug Delivery (UK) Ltd.
A business of Philips Electronics UK Limited
Chichester, West Sussex, United Kingdom

Joshua J. Reineke
Pharmaceutical Sciences
South Dakota State University
Brookings, South Dakota

Alexandria Ritchie
Department of Biomedical Engineering
Virginia Commonwealth University
Richmond, Virginia

Thomas D. Roper
Department of Chemical and Life Science Engineering
Virginia Commonwealth University
Richmond, Virginia

Dennis Sandell
S5 Consulting
Blentarp, Sweden

William Craig Stagner
Department of Pharmaceutics
Campbell University
Buies Creek, North Carolina

Nicole Schneider-Daum
Helmholtz Institute for Pharmaceutical Research Saarland (HIPS)
Helmholtz Center for Infection Research (HZI)
Saarland University
Saarbrücken, Germany

Martina Steinmaurer
Department of Pharmacy
Ludwig-Maximilians Universität München
Munich, Germany

Helen N. Strickland
GlaxoSmithKline
Zebulon, North Carolina

David C. Thompson
Department of Clinical Pharmacy
University of Colorado Health Sciences Center
Denver, Colorado

S. van den Ban
GlaxoSmithKline Global Manufacturing and Supply
Ware, United Kingdom

Reinhard Vehring
Department of Mechanical Engineering
University of Alberta
Edmonton, Alberta, Canada

Dirk von Hollen
Respironics, Inc.
A Philips Healthcare Company
Murrysville, Pennsylvania

Herbert Wachtel
Boehringer Ingelheim Pharma GmbH and Co. KG
Analytical Development
Ingelheim am Rhein
Germany

Lin Yang
Aurobindo Pharma USA Inc.
Durham, North Carolina

Hao Yin
Medical Research Institute
Wuhan University
Wuhan, China

Bethany M. Young
Department of Biomedical Engineering
Virginia Commonwealth University
Richmond, Virginia

Ying Zhang
Medical Research Institute
Wuhan University
Wuhan, China

1

Introduction

Anthony J. Hickey and Sandro R.P. da Rocha

A number of outstanding texts on foundational elements of the topics discussed in this book exist, and the reader is encouraged to familiarize themselves with these materials, as they describe basic principles (Finlay, 2001), specific (Purewal and Grant, 1997, Srichana, 2016 and Zeng et al, 2000) and general dosage forms (Colombo et al., 2013, Hickey, 2007, Newman, 2009, Smyth and Hickey, 2011), and analytical methods (Tougas et al., 2013).

The advances in pharmaceutical inhalation aerosol technology occurring since the turn of the millennium have increased the potential of pulmonary drug delivery substantially. While some of the new developments had their origins in earlier work, we have seen the appearance of new propellants and new regulations considering the phase out of what we still consider new propellants, new dry powder inhalers, nebulizers, and a new category of product, soft mist inhalers.

In parallel with these new products, the breadth of application has increased to include the treatment of chronic obstructive pulmonary disease, a range of infectious diseases, diabetes, idiopathic pulmonary fibrosis, and pulmonary arterial hypertension. Pre-clinical studies and clinical trials covering yet a range of other potential applications of orally inhaled products include the use of a broader range of biologics and also nanomaterials that may help further advance the pulmonary drug delivery market.

Successful aerosol therapy has given research and development a boost, and the prospects of even greater opportunities for disease management is emerging from patient compliance, adherence tools, and new classes of drugs for local and systemic delivery through the lungs.

This text is focused on the active pharmaceutical ingredient, formulation development, device design, process and product engineering, and analytical methods to assess critical quality attributes underpinning safe and efficacious dosage forms.

Figure 1.1 depicts the sequence in which these topics will be presented, which follows the product development pathway. The conclusion of the volume is a discussion of bioequivalence testing and the interface between the dosage form and the patient. This reflects the point at which design and engineering controls, which are embedded in a regulated environment of quality by design, give way to biological factors.

It is intended that the materials covered in subsequent sections familiarize the reader with the underlying science and engineering associated with the design and characterization of complex dosage forms required to deliver orally inhaled aerosols. The platform of knowledge will be useful in considering options for specific applications and is a point from which to launch new technologies that will frame future developments in the field as described in a companion text (Hickey and Mansour, in press).

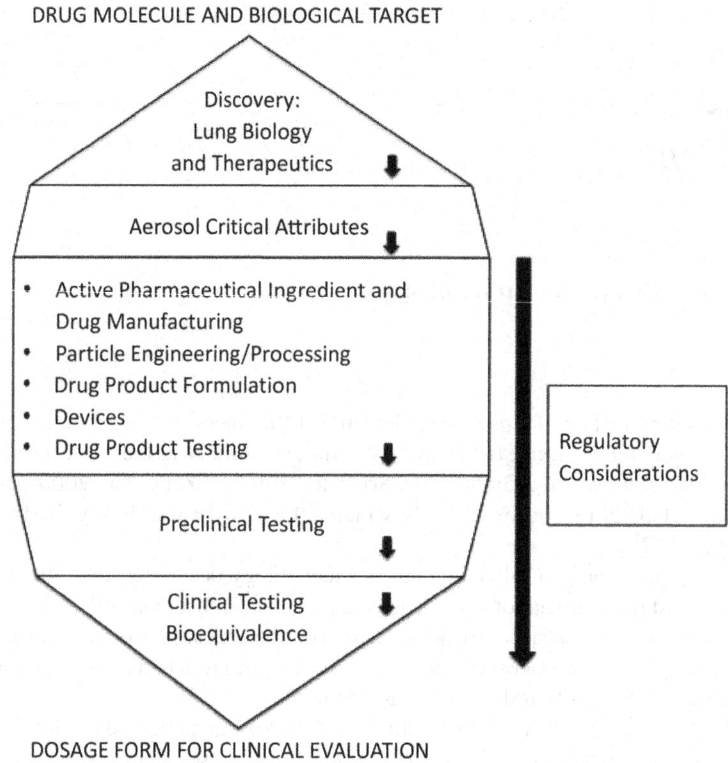

FIGURE 1.1 Product development themes in pharmaceutical inhalation aerosol technology.

REFERENCES

Colombo P, Traini D, Buttini F. *Inhaled Drug Delivery: Techniques and Products.* New York: Wiley-Blackwell; 2013.

Finlay W. *The Mechanics of Inhaled Pharmaceutical Aerosols: An Introduction.* New York: Academic Press; 2001.

Hickey A. *Inhalation Aerosols, Physical and Biological Basis for Therapy.* 2nd ed. New York: Informa Healthcare; 2007.

Hickey A J, Mansour H H, Eds. *Inhalation Aerosols, Physical and Biological Basis for Therapy*, Third Edition. Boca Raton, FL: CRC Press; in press.

Newman S. *Respiratory Drug Delivery: Essential Theory and Practice.* Richmond, VA: RDD Online; 2009.

Purewal T, Grant D. *Metered Dose Inhaler Technology.* Boca Raton, FL: CRC Press; 1997.

Smyth H, Hickey A. *Controlled Pulmonary Drug Delivery.* New York: Springer; 2011.

Srichana T. *Dry Powder Inhalers: Formulation, Device and Characterization.* Hauppauge, NJ: Nova Science Publishers; 2016.

Tougas T, Mitchell J, Lyapustina S, Eds. *Good Cascade Impactor Practices, AIM and EDA for Orally Inhaled Products.* New York: Springer; 2013.

Zeng X, Martin G, Marriott C. *Particulate Interactions in Dry Powder Formulations for Inhalation.* New York: CRC Press; 2000.

Section I

Discovery

2

Physiology of the Airways

Anthony J. Hickey and David C. Thompson

CONTENTS

2.1 Introduction

The airways represent a unique organ system in the body, their structure allowing air to come into close contact with blood, is one of the principal adaptions permitting the existence of terrestrial life. This adaptation also makes the airways a useful route of administration of drugs in the inhaled or aerosol form. This chapter provides an overview of the physiology of the airways excluding that of the nasopharyngeal regions of the airways. Aspects considered relevant to the practical and theoretical application of inhaled substances are emphasized.

2.2 Anatomy of the Airways

The airways (constituting the lungs) may be viewed as a series of dividing passageways originating at the trachea and terminating at the alveolar sac. In the context of aerosol design and delivery, such a "static" overview represents a satisfactorily simple model. However, many factors beyond the anatomy of the airways are relevant to the therapeutic use of aerosols.

2.2.1 Structure

The airways are often described as the pulmonary tree in that their overall form resembles a tree. The tree trunk is analogous to the trachea of the airways that bifurcates to form main bronchi. These divide to form smaller bronchi that lead to individual lung lobes: three lobes on the right side and two on the left side. Inside each lobe, the bronchi undergo further divisions to form new generations of smaller caliber airways: the bronchioles. This process continues through the terminal bronchioles (the smallest airway not involved with an alveolus), the respiratory bronchioles (which exhibit alveoli protruding from their walls), alveolar ducts, and terminates with the alveolar sacs. In the classic model of the airways, as described by Weibel (1963), each airway divides to form two smaller "daughter" airways (Figure 2.1), and, as a result, the number of airways at each generation is double that of the previous generation. The model proposes the existence of 24 airway generations in total, with the trachea being generation 0 and the alveolar sacs being generation 23.

In passing from the trachea to the alveolar sac, two physical changes occur in the airways that are important in influencing airway function. Firstly, the airway caliber decreases with increasing generations, for example, tracheal diameter ≈ 1.8 cm versus alveolar diameter ≈ 0.04 cm (Figure 2.2). This permits

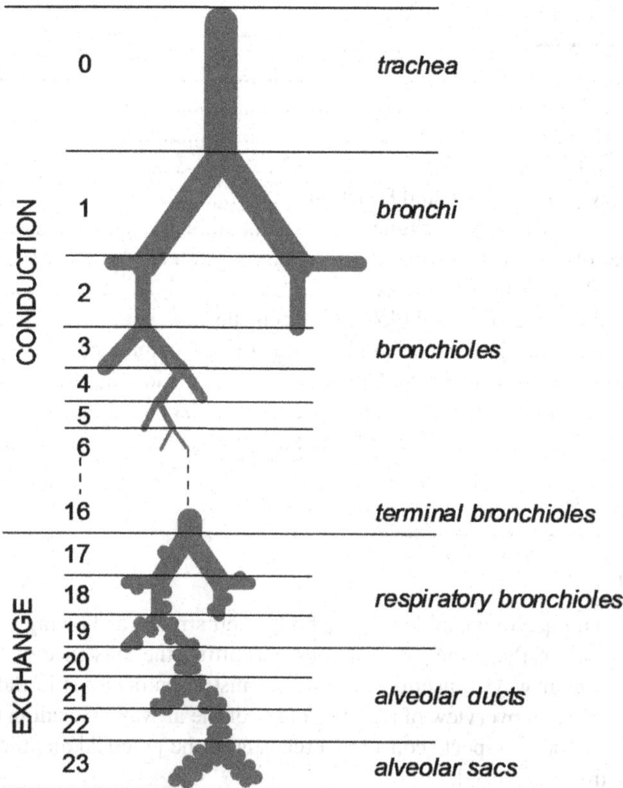

FIGURE 2.1 Model of airway. (With kind permission from Taylor & Francis: *Morphometry of the Human Lung*, Berlin, Germany, Springer-Verlag, 1963, Weibel, E.)

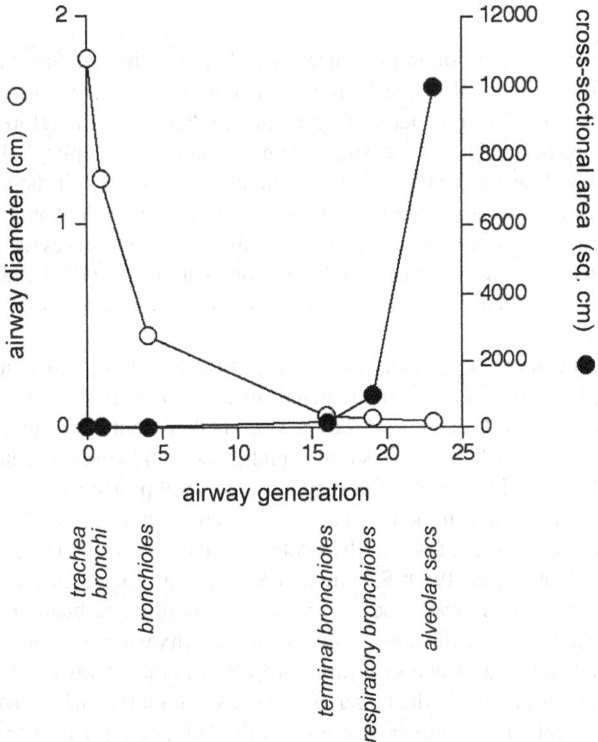

FIGURE 2.2 Graph of airway diameter and cross-sectional are as a function of airway generation.

adequate penetration of air to the lower airways for a given expansion of the lungs. Secondly, the surface area of the airways increases with each generation to the extent that the total area at the level of the human alveolus is in the order of 140 m^2 (Gehr et al., 1978). The alveolus is the principal site of gas exchange in the airways, a function compatible with the increased surface area that promotes extensive and efficient diffusional gas exchange between the alveolar space and the blood in alveolar capillaries (*vide infra*). The relatively small change in cross-sectional area that occurs over the 19 generations of airways between the trachea and the terminal bronchiole (from 2.5 cm^2 to 180 cm^2) (Bouhuys, 1974) fosters the rapid, bulk flow of inspired air down to the terminal bronchiole. By contrast, the cross-sectional area increases greatly in the four generations between the terminal bronchiole and the alveolar sac (from 180 cm^2 to 10,000 cm^2) (Bouhuys, 1974), which results in a significant decrease in the velocity of airflow to the extent that the flow velocity fails to exceed that of diffusing oxygen molecules (Weibel, 1984). Accordingly, diffusion assumes a greater role in determining the movement of gases in these peripheral airways.

The various levels of the airways may be categorized functionally as being either conducting or respiratory airways. Those airways not participating in gas exchange constitute the conducting zone of the airways and extend from the trachea to the terminal bronchioles. This region is the principal site of airway obstruction in obstructive lung diseases, such as asthma. The respiratory zone includes airways involved with gas exchange and comprises respiratory bronchioles, alveolar ducts, and alveolar sacs. As such, conducting and respiratory zones of the airways may be distinguished simply by the absence or presence of alveolar pockets (which confer gas exchange function). Regions within each zone may be classified further on a histological basis. For example, the contribution of cartilage to the airway wall is one means of differentiating the trachea from bronchi and bronchioles because cartilage exists as incomplete rings in the trachea, regresses to irregularly shaped plates in bronchi, and is absent from bronchioles. Also, respiratory bronchioles may be discriminated from terminal bronchioles by the presence of associated alveoli.

Other histological changes are evident downward throughout the pulmonary tree, and the cellular profile of each region has distinctive effect on functional aspects of the airways under physiological and pathophysiological conditions.

2.2.1.1 Epithelium

The epithelium of the airways is a continuous sheet of cells lining the lumenal surface of the airways. It separates the internal environment of the body (i.e. subepithelial structures) from the external environment (i.e. airway lumen). The lumenal surface of the epithelium is, therefore, exposed to inhaled substances, such as gases, particulates, or aerosols. Connecting adjacent epithelial cells are specialized tight junctional processes (Inoue and Hogg, 1974; Williams, 1990) that limit the penetration of inhaled substances by the intercellular route of administration. Under normal or physiological conditions, larger molecules must past through the epithelial cell. Therefore, the epithelium serves the important function of limiting access of inhaled substances to the internal environment of the body. Under pathophysiological conditions, the epithelium may be damaged, enhancing penetration of substances present in the airway lumen (Godfrey, 1997).

The airway epithelium comprises a variety of cell types (Table 2.1), the distribution of which confers different functions on the airways region. The lumenal surface of the airways are lined by ciliated cells from the trachea to the terminal bronchus. Mucus, a viscous fluid containing mucin glycoproteins and proteoglycans, floats on a watery layer of periciliary fluid (or sol) and covers the lumenal surface of the epithelium. The secretions fulfill four important functions. Firstly, it protects the epithelium from becoming dehydrated. Secondly, the water in the mucus promotes saturation of inhaled air. Thirdly, the mucus contains antibacterial proteins and peptides, such as defensins and lysozyme that suppress microbial colonization of the airways (Finkbeiner, 1999; Schutte and McCray, 2002). Fourthly, the mucus is involved in airway protection from inhaled xenobiotics or chemicals. Coordinated beating of the epithelial cilia propels the blanket of mucus towards the upper airways and pharynx where the mucus may either be swallowed or ejected. The rate of mucus propulsion varies according to the airway region such that movement in the smaller airways is slower than in the larger airways, a situation that arises from the proportionally larger number of ciliated cells in the larger airways and the higher ciliary beat frequency in the larger airways (Gail and L'enfant, 1983). Syllogistically, this process is advantageous, given that many small airways converge on the larger, more central airways whose mucus clearance rate would have to be greater to accommodate the large volumes of mucus being delivered by the smaller distal airways. This process of

TABLE 2.1
Cells of the Airway Epithelium

Cell	Putative Function
Ciliated columnar	Mucus movement
Mucous (goblet)	Mucus secretion
Serous	Periciliary fluid; mucus secretion
Clara (nonciliated epithelial)	Xenobiotic metabolism; surfactant production
Brush	Transitional form of ciliated epithelial cell
Basal	Progenitor for ciliated epithelial and goblet cells
Dendritic	Immunity
Intermediate	Transitional cell in differentiation of basal cell
Neuroendocrine (Kultschitsky or APUD)	Chemoreceptor; paracrine function
Alveolar type I	Alveolar gas exchange
Alveolar type II	Surfactant secretion; differentiation into type I cell
Alveolar macrophage	Pulmonary defense
Mast	Immunoregulation

Sources: Holt, P. et al., *Clin. Exp. Allergy*, 19, 597–601, 1989; Jeffrey, P., *Am. Rev. Respir. Dis.*, 128, S14–S20, 1983; Scheuermann, D., *Microsc. Res. Tech.*, 37, 31–42, 1997.

the movement of mucus up the pulmonary tree, known as the mucociliary escalator, serves the defensive function of clearing inhaled particles that become trapped in the mucus from the lung.

The significance of mucus trapping of aerosolized particles is emphasized by the fact that radiolabeled aerosols have been used in the measurement of mucociliary transport (Morrow, 1973). Coughing increases clearance of mucus from the airways, which rapidly propels the mucus towards the pharynx. Failure to clear mucus from the airways resulting from ciliary dysfunction or mucus hypersecretion (as may occur in cystic fibrosis or chronic bronchitis) can result in airway obstruction and infection. Such a situation may adversely affect the therapeutic activity of an inhaled drug by increasing the thickness of the mucus layer through which the drug must diffuse to reach its site of action and retard penetration of the aerosolized particles throughout the airways resulting from mucus plugging of the airway lumen. Goblet cells (and mucous glands) are not present in airways distal to the bronchi (Tyler, 1983), and, therefore, a mucus layer does not line the peripheral airways.

Alveolar type I cells represent the principal cell type lining the lumenal surface of the alveoli (Crapo et al., 1983; Gail and L'enfant, 1983), and it is through these cells that gases must diffuse for oxygen and carbon dioxide exchange to occur with blood in the pulmonary capillaries. Alveolar type II cells are also present in the alveoli. Cuboidal in nature, these cells possess microvilli and serve the important function of secreting surfactant (Gail and L'enfant, 1983), a mixture of carbohydrates, proteins, and lipids essential in reducing alveolar surface tension, which diminishes the work of alveolar expansion during inspiration. In addition, type II cells serve as progenitor cells in the regeneration of the alveolar epithelium. For example, type II cells differentiate into type I cells after type I cell damage (Gail and L'enfant, 1983; Voelker and Mason, 1989).

Epithelium of the central and peripheral airways have the capacity to produce and release pro-inflammatory mediators, such as arachidonic acid metabolites, nitric oxide, cytokines, and growth factors, and thereby modulate the progression of airway diseases (Mills et al., 1999). In addition, substances released from central airway epithelium can influence the ability of adjacent smooth muscle to contract (Spina, 1998).

2.2.1.2 Smooth Muscle Cells

Smooth muscle is separated from the epithelium by the lamina propria, a region of connective tissue containing nerves and blood vessels. In the trachea, the smooth muscle connects the open ends of the incomplete cartilage rings and, therefore, constitutes only a fraction of the circumference of this component of the airways. Further down the pulmonary tree, through the bronchi and bronchioles, the contribution of the smooth muscle to the airway wall increases to the point of completely encircling the airway. Contraction or relaxation of the smooth muscle has a direct influence on airway caliber and, thereby, affects airflow in the airways. Bronchoconstriction is the result of smooth muscle contraction and is the principal cause of airway obstruction in reversible obstructive airway diseases, such as asthma. The tone or state of contraction of airway smooth muscle is subject to control by neurotransmitters released from innervating nerves, hormones, or mediators released from activated inflammatory cells.

2.2.1.3 Gland Cells

Located in the submucosa of cartilage-containing airways and in the lamina propria of the trachea are glands that secrete mucus into the airway lumen (Reid, 1960). Each mucous gland consists of four regions: the ciliated duct, collecting duct, mucous tubules, and secretory tubules (Meyrick et al., 1960). The ciliated duct opens to the lumen of the airways and is lined by ciliated epithelial cells. It merges with the collecting duct, the walls of which comprise columnar cells. Mucous cells line the mucous tubules that lead from the collecting duct. Serous cells (which contribute to the more liquid component of mucus) line the blind-ended serous tubules that are located at the distal ends of the mucous tubules. Several secretory tubules feed into the collecting duct. Mucus is secreted *via* the collecting and ciliated ducts into the lumen of the airways. Goblet cells, located in the epithelium of the larger central airways, secrete mucus directly into the airway lumen (Rogers, 1994). Mucus hypersecretion results from an increase in the number and/or size of mucous glands and goblet cells in disease states, such as chronic bronchitis (Finkbeiner, 1999; Rogers, 1994).

2.2.1.4 Nerves

In the central nervous system regulation of airway function, afferent and efferent nerves serving sensory and effector functions, respectively, innervate the airways (Table 2.2, Figure 2.3) (Widdicombe, 2001). Slowly adapting receptors (or pulmonary stretch receptors) are located in the smooth muscle of the central airways (trachea to larger bronchi), respond to airway stretch, and are thought to be involved in the reflex control of ventilatory drive. Rapidly adapting receptors (or irritant receptors) ramify within the epithelium of the central airways and are sensitive to chemical or irritant stimuli (e.g. inflammatory mediators), mechanical stimuli, and interstitial edema. Activation of these receptors results in an increase in the rate or depth of breathing and in bronchoconstriction mediated through a central nervous system reflex in efferent cholinergic nerve activity. Inhalation of foreign substances, such as particulates, can activate these receptors to elicit reflex bronchoconstriction. Afferent C-fibers are tachykinin-containing nerves that ramify within the epithelium and between smooth muscle cells (Lundberg et al., 1984). Chemical (e.g. inflammatory mediators), particulate, and mechanical stimuli activate afferent C-fibers to cause rapid, shallow breathing or apnoea and to evoke central reflex bronchoconstriction through increased efferent cholinergic nerve activity (Coleridge and Coleridge, 1984; Widdicombe, 2001).

Under conditions of cholinoceptor blockade, central reflex bronchodilation through activation of efferent nonadrenergic noncholinergic nerves may be observed (Michoud et al., 1088). Stimulation of afferent C-fibers can result in the release of tachykinins at the site of stimulation and alter airway function independently of the central nervous system, e.g. by inducing mucosal edema (McDonald et al., 1996). These nerves are thought to be important sensory modalities for conveying retrosternal discomfort induced by inhaled irritants. Neuroepithelial bodies are located in the epithelium of the central airways and are intimately associated with the endings of nerves, which are primarily afferent in nature (McDonald et al., 1996; Widdicombe, 2001). Each neuroepithelial body comprises groups of neuroendocrine cells that contain biogenic amines, such as serotonin, and peptides, such as calcitonin gene-related peptide (cGRP) (Cutz and Jackson, 1999). Hypoxia induces the release of these biologically active substances which can then activate the sensory nerve endings to elicit a central reflex or act locally on adjacent tissues, such as blood vessels or airway smooth muscle (Cutz and Jackson, 1999; Widdicombe, 2001). Cholinergic nerves are carried to the airways in the vagus nerve and innervate airway smooth muscle and submucosal glands. The neurotransmitter, acetylcholine, released from cholinergic nerves promotes bronchoconstriction (Widdicombe, 1963) and mucus secretion (Baker et al., 1985; Ueki et al., 1980). Nonadrenergic noncholinergic inhibitory nerves, also carried in the vagus nerve, are the sole bronchodilator innervation of airway smooth muscle (Diamond and Altiere, 1989). These nerves may also inhibit airway mucus secretion (Rogers, 2000). Adrenergic nerves do not innervate human airway smooth muscle (Richardson, 1977) and have little effect on mucus secretion in human airways (Baker et al., 1985; Richardson, 1977).

TABLE 2.2
Innervation of the Airways

Nerve Type	Putative Function
Afferent	
slowly adapting receptor (pulmonary stretch receptor)	Breuer-Hering reflex (inhibition of inspiration; prolongation of expiration)
Rapidly adapting receptor	Responds to airway irritants, mechanical stimuli, Interstitial edema
C-fibers	Responds to airway irritants, mechanical stimuli
Neuroepithelial body	Responds to hypoxia
Efferent	
Adrenergic	Vasoconstriction
Cholinergic	Bronchoconstriction, mucus secretion
Nonadrenergic noncholinergic inhibitory	Bronchodilation, mucus secretion

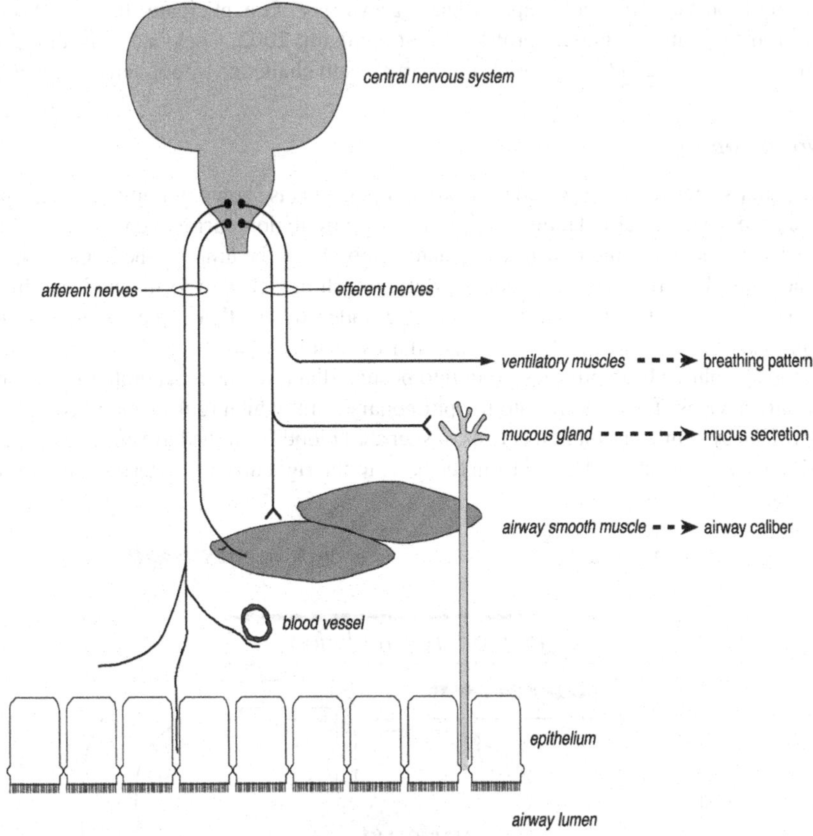

FIGURE 2.3 Role of afferent and efferent nerves in altering airway function. Stimulation of afferent (or sensory) nerves, such as afferent C-fibers, rapidly adapting receptors, or slowly adapting receptors, results in an increase in electrical impulse traffic to the central nervous system. Depending on the afferent nerve activated, processing and integration in the central nervous system may result in an increase in the activity of: (1) efferent motor nerves governing muscles that regulate breathing (i.e. affect the rate and depth of ventilation) or (2) efferent autonomic nerves, such as cholinergic and nonadrenergic noncholinergic inhibitory nerves, that modify mucus secretion or airway caliber through changes in smooth muscle tone. Afferent C-fibers may also serve an efferent function insofar as impulses can spread throughout the C-fiber network from the size of C-fiber stimulation to result in the release of tachykinins (such as substance P and neurokinin A). These released substances may then act on blood vessels to increase permeability or on smooth muscle to increase vascular permeability and elicit bronchoconstriction, respectively.

2.2.1.5 Defensive Cells

Alveolar macrophages are migrating mononuclear cells present in the interstitium and lumenal surface of the alveoli (Crapo et al., 1982). These cells phagocytize (envelop and, when possible, enzymatically degrade) foreign substances, particles, or microorganisms in the alveoli, after which they remain in the alveolus or migrate to the mucociliary escalator or into lymph tissue. Upon activation, macrophages release a variety of enzymes and biologically active mediators (Laskin and Laskin, 2001; Sibile and Reynolds, 1990) that may influence airway function. The synthesis and release of matrix metalloproteinases (MMPs) by activated alveolar macrophages can contribute to lung tissue remodeling (Parks and Shapiro, 2001; Shapiro, 1999).

Mast cells are located in the walls of the central and peripheral airways and may be found free in the lumen of the airways (Cutz and Orange, 1977). Activation by antigen cross-bridging of surface antibodies elicits cellular degranulation of the mast cell and the release of biologically active preformed and newly generated mediators. Also released are proteases, including chymase and tryptase, which can modify airway function by degrading biologically active proteins and peptides (Caughey, 1991). In addition, tryptase activates protease-activated receptors, leading a variety of unanticipated biological actions, such as induction of airway smooth muscle proliferation (Abraham, 2002; Cocks and Moffatt, 2001). Mast cells serve an important role in the response of the airways to challenge by antigens (or allergens).

2.2.1.6 Blood Supply

The cardiovascular system can be divided into two components (as shown in Figure 2.4): the pulmonary circulation and the systemic circulation. The pulmonary circulation carries deoxygenated blood from the right ventricle to the lungs and returns oxygenated blood from the lungs to the left atrium. Emerging from the right ventricle is the main pulmonary artery, which branches to form smaller pulmonary and intrapulmonary arteries. This pulmonary arterial tree undergoes further rapid subdivision in parallel with the pulmonary tree to form pulmonary capillaries, a fine network of blood vessels in intimate contact with the alveolus. The capillaries drain into postcapillary venules that unite to form small veins and, distally, larger veins. These drain into the pulmonary vein, which returns blood from the lungs to the left atrium. The systemic circulation carries oxygenated blood from the left ventricle to the tissues of the body and returns deoxygenated blood from the body to the right atrium. Arteries and arterioles carry

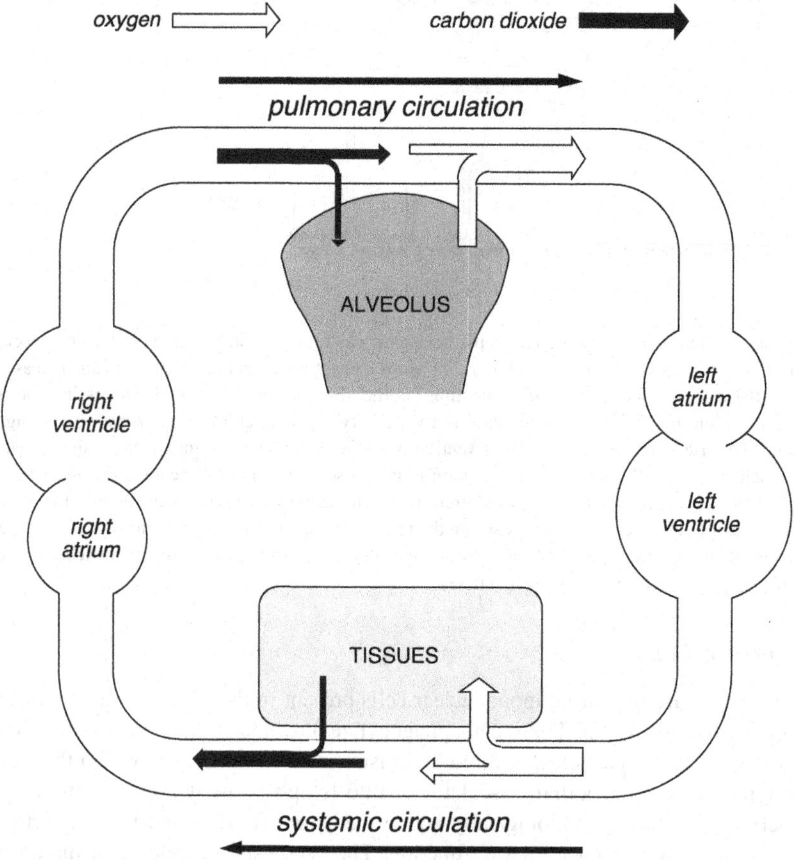

FIGURE 2.4 Cardiovascular system in the body. Oxygen diffuses from the oxygen-rich environment of the alveolus into the deoxygenated blood of the pulmonary circulation. The newly oxygenated blood returns by the pulmonary vein to the left atrium and ventricle: contraction of the latter provides the driving force for circulation of oxygen-rich blood to the organs and tissues of the body. Cells of the body use oxygen for energy-producing processes that result in the formation of carbon dioxide. Depleted of oxygen and richer in carbon dioxide, blood leaving the tissues returns by the venous circulation to the right atrium. The right ventricle pumps the carbon dioxide-rich blood into the pulmonary circulation from whence the carbon dioxide may diffuse into the alveolus. Arrows indicate the direction of blood flow.

blood to capillary networks within tissues, and venules and veins return blood from tissues to the heart. There are several important differences between the systemic and pulmonary circulations. First, blood pressure is lower in the pulmonary circulation than in the systemic circulation, for example, mean pressures in the pulmonary artery (emerging from the right ventricle) and aorta (artery emerging from the left ventricle) are 15 mmHg and 100 mmHg, respectively. As a result, the walls of the various pulmonary arterial vessels are thinner and are invested with less smooth muscle than their systemic counterparts, presumably resulting from the differences in stress borne by the vessel wall. Secondly, the pulmonary vessels are subject to different transmural pressures than are systemic vessels, such as those caused by changes in pressure in the alveolus and thoracic cavity, together with the stresses applied to the vessel wall through movement of adherent lung tissue. For example, during inspiration, alveoli expand and tend to compress the pulmonary capillaries, located in the walls of the alveoli. At the same time, large vessels are subject to distention caused by the negative intrapleural pressure during inspiration.

Blood vessels supplying the conducting or central airways (i.e. the bronchial circulation) are part of the systemic circulation. By contrast, the blood supply to the airways of the respiratory zone involves the pulmonary circulation. The separation of these vascular networks can be almost complete. For example, in the cat with separately perfused systemic (bronchial) and pulmonary circulations, infusion of Evans blue dye into the systemic circulation results in staining of the central airways (distal trachea to fourth generation intralobar bronchus) and no staining of parenchymal tissue (Figure 2.5). This circulation is part of the systemic circulation since 75%–80% of the dye returns to the right ventricle. The remainder of the dye returns to the left ventricle. This result taken together with the absence of staining of parenchymal tissue suggests that part of the bronchial circulation drains into the venous return of the pulmonary circulation. Recent studies demonstrate the ability to independently perfuse these two circulations in

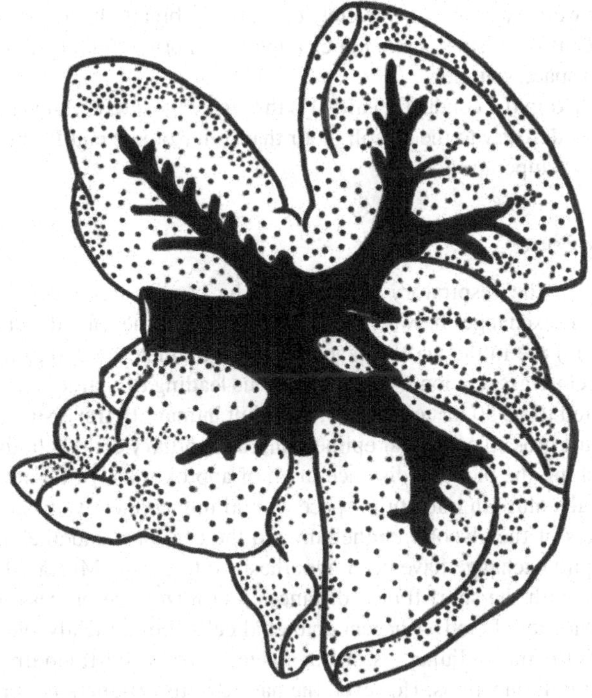

FIGURE 2.5 Diagram of staining of the bronchial circulation in the cat. The bronchial and pulmonary circulations of the cat were perfused separately with aerated physiological salt solution containing bovine serum albumin (4% wt/vol) maintained at 37°C. Perfusates from the bronchial and pulmonary circulations were collected from cannulae positioned in the right and left ventricles, respectively. Infusion of Evans blue dye (30 mg/Kg) into the systemic circulation resulted in deep blue staining of the central airways (black) with no staining of the parenchymal tissues (dotted). Further 75%–80% of the dye was collected from the cannula in the right heart.

larger animals (Serikov and Fleming, 2001). In studying the absorption of an aerosol from the central versus the peripheral airways, it is therefore prudent to be cognizant of the nature of the circulation servicing the site of expected deposition and sample from the appropriate sites, namely, right ventricle or left ventricle.

2.2.2 Zones of the Airways

The different zones of the airways, i.e. conducting and respiratory zones, possess different physiological functions and are distinguished by their roles in the exchange of gases.

2.2.2.1 Conducting Zone

Conducting airways do not contribute to the gas exchange and may be considered merely a conduit between the external environment and the respiratory zone (*vide infra*). The volume of air accommodated by the conducting airways represents the anatomic dead space and is air not directly available for gas exchange. Aside from serving as a conduit to the respiratory zone, the conducting airways perform two other functions: gas buffering and humidification.

The dead space (the volume of airway not involved indirectly in gas exchange) confers a buffering capacity on the airways in that, for each breath, air taken in from the external environment or alveolar air must mix with dead space air. This process, although decreasing the efficiency with which oxygen is delivered to and carbon dioxide is removed from the alveolar space (e.g. dead space oxygen concentration will be determined by the oxygen concentration of air inhaled from the external environment and of that in the alveolar space that was shunted into the dead space in the previous breath), serves to even out the alveolar gas concentrations by preventing dramatic swings in alveolar gas concentrations that would occur if the alveolar air were exchanged completely during each breath. It should be recognized that the volume of the dead space is not insignificant. For example, in a normal tidal breath of 500 mL–600 mL, 150 mL represents dead space volume.

Inhaled air is humidified in the conducting airways through exposure to fluids lining these airways, a process that results in the delivery to the alveoli of air that is in isotonic equilibrium of 99.5% or greater relative humidity at body temperature.

2.2.2.2 Respiratory Zone

The relationship between the respiratory system and the cardiovascular system is ideally suited for the process of gas exchange between the alveolus and the blood. Pulmonary capillaries (diameter = 6 μm–15 μm) are in the walls of each alveolus (diameter = 250 μm) (Simionescu, 1980). Many capillaries are in close association with each alveolus leading to a large "common" area for gas or solute exchange estimated to be 50 m^2 to 120 m^2 in an adult human. In traversing the air-blood barrier, gases in the alveolus must cross the alveolar epithelium, the capillary endothelium, and their basement membranes before reaching the blood, a distance in all of approximately 500 nm (Simionescu, 1980). In some regions of the alveolus, an interstitial space (containing connective tissue elements) separates the basement membranes of the alveolar epithelium and the capillary endothelium, and it is in these loci that solutes and liquid exchange have been hypothesized to occur (Murray, 1986). The large area for absorption, together with the short transit distances, optimizes the process of diffusion of gases between the alveolar space and blood. Adjacent epithelial cells lining the alveolus are connected by a tight junction that limits the intercellular passage of solutes (Effros, 1991; Godfrey, 1997). Pulmonary endothelial cells exhibit tight junctions. However, the nature of these junctional processes differs from that in the epithelium insofar as interruption of the junctions in the endothelium may occur and permit the intercellular passage of large solutes to and from the interstitium (Effros, 1991). Lipophilic solutes readily diffuse across epithelial and endothelial cells. Other solutes pass through the alveolar epithelium and capillary by transcellular paths (e.g. pores, transcytosis) in a manner related inversely to their size and lipophobicity (Effros, 1991).

2.3 Function of the Airways

2.3.1 Gas Exchange

The principal function of the airways is to permit exchange of gases between blood and the atmosphere that surrounds us, specifically, the supply of oxygen to the blood and the removal of carbon dioxide from the blood. This is accomplished by: (a) exchanging gases between the external environment and the alveolar space through breathing or ventilation and (b) exchanging gases between the alveolar space and the blood by diffusional processes. The structural features of the pulmonary tree optimize these two processes. Firstly, the caliber of the airways decreases from the trachea to the alveolus, thereby reducing the dead space volume. For a given tidal volume (volume of air inspired), decreasing the dead space volume enhances exchange of atmospheric gases with alveolar gases and results in higher levels of oxygen in the alveolar space and enhanced removal of carbon dioxide from the alveolar space. Secondly, the large surface area shared by the alveoli and the pulmonary capillaries and the short transit distance required for the passage of gases between the alveolar space and the blood enhance gas diffusion.

The direction and extent of passage of gases between the blood in the pulmonary capillary and the alveolar space is determined principally by the gas concentration or partial pressure gradient between these two sites. For example, the partial pressure of oxygen in the alveolus (104 mmHg) normally exceeds that in the deoxygenated blood of the pulmonary capillaries (40 mmHg), and, therefore, oxygen tends to diffuse from the alveolus to the blood (Figure 2.2). The opposite is true for carbon dioxide, which has a higher partial pressure in the blood of pulmonary capillaries (45 mmHg) than in the alveolus (40 mmHg), resulting in the diffusion of this gas from the blood into the alveolus. Under optimal conditions for gas exchange, all alveoli would be well ventilated and all pulmonary capillaries would be well perfused. However, not all alveoli are ventilated equally, and, similarly, not all pulmonary capillaries are perfused to the same degree. An alveolus may be well ventilated, but the associated capillaries may be poorly perfused or not perfused, a situation that may occur resulting from thrombosis, embolization, or compression of pulmonary vessels by high alveolar pressures. The volume of air ventilating unperfused alveolar units during each breath is the alveolar dead space. This volume, together with the anatomic dead space, is known as the physiological dead space. An alveolus may be poorly ventilated (resulting from bronchoconstriction, mucus obstruction, or atelectasis [peripheral airway closure]), and the associated capillaries may be well perfused. In this situation, deoxygenated blood coursing through the pulmonary capillaries is not subject to oxygenation and forms part of a physiological shunt that delivers inadequately oxygenated (or deoxygenated) blood to the left heart. Low alveolar or pulmonary arterial oxygen concentrations induce vasoconstriction (Marshall and Marshall, 1983), which diverts blood away from underventilated alveoli. This process could be viewed as an intrinsic one serving to optimize ventilation-perfusion relationships. Mismatching of ventilation and perfusion can result in less efficient gas exchange between the alveolus and blood. Under normal conditions, ventilation-perfusion of the airways is adequate to maintain the important function of gas exchange and is a composite of the previously mentioned situations.

2.3.2 Acid-Base Balance

Carbon dioxide is continually produced by cellular aerobic metabolism of glucose and fatty acids. Carbon dioxide diffuses down its concentration gradient from the cell to the blood, which carries it to the lungs. It can interact with water to form carbonic acid (H_2CO_3), a process catalyzed by carbonic anhydrase, an enzyme in erythrocytes. Carbonic acid can then dissociate to liberate bicarbonate ion (HCO_3^-) and hydrogen ion (H^+) as follows:

$$CO_2 + H_2O \rightarrow H_2CO_3 \rightarrow HCO_3^- + H^+$$

This process reverses in the lung where hydrogen ion and bicarbonate ion combine to form carbonic acid, which then breaks down to form water and carbon dioxide, the latter diffusing into the alveolar space down its concentration gradient for removal by ventilation.

A close relationship exists in the blood between carbon dioxide levels and hydrogen ion concentrations, such that increases in carbon dioxide cause increases in blood hydrogen ion levels and, as a result, decreases in blood pH. Ventilation has a direct influence on blood carbon dioxide concentrations, and thereby affects blood pH as shown:

$$\uparrow \text{ventilation} \rightarrow \downarrow [\text{blood } CO_2] \rightarrow \downarrow [\text{blood } H^+] \rightarrow \uparrow \text{blood pH} \rightarrow \text{respiratory alkalosis}$$

$$\downarrow \text{ventilation} \rightarrow \uparrow [\text{blood } CO_2] \rightarrow \uparrow [\text{blood } H^+] \rightarrow \downarrow \text{blood pH} \rightarrow \text{respiratory acidosis}$$

Alterations in ventilation, therefore, influence blood pH. Impaired ventilation, as may occur during central nervous system depression or airway obstruction, can result in respiratory acidosis. Conversely, respiratory alkalosis can be caused by hyperventilation, as might occur during ascent to high altitude or by fever. In general, renal mechanisms function to compensate for inordinate respiratory alternations in blood pH. In addition, feedback control mechanisms exist in the body that alter respiration in the face of changes in blood pH. For example, changes in blood pH resulting from nonrespiratory (such as may occur in severe diarrhea, altered renal function, and ingestion of acids or bases) or respiratory mechanisms may be returned towards normal (pH = 7.4) by altering the rate and depth of ventilation. Increases in blood hydrogen ion (and carbon dioxide) concentration stimulate carotid chemoreceptors (located in the bifurcation of the common carotid arteries) to elicit a central nervous system reflex in ventilation. A decrease in the blood concentration of hydrogen ions depresses ventilation through the same central nervous system reflex. In addition, ventilation is also regulated by chemoreceptors in the medulla of the brainstem sensitive to changes in hydrogen ion and carbon dioxide concentrations in the cerebrospinal fluid.

2.3.3 Endocrine

Cells of the lung produce and secrete substances that may exert a local action (i.e. autocrine or paracrine function) or, through passage into the pulmonary circulation, a systemic action (i.e. endocrine function). Prostacyclin, a potent vasodilator and inhibitor of platelet aggregation, is generated by pulmonary endothelium (Gryglewski, 1990). Antigenic challenge of sensitized airways induces the release of bronchoactive and vasoactive mediators from the airways, including histamine, prostaglandins, and leukotrienes (Wasserman, 1983), that, aside from exerting local bronchoconstrictor and vascular actions, can spill over into the pulmonary circulation to have actions in organs other than the lungs.

2.3.4 Metabolism

In passage through the pulmonary circulation, a variety of blood-borne substances are subject to metabolism by enzymes associated with the pulmonary endothelium (Table 2.3). The metabolic processes appear to be very selective as exemplified by the ability of the lung to metabolize norepinephrine, but no other catecholamines, such as epinephrine or dopamine. For many of the compounds, uptake into the endothelial cell is required before enzymatic degradation occurs, and it is the substrate selectivity of these processes that appear to govern metabolic selectivity. Substances that are taken up into the endothelial cells include 5-hydroxytryptamine, norepinephrine, and prostaglandins E_2 and $F_{2\alpha}$. The external surface of the endothelium bears several enzymes that serve to inactivate or biotransform blood-borne substances. These include phosphate esterases, which metabolize the adenosine phosphate compounds, and angiotensin-converting enzyme, which cleaves bradykinin to inactive fragments. The latter enzyme has been studied extensively primarily because it is responsible for the bioactivation of angiotensin I to form angiotensin II (a potent vasoconstrictor), and the lungs represent the principal site of this conversion. Other peptidases have been identified on the pulmonary endothelium, but their physiological relevance remains to be established (Ryan, 1989). A fair amount is known about the metabolic properties of the pulmonary endothelium, in large part because of the relative ease of studying the pulmonary circulation, and the ability to study endothelium grown in cell culture. Considerably less is known about the metabolic properties of the airway epithelium, save that related to neutral endopeptidase or endothelin-converting enzyme activity (Baraniuk et al., 1995; Battistini and Dussault, 1998; Martins et al., 1991). In both areas,

TABLE 2.3

Fate of Substances Passing Through the Pulmonary Circulation

Removal
5-Hydroxytryptamine
Norepinephrine
Prostaglandins E_2, $F_{2\alpha}$
Leukotrienes C_4, D_4
Adenosine monophosphate, diphosphate, triphosphate
Bradykinin
Tachykinins
Endothelin
Unaffected
Epinephrine
Dopamine
Isoproterenol
Histamine
Prostaglandin A_2
Prostacyclin
Oxytocin
Vasopressin
Angiotensin II
Activation
Angiotensin I

Source: From Battistini, B. and Dussault, P., *Pulm. Pharmacol. Ther.*, 11, 79–88, 1998; de Nucci, G. et al., *Proc. Natl. Acad. Sci. U.S.A.*, 85, 9797–9800, 1988; Ferreira, S. et al., *Metabolic Activities of the Lung—Ciba Foundation Symposium 78*, (p. 129). Amsterdam, the Netherlands, Excerpta Medica, 1980; Ferreira, S. and Vane, J., *Br. J. Pharmacol. Chemother.*, 30, 417–424, 1967; Hyman, A. et al., *Am. Rev. Respir. Dis.*, 117, 111–136, 1978; Martins, M. et al., *Int. Arch. Allergy. Appl Immunol.*, 94, 325–329, 1991; Piper, P. et al., *Bull. Eur. Physiopathol. Respir.*, 17, 571–583, 1981; Ryan, J. and Ryan, U., *Fed. Proc.*, 36, 2683–2691, 1977; Schuster, V. *Annu. Rev. Physiol.*, 60, 221–242, 1998; Sole, M. et al., *Circulation*, 60, 160–163, 1979; Thomas, D. and Vane, J. *Nature*, 216, 335–338, 1967.

more research is needed to allow a more comprehensive understanding about how the lung metabolizes substances perfused through or depositing in it. In the context of aerosol administration to the peripheral airways, it should be evident from the foregoing that compounds delivered to the alveoli and absorbed into the pulmonary circulation will be subject to endothelial metabolic processes.

2.4 Evaluation of Airway Physiology and Function

Previously, the anatomy and physiology of the airways were considered. In clinical practice, the assessment of pulmonary function is important in diagnosis of the airway disease, in determination of appropriate therapy, and in evaluation of the success of therapy.

2.4.1 Measures of Pulmonary Volumes

Spirometry is the measurement of the volume of air moving into or out of the airways. In this process, various ventilatory maneuvers are undertaken that permit an estimation of pulmonary volumes and capacities (Figure 2.6). Such measurements are valuable for diagnosis of airway disease because

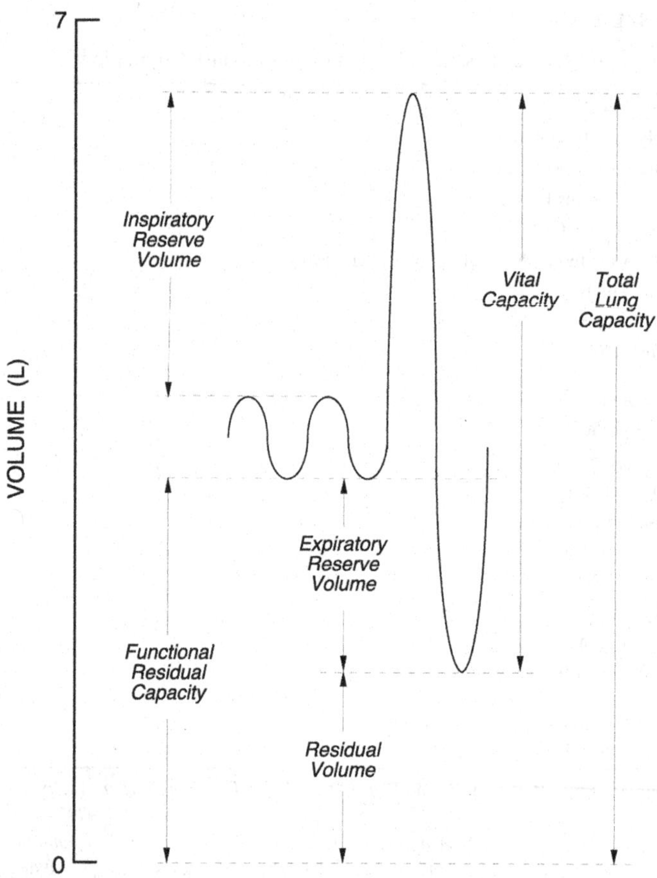

FIGURE 2.6 Spirometric representation of lung volumes.

pathological conditions can modify specific pulmonary volumes. Definitions of the specific lung volumes are provided in Table 2.4. Measurements of lung volumes are generally normalized for a subject's body size (weight, height, or surface area), age, and gender. This process permits a comparison with standardized or predicted lung volumes, thereby allowing identification of lung pathophysiologies using a simple procedure. Some examples of the way in which airway disorders alter lung volumes are described in the following. During an episode of airway obstruction (as in asthmatic bronchospasm), expiration of air is difficult, and air becomes trapped in the lower airways. This results in an increase in the residual volume and functional residual capacity and a decrease in vital capacity. In conditions that adversely affect respiratory muscles, such as poliomyelitis or spinal cord injuries, voluntary control of inspiratory or expiratory movement is diminished (or absent) and vital capacity is reduced.

Lung volumes can be determined by spirometry and reflect the volume of air remaining in the airways after various inspiratory or expiratory maneuvers. Lung capacities encompass two or more lung volumes (as shown by the provided formulas).

2.4.2 Measures of Airway Caliber

The diameter or caliber of the airways is of great value in the investigation or diagnosis of obstructive airways diseases. Techniques used to evaluate airway caliber generally centre on analysis of the rate of expiratory airflow because airway obstruction tends to diminish expiratory flow.

TABLE 2.4
Definitions of Lung Volumes

Volume	Definition
Tidal volume (TV)	Air inspired or expired during a normal breath
Inspiratory reserve volume (IRV)	Volume maximally inspired after a normal tidal inspiration
Expiratory reserve volume (ERV)	Volume maximally expired after a normal tidal expiration
Residual volume (RV)	Volume remaining in the airways after completion of a maximal expiratory effort
Inspiratory capacity	Volume inspired maximally after a normal expiration = TV + IRV
Functional residual capacity (FRC)	Volume remaining in the airways after a normal expiration = ERV + RV
Vital capacity	Volume maximally expired from the lungs after a maximal inspiration = IRV + TV + ERV
Total lung capacity	Volume in the airways after a maximal inspiration = IRV + TV + ERV + RV

2.4.2.1 Peak Flow Measurements

Perhaps the simplest measurement of expiratory airflow involves the use of a peak flowmeter. Subjects inspire maximally (i.e. to total lung capacity) and expire rapidly and maximally to residual volume into the mouthpiece of the instrument that provides a measurement of the peak expiratory flow. These instruments are simple to operate and often are provided to asthmatic patients for self-measurement and documentation of their ventilatory function.

2.4.2.2 Forced Expiratory Flow Measurements

Spirometric techniques are used to measure the time course of expired volumes. The same ventilatory maneuvers are conducted as those described for peak flow measurements. The subject exhales rapidly and maximally into the mouthpiece of the spirometer. This results in a trace similar to that shown in Figure 2.7. The volume expired in the first second is termed the forced expiratory volume ($FEV_{1.0}$), and the total volume expired is the forced vital capacity (FVC). $FEV_{1.0}$ may be normalized to account for the body size, sex, and age of the subject and, thereby, permit comparison with "normal" estimates. Alternatively, the ratio of $FEV_{1.0}$:FVC can be calculated. In subjects with normal airways, this ratio is approximately 0.8; under conditions of airway obstruction, the ratio is less than 0.8.

2.4.2.3 Airways Resistance and Dynamic Lung Compliance

Measurement of expiratory flow represents a simple, noninvasive means of estimating airway caliber. However, these measurements are relatively insensitive to changes in peripheral airway caliber. More complicated measures of caliber include airways resistance (R_L) and dynamic lung compliance (C_{dyn}). Airways resistance is thought to measure the caliber of the larger airways, such as the bronchi and bronchioles. Dynamic lung compliance measures the elasticity of the peripheral airways and is given as the change in volume of the lungs for a given change in pressure distending the alveoli. Measurement of these parameters in subjects involves highly specialized equipment (e.g. whole-body plethysmograph and pneumotachygraph) and can be invasive, i.e. requiring the placement of an intraesophageal balloon for intrathoracic pressure measurements. A precise description of the means of estimating these parameters is beyond the scope of the present discussion, but interested readers are directed to reference (Miller et al., 1987).

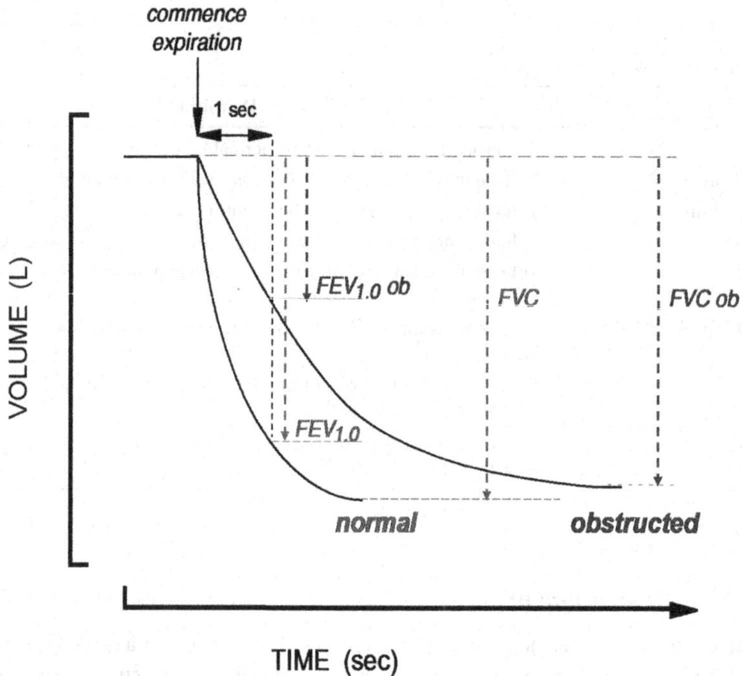

FIGURE 2.7 Forced expiratory flow maneuvers in normal and obstructed airways. A maximal expiratory effort from total lung capacity results in a rapid expiration of air from the lungs, the volume of which is equivalent to the FVC, and the rate of which is dependent on the caliber of the airways. The volume of air expired in the first second of a maximal expiratory effort is the $FEV_{1.0}$. In subjects with obstructed airways, air flow is retarded as reflected in a smaller $FEV_{1.0}$ ($FEV_{1.0}$ob) than in subjects with normal airways ($FEV_{1.0}$).

2.5 Aerosol Deposition and Airway Physiology

In considering the mechanisms of aerosol deposition within the lung and the factors that may influence them, it is of some importance to consider first the anatomy and air velocities within the respiratory tract. The temporal aspects of the passage of air through the various anatomic regions and the point during the breathing cycle are also relevant factors.

The angles of branching, the diameter and lengths of different elements of the airways, and the pulmonary air spaces must be visualized in an arbitrary and oversimplified form to make practical use of anatomic data. Some of the details of the divisions of the respiratory system that have been assumed by Landahl (1950a), and the anatomic flow rate and transitional features in these areas are shown in Table 2.5.

For a specific minute volume, the actual rate of airflow throughout the ventilatory cycle varies from zero to a maximum and back to zero. Thus, as air velocity and time of air transit within the system determine the effectiveness of particle deposition, it is evident that this must vary over a considerable range within the cycle.

At least two regions of the respiratory tract are ventilated at different rates. Of the total inspired air, 40% ventilates 17% of the lung, and the remaining 60% ventilates the other 83% of the lung. Consequently, such unequal distribution of ventilation, air velocity, and times of air passage produce different probabilities of deposition of the inhaled particles from one site to another at the same structural depth.

The volume of the nasopharyngeal chamber and airways is 150 mL, that is, dead space volume. Thus, with a resting tidal volume of 600 mL, only 75% of the air reaches the pulmonary air spaces. There is evidence to suggest that sequential breathing patterns occur that result in poorly ventilated regions (Bums et al., 1985; Frazer et al., 1985; Maxwell et al., 1985).

TABLE 2.5

Schematic Representation of the Respiratory Tract

Region	Diameter (cm)	Length (cm)	Velocity (cm s^{-1})	Passage Time (s)
Mouth	2	7	100	0.07
Pharynx	3	3	45	0.07
Trachea	1.4	11	150	0.07
Bronchi				
Primary	1.0	6.5	190	0.03
Secondary	0.4	3	200	0.015
Tertiary	0.2	1.5	100	0.015
Quarternary	0.15	0.5	22	0.02
Terminal bronchioles	0.06	0.3	2	0.15
Respiratory	0.05	0.15	1.4	0.1
Alveolar ducts	0.02	0.02	—	—
Alveolar sacs	0.03	0.03	—	—

Source: Landahl, H., *Bull. Math. Biophys.*, 12, 43–56, 1950a; Landahl, H., *Bull. Math. Biophys.*, 12, 161–169, 1950b.

The complexity of the anatomic and dynamic factors involved in deposition can readily be appreciated from the brief outline of factors involved.

The physiological factors that influence aerosol deposition in the lung have been investigated experimentally (Chan and Lippman, 1980; Chan et al., 1980; Ferron, 1977a, 1977b; Martonen, 1983; Schlesinger et al., 1977) and theoretically (Davies, 1980; Gerrity et al., 1979; Horsfield, 1976; Lee and Wang, 1976; Rudolph, 1984; Yeh and Schum, 1980; Yeh et al., 1979; Yu and Diu, 1983). Flow rates within the lung affect deposition. Airway obstruction (Dubois et al., 1956), breathing rate (Emmett et al., 1979; Williams, 1982), and breath holding (Lawford and McKenzie, 1982; Palmes et al., 1973; Yu and Thiagarajen, 1979) determine these rates. Because species variations (Brain et al., 1984; Taylor et al., 1984) and the state of the lung, whether healthy or diseased (Brain et al., 1984; Stahlhofen et al., 1984), influence the physiological factors, they are being investigated with a view to establishing predictable patterns in deposition.

The nature of particle deposition forces and their relationship to aerodynamic particle size have been the subject of many studies and reports. A variety of models for aerosol deposition in the respiratory tract have been proposed. The most notable are those of Findeisen (1935), Landahl (1950a, 1950b), and Weibel (1963).

Rohrer (1955) measured the diameter and length of the elements of the bronchial tree and constructed a dimensional model on which he based his reasoning on flow resistance in the human airways.

Findeisen was the first to examine the problem of respiratory deposition of aerosols in physical-mathematical terms. After dividing the airways into nine successive sections, starting with the trachea, he assumed a constant rate of respiration (frequency = 15 breaths/min, tidal volume = 200 mL) from which the air velocities and times of air passage through successive zones were calculated. With these parameters, the average angles of branching from one order to the next could be postulated. Landahl modified the assumed anatomic arrangement in some respects. In this model, the airways were divided into 12 sections by including the mouth and pharynx and two orders of alveolar ducts. The parameters adopted in this model were a tidal volume of 450 mL, a breathing frequency of 15 breaths/min, pauses of half seconds at the beginning and middle of each cycle, and a constant respiration rate of 300 mL/sec. The local velocities and times of air passage through the successive sections were obtained using this flow rate and a variety of breathing frequencies and tidal volumes in Landahl's calculation of respiratory deposition. In all cases, the inspiratory and expiratory phases were assumed to consist of a constant airflow rate. Work based on this model has been performed by Beeckmans (1965).

Weibel (1963) criticized the Findeisen-Landahl model as being based on insufficient clinical data, and, thus, the dimensions of even the proximal airways were not correct. The zones consisting of different branching factors were also criticized as inadequately representing the pulmonary architecture. Weibel proposed two alternative models: the first emphasized the regular features of the airways, and the second accounted for some irregularities. The fundamental geometry of dichotomy was the basis for these models: this refers to the average adult lung and includes the airway of the conductive, transitory, and respiratory zones, as well as the blood vessels (alveolar capillaries) of the respiratory zone.

Lipmann and colleagues described experimental data on the deposition of aerosols in vivo (Lippman, 1970; Lippman and Albert, 1969; Lippman et al., 1971). They noted that, among normal subjects and nonbronchitic smokers, each individual has a characteristic and reproducible deposition pattern with respect to particle size. This contrasts with the great variation from subject to subject among cigarette smokers and patients with lung disease. Other studies pertaining to alveolar penetration, deposition, and mixing have been performed (Altschuler et al., 1959; Beeckmans, 1965; Lippman, 1970). Davies and colleagues described deposition studies directed at particles with minimal settling and diffusional deposition tendencies, that is, 0.1 μm to 1.0 μm (Davies, 1970; Davies et al., 1972). Particulate deposition by the nasal airways has been reported (George and Breslin, 1967; Heyder and Rudolph, 1977; Hounam, 1971), as has deposition by mouth inhalation (Gonda and Byron, 1978). Other studies have emphasized deposition of highly diffusive aerosols (Yu and Thiagarajen, 1979).

In 1966, the ICRP Task Group on Lung Dynamics examined the models and experimental data in the literature and described the deposition of aerosols in three areas of the lung: the nasopharyngeal, tracheobronchial, and pulmonary regions (Dynamics, 1966). The investigators' major concern was the deposition of hazardous aerosols. The Task Group's predictive model uses Findeisen's simplified anatomy and his impaction and sedimentation equations (Findeisen, 1935). For diffusional deposition, the equations of Gormley and Kennedy (1949) were adopted, and the nasal route of entry was assumed. For a tidal volume of 1,450 mL, there were relatively small differences in estimated deposition over a wide range of geometric standard deviations ($1.2 < g < 4.5$). The comparison of this model with earlier predictive models indicated that Landahl's model was the closest, but overestimated alveolar deposition for particles with aerodynamic diameters larger than 3.5 μm. The major conclusion of the Task Group was that regional deposition within the respiratory tract may be estimated using a single aerosol measurement: the mass median diameter. Subsequently, investigators (Morrow, 1981) have reaffirmed the importance of the geometric standard deviation, taken in conjunction with the mass median diameter, in-mouth breathing, for describing the character of the aerosol. This observation may be of relevance because of the heterodispersed nature of therapeutic aerosols (Mercer et al., 1968). The degree of polydispersity of an aerosol, which may be described by the geometric standard deviation, has been shown to influence significantly aerosol deposition in the respiratory tract. Models have been developed for mouth inhalation where the complex nasal filtration and deposition does not occur (Gonda, 1981; Mercer et al., 1968).

From the Task Group model, it was suggested that particles must have a diameter less than 10 μm before deposition occurs in regions below the nasopharynx. Aerosols with diameters between 1 μm and 5 μm are deposited primarily in the tracheobronchial and pulmonary regions, and aerosols with diameters less than 1 μm are deposited predominately in the pulmonary region. This guide to the deposition of aerosol particles may be explained in terms of physicochemical parameters governing aerosol particle behavior.

2.6 Conclusion

The primary function of the lungs is gaseous exchange supplying oxygen to support life and eliminating carbon dioxide, the product of metabolism. The flow of air into and from the lungs is supported by a complex anatomical structure and demands a variety of physiological properties that support pulmonary function. The molecular and cellular structural elements of the lungs support specific biochemical and biophysical processes that maintain the integrity of the lungs. Biochemical mediators interact with cells to promote action at the macro-scale to move air and on micro-scale to facilitate transport of oxygen and a number of other important biomolecules and ions. The healthy lung is a finely tuned organ system that is essential to life. The diseased lung fails to a greater or lesser degree based on the ability to adequately support gaseous exchange and as a potential site for the dissemination of disease to other sites in the body, whether through inflammation, infection, or malfunctioning autologous cells. Understanding normal lung physiology and the influence of disease is a foundational component to using pharmaceutical aerosol treatment.

REFERENCES

Abraham, W. (2002). Trypase: Potential role in airway inflammation and remodeling. *American Journal of Lung Cell Molecular Physiology, 282*, L193–L196.

Altschuler, B., Palmes, E., Yarmus, L., & Nelson, N. (1959). Intrapulmonary mixing of gases studied with aerosols. *Journal of Applied Physiology, 14*, 321–327.

Baker, B., Peatfield, A., & Richardson, P. (1985). Nervous control of mucin secretion into human bronchi. *Journal of Physiology (London), 365*, 297–305.

Baraniuk, J.N., Ohkubo, K., Kwon, O.J., Mak, J., Ali, M., Davies, R., Twort, C., Kaliner, M., Letarte, M., & Barnes, P.J. (1995). Localization of neutral endopeptidase (NEP) mRNA in human bronchi. *European Respiratory Journal, 8*, 1458–1464.

Battistini, B., & Dussault, P. (1998). Biosynthesis, distribution and metabolism of endothelins in the pulmonary system. *Pulmonary Pharmacology and Therapeutics, 11*, 79–88.

Beeckmans, J. (1965). The deposition of aerosols in the respriatory tract. I. Mathematical analysis and comparison with experimental data. *Canadian Journal of Physiology and Pharmacology, 43*, 157–172.

Bouhuys, A. (1974). Breathing: Physiology, environment and lung disease. In A. Bouhuys (Ed.), (p. 25). New York: Grune & Stratton.

Brain, J., Sweeney, T., Tryka, A., Skomik, W., & Godleski, J. (1984). Effects of pulmonary fibrosis on aeroosl deposition in hamsters. *Journal of Aerosol Science, 15*, 217–218.

Bums, C., Taylor, W., & Ingram, R. (1985). Effects of a deep inhalation in ashtma: Relative airway and parenchymal hysteresis. *Journal of Applied Physiology, 59*, 1590–1596.

Caughey, G. (1991). The structure and airway biology of mast cell proteinases. *American Journal of Respiratory and Critical Care Medicine, 282*, 387–394.

Chan, T., & Lippman, M. (1980). Experimental measurements and empirical modelling of the regional deposition of inhaled particles in humans. *American Industrial Hygiene Association Journal, 41*, 399–409.

Chan, T., Schrenck, R., & Lippman, M. (1980). Effect of laryngeal jet on particle deposition in the human trachea and upper bronchial airways. *Journal of Aerosol Science, 11*, 447–459.

Cocks, T., & Moffatt, J. (2001). Protease-activated receptors-2 (PAR2) in the airways. *Pulmonary Pharmacology and Therapeutics, 14*, 183–191.

Coleridge, J., & Coleridge, H. (1984). Afferent vagal C fiber innervation of the lungs and airways and its functional significance. *Reviews in Physiology Biochemistry and Pharmacology, 99*, 1–110.

Crapo, J., Barry, B., Gehr, P., Bachofen, M., & Weibel, E. (1982). Cell number and cell characteristics of the normal human lung. *American Review Respiratory Disease, 125*, 332–337.

Crapo, J., Young, S., Fram, E., Pinkerton, K., Barry, B., & Crapo, R. (1983). Morphometric characteristics of cells in the alveolar region of mammalian lungs. *American Review Respiratory Disease, 128*, S42–S46.

Cutz, E., & Jackson, A. (1999). Neuroepithelial bodies as airway oxygen sensors. *Respiration Physiology, 115*, 201–214.

Cutz, E., & Orange, R. (1977). Mast cells and endocrine (APUD) cells of the lung. In L. Lichtenstein & K. Austen (Eds.), *Asthma: Physiology, Immunopharmacology and Treatment* (pp. 51–74). New York: Academic Press.

Davies, C. (1970). In T. Mercer, P. Morrow, & W. Stober (Eds.), *Assessment of Airborne Particles: Rochester Third International Conference on Environmental Toxicity* (p. 371). Springfield, IL: Charles C Thomas.

Davies, C. (1980). An algebraic model for the deposition of aerosols in the human respiratory tract during steady state breathing-Addendum. *Journal of Aerosol Science, 11*, 213–224.

Davies, C., Heyder, J., & Subba-Ramu, M. (1972). Breathing of half-micron aerosols. I. Experiment. *Journal of Applied Physiology, 32*, 591–600.

de Nucci, G., Thomas, R., D'Orleans-Juste, P., Antunes, E., Walder, C., Warner, T., & Vane, J. (1988). Pressor effects of circulating endothelin are limited by its removal in the pulmonary circulation and by the release of prostacyclin and endothelium-derived relaxing factor. *Proceedings of the National Academy of Sciences (USA), 85*, 9797–9800.

Diamond, L., & Altiere, R. (1989). Airway nonadrenergic noncholinergic inhibitory nervous system. In M. Kaliner & P. Barnes (Eds.), *The Airways: Neural Control in Health and Disease* (pp. 343–394). New York: Marcel Dekker.

Dubois, A., Botelho, S., & Comroe, J. (1956). A new method for measuring airway resistance in man using a body plethysmograph: Values in patients with respiratory disease. *Journal of Clinical Investigation, 35*, 327–335.

Dynamics, ICRP. Task Group on Lung (1966). Deposition and retention models for internal dosimetry of the human respiratory tract. *Health Physics, 12*, 173–207.

Effros, R. (1991). Permabulity of the blood gas barrier. In R. Crystal & J. West (Eds.), *The Lung: Scientific Foundations, Volume 1* (pp. 1163–1176). New York: Raven Press.

Emmett, P., Aitken, R., & Muir, D. (1979). A new apparatus for use in studies of the total and regional deposition of aerosol particles in the human respiratory tract during steady breathing. *Journal of Aerosol Science, 10*, 123–131.

Ferreira, S., Greene, L., Salgado, M., & Krieger, E. (1980) *Metabolic Activities of the Lung—Ciba Foundation Symposium 78* (p. 129). Amsterdam, the Netherlands: Excerpta Medica.

Ferreira, S., & Vane, J. (1967). The disappearance of bradykinin and eledoisin in the circulation and vascular beds of the cat. *British Journal of Pharmacology and Chemotherapy, 30*, 417–424.

Ferron, G. (1977a). Deposition of polydisperse aerosols in two glass models. Representing the upper human airways. *Journal of Aerosol Science, 8*, 409–427.

Ferron, G. (1977b). The size of soluble aerosol particles as a function of the humidity of the air. Application to the human repsiratory tract. *Journal of Aerosol Science, 8*, 251–267.

Findeisen, W. (1935). Uber sa absetzen kleiner, in der luft suspendierten teilchen in der menschlichen lunge bei der atmung. (Concerning the deposition of small airborne particles in the human lung during breathing.) *Pfluegers Arch Ges Physiol, 236–379*, 367.

Finkbeiner, W. (1999). Physiology and pathology of tracheobronchial glands. *Respiration Physiology, 118*, 77–83.

Frazer, D., Weber, K., & Franz, G. (1985). Evidence of sequential opening and closing of lung units during inflation-deflation of excised rat lungs. *Respiration Physiology, 61*, 277–288.

Gail, D., & L'enfant, C. (1983). Cells of the lung: Biology and clinical implications. *American Review Respiratory Disease, 127*, 366–387.

Gehr, P., Bachofen, M., & Weibel, E. (1978). The normal human lung: Ultrastructure and morphometric estimation of diffusion capacity. *Respiration Physiology, 32*, 121–140.

George, A., & Breslin, A. (1967). Deposition of natural radon daughters in human subjects. *Health Physics, 13*, 375–378.

Gerrity, T., Lee, P., Hass, F., Marinelli, A., Werner, P., & Lourenco, R. (1979). Calculated depotiionof inhaled particles in the airway generations of normal subjects. *Journal of Applied Physiology: Respiratory, Environmental and Exercise Physiology, 47*, 867–873.

Godfrey, R. (1997). Freeze fracture electron microscopy has been used to investigate the structure of human airway tight junctions and their morphology. *Microscopy Research Techniques, 38*, 488–499.

Gonda, I. (1981). A semi-empirical model of aerosol deposition in the human respiratory tract for mouth inhalation. *Journal of Pharmacy and Pharmacology, 33*, 692–696.

Gonda, I., & Byron, P. (1978). Perspectives on the biopharmacy of inhalation aerosols. *Drug Development and Industrial Pharmacy, 4*, 243–259.

Gormley, P., & Kennedy, M. (1949). Diffusion from a stream flowing through a cylindrical tube. *Proceedings of Royal Irish Academy, 52A*, 163–169.

Gryglewski, R. (1990) *Metabolic Activities of the Lung—Ciba Foundation Symposium 78* (p. 147). New York: Excerpa Medica.

Heyder, J., & Rudolph, G. (1977). Deposition of aerosol particles in the human nose. In W. Walton (Ed.), *Inhaled Particles, Volume IV* (p. 107). Oxford, UK: Pergamon Press.

Holt, P., Schon-Hegrad, M., Phillips, M., & McMenamin, P. (1989). Ia-positive densdritic cells form a tightly meshed network within the human airway epithelium. *Clinical and Experimental Allergy, 19*, 597–601.

Horsfield, K. (1976). Some mathematical properties of branching trees with application to the respiratory system. *Bulletin of Mathematical Biophysics, 38*, 305–315.

Hounam, R. (1971). In W. Walton (Ed.), *Inhaled Particles, Volume III* (p. 71). Oxford, UK: Pergamon Press.

Hyman, A., Spannhake, E., & Kadowitz, P. (1978). Prostaglandins and the lung. *American Review Respiratory Disease, 117*, 111–136.

Inoue, S., & Hogg, J. (1974). Intercellular junctions of the tracheal epithelium in guinea pigs. *Laboratory Investigation, 31*(68–71).

Jeffrey, P. (1983). Morphologic features of airway surface epithelial cells and glands. *American Review of Respiratory Disease, 128*, S14–S20.

Landahl, H. (1950a). On the removal of air-borne droplets by the human respiratory tract: I. The lung. *Bulletin of Mathematical Biophysics, 12*, 43–56.

Landahl, H. (1950b). On the removal of airborne droplets by the human respiratory tract II. The nasal passages. *Bulletin of Mathematical Biophysics, 12*, 161–169.

Laskin, D., & Laskin, J. (2001). Role of macrophages and inflammatory mediators in chemically induced toxicity. *Toxicology, 160*, 111–118.

Lawford, P., & McKenzie, D. (1982). Pressurized bronchodilator aerosol technique: Influence of breath-holding time and relationship of inhaler in mouth. *British Journal of Diseases of the Chest, 76*, 229–233.

Lee, W.C., & Wang, C.S. (1976). Particle deposition in systems of repeatedly bifurcating tubes. In W. Walton (Ed.), *Inhaled Particles* (pp. 49–53). Oxford, UK: Pergamon Press.

Lippman, M. (1970). Assessment sampling for hazard evaluation. In T. Mercer, P. Morrow, & W. Stober (Eds.), *Assessment of Airborne Particles. Rochester Third International Conference in Environmental Toxicity* (p. 449). Springfield, IL: Charles C Thomas.

Lippman, M., & Albert, R. (1969). The effect of particle size on the regional deposition of inhaled aerosols in the human respiratory tract. *American Industrial Hygiene Association Journal, 30*, 257–275.

Lippman, M., Albert, R., & Peterson, H. (1971). In W. Walton (Ed.), *Inhaled Particles, Volume III* (p. 105). Oxford, UK: Pergamon Press.

Lundberg, J., Hokfelt, T., Martling, C.R., Saria, A., & Cuello, C. (1984). Substance P-immunoreactive sensory nerves in the lower respiratory tract of various mammals including man. *Cell and Tissue Research, 235*, 251–261.

Marshall, C., & Marshall, B. (1983). Site and sensitivity for stimulation of hypoxic pulmonary vasoconstriction. *Journal of Applied Physiology: Respiratory, Environmental and Exercise Physiology, 55*, 711–716.

Martins, M., Shore, S., & Drazen, J. (1991). Peptidase modulation of the pulmonary effects of tachykinins. *International Archive of Allergy and Applied Immunology, 94*, 325–329.

Martonen, T. (1983). Measurement of particle dose distribution in a model of a human larynx and tracheobronchial tree. *Journal of Aerosol Science, 14*, 11–22.

Maxwell, D., Cover, D., & Hughes, J. (1985). Effect of respiratory apparatus on timing and depth of breathing in man. *Respiration Physiology, 61*, 255–264.

McDonald, D., Bowden, J., Baluk, P., & Bunnett, N. (1996). Neurogenic inflammation. A model for studying efferent actions of sensory nerves. *Advances in Experimental Medicine and Biology, 410*, 453–462.

Mercer, T., Goddard, R., & Flores, R. (1968). Output characteristics of three ultrasonic nebulizers. *Annals of Allergy, 26*, 18–27.

Meyrick, B., Sturgess, J., & Reid, L. (1960). A reconstruction of the duct system and secretory tubules of the human bronchial submucosal gland. *Thorax, 24*, 729–736.

Michoud, M.C., Jeanneret-Grosjean, A., Cohen, A., & Amyot, P. (1088). Refex decrease of histamine-induced bronchoconstriction after laryngeal stimulation in asthmatic patients. *American Review Respiratory Disease, 138*, 1548–1552.

Miller, W., Scacci, R., & Gast, L. (1987). *Laboratory Evaluation of Pulmonary Function*. New York: JD Lippincott.

Mills, P., Davies, R., & Devalia, J. (1999). Airway epithelia cells, cytokines and pollutants. *American Review Respiratory Disease and Critical Care Medicine, 160*, S38–S43.

Morrow, P. (1973). Alveolar clearance of aerosols. *Archives of Internal Medicine*, 101–108.

Morrow, P. (1981). An evaluation of the physical properties of monodisperse and heterodisperse aerosols used in the assessment of bronchial function. *Chest, 80*, 809–813.

Murray, J. (1986). Metabolic functions and liquid and solute exchange. In J. Murray (Ed.), *The Normal Lung: The Basis for Diagnosis and Treatment of Disease* (pp. 283–312). Philadelphia, PA: EB Saunders.

Palmes, E., Wang, C.-S., Goldring, R., & Altshuler, B. (1973). Effect of depth of inhalation on aerosol persistence during breaht holding. *Journal of Applied Physiology, 34*, 356–360.

Parks, W., & Shapiro, S. (2001). Matrix metalloproteinases in lung biology. *Respiration Physiology, 2*, 10–19.

Piper, P., Tippiins, J., Samhoun, M., Morris, H., Taylor, G., & Jones, C. (1981). SRS-A and its formation by the lung. *Bulletin Europeen Physiopathologie Respiratoire, 17*, 571–583.

Reid, L. (1960). Measurement of the bronchiual mucous gland layer: A diagnostic yardstick in chronic bronchitis. *Thorax, 15*, 132–141.

Richardson, J. (1977). The neural control of human tracheobronchial smooth muscle. In L. Lichtenstein & K. Austen (Eds.), *Asthma: Physiology, Immunopharmacology and Treatment* (pp. 237–245). New York: Academic Press.

Rogers, D. (1994). Airway goblet cells: Responsive and adaptable front-line defenders. *European Journal of Respiration, 7*, 1690–1706.

Rogers, D. (2000). Motor control of airway goblet cells and glands. *Respiration Physiology, 125*, 129–144.

Rohrer, F. (1955). In J. West (Ed.), *Translations in Respiratory Physiology* (p. 3). Stroudsberg, PA: Dowden, Hutchison and Ross.

Rudolph, G. (1984). A mathematical model for the deposition of aerosol particles in the human respiratory tract. *Journal of Aerosol Science, 15*, 195–199.

Ryan, J. (1989). Peptidase enzymes of the pulmonary vascular surface. *American Journal of Physiology: Lung celular and Molecular Physiology, 257*, L53–L60.

Ryan, J., & Ryan, U. (1977). Pulmonary endothelial cells. *Federal Proceedings, 36*, 2683–2691.

Scheuermann, D. (1997). Comparative histology of pulmonary neuroendocrine cell system in mammalian lungs. *Microscopy Research Techniques, 37*, 31–42.

Schlesinger, R., Bohning, D., Chan, T., & Lippman, M. (1977). Particle deposition in a hollow case of the human tracheobronchial tree. *Journal of Aerosol Science, 8*, 429–445.

Schuster, V. (1998). Molecular mechanisms of prostaglandin transport. *Annual Review of Physiology, 60*, 221–242.

Schutte, B., & MCCray, P.M., Jr. (2002). [beta]-defensins in lung host defense. *Annual Review of Physiology, 64*, 709–748.

Serikov, V., & Fleming, N. (2001). Pulmonary and bronchial circulations: Contributions to heat and water exchange in isolated lungs. *Journal of Applied Physiology, 91*, 1977–1985.

Shapiro, S. (1999). The macrophage in chronic obstructive pulmonary disease. *American Review Respiratory Disease and Critical Care Medicine, 160*, S29–S32.

Sibile, Y., & Reynolds, H. (1990). Macrophages and polymorphonuclear neutrophils in lung defense and injury. *American Review Respiratory Disease, 141*, 471–501.

Simionescu, M. (1980). *Metabolic Activities of the Lung: Ciba Foundation Symposium 78*. New York: Excerpta Medica.

Sole, M., Dobrac, M., Schwartz, L., Hussain, M., & Vaughn-Neil, E. (1979). The extraction of circulating catecholamines by the lungs in normal man and in patients with pulmonary hypertension. *Circulation, 60*, 160–163.

Spina, D. (1998). Epithelium smooth muscle regulation and interactions. *American Review Respiratory Disease and Critical Care Medicine, 158*, S141–S145.

Stahlhofen, W., Gebhart, J., Heyder, J., Scheuch, G., & Juraske, P. (1984). Particle deposition in extrathoracic airways of healthy subjects and of patients with early stages of laryngeal carcinoma. *Journal of Aerosol Science, 15*, 215–217.

Taylor, S., Pare, P., & Schellenberg, R. (1984). Cholinergic and nonadrenergic mechanisms in human and guinea-pig airways. *Journal of Applied Physiology, 56*, 958–965.

Thomas, D., & Vane, J. (1967). 5–Hydroxytrypatamine in the circulation of the dog. *Nature, 216*, 335–338.

Tyler, W. (1983). Comparative subgross anatomy of the lungs. Pleuras, interlobular septa, and distal airways. *American Review Respiratory Disease, 128*, S32–36.

Ueki, I., German, V., & Nadel, J. (1980). Micropipette measurement of airway submucosal gland secretion. Autonomic effects. *American Review Respiratory Disease, 121*, 351–357.

Voelker, D., & Mason, R. (1989). Lung cell biology. In D. Massaro (Ed.), *Lung Cell Biology* (pp. 487–538). New York: Marcel Dekker.

Wasserman, S. (1983). Mediators of immediate hypersensitivity. *Journal of Allergy and Clinical Immunology, 72*, 101–115.

Weibel, E. (1963). *Morphometry of the Human Lung*. Berlin, Germany: Springer-Verlag.

Weibel, E. (1984). *The Pathway for Oxygen*. Cambridge, MA: Harvard University Press.

Widdicombe, J. (1963). Regulation of tracheobronchial smooth muscle. *Physiological Reviews, 43*, 1–37.

Widdicombe, J. (2001). Airway receptors. *Respiration Physiology, 125*, 3–15.

Williams, M. (1990). In D. Schraufnagel (Ed.), *Electron Microscopy of the Lung* (p. 121). New York: Marcel Dekker.

Williams, T. (1982). The importance of aerosol technique: Does speed of inhalation matter? *British Journal of Diseases of the Chest, 76*, 223–229.

Yeh, H.C., & Schum, G. (1980). Models of human lung airways and their application to inhaledpartile deposition. *Bulletin of Mathematical Biology, 42*, 461–480.

Yeh, H.C., Schum, G., & Duggan, M. (1979). Anatomic models of the tracheobronchial and pulmonary regions ofthe rat. *Anatomical Record, 195*, 483–492.

Yu, C.P., & Diu, C. (1983). Total and regional deposition of inhaled aerosols in humans. *Journal of Aerosol Science, 14*, 599–609.

Yu, C.P., & Thiagarajen, C. (1979). Decay of aerosols in the lung during breath holding. *Journal of Aerosol Science, 10*, 11–19.

3

Drug Targeting to the Lung: Chemical and Biochemical Considerations

Peter A. Crooks, Narsimha R. Penthala, and Abeer M. Al-Ghananeem

CONTENTS

3.1 Introduction and General Considerations

Since the 1950s, most drugs that were targeted to the respiratory tract were used for their local action, that is, nasal decongestion, bronchodilation, and so on. It has become apparent that the lining of the upper respiratory tract (i.e. the nasal mucosa) and the airways can also be used for the absorption of a drug for its systemic effect, particularly if this route of administration avoids the metabolic destruction observed with alternative routes of administration (Crooks and Damani 1989, Brown et al. 1983). This area has attracted considerable interest, particularly with regard to the delivery of peptides and proteins, which suffer from rapid degradation by peptidases by the oral route. Numerous studies have demonstrated that such drugs can be administered systemically by application to the respiratory tract, either to the nasal mucosa or to the lungs.

The lung provides substantially greater bioavailability for macromolecules than any other port of entry to the body (Byron and Patton 1994, Patton and Platz 1992). Large proteins (18 kDa–20 kDa), such as human growth hormone, show pulmonary bioavailability approaching or exceeding 50% (Colthorpe et al. 1995), while bioavailability might approach 100% for small peptides and insulin (<6 kDa) placed in the lung compared to delivery by subcutaneous injection. The lung has several dynamic barriers, the first of which is the lung surfactant layer, which is probably a single molecule thick. Spreading at the air/water interface both in airway and alveolar surface, this surfactant layer may cause large molecules to aggregate, which might enhance engulfment and digestion by air space macrophages. Interaction of some drug molecules administered by inhalation may interfere with surfactant function and lead to an increase in local surface tension, which could produce either collapse of the alveoli or edema through altered transpulmonary pressures (Possmayer et al. 1984). Below the molecular layer(s) of lung surfactant lie the epithelial surface fluids. Macromolecules must defuse to get to the epithelial cell layer. It has been shown that the volume and composition of the surface liquids in this layer are regulated by ion transport in pulmonary epithelium (Boucher 1994). Patton (1996) mentioned in his review that in the airway, the thickness of the surface fluid is thought to average about 5 μm–10 μm, gradually decreasing distally until the vast expanse of the alveolar is reached, covered with a very thin layer of fluid that averages about 0.05 μm–0.08 μm thick. This layer may be several microns thick in pooled areas and as thin as 15 nm–20 nm in other areas. The lining fluid of the airway contains various types and amounts of mucus, except on the alveoli, which concentrate on top of the surface. This mucus blanket, which covers the conducting airways, and which is moved by ciliated cells in an upwards direction to the pharynx, may affect pulmonary drug delivery. Drug transport may be affected as a result of drug binding to mucus compounds; increases in the thickness of the mucus layer may reduce the rate of drug absorption, and a change in the diameter of the airways may also affect the sites of drug deposition.

The ultrastructure of the respiratory membrane is unique by virtue of its function. A diagrammatic representation of the respiratory membrane is shown in Figure 3.1. The respiratory membrane basically

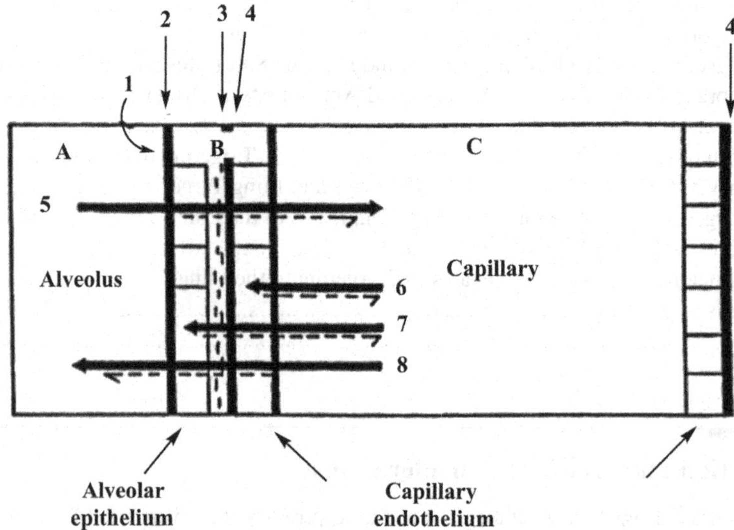

FIGURE 3.1 Diagrammatic representation of the ultrastructure of the respiratory membrane. Arrows indicate the passage of drugs (horizontal heavy lines) through the respiratory membrane after alveolar or capillary *exposure, or* of metabolites (horizontal broken lines) generated in the epithelial or endothelial layers. Key: (1) monomolecular surfactant layers, (2) thin fluid film, (3) interstitial space, (4) endothelial capillary basement membrane, (5) drug transport from the alveoli, (6) absorption of drug into endothelial cells from the circulation, (7) transport of drug from the circulation to alveolar epithelium, and (8) transport of drug from the circulation to the alveoli. (Reproduced by permission, FDC Report, May 22 1989, CRC Press.)

comprises two main layers. The first layer is the alveolar epithelium, which consists of at least three different cell types: alveolar types I, II, and III or brush cells and migratory alveolar macrophages. The epithelial layer has a thin fluid film that is covered by a monomolecular layer of surfactant. Unlike the endothelium, the epithelial basement membrane is not distinct, but is usually observed to be fused into one layer with the epithelial cells. The second layer, the capillary endothelium, with its basement membrane, is separated from the endothelial layer by an interstitial space. The overall thickness of these layers is less than 0.1 μm and in some areas of the respiratory tract is as thin as 0.1 μm. Exposure of the respiratory tract to drugs or xenobiotics can occur by either the airways or the vasculature. Because the venous drainage from the entire body perfuses through the alveolar capillary unit, drugs that are administered at sites other than by direct application to the respiratory tract may still find their way into lung tissue, either by unique lung uptake (endothelial) mechanisms or by designed targeting. In this case of drug delivery by inhalation administration, several factors can affect drug absorption and clearance from the respiratory tract.

The absorption of drug molecules through lung epithelium has received more attention in recent years. The lung is lined by a layer of epithelial cells that extends from the ciliated columnar cells of the conducting airways by an abrupt transition to the flattened cells of the alveolar region. Earlier studies by Schanker (1978) and Schanker et al. (1986) showed that most xenobiotics are absorbed by passive diffusion at rates that correlate with their apparent partition coefficients at pH 7.4. Thus, like the gastrointestinal membrane, the endothelial membrane appears to behave like a typical phospholipid membrane. However, poorly lipid-soluble compounds generally diffuse more rapidly than would be expected, suggesting that pulmonary epithelial diffusion may occur through aqueous pores. In addition, certain drugs (e.g. disodium cromoglycate) are known to undergo carrier-mediated transport, which is unique for lung epithelial cells. Pulmonary microvascular endothelial cells form a restrictive barrier to macromolecular flux, even more so than arterial cells. The mechanisms responsible for this intrinsic feature are unknown. However, cyclic adenosine monophosphate (cAMP) improves endothelial barrier function by promoting/regulating cell-cell and cell-matrix association (Adamson et al. 1998, Walter et al. 1995, Cullere et al. 2005, Sayner and Stevens 2006, Sayner et al. 2006), but prolonged activation of cAMP signaling leads to endothelial barrier disruption via transcriptional repression of the small guanosine triphosphate hydrolase Ras-related protein (R-)RAS (Perrot et al. in press). Endothelial cells form a semipermeable barrier to fluid and protein transudation in the non-inflamed lung that limits accumulation in interstitial spaces (Taylor et al. 1997). Inflammatory mediators increase pulmonary macrovascular permeability (Chetham et al. 1999, Townsley et al. 1988, Gavard and Gutkind 2006).

Significant emphasis has been placed on elucidating the cellular and molecular mechanisms governing the pulmonary microvascular endothelial cell response to inflammatory stimuli (Moore et al. 1998, Schlegel and Waschke 2014, Parnell et al. 2012). Constituent protein flux is greatly attenuated in response to inflammation (del Vecchio et al. 1992, Schaeffer and Bitrick 1995, Parnell et al. 2012). This enhancement in barrier property is associated with increased expression of focal adhesion complexes that promote cell-cell contact (Schnitzer et al. 1994, Seibert et al. 1992, Stevens et al. 1999, Sawada et al. 2012). Increases in cAMP may account for enhanced barrier properties of pulmonary endothelial cells, since elevating cAMP may reduce inflammation permeability by promoting cell-cell contact. When an aerosolized drug is administered to the respiratory tract, it must cross the epithelial cell barrier to enter either the lung tissue (topical effect) or the circulation (systemic effect). The pulmonary epithelium has a high resistance to the movement of water and lipid-insoluble compounds, which usually diffuse through the tissue very slowly, either by a vesicular mechanism or by leaks in the intercellular tight junctions. The characteristic feature of this type of junction bestows on the epithelium a 10-fold greater resistance to the permeation by hydrophilic probe molecules than that of the pulmonary vascular endothelium. For the delivery of macromolecules, such as peptides and oligonucleotides, an understanding of these mechanisms of epithelial transport is crucial.

Enhancement of drug uptake by altered junctional (paracellular) or vesicular (transcellular) transport (Figure 3.2) is an active area of research. The paracellular transport mechanism provides an explanation for the pulmonary absorption of peptides and proteins ≤ 40 kDa.

The pore radius of paracellular channels between epithelial cells is about 1 nm, which is a quarter of the pore radius found between the adjacent endothelial cells. Thus, macromolecules with molecular radii greater

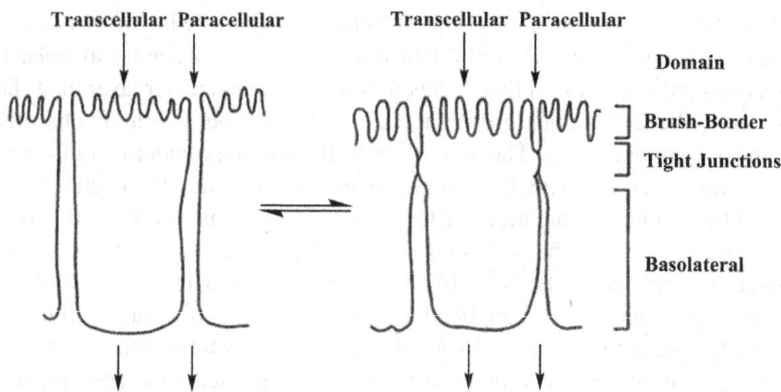

FIGURE 3.2 Transcellular and paracellular transport pathways across lung epithelial cells.

than 2 nm are completely excluded from paracellular transport (e.g. horseradish peroxidase, MW 40,000; molecular radius >3 nm). This implies that the main mechanism of transport of large particles across normal pulmonary epithelium is either by endocytosis by the epithelium itself or by phagocytosis and subsequent penetration of the epithelium. Of note, the epithelial tight junction is characterized by a network of sealing strands made up of a row of protein molecules on each adjacent cell wall; these molecules interlock like a zipper. The greater the number of strands, the more impermeable is the junction. However, it is hypothesized that the intercellular strands can reversibly "unzip" to permit lymphocytes, phagocytic macrophages, and polymorphonuclear leukocytes to enter or leave the airspace. Tight junction structure and function is now a very active area of research. They used to be thought of as simple cell adhesions composed of lipid structures (Schneeberger and Lynch 1992); however, it is now known that these junctions consist of a complex structure of multiple proteins that serves as a dynamic mechanism for the fastening of cells to each other. In fact, there are around 60 miles of cell junctions in human airways and over 2000 miles in the alveolar region. The pulmonary endothelial cell barrier is relatively permeable to macromolecules as compared to the epithelium.

Vesicular transport (endocytosis) of drugs may well depend on molecular structure and size. In this respect, the ionic structure of the pulmonary membrane may be an important factor to consider. The predominance of negative charge in the basement membrane structure and the interstitia of the lung (Vaccaro and Brody 1981) will no doubt influence the rate of transport of charged molecules by dipolar interactions. It has been observed that pulmonary absorption of similarly macromolecular fluorophore-labeled poly(hydroxyethylaspartamide) derivatives, either neutral or positively or negatively charged, occurs via both carrier-mediated and diffusive mechanisms. The highest rate of absorption was observed with the polyanionic derivative (Sun et al. 1999). An earlier study has also shown that pulmonary absorption of some peptidase-resistant polypeptides [poly-(2-hydroxyethy I)-aspartamides] administered intratracheally to the airways in isolated rat lung is molecular weight dependent (Niven et al. 1990). Approximately 70% absorption of a 0.2-mg dose of a 3.98-kDa polymer occurred in 100 minutes, whereas for larger polymers, the absorption rates appeared to be slower and suggested a molecular weight cut-off point between 4 kDa and 7 kDa. Nevertheless, according to the investigators, the results strongly suggest that systemic protein and peptide delivery by aerosol is feasible because even the largest polymers (11.65 kDa) were absorbed at finite rates. Intratracheally administered cytochalasin D and calcium ions are known to alter junctional transport by disruption of parts of the cytoskeleton that are attached to tight junctions. Airway epithelium appears to actively secrete chloride ions coupled with sodium ion; the exact organization of these ion pumps remains to be established, but they appear to be dependent on intracellular levels of cAMP. In this respect, target receptors on epithelial cell membrane surfaces may be exploitable in the development of bioadhesive carriers conjugated to a drug molecule, resulting in selective binding and rapid internalization. In addition, the observed specific uptake of certain drugs into pulmonary tissue is an intriguing area of study, particularly as it relates to the development of lung-targeting strategies. Both of these approaches to pulmonary targeting of drugs are discussed in later sections of this chapter.

A final, and not insignificant, consideration is the problem of drug metabolism in the respiratory tract. Although a large body of data indicate that pulmonary metabolism is generally relatively lower than hepatic metabolism (Benford and Bridges 1986, Powley and Carlson 1999), it is clear that nearly all of the drug metabolism activities found in the liver are present in the respiratory tract (Crooks and Damani 1989, Vaccaro and Brody 1981). In addition, some respiratory tissues contain enzyme activities much higher than corresponding activities found in the liver. Metabolism of drugs in respiratory tract tissue will most likely lead to the formation of more than one metabolite because of the variety of enzymes and their differential location throughout the respiratory tract. The metabolic profile of a particular drug will depend on a number of factors, which include ease of access of the drug to the enzyme active site, availability of cofactors, V_{max} and K_m of the enzyme(s), and possible competition at the active site with other exogenous or possible endogenous substrates and inhibitors, inducers, activators, and so on. Other factors are cell type, age, and health. The localization of drug-metabolizing enzymes in the respiratory tract has been addressed (Crooks and Damani 1989). Although pulmonary metabolism may be seen as a disadvantage, particularly in the case of peptides and proteins, because of the wide variety of peptidases and proteinases found in respiratory tract tissues, pulmonary activation of drugs by site-specific metabolism of a prodrug form is a possible way to increase selectivity and duration of action. For example, the bronchodilator bitolterol is converted into its active metabolite by hydrolysis in the respiratory tract (see the section on prodrug approaches), and the anti-tumor drug hexamethylmelamine owes its activity to pulmonary activation by *N*-demethylation (Harpur and Gonda 1987).

Because the main goal of drug delivery is to direct the drug to the target receptors while minimizing interactions with other possible sites of action, the question of receptor specificity is of primary importance in drug design. Although other factors that may affect receptor targeting, such as rate of delivery regional distribution and pharmacodynamics, are of significance, this chapter focuses on structure-activity considerations associated with receptor targeting in the lung.

3.2 Design of Drug Molecules for Pulmonary Receptor Targeting

The use of inhalation therapy has been applied mainly to the treatment of asthma and bronchitis. There is an increasing awareness that current treatment is inadequate and that the incidence of asthma is on the rise (Sly 1989, Buist 1989, Greenwood 2011). Indeed, it has been shown that an apparent increase in the prevalence of asthma at childhood has occurred in recent years (Lenny et al. 1994). Of particular interest is the structure-activity relationships associated with drug residence times in the respiratory tract.

3.2.1 β_2-Adrenoceptor Agonists

Drugs acting at β-adrenoceptors are the most common group of agents used in the treatment of asthma and other related respiratory diseases. Although several drugs in this group, such as isoproterenol and salbutamol, have been used for many years in the symptomatic treatment of bronchospasms, subsequent research has focused on the use of β_2-adrenergic stimulants as prophylactic drugs because of their ability to inhibit the release of spasmogens and inflammagens from human mast cells; in fact, short-acting β_2-agonists represent an important treatment for the relief of asthma symptoms (Barnes 1997). Furthermore, asthmatics patients are known to have greater response to bronchodilators than do patients of chronic obstructive pulmonary disease (Chhabra and Bhatnagar 2002).

Early structure-activity studies designed to provide selective β_2-receptor drug-binding clearly established the value of *N*-substitution for enhancing the β_2 selectivity of norepinephrine analogues (Lands et al. 1967), and subsequent work also highlighted the importance of uptake mechanisms and biotransformation by catechol-o-methyltransferase (COMT) in the metabolic inactivation of both natural and synthetic catecholamines (Iversen 1971). These advances have led to the development of potent, β_2 selective bronchodilators, which, when administered by inhalation aerosols, are practically devoid of any major side effects. However, it is generally accepted that aerosol administration of such drugs generally leads to deposition at sites other than the target receptors. In addition, it may be appropriate, for example, in the case of an acute asthmatic attack, to attain a rapid, prolonged, and effective concentration of the drug at the desired receptor site. Unfortunately, in this respect, relatively little progress has been made in establishing the regional distribution of β_2-receptors in the lung. Autoradiographic studies in human lung (Carstairs et al. 1985) indicated that β_2-receptors are located in smooth muscle from the large and small airways, with a greater population in bronchioli than in bronchi. High densities of receptors were also observed in airway epithelial cells and in bronchial submucosal glands, from the large bronchi to the terminal bronchioli. β_2-Receptors appear to be most highly concentrated in the alveolar wall; however, the physiological role of such receptors is not clear.

Examples of drugs that exhibit improved affinity for exoreceptor binding in the lung have been reported. The drug salmeterol (**6**) was developed from molecular modification of salbutamol (**4**) (Ullman and Svedmyr 1988) and represents a β_2-receptor stimulant with high exoreceptor affinity in order to persist in the vicinity of the β_2-receptors in the respiratory tract. Salmeterol given by inhalation has a markedly prolonged bronchodilatory effect compared to salbutamol, exhibiting sustained bronchodilation over a 12-hour period, with no tachyphylaxis after 9 days of treatment (Bradshaw et al. 1987).

Both salmeterol and formoterol (7) agonists are structurally related to salbutamol, in that they have an aromatic moiety replacing the catechol group, but that is resistant to metabolism by catechol-O-methyl transferase. However, in place of the *N*-isopropyl group, these compounds bear a large lipophilic *N*-substituent that appears to be responsible for the high affinity in lung and prolonged duration of action of these drugs (Ullman and Svedmyr 1988, Ullman et al. 1990). Whether this is due to improved receptor-binding characteristics or is the result of a selective uptake mechanism by lung tissue is open to question. This issue is dealt with in detail in the section on structural factors. The drug formoterol, when given by inhalation, is 10 times more potent than salbutamol and produces clinically significant bronchodilation for 8 hours when administered at a dose of 6 μg (Lofdahl and Svedmyr 1988). In an attempt to obtain optimal control of asthma, a combination therapy of an inhaled long-acting β_2-agonist and an inhaled corticosteroid (i.e. salmeterol/fluticasone and formoterol/budesonide) has been utilized, where the corticosteroids suppresses chronic inflammation of asthma, while the β_2-agonist induces bronchodilation and inhibits mast cell mediator release. Furthermore, it has been found that there are more positive interactions between both drug types. Corticosteroids increase the expression of β_2-receptors by increasing gene transcription, while β_2-agonists may potentiate the molecular mechanism associated with corticosteroid action, leading to an additive or sometimes synergistic suppression of inflammatory mediator release (Barnes 2002).

In earlier studies, Chiarino et al. (1986) described some potent and remarkably selective β_2-adrenoceptor agonists in a series of l-(3-substituted-5-isoxazolyi)-2-alkyl-aminoethanol derivatives in which the isoxazole ring replaces the catechol moiety in the β-adrenergic compounds. From this series, the compound broxaterol (**1**) displayed a marked selectivity towards β_2-receptors of the trachea and was selected for further development as a potential bronchodilatory agent.

It is important to point out that a selective response in vivo does not always reflect selectivity at the receptor level, but may depend on organ selectivity. This is particularly true for partial agonists of low intrinsic efficacy, which may exhibit receptor-selective activity in a tissue containing a large receptor pool or may operate the receptor-effector coupling system more efficiently.

β_2-receptor agonists such as soterenol (**2**), fenoterol (**3**), and salbutamol (**4**) bind with approximately equal affinity to both β_1- and β_2-receptors, but apparently owe their selectivity to greater efficacy at the latter receptor (Minneman et al. 1979), whereas other agonists, such as procaterol (**5**), show greater affinity for β_2-receptors (Rugg et al. 1978). In fact, procaterol is a particularly selective β_2-adrenoceptor drug.

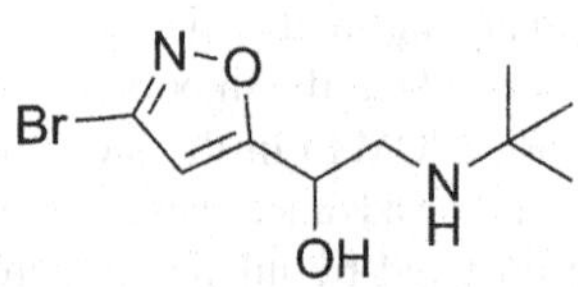

1 – broxaterol

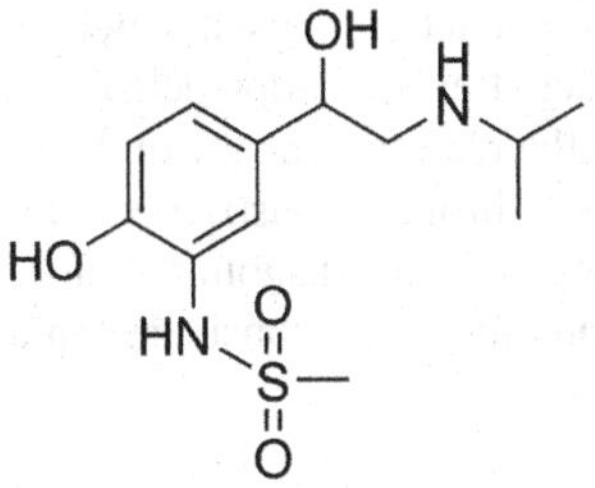

2 - soterenol

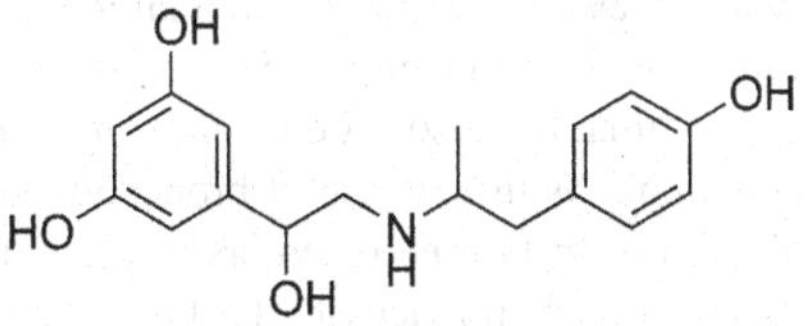

3 - fenoterol

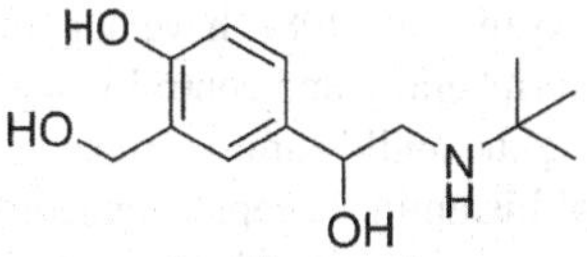

4 - salbutamol

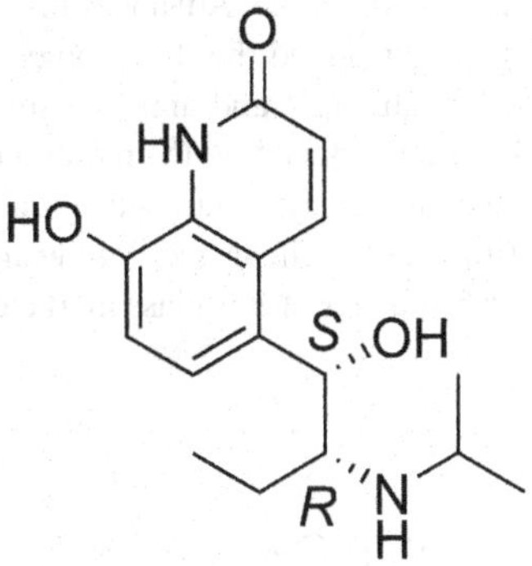

5 - procaterol

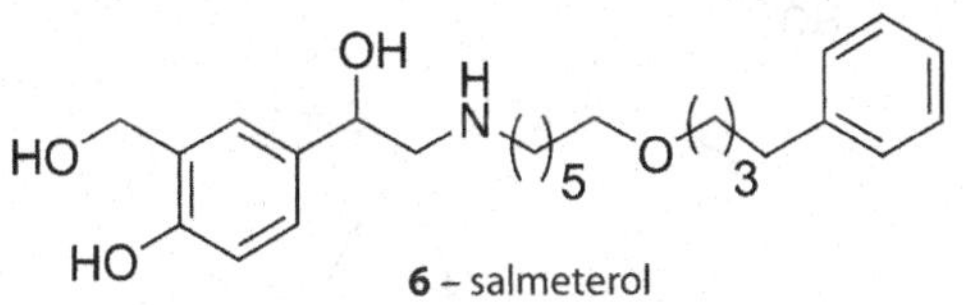

6 - salmeterol

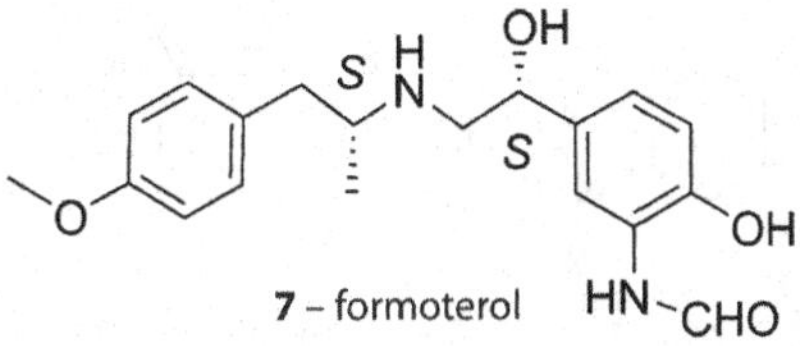

7 - formoterol

There is still a need to further improve the design of β_2-receptor stimulant drugs. Factors such as receptor selectivity, metabolic stability, and structural manipulation to prolong action are actively being investigated. Whether selectivity can ever be achieved is questionable, because skeletal muscle tremor in humans is β_2-receptor mediated (Levy and Apperley 1978), and the tachycardia exhibited by bronchodilator drugs appears to be mediated directly and indirectly through β_2-receptors (Gibson and Coltart 1971). When given by the inhalation route, the absorption characteristics of β_2-adrenoceptor stimulant drugs may well determine their duration of action; thus, a better understanding of the factors governing drug clearance from the respiratory tract after inhalation delivery is needed.

Another area for improvement is in the relative efficacy of β_2-bronchodilators. Compounds with low efficacy may be effective at low levels of bronchoconstriction. But as the severity of bronchoconstriction increases, such compounds will become partial agonists before those of greater efficacy. Therefore, the relative efficacies of new compounds should be considered in drug development decisions.

3.2.2 Antihistamines

H_1-receptors have been looked at with renewed interest as potential anti-asthmatic drugs (Bousquet et al. 1992, Wang et al. 2011). Such compounds, when given in adequate dosage, not only protect significantly against antigen and exercise-induced asthma, but also produce bronchodilation comparable with that seen after inhaled isoproterenol and salbutamol. As in the case of bronchodilator receptors, few attempts have been made to determine the distribution of histamine receptors in the human respiratory tract. It is well known that histamine is used in tests of bronchial reactivity. Histamine receptors are generally thought to reside in the large airways because centrally deposited aerosolized histamine results in significant histamine receptor-mediated responses. However, Ryan et al. (1981) have not confirmed this, although it is not known whether adequate differences between peripherally and centrally deposited aerosols were achieved in their studies. Previously, the drawback to using the antihistamines included their marked individual variation in response between patients, specificity of histamine receptor antagonism, and dose and route given. More importantly, the H_1-receptor antagonists were unsuitable for diurnal use because of their marked sedation as a consequence of central nervous system (CNS) uptake. Advances in this drug discovery area (Shaw 1989, Canonica and Blaiss 2011, Jones 2016) have included the development of H_1 antagonists with no H_2-, α-, β-receptor activity, no demonstrable anti-cholinergic and anti-5-hydroxytryptamine activity, and no ability to cross the blood-brain barrier. The drug terfenadine (**8**) represents the first example of this class of non-sedating antihistamine possessing the previously mentioned characteristics and exhibits no significant sedation in dosages up to 200 mg three times daily (Cheng and Woodward 1982). Terfenadine and the related drug astemizole (**9**) represent two established drugs of this class marketed in the United States.

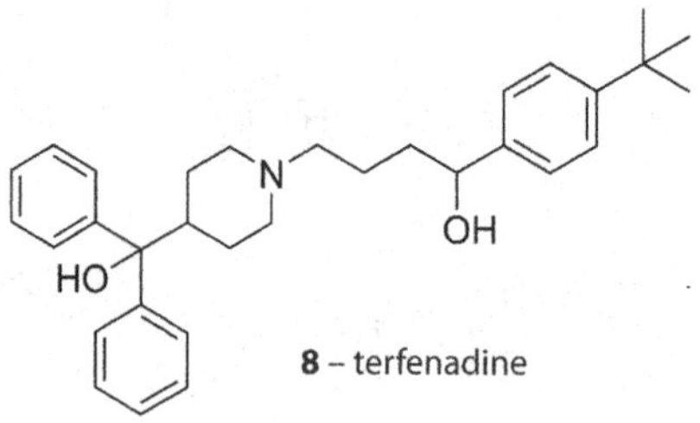

8 – terfenadine

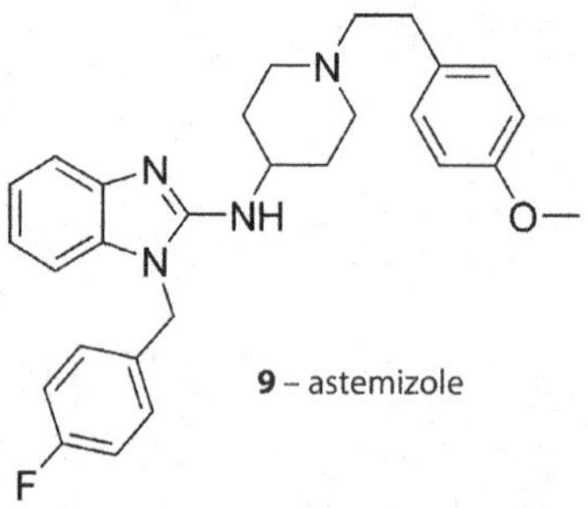

9 – astemizole

Structural modification of the antihistamine azatadine (**10a**) by replacing the *N*-methyl group with various carbamate groups eliminates CNS activity (Villani et al. 1986). Loratidine (**10b**), the most potent compound in this series of carbamates, shows no sedation liability in experimental animals and binds selectively to peripheral histamine receptors (Ahn and Barnett 1986). Other non-sedatory H_1 antihistamines are temelastine **(11)**, tazifylline **(12)**, cetrizine **(13)**, levocabastine **(14)**, and epinastine **(15)** (Brown et al. 1986, Nicholson and Stone 1986, deVos et al. 1986). Tazifylline is reported to have ten times the bronchodilator activity exhibited by either astemizole or terfenadine. The pre-clinical pharmacology of AHR-11325 **(16)** and PR 1036-654 **(17)** suggests that both these new compounds are potent, non-sedating, long-acting H_1 antagonists (Nolan et al. 1989, Palmer et al. 1989). Ebastine **(18a)**, a structural analogue of terfenadine, has been reported to be a potent, selective, long-lasting antihistamine devoid of sedation at an oral dose of 10 mg (Vincent et al. 1988). Its mode of action is thought to be due to metabolism to the active form **(18b)** (Vincent et al. 1988).

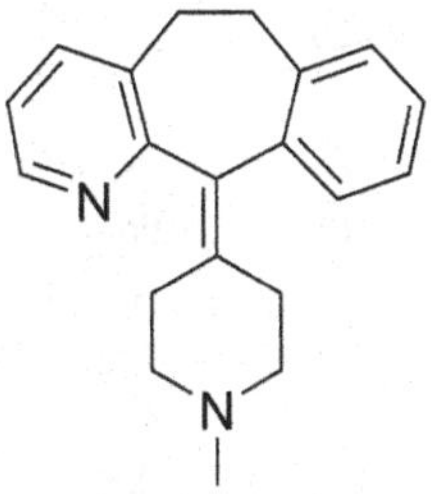

10a - azatadine

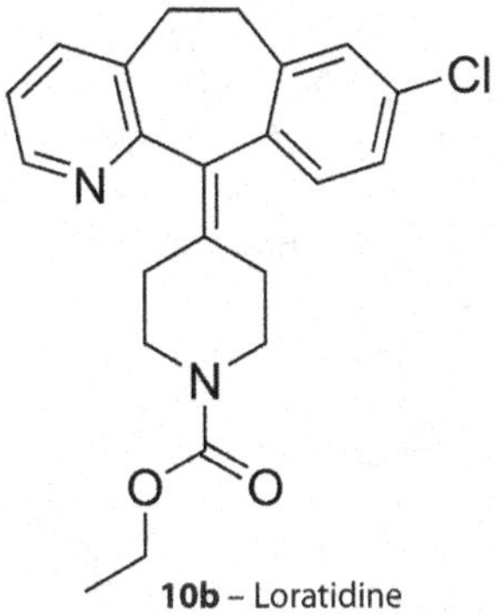

10b - Loratidine

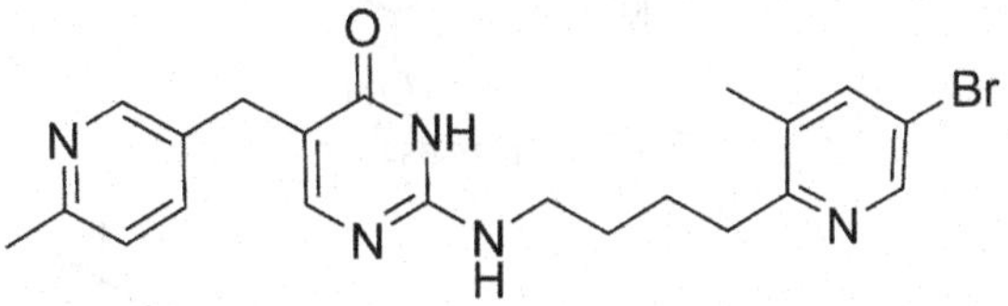

11 - temelastine

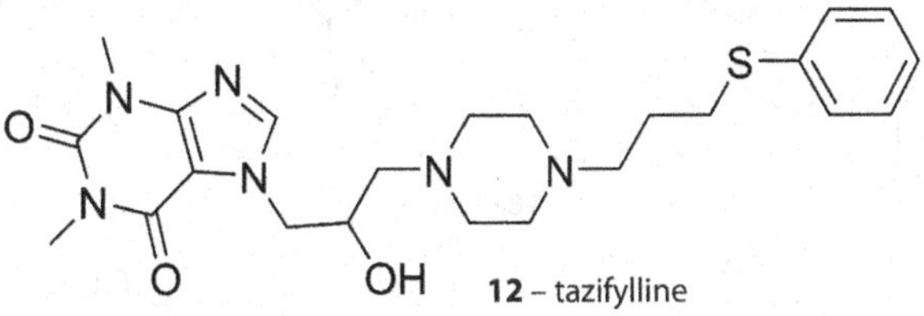

12 - tazifylline

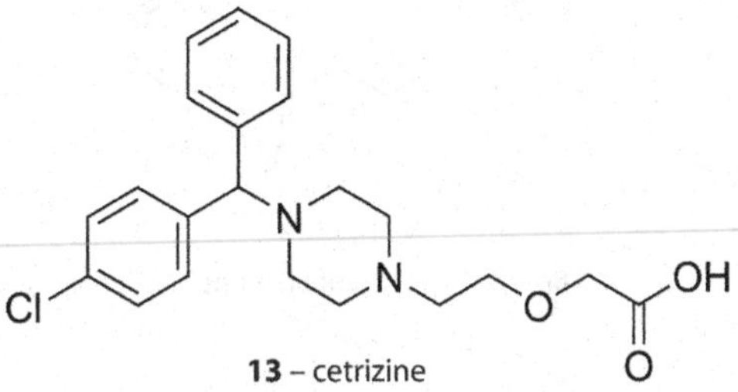

13 - cetrizine

N
N
OH
O
F
14 – levocabastine

N
NH2
N
15 – epinastine

N
N
O
N
S
16 – AHR-11325

O
N
OH
17 – PR 1036-654

N
O
O
18a – Ebastine

COOH
N
O
O
18b – Active form of Ebastine

It is clear that these agents will most likely benefit from being delivered locally into the respiratory tract in therapeutic concentrations that can avoid undesirable systemic side effects.

3.2.3 Anticholinergics

The lung expresses at least three subtypes of muscarinic acetylcholine receptor. M1 receptors are located primarily in the parasympathetic ganglia, where their activation facilitates transmission through the ganglia, whereas M2 receptors are found on presynaptic cholinergic nerve terminals and function to inhibit acetylcholine release, and M3 receptors are present on the smooth muscle and elicit contraction (Zaagsma et al. 1997). Although anti-cholinergic drugs have had a long history of use in the treatment of asthma, the development of a successful anti-asthmatic drug in this case has been slow. The major obstacle has been the lack of availability of compounds that produce optimal bronchodilation without accompanying side effects. Two drugs of this class, ipratropium bromide **(19)** and oxitropium bromide **(20)**, which are structural analogues of atropine **(21)**, have been studied extensively as alternatives to β_2 stimulant drugs (Buckle and Smith 1984, Rominger 1979, Frith et al. 1978). Although the distribution of cholinergic receptors in the human respiratory tract is not well understood, these quaternary ammonium drugs appear to exert their bronchodilatory activity mainly on the large airways, in contrast to β-adrenoceptor agonists, and probably produce bronchodilation by competitive inhibition of cholinergic receptors on bronchial smooth muscle, by antagonizing the action of acetylcholine at its membrane-bound receptor site. Thus, they block the bronchoconstrictor action of vagal efferent impulses; lung irritant receptors provide the chief efferent input for this vagal reflex. Because **19** and **20** are water-soluble quaternary ammonium derivatives, they lack the CNS stimulatory properties of atropine **(21)**.

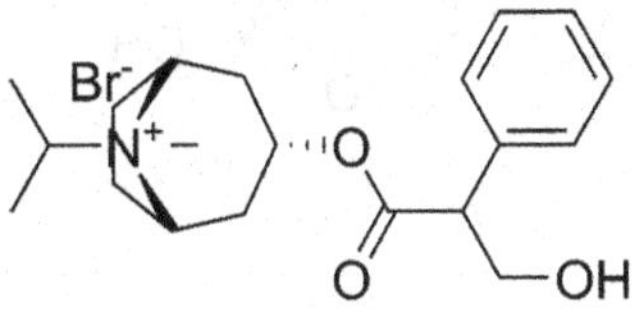

Br⁻ N⁺ O O OH

19 – ipratropium bromide

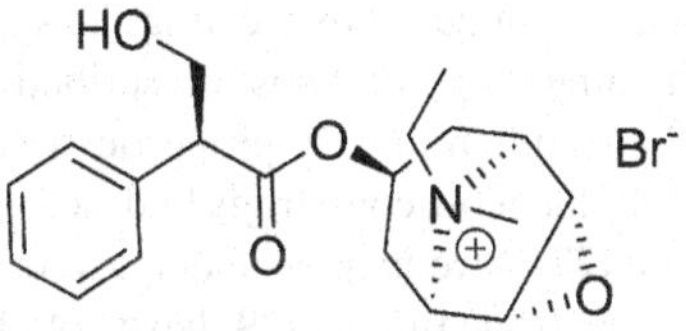

HO O O N⁺ Br⁻ O

20 – oxitropium bromide

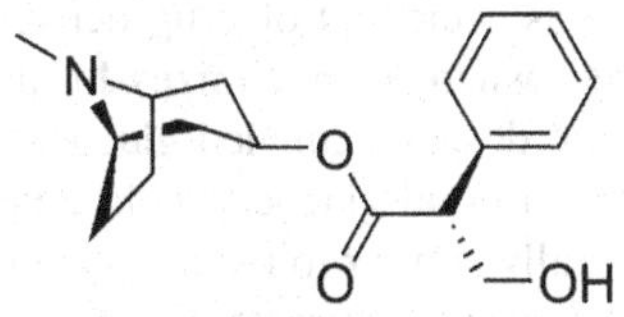

N O O OH

21 – atropine

When given by inhalation, ipratropium bromide and oxitropium bromide are slower acting than β_2-receptor stimulants, but have a longer duration of action (Storms et al. 1975, Schlueter and Neumann 1978). Both drugs are considerably more broncho-selective than atropine when given by inhalation and exhibit significantly less systemic anti-cholinergic side effects.

There is significant interest in identifying and developing either longer-acting, more potent non-selective muscarinic receptor antagonists than ipratropium, such as tiotropium **(22)** and oxitropate **(23)** or more subtype-selective muscarinic receptor antagonists, such as darifenacin and revatropate **(24)**. Revatropate is an M1/M3 receptor-selective muscarinic antagonist with about 50-fold lower potency against M2 receptors. In animal models, revatropate **(24)** inhibits acetylcholine-induced bronchoconstriction, but, unlike ipratropium, does not potentiate vagally induced bronchoconstriction (Tamaoki et al. 1994, Alabaster 1997).

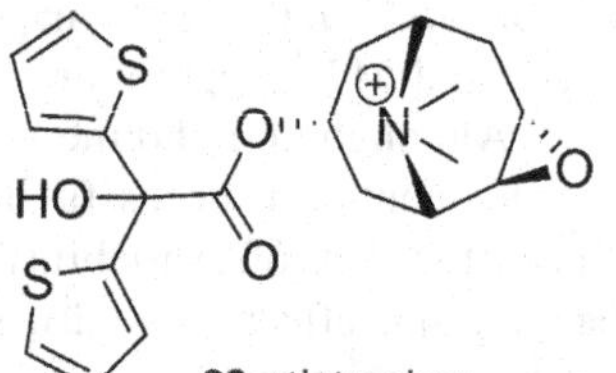

22 – tiotropium

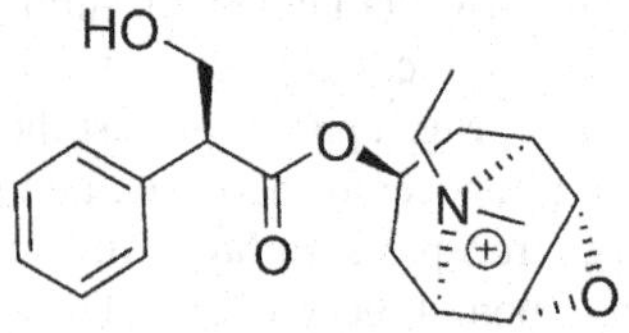

23 – oxitropate

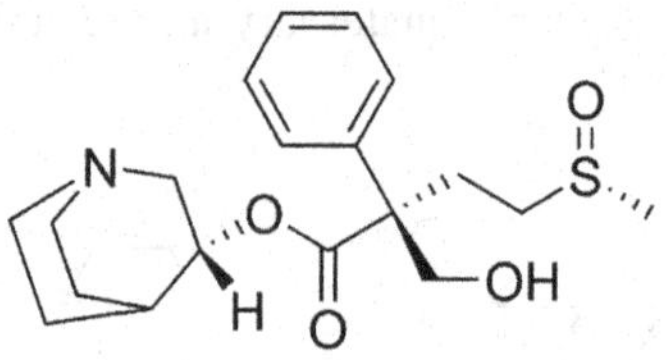

24 – revatropate

3.2.4 Glucocorticoids

Current effective therapies for asthma have focused on treating the symptoms of the disease. Asthma is characterized by inflammation of the lung; thus, the most prescribed agents to date are the glucocorticoids (GC), due to their widespread anti-inflammatory properties (Kelly 1998, Pedersen and O'Byrne 1997, Allen 1998, Alangari 2014). The glucocorticoid drugs budesonide **(25)**, beclomethasone dipropionate **(26)**, and triamcinolone acetonide **(27)** have long been employed for use in treating asthma.

Fluticasone propionate **(28)** and mometasone furoate **(29)** have both been formulated for use in asthma (Bernstein et al. 1999). Many of the adverse effects of elevated systemic glucocorticoid levels have been reduced through the use of inhalation as a method of drug delivery (Barnes et al. 1998). Inhalation therapy targets the local affected area, where it maximizes local efficacy, while reducing systemic bioavailability. Therefore, at therapeutic doses of inhaled glucocorticoids, the risk of systemic effect is considerably reduced when compared to oral glucocorticoid therapy. Mometasone furoate **(29)** is a synthetic glucocorticoid that is structurally similar to the adrenocorticosteroids and prednisolone. The structure was designed to optimize potency; the furoate group at position C17 greatly increases lipid solubility, while the 21-chloromoiety is important for maximum potency and topical activity (Onrust and Lamb 1998).

It has been shown that intact budesonide **(25)** after inhalation binds primarily to available steroid receptors, and mainly excess unbound budesonide is esterified (Petersen et al. 2001, Sorkness 1998, Miller-Larsson et al. 1998). Esterification of budesonide is a rapid process. Thus, in the rat, within 20 minutes of inhalation of radiolabeled budesonide, approximately 80% of the radioactivity within the trachea and main bronchi was associated with budesonide esters, primarily budesonide oleate (Sorkness 1998). The efficacy of topical glucocorticoids in rhinitis and asthma is likely to depend on drug retention in the airway mucosa. With fluticasone propionate (**28**), retention may be achieved exclusively by its inherent lipophilicity, whereas for budesonide, an additional possibility may be provided by its ability to form fatty acid esters in the airway mucosa that release the active drug (Petersen et al. 2001). A recent review on the use of corticosteroids in the treatment of acute asthma addresses the role of systemic and inhaled delivery in the management of symptoms (Alangari 2014). Studies have investigated the role of inhaled corticosteroids in the long-term management of chronic obstructive pulmonary disease (COPD) (van Grunsven et al. 1999, Hay and Barnette 1999). This disease is characterized by the presence of airflow obstruction due to chronic bronchitis or emphysema; in this respect, the airflow obstruction may be partially reversible, in contrast with asthma, which is largely a reversible disease. Although inflammation seems to be present in the airway of patients with COPD, the specific immunopathology is thought to be different from that of asthma (Lacoste et al. 1993). There is conflicting information on the ability of glucocorticoids to modulate the progression of COPD (Ziment 1990). Short-term treatment with both inhaled and systemic glucocorticoids may have beneficial effects on symptoms and lung function in subgroups of COPD patients, in particular, those with partially reversible airways obstruction (van Schayck et al. 1996).

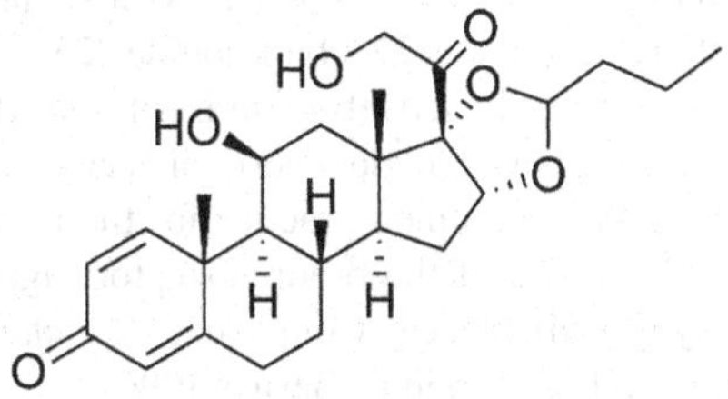

25 – budesonide

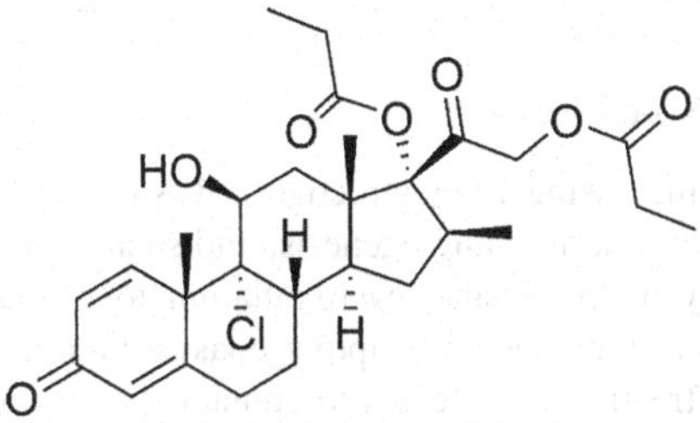

26 – beclomethasone dipropionate

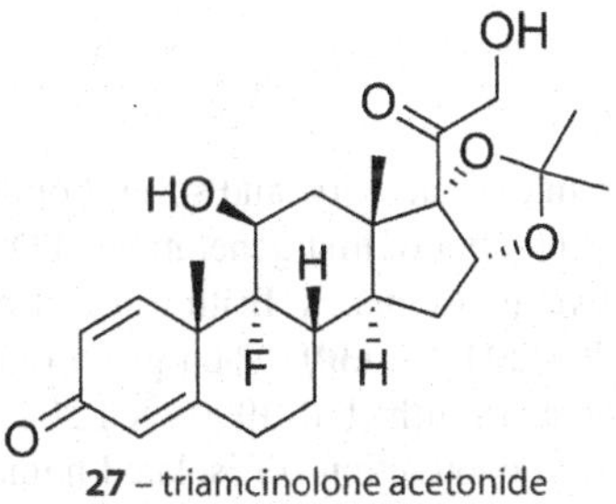

27 – triamcinolone acetonide

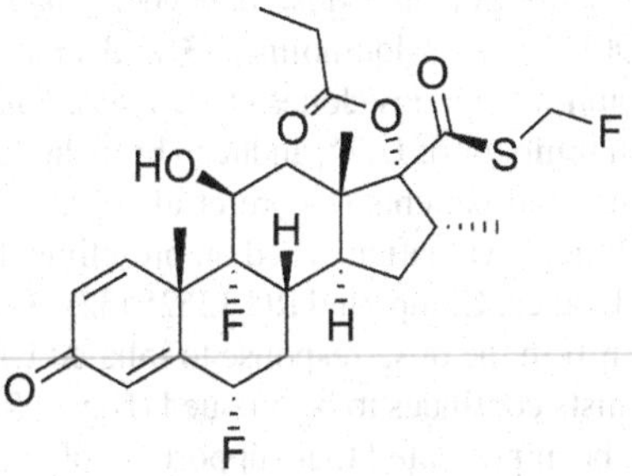

28 – Fluticasone propionate

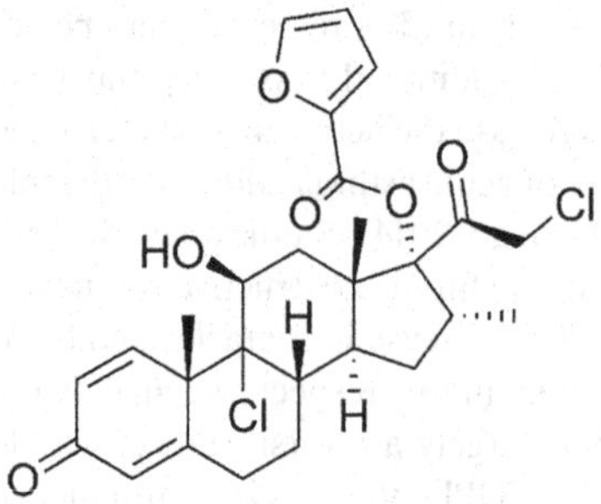

29 – mometasone furoate

Glucocorticoid mimics the action of the endogenous hormones (i.e. cortisol) that are involved in the regulation of the inflammatory response in the airway. The sequence of events in glucocorticoid action begins when this lipophilic corticosteroid molecule crosses the cell membrane and binds to the intracellular GR receptor which is located in the cytoplasm. Glucocorticoids bind to GR receptor with different affinities, for example, triamcinolone acetonide **(27)**, budesonide **(25)**, and dexamethasone are 10- to 90-fold less potent than mometasone furoate in activating transcription (Barnes et al. 1998, Wilson et al. 1996). Thus, large differences in potency between glucocorticoids can be observed in in vitro systems.

Combinations of medications have been common practice for the treatment of COPD. There is evidence of increased efficacy of combinations of the β-adrenoceptors agonists and cholinergic receptor antagonists. Such combined therapy is available, e.g. Combivent®, which is an aerosol formulation of the β-adrenoceptor agonist, salbutamol, and ipratropium (Barnes 1996).

3.3 Regulators of Lipid Mediators

Endogenous lipid mediators are increasingly being recognized as important regulators of cell activation, signaling, apoptosis, proliferation, and neo-angiogenesis, and such endogenous compounds can play a major role in the pathophysiology of chronic and severe inflammatory lung diseases. Counter-regulatory lipid mediators, such as leukotriene antagonists, 5-lipoxygenase inhibitors, thromboxane receptor antagonists, etc., have provided new treatment strategies to counter the morbidity and mortality associated with common diseases of the respiratory tract.

3.3.1 Leukotriene Antagonists

This area of drug discovery has seen intense activity, and several orally active leukotriene (LT) antagonists have been clinically evaluated. A number of first-generation LTD_4 antagonists were found to have an activity that was too weak to be effective in asthmatics (Britton et al. 1987, Barnes et al. 1988, Fleisch et al. 1988). Clinical studies showed that ICI 204,219 **(30)**, when given orally, could reduce antigen-induced bronchoconstriction in asthmatic patients (Smith et al. 1990). ICI 204,219 was reported to be a selective, competitive antagonist of LTD_4-induced contractions of isolated human bronchioli and was effective in reversing LTD_4-induced bronchoconstriction in a dose-dependent manner in guinea pigs by both oral and aerosol routes (Krell et al. 1990). The styrylquinolines **(31a–31c)** are another class of LTD_4-receptor antagonist with good potential as anti-asthmatics (Jones et al. 1989). One of these, MK-571, is a racemic compound that was evaluated as an inhibitor of LTD_4-induced bronchoconstriction following intravenous administration to healthy volunteers and patients (Depre et al. 1992). Development of the R-isomer of MK-679, which was selected for clinical evaluation based on pre-clinical in vitro and in vivo pharmacology, was terminated due to poor tolerance. Compound RG 12525 **(32)**, when dosed orally to mild asthmatics, was found to cause a 7.5-fold shift in the dose-response to inhaled LTD_4 (Jacobs et al. 1992).

The clinical use of LTD_4 antagonists continues to be pursued (Hay 1997, Balzano et al. 2002), although no definitive clinical evidence has been presented that supports a role for the peptide LTs in asthma and allergy. With respect to aerosolized drug studies, SKF 104353-22 **(33)** has been shown to block LTD_4- and antigen-induced bronchoconstriction in asthmatics on aerosol administration (Joos et al. 1989, 1991, Creticos et al. 1989). L-648051 **(34)** represents another aerosol-administered antagonist; however, relatively large doses (~12 mg) are required to inhibit LTD_4 bronchoconstriction (Evans et al. 1989).

3.3.2 5-Lipoxygenase Inhibitors

An interesting correlation between pseudoperoxidase activity and 5-lipoxygenase inhibitory potency has been observed for a series of *N*-hydroxyureas, suggesting that the redox properties of this class of drug contribute to their ability to inhibit 5-lipoxygenase (Jacobs et al. 1992). Some compounds has been investigated; the Zileuton (A-64,077) **(35)** shows activity in humans (Brooks et al. 1989). A series of quinoline-containing inhibitors of LT biosynthesis—WY-49,232 **(36)**, L-674,573 **(37)**, and REV-5,901 **(38)**—have been found to bind to the 5-lipoxygenose-activating protein (FLAP); their ability to interact with 5-lipoxygenose-activating protein correlated well with inhibition of LT biosynthesis.

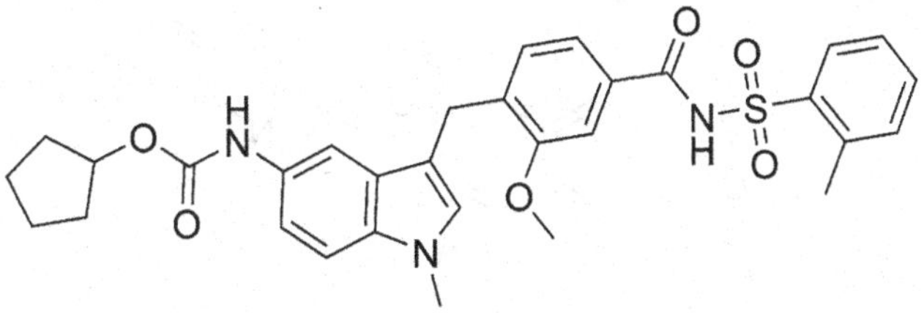

30 - ICI 204,219

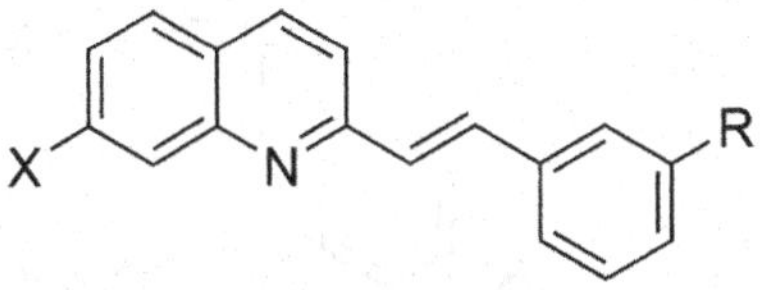

31a–31c - styrylquinolines

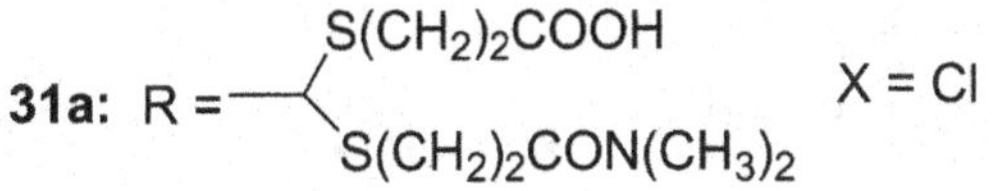

31a: R = $CH[S(CH_2)_2COOH][S(CH_2)_2CON(CH_3)_2]$; X = Cl

31b: R = $N(OH)CO(CH_2)_2CO_2CH_3$; X = H

31c: R = $NHSO_2CF_3$; X = H

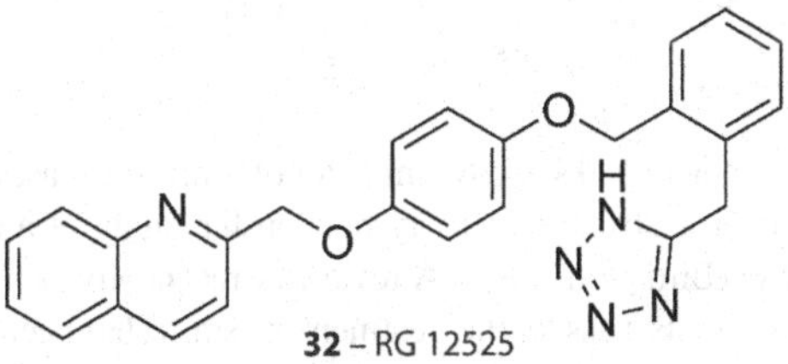

32 - RG 12525

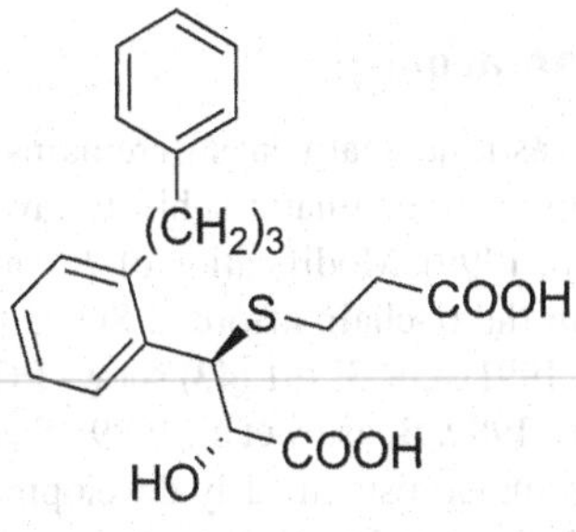

33 - SKF 104353-22

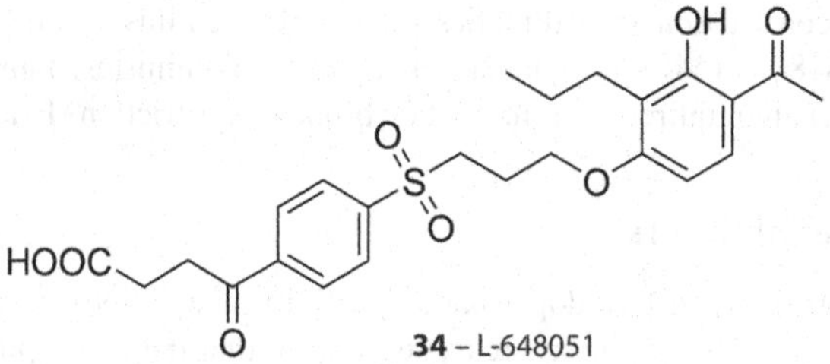

34 – L-648051

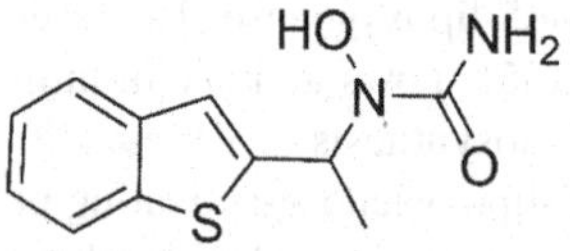

35 – Zileuton (A-64,077)

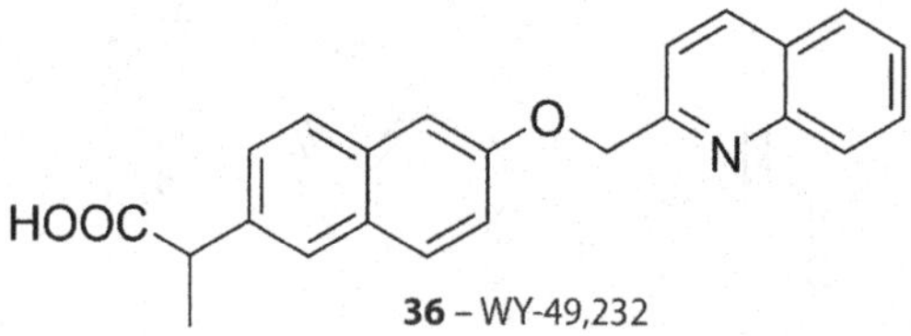

36 – WY-49,232

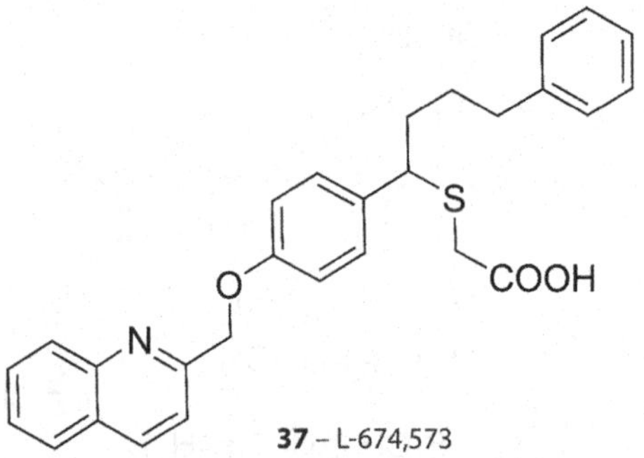

37 – L-674,573

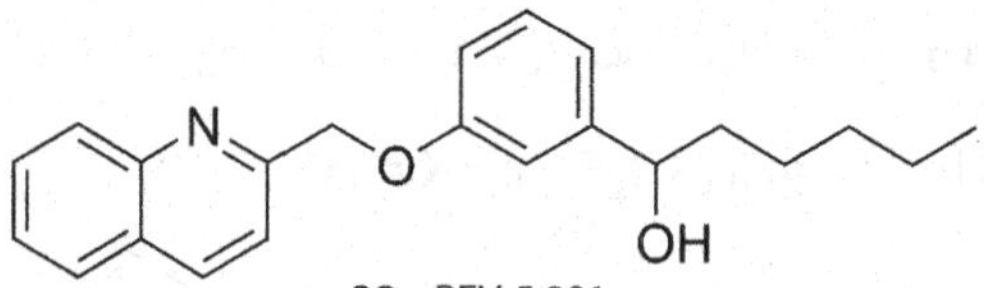

38 – REV-5,901

A-69,412 **(39)** was reported to be a potent and selective inhibitor of 5-lipoxygenase with a long duration of action, and 1C1-211,965 **(40)** emerged from a structure-activity relationship study of a (methoxyalkyl)thiazole series designed to inhibit 5-lipoxygenase (Bird et al. 1991). A review of recent advances in 5-lipoxygenase inhibition and the design of newer molecules of this class for the treatment of asthma has been published (Bruno et al. 2018).

3.3.3 Thromboxane-Receptor Antagonists

The role of thromboxane antagonists is asthma treatment still remains uncertain (Santus and Radovanovic 2016). AA-2414 **(41)** oral administration to asthmatic subjects favorably attenuated their response to methacholine challenge (Hoshino et al. 1999). Modification of 7-oxabicyclo heptane drug candidates by incorporation of a phenylene spacer in the α-chain afforded SQ 35,091 **(42)**, which shows longer duration of action ($t_{1/2}$ = 16 hr) (Misra et al. 1991). GR 32191 **(43)** shows PGD_2-induced bronchoconstriction in asthmatics at 80 mg PO (Hubbard et al. 1989, Beasley et al. 1989). Santus and Radovanovic have recently published a review on PGD_2 receptor antagonists in early development as potential therapeutic options for treatment of asthma (Santus and Radovanovic 2016).

3.3.4 Platelet Activating Factor Antagonists

These agents may be useful in platelet activating factor-induced bronchoconstriction (Kasperska-Zajac et al. 2008). In the hetrazepine class of platelet activating factor antagonist, apafant (WEB-2086) **(44)** has been shown to be rapidly absorbed following oral administration and produced no significant adverse effects (Jacobs et al. 1992). Two other compounds—WEB-2347 **(45)** and E-6123 **(46)**—also from the hetrazepine class, have emerged as orally active derivatives with profiles superior to WEB-2086 **(44)**.

3.3.5 Elastase Inhibitors

Strategies for designing inhibitors of human neutrophil elastase (HNE), the enzyme whose unrestrained action may result in the lung damage underlying the development of emphysema, has been under active research (Eriksson 1991, Ohbayashi 2002, Polverino et al. 2017). Prolastin, the natural human α_1-antitrypsin that inhibits HNE, was administered by aerosol, with demonstrated effectiveness in restoring the protease-antiprotease balance in genetic emphysema (Hubbard et al. 1989). Several other peptide drugs when administered intratracheally appear to have good residence times in the lung. Intratracheally administered L-6592866 **(47)**, a modified β-lactam **HNE** inhibitor, showed selective inhibition of lung **HNE** and blocked **HNE** damage to hamster lung (Bonney et al. 1989). ICI 200,880 **(48)** also showed a long residency time in the lung and potent HNE inhibition after intratracheal administration (Williams et al. 1981). To reduce the excess inflammatory response, various inhibitors of neutrophilic elastase (NE), ranging from nebulized α1-AT to systemic (oral or intravenous) or nebulized NE inhibitors (ONO-5046 [sivelestat]; AZD9668; engineered protease inhibitor, human NE 4 [EPI-hNE4 (depelstat; Debiopharm S.A.)]; monocyte NE inhibitor (MNEI); KRP-109, pre-elafin; BAY 85-8501; POL6014; and DX-890) have been tested in different diseases (Yamada et al. 2011, Toda et al. 2007).

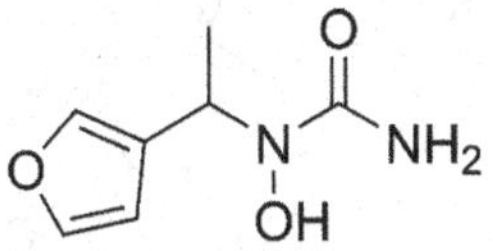

39 - A-69,412

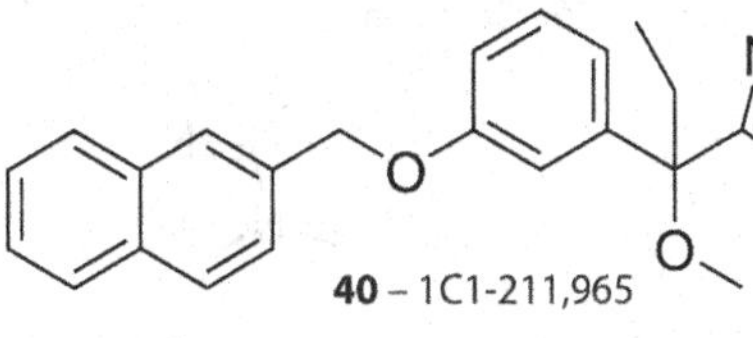

40 - 1C1-211,965

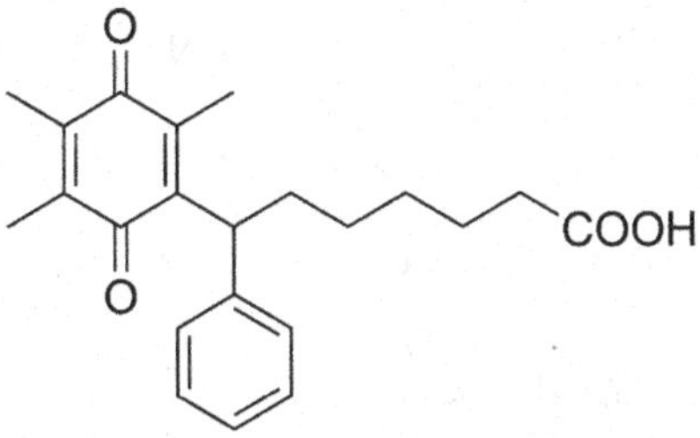

41 - AA-2414

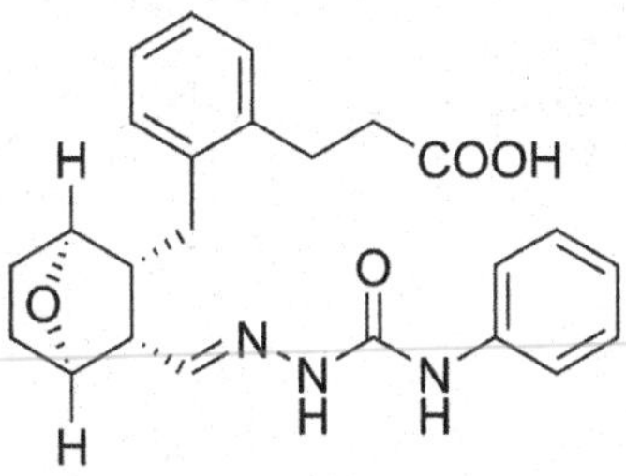

42 - SQ 35,091

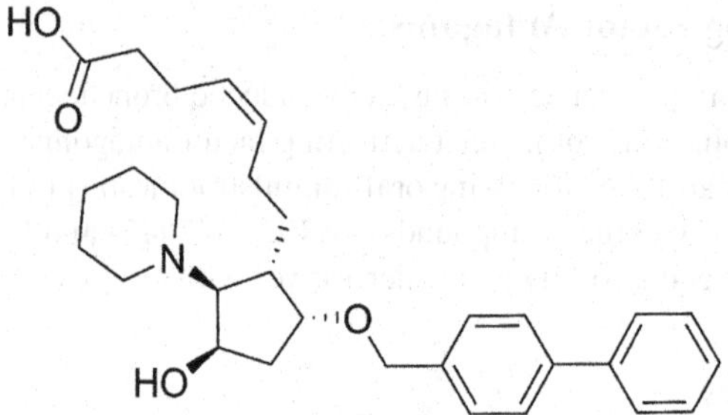

43 – GR 32191

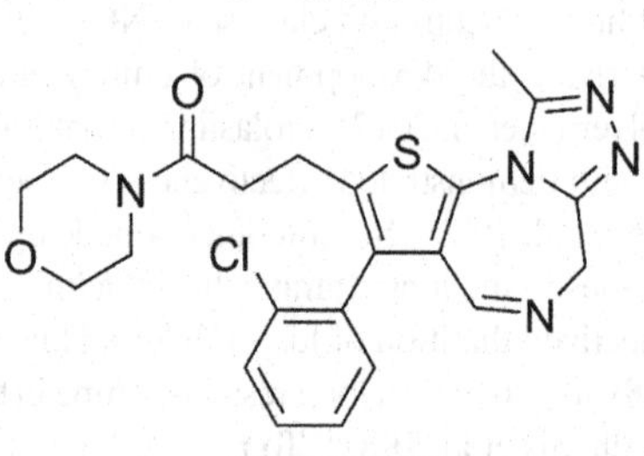

44 – WEB-2086

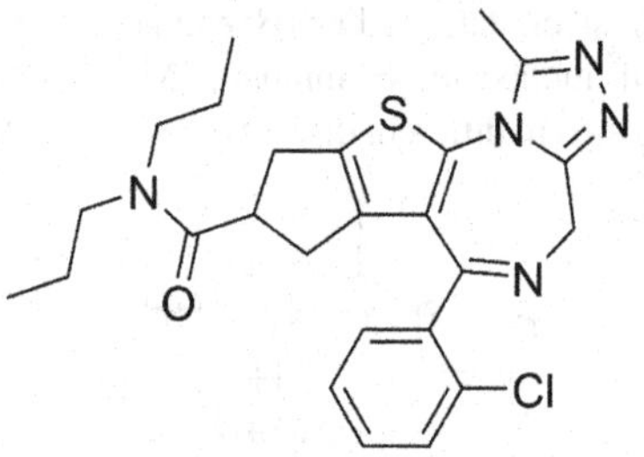

45 – WEB-2347

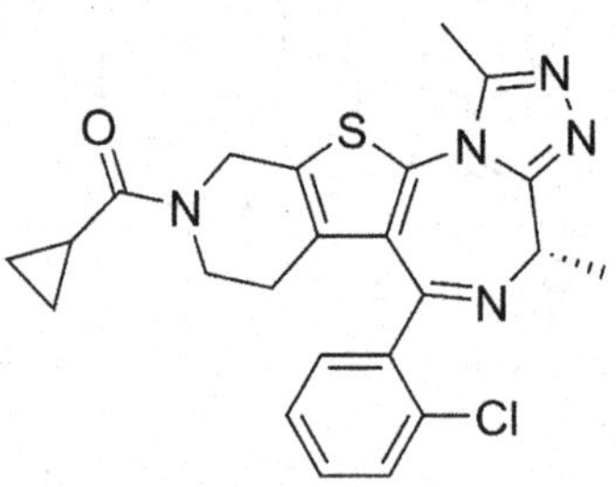

46 – E-6123

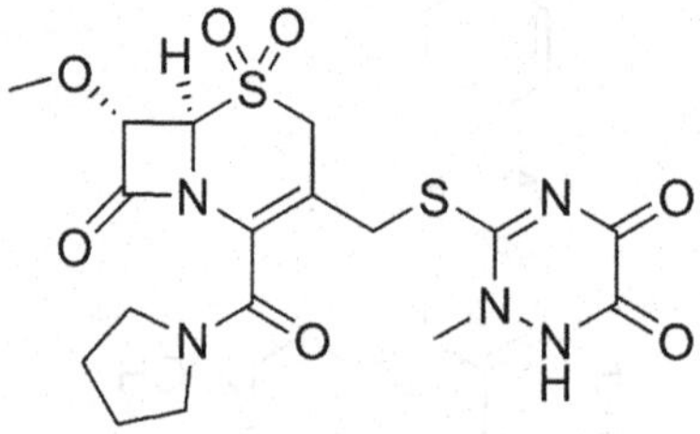

47 – L-6592866

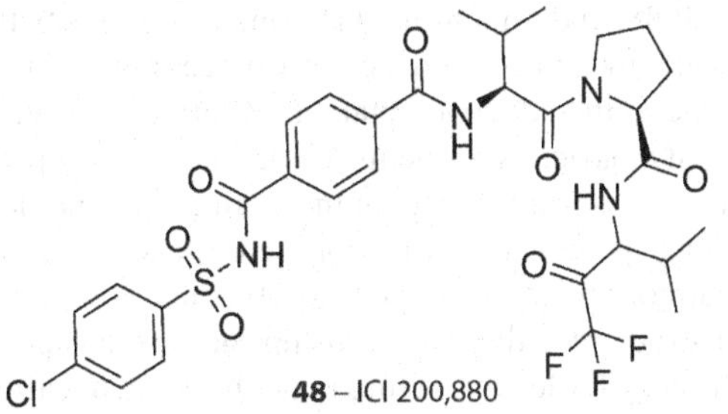

48 – ICI 200,880

3.3.6 Recent Studies on New Targets for Treating Pulmonary Arterial Hypertension and Idiopathic Pulmonary Fibrosis

Pulmonary arterial hypertension (PAH) is a progressive lung disease characterized by an increase in blood pressure in the small arterioles that supply blood to the lungs. The underlying molecular and cellular mechanisms involved in PAH appear to be complex, with the pathophysiology suggesting a multifaceted disease in which cellular proliferation and vascular remodeling occurs, along with several other additional cellular mechanisms (Vaidya and Gupta 2015, Gaine and McLaughlin 2017). Combination therapy is now commonly used as the standard of care approach, with therapies that target three different pathogenic pathways. These therapies involve the use of drugs that target the endothelin and nitric oxide pathways, as well as the prostacyclin pathway (Malenfant et al. 2013, Lang and Gaine 2015). In recent studies (Bertero et al. 2016), it has been shown that in PAH-diseased lung tissue, dysregulation of vascular stiffness and cellular metabolism mechanoactivates the transcriptional coactivators Yes-associated protein (YAP) and transcriptional co-activator with PDZ-binding motif (TAZ)-dependent glutaminolysis, to drive PAH. These studies indicate that targeting this pathology with drugs such as the glutaminase inhibitor, CB-839 (Gross et al. 2014) or the YAP inhibitor, verteporfin (King et al. 2014) may prove beneficial in this disease. CB-839 is currently undergoing active clinical development in early clinical trials for cancer therapy, and verteporfin is already approved by the FDA for treatment of age-related macular degeneration (Kent 2014).

Idiopathic pulmonary fibrosis (IPF) is a fatal lung disease with few options for treatment (Kim et al. 2006), since the aetiology of the disease is poorly understood. It has a 5-year survival rate of 30%–50%. Recent studies have shown that accumulation of extracellular matrix plays an important role in IPF, and repeated alveolar injury causes fibroblast activation, proliferation, and differentiation myofibroblasts (Wolters et al. 2014, Blackwell et al. 2014). The myofibroblasts overgrow the alveolar lung tissue, and this results in an irreversible increase in the amounts of extracellular matrix (Parker et al. 2014). Current therapeutic interventions involve targeting matrix and matrix-processing enzymes, and inhibition of the collagen cross-linking enzyme, lysyl oxidase-like 2 is currently being investigated as a treatment option for IPF (Ahluwalia et al. 2014). The FDA approved drugs pirfenidone and nintedanib are also being utilized to treat IPF (King et al. 2014, Richeldi et al. 2014). It is known that a deficiency in the chaperone protein, FK506-binding protein 10 can attenuate collagen secretion and decrease extracellular collagen cross-linking, and this might provide a potentially specific and effective drug for treatment of IPF (Staab-Weijnitz et al. 2015).

3.4 Some Structural Factors Governing the Uptake of Drugs

It has been known for many years that the lung is capable of active uptake of a number of endogenous and exogenous compounds. These include the neurotransmitters norepinephrine and 5-hydroxytryptamine, which are sequestered by lung endothelial cells (Iwasawa et al. 1973, Pitt et al. 1982) and the lung toxins paraquat (Baron et al. 1988) and 4-ipomeanol (Forman et al. 1982). Paraquat is selectively accumulated in type II alveolar cells by an energy-dependent process, whereas the site-specific toxicity of 4-ipomeanol appears to be due to the selective uptake by Clara cells that, because of the presence of cytochrome P-450 PB-B activity, bioactivates the molecule into a toxic species. In the case of the neurotransmitters norepinephrine and 5-hydroxy tryptamine, both compounds have been shown to be avidly sequestered by the canine lung; pulmonary extraction percentages after intravenous injection in the nanomolar range into the pulmonary artery amount to 70% and 50%, respectively (Pitt et al. 1982). Although it is not clear what structure-activity relationships govern the uptake of these compounds into lung endothelia, a possible strategy for lung targeting might be to chemically conjugate a drug molecule with either 5-hydroxytryptamine or norepinephrine or, better still, to conjugate the drug to pharmacologically inactive metabolites or analogues of these neurotransmitters that still retain the selective lung uptake properties. Generally, it is recognized that the lung has a mechanism for the high-affinity uptake of amines that are protonated at physiological pH and that also possess a hydrophilic moiety in their structure. In most cases, such compounds are metabolized by lung tissue and, therefore, do not accumulate. However, a select number of amines of this type that are resistant to lung metabolism have been observed to accumulate in lung tissue for prolonged periods (Wilson et al. 1979, Lullmann et al. 1973, Minchin et al. 1982). It is important to note that, generally, quaternary ammonium compounds, which are unable to dissociate into an unionized form, are not effectively taken up by lung tissue, although a notable exception is paraquat. Thus, the equilibrium between ionized and unionized drug is important and suggests that the unionized hydrophobic form may be required for transport, whereas the protonated form is necessary for binding to anionic sites in lung tissue. The exact nature of these anionic sites is not known, although they may be negatively charged phospholipid molecules, which are known to exist in high concentrations in lung tissue. Also, the uptake mechanism may involve a mechanism of preferential pH partitioning of the amine species into the lung or the involvement of a lipophilic ion-pair transport process. Several studies showed that lipophilic cationic drugs bound to anionic sites in the lung can be displaced by other lipophilic cationic drugs (Fowler et al. 1976).

The nature of the uptake site, or the involvement of any particular lung cell type in the uptake process, is as yet unknown. It seems possible that drugs conjugated to lipophilic amines of the types described previously can undergo efficient pulmonary targeting. Several amines may be useful in this respect; that is, the compounds chlorphentermine, amiodarone, desethylamiodarone, and desmethylimipramine all exhibit high affinity to lung tissue. Thus, drugs that normally have poor access to the lung may be targeted to this tissue through appropriate chemical combination of an available functional group (i.e. OH or COOH) with the amino function of the carrier molecule (Figure 3.3). Of course, the success of this drug design also depends on the ability of lung tissue to release the bound drug from the carrier molecule by some enzymic process; in other words, the approach basically would have to be a targeted prodrug design. Kostenbauder and Sloneker have investigated the usefulness of chlorphentermine as a carrier for lung targeting by conjugating it to an unspecified pulmonary drug to give a conjugate of general structure **49** (Figure 3.4) (Kostenbauder and Sloneker 1990). In this design, the released carrier molecule is anionic and would be predicted to be rapidly washed out of the lung. Isolated, perfused lung experiments indicated that the prodrug was able to displace chlorphentermine from lung-binding sites, and that subsequent prodrug hydrolysis occurred with carrier wash out from the lung. However, the in vivo activity of the prodrug could not be evaluated because of its extreme toxicity.

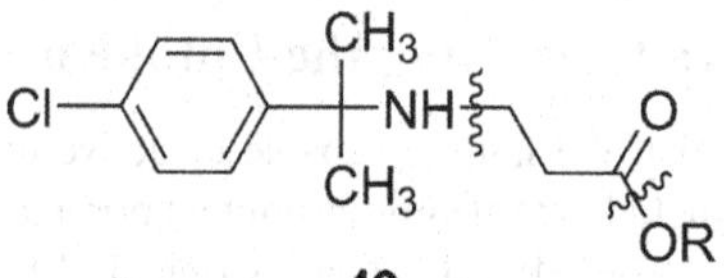

CH3
Cl NH O
CH3
OR

49

It has been argued that, because many strongly basic lipophilic amines have been found to exhibit high uptake, but only very few truly sequester in the lung and exhibit slowly effluxable pools in vivo, prodrug design should focus on simply achieving high concentrations of prodrug in the lung rather than

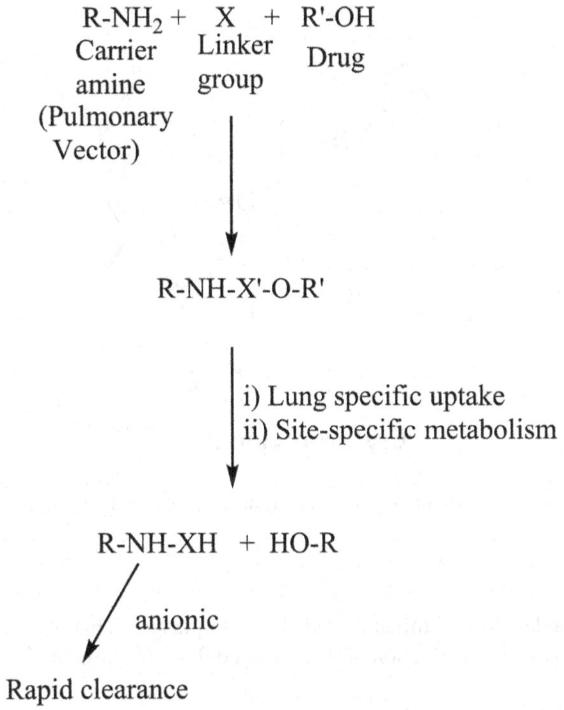

FIGURE 3.3 Basic design of a drug-amine carrier conjugate for lung targeting.

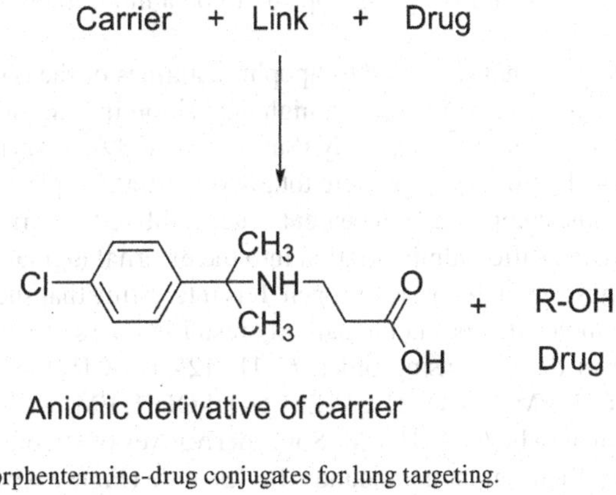

FIGURE 3.4 Design of chlorphentermine-drug conjugates for lung targeting.

developing conjugates that would establish amine effluxable pools in lung tissue (Kostenbauder and Sloneker 1990). In this respect, simple alkyl amines, such as octylamine, could be used because these compounds show high affinity for lung tissue, which correlate with their octanol-water partition coefficients. This approach has the added advantage of keeping conjugate structures as simple as possible to avoid pharmacological problems.

Of interest are the β_2 agonists salmeterol (6) and formoterol (7), both of which exhibit plasma half-lives similar to that of salbutamol (4), although the latter compound has a much shorter duration of action. Thus, in these cases, replacing the *N-t*-butyl group in salbutamol with a highly lipophilic group results in a drug with high affinity for lung tissue and long duration of drug action. It is puzzling, however, that the bronchodilator effects of these drugs are still present even when the drug is no longer detectable

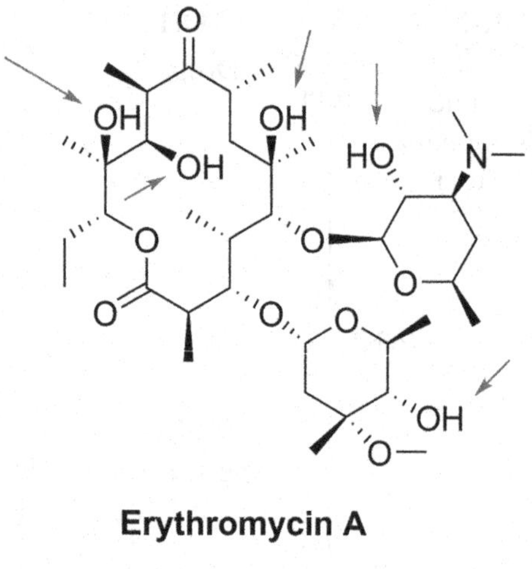

Erythromycin A

FIGURE 3.5 Erythromycin structure and position of O-methylation for obtaining increased lung uptake.

or, indeed, even predictable, from elimination half-lives, in plasma. This observation may relate to the possible retention in lung of a microfraction of the absorbed dose, presumably in the vicinity of the drug-receptor site.

Salmeterol (6) was designed by modifying salbutamol to obtain a drug with much greater affinity for its receptors because of increased "exoreceptor" binding (Brittain et al. 1976) and, consequently, a persistent localization in the vicinity of β_2-receptor. However, there is no evidence for this hypothetical mechanism, and the alternative suggestion that the drug is able to diffuse into the airway epithelium, which then acts as a reservoir for the drug, appears to be a more likely mechanism (Ullman and Svedmyr 1988).

Specific uptake by lung tissue is not restricted to lipophilic amines of the type previously mentioned. Certain antibiotics, such as leucomycin A3, show a high deposition in lung tissue at low concentration of drug (Kostenbauder and Sloneker 1990). A study (Suwa et al. 1989) on erythromycin derivatives, in which the 6′-, 11′-, 12′-, and 4′-hydroxyl groups were totally or partially replaced with *O*-methyl groups, indicated that these compounds, compared to the parent drug, exhibited a marked increase in lung tissue uptake (four to five times greater) after administration into the external jugular vein of rats (Figure 3.5). Of note, erythromycin also has a strongly basic nitrogen. It is interesting that such a significant structural change to the erythromycin molecule does not apparently result in a loss of anti-microbial activity. The tissue levels obtained were in the decreasing order: 6′-,11′-,12′-,4′-OCH_3 EM >6′-,11′-,4′-OCH_3 EM > 6′-,4′-OCH_3 EM = 6′-,11′-OCH_3 EM = 6′-OCH_2CH_3EM > 11′-OCH_3 EM > EM. The most potent anti-microbial derivative was shown to be 6′-OCH_3 EM. Some derivatives of steroidal drugs also exhibit better uptake in lung tissue than their parent compounds. Budesonide (Figure 3.6) is a glucocorticosteroid that has been used in inhalation therapy for many years (Clissold and Heel 1984). It possesses a 16α, 17α-acetal group that makes the molecule less polar and confers on the molecule better uptake properties in lung tissue. (Note: budesonide is used as a 1:1 mixture of the 22R- and 22S-epimers.) Budesonide is not metabolized in lung tissue and is slowly released from the lung to the systemic circulation. However, it is rapidly metabolized to the 23-hydroxylated 22S-epimer and 16α-hydroxyprednisolone, which is selectively formed from the 22R-epimer. The rapid inactivation of systemic budesonide by the liver minimizes the potential for systemic side effects (Edsbacker and Andersson 2004, Andersson et al. 1987, Ryrfeldt et al. 1984). In isolated lung perfusion studies, a difference in the distribution between lung tissue and perfusion medium for the two epimers of budesonide was found. Interestingly, the pharmacodynamically more potent 22R epimer showed an uptake in lung tissue that was 1.4 times higher than that of the 22S epimer. This property may be due to the fact that the 22R epimer is less water-soluble than the 22S epimer (Ryrfeldt et al. 1984).

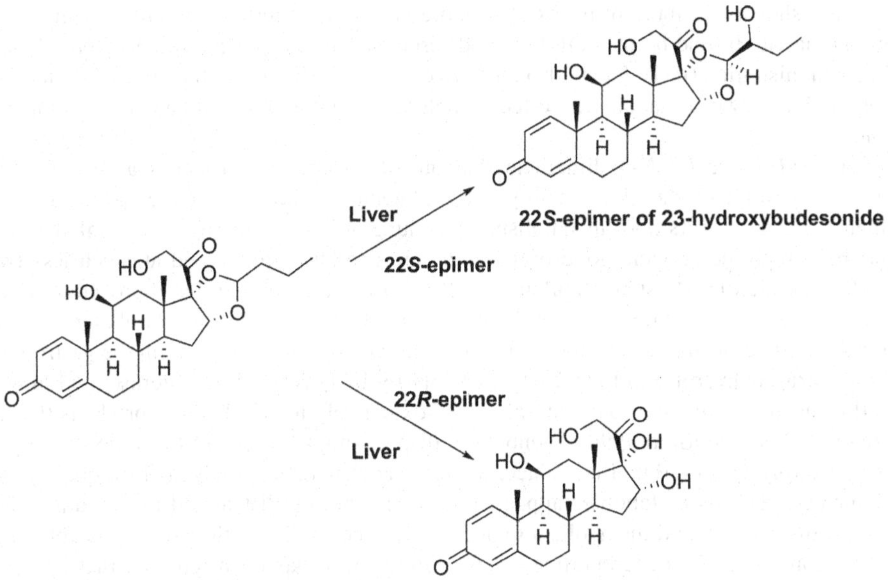

Liver

22*S*-epimer

22*S*-epimer of 23-hydroxybudesonide

22*R*-epimer

Liver

FIGURE 3.6 Stereoselective metabolism of budesonide.

3.5 Prodrug Approaches to Extending Drug Activity in the Lung

Most of the research centered on the targeting of drugs by the prodrug approach has been carried out on β_2 stimulants structurally related to isoproterenol and similar drugs. The basic approach has been to esterify the catechol functions of isoproterenol to achieve better uptake in lung tissues of the resulting inactive lipophilic drug, which may then be metabolically cleaved by lung esterases to release the active parent compound (Hussain and Truelove 1975, Shargel and Dorrbecker 1976). In addition, esterification of the catechol function acts to protect the drug from deactivation by metabolic conjugation. The elimination of cardiovascular side effects using this approach depends on the preferential uptake of the prodrug by the lung and the greater esterase activity in lung tissue relative to heart tissue. However, a prolonged therapeutic effect may also be obtained simply by increasing drug residence time in the body through reduced renal clearance. This can be achieved by conjugation of the drug to form a lipophilic prodrug containing a slowly hydrolysable linker group (e.g. a carbamate) (Olsson and Svensson 1984).

A few drugs have been investigated that are members of this class **(50–51)**. Bitolterol **(50a)** is the di-β-toluolyl ester of *N*-*t*-butylarterenol **(50b)** and is an effective long-lasting bronchodilator when given by intravenous injection, aerosol, or intraduodenal administration (Friedel and Brogden 1988); it is rapidly hydrolyzed after oral administration. Although the improved activity of this compound compared to the parent compound was thought to be due to its avid uptake by the lung followed by slow hydrolytic release of the active drug, lung perfusion studies in rabbits have shown that this is not the case (Small and Kostenbauder 1985). These studies indicate rapid pulmonary hydrolysis of prodrugs such as bitolterol; however, it was pointed out the rabbit lung has greater esterase activity than that of dogs or humans. Nevertheless, it is hard to rationalize that the effect of the drug persists long after any drug remains in the lung. The β_2 drugs ibuterol **(51a)** and bambuterol **(51b)** are further examples of pulmonary prodrugs. Ibuterol **(51a)** is the di-isobutyryl ester of the resorcinol function of terbutaline **(51c)**. After inhalation, ibuterol is three times as effective as terbutaline in the inhibition of bronchospasm (Andersson 1976). Five minutes after inhalation, ibuterol has been shown to exhibit a greater pulmonary pharmacological effect or potency than does terbutaline when administered by this route.

Studies have shown that ibuterol is absorbed more rapidly than terbutaline after administration to the lung, but that at all time points both lung and serum terbutaline concentrations were higher after terbutaline administration (Ryrfeldt and Bodin 1975). Thus, it appears that the prodrug ibuterol exhibits a greater pulmonary pharmacological effect or potency than does terbutaline when administered by inhalation.

Bambuterol **(51b)**, the *bis-N-N*-dimethylcarbamate of terbutaline, produces a sustained release of terbutaline, a result of the slow, mainly extrapulmonary hydrolysis of the carbamate linkage. Unfortunately, because of its poor metabolism in the lung, it is not effective by the inhalation route. But it has been reported to yield good oral results and can be administered at much less frequent intervals than terbutaline (Holstein-Rathlou et al. 1986). In fact, bambuterol is approved for treatment of asthma in more than 28 countries, in oral tablets as the hydrochloride salt. Bambuterol is stable to pre-systemic elimination and is concentrated by lung tissue after absorption from the gastrointestinal tract. The prodrug is hydrolyzed to terbutaline primarily by butyryl cholinesterase, and lung tissue contains this metabolic enzyme. Bambuterol is also oxidatively metabolized to products that can be hydrolyzed to terbutaline (Sitar 1996). Bambuterol displays high first-pass hydrolytic stability and is only slowly hydrolyzed to terbutaline; hence, it can be administered orally, as infrequently as once a day. Bambuterol and its metabolites appear to be preferentially distributed to the lung, where an advantageous distribution and metabolism to active drug occurs. Thus, the prodrug is able to generate adequate concentrations of terbutaline levels in the lung. It has been reported that bronchodilator effects at low dosage are greater than can be predicted by plasma concentrations of terbutaline (Svensson 1987). This may explain the significantly reduced systemic side effects compared to other oral bronchodilators. A study (Svensson 1985) has postulated that several explanations can account for the disparity between plasma levels and drug effects as observed for several of the pulmonary products: (a) the prodrug is metabolized in lung to an unknown, but potent and long-acting pharmacological agent, (b) the prodrug releases small amounts of the parent drug at sites in lung from which it does not readily efflux, and (c) small amounts of the prodrug not reflected by bulk concentrations of prodrug in lung or plasma may sequester specific sites in the lung.

A related approach to the design of prodrugs of terbutaline is the cascade ester approach. In this design, the phenolic functions of terbutaline are esterified with 4-*O*-(2,2-dimethylpropionyloxy)-benzoic acid **(51d)**. The cascade effect is postulated initially to involve cleavage of the pivalate ester and *O*-conjugation during first-pass metabolism to protect the terbutaline phenolic groups; the subsequent hydrolysis of the hydroxybenzoyl link would, therefore, be delayed. However, data indicate that in dogs and humans this type of prodrug has no advantage over bambuterol, because both compounds are very slowly hydrolyzed in plasma, and significant plasma concentrations of the monoester of these prodrugs are not seen in vivo (Svensson 1985). Another related approach to the design of prodrugs to target alveolar macrophages has been carried out using microspheres as a primary carrier of the prodrug (Sharma et al. 2001). The drug isoniazid has been used in this fashion, it has been structurally modified into an ionizable form suitable for hydrophobic ion-pairing. The charged prodrug, sodium isoniazid methanesulfonate, was then ion-paired with hydrophobic cations, such as alkyltrimethyl ammonium ion. The drug was then encapsulated into polymeric microspheres to form hydrophobic ion-paired complexes. The ion-pair complex and polymer were then coprecipitated using supercritical fluid methodology (Zhou et al. 2002).

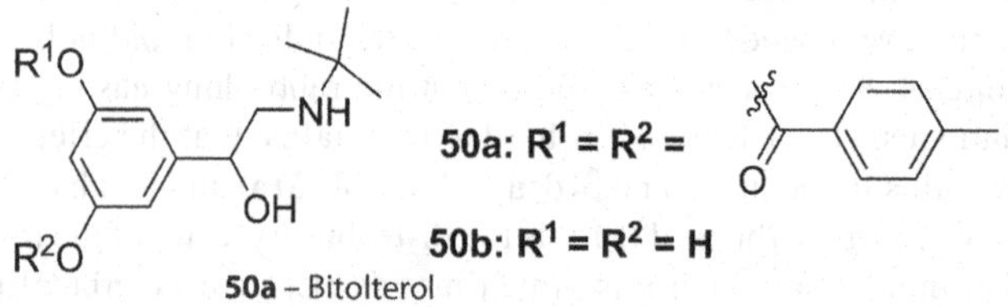

R^1O NH OH R^2O

50a: $R^1 = R^2 =$ O

50b: $R^1 = R^2 = H$

50a – Bitolterol
50b – N-t-butylarterenol

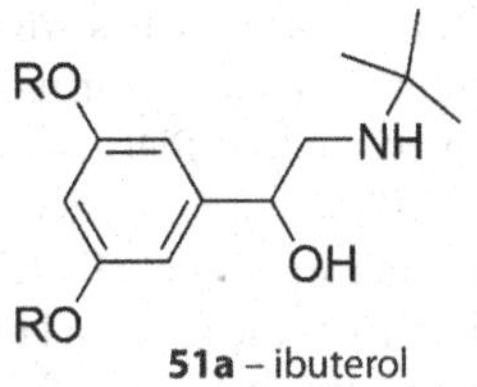

RO NH OH RO

51a: R = -CO-CH$(CH_3)_2$
51b: R = CO-N$(CH_3)_2$
51c: R = H
51d: R = CO-ph-OCO-C$(CH_3)_3$

51a – ibuterol
51b – bambuterol
51c – terbutaline
51d – benzoic acid

3.6 Potential Usefulness of Cell Membrane-Bound Enzyme Substrates and Inhibitors, and Cell Membrane-Bound Receptor Agonists and Antagonists as Drug Carriers with Lung Specificity

Ranney (1986, 1988) has postulated that pulmonary clearance of drug molecules from the systemic circulation may be achievable by targeting selective binding sites on the pulmonary endothelial membrane. In this regard, a possible strategy may be to link drug molecules to ligands that have high affinity for these endothelium binding sites. For example, several hydrolytic enzymes, such as peptidases and phosphorylases, are known to be located on the surface membrane of lung epithelium and endothelium (Krepela et al. 1985, Pitt et al. 1981, Ryan et al. 1976, Ryan 1989). Such enzymes may be targetable by designing drug conjugates with appropriate substrates or tight-binding inhibitors (i.e. non-hydrolysable substrates). Table 3.1 illustrates the number and types of peptidase enzymes that are known to be bound to pulmonary endothelial or epithelial membranes. The existence of a selection of membrane-bound epithelial enzymes may well be useful in designing appropriate drug conjugates with multiple ligands for these enzyme-active sites as bioadhesive targeting agents. Ranney (1986) pointed out that ligands that bind multiple active sites may be more useful as drug carriers on the grounds that populations of some receptors may be significantly decreased or lost entirely in some diseased states, for example, membrane-bound dipeptidyl aminopeptidase (angiotensin-converting enzyme) and phosphodiesterase

TABLE 3.1
Membrane-Bound Enzymes on Lung Endothelial and Epithelial Cells

Enzyme	Location
Dipeptidyl carboxypeptidase (ACE) (EC 3A.15.1)	Endothelial membrane
Dipeptidyl aminopeptidase IV (EC 3.4.14.5)	Endothelial membrane
Carboxypeptidase N (Arginine carboxypeptidase) (EC 3.4.17.3)	Endothelial membrane
Aminopeptidase M (EC 3.4.11.1)	Endothelial membrane
Aminopeptidase A (Microsomal aminopeptidase) (EC 3.4.11.2)	Endothelial membrane
Aminopeptidase P (aminoacyl-peptide hydrolase) (EC 3.4.11.9)	Endothelial membrane
Neutral metallo endopeptidase (enkephalinase) (EC 3.4.24.11)	Epithelial membrane
5′-Nucleotidase (EC 3.1.3.5)	Endothelial membrane
Adenyl cyclase	Endothelial and epithelial membrane
Carbonic anhydrase	Endothelial membrane
ATPase (EC 3.6.1.8)	Endothelial membrane
ADPase (EC 3.6.1.5)	Endothelial membrane

Source: Crooks, P.A., and Damani, L.A., Respiratory drug delivery, Chapter 3: Drug application to the respiratory tract: Metabolic and pharmacokinetic considerations, In *Respiratory Drug Delivery*, edited by P. R. Byron, pp. 61–90, Boca Raton, FL, CRC Press, 1989.

enzymes (PDEs). The cyclic nucleotide PDEs comprise a family of enzymes whose role is to regulate cellular levels of the second messengers, cAMP and Current good manufacturing practices (cGMP), by hydrolyzing them to inactive metabolites. PDE IV is the predominant PDE isozyme in inflammatory and immune cells and thus regulates a major pathway of cAMP degradation. Elevation of cAMP levels suppresses cell activation in a wide range of inflammatory and immune cells (Dent et al. 1991). The attraction of PDE IV inhibition as a therapy for asthma derives from the potential of selectively elevating cAMP levels in the airway smooth muscles and the inflammatory response (Stafford and Feldman 1996).

In order to achieve the desired pharmacological effects without unwanted side effects, it is likely that selective targeting of specific enzymes will be necessary. Selective inhibition of a specific target enzyme has been achieved using Rolipram (**52**), a selective PDE IV inhibitor, which shows reduction in allergen-induced bronchiole hyperreactivity in guinea pigs dosed at 75 μg/kg intraperitoneal (i.p.) (Santing et al. 1995) and cell adhesion molecules, constitutively expressed on the endothelial cell surface, i.e. angiotensin-converting enzyme (ACE) and aminopeptidase P (APP), have been targeted and show promising results in animal studies (Muzykantov 2013).

In a structure-activity correlation study, a number of *N*-substituted derivatives of rolipram (**52**) were prepared and evaluated (Tanaka et al. 1995). A carbamate ester of rolipram was found to be approximately 10-fold more potent than rolipram itself at inhibiting human PDE IV. A methyl ketone derivative of rolipram showed more potent inhibition of PDE IV compared to rolipram or its carbamate ester. Based on proton NMR spectroscopy and computer modeling studies, a pharmacophore model of the methyl ketone derivative was proposed (Stafford et al. 1995). This model showed that the ketone carbonyl oxygen atom is involved in an important interaction within the PDE IV active site. Sodium orthovanadate, a phosphotyrosine phosphate inhibitor, exhibits dose- and time-dependent suppression of Lewis lung carcinoma A11 cell spreading. Protein tyrosine phosphorylation levels in A11 cells were elevated after treatment with ortho vanadate; this increase was partially diminished by the tyrosine kinase inhibitor ST 638, concomitantly with restoration of the suppressed cell spreading, as well as invasive and metastatic ability (Takenaga 1996). These results suggest tyrosine phosphorylation influences adhesion of cancer cells to lung surface endothelia, and that a valid approach in treating cancer is inhibition of phosphotyrosine phosphatase.

Activity in the lung is known to be reduced by multiple diseases and by exposure to drugs and medical procedures, because of reversible endothelial damage (Catravas et al. 1983). Thus, the ideal carrier would be a non-pharmacological substrate (or inhibitor) with a broad spectrum affinity substrate for membrane-bound epithelial enzymes.

For such an approach to drug targeting to be effective, it is assumed that the drug and carrier are able to become internalized by transport across the contraluminal membrane and passage into the basement membrane tissues. In this respect, the use of macromolecule carriers, such as dextran (see later discussion) that can conjugate both drug and multiple-binding molecules may be an advantage. This approach can also be considered a viable strategy for the transendothelial route in the lung because several different peptidases are known to be bound to the endothelial membrane (Ryan and Ryan 1983, Ryan 1987a, Ryan 1987b) (Table 3.1).

Another strategy for obtaining an enhancement in pulmonary clearance of drugs is to conjugate the drug molecule to a chemical entity that binds to one or more surface receptors on endothelial or epithelial cells. Examples of the receptor agonists serotonin and norepinephrine have already been mentioned. However, there are examples of lung targeting that have used other pulmonary receptor substrates as targeting vectors (Geiger et al. 2010, Vallath et al. 2014, Korbelin et al. 2016, Orriols et al. 2017).

Human pulmonary carcinomas have been shown to contain high levels of opioid peptides and their corresponding membrane-bound receptors (Rigaudy et al. 1989). Rigaudy et al. (1989) targeted drugs to these receptors using modified metabolically stable enkephalins linked to cytotoxic drugs. These conjugates were expected to specifically internalize within opiate receptor-baring cells. Cell culture studies with NG 108-15 mouse tumor cells indicated that the peptide-ellipticinium conjugates **53a** and **53b** were internalized and were intracellularly stable, but showed much lower cytotoxicity than their parent drug towards the opioid receptor-bearing cells. Nevertheless, the study did indicate that enkephalin-derived peptides could be used as specific carriers to target cytotoxic agents towards opioid receptor-rich cells. A similar approach for targeting pulmonary epithelial membrane-bound enkephalinase (Table 3.1) may also be valid, using enkephalin drug or enkephalinase inhibitor-drug conjugates. One potential problem with the drug-targeting strategy is the likelihood that in disease states, membrane receptor populations may not be maintained. In this respect, an approach that uses a carrier capable of binding to multiple types of receptors may be more successful.

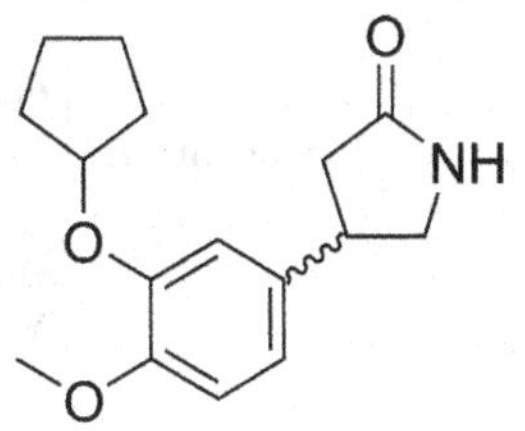

52 - Rolipram

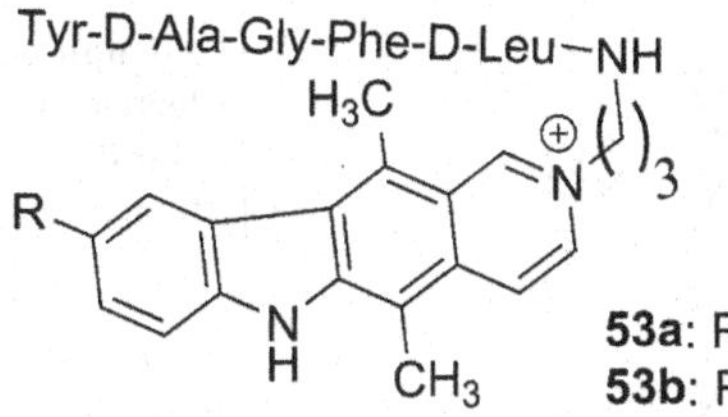

Tyr-D-Ala-Gly-Phe-D-Leu-NH

53

53a: R = H
53b: R = OH

A cell-based drug delivery system for lung targeting has been investigated. Doxorubicin was loaded into B16-F10 murine melanoma cells [a drug-loaded tumor cell (DLTC)]. The amount and rate of drug released from the DLTC mainly depended on the drug loading and carrier cell concentration. After a bolus injection of 30 μg doxorubicin either in the DLTC form or in free solution into the mice tail veins, drug deposition in the lung from DLTC was 3.6-fold greater than that achieved by free drug solution. This DLTC system demonstrated a lung-targeting activity that may be due to specific surface characteristics (Shao et al. 2001, Jones et al. 1988).

Other studies (Jones et al. 1988) indicate that insulin is efficiently absorbed from the lung when administered either by intratracheal instillation in the rat or by aerosol inhalation in the rabbit. Because insulin is also actively cleared from the systemic circulation (King and Johnson 1985) and has a lower potential for acute pharmacological effects, the conjugation of appropriate drug molecules to this polypeptide may also be a useful strategy for lung targeting.

3.7 Conjugation of Drugs with Macromolecules for Selective Targeting to the Lung

One approach to the selective targeting of drugs into those cells where their action is required is the conjugation of a pharmacologically active agent to a macromolecular vector that is recognized and actively taken up by the target cell, where bound drug can then be released in its active from. Several examples where macromolecules have been used as carriers in an effort to alter the tissue localization of a carrier-linked drug have been reported (Sezaki and Hashida 1984, Tram and Ee 2017). Selectivity of targeting is largely dependent on the properties of the macromolecular vector and usually results in an altered distribution of the free drug compared to the parent drug itself when administered by the same route.

It is clear that macromolecule-drug conjugates or, more accurately, macromolecular prodrugs may well alter the pharmacological and immunological activity of the parent compound. The macromolecular transport vector may vary considerably in size, electrical charges, hydrophobicity and hydrophilicity, and its ability to act as a substrate for transmembrane transport mechanisms.

Desirable properties of the macromolecular vectors are no intrinsic toxicity (e.g. nonantigenic), biodegradability with no accumulation in the body, and presence of functionalized moieties for drug

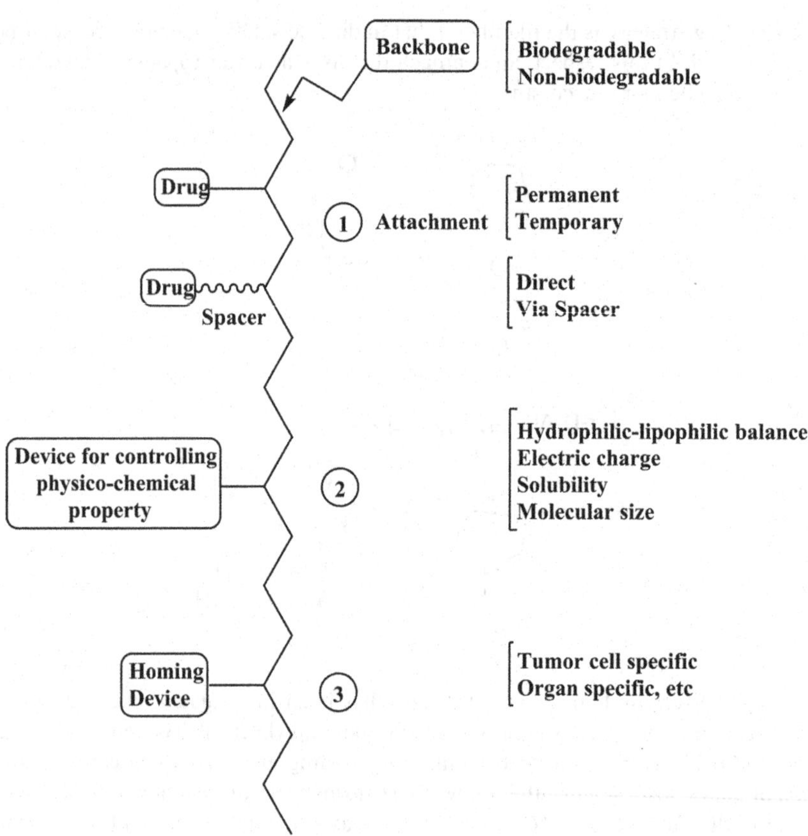

FIGURE 3.7 Model for macromolecule-drug conjugates. (With kind permission from Taylor & Francis: *J Pharmacol Exp Ther*, Carbon-11 labeled aliphatic amines in lung uptake and metabolism studies: Potential for dynamic measurements in vivo. 198, 1976, 133–145, Fowler, J.S. et al.)

conjugation. In addition, the macromolecule-drug conjugate must not possess the pharmacological activity of the parent drug, but the conjugate should retain the desirable targeting specificity of the parent macromolecular vector. With regard to the drug molecule, certain properties are also desirable for the formulation of an effective prodrug. For example, the therapeutic effect of the drug must be shown at relatively low doses to afford a reasonably low load of carrier macromolecule, and the macromolecule-drug conjugate structure must be chemically stable before drug release. Not all therapeutic drug molecules are capable of being conjugated to macromolecular vectors, simply because they lack adequate functional groups in their molecular structure for chemical fixation.

A variety of covalent linkages have been used in the design of macromolecule-drug conjugates, that is, esters, amides, hydrazones, imides, and disulfides. These linkages must be designed to be readily formed without chemical destruction of either the macromolecular vector or the drug during synthesis, and they must be readily broken by chemical or enzymatic hydrolysis. Figure 3.7 illustrates the various components of a macromolecule-drug conjugate.

3.7.1 In Vivo Fate of Macromolecular Prodrugs and Lung Targeting

The fate of macromolecular conjugates when administered by the systemic route is heavily dependent on the distribution and elimination properties of the prodrug. In addition, endothelial and epithelial membrane transport is of primary importance with regard to targeting and drug action. Distribution and elimination profiles are primarily determined by factors such as molecular size, charge, water solubility, and hydrophilic and lipophilic balance. Apart from the incorporation of specific targeting features into the conjugate (i.e. antibodies), such physiochemical factors can play an important role in tissue targeting. The administration of macromolecule-drug conjugates by inhalation has received relatively little attention, although some studies involving anti-cancer agents are available. If such conjugates are required to access the circulatory system, then initial diffusion or transport across the alveolar capillary membrane must take place. In addition, interaction will occur with other structures, such as the alveolar epithelial cells that face the air spaces, the capillary endothelial cells that are the major constituents of the pulmonary macrocirculation, and the phagocytic pulmonary intravascular macrophages.

The relationship between pulmonary sequestering of macromolecules and molecular weight or particle size is not clear. Hashida et al. (1984) showed that distribution of C-dextran-mitomycin C conjugates was dependent on molecular weight when given intravenously in rats, conjugates of MW 10,000–500,000 being sequestered mainly by spleen, liver, and lymph nodes, with no significant accumulation in the lung, heart, or muscle. Interestingly, cationic dextran conjugates of MW 70,000 or less are immediately distributed to the kidney and excreted, indicating that the glomerular capillary membrane is impermeable to polycationic macromolecules in excess of MW 70,000. There have been numerous studies in dogs and rats that indicate that particles exceeding 7 μm are retained in the lung after intravascular administration. However, other studies in ruminants have shown that liposomes, bacteria, and magnetic iron microaggregates are sequestered in the lung, even at particle sizes much smaller than 7 μm (Miyamoto et al. 1988, DeCamp et al. 1992, Warner et al. 1987). Studies have suggested that particulate trapping in the pulmonary circulation may not be solely dependent on size, but may also be determined by other factors, for example, the involvement of pulmonary intravascular macrophages (PIMs), because pulmonary sequestration is often associated with pulmonary hypertension and lung injury, conditions that increase the lung burden of pulmonary intravascular macrophages. Other studies (DeCamp et al. 1992) have shown that disruption of hepatic bacterial clearance mechanisms may also induce PIM formation in the lung; of importance in this connection, patients with impaired hepatic function often exhibit substantial pulmonary uptake of intravascular colloidal imaging agents that are normally localized in the liver, spleen, and bone marrow of healthy patients.

3.7.2 Targeting of Macromolecule-Drug Conjugates to the Lung

In general, the major problem in targeting macromolecules to the lung after intravascular administration is to overcome the biodistribution of such molecules to phagocytes in the reticuloendothelial organs (liver, spleen, and bone marrow). With a growing body of data on the nature of endothelial and epithelial receptors that enhance pulmonary drug clearance, the morphological factors governing transport of molecules through basement membranes, the effects of disease on endothelial and sequestered tissue receptors, and the availability of receptor-binding substrates that can be used for targeting entities in macromolecule-drug conjugates, the efforts to improve pulmonary targeting of drugs is already underway. Recent developments that have affected this progress have been due to new technologies, leading to an improvement in the design and production of drug-carrier molecules and coatings that afford circulating agents with specific affinity for lung endothelium and epithelium (Tram and Ee 2017, Muzykantov 2013). As previously mentioned in the section on structural factors governing drug uptake, several endogenous compounds are known to be actively taken up from the plasma by the pulmonary endothelium, for example, serotonin and norepinephrine. Drugs conjugated to these agents have been suggested to undergo pulmonary targeting; this has yet to be determined conclusively. A more rational approach is to use pharmacologically inactive analogues of these agents or their inactive metabolites, which would still retain their targeting abilities, in drug-drug or macromolecule-drug conjugates.

It is generally recognized that the use of liposomes, microparticulates, and colloidal carriers to achieve drug targeting has proven to be largely unsuccessful because of the difficulties in gaining access to targeted tissues, penetrating vascular barriers, and evading phagocytic capture by the reticuloendothelium system. However, the coating of microspheres and emulsions with block copolymers may overcome the latter problem. In some early studies, Illum et al. (Illum et al. 1987, Illum and Davis 1984), for example, coated model polystyrene microspheres with a poloxamine-980 block copolymer, and they observed a much longer circulatory half-life in the vascular compartment after intravenous injection, with little or no uptake by the reticuloendothelium system. Deposition of coated microspheres was observed to be significantly reduced in the liver and spleen, with high levels in the lungs. The conjugation of tissue-targeting vectors (e.g. sugar residues, lectins, monoclonal antibodies, apolipoproteins) to appropriate functionalities on a hydrophilic coating may allow colloidal carriers to be actively targeted to specific sites, either by systemic or intracavity administration (*N*-2-hydroxyporpyl)-methacrylamide copolymer macromolecules have also been used as targetable drug-carrier systems (Kopecek and Duncan 1987, Kopecek 1984). The advantages of these systems is that they can be tailor-made to include oligopeptide drug linkages that are stable in the circulation but are readily digested intracellularly by the lysosomal thiol-dependent (cysteine-) proteinases. They are readily synthesized and are efficiently internalized by cells via pinocytosis, and cleavage of linkages to drug can be controlled by appropriate structural manipulation. Thus, they provide good opportunities for controlled intracellular delivery of drugs. In addition, they can be synthesized to include potentially useful targeting residues, such as sugars, immunoglobulins, and antibodies.

Soluble macromolecule-drug carriers seem to offer greater potential because they can transverse compartmental barriers more efficiently and, therefore, gain access to a greater number of cell types and, in most cases, are not subject to clearance by the reticuloendothelial cells. Dextrans, human serum albumin, polysomes, and even tumor-specific antibodies (see the section on drug monoclonal-antibody conjugates) have all been evaluated as drug carriers for lung targeting (Kojima et al. 1980, Pimm 1988). Each system has advantages in terms of specificity or ease of chemical conjugation, but each also presents problems of limited body distribution or immunogenicity. Conjugation of methotrexate of poly-L-lysine has markedly increased the drug's tumoricidal activity in vitro (Ryser and Shen 1978), and intermittent administration of methotrexate-albumin conjugates has been shown to be more effective than free drug in reducing the number of lung metastases in mice after receiving subcutaneous inoculation of Lewis lung carcinoma (Chu and Whiteley 1980).

Mammalian macrophages contain a transport system that binds and internalizes glycoproteins with exposed mannose residues. It has been shown that small multivalent synthetic glycopeptides with mannose residues covalently linked through a spacer arm to the α- and ε-amino groups of lysine, dilysine, or trilysine are competitive inhibitors of rate alveolar macrophage uptake of the neoglycoprotein-bovine serum albumin with inhibition constants in the low micromolar range (Robbins et al. 1981) (Figure 3.8). Various compounds can be covalently attached to the α-carboxyl group of these glycopeptides without substantial loss of inhibition. TD-1792, a conjugate between glycopeptide and cephalosporin, is currently undergoing clinical trials for the treatment of skin infections and has yielded promising results and underpins the potential therapeutic value of such macromolecular conjugates (Stryjewski et al. 2012).

These synthetic substrates may be useful models for targeting pharmacological agents to alveolar macrophages, as well as other cell types. Monsigny et al. (1984) have conjugated the immunostimulant muramyldipeptide with neoglycoprotein and have shown that the conjugate was actively endocytosed by murine alveolar macrophages, leading to their dramatic activation, even at very low concentrations of the conjugate. Intravenous and intraperitoneal administration of the conjugate led to maximal activation of alveolar macrophages at 48 hours in mice and 72 hours in rats. This interesting example of drug targeting may have potential usefulness in the design of carrier-mediated anti-cancer, anti-parasitic, or anti-viral chemotherapy.

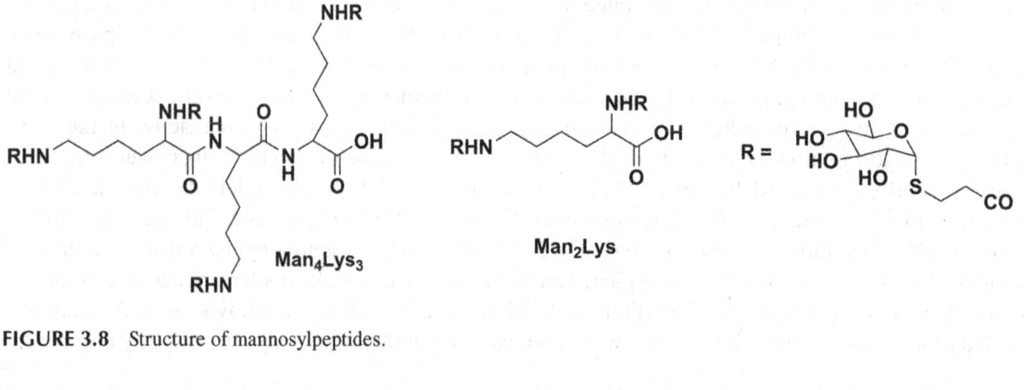

FIGURE 3.8 Structure of mannosylpeptides.

An attempt has been made to target the anti-tumor drug daunomycin to human squamous lung tumor cell monolayers by conjugating the drug with low-density lipoprotein. Although rapid uptake of the conjugate afforded equilibrium in 3 hours, the in vitro cytotoxicity of the conjugate was no different than that of the parent drug (Kerr et al. 1988). The high level of expression of high-affinity receptors for epidermal growth factor (EGF) on lung tumors may possibly be used as a target for ligand-complexed (conjugated) drugs (Veale et al. 1989). Antibodies to EGF have been shown to inhibit tumor growth (Masui et al. 1984), and ligand-complexed drugs can concentrate in receptor-positive cells by affinity targeting (Vollmar et al. 1987). More recent studies have utilized nanoparticle platforms for targeted delivery of daunomycin which can be exploited for efficient localization of this anti-cancer agent within the tumor microenvironment (Bazak et al. 2015).

The correct strategy for accomplishing the successful targeting and delivery of drugs using macromolecule-drug conjugates must be a judicious choice, based on the characteristics of the target tissue or cell type and the drug. Initially, the properties of the cell type, sites of complexation, transport, and internalization mechanisms, as well as the pharmacological and physicochemical properties of the drug molecule, its site of action (i.e. nature of interaction with receptors or enzyme active sites), and chemical stability, must be considered. The conjugation of the drug molecule to the carrier is also an important consideration because the bond must be stable enough to withstand cleavage before reaching the target site, but must be designed to release the drug at the site of action.

3.8 Bioadhesives and Drug Targeting to the Lung

The use of bioadhesive targeting as a means for specific delivery of drugs has gained some impetus since the late 1980s (Gu et al. 1988). The term *bioadhesion* refers to interactions involving multiple molecular and usually non-covalent bonds. However, a bioadhesive agent, to be effective as a drug carrier, must initially be trapped or sequestered by endothelial or epithelial cells, followed by multi-ligand binding of the surface material of the carrier particle to cell surface determinants, which then induces the rapid (10-minute to 15-minute) envelopment of the carrier by the cell either by transcytosis or migrational overgrowth mechanisms, followed by transfer to the proximal tissues. Bioadhesion targeting is, therefore, a combination of biophysical trapping and biochemical adherence. The carrier is usually a hydrophilic macromolecule or microparticulate, and, for systemic delivery, a particle size between 3 μm and 5 μm (non-embolizing) is preferable for pulmonary trapping, whereas larger particle sizes between 5 μm and 250 μm (embolizing) are also usable. Multivalent binding agents may comprise substance such as heparins, lectins, and antibodies to endothelial antigens, epithelial antigens, and glycosylated albumin.

Lectins are naturally occurring glycoproteins of non-immunological origin. They have the unique ability to recognize and bind to exposed carbohydrate residues on glycoproteins, such as those exposed at the surface of epithelial cells, and therefore have been classified as second-generation bioadhesives. In a study by Bruck et al. (2001), lectin-functionalized liposomes, in contrast to lectin-free liposomes, specifically bound to A 549, a tumor-derived cell line. This suggests that lectin-mediated bioadhesion and uptake of liposome-carriers may provide a useful technology for lung cancer treatment. The administration of liposome-encapsulated drugs by aerosols seems to be a feasible way of targeting these delivery systems to the lung. The tolerability and safety of liposome aerosols has been tested in animals as well as human volunteers, and no unwanted effects have been observed (Waldrep et al. 1997). Lectin-functionalized liposomes for pulmonary delivery may provide a useful technology for improved delivery of hydrophilic macromolecules to the alveolar epithelium (Bruck et al. 2001), and wheat germ agglutinin (WGA)-coated poly(lactide-co-glycolide) nanoparticles have been investigated as potential drug carriers for anti-tubercular drugs via both oral and aerosol delivery for treatment of Tuberculosis (TB) (Sharma et al. 2004, Sharma et al. 2004).

Both transendothelial and transepithelial migration of particles and molecular aggregates larger than about 2 nm in diameter have been shown to be accelerated by application of surface coatings that bind multiply to cell surface receptors or antigens (Ranney 1988). Such particles conjugate at least two molecules of drug or diagnostic agent and a multivalent binding agent (bioadhesive) that is specific for cell

TABLE 3.2
Composition of Bioadhesives

Carrier Particles	Multivalent Binding Agents	Endothelial and Epithelial Surface Determinants
Macromolecules	Heparin and heparin derivatives	Receptors
Microaggregates	Heparin fragments	Enzyme active sites
Microparticles	Lectins	Antigens
Microspheres	Antibodies	Endothelial and epithelial tissue factors
Nanospheres	Dextrans	Subcellular tissue moieties
Liposomes	Peptides	Fibrin D-D dimers
Microemulsions	Enzyme inhibitors	Glycoprotein complexes
	Receptor agonists; and antagonists	
	Albumins and glycosylated albumins	

surface determinants. Table 3.2 lists carrier particles, multivalent binding agents, and endothelial and epithelial cell surface determinants of potential usefulness in bioadhesive targeting to the lung. This list is by no means exhaustive. Carrier particles, preferably having a size between 1 nm and 250 μm or coatings comprising carbohydrates, oligosaccharides, or monosaccharides, proteins or peptides, and lipids or other biocompatible synthetic polymers are usually used. The chemical structure may be a simple single-chain polymer, a molecular microaggregate (i.e. a molecular carrier or aggregate that acts as both the cell target binding moiety and the backbone for linking prodrug moieties), or a more complex structure incorporating multiple matrix material or serial coating that is able to interact with multiple cell surface determinants, resulting in rapid sequestration and transport of the carrier. Substances from a wide range are known that bind to native endothelium and epithelium and to basement membrane constituents. All are promising candidates with potential usefulness as bioadhesive agents for lung-targeting studies. Laminin is a non-collagenous high-molecular-weight (10^6) protein that interacts with glycosaminoglycans and promotes adhesion of various cell types. Laminin is located in the lamina lucida of a cell's basal surface and the supporting matrix of type IV (basement membrane) collagen (Terranova et al. 1980, Vlodavsky and Gospodarowicz 1981, Foidart et al. 1980). Laminin receptors occur on cells that normally interact with basement membranes, as well as on cells that extravasate, for example, metastasizing cancer cells, macrophages, and leukocytes (Lopes et al. 1985). In vitro studies have clearly shown that laminin can mediate the attachment of a wide variety of epithelial and endothelial cells to type IV collagen (Terranova, et al. 1980, Vlodavsky and Gospodarowicz 1981), and a cell surface receptor protein for laminin has been isolated from murine fibrosarcoma cells that may mediate the interaction of the cell with its extracellular matrix (Malinoff and Wicha 1983). Aumailley (2013) has published a recent review on the Laminin family of glycoproteins.

Fibronectin, another constituent of basement membrane, may also be an effective constituent for promoting extravascular migration of particulate matter (Newman et al. 1985, Brown and Juliano 1985), and glycosylated serum albumins appear to undergo greater vesicular endothelial micropinocytosis by rat micro-vessels as compared to unmodified albumin, which may indicate a useful role for non-enzymatic glycosylated serum albumin in drug targeting (Williams et al. 1981). Fibronectin has been demonstrated to have potential applications as a material for clinical wound healing and tissue repair (Hsiao et al. 2017).

Heparin sulfates, the side-chain moieties of cell surface proteoglycans, are important factors in cell recognition phenomena. The proteoheparin sulfates are ubiquitous cell surface proteoglycan components of the cell coat or glycocalyx. They undergo chain-chain self-association in a structure-specific manner. Studies show that such compounds are useful bioadhesives (Fransson 1981). Lipoprotein lipase also attaches to endothelial cells through heparin sulfate interaction on the cell surface and is released by heparin through a detachment from this binding site (Shimada et al. 1981). Factor VIII antigen has been widely used as a marker for endothelial cells (Ordonez and Batsakis 1984), and studies have shown that *Ulex europaeus* 1 agglutinin (UEA-1), a lectin that is specific for α-L-fucose-containing glycol compounds, is also a marker for vascular endothelium in human tissues (Ordonez and Batsakis 1984). UEA-1 appears to be a more sensitive marker than factor VIII antigen for the factor VIII binding site and has a particularly high affinity for alveolar capillary endothelium and bronchial epithelium [194]. Furthermore, high factor VIII levels increase the risk of venous thromboembolism, but the cause of high factor VIII levels is unclear (Kamphuisen et al. 2001). In vivo studies indicate that intravenously injected fucose-blocked UEA-1-coated microspheres in CBA mice (derived from a cross of a Bagg Albino female mouse and a Dilute Brown Agouti male mouse) allowed approximately 90% of the injected dose to be concentrated in the lung after 20 minutes, with 80% of this amount being in extravascular locations (Ranney 1988). CBA is just genetic code no full form is required. The use of UEA-1 lectin as a diagnostic agent for tumors derived from human endothelial cells has previously been described (Miettinen et al. 1983).

Anionic sites on the lumenal surface of pulmonary microvascular endothelium have been shown to bind cationic ferritin in isolated, perfused rat lung studies (Pietra et al. 1983). The cationic ferritin is taken up by vesicles and discharged into the capillary membrane. Similar anionic sites are also present on alveolar epithelial surfaces (Vaccaro and Brody 1981).

In some cases, cell surface expression of certain species can be induced; for example, interleukin-1 has been shown to induce the biosynthesis and cell surface expression of procoagulant activity in human vascular endothelial cells (Bevilacqua et al. 1984). Such materials may also be exploitable as candidates for bioadhesion studies.

Millions of lives of patients with diabetes have been saved since the introduction of insulin therapy. However, several daily injections of insulin are required to maximize glucose control in diabetic patients. Insulin is administered by subcutaneous injection, but this route of administration has a slow onset and subsequent prolonged duration of action. These limitations show up more when higher doses of insulin are injected, which results in a long duration of action and forces the patients to consume additional amounts of food to limit the risk of hypoglycemia (Anderson et al. 1997). This limitation has been reduced by the availability of newer, short-acting insulin analogues (Lispro, Aspart, and Glulisine). However, these forms of insulin must be injected subcutaneously (Bode et al. 2011). Technosphere™ insulin is a formulation of regular human and a new drug-delivery system for pulmonary administration. The formulation is designed for efficient transport of insulin across the intact respiratory epithelium into the systemic circulation (Owens 2002); its duration of action is more than 3 hours, and maximal serum insulin levels can be reached within 13 minutes after inhalation (Steiner et al. 2002), which is considerably shorter than those observed with rapid-acting insulin analogues administered subcutaneously or other insulin inhalations (Skyler et al. 2001).

Other molecules have been suggested as being useful lung-specific bioadhesive agents (Ranney 1986, 1988), for example, insulin, transferrin, prostaglandins, hirudin-inhibited thrombin (which binds thrombomodulin), anionic polysaccharides, oligosaccharides (such as dextran sulfate, dermatan sulfate, chondroitin sulfate, hyaluronic acid), peptides (such as benzoyl-phe-ala-pro [BPAPI] that bind angiotensin-converting enzyme, 5′-nucleotides that bind 5′ nucleases, and inactive analogues of biogenic amines (such as 5-hydroxytryptamine) that interact with surface neuroreceptors. Such a list of compounds also includes antibodies directed against cell surface targets, such as factor VIII antigen and type IV collagen of the basement membrane, glycoproteins, and other antigens (see the later section on monoclonal antibody conjugates).

Bioadhesive agents have been hypothesized to interact with endothelial or epithelial cell surface determinants, inducing the cell to undergo transient separation or opening, thereby exposing subcellular determinants for which the agent may also have binding affinity. The interaction results in an acceleration of transport across at least one of the associated endothelial and epithelial structures or subcellular structures into a proximal tissue compartment. The basic premise is that this phenomenon will result in an improvement in the therapeutic index so that a reduced total dose of drug (or diagnostic agent) is required to obtain pharmacological effects comparable to significantly higher doses of free drug (or diagnostic agent).

Ranney (1988) showed that intravenously administered heparin-amphotericin Pluronic B-F108 nanospheres and microspheres in adult male CBA/J mice are specifically targeted to lung, endothelium uptake being complete within 15 minutes after injection (i.e. zero blood levels) (Table 3.3). The results indicate that preferential and rapid uptake in the lung occurs with both sub-embolizing and embolizing particle diameters. Such a rapid and efficient uptake was not observed for dextran and agarose placebo particles that lack the heparin surface coat.

TABLE 3.3

Organ Localization of Heparin-Amphotericin B Formulations after Intravenous Injection into Adult Male CBA/J Mice

	Organ Concentration (µg) Amphotericin/g Tissue) (%) 1 hr after Injection		
Tissue	Amphotericin B[a] (Unbound)	Heparin (Non-embolizing) (Nanospheres[b])	Heparin (Marginally Embolizing) (Microspheres[c])
Lung	4.0 (14)[d]	15.0 (52)[d]	25.7 (94)[d]
Liver	6.7 (24)	8.3 (29)	5.0 (18[d])
Kidney	2.5 (9.2)	1.1 (3.8)	0.4 (1.4)[d]
Spleen	11.0 (38.3)	6.2 (21)	2.2 (8.2)
Heart	0.3 (1.3)	0.2 (0.7)	0.3 (0.4)
Brain	0.0 (0)	1.4 (4.8)	0.2 (0.5)

[a] Biodistribution of fungizone (amphotericin β-deoxycholate nanoemulsion).
[b] Total body drug recovered, 70%.
[c] Total body drug recovered, 55%.
[d] Percent of injected dose localized per gram of tissue (wet weight).

Histochemical analysis of lung deposition showed the amphotericin B to be distributed in the alveoli, pulmonary interstitium, respiratory epithelium, and bronchial and tracheal lymph nodes, thus indicating extensive tissue percolation of the drug carrier; no significant kidney deposition was observed. (Note: This is a major site of amphotericin toxicity.) The results establish that it is possible to achieve high-efficiency endothelial bioadhesion, selective drug uptake, and retention in the lung using this approach.

In the same study, intravenous injection of *Ulex europaeus* 1 lectin microspheres were shown to be specifically taken up by lung endothelial cells and rapidly underwent migration into the extravascular tissues and into the airspace within 5 minutes–10 minutes after injection, with 90% of the injected dose being identified in the lung. Intratracheal administration of heparin nanospheres of 200-nm to 800-nm diameter containing iron oxide (Fe_3O_4) and ionic iron (Fe^{3+}) to pentobarbital-anesthetized adult male CBA/J mice indicated a very similar deposition profile to that observed after intravenous injection of amphotericin B-containing nanospheres (Table 3.3) (Ranney 1988).

Liver and kidney deposition was negligible to very low, showing that stabilized heparin nanosphere carriers with heparin surfaces are taken up by epithelial transport and that a high proportion of the dose becomes localized in lungs relative to other organs when administered by the airways. This novel example of epithelial uptake provides a rationale for administering drug-bioadhesive carrier conjugates by the inhalation route and may be particularly useful for the topical or systemic delivery of highly toxic drugs (e.g. anti-tumor drugs, anti-fungals, anti-virals, antibiotics), drugs that are very labile (e.g. peptides, proteins, oligonucleotides), or drugs that for one reason or another exhibit poor access by conventional formulations to pulmonary tissues. More recent studies have focused on optimizing the efficacy of amphotericin B through nanomodification with lipids as liposomes or complexes (Barratt and Bretagne 2007), and an oral delivery system of amphotericin B-loaded to PEGylated polylactic-polyglycolic acid copolymer-PEG nanoparticle formulation has been developed that affords significant oral absorption and improved bioavailability in rats (Radwan et al. 2017).

3.9 Drug-Monoclonal Antibody Conjugates for Targeting to the Lung

Another drug-carrier system that has been investigated as a means of achieving specific tissue targeting is the use of an antibody directed against the tissue that is the proposed site of action of the drug; although this approach is not new, because pioneering work in this area was carried out as early as 1958 (Mathe et al. 1958). Recently, it has become evident that monoclonal antibody (mAb) biotechnology is effective in a wide range of disease states. The current estimated market for these agents is more than $25 billion each year. The application of antibodies is broad ranging and includes therapeutics, diagnostic tools, and research tools. The first therapeutic antibodies were mouse monoclonal antibodies that were selected against cytokines and cell surface proteins of proinflammatory, immunologic, or cancer cells (Takács et al. 2001). The development of monoclonal antibodies to human tumor-associated antigens has been achieved, and this has led to a renewed interest in the use of drug-antibody conjugates for cancer therapy (Stephens et al. 1995, Pimm 1988, Diamantis and Banerji 2016, Kang et al. 2018, Patel et al. 2018, Lambert and Morris 2017).

There are several questions that need to be addressed before considering the use of drug-monoclonal antibody conjugates.

1. Are sufficiently lung-specific antibodies available?
2. Is there evidence that such antibodies will localize only in lung tissues and not in other tissues in vivo?
3. Do the antibodies contain appropriate functionalities to enable covalent linkage of drug molecules, and, if so, will the conjugated antibody exhibit targeting characteristics similar to those of the parent antibody?
4. Will the formation of an antibody-drug conjugate result in an immunologically active entity on repeated administration?

With regard to these considerations, it is important to determine whether, after either regional or systemic administration, a drug-antibody conjugate can deliver potentially therapeutic doses of the drug. This may depend on the loading of drug at multiple sites of conjugation on the antibody surface. In this respect, the greater the number of drug molecules conjugated to each antibody molecule, the more ineffective the resultant molecule might be, because attachment of drug molecules near or around the antibody-antigen binding site or at locations that compromise the three-dimensional integrity of the antibody will lead to decreased tissue specificity or increased immunological activity, respectively. Thus, an evaluation of the therapeutic index of the conjugate must be undertaken to determine whether it is superior to the free drug.

When considering the targeting of therapeutic agents to lung tissue by this approach, the choice of cell surface antigens would appear to be most appropriate, although there is evidence that antibodies that can recognize in vivo antigens that are expressed extracellularly (Chan et al. 1986) can also be used for specific tissue targeting. A recombinant humanized mAb to human IgE has been found to inhibit mast-cell-dependent airway narrowing and other components of the asthmatic inflammatory response (Milgrom et al. 1999). Currently, omalizumab is undergoing clinical testing for a number of indications, including asthma. Omalizumab (Xolair) is a monoclonal anti-IgE antibody that specifically recognizes human IgE (Easthope and Jarvis 2001, Belliveau 2005). It is used for the treatment of moderate to severe allergic asthma in adults and adolescents that is inadequately controlled by inhaled corticosteroids (Chipps et al. 2012).

The most commonly used route of administration for antibody-drug conjugates has been the intravenous route, but intracavity administration has also been investigated; and, generally, localization of antibody conjugates in the targeted tissue by this latter route appears to be superior to the intravenous route (Colcher et al. 1987). The mechanism of antibody-drug delivery at the cellular level is believed to involve initial binding to the specific cell surface antigen. This binding is followed by internalization and endocytosis into lysosomes, where digestion of the conjugate by lysosomal proteinases would release free drug from where it would diffuse to the site of action (de Duve et al. 1974).

As mentioned previously, a significant reduction in antibody reactivity is often observed after multiple sites of conjugation of drug with antibody. This has led to the development of carriers that, when covalently linked to antibody, are able in turn to covalently bind many drug molecules to appropriate carrier functionalities. Examples of carrier molecules that have been used include dextran (Pimm et al. 1982, Hurwitz et al. 1979, Tsukada et al. 1987), human serum albumin (Garnett et al. 1983), and poly-L-glutamate (Tsukada et al. 1984). Obviously, such a gross molecular modification of the parent antibody may well affect its overall properties, and this often leads to significant differences in biodistribution of an antibody-carrier-drug complex relative to the parent antibody. In addition, for reasons stated previously, such a structural derivatization may also result in lower tissue specificity and increased toxicity. Factors affecting the pharmacology of antibody-drug conjugates (ADCs) and the interaction between ADC carriers and biological systems has recently been reviewed (Lucas et al. 2018).

More innovative approaches to the targeting of drugs by antibody-drug complexes involve the use of hybrid-hybrid antibodies (Corvalan et al. 1987, Corvalan et al. 1987, Moran et al. 1990). This approach uses hybrid antibodies with dual specificity (bifunctional/bispecific antibodies), one site binding with, say, a cell surface antigen, and the other with drug or cytotoxic agent. Such bispecific antibodies are prepared by reassociation of enzyme-prepared fragments of two antibodies or by hybridization of two existing hybridomas, one producing antibody to cell antigen, and the other producing antibody to drug. The application of this strategy to the development of therapeutic agents could be twofold: bispecific antibody would be initially administered, resulting in specific tissue localization (i.e. pre-targeting), followed by drug, some of which would be taken up by the localized antibody; alternatively, binary complexes of both drug and antibody could be performed in vitro and then administered or drug and antibody could be given simultaneously. The concept of pre-targeting is not new and has been investigated for diagnostic tumor imaging with the high-affinity avidin-biotin system (Hnatowich et al. 1987). In this system, antibody conjugated to avidin was evaluated for localization in tumors followed by administration of radiolabeled biotin. It is conceivable that such a system may be useful for the pre-targeting of drugs to the lung, perhaps by using a biotin-drug conjugate in place of biotin.

The use of drug-antibody fragments has been examined as a means for tissue targeting (Andrew et al. 1988, Buchegger et al. 1983, Nelson 2010, Richards et al. 2017). Generally, fragments appear to be poorer targeting agents than intact antibody, although they do exhibit relatively faster overall clearance and catabolism, which may result in less systemic toxicity. However, studies indicate that the increased clearance and kidney metabolism of antibody fragments may lead to renal toxicity (Rowland et al. 1986). The use of antibody fragments lacking a more immunogenic portion of the intact antibody molecule has generally not resulted in a decrease in immunogenic properties.

Some earlier reports involving monoclonal antibodies directed against epithelial and endothelial cell surface components suggest that this approach to drug targeting in the lung may have good potential. For example, monoclonal antibodies to a glycoprotein involved in fibronectin-mediated adhesion mechanisms has been reported for fibroblasts (Brown and Juliano 1985), and the injection of rabbit antisera or purified antibodies against basement membrane proteins type IV collagen and laminin into inbred mice results in cellular infiltration of mainly lung and kidney tissue. Antibody location was shown to be on the basement membranes of glomeruli, alveoli (pronounced), choroids plexus, liver, and blood vessels and in epidermal junctions (Wick et al. 1982).

Developments in the cancer area are worthy of mention. In earlier studies, an immunotoxin consisting of a murine monoclonal antibody (B4G7) that recognizes EGF receptor conjugated with gelonin, a ribose-inactivating protein, was specifically cytotoxic to EGF receptor-hyperproducing cells in mice and was non-toxic at 250 μm conjugate per mouse (Hirota et al. 1989). The results suggested that this conjugate may be useful for targeted therapy to epidermal growth factor receptor-hyperproducing squamous carcinoma. Also, a ^{125}I-labeled monoclonal antibody directed against MW 48,000 human lung cancer-associated antigen may be useful in the diagnosis and treatment of lung cancer (Endo et al. 1987). Chan et al. (1986) reported that a set of mouse monoclonal antibodies directed against the c-myc oncogene product, a 62,000-d nuclear binding protein involved in cell cycle control, was constructed by immunization with synthetic peptide fragments. After intravenous administration, these monoclonal antibodies exhibited good tumor localization with primary bronchial carcinoma patients, thus indicating that monoclonal antibodies directed against oncogene products may provide novel selective tools for diagnosis and targeted therapy of cancer. Utilization of mAb to prevent cancer cell metastasis has been examined too. Studies have been done to utilize mAb, such as the inhibitor of lung endothelial cell adhesion molecule (anti-lu-ECAM-1) to inhibit colonization of the lung by lung metastatic murine B16 melanoma cells (Zhu et al. 1992). Lung endothelial cell adhesion molecule (Lu-ECAM-1) has been isolated and characterized (Elble et al. 1997); this molecule selectively binds lung-metastatic melanoma cells (Zhu and Pauli 1993). In a similar manner, mAb 6A3 selectively binds a membrane glycoprotein of rat lung capillary endothelia and has been shown to inhibit specific adhesion of lung endothelial vesicles to lung metastatic breast cancer cells.

Because most monoclonal antibodies that have been studied for tissue targeting are from mouse or, occasionally, from rat, the problem of antibody production to such foreign proteins always exists. While murine-derived mAbs are well tolerated for acute therapy, their use in chronic therapy has been limited, due to severe human anti-mouse antibody response (HAMA) (Schroff et al. 1985). The HAMA response is elicited due to the foreign nature of the antibody itself. Molecular engineering has therefore been utilized to replace the foreign components of the murine antibody with human antibody sequences to overcome their immunogenicity (Birch and Lennox 1995).

Numerous successful procedures have been developed for preparing humanized and fully human monoclonal antibodies (Takács et al. 2001, Chames et al. 2009, Mallbris et al. 2016), and to date, greater than 30 fully human antibodies are currently being profiled in clinical studies.

Future directions for the more effective utilization of monoclonal antibodies as drug targeting agents must focus on a more rational design of the antibody-drug conjugate. Earlier studies have focused on the development of bispecific antibodies combining the VH and VL of two different antibodies into one molecule to ensure cellular targeting constitutes an effective disease treatment (van Spriel et al. 2000). In particular, these studies have shown that the chemistry of the linker groups in relation to release mechanisms at the site of action must be carefully evaluated. In addition, chemical entities that could be incorporated into the conjugate structure that may influence its biodistribution should also be investigated. Also, more emphasis should be placed on determining the precise mechanism of action to avoid misinterpretation of in vivo data. In instances where a therapeutic effect has been observed, little attempt has been made to determine whether site specificity has been achieved by the proposed mechanism. Finally, with the increasing availability of human monoclonal antibodies, it is clear that drug-antibody conjugates have even greater potential for clinical therapy, although the cost of manufacturing and purifying monoclonal antibodies still limits their clinical utility.

3.10 Conclusions and Future Directions

The continuing development of targetable drugs to the respiratory tract looks promising. Much emphasis will continue to be focused on the respiratory tract as a suitable entry point for proteins and peptides for delivery into the systemic circulation. The use of macromolecule- and monoclonal antibody-drug conjugates will almost certainly increase with the advent of new nanoformulations (for some recent reviews see van Rijt et al. 2014, Yhee et al. 2016, El-Sherbiny et al. 2015, Loira-Pastoriza et al. 2014, Moreno-Sastre et al. 2015), liposomes (Rudokas et al. 2016, Wauthoz and Amighi 2014) and polymer technology (Liang et al. 2015, Loira-Pastoriza et al. 2014), and the availability and efficacy of human monoclonal antibodies (Lucas et al. 2018). However, these advances may well be tempered unless parallel progress is made in other important areas. An area that still requires attention is determining the distribution of metabolizing enzymes throughout the respiratory tract. An in-depth study of the distribution of pulmonary metabolizing enzymes is necessary to achieve a greater cellular selectivity by the activation of appropriately designed prodrugs or drug conjugates in the vicinity of the target cell or a more efficient inactivation to minimize the systemic absorption of the drug.

A greater emphasis will also need to be placed on elucidating epithelial membrane transport mechanisms, especially with regard to improving the epithelial transport of macromolecules. Studies are presently focusing on the microstructural aspects of macromolecular transport across pulmonary epithelia; the results of these investigations will certainly be of value in pulmonary drug-targeting strategies. The discovery of new epithelial and endothelium membrane receptors and proteins, the identification of selective materials for binding, or adhering to these receptors/proteins will also aid in the targeting of drugs to the respiratory tract.

Specific targeting of drugs to other pulmonary targets, such as the alveolar macrophages, which lie in contact with the surfactant lining of the alveoli (Weibel and Gil 1968) and which have well-defined surface membrane receptors for initiating particle attachment and phagocytosis (Rowlands and Daniele 1975), may also be exploitable for improving selectivity. If one considers the inhalation route as a means for delivery of drugs to the systemic circulation, then inhaled drugs must enter the circulatory system principally by diffusion or transport across the alveolar capillary membrane. Drug molecules will therefore come into contact with the alveolar membrane, the alveolar epithelial cells, the capillary endothelial cells, and other "residents" of the pulmonary circulation, such as the PIMs. In humans, these PIMs have been poorly studied, since PIMs are not constitutive in humans and other primates. Nevertheless, PIMS have been detected in human pulmonary capillaries (Dehring and Wismar 1989), and it is known that PIMs can be induced by hepatic disease in humans (Klingensmith et al. 1978), and may be an induced cellular target in pulmonary disease and of potential utility for inhaled drugs (Gillespie 1990, Lohmann-Matthes et al. 1994, Csukás et al. 2015, Schneberger et al. 2012). However, PIMS reside in "thick" portions of the pulmonary capillaries and are attached to the capillary endothelium by an electron-dense membrane-adhesive complex. It is likely that such cells would be exposed to high concentrations of inhaled drugs. The PIM cell density appears to increase with pathological stimuli; thus, acute lung injury or lung infection augments the lung burden of PIMs and raises the question of the role of this cell type in the development of lung injury.

It has been suggested that microparticulate delivery systems given by intravascular administration might be targeted to PIMs in pulmonary disease (Gillespie 1990). This suggestion is based on these investigators' observation that particles exceeding 7 μm are often retained in the lung, while smaller particles localize in the liver and spleen. The sequestering in the lung is associated with pulmonary hypertension and lung injury, and, in some cases, it is not related to particle size. Thus, lung sequestering of particles was speculated to be a result of phagocytosis by PIMs, and that this could be used as a means of targeting conventional drug entities, synthetic genes, or anti-sense oligonucleotides that could perturb PIM function. Any PIMs that have sequestered particulate drug-delivery systems may serve as depots for the release of drug entities into the circulation.

Thus, the future of pulmonary drug targeting remains promising, and although drug discovery efforts will no doubt lead to the development of agents with greater selectivity for pulmonary receptors, a greater emphasis will be placed on cell targeting and the development of new macromolecular vectors and cellular targets for this purpose.

REFERENCES

Adamson R.H., Liu B., Fry G.N., Rubin L.L., and Curry F.E. 1998. "Microvascular permeability and number of tight junctions are modulated by cAMP." *Am J Physiol*, 274 (6 Pt 2):H1885–H1894.

Ahluwalia N., Shea B.S., and Tager A.M. 2014. "New therapeutic targets in idiopathic pulmonary fibrosis. Aiming to rein in runaway wound-healing responses." *Am J Respir Crit Care Med*, 190 (8):867–878.

Ahn H.S., and Barnett A. 1986. "Selective displacement of [3H]mepyramine from peripheral vs. central nervous system receptors by loratadine, a non-sedating antihistamine." *Eur J Pharmacol*, 127 (1–2):153–155.

Alabaster V.A. 1997. "Discovery & development of selective M3 antagonists for clinical use." *Life Sci*, 60 (13):1053–1060.

Alangari A.A. 2014. "Corticosteroids in the treatment of acute asthma." *Ann Thorac Med*, 9 (4):187–192.

Allen D.B. 1998. "Influence of inhaled corticosteroids on growth: A pediatric endocrinologist's perspective." *Acta Paediatr*, 87 (2):123–129.

Anderson J.H., Jr., Brunelle R.L., Keohane P., Koivisto V.A., Trautmann M.E., Vignati L., and DiMarchi R. 1997. "Mealtime treatment with insulin analog improves postprandial hyperglycemia and hypoglycemia in patients with non-insulin-dependent diabetes mellitus. Multicenter insulin lispro study group." *Arch Intern Med*, 157 (11):1249–1255.

Andersson P. 1976. "Bronchospasmolytic and cardiovascular effects in anaesthetized cats of ibuterol and terbutaline given intravenously and after inhalation: Drug and prodrug compared." *Acta Pharmacol Toxicol (Copenh)*, 39 (2):225–231.

Andersson P., Lihne M., Thalen A., and Ryrfeldt A. 1987. "Effect of structural alterations on the biotransformation rate of glucocorticosteroids in rat and human liver." *Xenobiotica*, 17 (1):35–44.

Andrew S.M., Perkins A.C., Pimm M.V., and Baldwin R.W. 1988. "A comparison of iodine and indium labelled anti CEA intact antibody, F(ab)2 and Fab fragments by imaging tumour xenografts." *Eur J Nucl Med*, 13 (11):598–604.

Aumailley M. 2013. "The laminin family." *Cell Adh Migr*, 7 (1):48–55.

Balzano G., Fuschillo S., and Gaudiosi C. 2002. "Leukotriene receptor antagonists in the treatment of asthma: An update." *Allergy*, 57 Suppl 72:16–19.

Barnes N., Evans J., Zakrzewski J., Piper P., and Costello J. 1988. "Pharmacology and physiology of leukotrienes and their antagonists." *Ann N Y Acad Sci*, 524:369–378.

Barnes N.C. 1997. "Current therapy for asthma: Time for a change?" *J Pharm Pharmacol*, 49 Suppl 3:13–16.

Barnes P.J. 1996. "Molecular mechanisms of steroid action in asthma." *J Allergy Clin Immunol*, 97 (1 Pt 2):159–168.

Barnes P.J. 2002. "Scientific rationale for inhaled combination therapy with long-acting β2-agonists and corticosteroids." *Euro Respi J*, 19 (1):182–191.

Barnes P.J., Pedersen S., and Busse W.W. 1998. "Efficacy and safety of inhaled corticosteroids. New developments." *Am J Respir Crit Care Med*, 157 (3 Pt 2):S1–S53.

Baron J., Burke J.P., Guengerich F.P., Jakoby W.B., and Voigt J.M. 1988. "Sites for xenobiotic activation and detoxication within the respiratory tract: Implications for chemically induced toxicity." *Toxicol Appl Pharmacol*, 93 (3):493–505.

Barratt G., and Bretagne S. 2007. "Optimizing efficacy of Amphotericin B through nanomodification." *Int J Nanomedicine*, 2 (3):301–313.

Bazak R., Houri M., El Achy S., Kamel S., and Refaat T. 2015. "Cancer active targeting by nanoparticles: A comprehensive review of literature." *J Cancer Res Clin Oncol*, 141 (5):769–784.

Beasley R.C., Featherstone R.L., Church M.K., Rafferty P., Varley J.G., Harris A., Robinson C., and Holgate S.T. 1989. "Effect of a thromboxane receptor antagonist on PGD2- and allergen-induced bronchoconstriction." *J Appl Physiol (1985)*, 66 (4):1685–1693.

Belliveau P.P. 2005. "Omalizumab: A monoclonal anti-IgE antibody." *MedGenMed*, 7 (1):27.

Benford D.J., and Bridges J.W. 1986. "Xenobiotic metabolism in lung." *Prog Drug Metab* 9:53.

Bernstein D.I., Berkowitz R.B., Chervinsky P., Dvorin D.J., Finn A.F., Gross G.N., Karetzky M. et al. 1999. "Dose-ranging study of a new steroid for asthma: Mometasone furoate dry powder inhaler." *Respir Med*, 93 (9):603–612.

Bertero T., Oldham W.M., Cottrill K.A., Pisano S., Vanderpool R.R., Yu Q., Zhao J. et al. 2016. "Vascular stiffness mechanoactivates YAP/TAZ-dependent glutaminolysis to drive pulmonary hypertension." *J Clin Invest*, 126 (9):3313–3335.

Bevilacqua M.P., Pober J.S., Majeau G.R., Cotran R.S., and Gimbrone M.A., Jr. 1984. "Interleukin 1 (IL-1) induces biosynthesis and cell surface expression of procoagulant activity in human vascular endothelial cells." *J Exp Med*, 160 (2):618–623.

Birch J.R., and Lennox E.S. 1995. *Monoclonal Antibodies: Principles and Applications*. Edited by J. R. Birch and E. S. Lennox. New York: Wiley-Liss.

Bird, B.P., Crawley G.C., Edwards M.P., Foster S.J., Girodeau J.M., Kingston J.F., and McMillan R.M. 1991. "(Methoxyalkyl)thiazoles: A new series of potent, selective, and orally active 5-lipoxygenase inhibitors displaying high enantioselectivity." *J Med Chem*, 34 (7):2176–2186.

Blackwell T.S., Tager A.M., Borok Z., Moore B.B., Schwartz D.A., Anstrom K.J., Bar-Joseph Z. et al. 2014. "Future directions in idiopathic pulmonary fibrosis research. An NHLBI workshop report." *Am J Respir Crit Care Med*, 189 (2):214–222.

Bode B.W. 2011. "Comparison of pharmacokinetic properties, physicochemical stability, and pump compatibility of 3 rapid-acting insulin analogues-aspart, lispro, and glulisine." *Endocr Pract*, 17 (2):271–280.

Bonney R.J., Ashe B., Maycock A., Dellea P., Hand K., Osinga D., Fletcher D. et al. 1989. "Pharmacological profile of the substituted beta-lactam L-659,286: A member of a new class of human PMN elastase inhibitors." *J Cell Biochem*, 39 (1):47–53.

Boucher R.C. 1994. "Human airway ion transport. Part one." *Am J Respir Crit Care Med*, 150 (1):271–281.

Bousquet J., Godard P., and Michel F.B. 1992. "Antihistamines in the treatment of asthma." *Eur Respir J*, 5 (9):1137–1142.

Bradshaw J., Brittain R.T., Coleman R.A., Jack D., Kennedy I., Lunts L.H.C., and Skidmore I.F. 1987. "The design of salmeterol, a long-acting selective β2-Adrenoceptor agonist." *Bri J Pharmacol*, 92:590.

Brittain R.T., Dean C.M., and Jack D. 1976. "Sympathomimetic bronchodilator drugs." *Pharmacol Ther B*, 2 (3):423–462.

Britton J.R., Hanley S.P., and Tattersfield A.E. 1987. "The effect of an oral leukotriene D4 antagonist L-649,923 on the response to inhaled antigen in asthma." *J Allergy Clin Immunol*, 79 (5):811–816.

Brooks D.M., Summers J.B., Gunn B.P., Martin J.C., Martin M.B., Mazdiyasni H., Holms J.H. et al. 1989. 197th ACS Annual Meeting (abstr) (MEDI 69 1989).

Brown D., Marriott C., and Beeson M. 1983. "Antibiotic binding to purified mucus glycoproteins." *J Pharm Pharmacol*, 35:80P.

Brown E.A., Griffiths R., Harvey C.A., and Owen D.A. 1986. "Pharmacological studies with SK&F 93944 (temelastine), a novel histamine H1-receptor antagonist with negligible ability to penetrate the central nervous system." *Br J Pharmacol*, 87 (3):569–578.

Brown P.J., and Juliano R.L. 1985. "Selective inhibition of fibronectin-mediated cell adhesion by monoclonal antibodies to a cell-surface glycoprotein." *Science*, 228 (4706):1448–1451.

Bruck A., Abu-Dahab R., Borchard G., Schafer U.F., and Lehr C.M. 2001. "Lectin-functionalized liposomes for pulmonary drug delivery: Interaction with human alveolar epithelial cells." *J Drug Target*, 9 (4):241–251.

Bruno F., Spaziano G., Liparulo A., Roviezzo F., Nabavi S.M., Sureda A., Filosa R., and D'Agostino B. 2018. "Recent advances in the search for novel 5-lipoxygenase inhibitors for the treatment of asthma." *Eur J Med Chem*, 153:65–72.

Buchegger F., Haskell C.M., Schreyer M., Scazziga B.R., Randin S., Carrel S., and Mach J.P. 1983. "Radiolabeled fragments of monoclonal antibodies against carcinoembryonic antigen for localization of human colon carcinoma grafted into nude mice." *J Exp Med*, 158 (2):413–427.

Buckle D.R., and Smith H. 1984. *Development of Anti-Asthma Drugs*. Edited by Derek R. Buckle and Harry Smith. London, UK: Butterworth-Heinemann.

Buist A.S. 1989. "Asthma mortality: What have we learned?" *J Allergy Clin Immunol*, 84 (3):275–283.

Byron P.R., and Patton J.S. 1994. "Drug delivery via the respiratory tract." *J Aerosol Med*, 7 (1):49–75.

Canonica G.W., and Blaiss M. 2011. "Antihistaminic, anti-inflammatory, and antiallergic properties of the nonsedating second-generation antihistamine desloratadine: A review of the evidence." *World Allergy Organ J*, 4 (2):47–53.

Carstairs J.R., Nimmo A.J., and Barnes P.J. 1985. "Autoradiographic visualization of beta-adrenoceptor subtypes in human lung." *Am Rev Respir Dis*, 132 (3):541–547.

Catravas J.D., Lazo J.S., Dobuler K.J., Mills L.R., and Gillis C.N. 1983. "Pulmonary endothelial dysfunction in the presence or absence of interstitial injury induced by intratracheally injected bleomycin in rabbits." *Am Rev Respir Dis*, 128 (4):740–746.

Chames P., Van Regenmortel M., Weiss E., and Baty D. 2009. "Therapeutic antibodies: Successes, limitations and hopes for the future." *Br J Pharmacol*, 157 (2):220–233.

Chan S.Y., Evan G.I., Ritson A., Watson J., Wraight P., and Sikora K. 1986. "Localisation of lung cancer by a radiolabelled monoclonal antibody against the c-myc oncogene product." *Br J Cancer*, 54 (5):761–769.

Cheng H.C., and Woodward J.K. 1982. "Antihistaminic effect of terfenadine: A new piperidine-type antihistamine." *Drug Develop Res*, 2 (2):181–196.

Chetham P.M., Babal P., Bridges J.P., Moore T.M., and Stevens T. 1999. "Segmental regulation of pulmonary vascular permeability by store-operated Ca2+ entry." *Am J Physiol*, 276 (1 Pt 1):L41–L50.

Chhabra S.K., and Bhatnagar S. 2002. "Comparison of bronchodilator responsiveness in asthma and chronic obstructive pulmonary disease." *Indian J Chest Dis Allied Sci*, 44 (2):91–97.

Chiarino D., Fantucci M., Carenzi A., Della Bella D., Frigeni V., and Sala R. 1986. "New isoxazole derivatives with a potent and selective beta 2-adrenergic activity." *Il Farmaco; edizione scientifica*, 41 (6):440–453.

Chipps B.E., Figliomeni M., and Spector S. 2012. "Omalizumab: An update on efficacy and safety in moderate-to-severe allergic asthma." *Allergy Asthma Proc*, 33 (5):377–385.

Chu B.C., and Whiteley J.M. 1980. "The interaction of carrier-bound methotrexate with L1210 cells." *Mol Pharmacol*, 17 (3):382–387.

Clissold S.P., and Heel R.C. 1984. "Budesonide. A preliminary review of its pharmacodynamic properties and therapeutic efficacy in asthma and rhinitis." *Drugs*, 28 (6):485–518.

Colcher D., Esteban J., Carrasquillo J.A., Sugarbaker P., Reynolds J.C., Bryant G., Larson S.M. et al., 1987. "Complementation of intracavitary and intravenous administration of a monoclonal antibody (B72.3) in patients with carcinoma." *Cancer Res*, 47 (15):4218–4224.

Colthorpe P., Farr S.J., Smith I.J., Wyatt D., and Taylor G. 1995. "The influence of regional deposition on the pharmacokinetics of pulmonary-delivered human growth hormone in rabbits." *Pharm Res*, 12 (3):356–359.

Corvalan J.R., Smith W., Gore V.A., and Brandon D.R. 1987. "Specific in vitro and in vivo drug localisation to tumour cells using a hybrid-hybrid monoclonal antibody recognising both carcinoembryonic antigen (CEA) and vinca alkaloids." *Cancer Immunol Immunother*, 24 (2):133–137.

Corvalan J.R., Smith W., Gore V.A., Brandon D.R., and Ryde P.J. 1987. "Increased therapeutic effect of vinca alkaloids targeted to tumour by a hybrid-hybrid monoclonal antibody." *Cancer Immunol Immunother*, 24 (2):138–143.

Creticos PS., Bodenheimer S., Albright A., Lichtenstein L.M., and PS N. 1989. "Effects of Inhaled leukotriene antagonist on brochial challenge with antigen." *J Allergy Clin Immunol*, 83 (1):187.

Crooks P.A. 1990. "Lung peptidases and their activities." *Conference Proceedings*. Lexington, KY: Respiratory Drug Delivery II University of Kentucky, 50–103.

Crooks P.A., and Damani L.A. 1989. "Respiratory drug delivery; Chapter 3: Drug application to the respiratory tract: Metabolic and pharmacokinetic considerations." In *Respiratory Drug Delivery*, edited by P. R. Byron, pp. 61–90. Boca Raton, FL: CRC Press.

Csukás D., Urbanics R., Wéber G., Rosivall L., and Szebeni J. 2015. "Pulmonary intravascular macrophages: Prime suspects as cellular mediators of porcine CARPA." *European Journal of Nanomedicine*, 7 (1):27–36.

Cullere X., Shaw S.K., Andersson L., Hirahashi J., Luscinskas F.W., and Mayadas T.N. 2005. "Regulation of vascular endothelial barrier function by Epac, a cAMP-activated exchange factor for Rap GTPase." *Blood*, 105 (5):1950–1955.

de Duve C., de Barsy T., Poole B., Trouet A., Tulkens P., and Van Hoof F. 1974. "Commentary. Lysosomotropic agents." *Biochem Pharmacol*, 23 (18):2495–2531.

DeCamp M.M., Warner A.E., Molina R.M., and Brain J.D. 1992. "Hepatic versus pulmonary uptake of particles injected into the portal circulation in sheep. Endotoxin escapes hepatic clearance causing pulmonary inflammation." *Am Rev Respir Dis*, 146 (1):224–231.

Dehring D.J., and Wismar B.L. 1989. "Intravascular macrophages in pulmonary capillaries of humans." *Am Rev Respir Dis*, 139 (4):1027–1029.

del Vecchio P.J., Siflinger-Birnboim A., Belloni P.N., Holleran L.A., Lum H., and Malik A.B. 1992. "Culture and characterization of pulmonary microvascular endothelial cells." *In Vitro Cell. Dev. Biol Animal*, 28 (11):711–715.

Dent G., Giembycz M.A., Rabe K.F., and Barnes P.J. 1991. "Inhibition of eosinophil cyclic nucleotide PDE activity and opsonised zymosan-stimulated respiratory burst by 'type IV'-selective PDE inhibitors." *Br J Pharmacol*, 103 (2):1339–1346.

Depre M., Margolskee D.J., Van Hecken A., Hsieh J.S., Buntinx A., De Schepper P.J., and Rogers J.D. 1992. "Dose-dependent kinetics of the enantiomers of MK-571, and LTD4-receptor antagonist." *Eur J Clin Pharmacol*, 43 (4):431–433.

deVos C., Rihoux J.P., and Juhlin L. 1986. *In Proceedings of the Congress of the European Academy of Allergology and Clinical Immunology*. Budapest, Hungary.

Diamantis N., and Banerji U. 2016. "Antibody-drug conjugates—An emerging class of cancer treatment." *Br J Cancer*, 114 (4):362–367.

Easthope S., and Jarvis B. 2001. "Omalizumab." *Drugs*, 61 (2):253–260.

Edsbacker S., and Andersson T. 2004. "Pharmacokinetics of budesonide (Entocort EC) capsules for Crohn's disease." *Clin Pharmacokinet*, 43 (12):803–821.

El-Sherbiny I.M., El-Baz N.M., and Yacoub M.H. 2015. "Inhaled nano- and microparticles for drug delivery." *Glob Cardiol Sci Pract*, 2015:2.

Elble R.C., Widom J., Gruber A.D., Abdel-Ghany M., Levine R., Goodwin A., Cheng H.C., and Pauli B.U. 1997. "Cloning and characterization of lung-endothelial cell adhesion molecule-1 suggest it is an endothelial chloride channel." *J Biol Chem*, 272 (44):27853–27861.

Endo K., Kamma H., and Ogata T. 1987. "Radiolocalization of xenografted human lung cancer with monoclonal antibody 8 in nude mice." *Cancer Res*, 47 (20):5427–5432.

Eriksson S. 1991. "The potential role of elastase inhibitors in emphysema treatment." *Eur Respir J*, 4 (9):1041–1043.

Evans J.M., Barnes N.C., Zakrzewski J.T., Sciberras D.G., Stahl E.G., Piper P.J., and Costello J.F. 1989. "L-648,051, a novel cysteinyl-leukotriene antagonist is active by the inhaled route in man." *Br J Clin Pharmacol*, 28 (2):125–135.

Fleisch J.H., Cloud M.L., and Marshall W.S. 1988. "A brief review of preclinical and clinical studies with LY171883 and some comments on newer cysteinyl leukotriene receptor antagonists." *Ann N Y Acad Sci*, 524:356–368.

Foidart J.M., Bere E.W., Jr., Yaar M., Rennard S.I., Gullino M., Martin G.R., and Katz S.I. 1980. "Distribution and immunoelectron microscopic localization of laminin, a noncollagenous basement membrane glycoprotein." *Lab Invest*, 42 (3):336–342.

Forman H.J., Aldrich T.K., Posner M.A., and Fisher A.B. 1982. "Differential paraquat uptake and redox kinetics of rat granular pneumocytes and alveolar macrophages." *J Pharmacol Exp Ther*, 221 (2):428–433.

Fowler J.S., Gallagher B.M., MacGregor R.R., and Wolf A.P. 1976. "Carbon-11 labeled aliphatic amines in lung uptake and metabolism studies: Potential for dynamic measurements in vivo." *J Pharmacol Exp Ther*, 198 (1):133–145.

Fransson L.A. 1981. "Self-association of bovine lung heparan sulphates: Identification and characterization of contact zones." *Eur J Biochem*, 120 (2):251–255.

Friedel H.A., and Brogden R.N. 1988. "Bitolterol. A preliminary review of its pharmacological properties and therapeutic efficacy in reversible obstructive airways disease." *Drugs*, 35 (1):22–41.

Frith P.A., Ruffin R.E., Cockcroft D.W., and Hargreave F.E. 1978. "155. A comparison of the protective effect of sch 1000 and fenoterol against bronchoconstriction induced by histamine and methacholine." *J Allergy Clin Immunol*, 61 (3):175.

Gaine S., and Mc Laughlin V. 2017. "Pulmonary arterial hypertension: Tailoring treatment to risk in the current era." *Eur Respir Rev*, 26 (146):170095.

Garnett M.C., Embleton M.J., Jacobs E., and Baldwin R.W. 1983. "Preparation and properties of a drug-carrier-antibody conjugate showing selective antibody-directed cytotoxicity in vitro." *Int J Cancer*, 31 (5):661–770.

Gavard J., and Gutkind J.S. 2006. "VEGF controls endothelial-cell permeability by promoting the beta-arrestin-dependent endocytosis of VE-cadherin." *Nat Cell Biol*, 8 (11):1223–1234.

Geiger J., Aneja M.K., Hasenpusch G., Yuksekdag G., Kummerlowe G., Luy B., Romer T. et al. 2010. "Targeting of the prostacyclin specific IP1 receptor in lungs with molecular conjugates comprising prostaglandin I2 analogues." *Biomaterials*, 31 (10):2903–2911.

Gibson D.G., and Coltart D.J. 1971. "Haemodynamic effects of intravenous salbutamol in patients with mitral valve disease: Comparison with isoprenaline and atropine." *Postgrad Med J*, 47:Suppl:40–44.

Gillespie M.N. 1990. "Pulmonary intravascular macrophages: Cellular targets of opportunity for inhaled drugs." *Conference Proceedings*. Lexington, KY: Respiratory Drug Delivery II, University of Kentucky, 646–668.

Greenwood V. 2011. "Why are asthma rates soaring?" *Sci Am*, 304 (4):32–33.

Gross M.I., Demo S.D., Dennison J.B., Chen L., Chernov-Rogan T., Goyal B., Janes J.R. et al. 2014. "Antitumor activity of the glutaminase inhibitor CB-839 in triple-negative breast cancer." *Mol Cancer Ther*, 13 (4):890–901.

Gu J.M., Robinson J.R., and Leung S.H. 1988. "Binding of acrylic polymers to mucin/epithelial surfaces: Structure-property relationships." *Crit Rev Ther Drug Carrier Syst*, 5 (1):21–67.

Harpur E.S., and Gonda I. 1987. "Metabolism of hexamethylmelamine by rodent lung microsomes." *Xth Congress of Pharmacology (IUPHAR '87)*, Sydney, Australia. Conference paper 1045.

Hashida M., Kato A., Takakura Y., and Sezaki H. 1984. "Disposition and pharmacokinetics of a polymeric prodrug of mitomycin C, mitomycin C-dextran conjugate, in the rat." *Drug Metab Dispos*, 12 (4):492–499.

Hay D.W. 1997. "Pharmacology of leukotriene receptor antagonists. More than inhibitors of bronchoconstriction." *Chest*, 111 (2 Suppl):35S–45S.

Hay D.W.P., and Barnette M.S. 1999. "Chapter 11. Current and potential new therapies for chronic obstructive pulmonary disease." In *Annu Rep Med Chem*, edited by Annette M. Doherty, 111–120. Cambridge, MA: Academic Press.

Hirota N., Ueda M., Ozawa S., Abe O., and Shimizu N. 1989. "Suppression of an epidermal growth factor receptor-hyperproducing tumor by an immunotoxin conjugate of gelonin and a monoclonal anti-epidermal growth factor receptor antibody." *Cancer Res*, 49 (24 Pt 1):7106–7109.

Hnatowich D.J., Virzi F., and Rusckowski M. 1987. "Investigations of avidin and biotin for imaging applications." *J Nucl Med*, 28 (8):1294–1302.

Holstein-Rathlou N.H., Laursen L.C., Madsen F., Svendsen U.G., Gnosspelius Y., and Weeke B. 1986. "Bambuterol: Dose response study of a new terbutaline prodrug in asthma." *Eur J Clin Pharmacol*, 30 (1):7–11.

Hoshino M., Sim J., Shimizu K., Nakayama H., and Koya A. 1999. "Effect of AA-2414, a thromboxane A2 receptor antagonist, on airway inflammation in subjects with asthma." *J Allergy Clin Immunol*, 103 (6):1054–1061.

Hsiao C.T., Cheng H.W., Huang C.M., Li H.R., Ou M.H., Huang J.R., Khoo K.H. et al. 2017. "Fibronectin in cell adhesion and migration via N-glycosylation." *Oncotarget*, 8 (41):70653–70668.

Hubbard R.C., Casolaro M.A., Mitchell M., Sellers S.E., Arabia F., Matthay M.A., and Crystal R.G. 1989. "Fate of aerosolized recombinant DNA-produced alpha 1-antitrypsin: Use of the epithelial surface of the lower respiratory tract to administer proteins of therapeutic importance." *Proc Natl Acad Sci U S A*, 86 (2):680–684.

Hurwitz E., Schechter B., Arnon R., and Sela M. 1979. "Binding of anti-tumor immunoglobulins and their daunomycin conjugates to the tumor and its metastase. In vitro and in vivo studies with Lewis lung carcinoma." *Int J Cancer*, 24 (4):461–470.

Hussain A.A., and Truelove J.E. 1975. "Ester of 3,4-dihydroxy-alpha (isopropylamino) methyl benzyl alcohol, composition and anti-asthma use thereof. US patent number 3868461.

Illum L., and Davis S.S. 1984. "The organ uptake of intravenously administered colloidal particles can be altered using a non-ionic surfactant (Poloxamer 338)." *FEBS Lett*, 167 (1):79–82.

Illum L., Davis S.S., Muller R.H., Mak E., and West P. 1987. "The organ distribution and circulation time of intravenously injected colloidal carriers sterically stabilized with a block copolymer—Poloxamine 908." *Life Sci*, 40 (4):367–374.

Iversen L.L. 1971. "Role of transmitter uptake mechanisms in synaptic neurotransmission." *Br J Pharmacol*, 41 (4):571–591.

Iwasawa Y., Gillis C.N., and Aghajanian G. 1973. "Hypothermic inhibition of 5-hydroxytryptamine and norepinephrine uptake by lung: Cellular location of amines after uptake." *J Pharmacol Exp Ther*, 186 (3):498–507.

Jacobs R.T., Veale C.A., and Wolanin D.J. 1992. "Chapter 12. Pulmonary and anti-allergy agents." In *Ann Rep Med Chem*, edited by James A. Bristol, 109–118. Cambridge, MA: Academic Press.

Jones A., Kellaway I., and Taylor G. 1988. "Pulmonary absorption of aerosolised insulin in the rabbit." *J. Pharm. Pharmacol*, 40:92.

Jones A.W. 2016. "Perspectives in drug development and clinical pharmacology: The discovery of histamine H1 and H2 antagonists." *Clin Pharmacol Drug Dev*, 5 (1):5–12.

Jones T.R., Zamboni R., Belley M., Champion E., Charette L., Ford-Hutchinson A.W., Frenette R. et al. 1989. "Pharmacology of L-660,711 (MK-571): A novel potent and selective leukotriene D4 receptor antagonist." *Can J Physiol Pharmacol*, 67 (1):17–28.

Joos G.F., Kips J.C., Pauwels R.A., and Van der Straeten M.E. 1991. "The effect of aerosolized SK&F 104353-Z2 on the bronchoconstrictor effect of leukotriene D4 in asthmatics." *Pulm Pharmacol*, 4 (1):37–42.

Joos G.F., Pauwels R.A., and Van Der Straeten M.E. 1989. "The effect of nedocromil sodium on the bronchoconstrictor effect of neurokini A in subjects with asthma." *J Allergy Clin Immunol*, 83 (3):663–668.

Kamphuisen P.W., Eikenboom J.C., Rosendaal F.R., Koster T., Blann A.D., Vos H.L., and Bertina R.M. 2001. "High factor VIII antigen levels increase the risk of venous thrombosis but are not associated with polymorphisms in the von Willebrand factor and factor VIII gene." *Br J Haematol*, 115 (1):156–158.

Kang X., Zhou L., Jian Y.M., Lan S.A., and Xu F. 2018. "Effectiveness of antibody-drug conjugate (ADC): Results of in vitro and in vivo studies." *Med Sci Monit*, 24:1408–1416.

Kasperska-Zajac A., Brzoza Z., and Rogala B. 2008. "Platelet-activating factor (PAF): A review of its role in asthma and clinical efficacy of PAF antagonists in the disease therapy." *Recent Pat Inflamm Allergy Drug Discov*, 2 (1):72–76.

Kelly H.W. 1998. "Establishing a therapeutic index for the inhaled corticosteroids: Part I. Pharmacokinetic/pharmacodynamic comparison of the inhaled corticosteroids." *J Allergy Clin Immunol*, 102 (4 Pt 2):S36–S51.

Kent D.L. 2014. "Age-related macular degeneration: Beyond anti-angiogenesis." *Mol Vis*, 20:46–55.

Kerr D.J., Hynds S.A., Shepherd J., Packard C.J., and Kaye S.B. 1988. "Comparative cellular uptake and cytotoxicity of a complex of daunomycin-low density lipoprotein in human squamous lung tumour cell monolayers." *Biochem Pharmacol*, 37 (20):3981–3986.

Kim D.S., Collard H.R., and King T.E., Jr. 2006. "Classification and natural history of the idiopathic interstitial pneumonias." *Proc Am Thorac Soc*, 3 (4):285–292.

King G.L., and Johnson S.M. 1985. "Receptor-mediated transport of insulin across endothelial cells." *Science*, 227 (4694):1583–1586.

King T.E., Jr., Bradford W.Z., Castro-Bernardini S., Fagan E.A., Glaspole I., Glassberg M.K., Gorina E. et al. 2014. "A phase 3 trial of pirfenidone in patients with idiopathic pulmonary fibrosis." *N Engl J Med*, 370 (22):2083–2092.

Klingensmith W.C., 3rd, Yang S.L., and Wagner H.N., Jr. 1978. "Lung uptake of Tc-99m sulfur colloid in liver and spleen imaging." *J Nucl Med*, 19 (1):31–35.

Kojima T., Hashida M., Muranishi S., and Sezaki H. 1980. "Mitomycin C-dextran conjugate: A novel high molecular weight pro-drug of mitomycin C." *J Pharm Pharmacol*, 32 (1):30–34.

Kopecek J. 1984. "Synthesis of tailor-made soluble polymeric drug carriers." In *Recent Advances in Drug Delivery Systems*, edited by J. M. Anderson and S. W. Kim, 41–62. New York: Plenum Press.

Kopecek J., and Duncan R. 1987. "*N*-(2-hydroxypropyl) methacrylamide macromolecules as drug carrier systems." In *Polymers in Controlled Drug Delivery*, edited by L. Illum and S. S. Davis, 152–170. Bristol, England: Wright.

Korbelin J., Sieber T., Michelfelder S., Lunding L., Spies E., Hunger A., Alawi M. et al. 2016. "Pulmonary targeting of adeno-associated vral vectors by next-generation sequencing-guided screening of random capsid displayed peptide libraries." *Mol Ther*, 24 (6):1050–1061.

Kostenbauder H.B., and Sloneker S. 1990. "Prodrugs for pulmonary drug targeting." In *Respiratory Drug Delivery*, edited by P. R. Byron, 91–106. Boca Raton, FL: CRC Press.

Krell R.D., Aharony D., Buckner C.K., Keith R.A., Kusner E.J., Snyder D.W., Bernstein P.R. et al. 1990. "The preclinical pharmacology of ICI 204,219. A peptide leukotriene antagonist." *Am Rev Respir Dis*, 141 (4 Pt 1):978–987.

Krepela E., Viccar J., Zizkova L., Kasafirek E., Kolar Z., and Lichnovsky V. 1985. "Dipeptidyl peptidase IV in mammalian lungs." *Lung*, 163 (1):33–54.

Lacoste J.Y., Bousquet J., Chanez P., Van Vyve T., Simony-Lafontaine J., Lequeu N., Vic P., Enander I., Godard P., and Michel F.B. 1993. "Eosinophilic and neutrophilic inflammation in asthma, chronic bronchitis, and chronic obstructive pulmonary disease." *J Allergy Clin Immunol*, 92 (4):537–548.

Lambert J.M., and Morris C.Q. 2017. "Antibody-drug conjugates (ADCs) for personalized treatment of solid tumors: A review." *Adv Ther*, 34 (5):1015–1035.

Lands A.M., Luduena F.P., and Buzzo H.J. 1967. "Differentiation of receptors responsive to isoproterenol." *Life Sci*, 6 (21):2241–2249.

Lang I.M., and Gaine S.P. 2015. "Recent advances in targeting the prostacyclin pathway in pulmonary arterial hypertension." *Eur Respir Rev*, 24 (138):630–641.

Lenny W., Wells N., and BA O.N. 1994. Burden of childhood asthma. *Eur Respir Rev* 4, 49–62.

Levy G.P., and Apperley G.H. 1978. "*Recent Advances in the Pharmacology of Adrenoceptors: Proceedings of a Satellite Symposium of the 7th International Congress of Pharmacology Held at Owens Park, Manchester, on 24th–26th July, 1978*." International Congress of, Pharmacology, Amsterdam; New York; Amsterdam [etc.]; Oxford; New York, 1978, 403.

Liang Z., Ni R., Zhou J., and Mao S. 2015. "Recent advances in controlled pulmonary drug delivery." *Drug Discov Today*, 20 (3):380–389.

Lofdahl C.G., and Svedmyr N. 1988. "Inhaled formoterol, a new beta-adrenoceptor agonist, compared to salbutamol in asthmatic patients (abstract)." *Am Rev Respir Dis* 137 (4, Part 2), 330.

Lohmann-Matthes M., Steinmuller C., and Franke-Ullmann G. 1994. "Pulmonary macrophages." *Eur. Respir. J.*, 7 (9):1678–1689.

Loira-Pastoriza C., Todoroff J., and Vanbever R. 2014. "Delivery strategies for sustained drug release in the lungs." *Adv Drug Deliv Rev*, 75:81–91.

Lopes J.D., dos Reis M., and Brentani R.R. 1985. "Presence of laminin receptors in *Staphylococcus aureus*." *Science*, 229 (4710):275–277.

Lucas A., Price L., Schorzman A., Storrie M., Piscitelli J., Razo J., and Zamboni W. 2018. "Factors affecting the pharmacology of antibody–drug conjugates." *Antibodies*, 7, (10), 1–28.

Lullmann H., Rossen E., and Seiler K.U. 1973. "The pharmacokinetics of phentermine and chlorphentermine in chronically treated rats." *J Pharm Pharmacol*, 25 (3):239–243.

Malenfant S., Margaillan G., Loehr J.E., Bonnet S., and Provencher S. 2013. "The emergence of new therapeutic targets in pulmonary arterial hypertension: From now to the near future." *Expert Rev Respir Med*, 7 (1):43–55.

Malinoff H.L., and Wicha M.S. 1983. "Isolation of a cell surface receptor protein for laminin from murine fibrosarcoma cells." *J Cell Biol*, 96 (5):1475–1479.

Mallbris L., Davies J., Glasebrook A., Tang Y., Glaesner W., and Nickoloff B.J. 2016. "Molecular insights into fully human and humanized monoclonal antibodies: What are the differences and should dermatologists care?" *J Clin Aesthet Dermatol*, 9 (7):13–15.

Masui H., Kawamoto T., Sato J.D., Wolf B., Sato G., and Mendelsohn J. 1984. "Growth inhibition of human tumor cells in athymic mice by anti-epidermal growth factor receptor monoclonal antibodies." *Cancer Res*, 44 (3):1002–1007.

Mathe G., Tran Ba L.O., and Bernard J. 1958. "Effect on mouse leukemia 1210 of a combination of diazo-reaction of amethopterin and gamma-globulins from hamsters inoculated with such leukemia by heterografts." *C R Hebd Seances Acad Sci*, 246 (10):1626–1628.

Miettinen M., Holthofer H., Lehto V.P., Miettinen A., and Virtanen I. 1983. "*Ulex europaeus* I lectin as a marker for tumors derived from endothelial cells." *Am J Clin Pathol*, 79 (1):32–36.

Milgrom H., Fick R.B., Jr., Su J.Q., Reimann J.D., Bush R.K., Watrous M.L., and Metzger W.J. 1999. "Treatment of allergic asthma with monoclonal anti-IgE antibody. rhuMAb-E25 Study Group." *N Engl J Med*, 341 (26):1966–1973.

Miller-Larsson A., Mattsson H., Hjertberg E., Dahlback M., Tunek A., and Brattsand R. 1998. "Reversible fatty acid conjugation of budesonide. Novel mechanism for prolonged retention of topically applied steroid in airway tissue." *Drug Metab Dispos*, 26 (7):623–630.

Minchin R.F., Barber H.E., and Ilett K.F. 1982. "Effect of prolonged desmethylimipramine administration on the pulmonary clearance of 5-hydroxytryptamine and beta-phenylethylamine in rats." *Drug Metab Dispos*, 10 (4):356–360.

Minneman K.P., Hedberg A., and Molinoff P.B. 1979. "Comparison of beta adrenergic receptor subtypes in mammalian tissues." *J Pharmacol Exp Ther*, 211 (3):502–508.

Misra R.N., Brown B.R., Han W.C., Harris D.N., Hedberg A., Webb M.L., and Hall S.E. 1991. "Interphenylene 7-oxabicyclo[2.2.1]heptane thromboxane A2 antagonists. Semicarbazone omega-chains." *J Med Chem*, 34 (9):2882–2891.

Miyamoto K., Schultz E., Heath T., Mitchell M.D., Albertine K.H., and Staub N.C. 1988. "Pulmonary intravascular macrophages and hemodynamic effects of liposomes in sheep." *J Appl Physiol (1985)*, 64 (3):1143–1152.

Monsigny M., Roche A.C., and Bailly P. 1984. "Tumoricidal activation of murine alveolar macrophages by muramyldipeptide substituted mannosylated serum albumin." *Biochem Biophys Res Commun*, 121 (2):579–584.

Moore T.M., Chetham P.M., Kelly J.J., and Stevens T. 1998. "Signal transduction and regulation of lung endothelial cell permeability. Interaction between calcium and cAMP." *Am J Physiol*, 275 (2 Pt 1):L203-L222.

Moran T.M., Usuba O., Shapiro E., Rubinstein L.J., Ito M., and Bona C.A. 1990. "A novel technique for the production of hybrid antibodies." *J Immunol Methods*, 129 (2):199–205.

Moreno-Sastre M., Pastor M., Salomon C.J., Esquisabel A., and Pedraz J.L. 2015. "Pulmonary drug delivery: A review on nanocarriers for antibacterial chemotherapy." *J Antimicrob Chemother*, 70 (11):2945–2955.

Muzykantov V.R. 2013. "Targeted drug delivery to endothelial adhesion molecules." *ISRN Vascular Medicine*, 2013, 1–27.

Nelson A.L. 2010. "Antibody fragments: Hope and hype." *MAbs*, 2 (1):77–83.

Newman S.A., Frenz D.A., Tomasek J.J., and Rabuzzi D.D. 1985. "Matrix-driven translocation of cells and nonliving particles." *Science*, 228 (4701):885–889.

Nicholson A.N., and Stone B.M. 1986. "Antihistamines: Impaired performance and the tendency to sleep." *Eur J Clin Pharmacol*, 30 (1):27–32.

Niven R.W., Rypacek F., and Byron P.R. 1990. "Solute absorption from the airways of the isolated rat lung. III. Absorption of several peptidase-resistant, synthetic polypeptides: Poly-(2-hydroxyethyl)-aspartamides." *Pharm Res*, 7 (10):990–994.

Nolan J.C., Stephens D.J., Proakis A.G., Leonard C.A., Johnson D.N., Kilpatrick B.F., Foxwell M.H., and Yanni J.M. 1989. "Rocastine (AHR-11325), a rapid acting, nonsedating antihistamine." *Agents Actions*, 28 (1–2):53–61.

Ohbayashi H. 2002. "Novel neutrophil elastase inhibitors as a treatment for neutrophil-predominant inflammatory lung diseases." *IDrugs*, 5 (9):910–923.

Olsson O.A., and Svensson L.A. 1984. "New lipophilic terbutaline ester prodrugs with long effect duration." *Pharm Res*, 1 (1):19–23.

Onrust S.V., and Lamb H.M. 1998. "Mometasone furoate. A review of its intranasal use in allergic rhinitis." *Drugs*, 56 (4):725–745.

Ordonez N.G., and Batsakis J.G. 1984. "Comparison of *Ulex europaeus* I lectin and factor VIII-related antigen in vascular lesions." *Arch Pathol Lab Med*, 108 (2):129–132.

Orriols M., Gomez-Puerto M.C., and Ten Dijke P. 2017. "BMP type II receptor as a therapeutic target in pulmonary arterial hypertension." *Cell Mol Life Sci*, 74 (16):2979–2995.

Owens D.R. 2002. "New horizons—alternative routes for insulin therapy." *Nat Rev Drug Discov*, 1 (7):529–540.

Palmer G.C., Radov L.A., Napier J.J., Griffiths R.C., Stagnitto M.L., and Garske G.E. 1989. "CNS safety evaluation of PR 1036-654, a new antihistamine with a low potential for sedation." *FASEB J*, 3(3):A439.

Parker M.W., Rossi D., Peterson M., Smith K., Sikstrom K., White E.S., Connett J.E., Henke C.A., Larsson O., and Bitterman P.B. 2014. "Fibrotic extracellular matrix activates a profibrotic positive feedback loop." *J Clin Invest*, 124 (4):1622–1635.

Parnell E., Smith B.O., Palmer T.M., Terrin A., Zaccolo M., and Yarwood S.J. 2012. "Regulation of the inflammatory response of vascular endothelial cells by EPAC1." *Br J Pharmacol*, 166 (2):434–446.

Patel J., Amrutiya J., Bhatt P., Javia A., Jain M., and Misra A. 2018. "Targeted delivery of monoclonal antibody conjugated docetaxel loaded PLGA nanoparticles into EGFR overexpressed lung tumour cells." *J Microencapsul*, 35 (2):204–217.

Patton J.S. 1996. "Mechanisms of macromolecule absorption by the lungs." *Adv. Drug Deliv. Rev.*, 19 (1):3–36.

Patton J.S., and Platz R.M. 1992. "(D) Routes of delivery: Case studies: (2) Pulmonary delivery of peptides and proteins for systemic action." *Adv. Drug Deliv. Rev.*, 8 (2):179–196.

Pedersen S., and O'Byrne P. 1997. "A comparison of the efficacy and safety of inhaled corticosteroids in asthma." *Allergy*, 52 (s39):1–34.

Perrot C.Y., Sawada J., and Komatsu M. in press. "Prolonged activation of cAMP signaling leads to endothelial barrier disruption via transcriptional repression of RRAS." *FASEB J.*

Petersen H., Kullberg A., Edsbacker S., and Greiff L. 2001. "Nasal retention of budesonide and fluticasone in man: Formation of airway mucosal budesonide-esters in vivo." *Br J Clin Pharmacol*, 51 (2):159–163.

Pietra G.G., Sampson P., Lanken P.N., Hansen-Flaschen J., and Fishman A.P. 1983. "Transcapillary movement of cationized ferritin in the isolated perfused rat lung." *Lab Invest*, 49 (1):54–61.

Pimm M.V. 1988. "Drug-monoclonal antibody conjugates for cancer therapy: Potentials and limitations." *Crit Rev Ther Drug Carrier Syst*, 5 (3):189–227.

Pimm M.V., Jones J.A., Price M.R., Middle J.G., Embleton M.J., and Baldwin R.W. 1982. "Tumour localization of monoclonal antibody against a rat mammary carcinoma and suppression of tumour growth with adriamycin-antibody conjugates." *Cancer Immunolog Immunother*, 12 (2):125–134.

Pitt B.R., Gillis C.N., and Hammond G.L. 1981. "Influence of the lung on arterial levels of endogenous prostaglandins E and F." *J Appl Physiol Respir Environ Exerc Physiol*, 50 (6):1161–1167.

Pitt B.R., Hammond G.L., and Gillis C.N. 1982. "Comparison of pulmonary and extrapulmonary extraction of biogenic amines." *J Appl Physiol Respir Environ Exerc Physiol*, 52 (6):1545–1551.

Polverino E., Rosales-Mayor E., Dale G.E., Dembowsky K., and Torres A. 2017. "The role of neutrophil elastase inhibitors in lung diseases." *Chest*, 152 (2):249–262.

Possmayer F., Yu S.H., Weber J.M., and Harding P.G. 1984. "Pulmonary surfactant." *Can J Biochem Cell Biol*, 62 (11):1121–1133.

Powley M.W., and Carlson G.P. 1999. "Species comparison of hepatic and pulmonary metabolism of benzene." *Toxicology*, 139 (3):207–217.

Radwan M.A., AlQuadeib B.T., Siller L., Wright M.C., and Horrocks B. 2017. "Oral administration of amphotericin B nanoparticles: Antifungal activity, bioavailability and toxicity in rats." *Drug Deliv*, 24 (1):40–50.

Ranney D.F. 1986. "Drug targeting to the lungs." *Biochem Pharmacol*, 35 (7):1063–1069.

Ranney D.F. 1988. "Bioadhesion drug carriers for endothelial and epithelial uptake and lesional localization of therapeutic and diagnostic agents. Patent number: WO/1988/007365.

Richards D.A., Maruani A., and Chudasama V. 2017. "Antibody fragments as nanoparticle targeting ligands: A step in the right direction." *Chem Sci*, 8 (1):63–77.

Richeldi L., du Bois R.M., Raghu G., Azuma A., Brown K.K., Costabel U., Cottin V. et al. 2014. "Efficacy and safety of nintedanib in idiopathic pulmonary fibrosis." *N Engl J Med*, 370 (22):2071–2082.

Rigaudy P., Charcosset J.Y., Garbay-Jaureguiberry C., Jacquemin-Sablon A., and Roques B.P. 1989. "Attempts to target antitumor drugs toward opioid receptor-rich mouse tumor cells with enkephalin-ellipticinium conjugates." *Cancer Res*, 49 (7):1836–1842.

Robbins J.C., Lam M.H., Tripp C.S., Bugianesi R.L., Ponpipom M.M., and Shen T.Y. 1981. "Synthetic glycopeptide substrates for receptor-mediated endocytosis by macrophages." *Proc Natl Acad Sci U S A*, 78 (12):7294–7298.

Rominger K.L. 1979. "Chemistry and pharmacokinetics of ipratropium bromide." *Sca J respi dis. Supplementum*, 103:116–129.

Rowland G.F., Simmonds R.G., Gore V.A., Marsden C.H., and Smith W. 1986. "Drug localisation and growth inhibition studies of vindesine-monoclonal anti-CEA conjugates in a human tumour xenograft." *Cancer Immunol Immunother*, 21 (3):183–187.

Rowlands D.T., and Daniele R.P. 1975. "Surface receptors in the immune response." *N Engl J Med*, 293 (1):26–32.

Rudokas M., Najlah M., Alhnan M.A., and Elhissi A. 2016. "Liposome delivery systems for inhalation: A critical review highlighting formulation issues and anticancer applications." *Med Princ Pract*, 25 Suppl 2:60–72.

Rugg E.L., Barnett D.B., and Nahorski S.R. 1978. "Coexistence of beta1 and beta2 adrenoceptors in mammalian lung: Evidence from direct binding studies." *Mol Pharmacol*, 14 (6):996–1005.

Ryan G., Dolovich M.B., Obminski G., Cockcroft D.W., Juniper E., Hargreave F.E., and Newhouse M.T. 1981. "Standardization of inhalation provocation tests: Influence of nebulizer output, particle size, and method of inhalation." *J Allergy Clin Immunol*, 67 (2):156–161.

Ryan J.W. 1987a. "Assay of pulmonary endothelial surface enzymes in vivo." In *Pulmonary Endothelium in Health and Disease*, edited by Ryan U.S., 161–188. New York: Marcel Dekker.

Ryan J.W. 1989. "Peptidase enzymes of the pulmonary vascular surface." *Am J Physiol*, 257 (2 Pt 1):L53–L60.

Ryan U.S. 1987b. "Endothelial cell activation response." In *Pulmonary Endothelium in Health and Disease*, 3–33. New York: Marcel Dekker.

Ryan U.S., and Ryan J.W. 1983. "Endothelial cells and inflammation." *Clin Lab Med*, 3 (4):577–599.

Ryan U.S., Ryan J.W., Whitaker C., and Chiu A. 1976. "Localization of angiotensin converting enzyme (kininase II). II. Immunocytochemistry and immunofluorescence." *Tissue Cell*, 8 (1):125–145.

Ryrfeldt A., and Bodin N.O. 1975. "The physiological disposition of ibuterol, terbutaline and isoproterenol after endotracheal instillation to rats." *Xenobiotica*, 5 (9):521–529.

Ryrfeldt A., Edsbacker S., and Pauwels R. 1984. "Kinetics of the epimeric glucocorticoid budesonide." *Clin Pharmacol Ther*, 35 (4):525–530.

Ryser H.J., and Shen W.C. 1978. "Conjugation of methotrexate to poly(L-lysine) increases drug transport and overcomes drug resistance in cultured cells." *Proc Natl Acad Sci U S A*, 75 (8):3867–3870.

Santing R.E., Olymulder C.G., Van der Molen K., Meurs H., and Zaagsma J. 1995. "Phosphodiesterase inhibitors reduce bronchial hyperreactivity and airway inflammation in unrestrained guinea pigs." *Eur J Pharmacol*, 275 (1):75–82.

Santus P., and Radovanovic D. 2016. "Prostaglandin D2 receptor antagonists in early development as potential therapeutic options for asthma." *Expert Opin Investig Drugs*, 25 (9):1083–1092.

Sawada J., Urakami T., Li F., Urakami A., Zhu W., Fukuda M., Li D.Y., Ruoslahti E., and Komatsu M. 2012. "Small GTPase R-Ras regulates integrity and functionality of tumor blood vessels." *Cancer Cell*, 22 (2):235–249.

Sayner S., and Stevens T. 2006. "Soluble adenylate cyclase reveals the significance of compartmentalized cAMP on endothelial cell barrier function." *Biochem Soc Trans*, 34 (Pt 4):492–494.

Sayner S.L., Alexeyev M., Dessauer C.W., and Stevens T. 2006. "Soluble adenylyl cyclase reveals the significance of cAMP compartmentation on pulmonary microvascular endothelial cell barrier." *Circ Res*, 98 (5):675–681.

Schaeffer R.C., Jr., and Bitrick M.S., Jr. 1995. "Effects of human alpha-thrombin and 8bromo-cAMP on large and microvessel endothelial monolayer equivalent "pore" radii." *Microvasc Res*, 49 (3):364–371.

Schanker L.S. 1978. "Drug absorption from the lung." *Biochem Pharmacol*, 27 (4):381–385.

Schanker L.S., Mitchell E.W., and Brown R.A., Jr. 1986. "Species comparison of drug absorption from the lung after aerosol inhalation or intratracheal injection." *Drug Metab Dispos*, 14 (1):79–88.

Schlegel N., and Waschke J. 2014. "cAMP with other signaling cues converges on Rac1 to stabilize the endothelial barrier- a signaling pathway compromised in inflammation." *Cell Tissue Res*, 355 (3):587–596.

Schlueter D.P., and Neumann J.L. 1978. "Double blind comparison of acute bronchial and ventilation-perfusion changes to atrovent and isoproterenol." *Chest*, 73 (6):982–983.

Schneberger D., Aharonson-Raz K., and Singh B. 2012. "Pulmonary intravascular macrophages and lung health: What are we missing?" *Am J Physiol Lung Cell Mol Physiol.*, 302 (6):L498–L503.

Schneeberger E.E., and Lynch R.D. 1992. "Structure, function, and regulation of cellular tight junctions." *Am J Physiol*, 262 (6 Pt 1):L647–L661.

Schnitzer J.E., Siflinger-Birnboim A., Del Vecchio P.J., and Malik A.B. 1994. "Segmental differentiation of permeability, protein glycosylation, and morphology of cultured bovine lung vascular endothelium." *Biochem Biophys Res Commun*, 199 (1):11–19.

Schroff R.W., Foon K.A., Beatty S.M., Oldham R.K., and Morgan A.C., Jr. 1985. "Human anti-murine immunoglobulin responses in patients receiving monoclonal antibody therapy." *Cancer Res*, 45 (2):879–885.

Seibert A.F., Thompson W.J., Taylor A., Wilborn W.H., Barnard J., and Haynes J. 1992. "Reversal of increased microvascular permeability associated with ischemia-reperfusion: Role of cAMP." *J Appl Physiol (1985)*, 72 (1):389–395.

Sezaki H., and Hashida M. 1984. "Macromolecule-drug conjugates in targeted cancer chemotherapy." *Crit Rev Ther Drug Carrier Syst*, 1 (1):1–38.

Shao J., DeHaven J., Lamm D., Weissman D.N., Malanga C.J., Rojanasakul Y., and Ma J.K. 2001. "A cell-based drug delivery system for lung targeting: II. Therapeutic activities on B16-F10 melanoma in mouse lungs." *Drug Deliv*, 8 (2):71–76.

Shargel L., and Dorrbecker S.A. 1976. "Physiological disposition and metabolism of (3H)bitolterol in man and dog." *Drug Metab Dispos*, 4 (1):72–78.

Sharma A., Pandey R., Sharma S., and Khuller G.K. 2004. "Chemotherapeutic efficacy of poly (DL-lactide-co-glycolide) nanoparticle encapsulated antitubercular drugs at sub-therapeutic dose against experimental tuberculosis." *Int J Antimicrob Agents*, 24 (6):599–604.

Sharma A., Sharma S., and Khuller G.K. 2004. "Lectin-functionalized poly (lactide-co-glycolide) nanoparticles as oral/aerosolized antitubercular drug carriers for treatment of tuberculosis." *J Antimicrob Chemother*, 54 (4):761–766.

Sharma R., Saxena D., Dwivedi A.K., and Misra A. 2001. "Inhalable microparticles containing drug combinations to target alveolar macrophages for treatment of pulmonary tuberculosis." *Pharm Res*, 18 (10):1405–1410.

Shaw C.D. 1989. "Medical audit in Britain: What now and what next?" *Qual Assur Health Care*, 1 (1):61–63.

Shimada K., Gill P.J., Silbert J.E., Douglas W.H., and Fanburg B.L. 1981. "Involvement of cell surface heparin sulfate in the binding of lipoprotein lipase to cultured bovine endothelial cells." *J Clin Invest*, 68 (4):995–1002.

Sitar D.S. 1996. "Clinical pharmacokinetics of bambuterol." *Clin Pharmacokinet*, 31 (4):246–256.

Skyler J.S., Cefalu W.T., Kourides I.A., Landschulz W.H., Balagtas C.C., Cheng S.L., and Gelfand R.A. 2001. "Efficacy of inhaled human insulin in type 1 diabetes mellitus: A randomised proof-of-concept study." *Lancet*, 357 (9253):331–335.

Sly R.M. 1989. "Mortality from asthma." *J Allergy Clin Immunol*, 84 (4 Pt 1):421–434.

Small D., and Kostenbauder H.B. 1985. "Unpublished data."

Smith L.J., Geller S., Ebright L., Glass M., and Thyrum P.T. 1990. "Inhibition of leukotriene D4-induced bronchoconstriction in normal subjects by the oral LTD4 receptor antagonist ICI 204,219." *Am Rev Respir Dis*, 141 (4 Pt 1):988–992.

Sorkness C.A. 1998. "Establishing a therapeutic index for the inhaled corticosteroids: Part II. Comparisons of systemic activity and safety among different inhaled corticosteroids." *J Allergy Clin Immunol*, 102 (4 Pt 2):S52–S64.

Staab-Weijnitz C.A., Fernandez I.E., Knuppel L., Maul J., Heinzelmann K., Juan-Guardela B.M., Hennen E. et al. 2015. "FK506-binding protein 10, a potential novel drug target for idiopathic pulmonary fibrosis." *Am J Respir Crit Care Med*, 192 (4):455–467.

Stafford J.A., and Feldman P.L. 1996. "Chapter 8. Chronic pulmonary inflammation and other therapeutic applications of PDE IV inhibitors." In *Ann Rep Med Chem*, edited by James A. Bristol, 71–80. Cambridge, MA: Academic Press.

Stafford J.A., Veal J.M., Feldman P.L., Valvano N.L., Baer P.G., Brackeen M.F., Brawley E.S. et al. 1995. "Introduction of a conformational switching element on a pyrrolidine ring. Synthesis and evaluation of (R*,R*)-(+/-)-methyl 3-acetyl-4-[3-(cyclopentyloxy)-4-methoxyphenyl]-3-methyl-1-pyrrolidinecarboxylate, a potent and selective inhibitor of cAMP-specific phosphodiesterase." *J Med Chem*, 38 (26):4972–4975.

Steiner S., Pfutzner A., Wilson B.R., Harzer O., Heinemann L., and Rave K. 2002. "Technosphere/Insulin—Proof of concept study with a new insulin formulation for pulmonary delivery." *Exp Clin Endocrinol Diabetes*, 110 (1):17–21.

Stephens S., Emtage S., Vetterlein O., Chaplin L., Bebbington C., Nesbitt A., Sopwith M., Athwal D., Novak C., and Bodmer M. 1995. "Comprehensive pharmacokinetics of a humanized antibody and analysis of residual anti-idiotypic responses." *Immunology*, 85 (4):668–674.

Stevens T., Creighton J., and Thompson W.J. 1999. "Control of cAMP in lung endothelial cell phenotypes. Implications for control of barrier function." *Am J Physiol*, 277 (1 Pt 1):L119–L126.

Storms W.W., DoPico G.A., and Reed C.E. 1975. "Aerosol Sch 1000. An anticholinergic bronchodilator" *Am Rev Respir Dis.*, 111 (4):419–422.

Stryjewski M.E., Potgieter P.D., Li Y.P., Barriere S.L., Churukian A., Kingsley J., Corey G.R., and Group T.D.I. 2012. "TD-1792 versus vancomycin for treatment of complicated skin and skin structure infections." *Antimicrob Agents Chemother*, 56 (11):5476–5483.

Sun J.Z., Byron P.R., and Rypacek F. 1999. "Solute absorption from the airways of the isolated rat lung. V. Charge effects on the absorption of copolymers of N(2-hydroxyethyl)-DL-aspartamide with DL-aspartic acid or dimethylaminopropyl-DL-aspartamide." *Pharm Res*, 16 (7):1104–1108.

Suwa T., Kohno Y., Yoshida H., Morimoto S., and Suga T. 1989. "Uptake of O-alkyl erythromycin derivatives in the lung tissue and cells of rats." *J Pharm Sci*, 78 (9):783–784.

Svensson L.A. 1985. "Sympathomimetic bronchodilators: Increased selectivity with lung-specific prodrugs." *Pharm Res*, 2 (4):156–162.

Svensson L.A. 1987. "Bambuterol: a prodrug-prodrug with built-in hydrolysis brake." *Acta Pharm Suec*, 24 (6):333–341.

Takács L., Vazquez-Abad M.-D., and Elliott E.A. 2001. "Chapter 23. Therapeutic monoclonal antibodies: History, facts and trends." In *Annu Rep Med Chem*, 237–246. Cambridge, MA: Academic Press.

Takenaga K. 1996. "Suppression of metastatic potential of high-metastatic Lewis lung carcinoma cells by vanadate, an inhibitor of tyrosine phosphatase, through inhibiting cell-substrate adhesion." *Invasion Metastasis*, 16 (2):97–106.

Tamaoki J., Chiyotani A., Tagaya E., Sakai N., and Konno K. 1994. "Effect of long term treatment with oxitropium bromide on airway secretion in chronic bronchitis and diffuse panbronchiolitis." *Thorax*, 49 (6):545–548.

Tanaka T., Yamamoto A., and Amenomori A. 1995. "3-Phenylpyrrolidine derivatives. EP patent number: EP0671389.

Taylor A.E., Khimenko P.L., Moore T.M., and Adkins W.K. 1997. "Fluid balance." In *The Lung: Scientific Foundations*, edited by R. G. West Crystal et al., 1549–1566. New York: Lippincott-Raven.

Terranova V.P., Rohrbach D.H., and Martin G.R. 1980. "Role of laminin in the attachment of PAM 212 (epithelial) cells to basement membrane collagen." *Cell*, 22 (3):719–726.

Toda Y., Takahashi T., Maeshima K., Shimizu H., Inoue K., Morimatsu H., Omori E., Takeuchi M., Akagi R., and Morita K. 2007. "A neutrophil elastase inhibitor, sivelestat, ameliorates lung injury after hemorrhagic shock in rats." *Int J Mol Med*, 19 (2):237–243.

Townsley M.I., Parker J.C., Longenecker G.L., Perry M.L., Pitt R.M., and Taylor A.E. 1988. "Pulmonary embolism: Analysis of endothelial pore sizes in canine lung." *Am J Physiol*, 255 (5 Pt 2):H1075–H1083.

Tram N.D.T., and Ee P.L.R. 2017. "Macromolecular conjugate and biological carrier approaches for the targeted delivery of antibiotics." *Antibiotics (Basel)*, 6 (3):14.

Tsukada Y., Kato Y., Umemoto N., Takeda Y., Hara T., and Hirai H. 1984. "An anti-alpha-fetoprotein antibody-daunorubicin conjugate with a novel poly-L-glutamic acid derivative as intermediate drug carrier." *J Natl Cancer Inst*, 73 (3):721–729.

Tsukada Y., Ohkawa K., and Hibi N. 1987. "Therapeutic effect of treatment with polyclonal or monoclonal antibodies to alpha-fetoprotein that have been conjugated to daunomycin via a dextran bridge: Studies with an alpha-fetoprotein-producing rat hepatoma tumor model." *Cancer Res*, 47 (16):4293–4295.

Ullman A., Hedner J., and Svedmyr N. 1990. "Inhaled salmeterol and salbutamol in asthmatic patients. An evaluation of asthma symptoms and the possible development of tachyphylaxis." *Am Rev Respir Dis*, 142 (3):571–575.

Ullman A., and Svedmyr N. 1988. "Salmeterol, a new long acting inhaled beta 2 adrenoceptor agonist: Comparison with salbutamol in adult asthmatic patients." *Thorax*, 43 (9):674–678.

Vaccaro C.A., and Brody J.S. 1981. "Structural features of alveolar wall basement membrane in the adult rat lung." *J Cell Biol*, 91 (2 Pt 1):427–437.

Vaidya B., and Gupta V. 2015. "Novel therapeutic approaches for pulmonary arterial hypertension: Unique molecular targets to site-specific drug delivery." *J Control Release*, 211:118–133.

Vallath S., Hynds R.E., Succony L., Janes S.M., and Giangreco A. 2014. "Targeting EGFR signalling in chronic lung disease: Therapeutic challenges and opportunities." *Eur Respir J*, 44 (2):513–522.

van Grunsven P.M., van Schayck C.P., Derenne J.P., Kerstjens H.A., Renkema T.E., Postma D.S., Similowski T. et al. 1999. "Long term effects of inhaled corticosteroids in chronic obstructive pulmonary disease: A meta-analysis." *Thorax*, 54 (1):7–14.

van Rijt S.H., Bein T., and Meiners S. 2014. "Medical nanoparticles for next generation drug delivery to the lungs." *Eur Respir J*, 44 (3):765–774.

van Schayck C.P., van Grunsven P.M., and Dekhuijzen P.N. 1996. "Do patients with COPD benefit from treatment with inhaled corticosteroids?" *Eur Respir J*, 9 (10):1969–1972.

van Spriel A.B., van Ojik H.H., and van De Winkel J.G. 2000. "Immunotherapeutic perspective for bispecific antibodies." *Immunol Today*, 21 (8):391–397.

Veale D., Kerr N., Gibson G.J., and Harris A.L. 1989. "Characterization of epidermal growth factor receptor in primary human non-small cell lung cancer." *Cancer Res*, 49 (5):1313–1317.

Villani F.J., Magatti C.V., Vashi D.B., Wong J., and Popper T.L. 1986. "N-substituted 11-(4-piperidylene)-5,6-dihydro-11*H*-benzo-[5,6]cyclohepta [1,2-*b*]pyridines. Antihistamines with no sedating liability." *Arzneimittelforschung*, 36 (9):1311–1314.

Vincent J., Liminana R., Meredith P.A., and Reid J.L. 1988. "The pharmacokinetics, antihistamine and concentration-effect relationship of ebastine in healthy subjects." *Br J Clin Pharmacol*, 26 (5):497–502.

Vincent J., Sumner D.J., and Reid J.L. 1988. "Ebastine: The effect of a new antihistamine on psychomotor performance and autonomic responses in healthy subjects." *Br J Clin Pharmacol*, 26 (5):503–508.

Vlodavsky I., and Gospodarowicz D. 1981. "Respective roles of laminin and fibronectin in adhesion of human carcinoma and sarcoma cells." *Nature*, 289 (5795):304–306.

Vollmar A.M., Banker D.E., Mendelsohn J., and Herschman H.R. 1987. "Toxicity of ligand and antibody-directed ricin A-chain conjugates recognizing the epidermal growth factor receptor." *J Cell Physiol*, 131 (3):418–425.

Waldrep J.C., Gilbert B.E., Knight C.M., Black M.B., Scherer P.W., Knight V., and Eschenbacher W. 1997. "Pulmonary delivery of beclomethasone liposome aerosol in volunteers. Tolerance and safety." *Chest*, 111 (2):316–323.

Walter U., Geiger J., Haffner C., Markert T., Nehls C., Silber R.E., and Schanzenbacher P. 1995. "Platelet-vessel wall interactions, focal adhesions, and the mechanism of action of endothelial factors." *Agents Actions Suppl*, 45:255–268.

Wang Y., Wang J., Lin Y., Si-Ma L.F., Wang D.H., Chen L.G., and Liu D.K. 2011. "Synthesis and antihistamine evaluations of novel loratadine analogues." *Bioorg Med Chem Lett*, 21 (15):4454–4456.

Warner A.E., Molina R.M., and Brain J.D. 1987. "Uptake of bloodborne bacteria by pulmonary intravascular macrophages and consequent inflammatory responses in sheep." *Am Rev Respir Dis*, 136 (3):683–690.

Wauthoz N., and Amighi K. 2014. "Phospholipids in pulmonary drug delivery." *Eur J Lipid Sci Technol.*, 116 (9):1114–1128.

Weibel E.R., and Gil J. 1968. "Electron microscopic demonstration of an extracellular duplex lining layer of alveoli." *Respir Physiol*, 4 (1):42–57.

Wick G., Muller P.U., and Timpl R. 1982. "In vivo localization and pathological effects of passively transferred antibodies to type IV collagen and laminin in mice." *Clin Immunol Immunopathol*, 23 (3):656–665.

Williams S.K., Devenny J.J., and Bitensky M.W. 1981. "Micropinocytic ingestion of glycosylated albumin by isolated microvessels: Possible role in pathogenesis of diabetic microangiopathy." *Proc Natl Acad Sci U S A*, 78 (4):2393–2397.

Wilson A.G., Pickett R.D., Eling T.E., and Anderson M.W. 1979. "Studies on the persistence of basic amines in the rabbit lung." *Drug Metab Dispos*, 7 (6):420–424.

Wilson J., Serby C., Menjoge S., and Witek Jr T. 1996. "The efficacy and safety of combination bronchodilator therapy." *Eur Respir Rev*, 6 (39):287–289.

Wolters P.J., Collard H.R., and Jones K.D. 2014. "Pathogenesis of idiopathic pulmonary fibrosis." *Annu Rev Pathol*, 9:157–179.

Yamada K., Yanagihara K., Araki N., Harada Y., Morinaga Y., Izumikawa K., Kakeya H. et al. 2011. "In vivo efficacy of KRP-109, a novel elastase inhibitor, in a murine model of severe pneumococcal pneumonia." *Pulm Pharmacol Ther*, 24 (6):660–665.

Yhee J.Y., Im J., and Nho R.S. 2016. "Advanced therapeutic strategies for chronic lung disease using nanoparticle-based drug delivery." *J Clin Med*, 5 (9):82.

Zaagsma J., Roffel A.F., and Meurs H. 1997. "Muscarinic control of airway function." *Life Sci*, 60 (13–14):1061–1068.

Zhou H., Lengsfeld C., Claffey D.J., Ruth J.A., Hybertson B., Randolph T.W., Ng K.Y., and Manning M.C. 2002. "Hydrophobic ion pairing of isoniazid using a prodrug approach." *J Pharm Sci*, 91 (6):1502–1511.

Zhu D., Cheng C.F., and Pauli B.U. 1992. "Blocking of lung endothelial cell adhesion molecule-1 (Lu-ECAM-1) inhibits murine melanoma lung metastasis." *J Clin Invest*, 89 (6):1718–1724.

Zhu D., and Pauli B.U. 1993. "Correlation between the lung distribution patterns of Lu-ECAM-1 and melanoma experimental metastases." *Int J Cancer*, 53 (4):628–633.

Ziment I. 1990. "Pharmacologic therapy of obstructive airway disease." *Clin Chest Med*, 11 (3):461–486.

Section II

Aerosol Critical Attributes

4

Aerosol Physics and Lung Deposition Modeling

Warren H. Finlay

CONTENTS

4.1 Aerosol Physics

4.1.1 Aerodynamic Diameter

While the airborne behavior of an aerosol particle inhaled into the respiratory tract is affected by a number of parameters, for most pharmaceutical aerosols, this behavior is primarily determined by the value of the Stokes number Stk, defined as:

$$\text{Stk} = \rho d^2 U/(18\ \mu\ L) \tag{4.1}$$

where, ρ is particle density, d is particle diameter, U is a characteristic speed of the air carrying the aerosol, μ is the viscosity of air, and L is a characteristic dimension of the flow passage under consideration (e.g. airway diameter). From this equation, it is seen that as far as particle properties go, it is the value of ρd^2 that determines particle behavior. Because of the importance of ρd^2, it is common to define the aerodynamic diameter of a particle, d_{ae}, as:

$$d_{ae} = (\rho/\rho_{ref})^{1/2}\, d \tag{4.2}$$

where ρ_{re} is a reference density, commonly set to 1000 kg/m^3. This equation implies, for example, that a particle with twice the physical diameter, but ¼ the density of a reference particle, will have the same aerodynamic diameter (and therefore the same Stokes number) as the reference particle. Having the same Stokes number, the dynamics of these two particles will be the same (neglecting various effects that are usually small for pharmaceutical aerosols), despite their different densities and actual physical diameters. This means then, for example, that a small dense particle will have the same airborne motion as a large low density particle.

Equation 4.2 also implies that when specifying particle properties, it is not necessary to specify both particle diameter and particle density, but rather aerodynamic diameter alone is sufficient to characterize the diameter of a spherical aerosol particle (again neglecting various effects that are usually small for pharmaceutical aerosols). It is for this reason that aerodynamic diameter is commonly used when specifying the diameter of an inhaled aerosol formulation.

An inhaled aerosol typically consists of millions of particles whose diameters have a range of values. The distribution of particle diameters over this range is determined by the particle size distribution, which specifies the fraction of particles within each size range. The particle size distribution of many, but not all, inhaled pharmaceutical aerosols can often be approximated by a so-called lognormal distribution given by:

$$m(x) = [x\,(2\pi)^{1/2} \ln \sigma_g]^{-1} \exp[-(\ln x - \ln \mathrm{MMD})^2 (\ln \sigma_g)^{-2}/2] \tag{4.3}$$

where $m(x)\Delta x$ is the fraction of the aerosol mass in particles with diameters between x and $x + \Delta x$, MMD is the mass median diameter of the distribution (such that half the aerosol mass is contained in particles with diameter less than MMD), and σ_g is the geometric standard deviation. A commonly quoted diameter is the mass median aerodynamic diameter (MMAD), which is related to the MMD via Equation (4.2).

The concept of MMAD is not specific to an aerosol whose distribution is lognormal. Rather, the MMAD applies to any aerosol distribution and is simply the aerodynamic diameter for which half the aerosol mass is contained in particles whose aerodynamic diameter is less that this value.

4.1.2 Primary Factors Affecting Inhaled Aerosol Mechanics

4.1.2.1 Particle Inertia

As we have just noted, aerodynamic diameter is a primary determinant of the behavior of an aerosol particle. However, the motion of the air carrying the particle is also important, as can be seen by the parameter U appearing in the Stokes number in Equation 4.1. For low values of the Stokes number (i.e. corresponding to small aerodynamic diameter and/or low air speeds), aerosol particles closely follow the air motion, but for larger values of the Stokes number the two deviate, typically leading to aerosol particles depositing on walls, which is called inertial impaction. Such deposition is due to the inertia of the aerosol particles, whereby they are unable to follow the sharp curvature of the fluid streamlines. From Equation 4.1, it is clear that, all else being equal, deposition by inertial impaction can be expected to be higher for larger particles, as well as for higher flow speeds (i.e. higher inhalation flow rates). This is why orally inhaled aerosol particles that are too large, or inhaled at too high an inhalation flow rate, deposit by inertial impaction in the mouth-throat.

4.1.2.2 Gravity

Gravity acts on aerosol particles, which may also cause particle trajectories to deviate from fluid streamlines. Again, this may cause aerosol particles to deposit on walls and is referred to as gravitational sedimentation. Aerodynamic diameter is the relevant particle property that determines gravitational sedimentation, so that as expected, larger diameter particles settle faster than smaller particles and so have larger amounts of gravitational sedimentation. For inhaled aerosol particles, sedimentation is a major mechanism of deposition in the small airways and alveolar regions of the lung, since air speeds are often too low in these regions for inertial impaction to be a major factor.

4.1.2.3 Brownian Diffusion

Brownian motion can cause small aerosol particles to diffuse, also leading to deviation from fluid streamlines. Such diffusion may lead to particle deposition on walls. However, in many applications, diffusion typically becomes important only for particles smaller than a micrometer or so. Most pharmaceutical aerosols have particle size distributions with little mass contained in such small particles, so that diffusional deposition is usually a less important deposition mechanism than impaction and sedimentation for such aerosols (Finlay 2019).

4.1.2.4 Hygroscopic and Evaporative Effects

Given the importance of diameter in affecting the fate of airborne particles, any changes in particle diameter during a particle's motion can cause changes in that particle's trajectory. Evaporation or condensation of gas to or from an aerosol particle is a primary cause of changes in diameter. This can be an important effect for nebulized aqueous aerosols, since such aerosols may evaporate quickly if exposed to low humidity air or if heated without humidification, resulting in much smaller particle diameters, a common effect that occurs when cascade impactors are used incorrectly when measuring nebulized aerosols (Mitchell and Nagel 2003). Particle size changes due to evaporation or condensation of water are referred to as "hygroscopic."

Metered dose inhaler aerosols consist essentially of highly volatile propellant droplets when they first exit the nozzle, but then undergo rapid evaporation as they transit into and through the mouth-throat (or cascade impactor). The behavior of propellant aerosols close to the exit of the inhaler is thus affected by rates of evaporation (Sheth et al. 2017), since droplets change size as they evaporate. Such evaporation also causes cooling, resulting in aerosol particles that are much colder than ambient temperatures, which can lead to condensation of water onto such particles, giving a temporary increase in particle diameter that is reversed as the particles warm back up to ambient temperature (Martin and Finlay 2005). For some metered dose inhaler formulations, this can be followed by aqueous dissolution and water uptake, leading to the usual hygroscopic growth that occurs with water soluble particles inhaled into the humid air within the lungs (Davidson et al. 2017).

When significant evaporation or condensation of an aerosol occurs, the diameter of the aerosol particles can be predicted by consideration of the underlying physics (Finlay 2019), leading to an equation first derived by Maxwell (1890) for the rate of change of the diameter of a spherical droplet

$$\frac{dd}{dt} = -\frac{4D(c_s - c_\infty)}{\rho d} \tag{4.4}$$

where c_s is the concentration of vapor in the gas at the droplet surface (e.g. water vapor concentration, or propellant vapor concentration in the case of a metered dose inhaler, in air at the droplet surface), c_∞ is the ambient concentration of vapor in the gas phase, D is the diffusion coefficient of the vapor in the gas phase, and ρ is the particle density. The value of c_s depends on the droplet temperature, which is lower than ambient during evaporation due to the latent heat of evaporation, but can be determined by heat transfer considerations (Finlay 2019).

From Equation 4.4, it is apparent that droplets evaporate more quickly when the ambient phase contains low amounts of the volatile material making up the droplet, e.g. when the ambient humidity is low if considering aqueous droplets. If many evaporating droplets are present that are all exchanging mass with the air carrying them, then they can increase the ambient concentration leading to so-called two-way coupled hygroscopic effects that alter evaporation rates and require consideration of not just the changing droplet diameters, but also the changing conditions of the air (Finlay 2019). For metered dose inhaler droplets, a factor that throttles the rate of evaporation of propellant droplets is the rate of heat transfer into the droplets, rather than the ambient concentrations of propellant, since the latter is low already (the propellant concentration of room air is normally zero). Predicting the behavior of metered dose inhaler droplets in the vicinity of the nozzle exit is thus challenging, requiring consideration of heat and mass transfer to and from the carrier gas besides consideration of Equation 4.4 (Dunbar et al. 1997).

4.2 Lung Deposition Modeling

Inhaled pharmaceutical aerosols cannot act unless they deposit in the respiratory tract. However, the amount and location of such deposition is affected by particle aerodynamic diameter and breath pattern, as well as lung geometry. Since some control over aerosol properties and breath pattern is possible when

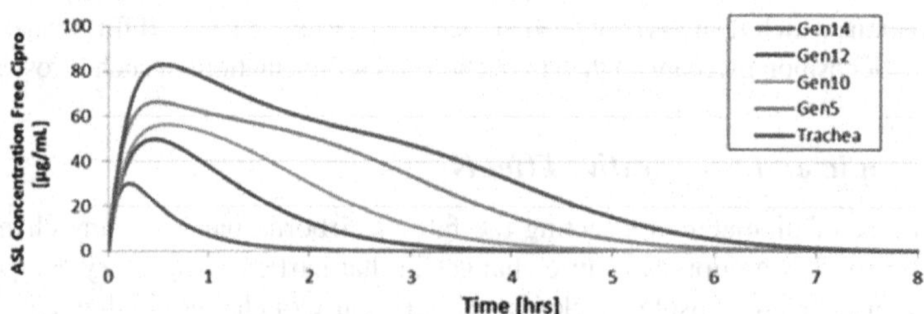

FIGURE 4.1 Model estimates of the concentration of free ciprofloxacin in the airway surface liquid are shown for different airway generations in the trachea-bronchial region when delivered by an inhaled aerosol liposomal formulation. (Reprinted from Martin, A.R. and Finlay, W.H., *J. Aerosol Med. Pulm. Drug Deliv.*, 31, 49–60, 2018. With permission.)

designing an inhaled aerosol formulation, access to tools that permit parametric exploration of lung deposition is useful in order to optimize these parameters and guide preclinical development. It is for this reason that methods allowing simulation of deposition in the lung have become increasingly common in the respiratory drug delivery arena.

An example of the kind of information that can be obtained with lung deposition models is given in Figure 4.1, where a one-dimensional Lagrangian dynamical model (see later in this chapter for an explanation of this term) is combined with a model of the mucous and periciliary layers to give estimates of drug concentration in the liquid lining the airways when a liposomal antimicrobial formulation is delivered as an inhaled aerosol (Martin and Finlay 2018). Combining these predictions with simulations of disposition of deposited drug yields pharmacokinetic models (discussed in Chapter 6) that are increasingly becoming part of the preclinical development process with inhaled pharmaceutical aerosols.

The purpose of the remainder of this chapter is to briefly outline some of the deposition models that have been used with inhaled pharmaceutical aerosols and their basis. The reader is referred to Finlay (2019) for a detailed treatment of the underlying mechanics.

It should be noted that throughout this chapter, the words "model" and "simulation" are used to mean a procedure that solves mathematical equations to represent reality. This may be a less common definition of the word "model" for some readers. However, since the equations governing aerosol and fluid motion are well established and represent reality exactly, such models have the ability to represent reality exactly, at least in principle.

It should be also be mentioned that much less attention has been paid to modeling deposition in lungs altered by disease, largely because the geometry of diseased lung airways has not been well characterized and is different for each disease, as well as being dependent on the progression of the disease. Application of the approaches discussed in this chapter to diseased lungs is thus not considered here.

4.2.1 The Need for Simplification

Most readers would probably intuitively agree that simulating the behavior of an aerosol as it is inhaled and dispersed throughout the entire respiratory tract is a difficult task. In fact, at the present time, it is impossible to precisely simulate this behavior because the geometry of the lung, including the time-dependent shape of all several hundred million alveoli, is not known. Even so, calculation of the detailed fluid and aerosol motion in every single airway and alveolar space of the lungs would require excessively large computing resources and result in far more information than is needed in most inhaled aerosol applications. Besides, deposition of aerosol particles in the respiratory tract is merely the first step in a series of relatively poorly characterized steps that lead to the onset of action of a drug. Simulation of the subsequent disposition of drug, including its dissolution, pharmacokinetics, and finally pharmacodynamics, requires an understanding at a cellular and molecular level that remains incomplete. As a result, although direct simulation of aerosol and fluid motion throughout the entire lung may be useful in developing and refining simpler deposition models, at present, it is not feasible from the perspective of aiding preclinical development. Instead, simplifications are used, to which we now turn.

4.2.2 Empirical Models

In terms of computational requirements, the simplest models that can be considered are empirical models. These models are usually based on parametric curve fits to *in vivo* data of aerosol deposition in humans or to data from more complicated lung deposition models or realistic airway replicas. The simplest of all such models is the rule-of-thumb that inhaled pharmaceutical aerosol should have particle diameters in some "fine particle" range of, e.g. 1 μm–5 μm, which is based on observations that lung deposition during tidal breathing (of monodisperse aerosols from tubes inserted partway into the mouth) decreases for particles with diameters on either side of this range (see e.g. Stahlhofen et al. 1989).

Several popular empirical models adopted for respiratory pharmaceutical use owe their existence to the need for radiological dose estimation of inhaled particulates, beginning with the International Commission on Radiological Protection (ICRP) Task Group on Lung Dynamics (1966), superseded by ICRP (1994), or alternatively National Council on Radiation Protection (NCRP) (1997). Yeh et al. (1996) compare the ICRP (1994) and NCRP (1997) models, with the largest differences between these models occurring for particles that are smaller than those used in respiratory drug delivery (i.e. <0.1 μm diameters). Other empirical models include e.g. Yu et al. (1992) and Davies (1982).

For the extrathoracic region, a number of empirical models have been developed using measurements of deposition in sets of extrathoracic airway replicas obtained from medical scans of subjects. These allow prediction of extrathoracic deposition (see the review by Carrigy et al. 2015). Recent work indicates that average *in vivo* extrathoracic deposition is well predicted by some of these models, but the ability to predict deposition in individual subjects with existing empirical models remains elusive (Yang et al. 2017). Prediction of not just average deposition, but also intersubject variability of this deposition is useful during development of inhaled formulations. In this regard, Ruzycki et al. (2017) present an empirical method that allows prediction of intersubject variability in extrathoracic deposition and which matches intersubject variability seen *in vivo*.

For inhaled pharmaceutical aerosols, the principal attractions of empirical models are the ease with which they can be programmed (requiring little more than entering a handful of algebraic equations into a spreadsheet) and the small amount of computation time they require. Compared to simply using some rule-of-thumb specifying that particle size must be in some range, empirical models give considerable additional information. In particular, they can provide predictions of doses depositing in various morphological regions (e.g. alveolar, tracheobronchial, and extrathoracic regions), and these predictions depend on the particle size distribution and inhalation parameters (e.g. flow rate and inhaled volume), which the user supplies as input. Thus, these models allow a degree of parametric optimization that a particle size rule-of-thumb does not allow.

However, empirical models must be used with caution for several reasons. First, the mouth-throat (oropharyngeal) deposition predictions of some older empirical models differ considerably from reality when inhaling from existing dry powder inhalers and metered dose inhalers (Clark and Egan 1994, Clark et al. 1998, DeHaan and Finlay 2004, Mellat et al. 2017). For metered dose inhalers, these errors occur partly due to the high speed of the aerosol relative to the inhaled air, an effect not present in the experimental data on which the empirical extrathoracic deposition models are based. These concerns are not minor, since correct prediction of lung deposition is entirely dependent on correct prediction of mouth-throat deposition. This is because with single breath inhalation devices there is typically negligible exhaled aerosol, especially with breath holding, so that any aerosol not depositing in the mouth-throat deposits in the lung. As a result, underestimation of mouth-throat deposition by 50% of the inhaled dose results in overestimation of the lung dose by a corresponding amount.

A partial solution to this failing of existing empirical models is to use them only to predict deposition distal to the mouth-throat, relying instead on bench-top measurements in mouth-throat replicas to give the particle size and dose delivered distal to the oropharynx (e.g. Weers and Clark 2017, Wei et al. 2017). Correct use of such a procedure requires realizing that mouth-throat deposition varies dramatically between different individuals (see Stahlhofen et al. 1989, Grgic et al. 2004) due not just to differences in the size of different individual's extrathoracic airways, but also geometric dissimilarities (Ruzycki et al. 2017), so that the mouth-throat replica being used should be chosen carefully in order to give representative particle size versus flow rate filtering properties of the given population. In addition, inhaler aerosols (and their deposition) are often flow rate dependent so that care must also be taken to ensure that the flow rates and breathing patterns used in the bench-top testing are similar to those used during delivery *in vivo*.

A second drawback of empirical models lies in the danger of extrapolating to parameter values outside the range of the experimental data on which they are based. In particular, existing empirical lung deposition models have typically been developed for tidal breathing of aerosols in healthy subjects. Using them for subjects with lung disease involves extrapolation with largely unknown error. In addition, except for nebulizers, inhaled pharmaceutical aerosols are not delivered with tidal breathing, but instead with a single large breath, often with a breath hold. This is a very different breathing pattern than tidal breathing. However, whether this causes significant errors in empirical models applied to single breath inhalation devices is difficult to determine, since there is a lack of rigorous methods for determining alveolar versus trachea-bronchial deposition *in vivo* (unknown amounts of slow clearance from the tracheobronchial region hamper the ability of standard 24 hour clearance methods to give these measurements, see e.g. ICRP 1994, Majoral et al. 2014). Thus, the ability of empirical models to predict regional deposition within the lung with single breath inhaled pharmaceutical devices remains largely untested. However, even if such data are obtained, it must be realized that to avoid extrapolation with empirical models, it is necessary to produce new data for every new situation not covered by existing data, a limitation that will always hamper the generality of empirical models.

One final point to bear in mind with existing empirical models is that they cannot normally be used when droplet size changes occur due to hygroscopic or evaporative effects. Droplet size changes in inhalation devices, which can be important in determining respiratory tract deposition, often involve two-way coupled hygroscopic effects (Finlay 2019), which are beyond the capabilities of existing empirical models.

4.2.3 Lagrangian Dynamical Models

To overcome some of the limitations mentioned above that are associated with purely empirical models, simulations that include various aspects of the inhaled aerosol dynamics have been developed. The simplest of these belong to a class of models called Lagrangian dynamical models (LDMs), meaning that the model simulates some of the dynamical behavior of the aerosol in a frame of reference that travels with the aerosol (i.e. a "Lagrangian viewpoint").

A complete Lagrangian dynamical model would be very difficult since it would follow all individual particles and air parcels as they travel through the entire lung. Instead, existing one-dimensional LDMs make the major simplifying assumption that the aerosol and air travel together at the same velocity, and this velocity is obtained by treating the lung as a sequence of branching circular pipes whose diameter is given by some idealized lung geometry. For example, if the inhalation flow rate is Q, then the flow rate in each airway in the 10th lung generation is $Q/2^{10}$, and the average velocity in these airways is $v = (Q/2^{10})/\pi R^2$, where R is the radius of the airways in the 10th generation of the idealized lung geometry being used. With the velocity in each airway known, the amount of time the aerosol spends traveling through each airway generation can be obtained by dividing the length of each airway in the idealized lung geometry by this velocity. With this information, then by treating each airway generation as an inclined circular tube, it is possible to predict how much aerosol will deposit due to gravitational sedimentation and by Brownian diffusion in each airway generation (by using exact solutions of the dynamical equations for sedimentation and diffusion in inclined circular tubes—see Finlay 2019 for these equations). Deposition in each airway by inertial impaction is dealt with empirically in one-dimensional LDMs (since simulation of the equations governing impaction requires full simulation of at least several lung branches at a time, which dramatically increases computation times). Many different empirical equations for impaction have been suggested, largely based on data from *in vitro* experiments in branched tubes, although those obtained using several generations probably represent reality more closely (Finlay 2019), since it is known that typically three or more generations of branches are needed before sensitivity to artificial inlet conditions is reduced (Comer et al. 2000). Although many LDMs assume each bifurcation is symmetric, this assumption can be removed using a stochastic Monte Carlo approach (Koblinger and Hofmann 1990, Horváth et al. 2017).

A major advantage of LDMs over empirical models is the ease with which they can capture droplet size changes (e.g. due to evaporation), and its effect on respiratory tract deposition, making them especially suitable for predicting drug delivery with nebulized aqueous aerosols (Finlay et al. 1998b). As noted earlier, many aqueous inhaled pharmaceutical aerosols that undergo hygroscopic size changes require two-way coupled heat and mass transfer modeling (Finlay et al. 1997), in which the air properties are affected by the droplets and vice versa. This is unfortunate, since two-way coupled hygroscopic effects complicate the model considerably, as well as increasing computation times. Various hygroscopic models (e.g. Martonen 1982, Persons et al. 1987, Ferron et al. 1988, ICRP 1994, Asgharian 2004, Grasmeijer et al 2016, Mellat et al. 2017) do not include such two-way coupled effects and are therefore limited to those cases where the inhaled air can be considered as an infinite source of water vapor, otherwise giving varying degrees of inaccuracy depending on the relevant parameters (Finlay et al. 1997).

A second advantage of one-dimensional LDMs over empirical models is that their inclusion of some of the aerosol dynamics (albeit semi-empirically) reduces the dangers of extrapolation, allowing, for example, prediction of deposition with breathing patterns that are quite different from normal tidal breathing. Indeed, Anderson et al. (1999) use a one-dimensional LDM to examine extremely slow inhalations consisting of inhalation flow rates of <2 L/min with a single inhalation duration of 10 seconds–20 seconds, which allows much larger particles to deposit in the small airways compared to normal tidal breathing.

The ability of different one-dimensional LDMs to predict the regional deposition of aerosols inhaled from pharmaceutical devices has been examined by several authors without inclusion of particle size changes due to evaporation (Finlay et al. 1998a, Hashish et al. 1998, Katz et al. 2013, Jókay et al. 2016), as well as with inclusion of two-way coupled hygroscopic effects (Finlay et al. 1996). These comparisons show that LDMs are sensitive to the dimensions of the idealized lung geometry being used, with the division of deposition between the alveolar and tracheobronchial regions matching *in vivo* data with some idealized lung geometries, but not others (Finlay et al. 2000). Such sensitivity of LDMs to the dimensions of the idealized geometry is a concern if a model remains untested in comparison to *in vivo* data, particularly since the commonly used Weibel A model is known to have narrower tracheobronchial airways than more recent models (Finlay et al. 2000).

Because one-dimensional LDMs include the aerosol dynamics by using solutions of the dynamical equations in simplified versions of parts of the lung geometry and by including empirical data from experiments on inertial impaction, they remain semi-empirical in nature. As a result, they share some of the drawbacks of purely empirical models mentioned earlier. In particular, one-dimensional LDMs use the same mouth-throat deposition models used with the purely empirical models and so suffer from the same inability to predict mouth-throat deposition with metered dose inhalers discussed earlier.

A second drawback with one-dimensional LDMs is associated with the major simplifying assumption that the air and aerosol travel together as a single plug which does not distort (other than splitting in half at each bifurcation). Although this assumption makes LDMs computationally inexpensive, it causes an inhaled aerosol to proceed through the lung without axial dispersion (i.e. stretching and distortion of the aerosol front). Models for axial dispersion suitable for one-dimensional LDMs have been developed (Sarangapani and Wexler 2000, Hofmann et al. 2008) that allow incorporation of irreversibility of dispersion between inhalation and exhalation. However, the effect of axial dispersion on aerosol deposition remains poorly characterized (Finlay 2019), so it is difficult to assess the magnitude of the errors associated with the lack of its presence. The reasonable agreement of one-dimensional LDMs with *in vivo* data would suggest that this effect may be minor for inhaled pharmaceutical aerosol deposition, but further research addressing this issue is needed.

Another drawback with one-dimensional LDMs is the difficulty they have in treating time-dependence of inhalation flow rates and aerosol properties (a situation which commonly occurs with single breath inhalers), as well as time-dependence of the lung geometry. This difficulty is due to their Lagrangian nature in which a single parcel of air and aerosol is tracked as it moves through an idealized lung geometry. In one-dimensional LDMs, once this parcel has left the mouth-throat, no further regard is paid to the conditions at the mouth so that the only way to capture time-dependence of the air and aerosol properties (e.g. MMAD, GSD, inhalation flow rate) is with a quasi-steady procedure whereby parcels released at different times in the breath are each tracked separately. However, such an approach increases computation times significantly and has not been pursued with inhaled pharmaceutical LDMs to the author's knowledge.

4.2.4 Eulerian Dynamical Models

To remove some of the limitations associated with one-dimensional LDMs, particularly their clumsiness with axial dispersion and time-varying breathing, more complex models can be considered. The next level of complexity beyond one-dimensional LDMs are the one-dimensional Eulerian dynamical models (EDMs).

With these models, the dynamical behavior of the aerosol is viewed by a stationary observer watching the aerosol's behavior in the entire respiratory tract at once (a so-called "Eulerian" viewpoint). To solve the equations governing the aerosol dynamics without simplification would mean doing a direct simulation of the full governing equations throughout the lungs, which is not practical as discussed earlier. Instead, the fluid flow is assumed known (e.g. parabolic or plug flow in an idealized lung geometry), and the equation governing the aerosol number density (i.e. number of aerosol particles/unit volume) is reduced to one-dimension by integrating over cross-sectional planes at each axial location in the respiratory tract (see Finlay 2019 for a detailed development of the basis of these models). The result is a single, partial differential equation for the aerosol concentration as a function of depth x into the respiratory tract and time t. This equation is solved numerically, giving the aerosol number density at a number of discrete depths, x, and times, t.

Particle deposition in one-dimensional EDMs is dealt with in the same manner as in LDMs by using exact solutions of the dynamical equations for sedimentation and diffusion in inclined circular tubes and using empirical equations for inertial impaction from experiments in branched airway replicas.

Because one-dimensional EDMs require the numerical solution of a partial differential equation (as opposed to simple algebraic equations with empirical models and one-dimensional LDMs or ordinary differential equations with hygroscopic LDMs), EDMs are more difficult to program, and require somewhat more computational resources. For these reasons, only a few examples exist of one-dimensional EDMs being used with inhaled pharmaceutical aerosols (e.g. Clark and Egan 1994), although they have been used to aid in the development of purely empirical models (e.g. the ICRP 1994 model is partly a curve fit to data from the one-dimensional EDM of Egan et al. 1989).

The principal attractions of one-dimensional EDMs are their ability to implement time-dependence of the aerosol properties at the respiratory tract entrance (e.g. variations in aerosol concentration and size associated with a burst or "bolus" of inhaled particles), the ease with which simple models of axial dispersion can be incorporated, as well as their ability to include time-dependence of the lung geometry associated with lung inflation during inhalation (Taulbee et al. 1978, Egan and Nixon 1985, Edwards 1995). When any of these effects are deemed important, then one-dimensional EDMs are advantageous over the other simpler approaches we have considered thus far.

Of course one-dimensional EDMs are not without their drawbacks. Indeed, they suffer from several of the same problems that plague empirical and one-dimensional LDMs. In particular, their use of flawed empirical mouth-throat deposition models can lead to errors when modeling of dry powder and metered dose inhalers, as discussed earlier with purely empirical models. As with one-dimensional LDMs, the use of simplified lung geometries and empirical impaction data for predicting deposition within each airway give an element of empiricism to one-dimensional EDMs that limits their generality.

Another drawback with one-dimensional EDMs lies in the information that is lost when the flow and aerosol properties are averaged over cross-sections at each depth in the lung in deriving these models. This missing information is crucial in determining axial dispersion (Finlay 2019), so that existing one-dimensional EDMs instead model axial dispersion using simple analogies with molecular diffusional transport. This is one of the least scrutinized aspects of one-dimensional EDMs, and although this has been previously examined (Lee et al. 2000), it remains to be seen how accurate axial dispersion models in one-dimensional EDMs must be in order to correctly predict deposition of inhaled pharmaceutical aerosols. It should be noted, however, that comparisons of regional deposition predictions of a one-dimensional EDM (Egan et al. 1989) to *in vivo* data of aerosols inhaled with tidal breathing from tubes show good agreement with *in vivo* data (ICRP 1994), so that such axial dispersion models may be adequate under these circumstances. Whether this is true for single breath inhaled pharmaceutical aerosols remains unknown.

4.2.5 Three-Dimensional Partial Lung Simulation

Some of the major limitations of existing one-dimensional LDMs and EDMs are caused by their consideration of only one spatial dimension. By removing this one-dimensional restriction, these limitations can be removed. This is normally done by simulating the airways instead in three spatial dimensions and performing numerical simulation of the fluid and aerosol equations on a three-dimensional grid placed in each lung airway. Since simulation of the whole respiratory tract in this manner is prohibitively demanding of computational resources, work to date in this direction has limited itself to simulations of small parts of the respiratory tract, which we refer to as three-dimensional partial lung simulations (abbreviated as "PLS," with "three-dimensional" implied). Since it is easier to solve the fluid flow equations in an Eulerian framework (using standard computational fluid dynamics (CFD) methods), while particle deposition is more naturally dealt with in a Lagrangian framework, most PLS researchers have used a mixed approach with Eulerian equations for the fluid and Lagrangian equations for the aerosol.

A host of authors have performed PLS in various idealized replicas of single, double, and multiple bifurcation segments of the lung, as well as parts of simplified alveolar ducts. Deposition in the particular respiratory tract segment being simulated can be predicted more accurately with this approach than with the simplified, one-dimensional LDMs or EDMs. While PLS can be used to simulate deposition in every one of the airways of the first few lung generations (e.g. Vos et al. 2016, Kannan et al. 2017), PLS studies whose domain extends to the distal parts of the trachea-bronchial tree typically instead simulate a single airway path through the trachea-bronchial airways (e.g. Walenga and Longest 2016, Ciciliani et al. 2017), since this is far less computationally demanding (Tian et al. 2011).

However, PLS is not without its drawbacks. A major limiting factor with PLS is the lack of knowledge of the three-dimensional geometry of the respiratory tract airways, particularly distal to the first few lung generations. Current imaging technology has been used to obtain this information for the mouth-throat and first few proximal tracheobronchial airways, so that at present, PLS in regions distal to the first few airway generations requires speculation as to the actual geometry of these airspaces. This is unfortunate, since the alveolar region is important because of its ability to give access to systemic delivery through the lungs. Imaging of the alveolar airspaces requires improvement in spatial resolution over present medical imaging technology. Since the alveoli change shape significantly during inhalation, temporal resolution well below 1 second is also required in these images. Such imaging demands are likely to remain beyond our technological capabilities for some time to come, so that PLS is not yet ready to completely supplant one-dimensional LDMs and EDMs in inhaled pharmaceutical aerosol design for predicting drug delivery, particularly in the alveolar region. However, PLS is commonly used to simulate the behavior of the extrathoracic and proximal conducting airways and has been extended to simulate idealized alveolar airways (Khajeh-Hosseini-Dalasm and Longest 2015), allowing it to be used for determination of the distribution and deposition of aerosol throughout the entire lung (e.g. Longest et al. 2016).

REFERENCES

Anderson, M., Svartengren, M. and Canmer, P. 1999. Human tracheobronchial deposition and effect of a cholinergic aerosol inhaled by extremely slow inhalations. *Exp. Lung Res.* 25:335–352.

Asgharian, B. 2004. A model of deposition of hygroscopic particles in the human lung. *Aerosol Sci. Tech.* 38:938–947.

Carrigy, N. B., Martin, A. R. and Finlay, W. H. 2015. Use of extrathoracic deposition models for patient-specific dose estimation during inhaler design. *Curr. Pharm. Des.* 21(27): 3984–3992.

Ciciliani, A.-M., Langguth, P. and Wachtel, H. 2017. In vitro dose comparison of Respimat® inhaler with dry powder inhalers for COPD maintenance therapy. *Int. J. Chron. Obstruct. Pulmon. Dis.* 12:1565–1577.

Clark, A. R. and Egan, M. 1994. Modelling the deposition of inhaled powdered drug aerosols. *J. Aerosol Sci.* 25:175–186.

Clark, A. R., Newman, S. P. and Dasovich, N. 1998. Mouth and oropharyngeal deposition of pharmaceutical aerosols. *J. Aerosol Med.* 11 (Suppl. 1):116–121.

Comer, J. K., Kleinstreuer, C. and Zhang, Z. 2000. Aerosol transport and deposition in sequentially bifurcating airways. *ASME J. Biomech. Eng.* 122:152–158.

Davidson, N., Tong, H.-J., Kalberer, M., Seville, P. C., Ward, A. D., Kuimova, M. K. and Pope, F. D. 2017. Measurement of the Raman spectra and hygroscopicity of four pharmaceutical aerosols as they travel from pressurized metered dose inhalers (pMDI) to a model lung. *Int. J. Pharm.* 520:59–69.

Davies, C. N. 1982. Deposition of particles in the human lung as a function of particle size and breathing pattern: An empirical model. *Ann. Occup. Hyg.* 26:119–135.

DeHaan, W. H. and Finlay, W. H. 2004. Predicting extrathoracic deposition from dry powder inhalers. *J. Aerosol Sci.* 35:309–331.

Dunbar, C. A., Watkins, A. P. and Miller, J. F. 1997. Theoretical investigation of the spray from a pressurized metered dose inhaler. *Atom. Sprays* 7:417–436.

Edwards, D. 1995. The macrotransport of aerosol particles in the lung: aerosol deposition phenomena. *J. Aerosol Sci.* 26:293–317.

Egan, M. J. and Nixon, W. 1985. A model of aerosol deposition in the lung for use in inhalation dose assessments. *Rad. Prot. Dos.* 11:5–17.

Egan, M. J., Nixon, W., Robinson, N. I., James, A. C., and Phalen, R. T. 1989. Inhaled aerosol transport and deposition calculations for the ICRP Task Group. *J. Aerosol Sci.* 20:1305–1308, 1989.

Ferron, G. A., Kreyling, W. G. and Haider, B. 1998. Inhalation of salt aerosol particles—II. Growth and deposition due to hygroscopic growth. *J. Aerosol Sci.* 19:611–631.

Finlay, W. H. 2019. *The Mechanics of Inhaled Pharmaceutical Aerosols: An Introduction.* 2nd Edition, Elsevier, Cambridge, UK.

Finlay, W. H., Lange, C. F., Li, W.-I. and Hoskinson, M. 2000. Validating deposition models in disease: What is needed? *J. Aerosol Med.* 13:381–385.

Finlay, W.H., Stapleton, K. W. and Zuberbuhler, P. 1998. Variations in predicted regional lung deposition of salbutamol sulphate between 19 nebulizer models. *J. Aerosol Med.* 11:65–80.

Finlay, W. H., Hoskinson, M. and Stapleton, K. W. 1998a. Can models be trusted to subdivide lung deposition into alveolar and tracheobronchial fractions? in *Respiratory Drug Delivery VI,* Eds. R. N. Dalby, P. R. Byron, and S. J. Farr (Eds.), pp. 235–242. Englewood, CO: Interpharm Press.

Finlay, W. H., Stapleton, K. W. and Zuberbuhler, P. 1997. Errors in regional lung deposition predictions of nebulized salbutamol sulphate due to neglect or partial inclusion of hygroscopic effects. *Int. J. Pharm.* 149:63–72.

Finlay, W. H., Stapleton, K. W., Chan, H. K., Zuberbuhler, P. and Gonda, I. 1996. Regional deposition of inhaled hygroscopic aerosols: In vivo SPECT compared with mathematical deposition modelling. *J. Appl. Physiol.* 81:374–383.

Grasmeijer, N., Frijlink, H. W. and Hinrichs, W. L. J. 2016. An adaptable model for growth and/or shrinkage of droplets in the respiratory tract during inhalation of aqueous particles. *J. Aerosol Sci.* 93:21–34.

Grgic, B., Heenan, A. F., Burnell, P. K. P. and Finlay, W. H., 2004. In vitro intersubject and intrasubject deposition measurements in realistic mouth-throat geometries. *J. Aerosol Sci.* 35:1025–1040.

Horváth, A., Balásházy, I., Tomisa, G. and Farkas, A. 2017. Significance of breath-hold time in dry powder aerosol drug therapy of COPD patients. *Eur. J. Pharm. Sci.* 104:145–149.

Hashish, A. H., Fleming, J. S., Conway, J., Halson, P., Moore, E., Williams, T. J., Bailey, A. G., Nassim, M. N. and Holgate, S. T. 1998. Lung deposition of particles by airway generation in healthy subjects: Three-dimensional radionuclide imaging and numerical model prediction. *J. Aerosol Sci.* 29:205–215.

Hofmann, W., Pawlak, E. and Sturm, R. 2008. Semi-empirical stochastic model of aerosol bolus dispersion in the human lung. *Inhal. Toxicol.* 20:1059–1073.

ICRP Task Group on Lung Dynamics, 1966. Deposition and retention models for internal dosimetry of the human respiratory tract. *Health Phys.* 12:173–207.

ICRP (International Commission on Radiological Protection) 1994. Human respiratory tract model for radiological protection. Annals of the ICRP, ICRP publication 66, Elsevier, New York.

Jókay, Á., Farkas, Á., Füri, P., Horváth, A., Tomisa, G. and Balásházy, I. 2016. Computer modeling of airway deposition distribution of Foster® NEXThaler® and Seretide® Diskus® dry powder combination drugs. *Eur. J. Pharm. Sci.* 88:210–218.

Kannan, R., Przekwas, A. J., Singh, N., Delvadia, R., Tian, G. and Walenga, R. 2017. Pharmaceutical aerosols deposition patterns from a dry powder inhaler: Euler Lagrangian prediction and validation. *Med. Eng. Phys.* 42:35–47.

Katz, I., Pichelin, M., Caillibotte, G., Montesantos, S., Majoral, C., Martonen, T., Fleming, J., Bennett, M. and Conway, J. 2013. Controlled, parametric, individualized, 2D, and 3D imaging measurements of aerosol deposition in the respiratory tract of healthy human subjects: Preliminary comparisons with simulations. *Aerosol Sci. Tech.* 47:714–723.

Khajeh-Hosseini-Dalasm, N. and Longest, P. W. 2015. Deposition of particles in the alveolar airways: Inhalation and breath-hold with pharmaceutical aerosols. *J. Aerosol Sci.* 79:15–30.

Koblinger, L. and Hofmann, W. 1990. Monte Carlo modelling of aerosol deposition in human lungs. Part I. Simulation of particle transport in a stochastic lung structure. *J. Aerosol Sci.* 21:661–674.

Lee, J. W., Lee, D. Y. and Kim, W. S. 2000. Dispersion of an aerosol bolus in a double bifurcation. *J. Aerosol Sci.* 31:491–505.

Longest, P. W., Tian, G., Khajeh-Hosseini-Dalasm, N. and Hindle, M. 2016. Validating whole-airway CFD predictions of DPI aerosol deposition at multiple flow rates. *J. Aerosol Med. Pulm. Drug Del.* 29:461–482.

Majoral, C, Fleming, J., Conway, J., Katz, I., Tossici-Bolt, L., Pichelin, M., Montesantos, S. and Caillibotte, G. 2014. Controlled, parametric, individualized, 2D, and 3D imaging measurements of aerosol deposition in the respiratory tract of healthy human volunteers: In vivo data analysis. *J. Aerosol Med. Pulm. Drug Del.* 27:349–362.

Martonen, T. B. 1982. Analytical model of hygroscopic particle behaviour in human airways. *Bull. Math. Biology* 44:425–442.

Martonen, T. B., Yang, Y., Xue, Z. Q. and Zhang, Z. 1994. Motion of air within the human tracheobronchial tree. *Particul Sci. Technol.* 12:175–188.

Martin, A. R. and Finlay, W. H. 2005. The effect of humidity on particle sizing from metered-dose inhalers. *Aerosol Sci. Technol.* 39:283–289.

Maxwell, J. C. 1890. *The Scientific Papers of Clerk Maxwell*, (W. D. Niven ed.), Cambridge University Press, London.

Martin, A. R. and Finlay, W. H. 2018. Model calculations of regional deposition and disposition for single doses of inhaled liposomal and dry powder ciprofloxacin. *J. Aerosol Med. Pulm. Drug Deliv.* 31:49–60.

Mellat, M., Borojeni, A. A. M., Sahebkar, A. and Ghanei, M. 2017. Adapting the ICRP model to predict regional deposition of the pharmaceutical aerosols inhaled through DPIs and nebulizers. *J. Drug Del. Sci. Tech.* 37:81–87.

Mitchell, J. P. and Nagel, M. W. 2003. Cascade impactors for the size characterization of aerosols from medical inhalers: Their uses and limitations. *J. Aerosol Med. Pulm. Drug Deliv.* 16:341–377.

NCRP (National Council on Radiation Protection). 1997. Deposition, retention and dosimetry of inhaled radioactive substances, Report No. 125, National Council on Radiation Protection and Measurement, Bethesda, MD.

Persons, D. D., Hess, G. D., Muller, W. J. and Scherer, P. W. 1987. Airway deposition of hygroscopic heterodispersed aerosols: Results of a computer calculation. *J. Appl. Physiol.* 63:1195–1204.

Ruzycki, C. A., Yang, M., Chan, H.-K. and Finlay, W. H. 2017. Improved prediction of intersubject variability in extrathoracic aerosol deposition using algebraic correlations. *Aerosol Sci. Technol.* 51:667–673.

Sarangapani, R. and Wexler, A. S. 2000. The role of dispersion in particle deposition in human airways. *Toxicol. Sci.* 54:229–236.

Sheth, P., Grimes, M. R., Stein, S. W. and Myrdal, P. B. 2017. Impact of droplet evaporation rate on resulting in vitro performance parameters of pressurized metered dose inhalers. *Int. J. Pharm.* 528:360–371.

Stahlhofen, W., Rudolf, G. and James, A. C. 1989. Intercomparison of experimental regional aerosol deposition data. *J. Aerosol Med.* 2:285–308.

Taulbee, D. B., Yu, C.P. and Heyder, J. 1978. Aerosol transport in the human lung from analysis of single breaths. *J. Appl. Physiol.* 44:803–812.

Tian G., Longest P. W., Su G., Walenga R. L. and Hindle M. 2011. Development of a stochastic individual path (SIP) model for predicting the tracheobronchial deposition of pharmaceutical aerosols: Effects of transient inhalation and sampling the airways. *J. Aerosol Sci.* 42:781–799.

Vos, W, Hajian, B., De Backer, J., Holsbeke, C. V., Vinchurkar, S., Claes, R, Hufkens, A., Parizel, P. M., Bedert, L. and De Backer, W. 2016. Functional respiratory imaging to assess the interaction between systemic roflumilast and inhaled ICS/lABA/LAMA. *Int. J. Chron. Obstruct. Pulmon Dis.* 11:263–271.

Walenga, R. L. and Longest, P. W. 2016. Current inhalers deliver very small doses to the lower tracheobronchial airways: Assessment of healthy and constricted lungs. *J. Pharm. Sci.* 105:147–159.

Weers, J. and Clark, A. 2017. The impact of inspiratory flow rate on drug delivery to the lungs with dry powder inhalers. *Pharm. Res.* 34:507–528.

Wei, X., Hindle, M., Delvadia, R. R. and Byron, P. R. 2017. In vitro tests for aerosol deposition. V: Using realistic testing to estimate variations in aerosol properties at the trachea. *J. Aerosol Med. Pulm. Drug Deliv.* 30:339–348.

Yang, M. Y., Ruzycki, C., Verschuer, J., Katsifis, A., Eberl, S., Wong, K., Golshahi, L., Brannan, J., Finlay, W. H. and Chan, H.-K. 2017. Examining the ability of empirical correlations to predict subject specific in vivo extrathoracic deposition during tidal breathing. *Aerosol Sci. Technol.* 51:363–376.

Yeh, H.-C., Cuddihy, R. G., Phalen, R. F. and Chang, I. Y. 1996. Comparisons of calculated respiratory tract deposition of particles based on the proposed NCRP model and the new ICRP66 Model. *Aerosol Sci. Technol.* 25:134–140.

Yu, C. P., Zhang, L., Becquemin, M. H., Roy, M. and Bouchikhi, A. 1992. Algebraic modeling of total and regional deposition of inhaled particles in the human lung of various ages. *J. Aerosol Sci.* 23:73–79.

5

Practical Aspects of Imaging Techniques Employed to Study Aerosol Deposition and Clearance

Myrna B. Dolovich

CONTENTS

5.1 Introduction

Since the last edition of this book in 2004, a number of changes have occurred in the areas of aerosol characterization and methods for imaging the lung. Techniques to measure aerosol performance characteristics, required to support, confirm, and correlate with imaging outcomes of dose and distribution have been further developed with improved accuracy in outcomes. However, the need by investigators for correlating in vitro sizing measurements with in vivo imaging outcomes and clinical response still remains an elusive goal for a number of reasons. The human lung is not a cascade impactor, the resolution of 2D and 3D imaging tools is far below the actual airway dimensions of the distal airways of the lung and, variables related to lung disease, which are not incorporated into any in vitro lung deposition model, play the major role in determining regional airway deposition and clearance of inhaled medicinal products. Currently, while some clinical scanners can differentiate airway diameters at the level of the 9th generation of airway (Figure A5.1), this is not typical of most 3D research scanners. Increased resolution is dependent on scanner design and cost of same. The issues listed in Table 5.2 of Chapter 5 remain pertinent when designing, planning, and implementing an imaging study, with procedures required to be validated prior to beginning an exposure of human subjects to a radioactive tracer aerosol further outlined in Table 5.1. Imaging studies are still not required by United States and Canadian regulatory agencies when pharmaceutical companies seek approval for a therapeutic aerosol to treat respiratory disease, but this could change with better substantiated procedures to support the imaging outcomes (Figure A5.1). In Europe, imaging studies are, however, considered supportive information.

The measurement of lung deposition of inhaled therapeutics and its interpretation have been debated within the field of inhaled drug delivery science for many years. Historically, two-dimensional gamma scintigraphy (planar imaging) has been used to demonstrate total and regional lung deposition of drugs inhaled from selected aerosol delivery systems [1–4]. Efforts have been made to link total lung deposition with the clinical parameters of efficacy and safety, though with limited success. Acquisition of 2D scintigraphic data can be confounded by several factors, such as poor radiolabeling of the study drug, use of inaccurate tissue attenuation factors applied when calculating absolute amounts of radioactivity in the lung, oropharynx, and gut, and poor delineation of the edge of the lung, leading to incorrectly defined lung regions. In addition, factors influencing the inhalation of the radiolabeled aerosols may not be well controlled, producing variability in deposition patterns. Intraindividual variability in data outcomes may result from a lack of adherence to inclusion/exclusion criteria for study subjects or the enrolment of subjects with too broad a range of disease severities. Furthermore, for deposition protocols with concurrent pharmacokinetic measurements, acquisition of imaging data may be constrained by the need to image immediately following inhalation of the labeled drug and to precisely measure plasma drug levels at the

TABLE 5.1

Aerosols Used in Clinical Investigations

Technique	Application	Aerosol Size	Disease or Condition
Mucociliary clearance (MCC)	Ciliary dysfunction, airway caliber, mucus production	>2 μm	Primary ciliary dyskinesia, bronchial disorders, lung transplantation
Inhalation challenge	Airway responsiveness, allergen challenge, sputum induction	1–6 μm	Asthma, COPD
Respiratory solute absorption	Epithelial permeability	<2 μm	Interstitial lung disease, lung injury, *Pneumocystis carinii* pneumonia, adult respiratory distress syndrome
Ventilation/perfusion	Vascular occlusion, presurgery evaluation	<1 μm	Pulmonary embolism, localized airway disease
Dosimetry	Drug dose and distribution/response to therapy	1–5 μm	Asthma, cystic fibrosis, COPD, bronchopulmonary dysplasia, respiratory syncytial virus, diabetes, adult respiratory distress syndrome

TABLE 5.2

Issues in Imaging with Radioaerosols

Characteristics of Aerosol System (particle size, drug output)
Standard Curves (impactor plates, filter, inlet, collection tube)
Radiolabeling of Drug
Types of tracers
Validation of radioaerosol
Particle size characterization: drug versus radioactivity
Measurement of emitted dose from inhaler
Drug versus radioactivity
Scanner selection
Scanner resolution and sensitivity
Type of collimator for gamma camera
Controls during administration and imaging of radioaerosol
Breathing technique
Mouthpiece seal
Gas flow rate
Subject movement during imaging
Subject characteristics
Age
Sex
Severity of disease
Stability of baseline pulmonary function
Data analysis
Defining the lung edge
Defining regions of interest within the lung
Correction for tissue attenuation of radioactivity
Calculation of dose deposited
Expression of results

same time and, therefore, possibly requiring correction factors to be applied to the data for any discrepancy in time between the two sets of measurements.

The response to a therapeutic aerosol is considered to be a function of the dose deposited at the target site in the lung [5–10]. The dose, in turn, is dependent upon the system producing the aerosol, the particle size characteristics of the inhaled aerosol, the mode of inhalation, and the caliber of the airways [11–16]. The influence of the pattern of deposition of the inhaled dose, that is, selective delivery to the central versus small, peripheral airways, on the response is not as well defined [17–19]. Direct measurements of deposition and distribution of therapeutic aerosols in the lung, mucociliary clearance (MCC), and lung epithelial permeability (LEP) have been made using a variety of tracer methods employing external imaging [4,20,21]. These diagnostic tests (Table 5.1) [20,21,24] measure the surface transport of secretions (mucociliary clearance) [22–24], transepithelial transport of fluid and hydrophilic solutes (respiratory clearance or epithelial permeability) related to the integrity of the lung epithelium [25–27], and the distribution of inhaled gases or extrafine (~1 μm) aerosols in the lung (ventilation) [28–33]; correlations with clinical response have been obtained in a limited number of these same studies. When properly conducted, the procedures are convenient and involve minimal radiation and risk. It should be understood that these tests are dependent on the production, characterization, and inhalation of aerosols within a particular size range [32–35].

While 2D imaging is easy to implement in practice, the blurring caused by structures overlying and underlying the structures of interest limits its usefulness for quantitation of the distribution of an inhaled dose within the lung [36]. However, over the last approximately 30 years, advances in imaging technology have enabled more sophisticated three-dimensional techniques to be utilized to image and provide greater detail about the regional deposition of drugs in the lung, e.g. single-photon-emission computed tomography (SPECT) [28,37–42] and positron-emission tomography (PET) [40,43–46]. Both PET and

SPECT provide accurate and highly specific information about the dose and distribution within the body of inhaled or injected tracers, and both are widely used as diagnostic tools in nuclear medicine. Of the two imaging techniques, PET provides greater resolution, with the advantage of utilizing radiolabeled molecular markers to obtain functional imaging of biologic processes in vivo [47–51]. Supporting these measurements are analytical methodologies that have allowed a more precise measure of the pharmacokinetic profiles of many inhaled drugs, enhancing understanding of their absorption, distribution, and clearance kinetics from the respiratory tract [52,53].

This chapter will discuss some of the practical issues to be aware of when performing radiolabeled deposition and clearance studies (Table 5.2). The considerations apply to both in vivo studies in man and, in animal models and, to some extent, in in vitro models. Nasal deposition and clearance studies and tracheal transport measurements will not be discussed in detail, although it should be understood that the importance of a valid radiolabeled test aerosol is key to the successful interpretation of the deposition data for both nasal and lung studies [54,55].

5.2 Issues in Using Radiolabeled Aerosols to Determine Drug Delivery to the Lung

5.2.1 Characterization of the Aerosol from the Delivery System

Systems used to provide unit doses of therapeutic aerosols are the pressurized metered-dose inhaler (pMDI), containing drug in a propellant formulation, the dry powder inhaler (DPI), and nebulizers for aqueous and ethanolic formulations [56,57]. Many inhaler systems now available to patients and dispensing a variety of therapies have been tested in vivo with radiolabeled drugs to measure their efficiency of delivery to the lung. These measurements of lung deposition have yielded values on the order of 5%–30%, even under optimal inhalation conditions. Newer nebulizer technologies, such as the metered-dose liquid inhalers currently in development, have much greater efficiencies, on the order of 70% or more of the drug dose deposited in the lung [58]. It is widely accepted that knowledge of the lung dose and distribution of inhaled aerosols from these various systems is critical for optimal development of the delivery system technology and for the assessment of the performance of these inhalers in vivo. The information provided is of interest not only to the pharmaceutical industry [30,59,60], but also to physicians prescribing inhalant therapy for a variety of diseases. If deposition from a particular aerosol dispensed from a delivery system is poor, it is likely that the response to therapy given from that aerosol will be suboptimal. The deposition measurements provide the physician with data on which to base the selection of an inhaler or mode of therapy for that particular patient.

5.2.2 Radiolabeling Methods for Aerosols

The first step when embarking on a series of experiments to measure lung deposition for an inhaled pharmaceutic is to produce the radioactive aerosol that mirrors the therapy dispensed from the inhaler being tested [61–63]. This may be a fairly straightforward radiopharmaceutical procedure, in particular for nebulizer and pMDI solution formulations, but it may also take months to produce and validate the tracer. Suspension formulations labeled with a tracer for 2D and SPECT imaging and drugs synthesized with a positron emitter can fall into the latter category. For 2D imaging and SPECT deposition studies, most labeled drugs produced are "association" products; that is, the label is associated with the drug, but is not firmly bound. Without firm binding, images must be acquired quickly before the dissociation of the label from the drug leads to a circulating level of absorbed radioactivity that would introduce an unacceptable error in the measurement of radioactivity in the lung. Knowing the effective half-life $\left(1/t^{1/2}_{\text{effective}} = 1/t^{1/2}_{\text{physical}} + 1/t^{1/2}_{\text{biological}}\right)$ of the tracer in the lung may allow a correction for the uptake, but this is not a desirable solution. Deposition studies using SPECT with these types of absorbable labeled drugs as the test agents are less accurate because the time required for imaging is often greater than the $t^{1/2}_{\text{effective}}$, although acquisition times with newer SPECT cameras are much shorter [64].

There are several protocols designed to measure mucociliary clearance. Which protocols are used are dependent upon the question being asked. To measure the acute effect of a pharmaceutic on clearance, the unlabeled drug is inhaled, followed by the nonabsorbable tracer aerosol [65,66]. In other protocols, designed to determine the effect of an intervention on MCC, the tracer aerosol is inhaled, and clearance is measured for 30 minutes–60 minutes to establish the control curve. The treatment or intervention is then administered for a fixed length of time while continuing to measure clearance. This period is usually followed by another series of clearance measurements to define changes from the control period postintervention [67,68]. Thus, it is important that there be little or no uptake of the inhaled tracer, more or less guaranteed, i.e. the $t_{1/2\ \text{effective}}$ of the tracer similar to the physical half-life of the isotope.

5.2.3 Production of Radiolabel

A number of methods have been developed to produce radioactive products for inhalation and use in lung deposition measurements. When imaging with 2D planar or 3D SPECT, the tracer most commonly used for diagnostic and research studies in humans is 99m-technetium, i.e. pertechnetate ($^{99m}TcO_4^-$). The short physical half-life of ^{99m}Tc (6.0 hours) and effective half-life of 0.16 hours–6.0 hours, dependent on the compound labeled, coupled with a low gamma emission energy (140 KeV) minimizes the radiation exposure and risk to the subject as well as to personnel handling or preparing the radioactive drugs for inhalation. With the exception of PET tracers, very few radiolabeled studies involve direct labeling of the drug [69]. As already mentioned for inhalation products used for imaging with either planar or SPECT, the tracer is associated with, but not part of, the drug formulation, whether the formulation is a drug in suspension, a drug in solution, or a drug powder. As stated earlier, unless firmly bound, the label and drug rapidly dissociate following deposition on the airway surface; the label then no longer provides a marker for the drug. For $^{99m}TcO_4$, a soluble tracer, the effective half-life in the lung, once separated from the drug, is of the order of 11 minutes–15 minutes, while that in the oropharynx is approximately 25 minutes. Thus, imaging must be done quickly and over a short period of time, with possible correction of the data for the loss of radioactivity due to absorption through the lungs, seen if the kidneys become obvious within minutes of administering the radioactive aerosol. Accumulation of pertechnetate in tissue may be detected by simultaneously imaging the thigh, although the sensitivity of this measurement will depend on the activity of the dose inhaled and the rates of absorption and excretion from the lungs and other compartments in the body. Measuring radioactivity in the blood by defining a region over the heart is possible with PET, but not with planar imaging.

Dose calibrators are standard equipment in all nuclear medicine facilities. They are used to measure the dose of radioactivity of all drugs administered. Because quantitative outcomes based on administered dose are dependent on the exactness of the dose measurement, the accuracy of the dose calibrator must be ensured with routine measurements using reference standards. Quality control and calibration of the scanners must also be scheduled on a regular basis to maintain proper performance. Because a variety of 2D and 3D scanners is used, variability in performance can be a major issue [70].

Deposited doses in the lung and oropharynx vary among infants, children, adults, geriatric patients, and patients being mechanically ventilated, the differences being mainly a function of breathing pattern and oropharyngeal and airway geometry [71–76]. Adjustments to the nominal dose of radioactivity must be made to avoid excessive radiation exposure, in particular when imaging is used to measure deposited dose in children [77]. For research deposition measurements of pMDI drugs in adults, we load approximately 200 mCi into the canister to obtain 150 μCi–200 μCi per actuation, for an effective radiation dose of less than 1 mSv [78]. When imaging children and small animals, approximately one-fourth of the adult dose is given. While these administered doses of radioactivity are much less than those used for nuclear medicine diagnostic procedures, counting statistics for the acquired images are well within acceptable limits.

5.2.3.1 pMDIs

Procedures for labeling some pMDI formulations are described in the literature [74,79–83]. The method varies with the category of drug and the excipients present in the formulation.

The first step in the preparation of a labeled canister is to extract the pertechnetate, using methylethylketone (MEK), into an empty canister. When the MEK has evaporated, the finishing steps must be carried out fairly quickly, aiming for 90 seconds or less to complete the cutting open of the frozen drug canister, the transfer of its contents to the fresh canister containing the radioactivity, and the crimping of a new metering valve onto the radioactive canister. If this procedure takes longer, there is a risk that a significant amount of propellant will evaporate, changing the vapor pressure of the newly sealed canister, and subsequently the unit dose and particle size characteristics of the dispensed tracer aerosol.

When the radioactive canister reaches room temperature, 15-unit (emitted or exactuator) doses should be dispensed. The first five doses are considered priming doses and are to be discarded, along with the actuator mouthpiece. The remaining ten doses are each collected into individual dose collection tubes (Figure 5.1) [84] using a fresh actuator mouthpiece. The radioactivity from the single sprays can be measured directly in the dose calibrator and the drug content assayed chemically afterwards. However, if the doses are inconsistent, another ten must be dispensed. The canister should be discarded if the unit doses fall outside of the allowable FDA limits [85]. It is not possible to accurately measure the dispensed dose for each individual subject inhaling a single puff from the pMDI by counting the canister before and after the subject has inhaled his/her dose. The total radioactivity in the labeled canister is much higher than the radioactivity contained in a single actuated dose, and the sensitivity of most dose calibrators is such that the detection of the difference of one dose from the total load tends to be unreliable. One should also not divide the total amount of radioactivity in the pMDI by the number of doses in the canister, for several reasons. The radioactivity that is adsorbed onto the walls of the canister and metering valve, and, hence, not available for inhalation, is counted as part of the total canister dose. In addition, the number of doses cannot be accurately known because there is usually overfill by the drug company and the evaporation of propellant when the can is opened during the radiolabeling procedure may result in loss of doses. Because the mean of the ten doses of radioactivity is used in the calculation of lung deposition when expressing the results as a percentage of the inhaled or emitted dose from the delivery system, the introduction of variability in the emitted dose of radioactivity should be minimized, aiming for a coefficient of variation of the measured single unit doses of less than 15%. Good labeling technique, reproducible dose-collection procedures, and correction of dose measurements for decay of isotope all contribute to minimization of error.

Suspension pMDIs are more difficult to label than solution pMDIs, but for both types of pMDIs, the label is soluble in the propellant and associated only with the drug or other excipients in the canister. Thus, 2D imaging must begin immediately after inhaling the dose. Radiolabeled pMDI suspensions should be shaken prior to use, particularly if they were prepared several hours earlier and at least three priming doses wasted before the subject inhales the radioactive dose.

5.2.3.2 Nebulizers

With nebulizer solution formulations, the labeling process to produce an aerosol for planar and SPECT imaging is fairly straightforward, in that the radioactivity, nonabsorbable tracers, such as ^{99m}Tc-HSA or ^{99m}Tc-SC or ^{99m}Tc-DTPA, are mixed into the drug product. These compounds, made either from commercial kits or by implementing approved radiopharmacy protocols, are also used as diagnostic agents in nuclear medicine. Each droplet will contain amounts of drug, carrier, and radioactivity in proportion

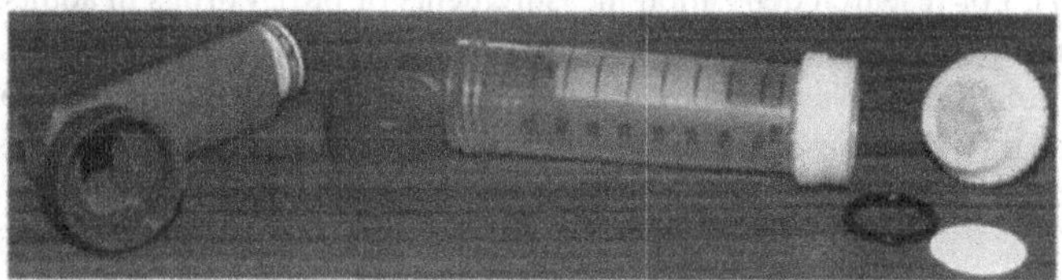

FIGURE 5.1 Unit Dose Collection Apparatus (UDA) for aerosol emitted from an aerosol delivery device. The setup is shown with a pMDI interface, but similar connecting pieces have been made in our laboratory for nebulizers. The sample is collected in the tube and solvent added to absorb the drug collected on the filter. (With kind permission from Taylor & Francis: *Respir. Care, Assessing nebulizer performance*, 47, 2002, 1290–1301, Dolovich, M.B.)

to the original concentrations. However, the radiolabel is not bound to the drug, but is associated with it, within the droplet. With the exception of DTPA in smokers and patients with interstitial lung disease, they all have effective $t^{1/2}$ comparable to the physical half-life of ^{99m}Tc, thus allowing imaging to occur over time and without loss of the tracer, other than from natural decay of the isotope and via mucociliary clearance from the lung. The drug particles in nebulizer suspensions cannot be labeled in this way; mixing the radioactivity into the nebulizer suspension means that only the carrier is labeled and not the drug. While it is the droplet size that determines the deposition distribution of the aerosol in the lung, one cannot infer deposited drug dose from these measurements without a parallel measurement of the drug content within the droplets.

5.2.3.3 Powders

Techniques for labeling drug powders are more complex than those used for pMDIs. As with pressurized aerosols, pertechnetate must first be extracted from saline. It is possible to apply a nonabsorbable ^{99m}Tc label onto the powder particles, but this technique is dependent on the category of drug being labeled [86]. Lactose, if a part of the formulation, is blended into the powder after the labeling and prior to loading of the labeled powder into capsules or blisters or to placing it in the DPI reservoir. A method devised by Newman et al. mixed radioactivity, following extraction and evaporation of solvent, into the dry powder [87]. While successful, the technique assumes an even mixing of the components and may explain why deposition values for budesonide in the Turbuhaler vary between laboratories [62]. The radioactivity is associated with the drug and is not a firm chemical or physical bond with the drug molecule.

With breath-actuated inhalers such as DPIs, the variability in dispensing the dose between individual places added importance on knowing the absolute amount of radioactivity actually inhaled. For DPIs designed to dispense multi- or single unit doses rather than dispensing from a reservoir, the amount can be obtained if the radioactivity in the inhaler is assayed in a dose calibrator pre- and then postinhalation for *each* study subject to give, respectively, the nominal or metered dose and the dose remaining in the DPI. The difference between these two measurements is the dose of drug emitted from the inhaler or inhaled at the mouth. Figure 5.2 shows a reasonable correlation between the deposited lung dose, measured with the gamma camera and expressed as a percentage of the nominal dose, and that portion of the nominal dose containing drug in particles of less than 5 μm (fine particle dose), measured by the dose calibrator [88]. The variability in the fine particle dose for both inspiratory flow rates tested contributed to differences in deposition between subjects, adding to other influencing factors, such as airway caliber. Therefore, it is important to account for dose differences by normalizing the data so as not to introduce additional error in the calculations. Accurate calculations of deposited dose, either as a percentage of the nominal or emitted dose or

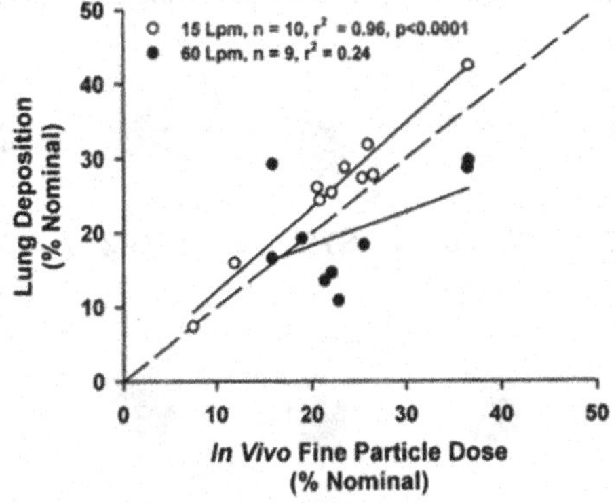

FIGURE 5.2 Relationship between deposition of a radiolabeled DPI aerosol and the measured fine particle dose of the labeled powder inhaled for each subject. Both variables are expressed as the percent of nominal dose. The correlation is higher for the lower flow rate used to inhale the powder, possibly due to the more consistent amount of drug deposited in the oropharynx. (With kind permission from Taylor & Francis: *Am. J. Respir. Crit. Care Med.*, Lung deposition of albuterol sulphate from the Dura Dryhaler in normal adults, 153, 1996, A62, Dolovich, M. et al.)

in absolute terms, i.e. as microcuries of radioactivity or micrograms of drug, cannot be made without the measurement of inhaled dose. When this is done, the fine particle dose of the inhaled aerosol can provide a good estimate for dose deposited below the larynx, as seen in mean data obtained for several other DPIs [89].

For deposition studies to be an accurate representation of the behavior of the drug inhaled, the aerosol produced from the tracer powder must be similar to the unlabeled aerosol, and validation of its performance characteristics must be demonstrated prior to use. This involves the same sizing and dosing measurements described earlier.

5.2.4 Validation of a Radiolabeled Aerosol Formulation: Particle Size and Unit Dose

Deposition is a function of the particle size characteristics of the aerosol, and the in vivo response is influenced by the dose of drug inhaled per actuation from the inhaler. Thus, prior to using a labeled aerosol product to measure lung deposition and response, confirmation that the aerosol characteristics have not been altered by the labeling procedure must be obtained, as well as demonstrating that the dose of active substance in the aerosol formulation is dispensed consistently, similar to the original nonlabeled formulation, and that the drug is viable. The latter is particularly important when using imaging and simultaneous pharmacokinetic measurements to assess the response to the radiolabeled drug postinhalation [90].

5.2.4.1 Particle Size Measurements for Validation

The validity of the radiolabeling process is confirmed by a three-way comparison of drug particle size distributions before and after labeling and to the size distribution of radioactivity in the drug product after labeling [61,63]. The characterization of the aerosols is typically performed using cascade impaction, counting the radioactivity deposited on the impactor stages (Figure 5.3), and then assaying the drug chemically. The unit spray content and consistency (drug, radioactivity) of the emitted doses from the aerosol inhaler, that is, a pMDI, DPI, or nebulizer, are assessed by comparing the amount and variability of drug (micrograms) and radioactivity (microcuries) emitted per actuation pre- and postlabeling, as well as the coefficient of variation for the unit doses in terms of drug and radioactivity. Limits for acceptability are specified in the U.S. FDA Guidance for Industry—Metered-Dose Inhalers (MDI) and Dry Powder Inhaler (DPI) Drug Products—Chemistry, Manufacturing and Controls Documentation, issued in 1998 [85]. For synthesis of drugs with positron emitters, the structure and purity of the radiotracer must be verified, using HPLC, in comparison to an authentic standard prior to administration to human subjects.

When validating whether a radiolabeled aerosol has the same properties as the original aerosol, one needs to use a sizing system that gives both the measurement of the drug substance and the radioactivity. While there are a number of instruments used for sampling and classifying aerosols, multistage cascade impactors

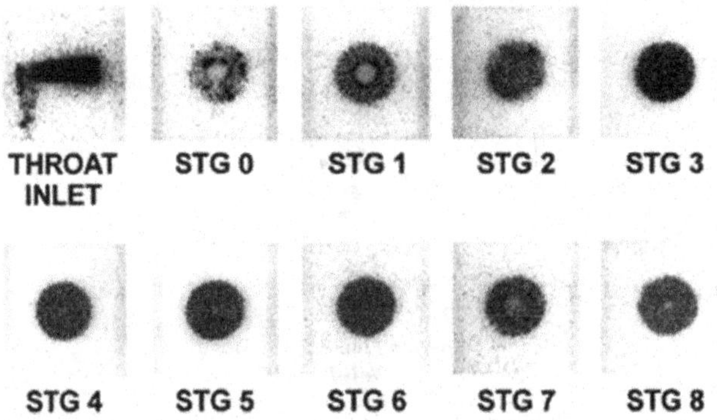

FIGURE 5.3 Individual stage plates and inlet from the Anderson Cascade Impactor showing the pattern of radioactivity on the plates following sizing of a radiolabeled pMDI formulation. The plates and inlet were placed on the planar gamma camera face and imaged to measure the amount of deposited radioactivity. The plates were subsequently washed with solvent and assayed using UV spectroscopy to obtain the amount of drug deposited.

are used for validation work because radioactivity can be measured on the individual stage plates, and then the drug can be dissolved off the plates and assayed chemically by UV spectroscopy or HPLC. The latter is particularly useful for single doses or small quantities of drug. Using these data allow the frequency distributions for particle diameter in terms of radioactivity and mass of drug to be plotted in parallel.

Figure 5.4a and b give examples of graphs plotted from sizing data obtained for a radiolabeled formulation in comparison to the unlabeled or control formulation. The graphs plotted are the frequency and cumulative mass distributions for drug mass and radioactivity [86]. Figure 5.4c gives the line of identity (LOI) between drug mass and radioactivity in this particular formulation. All the data from all the impactor stages from 19 sizing runs have been plotted. The deviation from the line of identity allows one to see the extent of the variability of the "match" within the aerosol. Statistically, the radiolabel was considered to be a match and reliable surrogate for the drug, and it was subsequently used in a deposition study in asthmatic subjects.

5.2.4.2 Measurement of Dose of Radioactivity and Drug to Be Administered

As described earlier, unit doses of dispensed aerosol—pressurized, powder, or liquid—can be collected in the apparatus shown in Figure 5.1 [84,91]. The single doses are dispensed into the tube, using a suction airflow matching that for the impactor sizings and the inspiratory flowrate to be used by the study subjects.

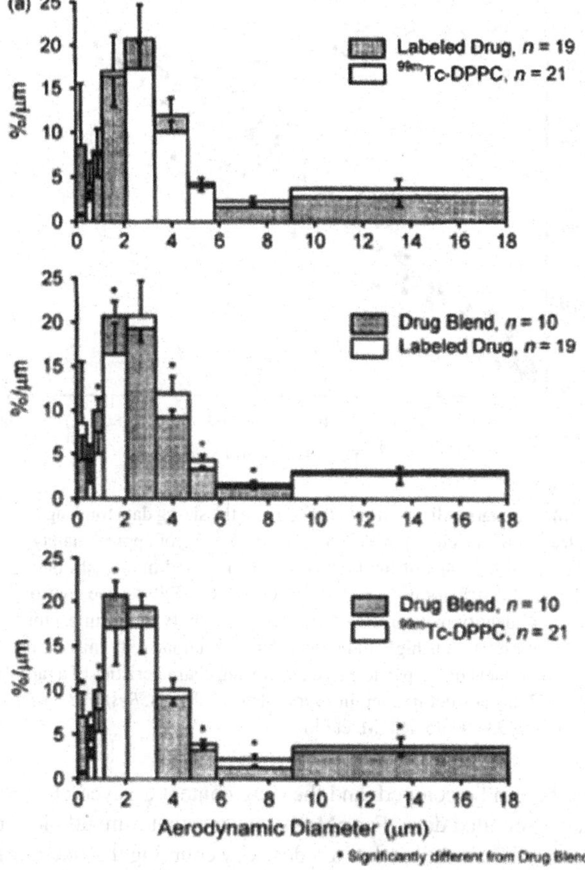

FIGURE 5.4 (a) Frequency distribution of drug mass and radioactivity for a radiolabeled powder and the drug in the original (control) powder versus aerodynamic particle diameter, obtained to validate the radiolabeled powder for deposition experiments. Measurements were obtained using the Anderson Cascade Impactor operated at 28 lpm. While the statistical comparisons showed significant differences between some of the amounts of drug and radioactivity on several of the stages, the differences were small and not sufficient to preclude the aerosol from being used in deposition studies. The drug was unchanged by the labeling process. *(Continued)*

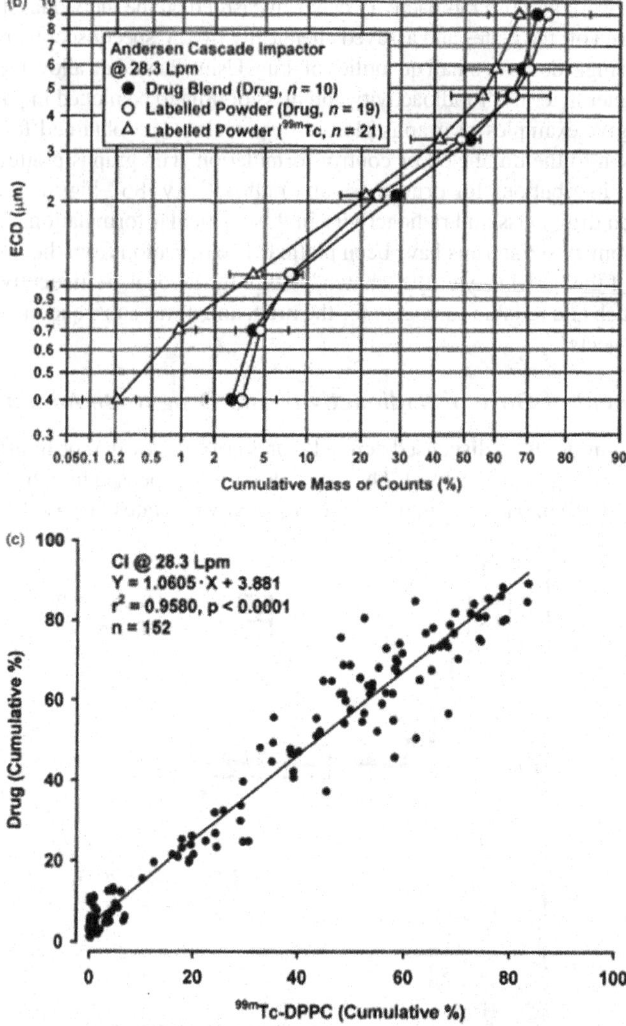

FIGURE 5.4 (Continued) (b) Cumulative distribution plotted from the sizing data for drug and radioactivity in the radiolabeled formulation and the drug in the original powder. A mean difference of approximately 3.0% was obtained between the radioactivity and drug on the lowest stage of the impactor. This resulted in a small, but significant difference in the FPF (% < 5.8 μm) between the three distributions ($p = 0.01$, ANOVA). The FPF for the control powder and the drug in the labeled powder were the same, (c) identity plot for the drug and radioactivity on all impactor plates from 19 sizings of a labeled powder formulation. The correlation is high, indicating that the radioactivity mirrors the drug. (With kind permission from Taylor & Francis: Measurement of the particle size and dosing characteristics of a radiolabeled albuterol-sulphate lactose blend used in the SPIROS7 dry powder inhaler, in: Byron, P.R. et al., eds, *Respiratory Drug Delivery V*, Interpharm Press, Buffalo Grove, IL, 1996, 332–335, Dolovich, M. et al.)

The radioactivity in the tube can be counted, and the drug content assayed chemically by UV spectroscopy or HPLC to provide the emitted dose. For pMDIs, mean actuator mouthpiece content of radioactivity and drug can be determined from the total of ten doses by counting the actuator in the dose calibrator, the drug is measured by dropping the actuator into a fixed volume of solvent and assaying the drug content chemically.

Figure 5.5 [86] shows an example of the mean unit spray content for drug and radioactivity for several study days using this labeled powder. Each bar of the graph represents a mean ± standard deviation of ten unit doses. While the coefficient of variation (CV) of the daily measurements for both drug and radioactivity must be within specified limits, it should be understood that the mean daily level of radioactivity

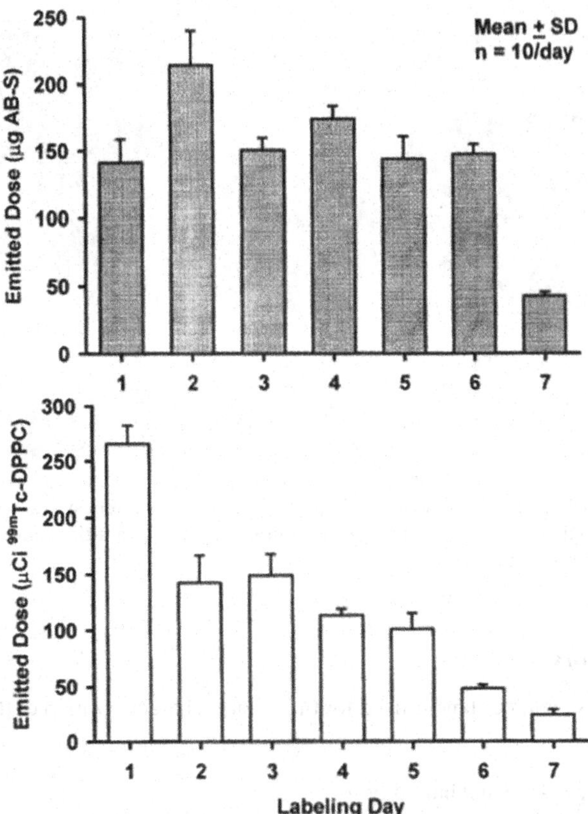

FIGURE 5.5 Graph demonstrating in vitro reproducibility of the emitted dose for a radiolabeled drug powder inhaled at two different inspiratory flowrates. Although the mean dose of drug and radioactivity varied between study days, the coefficient of variation for the emitted doses of drug or radioactivity on each study day was low. The amount of radioactivity used in the labeling of the powder varied with the specific activity of the $^{99m}TcO_4^-$ supply on each labeling day. (With kind permission from Taylor & Francis: Measurement of the particle size and dosing characteristics of a radiolabeled albuterol-sulphate lactose blend used in the SPIROS7 dry powder inhaler, in: Byron, P.R. et al., eds, *Respiratory Drug Delivery V*, Interpharm Press, Buffalo Grove, IL, 1996, 332–335, Dolovich, M. et al.)

in the formulation or nominal dose of radioactivity varies as a function of the level of the specific activity available from the generator on the day of the study. This variability in the amount of radioactivity affects only the absolute dose of radioactivity inhaled and not the measured deposition distribution. Deposition results should be normalized to account for these differences, even for the small, day-to-day variability in the supply of radioactivity.

Because radiolabeling techniques are not precise and specific activities of the isotopes can vary, validation and calibration should be done for each radiolabeled aerosol produced. In particular, the measurement of emitted doses provides the mean value for the dose of radioactivity administered, which must be further corrected for decay between the time of production and the time of use. This value is critical if calculating absolute doses inhaled rather than percentages of radioactivity distributed within the respiratory tract.

Provided that the radiolabeling process does not alter the particle size distribution of the emitted drug and that the size distribution of the radiotracer is similar, the radiolabeled formulation may be used to measure total lung deposition and distribution of the inhaled drug. If clinical response measurements are performed following inhalation of the radiolabeled pMDI aerosol, the particle size characteristics and dose of drug per actuation in the radiolabeled formulation must match those of the drug in the unlabelled or original formulation. A successful match is indicated by an equivalent in vivo clinical response to the labeled and unlabeled formulations. Useful information from these studies will be obtained only if the label accurately follows the drug during inhalation.

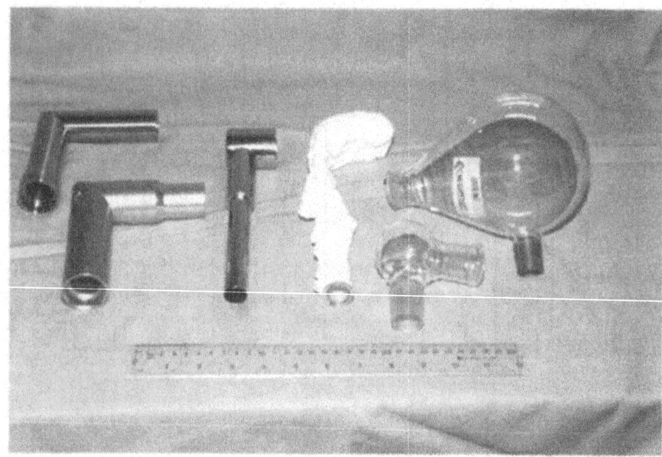

FIGURE 5.6 Different inlets used to couple a cascade impactor to an aerosol delivery system. The inlets range in volume from 66 mL to 1080 mL [92] and collect varying amounts of drug, depending on their volume. This in turn affects the amount of aerosol sampled by the impactor.

5.2.4.3 Other Factors

Additional factors that should be standardized for the in vitro characterization of the aerosol size distribution are:

- The ambient temperature and humidity
- The inlet stage or entry port for the sizing system (Figure 5.6 [92])
- The coupling of the inhaler to the inlet stage
- The number of priming doses to be "wasted" from the inhaler prior to sampling the aerosol
- The number of doses sampled
- The time between actuations
- Whether a pMDI is shaken between doses
- The type of pMDI actuator mouthpiece used
- The expression of the results

With a sensitive balance, it is possible to measure the actual weight of drug deposited on the various stages of the impactor. The weight, however, would include the weight of any excipients in the formulation as well as the drug. For any impactor sizing system used and where drug assays are required for analysis, reproducible standard curves must be produced for each drug tested. Standard curves for the drug on impactor plates, filters, impactor inlets, and the unit dose collection apparatus should be obtained to correct for the possibility of interference from extractables.

5.3 Control During Inhalation of a Radiolabeled Aerosol and Subject Variables

Lung deposition varies with the drug and the formulation. In addition, many of the 2D deposition studies have been performed in normal, healthy volunteers rather than in the patient groups intended for the therapy. This option of using normals is chosen for several reasons. The subject with normal pulmonary function provides the best possible outcome or the "envelope" for the deposition value obtained. Patients with lung disease may have greater or lesser deposition compared to normals, depending upon the particle size characteristics of the test aerosol and the inspiratory volumes and flow rates used during aerosol inhalation. The regional distribution of the inhaled therapy within the lung would, however, be abnormal [11,93–96]. It is often easier to solicit normal healthy volunteers for deposition studies, and certainly there is not the inevitable rescheduling due to variability in baseline lung function or exacerbations of the disease that occurs when doing studies in patients. However, the drugs being tested are to be prescribed for the treatment of respiratory and other diseases. Therefore, knowing the lung deposition and distribution in the various patient groups is more relevant to the assessment of the drug and the delivery device.

When designing protocols to measure deposition, a number of clinical factors need to be considered and incorporated into the study design: subjects' age, sex, smoking history, and current drug regimens, presence of a viral infection, severity of disease, stability of pulmonary function, and other outcome measures that could affect the inhalation of the radioaerosol, the measurement of deposition, and the results. Some of these also apply when using healthy volunteers as subjects for deposition studies. For example, we allow a 4- to 6-week recovery period between repeat studies for subjects who have suffered an exacerbation of their asthma or developed a chest cold or infection after enrolment.

The particle size of therapeutic aerosols range from <l- μm mass median aerodynamic diameter (MMAD) to 8 μm MMAD. However, the "effect" of particle size, once the inspiratory flowrate is taken into account, can be much greater, shifting the deposition pattern to more proximal airways, as does airway narrowing due to the presence of lung disease, effects demonstrated in a number of published deposition studies. Thus the inhalation variables—inspiratory flowrate, inspiratory volume, and time of breath hold—are important to control during the inhalation of the tracer aerosol [11,97,98]. This can be accomplished by either training the subject prior to the inhalation man oeuvre or using a monitoring system with or without visual feedback. While this level of control is rarely present during actual patient use of the inhaler, nonetheless, it is important to the interpretation of deposition results if the objective is to determine delivery efficiency under optimal conditions of use. Small changes in particle size and/or inspiratory flowrate can influence the deposition measurement (Figure 5.7, [99]). Control of these variables may contribute to a reduction in inter-subject variability in deposition and, perhaps, response to the therapy. Similarly, when measuring deposition in patients, clinical classification of their disease must be documented, and an attempt should be made to study patients with similar severities or extent of airway narrowing.

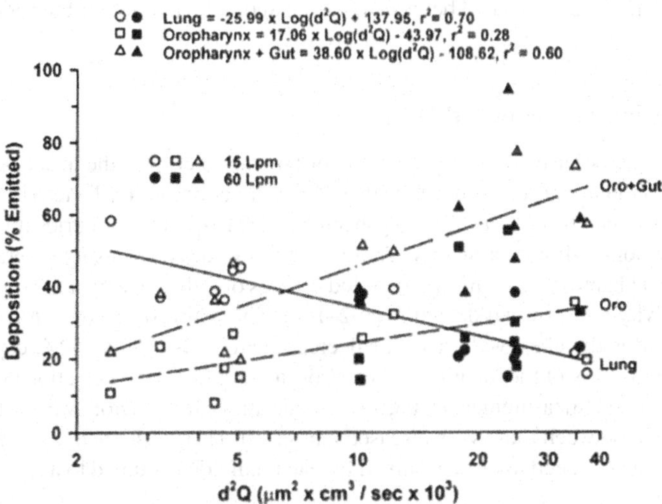

FIGURE 5.7 Deposition in the lung, the oropharynx, and the sum of the oropharynx and gut, expressed as the percent of nominal dose, plotted against the impaction parameter, d^2Q, where d is particle size and Q is inspiratory flow rate [99]. With this particular inhaler, a four-fold difference in Q caused a marked shift in the distribution of drug between lung and oropharynx and gut. Variability in deposition seen between subjects may be reduced by controlling the particle size of the inhaled drug and the inspiratory flowrate during the inhalation man oeuvre.

Other technical factors influencing the delivery and measurement of the radioactivity must be well controlled. Some of these are:

- Use of the same collimator for all studies.
- Position of the subject in front of the gamma camera and restriction of movement of the subject during imaging [100].
- Careful notation of image acquisition times and times of the in vitro emitted dose measurements prior to administration of the radiolabeled formulation in order that all data can be corrected for decay to a common time (time 0).
- Normalization of acquired counts for time to account for different imaging times between subjects. Images presented should have the same acquisition time because the scans can then be compared visually for differences in deposited radioactivity. This can be done, however, only if the nominal dose is similar between subjects. The use of color palettes can be misleading when presenting images of different subjects within a study, unless the scale relating count levels to color is kept the same for all images.
- Accurate measurement of the various calibration factors to be applied to both the in vivo data and any gamma camera images taken of inhalers and tubing. These latter calibration factors are different from those for the subject and need to be measured using sources or phantoms with known quantities of the same radioactivity as being inhaled.
- Ensuring a tight mouthpiece seal between the subject and the delivery system to avoid loss of aerosol inhaled and contamination of the room [101]. The use of a facemask is not recommended, except for infants.

5.4 Data Analysis

When imaging a subject after inhalation of a radiolabeled formulation, it is the radioactivity that is detected and measured; absolute amounts of deposited drug are inferred from the counts of radioactivity in the lung and other regions, based on the assumption that there is a 1:1 relationship between the two components. This relationship holds true for direct-labeled PET products or for those formulations where a firm bond can be demonstrated between the drug and radioactivity for the time taken to acquire all the images.

5.4.1 Determination of Deposited Dose

A number of investigators have addressed the issue of how to determine the absolute dose of radioactivity deposited in the lung and measured by either 2D or 3D imaging. Radioactivity counted over the lung field (counts/time) can be converted to megabecquerels (MBq) or microcuries (μCi) detected in the lung by applying various calibration factors. These factors are measured using several techniques that utilize either external phantoms containing calibrated sources of radioactivity or the injection of a known amount of radioactivity and external detection [102–107]. The main source of reduction in the level of radioactivity detected is the chest wall, and this decrease can be as high as 50%, depending upon the subject [107]. The sensitivity of the imaging detector/collimator affects the detection of radioactivity and should be factored into the measurements [108,109]. Tissue attenuation factors vary between individuals with normal lungs and between those with diseased lungs [110–112], with greater variability in the latter group. Hence, these factors need to be determined for each individual studied to accurately calculate the deposited lung dose.

It should be recognized that the deposited dose is a fraction of the dose inhaled and that the inhaled dose is, in turn, a fraction of the nominal, or label claim, dose of the inhaler. Estimates of inhaled doses correlate with the fine particle dose, calculated from the fine particle fraction (% particles < 4.7 μm or <5.8 μm in diameter) of the aerosol and the emitted ex-actuator or ex-device dose from the aerosol inhaler. The latter are measured in terms of radioactivity and drug prior to delivering the aerosol for deposition measurements. Drug deposition in the lung will further be reduced due to losses occurring in the inhaler device and in the oropharynx. This is particularly true for spacers attached to pMDIs, where upwards of 60% of the metered dose remains in the spacer. Figure 5.7 illustrates the losses on the actuator mouthpiece and in the spacer, showing how the emitted dose of radioactivity is calculated. When possible, the device should be assayed for radioactivity postinhalation, either using a dose calibrator to measure the absolute amount of radioactivity or imaging the inhaler using the gamma camera and applying the appropriate calibration factors to obtain an absolute dose of radioactivity in the device. If possible, the inhaler can then be assayed for drug. These measurements will allow an estimation of the dose of tracer and drug delivered to the mouth.

5.4.2 Defining Lung Borders and Regions of Interest

Defining the edge of the lung is critical to determining both total and regional deposited doses. Several methods used for delineating the outer lung boundary are described in the literature. The options are:

- A transmission scan with an external source of radioactivity
- Inhalation of a radioactive gas, i.e. ^{133}xenon (^{133}Xe) or ^{81m}krypton (^{81m}Kr)
- Inhalation of an extrafine aerosol (< 1 µm MMAD) of Technegas, ^{99m}technetium (^{99m}Tc), sulfide colloid, or albumin
- Measuring lung perfusion using an injection of ^{99m}Tc macroaggregated albumin

Figure 5.8 illustrates examples of images for all of these procedures, acquired using planar imaging and, with the exception of the transmission scan, obtainable with SPECT imaging. The assessment of ventilation, which usually tracks the edge of the lung, has traditionally been measured with radioactive gases, but the inhalation of extrafine aerosols has been shown to give comparable information both in normals and in patients with airways disease [34,113,114]. While perfusion scanning is considered the "gold" standard [104], all these methods provide an acceptable outline of the lung.

5.4.3 Tissue Attenuation of Radioactivity

Using planar imaging, expressing the dose deposited in the lung in absolute terms requires the measurement of global lung tissue attenuation factors (TAF) to correct for the reduction of activity due to chest wall absorption. These can be determined from a perfusion scan or a transmission scan or by measuring the thickness of the chest with calipers and calculating the factor from derived equations. The perfusion scan uses a known internal source of injected radioactivity,

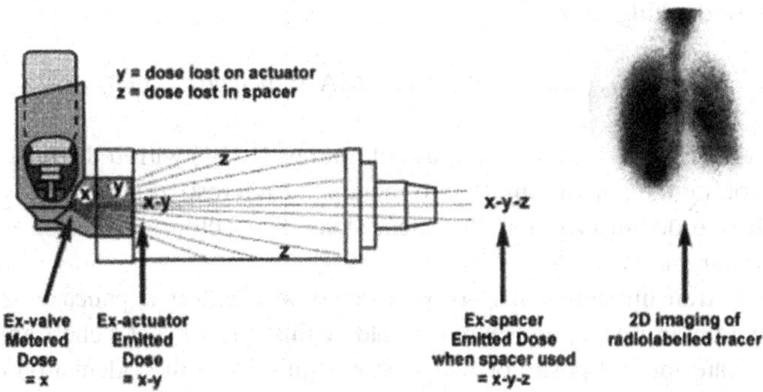

FIGURE 5.8 Schematic illustrating losses of radioactivity and drug in a pMDI and spacer delivery system. The emitted dose calculated when a spacer is used is reduced compared to when the spacer is not used, reflecting the loss of drug in the spacer. The radioactivity deposited in the oropharynx and stomach, shown in the 2D image, is from the coarse aerosol not collected by the spacer, but inhaled.

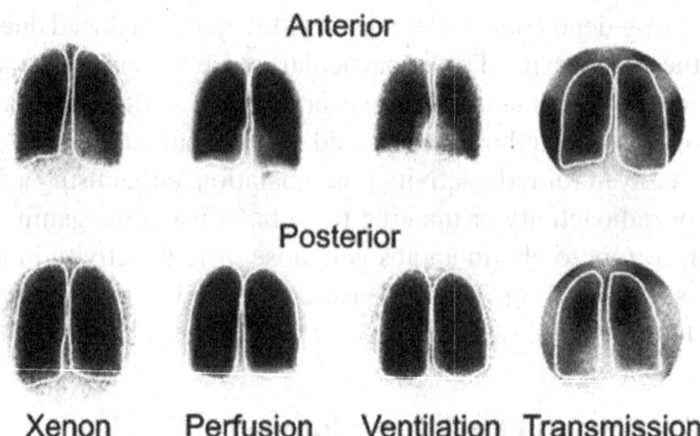

FIGURE 5.9 Methods for outlining the whole lung used in planar or 2D imaging. The area defined by the transmission scan appears to be approximately 10% smaller than with the other techniques. Scatter of low-energy gamma rays into the chest wall area is the most likely explanation for the larger lung seen with inhalation of xenon-133 gas. (With kind permission from Taylor & Francis: *Eur. Resp. J.*, Defining and quantitating peripheral lung deposition using radiolabeled tracers and 2D imaging, 16, 2000, 625, Dolovich, M.B. et al.)

namely, ^{99m}Tc-microaggregated albumin (MAA) particles. Anterior and posterior images of the lung (Figure 5.9) are obtained, the lung edge defined, followed by the calculation of the geometric mean count for the delineated lung. This last step is done to correct the acquired counts for the distance factor, i.e. the decrease in sensitivity of detection of activity emanating from the anterior lung when acquiring a posterior image. An error in the calculation of deposited dose of approximately 15% will be introduced if only the posterior image is acquired (M Dolovich, laboratory data). As the actual dose of injected radioactivity is known, a simple calculation can be made relating counts per minute per microcurie (or megabecquerel) of activity in the whole lung as follows:

Tissue attenuation factor (cpm/μCi) from the perfusion scan (Q):

$$\text{TAF}_Q = \left(N_A \times N_P\right)_Q^{1/2} \times \left(\frac{1}{A_{\text{injected}}}\right) \text{cpm/}\mu\text{Ci} \tag{5.1}$$

where:

N_A is the anterior perfusion cpm = sum of right and left lung cpm

N_P is the posterior perfusion cpm = sum of right and left lung cpm, and $\left(N_A \times N_P\right)^{\frac{1}{2}}$ is the geometric mean count for the lung, cpm

$$A_{\text{injected}} = \text{amount of } ^{99\text{m}}\text{Tc} - \text{MAA injected}, \quad \mu\text{Ci}$$

Factors for the right and left lung and other regions of interest (ROIs) within the lung can be calculated separately by apportioning the amount injected to the area of interest, although this step is not without assumptions, possibly introducing error into the calculations. The factors can then be applied to the emission data for that particular area.

For planar imaging, transmission scans are performed with external pancake sources of ^{58}Co or $^{99m}TcO_4^-$ [109]. To obtain an image, the source is held against the subject's chest and back for a fixed period of time. Both anterior and posterior images are acquired for the calculation of the attenuation factor. In addition, it is necessary to know precisely the dose of radioactivity in the source imaged by the gamma camera and the sensitivity of the gamma camera/collimator system for counting the particular isotope being used.

TAF from the transmission scan (TR):

$$\text{TAF}_{\text{TR}} = \left(N_O / N_T\right)^{1/2} \times 1/E \text{ cpm/}\mu\text{Ci} \tag{5.2}$$

where:

N_O is the geometric mean of flood source count rate with regions defined from the transmission scan
N_T is the geometric mean of count rate from transmission scan for the same regions $= \left(N_A \times N_P\right)_{\text{TR}}^{1/2}$
E is the *gamma* camera sensitivity, cpm/μCi

This procedure can also be applied to the oropharyngeal region using lateral scans of the head and outlining the oropharynx in the images.

5.4.4 Defining Regions of Interest in the Lung

Defining regions of the lung for determining deposition of an inhaled therapy to the small peripheral (P) versus large central (C) airways needs to accurately reflect lung geometry. This is especially true with 2D imaging. Because of the overlapping of airway structures, it is not possible to differentiate radioactivity emanating from small versus large airways [36,116], particularly when imaging immediately following inhalation of the tracer aerosol. Repeat imaging at 24 hours allows MCC to remove aerosol deposited on airway surfaces, leaving the remaining activity "representing" aerosol retained on peripheral airways. Aside from the need to align the subject in the same position in front of the scanner, this measurement is not always convenient to obtain. With 2D imaging, the peripheral region should be a narrow region, defined from the outer edge of the lung. Otherwise, the data are confounded by the detection of radioactivity from larger airways. As illustrated in Figure 5.10, a number of methods have been applied to planar images to define central and peripheral regions within the lung [114]; a comparison between planar imaging and SPECT, using similar definitions for the lung regions demonstrated greater discrimination between aerosol deposited in central versus peripheral regions for SPECT [117]. As described above, the outer boundary of the lungs must be defined in the gamma

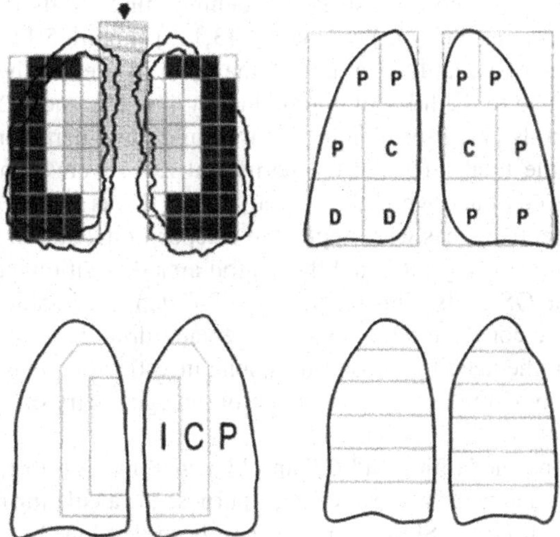

FIGURE 5.10 Various methods for defining regions of interest within the lung for images obtained with planar (2D) scanning. (With kind permission from Taylor & Francis: *Respir. Care*, Methods of calculating lung delivery and deposition of aerosol particles, 45, 2000, 695–711, Kim, C.S.)

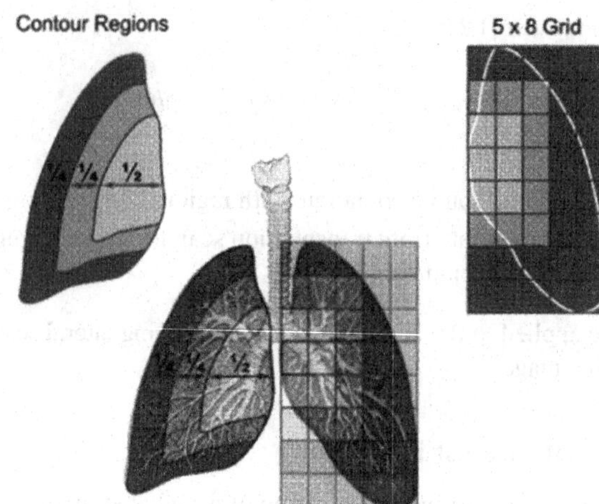

FIGURE 5.11 Illustration of two methods for defining regions of interest in the lung to calculate the distribution to the central and peripheral areas. For the 5 × 8 grid technique, rectangular grids, five sections wide by eight sections high, are placed over the right and left gas-filled lungs so that the perimeter of the grids enclose the lungs. The ROIs, containing different numbers of sections, are then drawn as nested rectangles, centered about the hilus, of varying height and width: outer border of C = 2 × 3, I = 3 × 5, and P = 5 × 8 sections. For regions defined by the onionskin contour method, right and left lung areas are drawn by following the outer contours of the gas-filled lungs. The C, I, and P regions are drawn as three concentric regions from the outer edge to the hilus of the lung, with P and I regions each representing one-fourth the width of the lung and C representing one-half the width of each lung. Significant differences were seen between the central and peripheral regions for the two methods affecting the calculation of the P/C ratio. (With kind permission from Taylor & Francis: *Am. J. Respir. Crit. Care Med.*, Defining lung regions for the purpose of calculating deposition to the small airways, 165, 2002, A190, Dolovich, M. et al.)

camera images—this is the first step in mapping regions within the lung. The whole lung (right and left lungs) region is then further divided into ROIs, which correspond to the large (central), medium, and small (peripheral) airways.

Two methods that have been used extensively for defining three ROIs in planar lung images are the 5 × 8 grid [118] and "onionskin" (OS) contours [113,119] (Figure 5.11). The former divides the lung into rectangular areas of variable size around the hilus, while for the latter, concentric rings are drawn from the lung edge to the hilus of approximately 1/4, 1/4, and 1/2 the lung width. A comparison of these two methods [113] for defining central, mid-, and peripheral lung showed that the cross-sectional areas for the total lung and the peripheral ROIs were significantly greater for the 5 × 8 grid than for the OS contours, while the central lung ROI was significantly smaller, as defined by the grid. When the respective areas were applied to a deposition data set, the values for peripheral lung deposition were significantly greater and the central area deposition significantly less applying the grid as compared to the OS ROIs. This resulted in a P/C deposition ratio significantly greater for the 5 × 8 template, with the conclusion that there was greater drug deposited in the peripheral lung. The comparison points out the need for consensus among investigators imaging the lung for the purposes of assessing drug deposition as to the most appropriate geometry on which to base deposition calculations.

For the other two imaging modalities, SPECT and PET, multiple (up to ten) concentric regions of interest or shells are used to define the geometry for the purpose of calculating regional drug distribution (Figure 5.12). The methods used for SPECT images have been developed by Fleming and colleagues and are described extensively in the literature [40,41,43,107,120,121]. For PET images, the shells are generated from the transmission scans for each transverse slice and applied to the specific emission slice (Figure 5.13). Because of the way PET data are acquired, absolute quantitation of drug dose is possible for discrete areas within the lung.

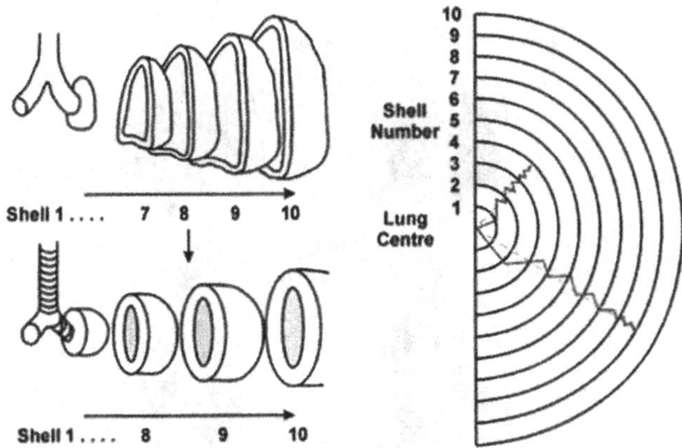

FIGURE 5.12 Illustration of shells constructed for a SPECT analysis. (With kind permission from Taylor & Francis: *J. Aerosol. Med.*, Description of pulmonary deposition of radiolabeled aerosol by airway generation using a conceptual three-dimensional model of lung morphology, 8, 1995, 341–356, Fleming, J.S. et al.)

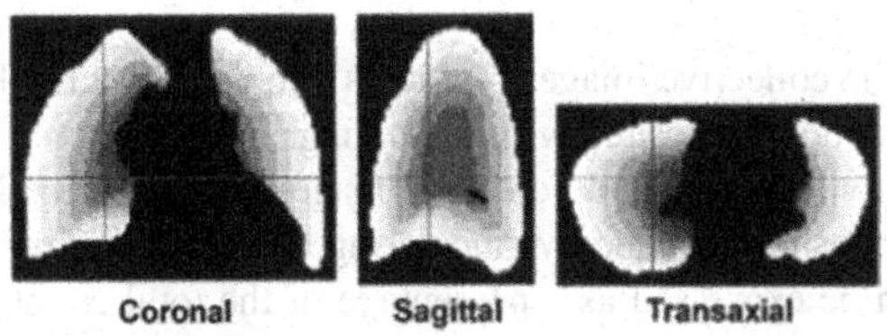

FIGURE 5.13 Applying the PET shell analysis program to the lung images. One transmission slice from each of the coronal, transaxial, and sagittal planes is illustrated. The number of shells will vary with the geometry (cross-sectional area) of the slice. The shell configurations, obtained for the transmission scan slices, are then superimposed on the emission scans, slice by slice, providing volume and activity information related to the distribution of drug within the lung.

5.5 Differences Between Imaging Modalities for the Detection and Measurement of Deposited Radioactivity

A number of steps need to be implemented when using two- and three-dimensional imaging to measure lung deposition. Protocols should be in place to define the edge of the lung and the regions of interest, the measurement of tissue attenuation correction factors that are applied to the scanner data, and the calculation and expression of the deposition results. If possible, the correlation of dose and distribution data with clinical outcome measurements obtained at the time of imaging should be undertaken. There is still no consensus regarding the methods and protocols that should be used for these, but there is general agreement that the steps outlined are necessary to obtain meaningful deposition data.

5.5.1 Planar (2D) Scintigraphy

Planar (or projection) imaging using a gamma scintillation camera is the conventional technique for imaging the lung, providing two-dimensional analogue/digital information on the inhaled radiotracer. It is widely used to measure the dose and distribution of inhaled drugs. Each pixel (picture element) does not provide information on depth, but represents the sum of the radioactivity along the axis perpendicular

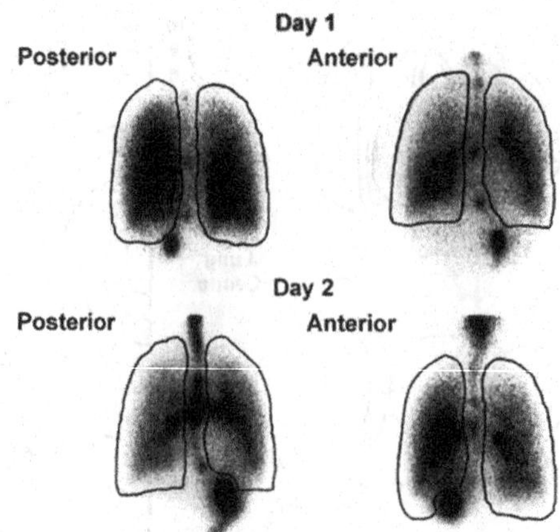

FIGURE 5.14 Planar anterior and posterior images obtained following inhalation of two different-size pMDI aerosols, with the outline of the lung drawn from the anterior and posterior perfusion scans. The difference in geometry and distribution of deposited radioactivity between the anterior and posterior images reflects the proximity of that area of the lung to the gamma camera face.

to the face of the camera. The collective images provide a good sense of total dose, but they are limited in offering information about dose deposited within the lung.

When measuring deposition, anterior and posterior images are obtained (Figure 5.14) and the determination of radioactivity deposited is made by calculating the geometric mean count rate of these two images. The result can then be expressed as a percentage of the total counts detected, or alternatively can be converted, using, as discussed earlier, tissue attenuation factors specific for the individual being imaged, to a deposited dose of radioactivity (μCi) or microgram quantities of drug. This value can be used to calculate inhaler deposition efficiency as a percentage of the emitted or inhaled dose of radioactivity or drug from the delivery system.

For example, when using a perfusion scan to outline the lung and to correct for tissue attenuation of radioactivity, the total lung dose deposited (TLD_d) is calculated as follows:

$$\mathrm{TLD}_d = \left(N_A \times N_P\right)^{1/2} / \mathrm{TAF}_Q, \quad \mu\mathrm{Ci} \tag{5.3}$$

where

N_A is the anterior cpm for the lung following radioaerosol inhalation
N_P is the posterior cpm for the lung following radioaerosol inhalation
TAF_Q is the tissue attenuation factor using perfusion method, cpm/μCi

The dose deposited in the lung (L) as a percentage of the emitted dose or metered dose is calculated as follows:

$$\%\mathrm{ED}_L = \text{dose deposited}_{\mathrm{ED}} = \mathrm{TLD}_d / \mathrm{ED} \times 100, \quad \% \tag{5.4i}$$

or

$$\%\mathrm{MD}_L = \text{dose deposited}_{\mathrm{MD}} = \mathrm{TLD}_d / \mathrm{MD} \times 100, \quad \% \tag{5.4ii}$$

where ED is the emitted dose or dose available at the mouth, in μCi, and MD is the metered dose from the inhaler, in μCi.

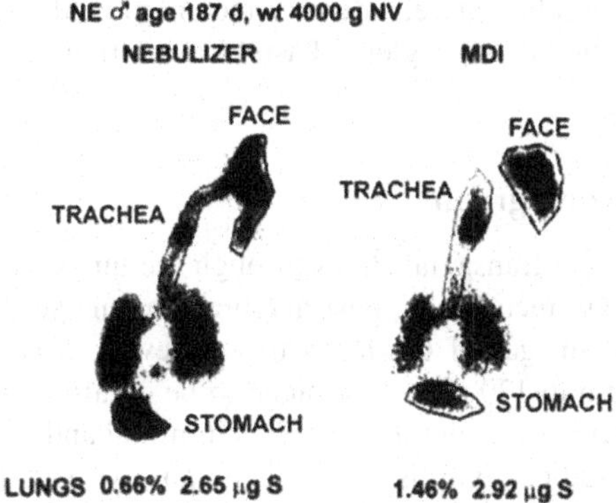

FIGURE 5.15 Deposition images obtained on two separate days for a 4-kg nonventilated neonate following inhalation of a pMDI radioaerosol, $^{99m}TcO_4^-$ salbutamol and a 99mTc-sulfide colloid plus salbutamol nebulizer solution. The lung deposition, expressed as percentages of the emitted dose, showed a two-fold difference between the inhalers, favoring the pMDI. However, a similar lung dose of drug was received from both inhalers when the percentages were converted to absolute doses of salbutamol by using the nominal dose for each delivery system. (With kind permission from Taylor & Francis: *Pediatr. Pulmonol.*, Efficiency of aerosol medication delivery from a metered-dose inhaler versus jet nebulizer in infants with bronchopulmonary dysplasia, 21, 1996, 301–309, Fok, T.F. et al.)

Similar calculations can be done for the different regions of interest in the lung or for the oropharynx and gut. The radioactivity deposited in specified regions of the lung is typically expressed as a percentage of the total lung dose of radioactivity or as a ratio of one region to another, such as the central to peripheral airways. To account for all the activity administered, mouthpieces, actuators, filters, etc. need to be imaged and/or measured in the dose calibrator. In the preceding calculations, the %ED will always be greater than the %MD, but the absolute values calculated for the dose in micrograms will be the same. There is merit in expressing the deposited dose in absolute terms. However, it is essential to measure the emitted dose also in micrograms, particularly when testing subjects with the same inhaler on different days, each day with varying amounts of loaded radioactivity, or when comparing different inhalers in the same subject. As shown in Figure 5.15, while the deposition percentages for the lung were vastly different, the absolute amounts of drug delivered were not, a function of different nominal doses.

5.5.2 Single-Photon-Emission Computed Tomography

SPECT imaging is more complex than planar imaging, in that rather than obtaining single anterior and posterior cumulative two-dimensional images of the thorax, the gamma camera rotates through a full 360° obtaining multiple images from different angles [122]. Subsequent manipulation of the data using computers permits tomographic images to be constructed. This approach has potential advantages in that it improves the accuracy of assessing the pattern of deposition within the lungs. However, it has the associated disadvantages of longer acquisition times and requiring relatively high doses to be administered to improve the counting efficiency per slice. Newer dual- and triple-headed cameras are now available with reduced acquisition times, and they have become the "work horse" camera in many nuclear medicine departments. The per-pixel resolution (8 mm–10 mm) is similar to or better than that of the gamma camera (10 mm–14 mm). To interpret the scans and obtain accurate data, a computed tomography (CT) scan or magnetic resonance imaging (MRI) is required to correct for attenuation and define the edge of the lung [123]. Protocols must be in place to coregister the data from the two machines or, alternatively, density factors are calculated for defined regions and applied to the SPECT emission data on a global basis. Calculation of deposited dose is then made from these data.

5.5.3 Positron-Emission Tomography

PET imaging provides a series of transaxial slices through the lungs, comparable to a CT scan. The transaxial information is used to reconstruct, postimaging, the lung activity for the other two planes, enabling coronal and sagittal images of the lungs to be viewed. PET resolution is approximately 4 mm–6 mm/slice, enabling up to 120 slices per plane to be obtained. Because of the nature of the emissions and the use of coincidence counting, scatter is minimal and location of the pixels or voxels (volume unit) containing the radioactivity is precise. The ability of PET to examine and quantitate regional or local deposition from the coronal, sagittal, or transaxial views has clear advantages over 2D planar imaging (Figure 5.16 [10]).

Correction for the natural decay of the PET isotope used is incorporated into the software protocols; correction for tissue attenuation of the radioactivity is made directly using PET and following each procedure by acquiring a transmission (density) scan with an external source of radioactivity. The advantages are that the geometry is constant, because the patient remains in the same position under the scanner as for the original investigation, and that the corrections are applied to each voxel in each slice of each plane. Applying attenuation correction to deposition data from the emission scans allows absolute amounts of radioactivity to be measured per cubic millimeter of lung tissue, giving the actual topographic distribution of drug throughout the lung. The transmission image also defines the lung borders for each slice, providing landmarks from which to delineate regions of interest in the emission scan (Figure 5.17). When the lungs are imaged over time, the kinetics of the drug can be described for the whole lung as well as for specific regions. As with SPECT, multiple regions of interest or shells (Figure 5.13), concentric about the hilus, can be defined and the deposition data per region of interest, reconstructed in all three planes. Both volume and dose information are obtained from the PET images. The information for deposited dose is obtained by summing the voxel data from the emission scan for designated regions (slices/shells) and applying the appropriate calibration factors, absolute volumes are obtained by summing the number of voxels in the particular regions and applying volume factors. Data can be expressed in a number of ways, including the dose per unit lung volume.

PET techniques offer the important advantage in that the drug under study can be firmly labeled with the appropriate positron emitting isotope, usually ^{11}C or ^{18}F. Thus, deposition reflects the pharmaceutical itself, without interference from free isotope. Fluticasone dipropionate, triamcinolone acetonide, and zanamivir have all been labeled, and their dose and distribution in the respiratory tract and/or the nasal cavity assessed with PET [48,50,124].

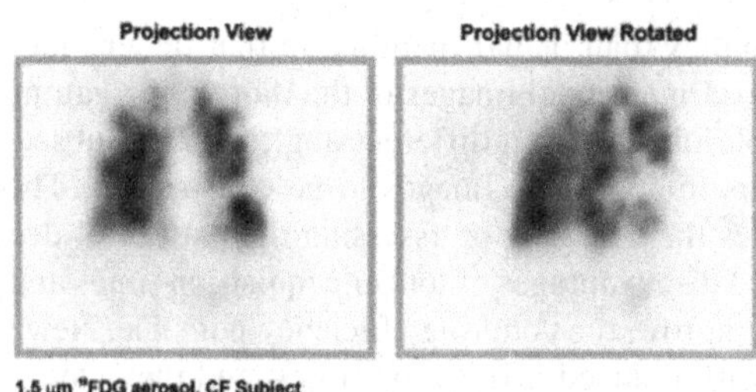

FIGURE 5.16 Projection view from a PET scan for one subject with cystic fibrosis. Rotation of the projection view, shown on the right, indicates that the location of aerosol deposited in both the right lung and left lung is posterior and basal, with some impaction of aerosol in the anterior of the left lung. This information is not apparent in the "head-on" view shown on the left. (With kind permission from Taylor & Francis: Aerosol delivery devices and airways/lung deposition, in: Schleimer, R. et al., eds., *Inhaled Steroids in Asthma: Optimizing Effects in the Airways,* Marcel Dekker, New York, 2002, 169–211, Dolovich, M.)

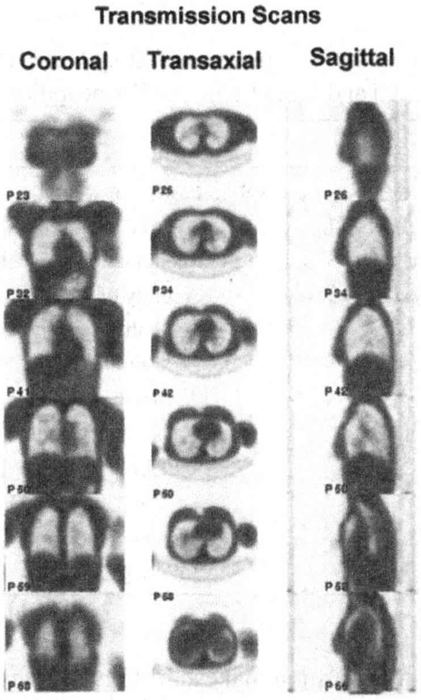

FIGURE 5.17 PET transmission scans for several slices of lung in the three planes showing the difference in geometry of the lung. During the reconstruction of the data, the tissue attenuation factors obtained from the transmission scan are applied to the absolute counts from the emission scan on a voxel-by-voxel basis. In the slice-by-slice analysis of the images, the emission scan of each slice is superimposed on its own transmission slice, allowing a more accurate location of the lung edge for the drawing of the shell regions, a distinct advantage over 2D imaging.

5.6 Aerosols Used in Clinical Investigations of Disease

Several diagnostic tests utilizing specific-size nonradioactive aerosols and also radioactive aerosols with standard nuclear medicine technology are practiced in respiratory medicine (Table 5.2). For example, inhalation of aerosols of methacholine and histamine is widely used to assess nonspecific bronchial responsiveness in asthma; the concentration of the challenge aerosol that provokes a specific fall in FEV1 gives an indication of the severity of the disease. Changes in the disease with treatment or with exposure to sensitizing agents can be monitored over time with repeated measurements. These measurements are coupled with clinical outcomes, such as spirometry and pharmacokinetic and pharmacodynamic measurements in the same group of subjects. In the research laboratory, measurements using radioactive aerosols of these challenge agents have determined the change in distribution effected with changes in airway caliber [125,126], as well as compared techniques and outcomes in inhalation challenge testing [127–129].

Mucociliary clearance, a measure of the surface transport properties of the lung, and lung epithelial permeability, a measure of the integrity of the alveolar-capillary membrane, can be assessed using radiotracers and imaging. MCC is determined from the rate of removal (from ciliated airways) of an inhaled tracer aerosol, while LEP is determined from the rate of removal of an inhaled tracer resulting from absorption across the alveolated surface of the lung and into the circulation. Table 5.3 lists the factors affecting these measurements, some of which need to be controlled when performing these studies [31].

MCC is measured by imaging the lung over time to obtain the retention of an inhaled radioaerosol. Planar imaging is used mainly and serial measurements are required. Because aerosol size and ventilatory parameters affect where aerosol is initially deposited in the lung and because the rate of transport is more rapid from proximal airways than peripheral airways, changes to the initial deposition pattern as a result of treatment or the factors listed in Table 5.3 will have a marked effect on MCC. In addition,

TABLE 5.3

Factors Affecting the Measurement of Lung Mucociliary Clearance (MCC) and Lung Epithelial Permeability (LEP)

MCC	LEP
Site of deposition of tracer aerosol	Molecular weight of solute probe
Particle size of aerosol	Site of deposition of labeled solute
Pattern of inhalation	Recirculation of labeled solute
Airway caliber	Stability of labeled solute in vivo
Lung capacity	Ventilation
Mucus/cilia interaction	Posture
Mucosal surface damage	Apex-base gradient in LEP
Spontaneous cough	Inspiratory volume
Exercise	PEEP
Disease	CPAP
Drugs	Exercise
	Smoking

inter- and intrasubject variability in deposition makes it difficult to do repeated measurements of MCC and to group subjects. The differences between subjects can be partly attributed to airway geometry and lung size [130]; therefore, measurements of lung volumes and expiratory flowrates should be obtained for each subject studied.

Submicronic aerosols of low molecular weight solutes are used to measure epithelial permeability [25,26]; the site of deposition of these tracers must be distal to the ciliated airway surfaces. LEP is measured by dynamic planar imaging of the lung for 15 minutes–30 minutes. Parallel blood samples can be obtained at the same time points to measure plasma radioactivity, but this is not critical to the determination of the rate of absorption of the radiotracer. MCC of the submicronic aerosol is extremely slow, with $t^{1/2}$ in excess of 24 hours. Because LEP is measured over 30 minutes, the error due to MCC is negligible. Peripheral lung regions of interest are usually chosen for analysis of uptake to avoid the contribution from any radioactivity deposited in the hilar regions [131].

Inhalation of hypertonic saline is a noninvasive diagnostic test using nonradioactive aerosols and results in expectoration of sputum. The cellular content of the sputum, related to the degree of inflammation present in the lung in asthma, is then measured using specific laboratory techniques and provides an objective means of monitoring the disease and the effectiveness of anti-inflammatory therapy. Scheduling of these tests, either pre- or postinhalation of the tracer aerosol, would be determined by the clinical question or the research objective.

5.7 Summary

The total and regional dose deposited in the lung obtained using two- or three-dimensional scintigraphic imaging is a useful measurement of topical drug delivery, made doubly useful when correlated with pharmacodynamic and/or and pharmacokinetic data and preferably in the same subjects that undergo imaging. While the accuracy, sensitivity, and resolution of current 2D detectors is high, the use of 3D imaging is to be encouraged [28,45,52]. Further support for the deposition data must be provided by efficacy and safety studies of the test aerosol in various types of patients that would be prescribed the test medications. Knowledge of the lung dose and distribution of inhaled aerosols from delivery systems is critical for the assessment of their performance in vivo and can provide a rationale for adjusting the therapeutic dose for different categories of patients. Arguments for using imaging as a means of predicting clinical response have been raised [120,132]; however, improved accuracy of both in vitro and in vivo data must be demonstrated before this approach is accepted by the medical community as a suitable substitution for biological data.

ADDENDUM

A5.1 Developments in *In Vitro* Measurements

A5.1.1 Standardized Measurement Equipment

Data generated from different laboratories providing comparative performance measurements of the same inhaler should ideally be done using standardized equipment or the same equipment positioned in the different laboratories. This is especially critical for multi-centre imaging studies where it is important to standardized impactor and emitted dose sampling equipment as well as the sampling and active pharmaceutical ingredient (API)/radioactivity detection methods to ensure that the radioactive drug aerosol delivered is validated and comparable between subjects with measurements made prior to exposing subjects (Figure A5.2). Sizing and dose results obtained can then be combined from different test sites. Similarly, implementation of uniform imaging and analysis protocols, in addition to validation of sizing and dosing measurements, are critical to the accuracy of the total and regional lung deposition data obtained.

A5.1.2 Changes in Methodologies to Measure Particle Size

A5.1.2.1 Impactor Inlets

The cascade impactor, for example, the Next Generation Impactor (Copley Scientific, United Kingdom) is used for (Figure A5.3) quality control measurements of the aerosol drug delivery system (A2). However, impactors have been, and increasingly are being used to simulate the delivered dose and predict the deposition pattern of aerosol in the lung, with limited success for a variety of reasons. Recently,

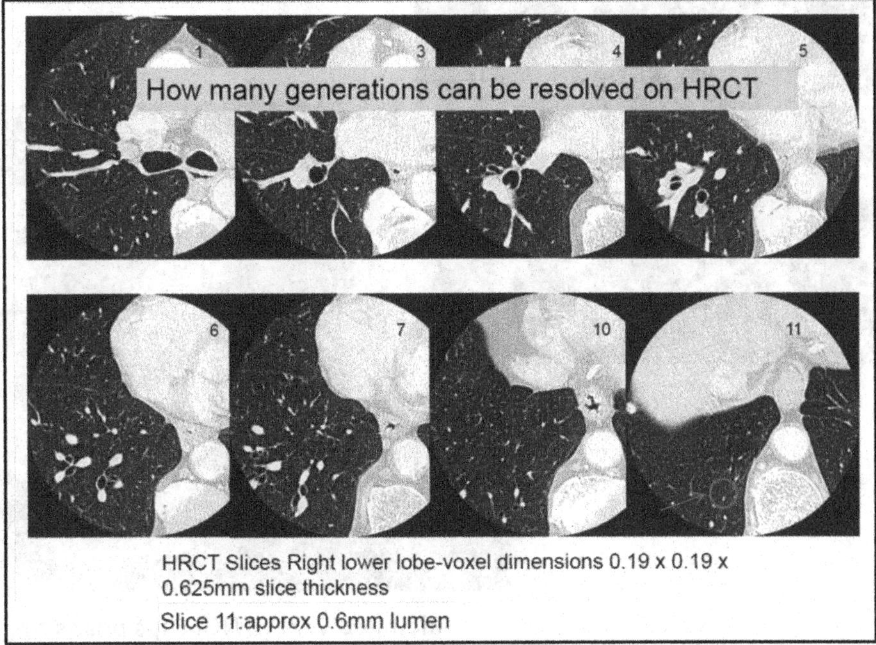

FIGURE A5.1 Eight slices from a high-resolution computed tomography (HRCT) clinical lung scan. One can follow the branching of the airways up until slice 11, which is from the 9th generation and with a luminal diameter of approximately 0.6 mm. Not all scanners have this high a resolution. (Courtesy of Department of Radiology, St Joseph's Healthcare, McMaster University, Hamilton, Ontario, Canada, 2017.)

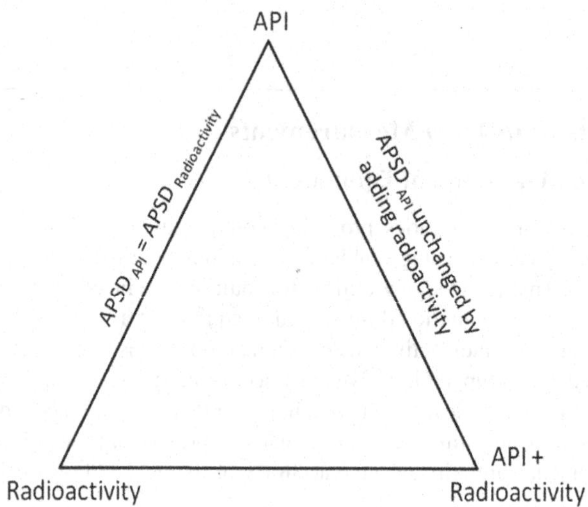

FIGURE A5.2 Cartoon illustrating the matching that needs to be obtained between the API and the radionuclide to produce a surrogate radiolabelled product for inhalation. (Courtesy of Dolovich, M., St Joseph's Healthcare, McMaster University, Hamilton, Ontario, Canada, 2018.)

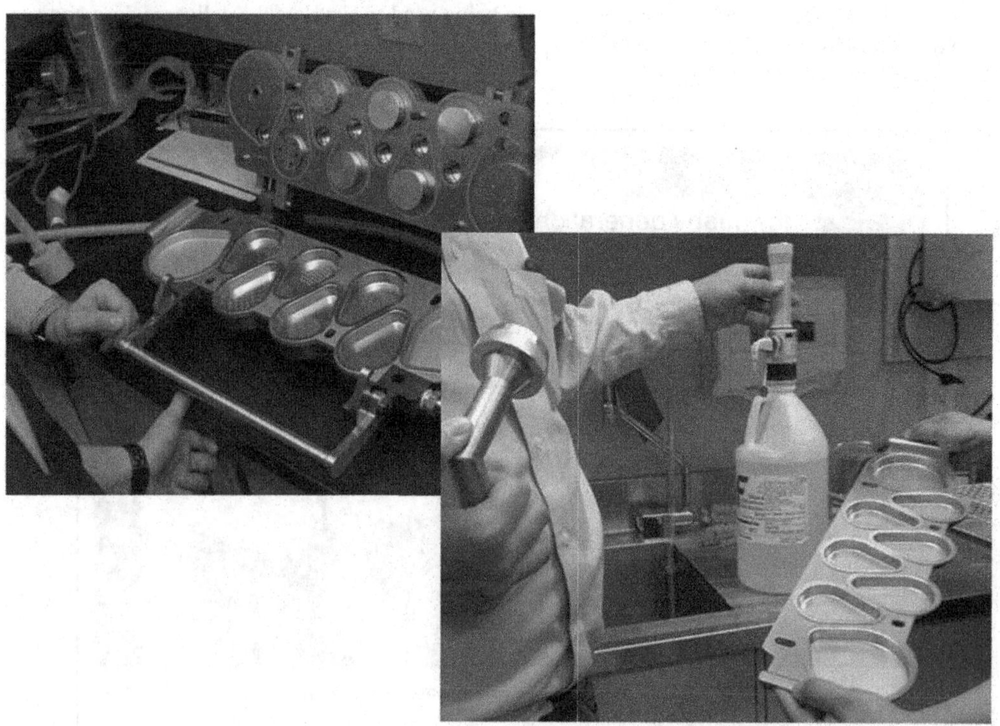

FIGURE A5.3 The Next Generation Impactor is opened after a sampling of powder, showing the stage cups. The distinct deposition pattern can be seen in each cup and is related to the number of holes in the particular stage nozzle. The second illustration shows how an aliquot of solvent is added to each cup to dissolve the drug deposited, allowing the quantities of drug on each stage to be measured.

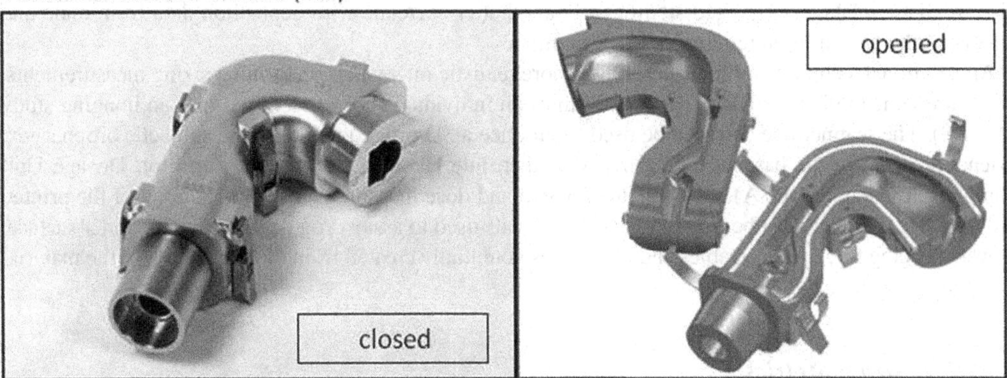

FIGURE A5.4 The adult AIT shown in the closed position and when opened. The channels collecting deposited drug particles or droplets representative of drug collected in the mouth and throat, can be removed easily from the inlet with added solvent. (Courtesy of Copley Scientific, Nottingham, UK.)

inlets that better match the human geometry are being used to introduce aerosol into the impactor system for these modeling purposes. The Alberta Idealized Throat (AIT) is designed for *in vitro* measurements of size and emitted dose. The dimensions of the AIT are based on the geometry of adult human subjects and there is now a pediatric version of this inlet. The performance of the AIT appears to be independent of airflow through the inlet and published results show improved correlation with *in vivo* measurements of deposited drug in the oropharynx compared to the United States Pharmacopeia (USP) inlet (A3,A4). A design benefit of the AIT is that it can be opened (Figure A5.4) along the vertical axis, allowing all of the deposited drug in the main channels of the inlet to be obtained and thus measured with increased accuracy.

Additionally, there are several manufacturers with "small, medium, and large" inlets (Figure A5.5) (A5) that have been compared to the standard USP inlet when performing particle size and dosing measurements, with some similarities and differences in outcome measures such as emitted dose and fine

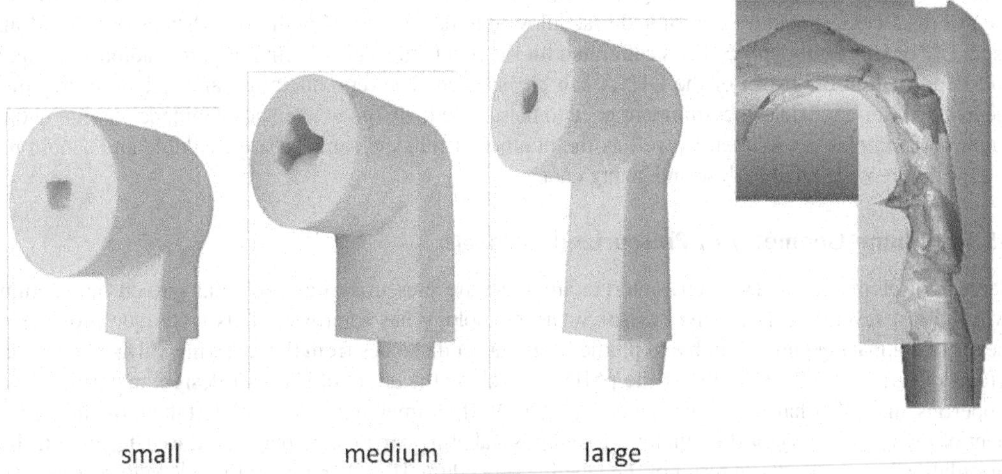

FIGURE A5.5 Small, medium, and large inlets developed by Emmace Consulting AB, Sweden to approximate a child, female adult, and male adult. The illustration on the right shows the internal geometry of the medium inlet. (Courtesy of Emmace Consulting AB, Sweden, www.emmace.se/.)

particle fraction of the test aerosol. Whether the results from these sizing measurements, using these more realistic inlets, are changed significantly and better correlate with deposition data from male and female adults and children remains to be determined.

An additional technique for incorporating a more realistic inlet when performing sizing measurements, for example, is to obtain a HRCT or MRI scan of an individual subject recruited into an imaging study (A6–A8). The scanned file can then be used to produce a 3D printed model of the subject's oropharynx, extending down to the base of the carina. It is then interfaced to the cascade impactor, Dosage Unit Sampling Apparatus (DUSA), or simulator for size and dose measurements. The material of the printed oropharyngeal model must be impervious to chemicals used to assay drug deposited on its inner surface, as well as being free of extractables and leachables potentially created from the interaction of the material with the assay chemicals.

A5.1.2.2 Sizing Metrics

Data from sizing measurements, such as the fine particle fraction, that percentage of the aerosol that is contained in particles or droplets less than 5 μm, is often used to predict the efficiency of delivery of the test aerosol to the distal lung. Its value is also often linked to the dose delivered to the lung, but can result in erroneous predictions. The emitted dose or dose presented to the mouth from the test inhaler can be less than anticipated, and, hence, the fine particle dose or that portion of the emitted dose that contains particles or droplets <5 μm will also be low, despite a high fine particle fraction. Calculating absolute values for doses delivered to the lung is to be preferred to relying on percentages as predictors of dose and should better correlate with imaging data and clinical outcomes.

A5.1.2.3 Emitted Dose Measurements

The DUSA (Copley Scientific, United Kingdom), an apparatus for collecting the dose of aerosol released from an inhaler and collected under fixed and calibrated conditions of airflow rate and "inhaled" volume, has become the standard piece of equipment for the purpose of measuring emitted dose from pMDIs, DPIs, and nebulizers. Its design, properties, and use are described fully in manufacturer's catalogues. Made of Teflon, the DUSA is impervious to chemicals used to dissolve drug particles. As with the connection to the impactor inlet for measuring particle size, interface connectors between the test inhaler and DUSA should be used to provide a firm seal and eliminate air leaks. Figure A5.6 shows the setup of the DUSA for use with a pMDI. For imaging studies, the radioactivity deposited on the removable internal filter of the DUSA should be determined first, allowed to decay over 24 hours, and then assayed for drug using UV or HPLC, both procedures calibrated for the API being studied. Similarly, the radioactivity and API deposited on the barrel of the DUSA can be assessed. The reproducibility and reliability requirements for the emitted dose measurement need to be satisfied with good statistics. Guidance outlining the number of samples per inhaler, as well as the number of inhalers sampled are available and should be followed to provide reliable dose and sizing data.

A5.1.3 Plume Geometry of Pressurized Aerosols

The use of plume geometry to characterize and compare pressurized aerosols has gained momentum over the last several years as this measurement technology has improved. This technique provides a means of comparing plume width and plume length at set distances from the metering valve exit nozzle, effects of different API strengths of the pMDI, as well as the effect of actuator design, metering valve properties, and other hardware components (A9,A10). If an imaging study is undertaken, the measurement of plume geometry of the inhaler pre-and post-labeling can also be performed to determine if the formulation has changed as a result of the labeling procedure. However, unless the radioactive spray can be fully contained, then the measurements should only be done when the radioactivity has decayed to background levels. Plume geometry measurements can also used be to compare properties of generic pMDI formulations versus the reference product of the drug.

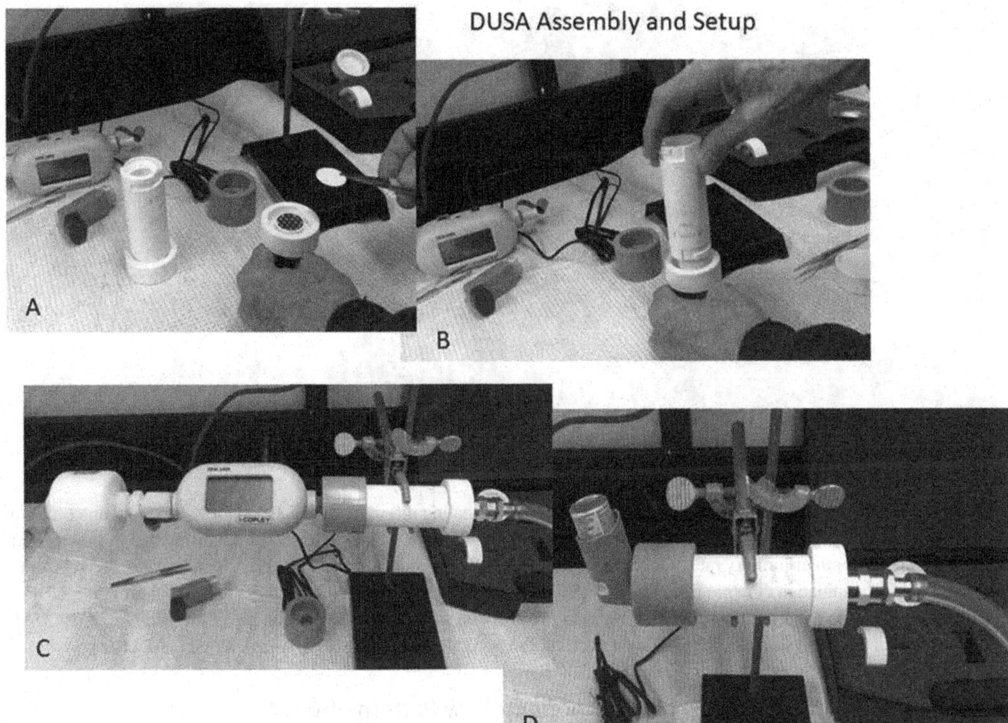

FIGURE A5.6 Preparing the DUSA for sampling A. DUSA components, including the endcaps. The filter to collect the drug is being placed on top of the support screen. B. Assembly of DUSA: the barrel is screwed onto the endcap containing the filter and filter housing. C. Experimental setup, with flow meter to adjust the flow rate through the DUSA. D. DUSA fully assembled with the pMDI inserted into the rubber endcap. Compressed air is turned onto the setting determined in panel C. DUSA Assembly and Setup.

A5.1.4 Flow-Volume Profiles

Obtaining subject flow-volume profiles generated when inhaling through a delivery device is useful information for evaluating the performance of the device when used with an individual subject (Figure A5.7) (A11). The inhalation profiles can be recorded and fed into a model circuit to estimate emitted dose and particle size under realistic inhalation conditions with the inhaler device. The outcome measurements from the simulation are dependent on the speed of inhalation and the volume of drug aerosol inhaled through the delivery device, variables which are subject dependent. Age and lung disease status contribute to the variability in dispersion of the aerosol and hence influence the dose inhaled from the device and the deposition and distribution pattern of the drug in the lung.

A5.1.5 CFD Measurements

This technique is used as a tool to provide information related to air flow patterns through an inhaler device and to help assess the influence of design features and performance following the introduction of a powder cloud or pressurized aerosol into a lung model. Additional areas of investigation using computational fluid dynamics (CFD) are capsule geometry and potentially API strength on airflow (A12,A13). Changes in particle traffic through an inhaler and/or the oropharynx or airway model, which potentially could influence deposition in proximal and distal airways have been investigated using CFD, providing a means of assessing changes during inhaler development and optimizing inhaler design (A14). An example of flow patterns through two different valved holding chambers was recently published by Sarkar et al. (A15) (Figure A5.8) showing the different tracks of airflow within the chamber immediately post

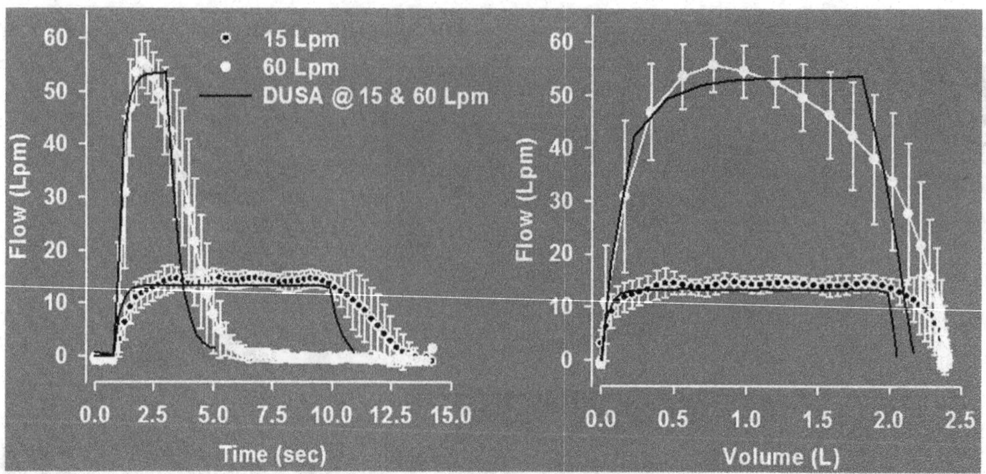

FIGURE A5.7 Flow-time and flow-volume curves from subjects inhaling through a radiolabeled DPI at 15 Lpm and 60 Lpm. The error bars are an indication of the variability between subjects. The solid black line shows the difference in flow pattern through the DUSA at both inspiratory rates. Once the target flow rate was achieved at either inspiratory flow rate, the DUSA rate was constant until the initiation of expiration. The DUSA flow pattern was applied for the *in vitro* measurements of emitted dose and particle size prior to exposing the subjects. (With kind permission from Taylor & Francis: *Am. J. Respir. Crit. Care Med.*, Lung deposition of albuterol sulphate from the Dura Dryhaler in normal adults, 153, 1996, A62, Dolovich, M. et al.)

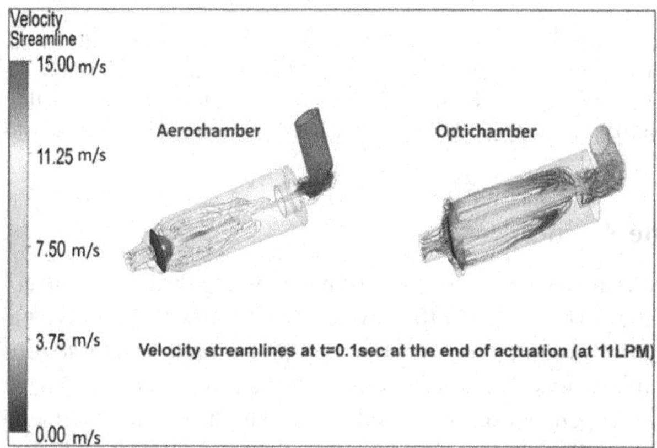

FIGURE A5.8 Multiphase multi-component flow patterns from pMDIs through two valved holding chambers. In addition to indicating the speed of the spray exiting the pMDI, the variable velocity streamlines show possible areas of deposition of drug within the two chambers. Multiphase Multicomponent Flow Patterns from MDIs Through Spacers. (With kind permission from Taylor & Francis: *Int. J. Pharm.*, Investigation of multiphase multicomponent aerosol flow dictating pMDI-spacer interactions, 529, 2017, 264–274, Sarkar, S. et al.)

actuation of the pMDI. The data obtained point to areas of losses of drug within the chamber and on the valved holding chamber (VHC) components and could possibly result in a lower measured emitted dose from the device, perhaps influencing further design features to minimize these losses (A15).

CFD simulation of the oropharynx and tracheobronchial airways has been used extensively to model drug delivery from various inhalers. The complexity of the models increases as more variables are added to achieve a more realistic representation of the human subject (A16,A17).

CFD coupled with CT scans has led to the development of an imaging procedure labeled functional respiratory imaging (A18,A19). This technique combines ventilation changes in the lung, modeled using

CFD, inputting parameters specific to the test aerosol and the subjects being studied. Morphologic airway properties are assessed by CT. The analysis can measure changes to specific airway generations >2 mm, namely, airways up to the 5th or 7th generation, depending on CT resolution and sensitivity. Predictive equations are then applied to calculate lobar deposition changes for smaller, distal airways.

A5.1.6 Second Entry Products or Generics

Measurements of emitted dose and particle size distribution of generic formulations follow the same protocols as for reference products. The determination of bioequivalence required that these metrics give the same results as for the reference products. Similarly, with imaging studies testing generic products, the *in vitro* determinations of size and dose must be compared to the reference inhaler. Including a control group of subjects receiving the reference inhaler on one day and then the generic on another, would likely satisfy most reviewers trying to assess similarity. Pharmacokinetic and pharmacodynamic (PD) studies should also be integrated into the imaging protocol.

The EMA/Health Canada 2006 Guideline for orally inhaled and nasal drug products (OINDPs) is currently being updated (A20). Topics to be addressed include dose proportionality, flow rate dependence, use of spacers, and holding chambers, all of which need to be considered and documented with *in vitro* measurements prior to beginning an imaging study.

A5.2 Developments in *In Vivo* Imaging Measurements

A5.2.1 Imaging Tools

Integrated commercial scanners, SPECT/CT, PET/CT, and also MRI/CT are scanners of choice today, compared to imaging with individual cameras and where the subject is likely moved from one room or floor of the imaging facility to another. Both types of scans are done sequentially on the same machine, eliminating the need to integrate two sets of imaging data to obtain the required information for correction of radioactive decay, tissue attenuation, and lung geometry, all factors applied to each voxel or pixel of the emission data. With hybrid cameras, these factors are built into the software, a major development in terms of reducing imaging time and errors, for example, due to subject movement and changed position from one camera to the other, both of which can result in misalignment of emission and transmission voxels, creating data errors (A21, A22). In centers where hybrid scanners are unavailable, investigators need to follow previous protocols for obtaining transmission scans and correction factors.

A5.2.2 Defining Lung Borders and Regions of Interest

With the improved resolution of newer 3D scanners with combined CT/SPECT, CT/PET, or PET/MRI features, coupled with greater accuracy in the methods for segmentation of the large, central airways as well as image analysis, the definitions of the lung border and regions of interest reflecting airway geometry should result in deposition results that improve correlation with clinical pharmacokinetic and pharmacodynamic outcomes. As demonstrated in the 2004 edition of this chapter, several methods are used to define regions of interest and provide the areas of radioactivity for the deposition calculations. Results are not always comparable for a variety of reasons, such as size of the lung regions, which should define as close as possible, the areas encompassing airways being investigated, inclusion of stomach radioactivity, and background radioactivity ex-lung. With 3D imaging, the latter two areas of activity are more easily defined and excluded, as in the case of the stomach. If required, a region distal from the lung can be outlined and analyzed for the rate and amount of background buildup from absorbed radioactivity.

In addition to Table 5.2 in the main text, the following should be considered when planning an imaging study.

ISSUES TO CONSIDER AND DOCUMENT WHEN IMAGING HUMAN SUBJECTS USING RADIOACTIVITY

- Objective of imaging study
- Camera options
  - 2D (planar) vs. 3D (SPECT, PET, CT)
  - Resolution of scanner
- Selection of tracer ($t_{1/2}$, compound)
- Delivery system
- Labeling procedure
- Lead shielding
- Dosimetry
  - Good signal-to-noise (S/N) ratio
  - Radiation exposure—organ dose and effective whole body (WB) dose
- Validation
  - Tracer versus active drug aerosol
  - Generic versus reference product
- Particle size distribution (MMAD, fine particle fraction, fine particle (WB) dose)
- Emitted dose from delivery system
- Ventilation pattern during inhalation of aerosol
- Segmentation of airways
- Definition of lung regions
- Calculation of regional dose and deposition pattern
- Calculation of pharmacokinetic metrics from inhaled drug (PET study)

ADDENDUM REFERENCES

A1. Evans C, Cipolla D, Chesworth T, Agurell E, Ahrens R, Conner D, Dissanayake S et al. 2012. Equivalence considerations for orally inhaled products for local action–ISAM/IPAC-RS European workshop report. *Journal of Aerosol Medicine and Pulmonary Drug Delivery* 25 (3): 117–139.

A2. Mitchell J, and Dolovich MB. 2012. Clinically relevant test methods to establish in vitro equivalence for spacers and valved holding chambers used with pressurized Metered Dose Inhalers (pMDIs). *Journal of Aerosol Medicine and Pulmonary Drug Delivery* 25 (4): 217–242.

A3. Zhang Y, and Finlay WH. 2005. Experimental measurements of particle deposition in three proximal lung bifurcation models with an idealized mouth-throat. *Journal of Aerosol Medicine* 18 (4): 460–473.

A4. Grgic B, Finlay WH, and Heenan AF. 2004. Regional aerosol deposition and flow measurements in an idealized mouth and throat. *Journal of Aerosol Science* 35 (1): 21–32.

A5. Lastow O, and Svensson M. 2014. Orally inhaled drug performance testing for product development, registration, and quality control. *Journal of Aerosol Medicine and Pulmonary Drug Delivery* 27 (6): 401–407.

A6. Grgic B, Finlay WH, Burnell PKP, and Heenan AF. 2004. In vitro intersubject and intrasubject deposition measurements in realistic mouth–throat geometries. *Journal of Aerosol Science* 35 (8): 1025–1040.

A7. Burnell PK, Asking L, Borgstrom L, Nichols SC, Olsson B, Prime D, and Shrubb I. 2007. Studies of the human oropharyngeal airspaces using magnetic resonance imaging IV—the oropharyngeal retention effect for four inhalation delivery systems. *Journal of Aerosol Medicine* 20 (3): 269–281.

A8. Bücking TM, Hill ER, Robertson JL, Maneas E, Plumb AA, and Nikitichev DI. 2017. From medical imaging data to 3D printed anatomical models. *PLoS One* 12 (5): e0178540.

A9. Farina DJ. 2010. CHAPTER 10–Regulatory aspects of nasal and pulmonary spray drug products. In *Handbook of Non-Invasive Drug Delivery Systems Personal Care & Cosmetic Technology* (Ed) Vitthal S. Kulkarni, pp. 247–290. Boston, MA: William Andrew Publishing.

A10. Li BV, Jin F, Lee SL, Bai T, Chowdhury B, Caramenico HT, and Conner DP. 2013. Bioequivalence for locally acting nasal spray and nasal aerosol products: Standard development and generic approval. *The AAPS Journal* 15 (3): 875–883.

A11. Dolovich M, Rhem R, Rashid F, and Bowen B. 1996. Lung deposition of albuterol sulphate from the Dura Dryhaler in normal adults. *American Journal of Respiratory and Critical Care Medicine* 153 (4(Part2)): A62.
A12. Longest PW, and Holbrook LT. 2012. In silico models of aerosol delivery to the respiratory tract–Development and applications. *Advanced Drug Delivery Reviews* 64 (4): 296–311.
A13. Ryans J, Welch B, Hyun S, Zhang Z, and Kleinstreuer C. 2010. Variations in tracheobronchial airway morphology for different age groups, ASME 2010 Summer Bioengineering Conference, Parts A and B, Naples, Florida, June 16–19, 667–668.
A14. Koullapis PG, Kassinos SC, Bivolarova MP, and Melikov AK. 2016. Particle deposition in a realistic geometry of the human conducting airways: Effects of inlet velocity profile, inhalation flowrate and electrostatic charge. *Journal of Biomechanics* 49 (11): 2201–2212.
A15. Sarkar S, Peri SP, and Chaudhuri B. 2017. Investigation of multiphase multicomponent aerosol flow dictating pMDI-spacer interactions. *International Journal of Pharmaceutics* 529 (1–2): 264–274.
A16. Kleinstreuer C, Zhang Z, and Li Z. 2008. Modeling airflow and particle transport/deposition in pulmonary airways. *Respiratory Physiology & Neurobiology* 163 (1–3): 128–138.
A17. Walenga RL, Tian G, and Worth Longest P. 2013. Development of characteristic upper tracheobronchial airway models for testing pharmaceutical aerosol delivery. *Journal of Biomechanical Engineering* 135 (9): 091010–091018.
A18. Forbes B, Backman P, Christopher D, Dolovich M, Li BV, and Morgan B. 2015. In vitro testing for orally inhaled products: Developments in science-based regulatory approaches. *The AAPS Journal* 17 (4): 837–852.
A19. De Backer LA, Vos WG, Salgado R, De Backer JW, Devolder A, Verhulst SL, Claes R, Germonpre PR, and De Backer WA. 2011. Functional imaging using computer methods to compare the effect of salbutamol and ipratropium bromide in patient-specific airway models of COPD. *International Journal of Chronic Obstructive Pulmonary Disease* 6 (November 28.): 637–646.
A20. Vincenzi C. 2017. Proceedings of DDL. EMA update on quality guidelines on inhalation and nasal products. In: The Aerosol Society, Proceedings of Drug Delivery to the Lungs (DDL 2017). p30.
A21. Dolovich MB, and Schuster DP. 2007. Positron emission tomography and computed tomography versus positron emission tomography computed tomography: Tools for imaging the lung. *Proceedings of the American Thoracic Society* 4 (4): 328–333.
A22. Dolovich MB. 2009. 18F-Fluorodeoxyglucose positron emission tomographic imaging of pulmonary functions, pathology, and drug delivery. *Proceedings of the American Thoracic Society* 6 (5): 477–485.

REFERENCES

1. O'Doherty MJ, Miller RF. Aerosols for therapy and diagnosis. *Eur J Nucl Med* 1993; 20(12):1201–1213.
2. Newman SP, Pitcairn GR, Hirst PH. A brief history of gamma scintigraphy. *J Aerosol Med* 2001; 14(2):139–145.
3. Gonda I. Scintigraphic techniques for measuring in vivo deposition. *J Aerosol Med* 1996; 9(suppl 1): S59–S67.
4. Newman SP. Scintigraphic assessment of therapeutic aerosols. *Crit Rev Ther Drug Carrier Syst* 1993; 10(1):65–109.
5. Kunka R, Andrews S, Pimazzoni M, Callejas S, Ziviani L, Squassante L et al. From hydrofluoroalkane pressurized metered-dose inhalers (pMDIs) and comparability with chlorofluorocarbon pMDIs. *Respir Med* 2000; 94(suppl B):S10–S16.
6. Selroos O, Pietinallo A, Riska H. Delivery devices for inhaled asthma medication. *Clin Immunother* 1996; 6(4):273–299.
7. Edsbacker S. Pharmacological factors that influence the choice of inhaled corticosteroids. *Drugs* 1999; 58(suppl 4):7–16.
8. Wilson A, Demsey O, Couties W, Sims E, Lipworth B. Importance of drug-device interaction in determining systemic effects of inhaled corticosteroids. *Lancet* 1999; 353:2128.
9. Taylor I, Hill A, Hayes M, Rhodes CG, O'Shaughnessy K, O'Connor BJ. Imaging allergen-invoked airway inflammation in atopic asthma with [18F]-fluorode-oxyglucose and positron emission tomography. *Lancet* 1996; 347:937–940.
10. Dolovich M. Aerosol delivery devices and airways/lung deposition. In: Schleimer R, O'Byrne P, Szefler SJ, Brattsand R, eds. *Inhaled Steroids in Asthma: Optimizing Effects in the Airways.* New York, NY: Marcel Dekker, 2002:169–211.

11. Dolovich MB. Influence of inspiratory flow rate, particle size, and airway caliber on aerosolized drug delivery to the lung. *Respir Care* 2000; 45(6):597–608.
12. Zanen P, Go LT, Lammers JW. Optimal particle size for beta 2 agonist and anticholinergic aerosols in patients with severe airflow obstruction [see comments]. *Thorax* 1996; 51(10):977–980.
13. Martin R, Szefler SJ, Chinchilli V, Kraft M, Dolovich M, Boushey HCR et al. Systemic effect comparisons of six inhaled corticosteroid preparations. *Am J Respir Crit Care Med* 2002; 165:1377–1383.
14. Byron PR, ed. *Pathophysiological and Disease Constraints on Aerosol Delivery.* Boca Raton, FL: CRC Press, 1990.
15. Heyder J, Gebbart J, Rudolf G, Stahlhofen W. Physical factors determining particle deposition in the human respiratory tract. *J Aerosol Sci* 1980; 11:505–515.
16. Everard ML, Dolovich M. In vivo measurements of lung dose. In: Bisgaard H, O'Callaghan C, Smaldone GC, eds. *Drug Delivery to the Lung.* New York, NY: Marcel Dekker, 2001:173–209.
17. Bennett WD, Brown JS, Zeman KL, Hu SC, Scheuch G, Sommerer K. Targeting delivery of aerosols to different lung regions. *J Aerosol Med* 2002; 15(2):179–188.
18. Laube BL, Jashnani R, Dalby RN, Zeitlin PL. Targeting aerosol deposition in patients with cystic fibrosis: Effects of alterations in particle size and inspiratory flow rate. *Chest* 2000; 118(4):1069–1076.
19. Smaldone GC, Führer J, Steigbigel RT, McPeck M. Factors determining pulmonary deposition of aerosolized pentamidine in patients with human immunodeficiency virus infection. *Am Rev Respir Dis* 1991; 143(4 Pt 1):727–737.
20. Anderson PJ, Dolovich MB. Aerosols as diagnostic tools. *J Aerosol Med* 1994; 7(1):77–88.
21. Dolovich M, Cockcroft D, Coates G. Aerosols in diagnosis: Ventilation, airway penetrance, airway reactivity, epithelial permeability and mucociliary transport. In: Moren F, Dolovich M, Newhouse M, Newman S, eds. *Aerosols in Medicine: Principles, Diagnosis and Therapy.* Amsterdam, the Netherlands: Elsevier Science, 1993:195–234.
22. Robinson M, Eberl S, Tomlinson C, Daviskas E, Regnis JA, Bailey DL et al. Regional mucociliary clearance in patients with cystic fibrosis. *J Aerosol Med* 2000; 13(2):73–86.
23. Robinson M, Bye PT. Mucociliary clearance in cystic fibrosis. *Pediatr Pulmonol* 2002; 33(4): 293–306.
24. Knowles MR, Boucher RC. Mucus clearance as a primary innate defense mechanism for mammalian airways. *J Clin Investig* 2002; 109(5):571–577.
25. Coates G, O'Brodovich H, Dolovich M. Lung clearance of 99mTc-DTPA in patients with acute lung injury and pulmonary edema. *J Thorac Imaging* 1988; 3(3):21–27.
26. Diot P, Galinier E, Grimbert D, Bugeon S, Valat C, Lemarie E et al. Characterization of 99mTc-DTPA aerosols for lung permeability studies. *Respiration* 2001; 68(3):313–317.
27. Effros R. Epithelial permeability. In: Moren F, Dolovich M, Newhouse M, Newman S, eds. *Aerosols in Medicine: Principles, Diagnosis and Therapy.* Amsterdam, the Netherlands: Elsevier Science, 1993:235–246.
28. Reinartz P, Schirp U, Zimny M, Sabri O, Nowak B, Schafer W et al. Optimizing ventilation-perfusion lung scintigraphy: Parting with planar imaging. *Nuklear-medizin* 2001; 40(2):38–43.
29. Tagil K, Evander E, Wollmer P, Palmer J, Jonson B. Efficient lung scintigraphy. *Clin Physiol* 2000; 20(2):95–100.
30. Davis SS, Hardy JG, Newman SP, Wilding IR. Gamma scintigraphy in the evaluation of pharmaceutical dosage forms. *Eur J Nucl Med* 1992; 19(11):971–986.
31. Dolovich MB, Jordana M, Newhouse MT. Methodologic considerations in mucociliary clearance and lung epithelial absorption measurements. *Eur J Nucl Med* 1987; 13(suppl):S45–S52.
32. Calmanovici G, Boccio J, Goldman C, Hager A, De Paoli T, Alak M et al. 99mTc-ENS ventilation scintigraphy: Preliminary study in human volunteers. *Nucl Med Biol* 2000; 27(2):215–218.
33. Walker PS, Conway JH, Fleming JS, Bondesson E, Borgstrom L. Pulmonary clearance rate of two chemically different forms of inhaled pertechnetate. *J Aerosol Med* 2001; 14(2):209–215.
34. Coghe J, Votion D, Lekeux P. Comparison between radioactive aerosol, technegas and krypton for ventilation imaging in healthy calves. *Vet J* 2000; 160(1):25–32.
35. Suarez S, Hickey AJ. Drug properties affecting aerosol behavior. *Respir Care* 2000; 45(6):652–666.
36. Martonen TB, Yang Y, Dolovich M. Definition of airway composition within gamma camera images. *J Thorac Imaging* 1994; 9(3):188–197.

37. Jaszczak R, Coleman RE, Lim C. SPECT: Single photon emission computed tomography. *IEEE Trans Nucl Sci* 1980; 27:1137–1153.
38. Fleming JS, Sauret V, Conway JH, Holgate ST, Bailey AG, Martonen TB. Evaluation of the accuracy and precision of lung aerosol deposition measurements from single-photon emission computed tomography using simulation. *J Aerosol Med* 2000; 13(3): 187–198.
39. Fleming JS, Hashish AH, Conway JH, Nassim MA, Holgate ST, Halson P et al. Assessment of deposition of inhaled aerosol in the respiratory tract of man using three-dimensional multimodality imaging and mathematical modeling. *J Aerosol Med* 1996; 9(3):317–327.
40. Fleming JS, Conway JH. Three-dimensional imaging of aerosol deposition. *J Aerosol Med* 2001; 14(2):147–153.
41. Eberl S, Chan HK, Daviskas E, Constable C, Young I. Aerosol deposition and clearance measurement: A novel technique using dynamic SPET. *Eur J Nucl Med* 2001; 28(9):1365–1372.
42. Chan HK, Eberl S, Daviskas E, Constable C, Young IH. Dynamic SPECT of aerosol deposition and mucociliary clearance in healthy subjects (abstr). *J Aerosol Med* 1999; 12:135.
43. Rhodes CG, Hughes JM. Pulmonary studies using positron emission tomography. *Eur Respir J* 1995; 8:1011–1017.
44. Dolovich MB. Measuring total and regional lung deposition using inhaled radiotracers. *J Aerosol Med* 2001; 14(suppl 1):S35–S44.
45. Musch G, Layfield JD, Harris RS, Melo MF, Winkler T, Callahan RJ et al. Topographical distribution of pulmonary perfusion and ventilation, assessed by PET in supine and prone humans. *J Appl Physiol* 2002; 93(5):1841–1851.
46. Dolovich M, Nahmias C, Coates G. Unleashing the PET: 3D imaging of the lung. In: Byron PR, Dalby R, Farr SJ, eds. *Respiratory Drug Delivery VII.* North Carolina, NC: Serentec Press, 2000:215–230.
47. Czemin J, Phelps M. Positron emission tomography scanning: Current and future applications. *Annu Rev Med* 2002; 53:89–112.
48. Bergstrom M, Cass LM, Valind S, Westerberg G, Lundberg EL, Gray S et al. Deposition and disposition of [11C]zanamivir following administration as an intranasal spray. Evaluation with positron emission tomography. *Clin Pharmacokinet* 1999; 36(suppl 1):33–39.
49. Bailey AG, Gilardi MC, Grootoonk S, Kinahan P, Nahmias C, Ollinger J et al. Quantitative procedures in 3D PET. In: Bendriem B, Townsend DW, eds. *The Theory and Practice of PET.* Dordrecht, the Netherlands: Kluwer Academic, 1998.
50. Lee Z, Berridge MS, Finlay WH, Heald DL. Mapping PET-measured triamcinolone acetonide (TAA) aerosol distribution into deposition by airway generation. *Int JPharm* 2000; 199(1):7–16.
51. Berridge MS, Lee Z, Heald DL. Regional distribution and kinetics of inhaled pharmaceuticals. *Curr Pharm Des* 2000; 6(16):1631–1651.
52. Aboagye EO, Price PM, Jones T. In vivo pharmacokinetics and pharmacodynamics in drug development using positron-emission tomography. *Drug Discov Today* 2001; 6(6):293–302.
53. Derendorf H, Lesko LJ, Chaikin P, Colburn WA, Lee P, Miller R et al. Pharmacokinetic/pharmacodynamic modeling in drug research and development. *J Clin Pharmacol* 2000; 40(12 Pt 2):1399–1418.
54. Cheng YS, Holmes TD, Gao J, Guilmette RA, Li S, Surakitbanham Y et al. Characterization of nasal spray pumps and deposition pattern in a replica of the human nasal airway. *J Aerosol Med* 2001; 14(2):267–280.
55. Boek WM, Graamans K, Natzijl H, van Rijk PP, Huizing EH. Nasal mucociliary transport: New evidence for a key role of ciliary beat frequency. *Laryngoscope* 2002; 112(3):570–573.
56. Dolovich MB. Aerosols. In: Barnes P, Grunstein M, Leff A, Woolcock A, eds. *Asthma.* Philadelphia, PA: Lippincott-Raven, 1997:1349–1366.
57. Fink JB. Metered-dose inhalers, dry powder inhalers, and transitions. *Respir Care* 2000; 45(6):623–635.
58. Dolovich M. New delivery systems and propellants. *Can Respir J* 1999; 6(3):290–295.
59. Chan HK, Daviskas E, Eberl S, Robinson M, Bautovich G, Young I. Deposition of aqueous aerosol of technetium-99m diethylene triamine penta-acetic acid generated and delivered by a novel system (AERx) in healthy subjects. *Eur J Nucl Med* 1999; 26(4):320–327.
60. Cass LM, Brown J, Pickford M, Fayinka S, Newman SP, Johansson CJ et al. Pharmacoscintigraphic evaluation of lung deposition of inhaled zanamivir in healthy volunteers. *Clin Pharmacokinet* 1999; 36(suppl 1):21–31.
61. Newman SP. Characteristics of radiolabeled versus unlabeled inhaler formulations. *J Aerosol Med* 1996; 9(suppl 1):S37–S47.

62. Warren S, Taylor G, Smith J, Buck H, Parry-Billings M. Gamma scintigraphic evaluation of a novel budesonide dry powder inhaler using a validated radiolabeling technique. *J Aerosol Med* 2002; 15(1):15–25.
63. Dolovich M. In vitro measurements of delivery of medications from MDIs and spacer devices. *J Aerosol Med* 1996; 9(suppl 1):S49–S58.
64. Chan HK, Eberl S, Daviskas E, Constable C, Young I. Changes in lung deposition of aerosols due to hygroscopic growth: A fast SPECT study. *J Aerosol Med* 2002; 15(3):307–311.
65. Bennett WD. Effect of beta-adrenergic agonists on mucociliary clearance. *J Allergy Clin Immunol* 2002; 110(suppl 6):S291–S297.
66. Sabater JR, Wanner A, Abraham WM. Montelukast prevents antigen-induced mucociliary dysfunction in sheep. *Am J Respir Crit Care Med* 2002; 166(11):1457–1460.
67. Oldenburg FA Jr, Dolovich MB, Montgomery JM, Newhouse MT. Effects of postural drainage, exercise, and cough on mucus clearance in chronic bronchitis. *Am Rev Respir Dis* 1979; 120(4):739–745.
68. Robinson M, Regnis JA, Bailey DL, King M, Bautovich GJ, Bye PT. Effect of hypertonic saline, amiloride, and cough on mucociliary clearance in patients with cystic fibrosis. *Am J Respir Crit Care Med* 1996; 153(5):1503–1509.
69. Spiro SG, Singh CA, Tolfree SE, Partridge MR, Short MD. Direct labeling of ipratropium bromide aerosol and its deposition pattern in normal subjects and patients with chronic bronchitis. *Thorax* 1984; 39(6):432–435.
70. Geworski L, Knoop BO, de Wit M, Ivancevic V, Bares R, Munz DL. Multicenter comparison of calibration and cross-calibration of PET scanners. *J Nucl Med* 2002; 43(5):635–639.
71. Mallol J, Rattray S, Walker G, Cook D, Robertson CF. Aerosol deposition in infants with cystic fibrosis. *Pediatr Pulmonol* 1996; 21(5):276–281.
72. Devadason SG, Everard ML, MacEarlan C, Roller C, Summers QA, Swift P et al. Lung deposition from the Turbuhaler in children with cystic fibrosis. *Eur Respir J* 1997; 10(9):2023–2028.
73. Fok TF, Monkman S, Dolovich M, Gray S, Coates G, Paes B et al. Efficiency of aerosol medication delivery from a metered-dose inhaler versus jet nebulizer in infants with bronchopulmonary dysplasia. *Pediatr Pulmonol* 1996; 21(5):301–309.
74. Fuller HD, Dolovich MB, Posmituck G, Pack WW, Newhouse MT. Pressurized aerosol versus jet aerosol delivery to mechanically ventilated patients. Comparison of dose to the lungs. *Am Rev Respir Dis* 1990; 141(2):440–444.
75. Anhoj J, Thorsson L, Bisgaard H. Lung deposition of inhaled drugs increases with age. *Am J Respir Crit Care Med* 2000; 162(5):1819–1822.
76. Salmon B, Wilson N, Silverman M. How much aerosol reaches the lungs of wheezy infants and toddlers? *Arch Dis Child* 1990; 98:401–404.
77. Everard ML. The use of radiolabeled aerosols for research purposes in paediatric patients: Ethical and practical aspects. *Thorax* 1994; 49(12):1259–1266.
78. Radiation dose to patients from radiopharmaceuticals. *A Report of a Task Group of Committees 2 and 3 of the International Commission on Radiological Protection* (ICRP). Oxford, UK: Pergamon Press, 1994.
79. Aug C, Perry RJ, Smaldone GC. Technetium 99m radiolabeling of aerosolized drug particles from metered dose inhalers. *J Aerosol Med* 1991; 4(2):127–138.
80. Farr SJ. The physicochemical basis of radiolabeling metered-dose inhalers with 99mTc. *J Aerosol Med* 1996; 9(suppl 1):S27–S36.
81. Fok TF, al Essa M, Monkman S, Dolovich M, Girard L, Coates G et al. Pulmonary deposition of salbutamol aerosol delivered by metered-dose inhaler, jet nebulizer, and ultrasonic nebulizer in mechanically ventilated rabbits. *Pediatr Res* 1997; 42(5):721–727.
82. Koehler D, Fleischer W, Matthys H. New method for easy labelling of (3-agonists in metered-dose inhalers with technetium 99m. *Respiration* 1988; 53:65–73.
83. Summers QA, Clark AR, Hollingworth A, Fleming JS, Holgate ST. The preparation of a radiolabeled aerosol of nedocromil sodium for administration by metered-dose inhaler that accurately preserves particle size distribution of the drug. *Drug Investig* 1990; 2:90–98.
84. Byron PR, Kelly EL, Kontny MJ, Lovering EG, Poochikian GK, Sethi S et al. Recommendations of the USP advisory panel on aerosols on the USP general chapters on aerosols [601] and uniformity of dosage units [905]. *Pharm Forum* 1994; 7:7477–7503. http://www.fda.gov/cder/guidance/index.htm.
85. Guidance for Industry Metered-Dose Inhaler (MDI) and Dry Powder Inhaler (DPI) Drug Products Chemistry, Manufacturing, and Controls Documentation. Center for Drug Evaluation and Research (CDER), 1998.

86. Dolovich M, Rhem R, Rashid F, Coates G, Hill M, Bowen B. Measurement of the particle size and dosing characteristics of a radiolabeled albuterol-sulphate lactose blend used in the SPIROS[7] dry powder inhaler. In: Byron PR, Dalby R, Farr SJ, eds. *Respiratory Drug Delivery V.* Buffalo Grove, IL: Interpharm Press, 1996:332–335.
87. Newman SP, Moren F, Trofast E, Talaee N, Clarke SW. Deposition and clinical efficacy of terbutaline sulphate from Turbuhaler, a new multidose powder inhaler. *Eur Respir J* 1989; 2(3):247–252.
88. Dolovich M, Rhem R, Rashid F, Bowen B. Lung deposition of albuterol sulphate from the Dura dryhaler in normal adults. *Am J Respir Crit Care Med* 1996; 153(4(Part 2)):A62.
89. Olsson B, Asking L, Borgstrom L, Bondesson E. Effect of inlet throat on the correlation between measured fine particle dose and lung deposition. In: Dalby RN, Byron PR, Farr SJ, eds. *Respiratory Drug Delivery V.* Buffalo Grove, IL: Interpharm Press, 1996:273–281.
90. Laube BL. In vivo measurements of aerosol dose and distribution: Clinical relevance. *J Aerosol Med* 1996; 9(suppl 1):S77–S91.
91. Dolovich MB. Assessing nebulizer performance. *Respir Care* 2002; 47:1290–1301.
92. Dolovich M, Rhem R. Impact of oropharyngeal deposition on inhaled dose. *J Aerosol Med* 1998; 11(suppl 1):S112–S115.
93. Laube BL, Links JM, LaFrance ND, Wagner HN Jr, Rosenstein BJ. Homogeneity of bronchopulmonary distribution of 99mTc aerosol in normal subjects and in cystic fibrosis patients. *Chest* 1989; 95(4):822–830.
94. Kim CS, Lewars GA, Sackner MA. Measurement of total lung aerosol deposition as an index of lung abnormality. *J Appl Physiol* 1988; 64(4):1527–1536.
95. Kim CS, Abraham WM, Garcia L, Sackner MA. Enhanced aerosol deposition in the lung with mild airways obstruction. *Am Rev Respir Dis* 1989; 139(2):422–426.
96. Kim CS, Kang TC. Comparative measurement of lung deposition of inhaled fine particles in normal subjects and patients with obstructive airway disease. *Am J Respir Crit Care Med* 1997; 155(3):899–905.
97. Farr SJ, Rowe AM, Rubsamen R, Taylor G. Aerosol deposition in the human lung following administration from a microprocessor-controlled pressurized metered dose inhaler. *Thorax* 1995; 50(6):639–644.
98. Smaldone GC. Deposition and clearance: Unique problems in the proximal airways and oral cavity in the young and elderly. *Respir Physiol* 2001; 128(1):33–38.
99. Dolovich M, Rhem R. Small differences in inspiratory flow rate (IFR) and aerosol particle size can influence upper and lower respiratory tract deposition. *J Aerosol Med* 1997; 10(3):238.
100. Mijailovich SM, Treppo S, Venegas JG. Effects of lung motion and tracer kinetics corrections on PET imaging of pulmonary function. *J Appl Physiol* 1997; 82(4):1154–1162.
101. Braga FJ, Souza JF, Trad CS, Santos AC, Ghillardi NT, Elias J Jr et al. An improved mouthpiece to prevent environmental contamination during radioaerosol inhalation procedures. *Health Phys* 1998; 75(4):424–427.
102. Bailey DL, Jones T, Spinks TJ. A method for measuring the absolute sensitivity of positron-emission tomographic scanners. *Eur J Nucl Med* 1991; 18(6):374–379.
103. Fok TF, al Essa M, Kirpalani H, Monkman S, Bowen B, Coates G et al. Estimation of pulmonary deposition of aerosol using gamma scintigraphy. *J Aerosol Med* 1999; 12(1):9–15.
104. Forge NI, Mountford PJ, O'Doherty MJ. Quantification of technetium-99m lung radioactivity from planar images [published erratum appears in Eur J Nucl Med 1993; 20(4):367]. *Eur J Nucl Med* 1993; 20(1):10–15.
105. Fleming JS. A technique for using CT images in attenuation correction and quantification in SPECT. *Nucl Med Commun* 1989; 10(2):83–97.
106. Ruffin R, Kenworthy M, Newhouse M. Response of patients to fenoterol inhalation: A method for quantifying the airway bronchodilator dose. *Clin Pharmacol Ther* 1978; 23:338–342.
107. Messina MS, Smaldone GC. Evaluation of quantitative aerosol techniques for use in bronchoprovocation studies. *J Allergy Clin Immunol* 1985; 75(2):252–257.
108. Fleming JS, Alaamer AS. Influence of collimator characteristics on quantification in SPECT. *J Nucl Med* 1996; 37(11):1832–1836.
109. Macey M, Marshall R. Absolute quantitation of radiotracer uptake in the lungs using a gamma camera. *J Nucl Med* 1982; 23:39–45.
110. Pitcairn G. Tissue attenuation corrections in gamma scintigraphy. *J Aerosol Med* 1997; 3:187–198.
111. Langenback EG, Foster WM, Bergofsky EH. Calculating concentration of inhaled radiolabeled particles from external gamma counting: External counting efficiency and attenuation coefficient of thorax. *J Toxicol Environ Health* 1989; 26:139–152.

112. Itoh H, Smaldone GC, Swift DL, Wagner HN Jr. Quantitative measurements of aerosol deposition: Evaluation of different techniques. *J Aerosol Sci* 1985; 16:367–371.
113. Dolovich M, Rhem R, Kish S, Saab C. Defining lung regions for the purpose of calculating deposition to the small airways. *Am J Respir Crit Care Med* 2002; 165:A190.
114. Kim CS. Methods of calculating lung delivery and deposition of aerosol particles. *Respir Care* 2000; 45(6):695–711.
115. Dolovich MB, Rhem R, Coates G. Defining and quantitating peripheral lung deposition using radiolabeled tracers and 2D imaging. *Eur Resp J* 2000; 16(suppl 31, P560):625.
116. Martonen TB, Yang Y, Dolovich M, Guan X. Computer simulations of lung morphologies within planar gamma camera images. *Nucl Med Commun* 1997; 18(9):861–869.
117. Phipps PR, Gonda I, Bailey DL, Borham P, Bautovich G, Anderson SD. Comparisons of planar and tomographic gamma scintigraphy to measure the penetration index of inhaled aerosols. *Am Rev Respir Dis* 1989; 139(6):1516–1523.
118. Newman SP, Hirst PH, Pitcairn GR, Clark AR. Understanding regional lung deposition in gamma scintigraphy. In: Dalby RN, Byron PR, Farr SJ, eds. *Respiratory Drug Delivery VI.* Buffalo Grove, IL: Interpharm Press, 1998:9–15.
119. Sanchis J, Dolovich M, Chalmers R, Newhouse M. Quantitation of regional aerosol clearance in the normal human lung. *J Appl Physiol* 1972; 33(6):757–762.
120. Fleming JS, Halson P, Conway J, Moore E, Nassim MA, Hashish AH et al. Three-dimensional description of pulmonary deposition of inhaled aerosol using data from multimodality imaging. *J Nucl Med* 1996; 37(5):873–877.
121. Newman SP. Can lung deposition data act as a surrogate for the clinical response to inhaled asthma drugs? *Br J Clin Pharmacol* 2000; 49(6):529–537.
122. Fahey FH. Positron-emission tomography instrumentation. *Radiol Clin N Am* 2001; 39(5):919–929.
123. Bailey DL. Transmission scanning in emission tomography. *Eur J Nucl Med* 1998; 25(7):774–787.
124. Rahman S, Rhodes CG, Constantinou M, Waters S, Aigbirho FOS, Osman S. Lung deposition of 18-F-fluticasone propionate in normal subjects using positron emission tomography. *Am J Respir Crit Care Med* 2000; 161(Part 2):A177.
125. Ruffin RE, Dolovich MB, Wolff RK, Newhouse MT. The effects of preferential deposition of histamine in the human airway. *Am Rev Respir Dis* 1978; 117(3):485–492.
126. Ruffin RE, Dolovich MB, Oldenburg FA Jr, Newhouse MT. The preferential deposition of inhaled isoproterenol and propranolol in asthmatic patients. *Chest* 1981; 80(suppl 6):904–907.
127. Ryan G, Dolovich MB, Roberts RS, Frith PA, Juniper EF, Hargreave FE et al. Standardization of inhalation provocation tests: Two techniques of aerosol generation and inhalation compared. *Am Rev Respir Dis* 1981; 123(2):195–199.
128. Schmekel B, Hedenstrom H, Kampe M, Lagerstrand L, Stalenheim G, Wollmer P et al. The bronchial response, but not the pulmonary response, to inhaled methacholine is dependent on the aerosol deposition pattern. *Chest* 1994; 106(6):1781–1787.
129. O'Riordan TG, Walser L, Smaldone GC. Changing patterns of aerosol deposition during methacholine bronchoprovocation. *Chest* 1993; 103(5):1385–1389.
130. Garrard CS, Gerrity TR, Yeates DB. The relationships of aerosol deposition, lung size, and the rate of mucociliary clearance. *Arch Environ Health* 1986; 41(1):11–15.
131. O'Doherty MJ, Page CJ, Croft DN, Bateman NT. Lung 99Tcm-DTPA transfer: A method for background correction. *Nucl Med Commun* 1985; 6(4):209–215.
132. Snell NJ, Ganderton D. Assessing lung deposition of inhaled medications. Consensus statement from a workshop of the British Association for Lung Research, held at the Institute of Biology, London, on April 17, 1998. *Respir Med* 1999; 93(2):123–133.
133. Fleming JS, Nassim MA, Hashish AH, Bailey AG, Conway J, Holgate ST et al. Description of pulmonary deposition of radiolabeled aerosol by airway generation using a conceptual three-dimensional model of lung morphology. *J Aerosol Med* 1995; 8:341–356.

6

Pharmacokinetics and Pharmacodynamics of Drugs Delivered to the Lung

Stefanie K. Drescher, Mong-Jen Chen, Jürgen B. Bulitta, and Günther Hochhaus

CONTENTS

6.1 Introduction

Pulmonary drug delivery has been successfully employed for the topical therapy of pulmonary diseases with the goal of achieving pron ounced pulmonary effects with reduced systemic side effects (Stein and Thiel 2017). Thus, inhalation therapy intends to obtain desired effects at smaller doses than those necessary after systemic administration, thereby reducing systemic side effects. This is often referred to as pulmonary targeting. The degree of pulmonary targeting is determined by several pharmacokinetic (PK) and pharmacodynamic (PD) factors. This chapter will discuss the relationships between pulmonary selectivity, pharmacokinetic and pharmacodynamic drug properties, including device and formulation related factors. In addition, various pharmacokinetic and pharmacodynamic approaches suitable to characterize the fate of inhalation drugs will be reviewed. These include non-compartmental, compartmental, and physiologically based pharmacokinetic approaches. An overview of selected studies evaluating pharmacokinetic/pharmacodynamic (PK/PD) relationships is provided as well.

6.2 Factors Important for Pulmonary Targeting

6.2.1 Pulmonary Targeting: As Seen through a Pharmacokineticists' Eye

Figure 6.1 illustrates the sequence of events occurring during and after pulmonary drug delivery. Once released from the device, a fraction (10%–60%) of the delivered dose will be deposited in the lung (respirable fraction), while particles not able to enter the lung will be deposited in the oropharynx or remain in the device. Drug deposited in the oropharynx will be swallowed and becomes subject to oral absorption. How much drug will be absorbed through the gastrointestinal (GI) tract will depend on how much drug is reaching the GI tract and the oral bioavailability of the drug. The drug passing through the oropharynx will be able to enter the lung.

The human lung can be divided into at least two major physiological zones differing in airway diameter and cellular composition (Patton 1996; Tronde et al. 2008; Verma et al. 2015). These are: (1) the conducting airways (generation 0–16) with 60 µm thick epithelium (Kumar et al. 2017), reaching from trachea, over bronchi, to terminal bronchioles, and expressing mucociliary clearance through ciliary cells (Kreyling and Scheuch 2000), as well as (2) the respiratory zone (generation 17–23), with alveolar epithelium being 0.2 µm thick (Patton 1996; Olsson et al. 2011). According to these zones, lung deposition of drug is often classified as either central or peripheral. The anatomy and physiology of the airways, together with drug formulation/device factors, will determine the fate of inhaled particles as specified by deposition efficiency, regional deposition, particle clearance, solubility, dissolution rate, metabolism, and permeability across central and peripheral lung regions (see in Figure 6.15) (Bhagwat et al. 2017).

For the treatment of asthma or chronic obstructive pulmonary disease (COPD), achieving high concentrations at the target site is crucial to induce a distinct clinical response with minimal systemic exposure (Labiris and Dolovich 2003a). Factors listed in Figure 6.15 present key biopharmaceutical aspects (deposited dose, regional deposition, dissolution, and permeability) which determine, together with systemic pharmacokinetic properties (systemic clearance, oral bioavailability), the degree of pulmonary effects and systemic side effects.

The PK/PD model used to evaluate the relevance of PK/PD parameters for pulmonary targeting essentially represents a mathematical translation of the scheme shown in Figure 6.1. A fraction of the released dose (generally particles larger than 5 µm [Heyder et al. 1986]) will deposit in the oropharynx from where it will be swallowed. The fraction of drug which is systemically available via absorption from the gastrointestinal (GI) tract depends on the oral bioavailability of the drug molecule.

Smaller particles (less than about 5 µm in diameter) will pass the oropharynx and reach the lung. Depending on the physicochemical properties of the inhaled dose, drug particles will deposit in central and peripheral portions of the lung with smaller particles depositing more peripherally. However, ultrafine particles, smaller than 1 µm, tend to be exhaled (Heyder et al. 1986). Deposited drug will subsequently dissolve and interact with relevant receptors to stimulate the desired drug effects. From there, drug molecules diffuse across pulmonary membranes into the systemic circulation, distribute into

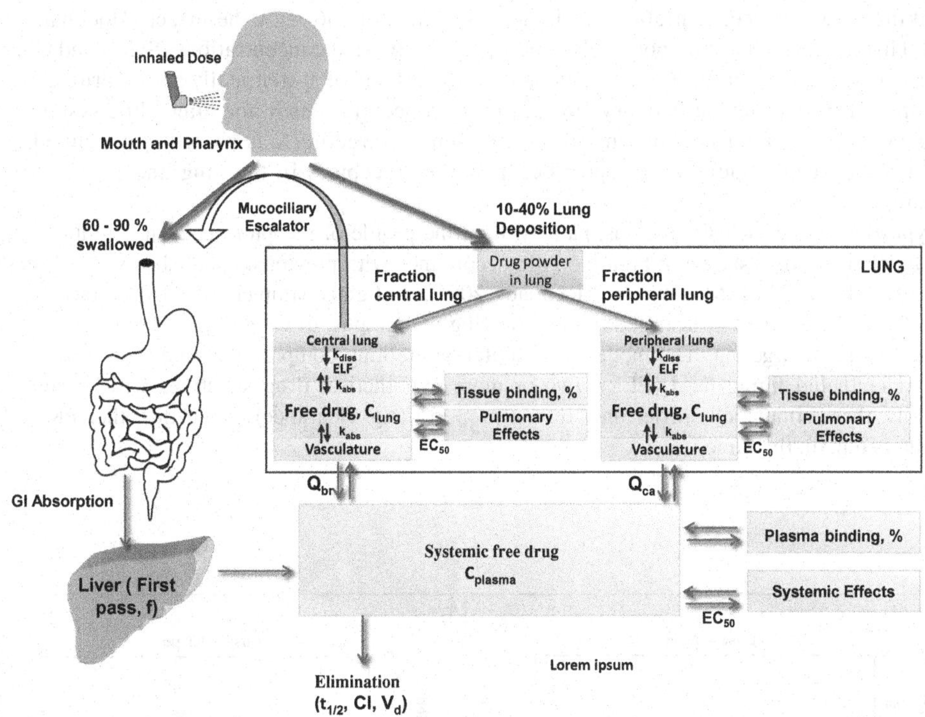

FIGURE 6.1 Pharmacokinetic/pharmacodynamic (PK/PD) model describing the fate of an inhaled drug. For a more detailed description see Section 6.2.1. After deposition in the central or peripheral lung, drug particles can dissolve in the epithelial lining fluid where the dissolution rate can be described by an empirical first-order dissolution constant or by the Nernst-Brunner equation (with solubility and particle surface area as input parameters). Free dissolved drug molecules are absorbed into the lung tissue via first-order absorption (affected by permeability and surface area). After absorption into the lung tissue the unbound drug fraction can induce pulmonary response or distribute into the vasculature from where it becomes systemically available by the cardiac output (Q_{ca}) in the peripheral lung or the bronchial blood flow (Q_{br}) in the central lung. The compartmentalization of the lung could be further extended by dividing it into trachea and large bronchi (BB), bronchioles (bb), and the alveolar interstitial space (AI) regions.

other parts of the body, and will subsequently be eliminated. Considering the above events, the questions listed in Table 6.1 are relevant for the performance, especially for explaining the degree of pulmonary specificity, referred to in the following as "pulmonary targeting."

In the case of glucocorticoids and a number of other inhalation drugs, a direct correlation between receptor occupancy and the degree of the pharmacological effects has been demonstrated; thus, receptor occupancies in either lung (as a marker for the desired effect) or systemic circulation (as a marker for undesired side effects) were derived from a simple E_{max} relationship. This was achieved

TABLE 6.1

Factors Relevant for Pulmonary Targeting

Pulmonary Components	Systemic Components
• How much drug is deposited in the lung? • Where is the drug deposited in the lung? • How long is the drug remaining in the lung (dissolution rate, mucociliary transport rate, pulmonary absorption rate, rates of cellular entrapment)? • What is the pulmonary tissue binding? • If a pro-drug, how efficient is the pulmonary activation? • How does the free pulmonary drug concentration relate to the pulmonary effect?	• How much drug is swallowed? • What is the oral bioavailability? • What is the systemic clearance? • What is the tissue binding? • What is the plasma protein binding? • If a prodrug, how efficient is the systemic activation? • How does the free systemic drug level relate to the systemic "side" effects?

by linking free drug concentrations in lung or systemic tissue with the effect (Hochhaus et al. 1997). This model is therefore not solely centerd around plasma concentrations (Sykes and Charlton 2012), as generally the case for models evaluating the effects of systemically acting drugs; instead, the proposed model links pulmonary effects to free concentrations in the lung while systemic side effects are related to plasma concentrations. Pulmonary targeting was accordingly defined as the difference between cumulative receptor occupancy of receptors in the lung and in the systemic circulation.

A typical result of such simulations, namely, the time profile of receptor occupancy in lung and the systemic circulation, is shown in Figure 6.2. In accordance with previously published work (Hochhaus et al. 1997, 1998, 2002; Mobley and Hochhaus 2001), a slightly simpler model than introduced in Figure 6.1 was utilized, as illustrated in the following paragraphs, to visualize how PK and PD factors affect pulmonary targeting. The model used contains one lung compartment and didn't include lung tissue or epithelial lining fluid (EFL). Two or more hypothetical drug situations will be compared. Generally, these simulations differ only in one property (e.g. clearance), while the other PK and PD parameters remain the same.

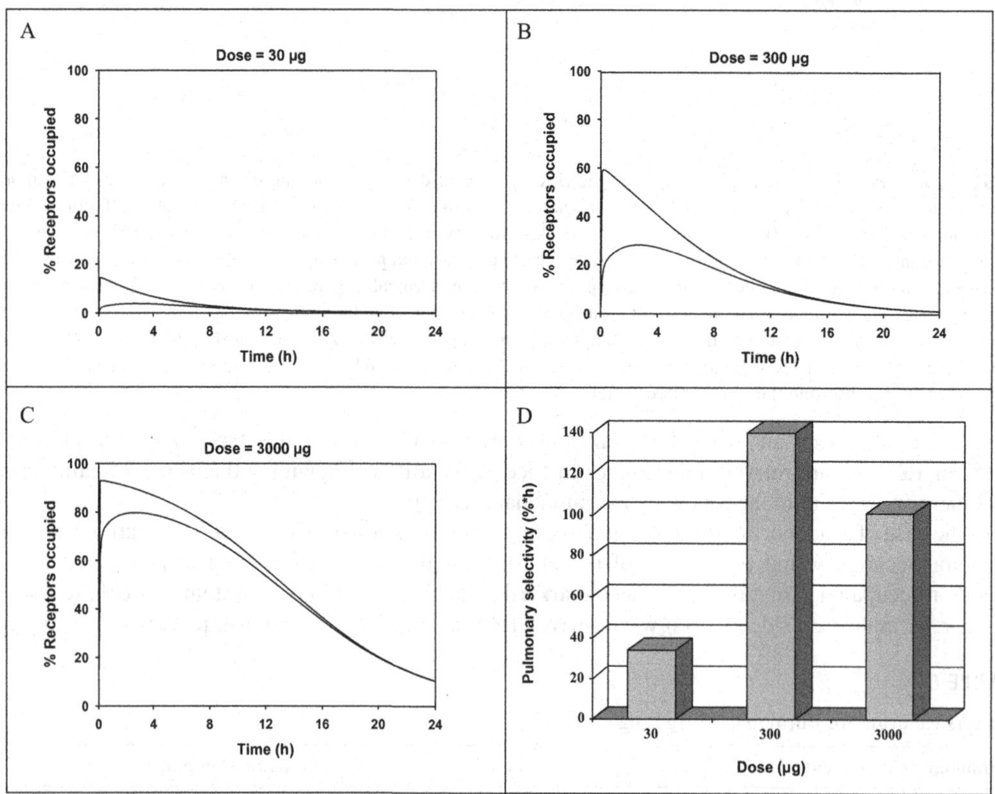

FIGURE 6.2 The effect of inhaled dose on pulmonary selectivity. The simulations illustrate pulmonary selectivity of an inhaled drug by utilizing PK/PD relationships and selecting receptor occupancy as a surrogate marker to predict the pulmonary and systemic effects. The pulmonary selectivity [area between pulmonary (upper line) and systemic (lower line) receptor occupancies] observed in A–C is compared in D. Simulations are shown for doses of 30, 300 and 3000 µg. At very low doses, relatively smaller pulmonary and systemic effects are observed, as most of the systemic and pulmonary receptors are unoccupied. With a subsequent increase in the dose, both the pulmonary and systemic effects increase and so does the difference between them (greater pulmonary selectivity). However, with a further decrease in the dose there is a loss in pulmonary targeting due to the saturation of both pulmonary and systemic receptors.

6.2.2 Pharmacokinetic Factors Important for Pulmonary Targeting

6.2.2.1 Biopharmaceutical Factors

Besides patient factors, key properties including the drug, formulation, and device will determine the amount of drug depositing in the lung and the regional drug deposition (Labiris and Dolovich 2003a; Tayab and Hochhaus 2005; Kandala and Hochhaus 2014). These biopharmaceutical factors such as the drug's particle size distribution, efficiency of the dry powder inhaler (DPI) system to de-agglomerate drug/carrier complexes, device resistance, droplet sizes generated by the metered dose inhaler (MDI) system, and other properties are listed in Figure 6.15. Once "landed," physicochemical properties will further contribute to the rates of dissolution and permeability across membranes.

These properties will consequently affect the time-course of pharmacologically relevant free drug concentrations in the lung and systemic circulation and, consequently, the degree of pulmonary targeting. In the following, the importance of biopharmaceutical properties (such as pulmonary deposition efficiency, delivered dose, dosing frequency, and pulmonary residence time) to enhance pulmonary targeting will be discussed.

6.2.2.2 Dose and Frequency of Dosing

Inhaled drugs are often used within a rather broad dose range, with low doses used in patients with light asthma and higher doses prescribed in patients with severe asthma. Therefore, it is of interest to evaluate whether pulmonary targeting depends on the prescribed dose. At very low doses of an inhaled drug, most of the pulmonary and systemic receptors are not occupied; thus, relatively smaller pulmonary and systemic effects are observed (Figure 6.2). As the dose increases, the differences between pulmonary and systemic receptor occupancies become more pronounced. However, with further increase in the dose, almost all the pulmonary receptors will be occupied, while systemic receptors continue to be occupied. The difference in cumulative receptor occupancy will therefore decrease at higher doses. The simulation suggests that there exists an optimal dose which provides maximal lung selectivity. If a patient needs higher doses to manage the asthma, pulmonary targeting decreases or is lost, and physicians should consider switching the patient from inhalation to oral drug treatment, because the cost/benefit ratio is improved.

Currently, there is a tendency to try to maintain patients on once daily doses. While the feasibility of the once-daily dosing depends on several drug specific factors and the disease state itself, one might ask what general relationships exist between dosing frequency and selectivity. As shown in Figure 6.3, pulmonary selectivity is improved if the same daily dose is administered in multiple smaller doses throughout the day; this intermittent dosing extends the time during that higher pulmonary (and presumably effective) drug concentrations are present (i.e. prolonging the pulmonary drug exposure time). Thus, increasing the dosing frequency will have a beneficial effect; this is most important for drugs which are absorbed relatively fast from the lung. This has been demonstrated in a clinical study, which showed that repeated dosing was beneficial in enhancing anti-asthmatic efficacy of budesonide (Toogood 1985). However, increasing the dosing frequency has its limitations because of problems with patient compliance; therefore, other ways of prolonging the contact time of the drug within the lung should be evaluated.

6.2.2.3 Pulmonary Deposition Efficiency

The efficiency of pulmonary drug delivery varies significantly across inhalation products. Key parameters for pulmonary particle deposition, such as aerodynamic particle size distribution, velocity of the droplets and particle density, among other factors, differ between inhalation products (Hastedt et al. 2016). It is likely that a pulmonary delivery device with higher pulmonary deposition will be more suitable for achieving pulmonary targeting. This is because the more efficient device not only increases the amount of drug in the lung, but also reduces the amount of drug that is available for absorption from the GI tract. In recent years, improvements in the design of inhalation drug products have increased pulmonary deposition from 10%–20% to up to 70% (Hill et al. 1996; Newman et al. 1998; Labiris and Dolovich 2003b). Simulation studies confirmed that high pulmonary deposition is beneficial for the degree of pulmonary targeting. This is especially true for a drug with high oral bioavailability, because an increase in pulmonary deposition will lead to a reduction in the fraction of the dose available for oral absorption

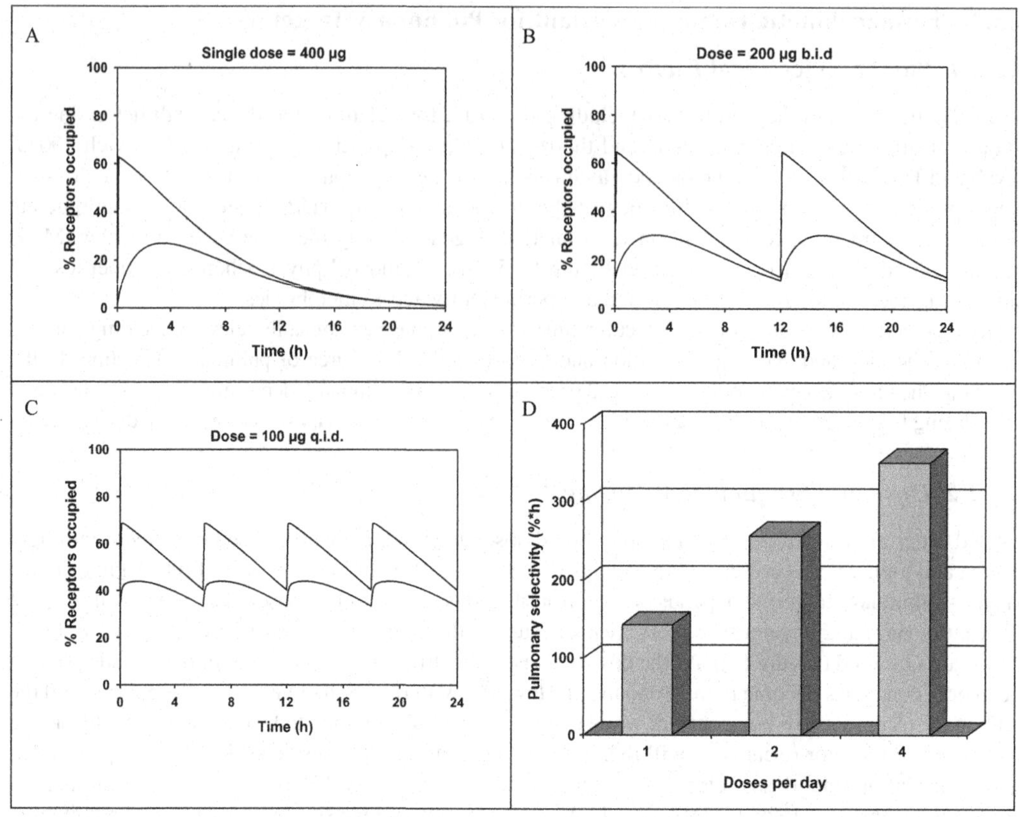

FIGURE 6.3 The effect of dosing regimen at steady state on pulmonary selectivity. Pulmonary selectivity (area between pulmonary (upper line) and systemic (lower line) receptor occupancies) observed in A–C are summarized in D. Additional doses are shown in D. A daily dose of 400 µg was administered as one single dose (A), 200 µg b.i.d (B), or 100 µg q.i.d. (C). Simulations show that a higher frequency of dosing results in greater pulmonary selectivity.

(Hochhaus et al. 1997). On the other hand, a high pulmonary deposition is less important for drugs with negligible oral bioavailability; for these compounds, drug entering the GI tract will not (or only minimally) be absorbed, and therefore will not lead to systemic side effects. In this case, however, using a device with higher pulmonary deposition would allow reducing the dose.

6.2.2.4 Pulmonary Residence Time

Pulmonary pharmacokinetics of an inhaled drug particle are mainly driven by drug dissolution and absorption across membranes. Both of these processes will affect lung targeting, since they determine the concentration-time profiles of free drug in the lung and the rate of drug absorption into the systemic circulation. Generally, the deposited drug particles will dissolve[1] in the pulmonary lining fluid (unless they are delivered as solution) or be removed as particles via mucociliary clearance in the upper parts of the lung.

After dissolution, drug molecules then penetrate across the lung lining fluid to the site of action. Relevant receptors may be on the cell membrane or in the cytosol of target cells. In addition to the dissolution rate, the rate of drug penetration across membranes to eventually reach the systemic circulation represents the second process, which controls the time of a drug to remain in the lung. The overall residence time of the drug will therefore be determined by the time required for the drug to dissolve and the time of the absorption across pulmonary membranes. Physicochemical properties of

[1] The release of drugs from delivery systems such as liposomes, nanoparticles or microsphere is the equivalent to the dissolution of solid particles.

the drug molecules (e.g. solubility C_s), as well as formulations factors (e.g. surface area S) are important for the dissolution rate; this is reflected in the Nernst-Brunner equation (Figure 6.4). Moreover, drug and membrane specific properties (such as diffusion coefficient, partition coefficient, permeability, membrane thickness, and membrane surface area) are essential for drug absorption across membranes, as governed by Fick's law (Figure 6.4) (Siepmann and Siepmann 2013).

It is assumed that for lipophilic corticosteroids the dissolution step is rate limiting, since their penetration (e.g. diffusion) across lipophilic membranes is fast (Lanman et al. 1973; Burton and Schanker 1974a, 1974b, 1974c; Gardiner and Schanker 1974). With absorption of low-molecular weight, hydrophilic drugs can also be very efficient, which leads to a short pulmonary residence time; these drug are often absorbed through water filled channels (Enna and Schanker 1972; Lanman et al. 1973; Burton et al. 1974; Schanker and Burton 1976). Facilitated transport might also be important for membrane permeability and drug absorption (Enna and Schanker 1973; Gardiner and Schanker 1974; Byron et al. 1994). For several less lipophilic drugs, including beta-2-adrenergics and antimuscarinics, membrane interactions seem to be more important for retaining the drug in the lung. This interaction might be specific, as in the case of retention via specific interactions of the drug molecule with lung components as seen for long acting beta-2-adrenergic drugs, trapping of drugs in lysosomes (Borghardt et al. 2016a); alternatively, formation of lipophilic esters may slow down or prevent absorption into the systemic circulation (Tunek et al. 1997).

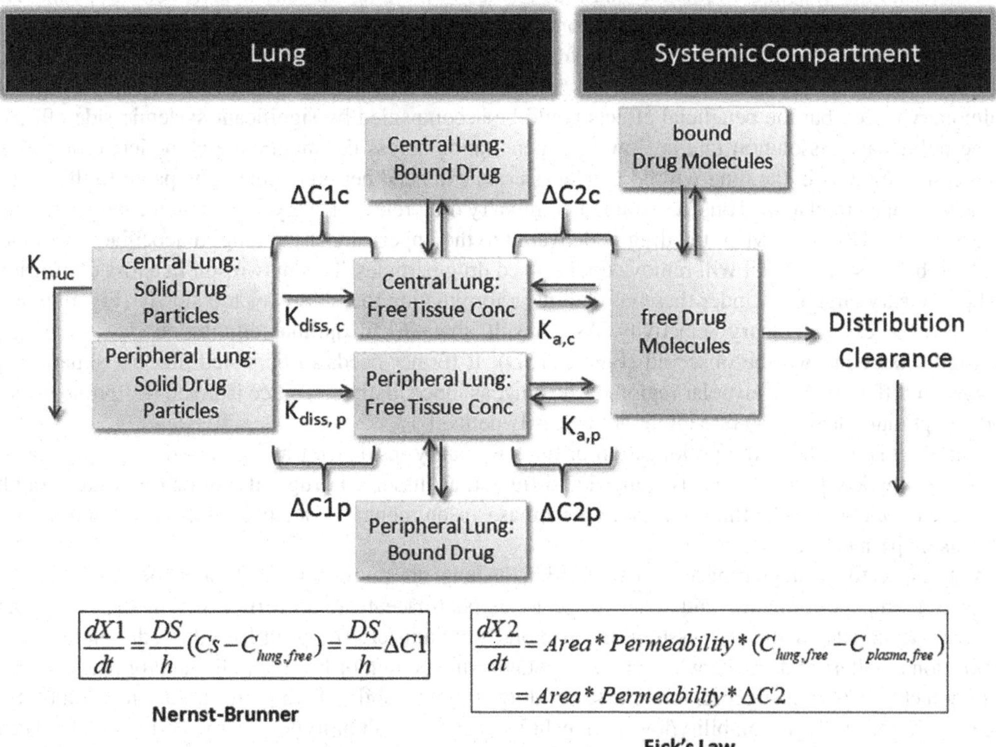

$$\frac{dX1}{dt}=\frac{DS}{h}(Cs-C_{lung,free})=\frac{DS}{h}\Delta C1$$

Nernst-Brunner

$$\frac{dX2}{dt}=Area*Permeability*(C_{lung,free}-C_{plasma,free})$$
$$=Area*Permeability*\Delta C2$$

Fick's Law

FIGURE 6.4 Scheme relevant for the prediction of free drug concentration-time profiles in the lung as determined by Nernst-Brunner equation and Fick's law. Drug particles are deposited in central or peripheral parts of the lung and will subsequently dissolve as described by the Nernst-Brunner equation. Besides physicochemical properties related to dissolution ($dX1/dt$: dissolution rate, D: diffusion coefficient, S: surface area of particles, and h: thickness of the stagnant diffusion layer, C_s solubility in dissolution medium), dissolution rate will also depend on the difference between solubility C_s and the free drug concentrations in the lung lining fluid $C_{\text{lung, free}}$ ($\Delta C1$). As $C_{\text{lung, free}}$ will also depend on the removal rate of dissolved drug through absorption across the lung membranes, as described by Fick's law, particles might dissolve more slowly in areas where the membrane permeability is smaller (e.g. central parts of the lung) and sink conditions are not achieved. Thus, dissolution rates will not only be affected by differences in the particle size distribution of particles depositing in central and peripheral parts of the lung, but also by differences in sink conditions observed in central and peripheral parts of the lung.

The above classification seems to suggest that either dissolution or membrane permeability will determine the pulmonary residence time, depending on the drug class. However, this black and white thinking is not always valid, especially for lipophilic drugs, for which the pulmonary residence time may be determined by the interplay between dissolution and membrane permeability (Figure 6.4); this interplay is affected by both the drug and the physiology of the lung (e.g. differences in thickness of membranes in central and peripheral areas of the lung). The dependence of the dissolution rate of lipophilic drugs on the region of the lung does not only depend on smaller particles depositing in the more peripheral regions; however, it also depends on the fact that membrane permeability will affect the free drug concentrations in the lung ($C_{\text{lung, free}}$), as indicated by Fick's law (Figure 6.4). The $C_{\text{lung, free}}$ will affect the dissolution rate as specified in the Nernst-Brunner equation (Figure 6.4),[2] and high free drug concentrations can considerably slow down the rate of dissolution. Dissolution rates of lipophilic drugs will therefore differ between central and peripheral areas of the lung, since these lung regions differ in their permeability towards drugs (Boger et al. 2015, 2016; Bäckman et al. 2017a). Likewise, differences in solubility and permeability can explain why the lack of sink conditions will be more pronounced for certain drugs than for others.

Figure 6.5 shows the relationship between the dissolution rate of inhaled drug particles and pulmonary selectivity. It was assumed that once the drug is dissolved, it will be absorbed relatively fast into the systemic circulation (no differences between central and peripheral lung were assumed). If the drug particles dissolve quickly (or the drug was given as a solution, Figure 6.5A), dissolved drug will be absorbed into the systemic circulation and thus resides in the lung for only a short period of time. As a result, lung selectivity (higher free drug concentrations in the lung than in the systemic organs) will only last for a short period of time, and the free unbound drug in the lung and the systemic circulation will be identical shortly after inhalation; this leads to a loss in targeting. This does not imply a lack of pulmonary effect, but the beneficial effects could be accompanied by significant systemic side effects. If the pulmonary dissolution rate is slow (and penetration across the membrane is moderate or slow), drug concentrations in the lung will be greater over an extended period of time, compared to the levels in the systemic circulation. Thus, a sustained pulmonary drug release is very beneficial for lung targeting (Figure 6.5B). However, when the drug is delivered to the upper part of the lung, mucociliary transport needs to be considered, as it will remove undissolved drug particles. This may result in a loss of efficacy and pulmonary targeting. Under these conditions, a formulation that dissolves too slowly (Figure 6.5C) will provide less pulmonary selectivity. As a result, there is an optimal dissolution rate for which maximum targeting will be observed (Figure 6.5D). It further needs to be stated that the situation is somewhat different in the alveolar region of the lung, as mucociliary clearance is much less pronounced, and an optimum dissolution rate might not be easily defined.

While not shown here, the prolongation of the pulmonary residence time by non-dissolution related events (e.g. by low permeability) is somewhat different, as dissolved drug will not be removed through mucociliary clearance. In this scenario, an increase in pulmonary selectivity will be observed with decreasing permeability.

With respect to the biopharmaceutical fate within the lung, one might consider systematic classifications to predict drug performance and relate these to biopharmaceutical properties within the lung. The biopharmaceutical classification system (BCS) of orally administered drugs utilizes dose, dissolution, and absorption numbers to describe whether a compound exhibits high or low solubility and/or permeability (Amidon et al. 1995). It suggests four classes of drugs (high solubility/high permeability; low solubility/high permeability, high solubility/low permeability, and low/solubility/low permeability) and relates these properties to the drug's oral bioavailability and dependence on drug formulation and physiological variables. Preliminary evaluation of such a system for classifying the post-deposition processes in the lung suggests that desired drug candidate inhalation products should either have a slow dissolution (i.e. low water solubility) or a low permeability.

As mentioned above, the absorption rate of many drugs is often too fast to achieve maximum pulmonary targeting. Thus, a significant body of work has concentrated on the design of drug delivery systems, which slow down this process and provide the drug with an increased pulmonary

[2] Under sink conditions (C_s-$C_{\text{lung, free}}$ is approaching C_s) dissolution is faster than under non-sink conditions (C_s-$C_{\text{lung, free}}$ much smaller than C_s). The drug's membrane permeability can therefore affect the drug's dissolution rate.

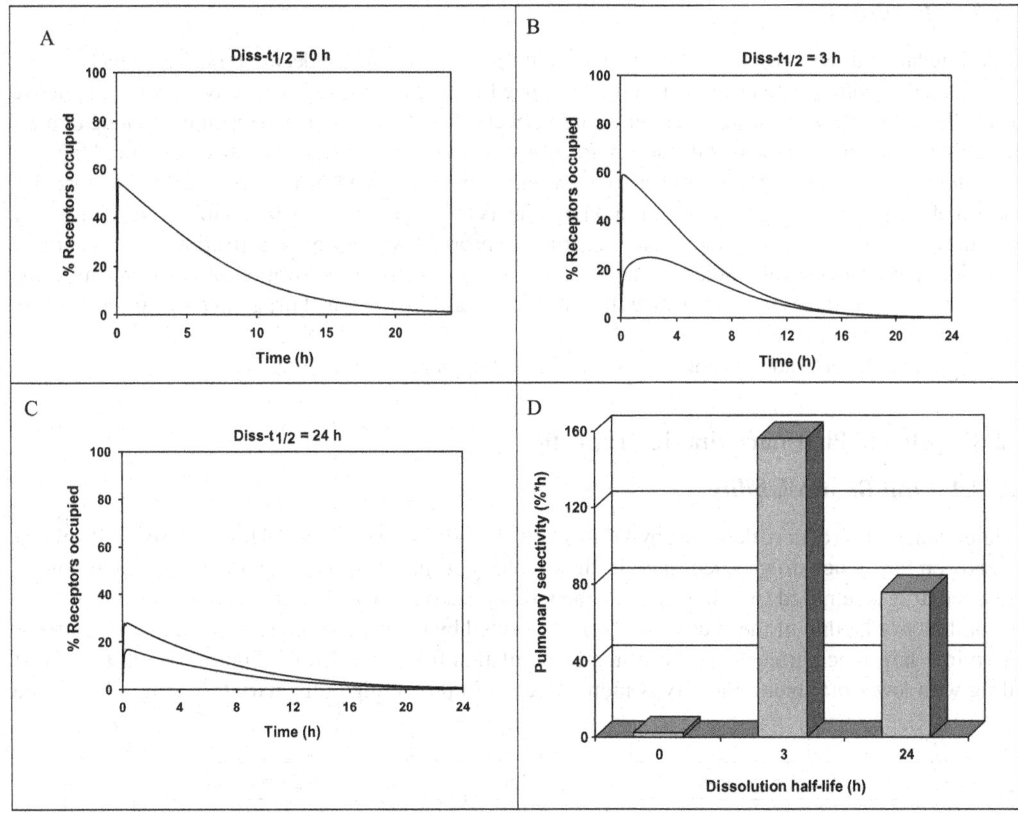

FIGURE 6.5 Effect of pulmonary dissolution rate on pulmonary selectivity. The dose of 300 µg was allowed to dissolve immediately (A), with a half-life of 3 hours (B), or with a half-life of 24 hours (C). Pulmonary selectivity (area between pulmonary (upper line) and systemic (lower line) receptor occupancies) observed in A–C are summarized in D. The dose was given once a day at steady state. A slower release/dissolution of the drug in the lung does significantly increase pulmonary selectivity, however, very slow dissolution rates further decrease pulmonary selectivity, as the undissolved drug particles are removed from the lung by the mucociliary transport system.

residence time. There have been several different approaches to improve the pulmonary residence time of inhaled drugs (Hardy and Chadwick 2000). These include the use of liposomes (Fielding and Abra 1992; Shek et al. 1994; Suarez et al. 1998), microspheres (Bot et al. 2000; Dellamary et al. 2000; Edwards et al. 1997, 1998), ultrathin coatings around drug dry powders (Talton et al. 2000), the use of new excipients such as oligolactic acid (Stefely et al. 1999) or trehalose derivatives (Hardy and Chadwick 2000), or simply the use of slow dissolving lipophilic drugs. There are also biological approaches to prolong the time the drug stays in the lung. For example, long acting beta-2-adrenergic drugs bind tightly to pulmonary cell membranes, and this fraction of drug provides a reservoir which "feeds" drug slowly to the receptor (Green et al. 1996). Similarly, reversible formation of fatty acid esters has been described for glucocorticoids. Glucocorticoids will enter the cell, and a fraction of the drug is converted into highly lipophilic inactive ester derivatives that are unable to leave the cell. The trapped ester can also act as depot for the active corticosteroid in the lung, as it can be slowly re-activated into the active glucocorticoid (Miller-Larsson et al. 1998; Thorsson et al. 1998; Wieslander et al. 1998; Nilsson et al. 2001). Such systems may serve as alternative mechanisms for enhancing pulmonary residence time, if a significant fraction of the drug deposited in the lung will be captured. Overall, a rational approach for identifying new molecules with improved pulmonary retention is still lacking and tools to streamlining this development are needed.

6.2.2.5 Prodrugs

A few inhalation drugs, such as beclomethasone dipropionate or ciclesonide, are prodrugs, which are not able to interact with the receptor themselves, but need to be metabolized (i.e. activated) into an active metabolite before they can stimulate their desired effects. This activation can happen in the lung or after absorption from the lung or the GI tract. A fraction of the prodrug dose is absorbed from the lung into the systemic circulation without prior activation and is then activated in the systemic circulation; this fraction of the prodrug dose can cause pulmonary effects only after redistribution into the lung. Targeting is reduced if a significant fraction of the prodrug is absorbed without prior activation. It is not trivial in clinical pharmacological studies to show the degree of pulmonary activation of such prodrugs; the associated clinical studies need to include the intravenous administration of drug. So far pharmacokinetic studies for beclomethasone propionate (Daley-Yates et al. 2001) and ciclesonide (Guo et al. 2006) indicate that the pulmonary activation is not complete and a certain degree of targeting is lost.

6.2.3 Systemic Pharmacokinetic Properties

6.2.3.1 Oral Bioavailability

A significant portion of drug delivered by MDI or DPI (40%–90%) reaches the GI tract. The overall amount depends on how much drug is deposited in the oropharynx and swallowed, and how much pulmonary deposited drug is removed from the lung by mucociliary clearance which ultimately reaches the GI tract. The oral bioavailability of the drug (*F*), which is affected by the hepatic or pre-hepatic first pass effect, determines how much drug enters the systemic circulation from the GI tract. Figure 6.6 illustrates that a drug with lower oral bioavailability is more effective in promoting pulmonary targeting. Fluticasone

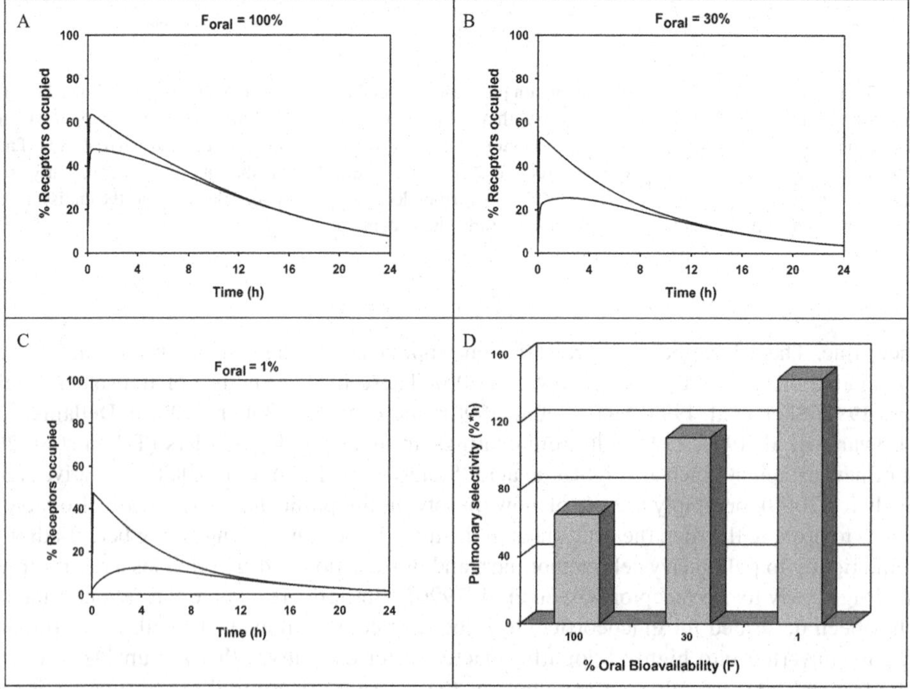

FIGURE 6.6 Effect of oral bioavailability (*F* value) on pulmonary (upper line) and systemic (lower line) receptor occupancies. The *F* value mainly determines the input of the swallowed drug (G.I.) into the systemic circulation. Simulations (A–C) are shown for 100%, 30%, and 1% oral bioavailability, whereas the other parameters like clearance, volume of distribution, and dose remain unchanged. With a decrease in the oral bioavailability, there was a significant increase in the degree of pulmonary targeting (see D).

propionate (FP), ciclesonide, fluticasone furoate, and mometasone furoate have been reported to have a low oral bioavailability of less than 1% (Ventresca et al. 1994; Falcoz et al. 1996). Bioavailabilities of currently used inhaled glucocorticoids range from <1% to 40% (Ryrfeldt et al. 1982; Hochhaus et al. 1992a; Derendorf et al. 1995; Dickens et al. 1999; Daley-Yates et al. 2001). Similarly, oral bioavailabilities of short-acting beta-2-adrenergic drugs vary significantly, from 1.5% to approximately 50% (Hochhaus and Möllmann 1995). These differences likely affect the degree of pulmonary selectivity. According to Rohatagi et al., oral bioavailabilities of approximately 25% or less should not induce clinically relevant systemic side effects as long as a large pulmonary deposition is responsible for a limited amount of drug being swallowed (Rohatagi et al. 1999).

6.2.3.2 Systemic Clearance

Systemic clearance describes the efficiency of the body to eliminate systemically absorbed drug. The cumulative systemic exposure, as indicated by the area under the drug concentration-time profile in plasma, is determined by the amount of drug entering the systemic circulation and the systemic clearance. If an inhaled drug shows pronounced systemic clearance, systemic exposure will be small. This is reflected in simulations shown in Figure 6.7 that indicate increased pulmonary targeting with increasing systemic clearance. Most inhaled glucocorticoids are predominantly cleared by hepatic metabolism so efficiently that their clearance values approach liver blood flow (Chaplin et al. 1980; Ryrfeldt et al. 1982; Derendorf et al. 1995; Mackie et al. 1996). This means for new drug developments in this field, that further improvements (i.e. increases) in the systemic clearance can only be achieved by incorporating

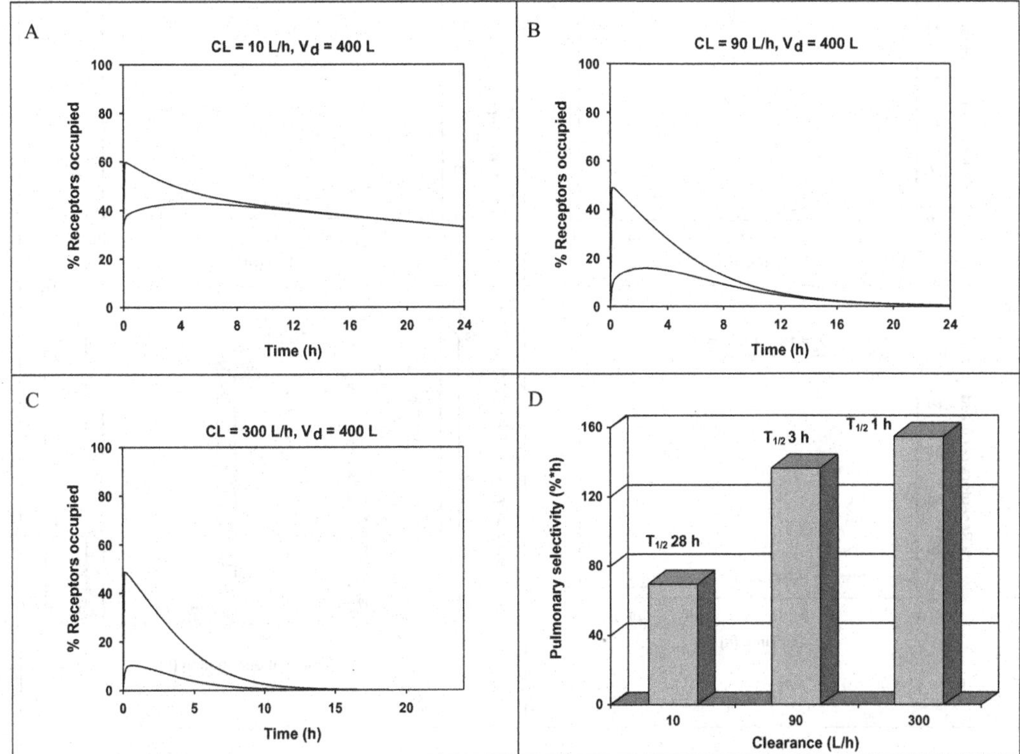

FIGURE 6.7 Effect of systemic clearance (CL) on pulmonary (upper line) and systemic (lower line) receptor occupancies. Simulations A, B, and C are shown for increasing CL values of 10, 90, and 300 L/h, respectively, whereas the other parameters like volume of distribution and dose remain unchanged. An increase in CL (10–300 L/h) produces a significant increase in the difference (AUC pulmonary–AUC systemic) between pulmonary and systemic receptor occupancies, thus indicating that CL is very beneficial in achieving pulmonary selectivity for an inhaled drug.

extra-hepatic clearance mechanisms, for example, by identifying glucocorticoids that are metabolized in the blood (Biggadike et al. 2000). The challenging aspect of such an endeavor is to find enzymatic systems that are present in the blood at sufficient concentrations, but are not (or only minimally) expressed in pulmonary cells; in the latter case, rapid pulmonary inactivation would result in very low pulmonary drug concentrations and likely insufficient pulmonary effects. It is therefore essential that such drugs are sufficiently stable in lung tissue to achieve effective pulmonary concentrations. So far, the development of corticosteroids with such properties have failed.

6.2.3.3 Volume of Distribution/Plasma Binding

Quite often, the half-life of a drug is used as an indicator for systemic exposure. Half-life is a secondary pharmacokinetic property, as it is determined by clearance and volume of distribution ($t_{1/2} = 0.693 \cdot V_d/\mathrm{CL}$). While clearance describes the ability of the body to eliminate the drug, volume of distribution (V_d) is the pharmacokinetic parameter that provides information on the extent of drug distribution into tissue compartments.

For lipophilic drugs, which can readily cross membranes and enter most of the tissue compartments, the volume of distribution (V_d) can be calculated by knowing the volume of the plasma (V_p), the volume of the tissue compartment (V_t), as well as the fraction of drug unbound in plasma (f_u) and in tissue (f_{uT}) (see Figure 6.8).

The more pronounced the tissue binding is over plasma protein binding, the larger will be V_d, thus, more drug will be in the peripheral compartment. A larger volume of distribution will increase the half-life ($t_{1/2}$)

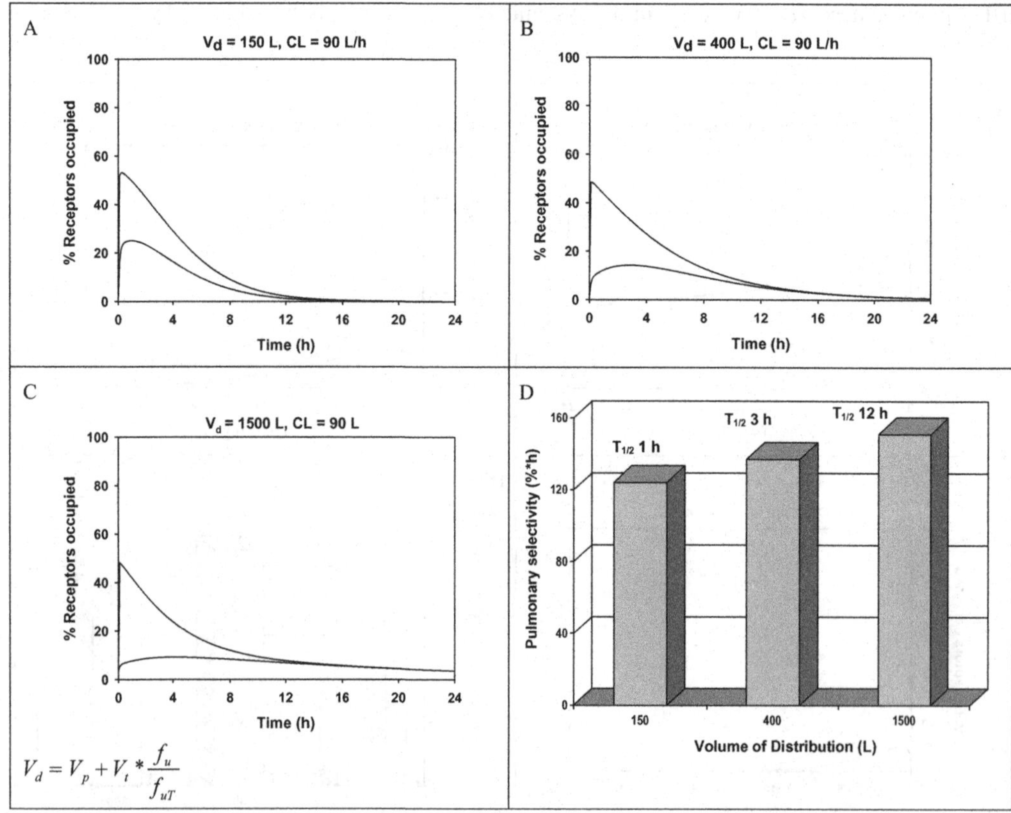

FIGURE 6.8 Effect of volume of distribution (V_d) on pulmonary (upper line) and systemic (lower line) receptor occupancies. Simulations, A, B, and C are shown for increasing V_d values of 150, 400, and 1500 L, respectively, whereas the other parameters like clearance and dose remain unchanged. An increase in V_d (100–1500 L) produces only a slight increase in the difference (AUC pulmonary–AUC systemic) between pulmonary and systemic receptor occupancies, thus indicating that V_d does not seem to be that significant in modulating pulmonary selectivity. As a result, drugs with similar clearance, but different half-lives due to differences in V_d will produce approximately equivalent degree of pulmonary and systemic effects.

of a drug, as less drug reaches the drug eliminating organs (liver or kidney) per time unit. While this leads to a longer half-life of the drug, the overall pulmonary effects,[3] the systemic side effects, and consequently the degree of pulmonary selectivity are not significantly affected (Figure 6.8). Therefore, drugs with a long half-life are not necessarily bad inhalation drugs, if the long half-life is due to a pronounced tissue binding.

Another aspect of tissue and plasma protein binding should be discussed. More lipophilic drugs are currently in development, which show both increased tissue and plasma protein binding. These compounds consequently have small f_u and f_{uT} values. Yet there are no dramatic increases in the estimates of volume of distribution and half-life when compared to other drugs, because f_u and f_{uT} are both higher (see Figure 6.8 for relevant equation). With a decrease in the overall fraction of free drug, the effects (local and systemic) will be smaller than those of a similar drug with equivalent volume of distribution, but lower tissue and plasma protein binding. In this case, the drug with the higher degree of binding, but otherwise identical properties, will show reduced systemic side effects and reduced pulmonary effects at a given concentration.

Systemic side effects are "hard" parameters in clinical studies, as concentration-response relationships can be rather readily detected; in contrast, pulmonary effects are generally "soft" parameters, since concentration-effect relationships are more difficult to detect. Such highly bound drugs given at identical doses might show very good safety profiles (due to low systemic effects) compared to less highly bound drugs. The anti-asthmatic effects of a highly bound drug may not be statistically significantly different, because of the soft pulmonary surrogate markers. In this case, the drug with a high plasma/tissue binding would suggest an improved safety profile. Animal experiments indicating a lower receptor occupancy in lung and non-pulmonary organs for drugs with higher plasma protein binding support this finding (Wu et al. 2009).

6.2.4 Pharmacodynamic Factors Important for Pulmonary Targeting

The effects and side effects of the majority of inhalation drugs are mediated through membrane or cytosolic receptors. For glucocorticoids, the activity at the site of action is related to the receptor binding affinity of the drug (Beato et al. 1972; Dahlberg et al. 1984; Druzgala et al. 1991). In the case of beta-2-adrenergic drugs, very good correlations were observed between *in vitro* indicators of drug activity in cell culture and the pharmacological activity *in vivo* (Hochhaus and Möllmann 1992, 1995). Therefore, receptor binding affinities or other *in vitro* parameters are often used in discussions describing the pharmacological properties of inhalation drugs at the site of action (e.g. in the lung). To evaluate the importance of the receptor potency of a drug on pulmonary targeting, two cases need to be differentiated. In the first case, such as for glucocorticoids,[4] pulmonary effects and systemic "side" effects are mediated through the identical receptors in pulmonary and systemic tissues. In the second case, such as for beta-adrenergic drugs, two receptor sub-types (β_1/β_2 adrenergic receptors) are involved in the pulmonary and systemic side effects.

If the "same" receptors are mediating pulmonary and systemic effects, simulations (Figure 6.9) show that pulmonary targeting (i.e. the difference between lung and systemic receptor occupancy) is not affected by different receptor binding affinities, as long as these affinities are being considered by a dose adjustment (i.e. the dose is doubled for a drug with two-fold lower receptor affinity). This means that a low receptor binding affinity can be compensated by an increase in the dose. Thus, the importance of a high receptor binding affinity for promoting pulmonary selectivity, which is often used to promote such high affinity drugs, should be questioned.

In the second case (Figure 6.10), where pulmonary and systemic effects are mediated through different receptors (e.g., beta-2-adrenergic drugs), a high binding selectivity (high affinity to the β_2 receptors, low affinity to the β_1 receptor) is important for the pulmonary selectivity; and drug candidates with the highest degree of selectivity are preferred.

[3] For simulations in Figure 6.8, drug binding in the lung and plasma stays constant across the simulations. Systemic receptor occupancy was estimating receptor occupancy from free plasma concentrations.

[4] Attempts to develop corticosteroids with improved safety profiles through pharmacodynamics properties (so called dissociated steroids) failed so far (Catley 2007)

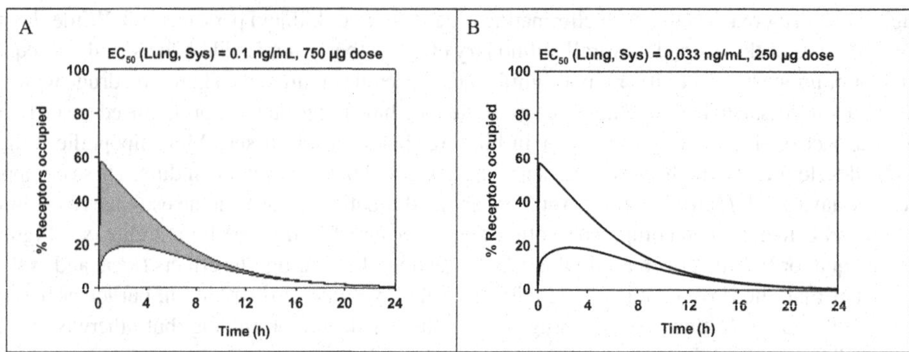

FIGURE 6.9 Effect of receptor affinity on pulmonary (upper line) and systemic (lower line) receptor occupancies. The simulations try to illustrate pulmonary selectivity of an inhaled drug by utilizing PK/PD relationships and selecting receptor occupancy as a surrogate marker to predict the pulmonary and systemic effects. The difference (shaded area) between the area under the curve for pulmonary and systemic receptor occupancy-time profiles indicates the degree of pulmonary targeting. Simulations A and B depict two hypothetical drugs with different receptor binding affinities, however, by adjusting their dose, the differences in their receptor binding affinities can be compensated. Both the drugs display the pulmonary and systemic side effects by interacting with the same sub-type of receptors. From the above figure, it is clear that by adjusting the dose of the drug displaying lower receptor binding affinity, identical pulmonary selectivity can be achieved. The EC50 value and the dose were modulated to obtain identical pulmonary selectivity, whereas other parameters (like clearance, volume of distribution) were fixed during the simulation.

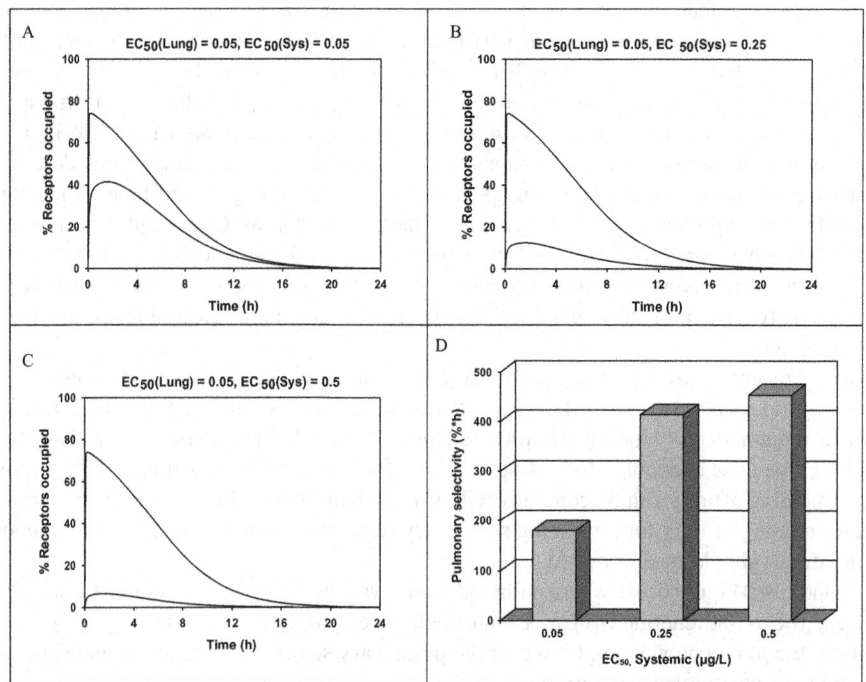

FIGURE 6.10 Simulations (A, B, and C) showing pulmonary (upper line) and (systemic (lower line) receptor occupancies for a hypothetical beta-2-adrenergic drug which display the desired (pulmonary) and undesired (systemic) effect by occupying two different types of receptors. Cases A, B, and C show the occupancy profiles for pulmonary and systemic effects when the receptor affinity of the drug in the lung (for beta-2 receptors) remains unchanged, but decreases (for beta-1 receptors) at the systemic organs (compare with A). Thus, pulmonary selectivity is achieved at the pharmacodynamic level. Pulmonary selectivity (area between pulmonary (upper line) and systemic (lower line) receptor occupancies) observed in A–C are summarized in D.

6.2.5 Summary: Factors Important for Pulmonary Targeting

In summary, a successful inhalation product should use a drug with high systemic clearance, low oral bioavailability, extended pulmonary residence time, and high receptor selectivity, if the mode of action allows the latter. Drug solubility as well as the rates of dissolution and membrane permeability are important contributors to the pulmonary residence time. Device/formulation properties should allow high pulmonary deposition and regional deposition profiles that favors deposition into pharmacodynamically relevant lung areas.

6.3 Methods to Assess Pharmacokinetic and Dynamic Properties of Inhalation Drugs

As outlined above, pharmacokinetic and dynamic properties of inhaled drugs are defining the degree of pulmonary effects and selectivity. Methods for identifying key pharmacokinetic and dynamic properties are therefore relevant for drug development and clinical practice. This section reviews several of the currently available tools in order of increasing complexity (Figure 6.11). These include *in vitro* approaches (e.g. cell lines, cell line constructs, lung isolated perfused lungs), animal models, and assessments in humans.

6.3.1 Cell Line Methods

Cell culture models are simple and efficient tools to study cellular drug uptake, membrane permeability, metabolism, pharmacodynamic and toxicological events, as well as toxicity at a molecular level (Ehrhardt et al. 2017; Ehrhardt and Kim 2008). The ideal *in vitro* model should be similar to the cellular phenotype of the lung barrier *in situ*. To be most realistic, it should be comprised of a mixed population of cell types including ciliated cells, mucus secreting cells, and surfactant producing cells depending on the airway generation. Moreover, these models should reflect the expression of drug transporters and metabolic enzymes (Ehrhardt et al. 2017). As mentioned previously, the cellular composition of the lung can roughly be divided into two completely different epithelia: conducting airways (trachea-bronchial region) and gas-exchanging airspaces (alveolar region); these regions differ in the cellular composition and thickness.

6.3.1.1 Airway Epithelial Cell Lines

The correlation between the permeability from respiratory epithelial cell lines in rats and the pulmonary absorption rate constant is well established (Bosquillon et al. 2017). The most commonly used human-derived cell lines (Calu-3 and 16HBE14o) show epithelial barrier-like properties in culture and permit the measurement of drug permeability.

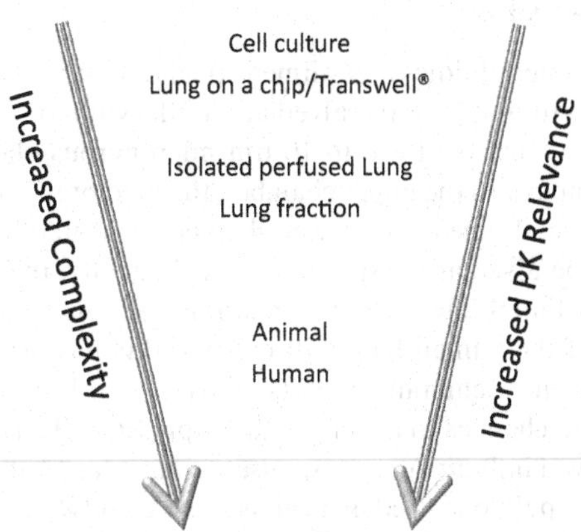

FIGURE 6.11 Methods to assess pharmacokinetics and pharmacodynamics of inhalation drugs.

The Calu-3 (American type culture collection ATCC HTB-55) derived from an adenocarcinoma in a 25-year-old male Caucasian has been applied and evaluated for drug absorption, metabolism, and transport (Ehrhardt and Kim 2008; Steimer et al. 2005). Calu-3 is the only human lung cancer derived cell line that exhibits similar mRNA and protein expression to the native epithelium (Steimer et al. 2005). Another bronchial epithelial cell line, 16HBE14o, was developed by transforming normal bronchial epithelium (of 1st bifurcation) from a 1-year-old male heart-lung transplant patient (Ehrhardt and Kim 2008; Steimer et al. 2005). The lung cells were infected with a SV40 large T-antigen containing a replication defective pSVori-plasmid (Ehrhardt and Kim 2008; Steimer et al. 2005). The 16HBE14o cells have been utilized as a model to examine transport and particle cell interactions, however, these cells are not commercially available (Ehrhardt and Kim 2008).

The culture conditions (i.e. air-liquid interface versus submerged culture) and barrier properties of these two cell lines have been reported by different permeability studies (Winton et al. 1998; Forbes 2000; Wan et al. 2000; Borchard et al. 2002; Ehrhardt et al. 2002; Patel et al. 2002; Pezron et al. 2002; Mathia et al. 2002; Fiegel et al. 2003; Forbes and Ehrhardt 2005). Drug permeability for a variety of drug compounds has been measured in Calu-3 and 16HBE14o cell lines, and a correlation with absorption from lungs *in vivo* and *ex vivo* has been shown (Bosquillon et al. 2017). In addition, *in vitro*/*in vivo* correlations between permeability and absorption data of intratracheally administered drugs in rats have been reported (Forbes and Ehrhardt 2005; Bosquillon et al. 2017).

The human bronchial epithelial cell line BEAS-2B, obtained from autopsy of non-cancerous individuals, and infected with a hybrid virus of adenovirus 12 and simian virus 40 (Ad12AV40), has limitations in modelling drug absorption; however, this cell line has been very popular in studies of airway epithelial cell structure, function, and cell biology, such as phenotyping and mechanistic investigation of cytokine regulation (Ehrhardt and Kim 2008; Steimer et al. 2005).

More recent human bronchial epithelial cell lines, such as NuLi-1, UNCN1T-3T, VA10, BCi-NS1.1, and hAELVi are more similar to the naive cells *in situ*; however, these cell lines have not yet been established for biopharmaceutical applications (Ehrhardt et al. 2017).

6.3.1.2 Alveolar Epithelial Cell Lines

For the alveolar epithelial region, there is no suitable cell line available. Most of the primary alveolar epithelial cell lines arise from the alveolar type II cells (Forbes and Ehrhardt 2005). The well-known and widely used human cell line A549 is derived from a human pulmonary adenocarcinoma of a 58-year-old Caucasian man (Ehrhardt and Kim 2008; Steimer et al. 2005). This cell line lacks functional tight junctions which limits its use for absorption studies; however, the A549 cell line reveals biological characteristics of alveolar epithelial type II cells (Forbes and Ehrhardt 2005; Steimer et al. 2005). The A549 models are accepted to access pulmonary toxicity and have been used in metabolism, cytotoxicity, and gene delivery studies (Ehrhardt and Kim 2008; Steimer et al. 2005).

6.3.2 Breathing Lung-on-a-Chip

Breathing lung-on-a-chip is a microfluidic three-dimensional device that reconstructs the microarchitecture and dynamic microenvironment of the alveolar-capillary unit of the living human lung. This micro-engineered lung model consists of a thin 10 μm microporous elastomeric membrane, which divides the air and blood chambers. In the upper chamber, the membrane is covered by human alveolar epithelial cells, whereas the membrane of the lower chamber is coated by pulmonary microvascular endothelial cells. To mimic the alveolar air space more realistically, the alveolar epithelial cells are exposed to air creating an air-liquid interface and breathing movements are introduced. During normal inspiration, the alveoli of the human lung will expand; this has been mimicked by a computer controlled cyclic stretching of the membrane with its adherent cell layer (Esch et al. 2015); however, this model lacks to incorporate changes in air flow and air pressure (Huh et al. 2010; Huh 2015). The lung-on-a-chip approach showed inflammatory responses to an induced alveolar bacterial infection. In addition, lung diseases such as pulmonary edema can be emulated (Huh et al. 2010; Esch et al. 2015). The suitability of this model to also probe for biopharmaceutical aspects of inhalation drug therapy still needs to be demonstrated.

6.3.3 Isolated Lung Perfusion Models

In the isolated perfused lung (IPL) model, the lung (usually obtained from an animal) is isolated from the systemic circulation, while keeping the structural and cellular integrity (Ehrhardt and Kim 2008). The lung is perfused via pulmonary circulation and ventilated via the trachea. The IPL has been instrumental in accessing the pulmonary fate of inhaled drugs by employing lungs mostly of rats, but also of mouse, sheep, pig, and lobes of human lungs (Ehrhardt et al. 2017). These models permit investigation of surfactant secretion, permeability measurements, pulmonary dissolution, absorption, lung tissue binding, transport phenomena, and metabolism; as one of its strengths, this model maintains the physiological properties of the lung (Steimer et al. 2005). Drug is delivered into the ventilated lung either by intratracheal injection or via a modified MDI. These experiments result in typical absorption profiles (drug absorbed as a function of time) of drug and its metabolites (if applicable, see Figure 6.12). The IPL was one of the models that indicated that a fraction of budesonide is captured in the lung. In addition, this model allows us to estimate the mucociliary clearance.

A strong correlation between the logarithm of the *in vivo* absorption half-life ($\log_{T50\%}$) and the absorption half-life ($t_{1/2}$) of an *ex vivo* rat ILP model has been shown (Bosquillon et al. 2017). The ILP became a well-established model, which has been explored for screening the pulmonary absorption of compounds by AstraZeneca and GlaxoSmithKline (Bosquillon et al. 2017). It has been used to generate quantitative structure activity relationships (QSAR). This novel QSAR approach identified physicochemical descriptors (for e.g. lipophilicity, size, shape, charge, hydrogen bounding) to predict the ability of the parent drug to penetrate the lung epithelium and appear in the perfusate once it is in solution. For this approach, 108 compounds were tested by utilizing an *in situ* isolated perfused rat lung model. The observed factors which influenced the pulmonary absorption were diverse; however, solubility was a very important characteristic. While measurements of permeability and hydrophobicity were found to positively correlate with pulmonary absorption, negative correlations were observed for ionization and molecule size (Edwards et al. 2016).

6.3.3.1 Drug Content in Lung Tissue

Determinations of drug levels in the lung and comparison with plasma levels have been used for the pharmacokinetic assessment of inhalation drugs. In such a scenario, drug is typically delivered to the lung of animals or patients who have to undergo lung resection. Subsequently, the lung or lung sections are removed at different time points, and the drug concentration-time profile is compared with that in the plasma.

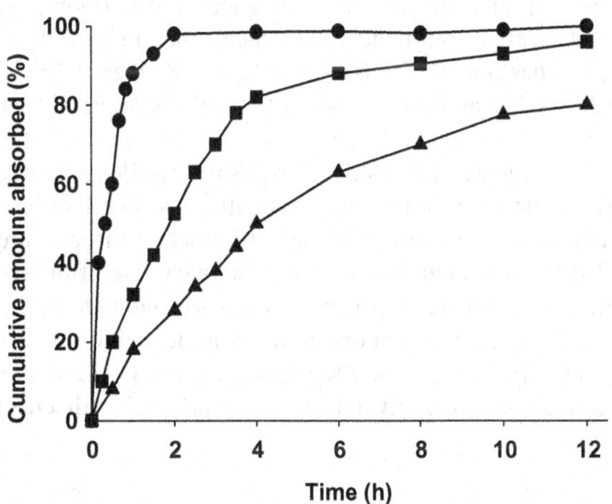

FIGURE 6.12 Possible absorption profiles obtained from experiments with isolated perfused lung or absorption profiles obtained after proper deconvolution from inhalation studies. Lines present drugs with different absorption rates. Circles = fast, square = intermediate, and triangle = slow absorption rates, respectively.

Studies were performed in patients undergoing lung resection surgery (Van den Bosch et al. 1993; Esmailpour et al. 1997), where lung cancer patients were dosed pre-operatively. The drug concentration was determined in the peripheral and central lung tissues and was compared to the blood samples taken during surgery. This enabled calculation of drug ratios between lung and plasma and of the pulmonary half-life of the drug. In general, this pharmacokinetic approach can evaluate the time profile of disappearance of drug from the lung, especially if advanced pharmacokinetic modelling approaches (such as population modelling) are employed. However, it needs to be taken into consideration that drug concentrations in the lung reflect undissolved drug, drug bound to pulmonary tissue components, and pharmacodynamically relevant free drug concentrations. In addition, higher drug concentrations in the lung than those in plasma are not *per se* indicative of pulmonary targeting. Even after intravenous administration for a drug with a large volume of distribution (i.e. high tissue binding), total tissue concentrations are often higher than the plasma concentrations. Thus, a careful study design (administration of the drug via the lung and intravenously) needs to be employed, if one seeks to use this approach to assess the pulmonary selectivity.

6.3.3.2 Imaging Studies

In vivo radiographic imaging techniques are proving extremely useful in assessing drug deposition (Digenis et al. 1998; Newman and Wilding 1999). These methods include gamma scintigraphy (e.g. gamma emitting nuclide 99mTc), single photon emission tomography (SPECT), and positron emission tomography (PET). For some applications, magnetic resonance imaging, which does not require radioactive labeling can be employed. These techniques, as discussed in more detail in other chapters of this book, can provide detailed information on the degree and location of pulmonary deposition, especially if they are combined with x-ray computed tomography (Darquenne et al. 2016). In addition, pulmonary pharmacokinetics can be assessed if the drug particles are labeled and can be followed over an extended period of time (Berridge et al. 1998; Chen and Kinahan 2010).

6.3.3.3 Animal/Human Studies

With the availability of highly sensitive analytical procedures, capable of detecting drug in the sub-picogram per mL range, pharmacokinetic studies allow a detailed characterization of the fate of inhaled drugs. Pharmacokinetic studies in animals (such as mice, rats, dogs, pigs, sheep, primates, for review see [Guillon et al. 2018]) and humans provide significant information for inhalation drugs. Important parameters to be obtained from PK studies (often in combination with iv PK data) include the pulmonary deposition efficiency and the pulmonary available dose (i.e. pulmonary deposited dose minus drug that is removed through mucociliary clearance). Furthermore, this includes parameters assessing the pulmonary absorption, pulmonary residence time, and the overall degree of systemic exposure (Table 6.2). Approaches suitable for assessing these and other pharmacokinetic properties are discussed below. Table 6.2 lists data analysis methods of different complexity and potential information provided by these methods.

PK studies allow one to evaluate the systemic exposure profiles of inhalation therapy, as the sum of drug absorbed from the lung and GI tract. For drugs which lack oral bioavailability or in studies where the oral absorption process is effectively blocked via a charcoal block, traditional pharmacokinetics will also allow conclusions on the pulmonary fate of inhalation drugs (Table 6.1). Resulting information includes estimates of the pulmonary available dose, the pulmonary residence time, and, in special cases, even information on the regional deposition (Goyal and Hochhaus 2010; Weber and Hochhaus 2015). The ability of PK studies to assess these important processes and parameters relevant for pulmonary bioequivalence is currently being discussed as an alternative to clinical efficacy studies.

6.3.3.3.1 Animal Studies

Guillon et al. (2018) reviewed recently the use of animal studies in the assessment of inhalation drugs. While important during drug development, differences in the pulmonary anatomy and physiology make interpretation of animal PK studies challenging. As an example, differences in the lung geometry,

TABLE 6.2

Information Relevant for Bioequivalence Decisions Extractable from PK Studies for Inhalation Drugs Showing ($F \gg 0$) or Lacking Oral Bioavailability ($F = 0$)

	Oral Bioavailability $F = 0$	Oral Bioavailability $F \gg 0$
% Pulmonary deposition	Yes	Not without blocking[a] oral absorption
Systemic exposure (AUC)	Yes	Yes
Pulmonary residence time	Yes	Not without blocking oral absorption
Pulmonary absorption rate	Yes	Only if oral absorption can be blocked or deconvolution is able to differentiate
Central/peripheral deposition	Potentially for slowly dissolving drugs or drugs showing distinct differences in the absorption rate	Not without blocking oral absorption
Absorption through GI Tract	Not applicable	Yes, if PK is assessed with or without blocking

[a] Or other methods able to differentiate between absorption through the lung and gastrointestinal tract.

breathing pattern, and nose versus oral inhalation will affect the efficiency and regional deposition across animal species, subsequently the pulmonary fate of drugs post-depositing may be affected. As animals will spontaneously inhale, methods of drug delivery will be different from human use. Instillation, chamber inhalation, and invasive mechanical ventilation in animals have been suggested. Despite the limitations, animal studies allow one to assess the pulmonary fate of inhalation drugs in more detail, resulted in assessing the degree of pulmonary selectivity (Suarez et al. 1998), and supported the development of physiologically based PK/PD models (Boger et al. 2016).

Pulmonary models have been developed for rats and mice, which allow the assessment of anti-inflammatory properties of a drug after antigen challenge. Alternatively, pulmonary eosinophilia can be induced by non-allergic modes, e.g. by administering sephadex (Hochhaus et al. 1992b; Bjermer et al. 1994a; Haddad et al. 2002). This results in an increase in lung weight. The topical activity of inhaled glucocorticoids has been tested in such models by administering the glucocorticoid into the left lung lobe of rats, followed by administration of sephadex to the whole lung. Observing the differential effects of the glucocorticoid on left and right lobe weight can be used to assess pulmonary targeting. Targeting is observed when the effects on the left lobe are more pronounced than the effects on the right lobe; the latter will only be exposed to systemic glucocorticoid concentrations (Bjermer et al. 1994b). Alternatively, systemic effects of glucocorticoids have been assessed by monitoring the effects on thymus weight, and these weights compared to those with the local effects in the sephadex assay with the drug administered to the whole lung (Bjermer et al. 1994b).

Other targeting models in rats or mice are based on the *ex vivo* monitoring of receptor occupancy after intratracheal administration of the drug, described here for glucocorticoids (Hochhaus et al. 1995; Arya et al. 2005; Boger et al. 2015). Such models are based on the finding that the glucocorticoid receptors are similar in different tissues, resulting in identical receptor occupancy time profile when free drug concentrations in different tissues are identical, e.g. after systemic administration of a drug. Pulmonary targeting after intratracheal administration can then be assessed by comparing the receptor occupancy in the lung to a systemic organ, such as the liver or kidney. A more pronounced receptor occupancy profile in the lung after intratracheal administration indicates pulmonary targeting. Importantly, this approach can provide quantitative data on the time-course of receptor binding *in vivo* which provides valuable insights. Similar approaches could be designed for cell membrane receptors, for example, for the beta-adrenergic receptors, using *ex vivo* receptor binding approaches developed for other membrane receptors (Sadée et al. 1983).

Pre-clinical *in vivo* models have been suggested for dose predictions in humans using empirical scale-up approaches mainly based on Ericsson et al. (2017) and Phillips (2017), although more sophisticated approaches should be developed that consider physiological and anatomical differences in the lungs between species in more detail (e.g. absorption kinetics, tissue binding).

6.3.3.3.2 Studies in Humans

Efficacy studies in humans are the cornerstone of virtually all drug development programs. It is beyond the scope of this chapter to provide a detailed description of all possible approaches. As outlined in a recent FDA guidance, clinical studies for COPD will include pulmonary function tests and exercise capacity ("Chronic Obstructive Pulmonary Disease: Developing Drugs for Treatment Guidance for Industry-Draft Guidance." FDA. Gov. n.d.). Lung function, airway hyper-responsiveness, and challenge tests have been suggested by the European Medicines Agency for clinical investigations of anti-asthma medications. A detailed review of clinical assessment tools was provided by the American Thoracic Society (Reddel et al. 2009).

Pharmacokinetic studies in humans have been often performed in healthy volunteers. This is an over-simplification if conclusions for patient are to be drawn, as lung disease will affect deposition and the pulmonary fate of inhaled drugs, especially for more severe disease states. It is therefore important to realize that pharmacokinetics, particularly in the lung, may differ between patients and healthy volunteers (Wang et al. 2014).

The systemic bioavailability of fluticasone propionate has been reported to be lower in asthma patients compared to healthy volunteers; this leads to a significantly lower area under the curve (AUC) and maximum concentration (C_{max}) in asthma patients (Mortimer et al. 2007; Wang et al. 2014). Diderichsen et al. (2013) showed that the maximum concentration (C_{max}) is reduced by 52% in asthma patients and 31% in COPD patients, as compared to that in healthy volunteers. Falcoz et al. (n.d.) and Daley-Yates et al. (2000) reported a 2–3 times reduced systemic availability for inhaled fluticasone propionate in asthmatics, while there was no significant difference in the kinetic parameters after intravenous administration between healthy volunteers and asthmatic patients. This indicates that differences after inhalation between healthy volunteers and asthmatics are likely caused by differences in the pulmonary factors.

Mortimer et al. (2006, 2007) linked reduced systemic availability of fluticasone propionate to a reduced lung function, as a linear relationship could be identified between reduction in systemic exposure and airway function (FEV1). Patients with impaired lung functions caused by lung diseases, such as COPD and asthma, not only have a different breathing pattern leading to a lower total lung deposition; however, these patients also have a thicker (i.e. more viscous) epithelial lining fluid (ELF), a slower mucociliary clearance, and an enhanced macrophage phagocytosis (Wang et al. 2014). The decreased systemic availability in asthmatics seems to depend on the severity of the disease. Moderate to severe asthmatics exhibited marked PK differences when compared to healthy volunteers, while PK properties were more comparable between healthy volunteers and mild asthmatics (Thorsson et al. 2001). These findings suggest that pharmacokinetic studies should be performed in the patient population of interest. This would also include children, as differences in the pharmacokinetics between adults and children have also been observed (Agertoft and Pedersen 1993; Wildhaber et al. 1998; Agertoft et al. 1999).

6.4 Pharmacokinetic Assessment Tools

6.4.1 General Considerations

This chapter briefly reviews the design of pharmacokinetic studies. It will not discuss studies that evaluate clinical efficacy. Pharmacokinetic studies which assess plasma concentrations solely after inhalation (i.e. without an intravenous dose as reference) will allow conclusions on the rate of absorption and general parameters, such as terminal half-life. However, studies with this design will only provide limited information on the systemic pharmacokinetic properties, such as systemic bioavailability, clearance, and volume of distribution. This issue is especially problematic with new drugs for limited or no information is available in the literature.

For proper characterization of an inhalation drug, information on the systemic pharmacokinetic properties should be provided through studies after intravenous and oral administration. This enables the estimation of clearance, volume of distribution, oral and overall systemic bioavailability. For prodrugs, this would include assessing the pharmacokinetics of the prodrug and of active metabolite as separate treatments with the respective compound being dosed intravenously. A major challenge for such studies is to provide a suitable formulation for intravenous dosing, especially as new drug candidates are often very lipophilic. The resulting parameters of such studies (including systemic clearance, volume of distribution, half-life, mean residence time) can then be readily calculated from the concentration-time profiles after intravenous administration via standard pharmacokinetic analysis by non-compartmental approaches. In addition, a detailed compartmental modelling analysis based on concentration-time profiles will be useful in evaluating the systemic distribution processes in more detail. This will be especially important if deconvolution procedures are included for the assessment of the pulmonary absorption profiles (see below).

Pharmacokinetic studies evaluating the dose linearity or the comparison of different drug strengths are greatly helpful to characterize the pharmacokinetic of inhaled drugs. Pharmacokinetics in relevant patient groups and the search for co-variates through population pharmacokinetic approaches, further inform about potentially altered pharmacokinetics in special patient groups. As an example, systemic exposure is reduced for fluticasone propionate in patients with reduced lung function (Mortimer et al. 2006). Estimates of the oral bioavailability of the drug are required to fully understand the plasma concentrations after inhaled dosing, since a part of the dose is swallowed.

For glucocorticoid studies, often very large doses of steroid often have to be given to obtain quantifiable drug concentrations after oral administration. The oral bioavailability can then be readily calculated by comparing the dose-adjusted area under the concentration-time profiles after oral and iv administration. An elegant way of obtaining information on iv and oral dosing at the same time (with the advantage of reducing the variability of such estimation by deleting the inter-assay variability) is to use unlabelled drug for one form of administration and to dose at the same time a deuterated form of the drug for the other form of administration (Lundin et al. 2001).

When using systemic (plasma, serum, or urine) drug concentrations for the evaluation of inhalation drugs, one must take into consideration that these concentrations are comprised of drug absorbed via the lung and the GI tract. Thus, these studies cannot be used *a priori* to characterize the pulmonary fate of inhalation drugs (see Table 6.2). To better interpret such data, the oral bioavailability should be known.

In the case of drugs that show negligible oral bioavailability (e.g. fluticasone propionate, mometasone furoate, or ciclesonide), systemic concentration-time profiles mirror the pharmacokinetic processes in the lung. In this case, pharmacokinetic parameters (See Table 6.2) will directly reflect and describe the pulmonary fate of the drug.

For drugs that show significant oral bioavailability (e.g. salbutamol [Chege and Chrystyn 2000], terbutaline sulfate [Borgström and Nilsson 1990], budesonide [Thorsson et al. 1994]), different approaches like the charcoal-block technique or the knowledge of differences in the pulmonary and GI absorption lag times can be utilized to determine the pulmonary fate of the inhaled drug.

The rationale for the charcoal block-design is that for a number of drugs, oral absorption of swallowed drug can be blocked by co-administered charcoal. Activated charcoal provides a very large surface area to adsorb drug molecules, and thereby the absorption of swallowed drug can be greatly minimized. For this technique, a subject typically ingests charcoal slurry both at the time of drug administration and one or two hours after drug administration; depending on the drug, the time points of charcoal dosing may need to be optimized. Thus, accurate delineation of pulmonary absorption can be achieved because the absorption of the orally swallowed fraction of the inhaled product is blocked by charcoal. Comparison of drug concentrations with and without charcoal dosing allows one to assess the degree of orally absorbed drug (Thorsson et al. 1994). Such approaches have been described for terbutaline (Borgström and Nilsson 1990), triamcinolone acetonide (Argenti et al. 1999), budesonide (Thorsson et al. 1994), and other glucocorticoids (Möllmann et al. 1997). It is, however, vital for this approach to ensure the efficacy of the charcoal treatment by assessing the charcoal block after oral administration of drug (Thorsson et al. 1994).

Another approach to handle drugs with significant oral bioavailability is based on the finding that the absorption rates from the lung and the GI tract differ for a number of drugs, with the pulmonary absorption being much faster. Thus, drug reaching the systemic circulation rapidly after the inhalation represents drug absorbed from the lung. Such differences in the absorption lag times (and absorption rates) from the lung and the GI tract have been utilized to determine the pulmonary deposition of salbutamol (Hindle and Chrystyn 1992). Hindle et al. showed that under these conditions, the collection of urine rather than blood, is sufficient. For example, negligible amounts of unchanged salbutamol were excreted in the urine within the first 30 minutes when given orally (Hindle and Chrystyn 1992). In contrast, salbutamol can be detected in the urine within the first 30 minutes when given as inhalation, indicating that the pulmonary absorption is fast. This method was validated in clinical trials indicating that 30 minute urinary excretion of salbutamol following a variety of inhalation maneuvers reflects the pulmonary absorbed fraction of the dose (Hindle et al. 1993). Monitoring the urine concentrations over long time can then be used as a marker for the total systemic drug exposure. The time lag between the oral and pulmonary absorption has been observed for other drugs, such as nedocromil (Aswania et al. 1998), sodium cromoglycate (Aswania et al. 1997), and gentamicin (Nasr and Chrystyn 1997). One needs, however, to consider that this approach is drug specific and cannot be applied to all classes of drugs, and that the time resolution is limited when urine is collected, especially if only done once.

6.4.2 Pharmacokinetic Analysis Tools

A range of analysis tools is available for the assessment of pharmacokinetic studies. These differ in the complexity and information possible to be extracted from PK studies. An overview of currently employed methods is shown in Table 6.3. These include: (a) non-compartmental analysis, that is able to derive key pharmacokinetic properties (clearance, volume of distribution, bioavailability, peak concentrations, time to reach peak concentrations (t_{max}) and (b) compartmental pharmacokinetic approaches, that empirically describe concentration-time profiles with suitable mathematical relationships in average or individual subjects. Furthermore, (c) population pharmacokinetic approaches, which allow a more statistical evaluation with the goal of quantifying and explaining variability by identifying co-variates and sub-populations of subjects with certain pharmacokinetic properties. And, finally, (d) physiologically based pharmacokinetic models (PBPK) can be applied which seek to predict concentration-time profiles in plasma and tissues by "re-creating physiological events" within the mathematical model, thus considering anatomical, physiological, physical, and chemical processes within the mathematical prediction of the drug's absorption, distribution, metabolism and elimination.

6.4.2.1 *Non-compartmental Analysis*

When assessing pharmacokinetic data, one either fits data to a proposed compartmental model (e.g. assuming the time-dependent transfer of drug from a central to a peripheral compartment or multiple peripheral compartments) or employs the so-called non-compartmental analysis which does not

TABLE 6.3

Pharmacokinetic Analysis Approaches (Extractable Information Over Less Complex Approach)

Increased Complexity (↓)	• Non-compartmental Analysis
	  • Bioavailability, Bioequivalence, half-life, clearance, volume of distribution, t_{max}, variability
	• Compartmental Analysis
	  (Additional Information over less complex method)
	  • More detailed Absorption kinetics,
	  • Mathematical description of plasma concentration-time profiles. Simulation and predictions possible
	• Population Pharmacokinetic Approaches
	  (Additional Information over less complex method)
	  • Variability, co-variates
	• Physiologically based Pharmacokinetic Models
	  (Additional Information over less complex method)
	  • Prediction of pharmacokinetic profiles in lung and plasma
	  • link to physicochemical drug properties (dissolution, permeability) to *in vitro* properties
	  • less information on variability, co-variates

rely on the assumption of such a specific compartmental model structure. Non-compartmental analysis (Table 6.3) represents a pharmacokinetic analysis approach that focuses on the overall exposure after drug administration and extracts key pharmacokinetic properties from pharmacokinetic data (Gabrielsson and Weiner 2012) by providing information on maximum observed concentrations (C_{max}), time at maximum concentrations (t_{max}), area under the concentration time profile, and area under the first momentum curve (AUMC, a relationship between product of concentration and time on the y-axis versus time as independent parameter on the x-axis). Based on these parameters, the main pharmacokinetic parameters clearance (Dose/AUC), mean residence time (MRT = AUMC/AUC), and volume of distribution at steady state (Vdss = MRT*CL)[5] can be derived by applying simple mathematical tools (e.g. the trapezoidal rule to determine the area under the concentration-time profile or the area under the first momentum curve).

The overall degree of drug absorbed into the systemic circulation is a parameter quantifying the systemic exposure after inhalation. The difference of systemic drug exposure between inhalation and intravenous administration (systemic availability) can be readily calculated via non-compartmental approaches by comparing the area under the plasma concentration-time profile extrapolated to infinity, (AUC_{∞}) observed after intravenous administration of the drug (AUC_{iv}) with that after inhalation (AUC_{inh}). To calculate these parameters, standard techniques for the determination of the AUC_{∞} (trapezoidal rule and extrapolation to infinity) can be used. Comparison of the AUC_{∞} obtained after inhalation with that after iv administration allows calculation of the systemic availability after inhalation.

For drugs with zero oral bioavailability, this method also provides a direct estimate of the pulmonary deposition efficiency. For drugs with distinct oral bioavailability, a clinical trial including a charcoal block enables the calculation of both pulmonary and oral availabilities (Borgström 1998).

Urine data, as previously described, might also be used for the assessment of the degree of systemic absorption through the lung (early urine data); and the total systemic exposure (total urine excretion); of note, for inhaled drugs, pulmonary absorption is generally faster than the absorption of swallowed drug as reported for beta-2-adrenergic drugs (Hindle and Chrystyn 1992). Resolution of such data will, however, depend on the correct cut-off time points defining pulmonary and oral absorption.

6.4.2.1.1 The Maximum Observed Concentration

C_{max} is a parameter which is affected by the dose reaching the systemic circulation, absorption, and distribution kinetics. Since C_{max} is affected by a number of parameters, the interpretation of C_{max} results depends on the nature of the study performed. For example, the differences in C_{max} between two devices delivering a solution-based drug with negligible oral bioavailability might indicate differences in the respirable fraction between the two devices. In other studies (that evaluate immediate release and sustained release preparations, but similar deposition efficiencies), differences in C_{max} might indicate differences in the pulmonary absorption processes if the same doses are compared. Moreover, additional information, such as deposition efficiency, delivered dose and others, are suggested to be taken into consideration to ensure the results are interpreted properly.

Achieving a sustained character of lung absorption is vital for pulmonary selectivity. It is therefore important to evaluate lung absorption with pharmacokinetic assessments. Several assessments have been used to provide this information, including the time to reach the maximum plasma concentration (t_{max}), the mean absorption time (MAT), consideration of flip-flop kinetics, and deconvolution. These approaches are described below.

6.4.2.1.2 The Time to Reach Maximum Concentrations

T_{max} has been used to evaluate how fast the drug is absorbed. The slower the absorption from the lung, the later t_{max} will be. Thus, for a given drug, a formulation with a slower absorption rate k_a should show an increased t_{max} value. Because of the relatively fast absorption often seen after inhalation, intensive sampling at early time points is suggested in order to obtain a reliable estimate of t_{max}. However, one cannot solely use t_{max} to determine whether two different drug entities are being absorbed with different

[5] If the systemic bioavailability (f) is not known, as often the case in inhalation studies, only estimates of Cl/f or V_d/f can be obtained.

rates, as t_{max} is not only determined by k_a, but also by k_e (which likely differs between different drugs). It is even more complicated for drugs with multi-compartmental distribution properties. In these cases, t_{max} is determined by the absorption process and the elimination rate of systemically available drug and by rate constants governing the distribution among all systemic compartments. Also, in this case, an early t_{max} might not always indicate a fast absorption, and a later t_{max} might not indicate a slow absorption process if two drugs differ in their systemic compartmental distribution pattern (differences in the rate constants among systemic compartments) (Krishnaswami et al. 2000). Thus, the use of t_{max} to characterize the absorption pattern must be carefully considered. In addition, the discrete character of t_{max} makes it less suitable for use in bioequivalence assessments.

6.4.2.1.3 Mean Absorption Time

A much more robust parameter than t_{max} seems to be the estimation of the mean absorption time. This parameter can be readily calculated via non-compartmental analysis by estimating the mean residence time after inhalation (MRT_{inh}) and subtracting the mean residence time after iv administration (MRT_{iv}). This approach is relatively robust, as long as the terminal half-life can be reliably determined. Also, the mean absorption time allows one to characterize the absorption processes among different drugs if iv data are available. For example, differences in the absorption profiles between fluticasone propionate and budesonide can be easily identified with this method, while differences in t_{max} were not able to readily provide this information. The mean residence time without availability of intravenous data should not be used to compare absorption profiles of different drug entities, as it is also determined by the systemic elimination of the drug. The use of the mean residence time is, however, suitable for evaluating the differences in absorption of different formulations of the same drug.

6.4.2.1.4 The "Flip-Flop" Approach

Assuming that the absorption rate is much slower than the elimination rate, concentration-time profiles of an inhaled drug will show a terminal slope (slope of the semi-logarithmic plot at late time points) that reflects k_a rather than k_e. This phenomenon is called "flip-flop" (Falcoz et al. 1996). For drugs that are absorbed slowly from the lung, the terminal elimination phase after inhalation should be slower than that after iv administration. Monitoring the occurrence of flip-flop has been used to prove or disapprove the distinct slow absorption of pulmonary drugs (Krishnaswami et al. 2005). While the concept is correct for drugs that are absorbed much slower than they are eliminated, drugs with a small k_e (long half-life) can show similar terminal slopes after iv administration and inhalation, despite the fact that the drug is slowly absorbed from the lung. In this case, other PK parameters, such as the mean absorption time are more suitable for assessing the absorption properties.

6.4.2.1.5 Bioequivalence Assessment

Non-compartmental analysis plays a critical role in assessing the pharmacokinetic equivalence of generic drug products. While the lung is upstream of the blood, plasma concentrations measured in pharmacokinetic studies can provide important information on the bioequivalence of inhalation products by comparing the area under the plasma concentration-time profile and the maximum concentration (C_{max}).

Bioequivalence studies should ensure that test and reference drug products are equivalent in the dose delivered to the lung by test and reference products, the time the drug resides in the lung, and the regional deposition. In addition, systemic exposure needs to be equivalent. Thus, the equivalence in the pulmonary deposition and retention, as well as in the systemic exposure has to be investigated. The United States FDA has established an aggregate weight-of-evidence approach (Lee et al. 2015), which employs: (1) *in vitro* studies (including cascade impactor studies), (2) PK equivalence studies, and (3) PD or therapeutic equivalence studies. Non-compartmental analysis for the pharmacokinetic comparison of test and reference products has been judged to provide important information within the approval process (Apiou-Sbirlea et al. 2013). However, the necessity to assess equivalence in clinical end point studies for drugs with flat dose-response curves has been criticized (Hendeles et al. 2015). The European Medicine Agency uses similar tests for the evaluation of bioequivalence, but allows a step-wise approach asking for pharmacokinetic studies when *in vitro* tests fail (Lu et al. 2015).

In the following, the usefulness of pharmacokinetic studies in combination with non-compartmental analysis to evaluate the bioequivalence of inhalation drugs is discussed. If the absorption from the GI tract is negligible, e.g. for drugs with zero oral bioavailability (such as mometasone furoate, fluticasone propionate) or if oral absorption is blocked through co-administration of charcoal (Thorsson et al. 1994), a number of parameters important for bioequivalence testing can be extracted from non-compartmental pharmacokinetic studies. Table 6.1 indicates potential questions relevant to the generic approval process and the role non-compartmental analysis of pharmacokinetic studies can play.

Assessment of the area under the concentration-time profile as outlined above provides information on the dose deposited in the lung, if drug absorption from the GI tract is negligible or prevented by charcoal block. Differences in the pulmonary residence can be judged by comparison of the C_{max} values. While the above properties have been accepted by the scientific community to be investigated by pharmacokinetic studies, the ability of pharmacokinetics to probe for differences in the regional deposition is still under discussion. Weber and Hochhaus suggested that for slowly dissolving drugs such as fluticasone propionate, removal of undissolved particles through mucociliary clearance in the central parts of the lung and the resulting reduction in systemically absorbed drug can provide valuable information (Weber and Hochhaus 2015). This might allow detection of differences in the regional deposition of test and reference products. In addition, the dissolution rate of drug particles might be slower in more central areas of the lung, where lower permeability might be responsible for a lack of sink conditions, While a faster dissolution might occur in more peripheral areas of the lung because of sink conditions allowing a higher concentration gradient with a higher membrane permeability (see also discussion related to Figure 6.4).

6.4.3 Descriptive Compartmental Models

Compartmental models (Table 6.3) have been routinely used in pharmacokinetic studies after different forms of administration, and they also represent the basis for population pharmacokinetic assessments (Table 6.3). Advantage of compartmental approaches over non-compartmental analysis is that they are more versatile for simulation and prediction purposes, once properly validated, as the impact of various doses, absorption, and elimination rates on drug concentration-time profiles can be easily predicted with the developed mathematical relationships. Compartmental models seek to describe the data by providing a mathematical model that will fit the data and are therefore empirical in nature. They often referred to a top-down approach by extracting pharmacokinetic key properties from concentration-time profiles. They generally do not integrate *in vitro* characteristics, physicochemical properties relevant for dissolution, permeability, protein binding, and metabolism. However, compartmental models can integrate to a certain degree physiology, if necessary for describing the data (e.g. use of multiple absorption rates).

Applied models differ in complexity, based on the quality of the data (e.g. number of data points) and the pharmacokinetic properties of the drug molecule. Plasma concentration-time profiles have been described by models in which used one to three non-pulmonary compartments are used (Figure 6.13 shows a range of three compartmental models). Within the literature, analysis of the data has been performed with average concentration time profiles, although this approach is nowadays rarely used or performed for individual subjects. The latter approach can provide estimates of the between subject variability across the study population, but is less robust than analyzing the plasma concentration-time profiles of each subject separately as done in a standard-two-stage method (see also population pharmacokinetic models).

The absorption process after inhalation of drugs has often been modeled with a single first-order (Hochhaus et al. 1992b; Minto et al. 2000; Rohatagi et al. 2003; Krishnaswami et al. 2005; Wu et al. 2008; Xu et al. 2010; Okusanya et al. 2014; Borghardt et al. 2015) or single zero-order absorption for inhalation through nebulizers or chamber/masks (Maier et al. 2007; Blake et al. 2012). (Figure 6.13D); with systemic model structures ranging from one to three compartments. Other authors were able to identify three different absorption processes (Avram et al. 2009; Bartels et al. 2013) that might be related to one oral and two pulmonary absorption routes (Figure 6.13A). Variations of the absorption model were necessary for other drug/device combinations. These variations include pulmonary metabolic degradation (Sakagami 2004) or clearance from the lung absorption compartment, modeled as a first-order removal of undissolved drug particles from the lung to account for mucociliary clearance (Weber et al. 2013). In another modification, a descriptive transit compartment was introduced before the lung absorption compartment (Diderichsen et al. 2013) to

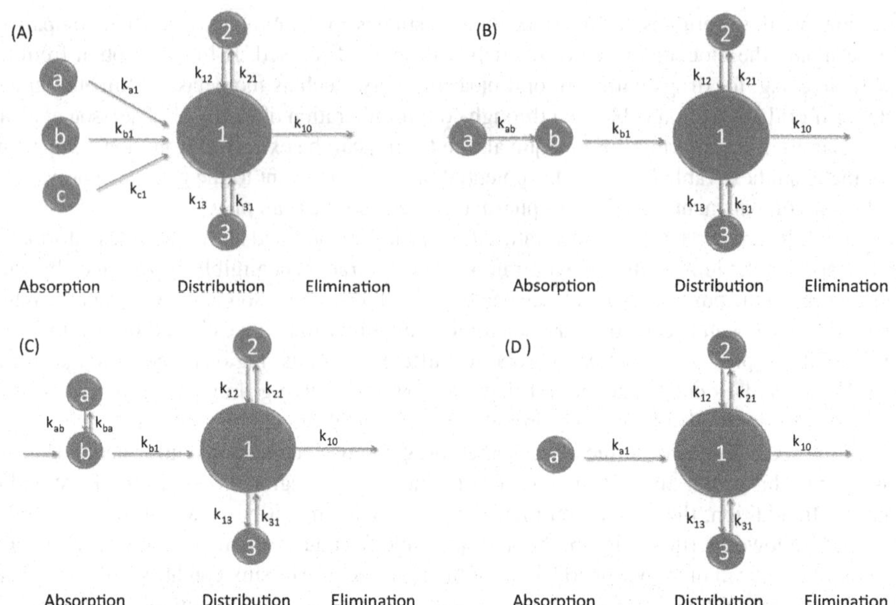

FIGURE 6.13 Absorption models employed within compartmental models. A three compartment body model is pictured; however, less complex body compartmental structures can be employed depending on PK data. (A) Multiple parallel absorption processes to the systemic circulation with different first-order absorption rates: Up to three parallel absorption processes have been used for modelling. While not fully identifiable within this approach, one of the absorption routes might represent oral absorption (Avram et al. 2009; Bartels et al. 2013). (B) Transit absorption process, similar to the ones used for oral absorption, has been employed for modelling a delay in absorption for the long-acting b2-agonist PF-00610355, while a lung depot compartment was used to model the prolonged residence time of inhalation drugs (Diderichsen et al. 2013). (C) Depot arrangement of two lung compartments has also been employed to capture retention of drug in the lung (Dershwitz et al. 2000; Hendrickx et al. 2017). (D) Basic single lung absorption compartment with either first order (Hochhaus et al. 1992b; Minto et al. 2000; Rohatagi et al. 2003; Krishnaswami et al. 2005; Wu et al. 2008; Xu et al. 2010; Okusanya et al. 2014; Borghardt et al. 2015) or zero order (Maier et al. 2007; Blake et al. 2012) absorption.

model the absorption process observed for the long-acting b2-agonist PF-00610355 (Figure 6.13B), which exhibits pulmonary and oral absorption. Other approaches to describe sustained release of drug from the lung were modelled from a pulmonary depot compartment (Dershwitz et al. 2000; Hendrickx et al. 2017) (Figure 6.13C). This deep lung compartment represents lysosomal trapping for basic drugs, slower passive cellular permeability, or active epithelial cell uptake by transporters.

Deconvolution approaches: to characterize absorption after inhalation in more detail, deconvolution techniques have been applied. These approaches allow one to visualize the absorption process more directly (Kaellen and Thorsson 1999). This can be performed with commercially available pharmacokinetic software. Application of deconvolution methods to inhalation drugs should consider the multi-compartmental drug disposition observed for most inhalation drugs. This makes it necessary to use PK estimates after intravenous administration within the deconvolution process. Thus, deconvolution of concentration-time profiles is based on the comparison of data obtained after iv administration and inhalation. This allows the generation of a drug input profile for inhalation, which describes the systemic absorption process and will generate full absorption profiles similar to those obtained from the isolated perfused lung preparations. Because of the compartmental approach used in these deconvolution processes, this method provides information not readily available from the non-compartmental analysis.

Using deconvolution, Falcoz and co-workers (Kaellen and Thorsson 1999) were able to identify that 50% of the pulmonary deposited dose of fluticasone propionate is absorbed within 2 hours, while the rest is absorbed more slowly, with 90% being absorbed by 12 hours. It is likely that differences in the absorption processes might reflect drug deposited in different regions of the lung (central or peripheral). Brindley and co-workers were able to show that, independent of the inhalation device, the absorption of fluticasone propionate is multi-exponential and that a slow absorption into the systemic circulation provides a long pulmonary residence time (Brindley et al. 2000). For the inhalation of fenoterol, similar approaches were used to show that parts of the delivered dose were absorbed relatively fast, while the remaining drug was absorbed more slowly. This observation might be linked to differences in the absorption rate of a drug deposited into the lung or in the GI tract. In summary, deconvolution of inhalation data has the potential of characterizing the absorption processes in more detail and with higher resolution. This approach depends, however, on the availability of intravenous data and may also be useful to evaluate differences in the regional absorption, if absorption rates differ between central and peripheral lung.

6.4.4 Population Pharmacokinetic Approaches

Pharmacokinetic models employed in population pharmacokinetic analyses (Table 6.3) using non-linear mixed-effects models (NLME) are an extension of traditional compartmental modelling approach outlined in Figure 6.13. These models have been used as backbone for population pharmacokinetic analyses (Rohatagi et al. 2003; Yang et al. 2017). The main advantage of population pharmacokinetic models is their ability to estimate between and within subject variability and identify co-variates which contribute to the variability. Population pharmacokinetic methods represent usually empirical and top-down approaches, which utilize compartmental model structures described above (Figure 6.13). They generally do not capture the physiological processes responsible for the fate of the drug after delivery. The use of population pharmacokinetic approaches for describing pharmacokinetics of inhalation drugs was recently reviewed (Borghardt et al. 2015) and two studies are highlighted in the following.

Borghardt et al. published a population PK model for olodaterol, as shown in scheme (A) in Figure 6.13. The best fit of plasma and urine samples of 148 subjects was achieved by assuming three distinct absorption processes. Smoking was found to be a co-variate on the fast and slow absorption rate constant. It increases the absorption rate constant of the fast lung absorption compartment, while decreasing the absorption rate constant of the slow lung absorption compartment (Borghardt et al. 2016a). This model has been used to evaluate the differences in pulmonary pharmacokinetics of asthmatic and COPD patients. COPD and asthma were found to influence the pulmonary bioavailable fraction and the absorption rate constant of the slow and fast lung absorption compartment (Borghardt et al. 2016b).

Diderichsen et al. developed a population pharmacokinetic model employing a three-compartment disposition model with first-order absorption occurring through a transit compartment for the modelling of the systemic exposure of the long-acting beta-2-agonist PF-00610355. Patient status (asthmatic or COPD patients, or healthy volunteers), inhalation device (2 devices were used), and demographic factors were identified as influential co-variates (Diderichsen et al. 2013).

6.4.4.1 Physiologically Based Pharmacokinetic or Semi-mechanistic Models

Physiologically based pharmacokinetic as shown in Figure 6.14 or semi-mechanistic modelling approaches have been used as an emerging tool within drug development for predicting the *in vivo* fate of drugs from *in vitro*/*in silico* assessments of the drug candidate with the goal of predicting absorption, distribution, metabolism, and excretion of a drug candidate (ADME) (Barnes et al. 1998; Rowland et al. 2011; Zhao et al. 2011; Gaohua et al. 2015). The mechanistic basis of this approach allows predictions considering the effects of the patient's age, genetics, and disease or characteristics of the drug formulation on ADME characteristics. This has been accomplished by building up a mathematical model that can describe the fate of the drug as close as possible to the actual processes responsible for absorption, distribution, metabolism, and elimination. The ultimate goal is to provide a broader physiological understanding of the drug's fate via a compartmental modelling approach. Semi-mechanistic approaches are somewhat less complex and attempt only to model part of the drug's ADME within the physiological context. The main purpose of this approach, once established, is to predict the drug's fate including drug-drug interactions, effects of formulations on drug absorption, thereby facilitating drug development, e.g. by facilitating the design of clinical studies.

The strength of such an approach within the inhalation field is to integrate drug/device/patient information generated from *in vitro* and/or *in silico* assessments and lung physiological characteristics into an integrated model. Figure 6.15 lists variables for metered dose and dry powder inhalers influencing

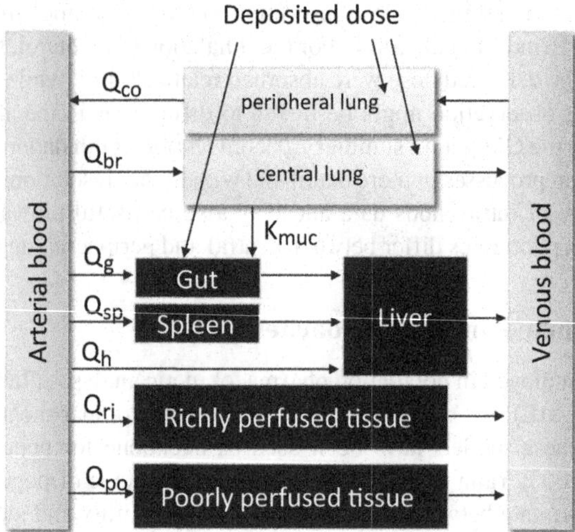

FIGURE 6.14 PBPK model with orally inhalation as route of administration. Following inhalation, drug can deposit in the central or peripheral lung as well as swallowed into the GI tract. The blood flow through the peripheral lung is similar to the cardiac output (Q_{co}), while the blood flow through the central lung is described by the bronchial blood flow (Q_{br}). Undissolved deposited drug particles can be cleared by the mucociliary clearance (Kmuc). The remaining organs are hold gastrointestinal (Q_g), splenic (Q_{sp}), hepatic (Q_h), the richly perfused (Q_{ri}) and the poorly perfused blood flow.

pulmonary deposition, dissolution, and permeability. Capturing relevant characteristics and integrating them into pharmacokinetic models might predict the fate of inhaled drugs in the lung and the systemic circulation. Relating drug/formulation/device characteristics extracted from *in silico* and *in vitro* methods to the *in vivo* characteristics is one of the main reasons for applying PBPK approaches with the ultimate goal of streamlining drug development.

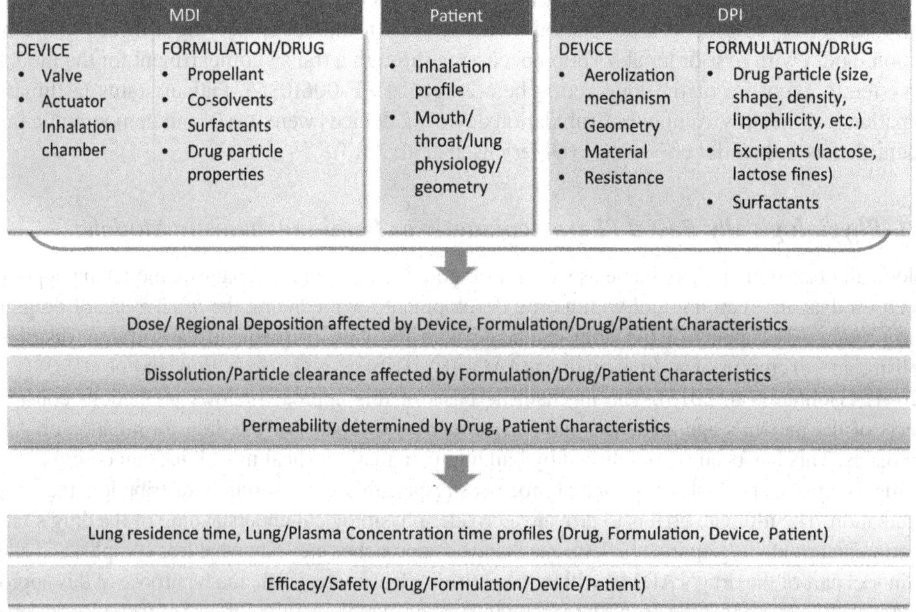

FIGURE 6.15 Device/Formulation/Drug/Patient characteristics that affect (A) biopharmaceutical properties (a) dose related (deposited lung dose, regional deposition), (b) dissolution, and (c) permeability; (B) pharmacokinetic concentration time profiles in lung and systemic circulation and consequently; (C) efficacy and safety. Potential factors affecting MDI and DPI performance are listed. List is not intended to be complete.

In vitro and *in silico* methods used to predict the deposited dose, regional deposition, dissolution, and permeability are summarized in Figure 6.16. *In vitro* methods to predict the lung dose have been achieved with set-ups consisting of an anatomical throat replica that is linked through a filter holder to a pump system that mimics an realistic inhalation profile. Such set-ups have been shown to be good predictors of the pulmonary deposited dose (Delvadia et al. 2013; Olsson et al. 2013; Olsson and Bäckman 2014). Similar approaches combined anatomical throats with realistic breathing profiles and cascade impactor systems (Olsson et al. 2013). These systems can further analyse the inhalable fraction with respect to the aerodynamic particle size distribution, a parameter suitable as input parameter for additional *in silico* predictions. Cascade impactor methods using constant flow rates throughout the system, such as those described in the United States Pharmacopeia, are currently used to determine aerodynamic particle size distribution. However, it needs to be considered that de-agglomerization of dry powder inhaler formulations depends on the inhalation flow. Mimicking realistic flow profiles within the *in vitro* assessment might be of advantage to obtain more realistic estimates of *in vivo* deposition, especially if particle size distributions are consequently used in computation fluid dynamic evaluations of the regional deposition profiles (Longest et al. 2016).

In silico methods of varying complexity from one-dimensional to three-dimensional approaches have been proposed to predict the pulmonary deposited dose and regional deposition of inhalation drugs (Figure 6.16). Most in-silico methods of one-dimensional deposition models are based on Weibel's lung model and require the aerodynamic particle size distribution and the inhalation profile information as input parameters. Available programs include the MPPD® model (Ginsberg et al. 2008; Price n.d.), ICRP 66 (Wang 2005; Rostami 2009; Hofmann 2011), and Mimetikus Preludium® (Olsson n.d.), a software specifically developed for clinical inhalation products, as it allows to incorporate realistic inhalation profiles into the calculations. The more complex and calculation intensive computational fluid dynamic models show 3D resolution (Tu et al. 2013; Feng et al. 2016). Whole lung computational fluid dynamic (CFD) simulations have been used to obtain the local drug deposition after inhalation (Longest et al. 2016). Recent comparisons of the predictions of CFD models with *in vitro* experimental measurements

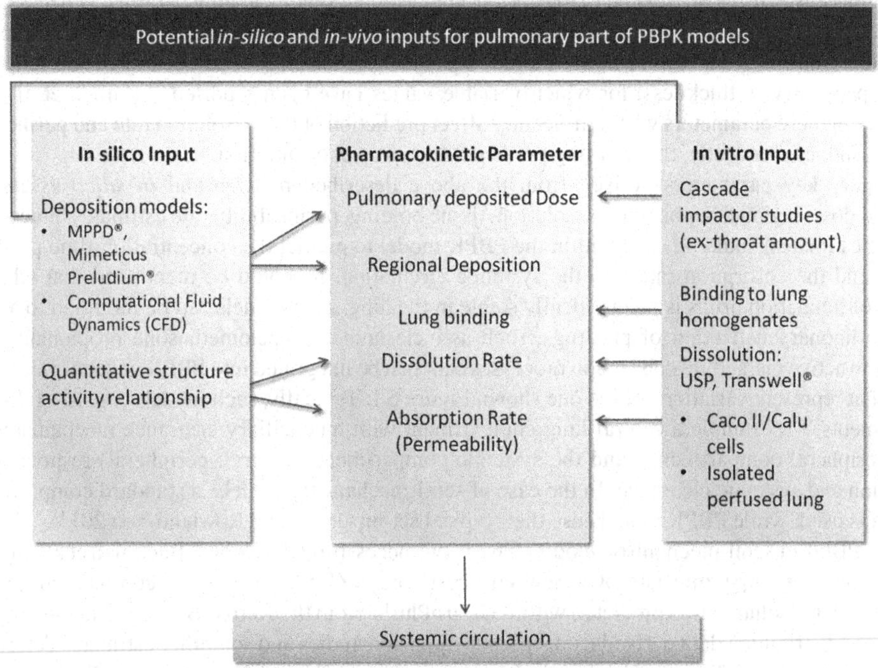

FIGURE 6.16 *In silico* and *in vitro* input for PBPK models relevant for pulmonary deposition, dissolution, and permeability.

indicate good agreement (Matida et al. 2006; Longest et al. 2007, 2016; Longest and Holbrook 2012). CFD modelling approaches have been used within PBPK models to predict lung dose and regional deposition (Feng et al. 2016).

In vitro methods to assess the dissolution of deposited particles have been described in the literature (Davies and Feddah 2003; Arora and Sakagami 2007; Son and McConville 2009; May et al. 2012, 2013; Riley et al. 2012; Rohrschneider et al. 2015; Gerde et al. 2017) using standard dissolution systems described in the USP or alternative approaches, such as the Transwell® system. Alternatively, prediction of the dissolution rate from particle size distribution and solubility has been suggested (Bhagwat et al. 2017). Physiologically based pharmacokinetic models could include dissolution processes by incorporating relevant physicochemical relationships between dissolution rate, particle surface area, and solubility as described in the Nernst-Brunner equation (Figure 6.4).

Pulmonary permeability has been measured with cell lines such as Caco II or Calu (Bosquillon et al. 2017) or in isolated perfused lung systems (Tronde et al. 2008; Eriksson et al. 2018). As alternative *in silico* approaches, employing quantitative structure-activity relationships have been proposed as alternative to isolated perfused lung systems (Edwards et al. 2016). The absorption process, initiated after deposition of drug particles, can be integrated into a PBPK model by considering relevant relationships for dissolution (k_{diss}, e.g. using the Nernst-Brunner equation) and diffusion processes across lung membranes (e.g. Fick's law). Figure 6.4 depicts the interplay between dissolution and diffusion processes in determining the pulmonary residence time of an inhaled drug.

As driving forces for dissolution and diffusion are based on the free drug concentration gradient (Figure 6.4), it is recommended to take pulmonary tissue binding into consideration during the development of PBPK model. The binding of drug in lung has been determined through dialysis experiments with lung homogenate or in isolated perfused lung systems (Tronde et al. 2003). Microdialysis (Feurstein and Zeitlinger 2011) has also been evaluated, but is currently hampered by the fact that it is a highly invasive technique. Improvement of related techniques (e.g. determination of lung binding without destruction of the lung structures by homogenization), identification of lysosome trapping, specific interaction with lung components is incumbent.

Other challenges for predicting the pulmonary concentration-time profiles, whether it is dissolved, free, or undissolved drug, are related to the correct choice of physiological lung parameters necessary for the calculations. These include parameters such as surface area of defined regions of the lung, pulmonary distribution volumes (lung lining fluid volume, aqueous volume of defined section of the lung-intracellular space, airway thickness) for which variable values have been reported (Fröhlich et al. 2016). Variability in these parameters will significantly affect prediction of the dissolution rate and permeability estimates and, consequently, the resulting predicted free drug concentration.

Pulmonary key parameters derived from the above described *in vitro* and *in silico* assessments (deposited dose, regional deposition, dissolution, tissue binding, permeability rate estimates, mucociliary clearance estimates) could be used within the PBPK model to predict the concentration-time profiles in the lung and the absorption rate into the systemic circulation. It should be mentioned that while the majority of inhalation drugs is metabolically stable in the lung, such models can be modified to account for the pulmonary activation of prodrugs, such as ciclesonide or beclomethasone propionate. These prodrugs to active metabolite conversion processes can then be integrated into PBPK or semi-mechanistic models that represent variations of the one shown Figure 6.1. Typically, such models consist of 2–3 lung compartments, for example a central lung compartment with mucociliary clearance mechanisms, one to two peripheral compartments, and the systemic compartments (central, peripheral) responsible for distribution and systemic clearance. In the case of semi-mechanistic models, a standard compartmental approach is used, while PBPK models use their typical set-up (Jones and Rowland-Yeo 2013).

Several PBPK or semi-mechanistic models have been successfully developed. Bäckman et al. predicted the pulmonary and systemic fate of a new corticosteroid AZD5423 using the commercial software GastroPlus™. Dissolution was predicted within GastroPlus™ from the Nernst-Brunner equation by using particle size distribution data derived from cascade impactor studies and solubility estimates determined for the "lung lining fluid" (water solubility). Permeability was calculated within GastroPlus™ from the molecular weight considering the differences in epithelial thickness across the lung (Bäckman et al. 2017b). Similar approaches were used to predict the absorption rate of fluticasone propionate from the particle size distribution of the DPI formulation, assuming that the dissolution process is the rate limiting step (Bhagwat et al. 2017). To identify a suitable dissolution medium within this approach, a pharmacokinetic concentration-time profile of a "calibrator" substance was deconvoluted, and the solubility necessary to obtain dissolution profiles similar to the observed absorption profile were determined. A surfactant containing solvent providing the same solubility was identified and used for subsequent solubility determinations of test substances. Alternative approaches predicted the overall absorption rate of glucocorticoids from Transwell®-based *in vitro* models that integrated dissolution and diffusion processes. This is done via a linear relationship between the mean dissolution time in a Transwell® dissolution model and the mean absorption time from a pharmacokinetic study (Bhagwat et al. 2017). Absorption rate constants for "unknown" compounds could be derived from these linear relationships between mean dissolution and absorption times.

Bhagwat et al. (2017) utilized a model similar to that shown in Figure 6.1 to predict the pulmonary PK of dry powder inhalers from *in vitro* properties. This study aimed to predict the systemic exposure after inhalation of fluticasone propionate, budesonide, and mometasone furoate. No attempts were made to predict the pulmonary drug concentrations. Drug dissolution was presumed to be the rate-limiting step of the absorption for these low solubility drugs, and permeability was consequently not incorporated into the model. The total lung dose was predicted from cascade impactor studies using realistic breathing profiles and anatomical throats. And the central to peripheral lung ratio (c/p) was estimated by utilizing the previously described MPPD® particle deposition model. Dissolution was integrated into the model as described above. The PK predictions of both approaches were in agreement with clinically observed data. Approach 2 has a simpler structure and performs equally well than the more mechanistic approach 1 (Bhagwat et al. 2017). Baeckman et al. used a similar overall model to predict the performance of a new corticosteroid AZD5423 (Bäckman et al. 2017b).

Boger et al. (2015) linked a physiologically based PK model with receptor occupancy as biomarker to evaluate the pulmonary targeting of fluticasone propionate using an animal PK/PD approach. With this PBPK model, it could be shown that lung-selectivity defined as the difference of pulmonary and systemic receptor occupancy could not be achieved for the peripheral lung.

Hendrickx et al. (2017) developed a semi-physiological model in rats for inhaled bronchodilators and explored inter-species translations to male Beagle dogs and humans. This model captured the pulmonary and systemic PK after iv and pulmonary administration of 12 bronchodilators (salmeterol, formoterol, salbutamol, terbutaline, indacaterol, tiotropium, ipratropium, glycopyrronium, AZD2115, batefenterol, AZD4518, and AZD3199) (Hendrickx et al. 2017) and demonstrated the usefulness of such models to translate between animal species and predict drug concentrations in the human lung.

Physiologically based PK model components have also been integrated into commercial software such as GastroPlus™, SimCyp Simulator™, or Pfizer's PulmoSim™.

6.4.4.1.1 GastroPlus™

The modelling and simulation software GastroPlus™ combines a PBPK model with deposition, dissolution, and pulmonary clearance mechanism. The nasal-pulmonary compartmental absorption and transit module in GastroPlus™ is based on Weibel's lung model and consists of five compartments: (1) optional nose, (2) extra thoracic (naso-oro-pharynx and larynx), (3) thoracic (trachea and bronchi), (4) bronchiolar (bronchioles and terminal bronchioles), and (5) alveolar-interstitial (respiratory bronchioles, alveolar ducts, alveolar sacs, and interstitial connective tissue). Since a fraction of drug can be swallowed, the lung compartments are linked to the advanced compartmental absorption and transit (ACATTM) gastrointestinal module. One can choose among the following pharmaceutical formulations: solution, powders, intratracheal administration, or nasal spray (solution or powder) ("Drug Administration Routes | Dermal Delivery | Inhaled Products | Injection" n.d.).

After inhalation, a fraction of the administered dose is either deposited in the mucus/surfactant layer of the airway system, swallowed, or exhaled. The user can choose to specify the fraction of dose deposited in each compartment. Alternatively, if the pulmonary particle deposition pattern is unknown, one can predict this pattern by the previously described ICRP 66 deposition model (Chaudhuri and Lukacova 2010). When using the ICRP model, the input parameters for monodisperse formulations are radius and shape factor; while for poly-disperse formulations, the entire particle size distribution is required (Chaudhuri and

Lukacova 2010). After deposition, particles can either dissolve and be absorbed into the systematic/lymphatic circulation or transported toward the extrathoracic compartment by mucociliary clearance.

Different user options for the dissolution rate kinetics are available, like the traditional Noyes-Whitney equation, which depends on the water diffusion coefficient, particle size, shape, and density, as well as solubility of the drug at pH of 6.9 (physiological mucus pH) (Chaudhuri and Lukacova 2010). The absorption rate is defined by passive diffusion, following a concentration gradient, and carrier mediated transport on the apical side. Mucociliary clearance is described as a first-order process with a constant ciliary motion, and metabolism degrades inhaled particles from the respiratory epithelium (Bäckman et al. 2017a). Published human lung physiological parameters, like surface area, thickness, and volume for the mucus and cells were incorporated into this model.

Input parameters for describing pulmonary absorption are pulmonary permeability, as well as drug specific parameters. The latter include logP, pKa, water solubility, particle radius, plasma protein binding, blood/plasma ratio, first pass extraction (liver and gut, for assessing oral absorption), lung fluid solubility, and systemic PK parameters.

Miller et al. (2010) developed an inhaled budesonide PBPK model based in GastroPlus™. Input parameters of budesonide were obtained from the literature; i.e. plasma concentration-time profiles of budesonide in six healthy subjects. It was concluded that the predicted plasma concentration-time profiles reflected the observations reasonable well. Since no input parameter were fitted, the authors concluded that PBPK-based prediction of the fate of inhalation drugs can serve as a valuable tool in the development of new inhaled and intranasal drug candidates (Miller et al. 2010).

6.4.4.1.2 PK-Sim™

PK-Sim™ represents a semi-mechanistic model that is somewhat restricted, as it does not allow prediction of deposition and dissolution from physicochemical characteristics of the device/formulation. Stass et al. (2013) used PK-Sim™ to investigate the pulmonary fate of ciprofloxacin dry powder after deconvolution to describe the contribution of regional pulmonary absorption (oral cavity, trachea and bronchi, and deep alveolar space) to the systemic exposure.

6.4.4.1.3 SimCyp Simulator™

The SimCyp Simulator™ contains a multiple-compartment permeability-limited lung model (Gaohua et al. 2015) to model active and passive drug disposition in the lung. It shows similar limitations as PK-Sim and does not allow one to predict lung deposition and dissolution rates. This non-mechanistic PBPK model, therefore, assumes instantaneous dissolution and controls lung concentrations within defined regions of the lung solely through the choice of defined first-order absorption rate processes (Borghardt et al. 2015).

Particles deposited in the airway lining fluid in the central region of the lung can be either absorbed or cleared via mucociliary clearance into the GI tract. Both processes are described by a respective first-order rate constant. Once absorbed into lung tissue, the unbound fraction can diffuse into the systemic circulation (Bäckman et al. 2017a). The compartmental absorption and transit model, the advanced dissolution, absorption and metabolism model, or a simple first-order absorption process can be employed to describe the oral absorption of the swallowed proportion. Gaohua et al. (2015) employed the SimCyp Simulator™ to investigate pulmonary PK after oral administration of the anti-tuberculosis treatment with rifampicin.

6.4.4.2 PK/PD Modelling of Inhaled Drugs

Up to this point, the discussion focused on pharmacokinetic relationships; however, models have not been discussed which evaluate pharmacodynamic effects over time.

6.4.4.2.1 Biomarkers

A number of systemic and topical pharmacodynamic endpoints which are potentially suitable to be incorporated into PK/PD models have been described for a range of inhalation drugs. The arsenal of pharmacodynamic studies for evaluation of topical effects has been recently reviewed by Hendeles et al. (2015). It should be possible to use any one or multiple of these markers within PK/PD models of pulmonary effects. However, the flat dose response curves (i.e. low doses already achieve near-maximal effects) observed for corticosteroids may represent a challenge. Various parameters associated with pulmonary function including forced expiratory volume in one sec (FEV1), peak expiratory flow rate (PEFR), forced vital capacity (FVC), mid-expiratory flow rate (MEFR), and use of airway hyper-responsiveness have been used to measure the degree of pulmonary effects in asthmatics using the spirometer or body phlethysmography. Additionally, biomarkers of local effects, such as the reduction in certain cytokines, or modulation of nitric oxide (Holford and Sheiner 1981; Derendorf and Meibohm 1999) can be useful.

Moreover, the use of more traditional clinical parameters such as diary scores, the need of rescue medication, treatment failures, progression of disease, and other routinely measure clinical parameters are useful. These include for corticosteroids effects on sputum eosinophils, exhaled nitric oxide, challenge models with histamine, denosine-5′-monophosphate, or methacholine. One of the challenges for evaluating corticosteroids is the rather flat dose response relationship is generally seen for this drug class. Some data seem to suggest that pulmonary effects after exercise-induced asthma or stimulation with adenosine phosphate (Geller et al. 1993; Byrnes et al. 1997) are more sensitive and dose response curves are easier to obtain (van den Berge et al. 2001).

For the assessment of beta-2-adrenergic or muscarinic drugs, i.e. drug classes with steeper dose response relationships, several clinical study designs ranging from direct measurements of lung function improvements (using forced expiratory volumes) to challenge models employing methacholine or histamine have been described (Hendeles et al. 2015). Systemic side effects used for assessing safety include cortisol suppression, reduction in lymphocytes (142), growth reduction (Daley-Yates and Richards 2004) for corticosteroids, effects on potassium (Jonkers et al. 1995), and increase in heart rate for beta-2-adrenergic drugs (Hochhaus et al. 1992b).

6.4.4.2.2 Modelling

PKPD models allow, once validated, to predict the time-course of effect(s) by linking the drug concentration profile over time at the site of action with the concentration-effect relationships (Meibohm and Derendorf 1997). A major challenge for modelling pulmonary effects after inhalation is the fact that drug effects are up-stream of the blood, in which drug concentrations are measured, and prediction of pulmonary free drug concentrations depend on a good estimation of dissolution, permeation, and tissue binding processes within this pulmonary "black box" (see physiologically based PK section). Thus, the majority of PK/PD reports, with few exceptions, focused on the evaluation of systemic effects of inhaled drugs or the PK/PD modelling of pulmonary effects after systemic administration.

PK/PD models are based on linking drug concentrations-time profiles with the concentration/effect relationships via compartmental approaches. Several pharmacodynamic models have been applied ranging from simple linear relationships between plasma concentration and effect or E_{max} models (Figure 6.17) that often can describe receptor mediated processes. A challenge during the early days of PK/PD modelling was to identify models that can capture time delays between drug concentrations and effects. Indirect response models are often well suitable to capture the time-course of effects via a differential equation quantifying the change in the biomarker over time (dMarker/dt) and as a function of the drug concentration. Alternatively, so-called effect compartment models have been defined. The latter assume that a small (i.e. negligible) amount of drug penetrated into an effect site and elicits the response in the effect compartment. Both of these approaches can model a time delay between plasma concentrations and effect (Meibohm and Derendorf 1997). As an example, the time delay in blood lymphocyte production by hydrocorticone was modeled.

Major advantage of such models is that they enable the optimization of dosage regimens with the desired effect profiles over time. They also allow the identification of equivalent doses of different drugs, as shown by Derendorf for corticosteroids (Derendorf et al. 1993) or the prediction of how changes in doses and delivery devices will affect the systemic side effects.

Basic PK/PD models as described in Figure 6.17 have been used to describe the effects of beta-2-adrenergic drugs on airway resistance for which no delay between drug concentrations and the effect was present. Other modelling approaches are necessary when a time delay between drug concentrations and effects are observed. Effect compartment (Rohatagi et al. 1995b) or indirect response models (Rohatagi et al.

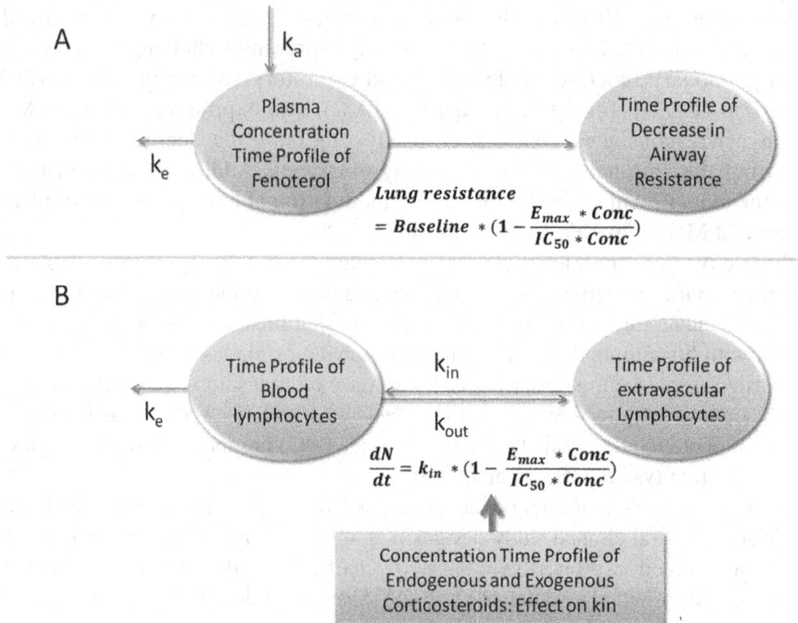

FIGURE 6.17 (A) Simple PK/PD model linking plasma concentration directly to the effect. In this case, airway resistance is reduced by a beta-2 adrenergic drug which was given orally. Plasma concentrations describe sufficiently well the drug concentration at the site of action. The decrease of airway resistance from baseline level could be properly described through an E_{max} model. E_{max}: maximum effect, E_{max} will be a value between 0–1. E_{max} of 0.5 would reduce the lung resistance by 50%. Conc: Drug concentration at the site of action (in this case in plasma), IC50: Drug concentration necessary to induce 50% of the maximum effect. This model provides a direct link between drug concentrations and effect on biomarker. There is no time-delay between change in drug concentrations and effect. (B) Indirect response model. Lymphocytes in blood and extravascular space are in equilibrium. Movement of lymphocytes from the blood into the extra-cellular space is described by a first-order process (rate is dependent on the number of lymphocytes in the blood), with k_{out} being the first-order rate constant. Movement of lymphocytes from the extra-vascular space into the blood is described by a zero-order process with the zero-order rate constant k_{in} (rate with which lymphocytes move into the blood does not depend on lymphocyte numbers). Exogenous or endogenous corticosteroids can reduce k_{in}. Lymphocyte numbers in the blood will be reduced with increasing corticosteroids concentrations in the blood. There is a delay between changes in drug concentrations and changes in blood lymphocyte numbers.

1996) have been employed in these cases, such as models describing the effects of glucocorticoids on lymphocytes (Figure 6.17) or endogenous cortisol (for a review, see [Rohatagi et al. 1995a]).

PK/PD models for the evaluation of systemic side effects have been reported for a number of drug classes including beta-2-adrenergic drugs (effects on potassium [Brattsand and Axelsson 1997]), increase in heart rate and glucocorticoids (cortisol suppression [Szefler and Martin 2002], as well as effects on lymphocytes and granulocytes [Boulet 2002]). An indirect response modelling approach for the cortisol suppression induced by exogenous corticosteroids and the combined effects of endogenous cortisol and exogenous corticosteroid on lymphocytes could explain why dosing of corticosteroids in the evening might be more efficacious (142). PK/PD models for evaluating the pulmonary effects of beta-2-adrenergic drugs after systemic forms of administration have been reported using airway resistance or changes in FEV1 as biomarker by applying an E_{max} model (Hochhaus et al. 1922b, 1993). Equivalent doses for systemically administered fenoterol, albuterol, and terbutaline could be established purely based on PK/PD assessments (Hochhaus and Möllmann 1992).

Predicting the pulmonary effects after inhalation represents a somewhat larger challenge, as concentrations at the site of action after inhalation are not readily available. Considering the challenges associated with pulmonary drug concentrations, Wu and colleagues (2011) applied the "K-PD" model approach (Jacqmin et al. 2007) that "extracts" the pharmacokinetic component from the PD data only, thereby allowing to link the kinetics of the drug effect to the drug amount in a hypothetical biophase, i.e. the lung. This enables using clinical trial simulations to streamline drug development.

Using animal models, Hendrickx et al. established a compartmental model for describing the lung and plasma concentrations after iv and it administrations. He then linked the lung concentrations to the PD model that utilised *in vitro* information from the guinea ileum test (Hendrickx et al. 2017) to describe the activity at the site of action.

6.4.4.3 Methods for Assessing Pulmonary Targeting

Inhalation therapy aimed to improve pulmonary effects with reduced systemic side effects. During drug development, methods should be available that can assess this property. Animal and human studies for assessing pulmonary targeting are summarized below.

6.4.4.3.1 Assessment of Pulmonary Targeting in Animal Models

Animal models are important tools in assessing the pharmacodynamic performance of anti-asthma drugs. Pulmonary models have been developed for rats and mice, which allow the assessment of anti-inflammatory properties of a drug after antigen challenge. Alternatively, pulmonary eosinophilia can be induced by non-allergic modes, e.g. by administering sephadex (Hochhaus et al. 1992b; Bjermer et al. 1994a; Haddad et al. 2002). This results in an increase in lung weight. The topical activity of inhaled glucocorticoids has been tested in such models by administering the glucocorticoid into the left lung lobe of rats, followed by administration of sephadex to the whole lung. Comparing the differential effects of the glucocorticoid on left and right lobe weight can assess targeting. Targeting is observed when the effects on the left lobe are more pronounced than the effects on the right lobe, which will be exposed only to systemic glucocorticoid concentrations (Bjermer et al. 1994b). Within a variation of this approach, the pulmonary effects measured in the sephadex model after pulmonary administration of corticosteroids are related to systemic effects, e.g. the effects of the systemically absorbed corticosteroid on thymus weight. A drug with the more pronounced targeting will produce the same activity in the sephadex model with reduced effects on the thymus weight (Brattsand and Axelsson 1997).

Other targeting models in rats or mice are based on the *ex vivo* monitoring of receptor occupancy after intratracheal administration of the drug, described here for glucocorticoids (Hochhaus et al. 1995; Arya et al. 2005; Boger et al. 2015). Such models are based on the finding that the glucocorticoid receptors are similar in different tissues, resulting in identical receptor occupancy time profile when free drug concentrations in different tissues are identical (or similar), e.g. after systemic administration of a drug. Pulmonary targeting after intratracheal administration can then be assessed by comparing the receptor occupancy in the lung to a systemic organ, such as the liver or kidney. A more pronounced receptor occupancy in the lung after intratracheal administration indicates pulmonary targeting. Similar approaches could be designed for cell membrane receptors, for example, for the beta-adrenergic receptors, using *ex vivo* receptor binding approaches developed for other membrane receptors (Sadée et al. 1983).

6.4.4.3.2 Assessment of Pulmonary Targeting in Humans

The direct assessment of pulmonary targeting in humans is anything but trivial. Generally, it is reduced to separately monitor pharmacodynamic effects in the lung (desired effects) and systemic circulation (undesired side effects). Comparing these properties with other drugs or dosage regimens often allows one to draw some conclusion on pulmonary selectivity.

In one semi-quantitative approach, the drug of interest is given either systemically or through inhalation. Doses are selected in such a way that systemic side effects (and plasma concentrations) are similar. Pulmonary effects are then quantified after systemic administration and inhalation. If inhalation therapy induces a local targeted effect, pulmonary effects after systemic administration and inhalation will differ, with more pulmonary effects observed after inhalation (Figure 6.18). Using a similar approach, one also can compare potential differences in targeting between two drugs. In this case, both drugs are dosed in such a way that systemic effects are equivalent. The drug with the more pronounced pulmonary effects shows then a more pronounced pulmonary selectivity (Figure 6.18).

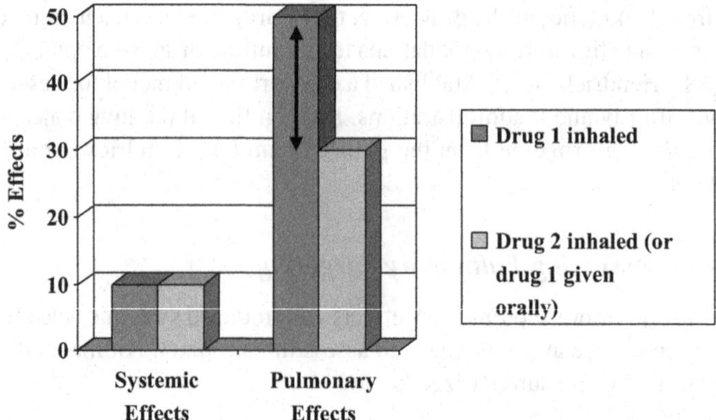

FIGURE 6.18 Clinical differences in pulmonary targeting. Doses of inhaled drugs are identified that will produce equivalent systemic effects. The drug with the higher degree of pulmonary effects will show more pronounced targeting. In a similar design, the same drug could be given orally and through inhalation. More pronounced pulmonary effects after inhalation show targeting.

PK/PD modelling approaches can also be useful in demonstrating pulmonary targeting after inhalation. In one example, pharmacokinetics, heart rate as systemic side effect and airway resistance, were measured after systemic administration of fenoterol (iv bolus, infusion, nasal administration) to asthmatics (Hochhaus et al. 1992b). This allowed the authors to establish a PK/PD model linking plasma fenoterol concentrations to systemic side effects and desired pulmonary effects. Once validated, PKPD model can be used to predict systemic effects and pulmonary effects after inhalation of fenoterol, assuming that only plasma fenoterol was responsible for inducing the effect. The pulmonary effects measured after inhalation were more pronounced than the one's predicted from the plasma concentration time profiles (Figure 6.19). The difference is due to pulmonary targeting after inhalation (Hochhaus et al. 1992b).

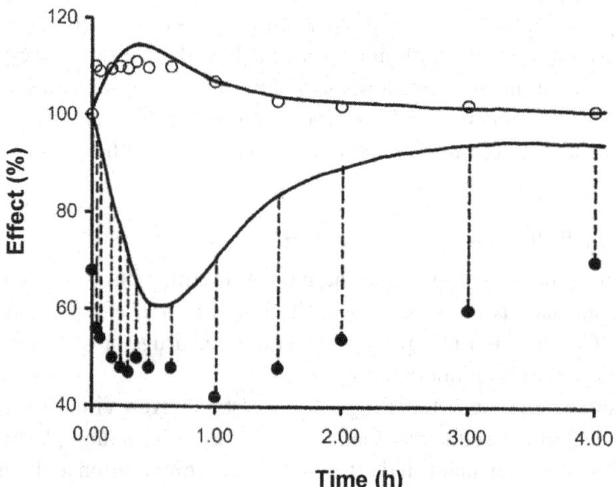

FIGURE 6.19 The effects of inhaled fenoterol (400 μg) on the heart rate (HR, open circles) and on reduction in pulmonary resistance (closed circles). Although the plasma levels of fenoterol are a good descriptor for systemic effects (HR), plasma levels cannot be used to predict effect on the pulmonary resistance. The dashed line between the closed circles and lower smooth line represents pulmonary selectivity.

6.5 Conclusions

Our understanding of pharmacokinetic and pharmacodynamics relationships for inhalation drugs has made a significant step forward over the past years. A robust understanding of necessary drug properties for achieving pulmonary selectivity has been generated. Pharmacokinetic modelling tools have greatly improved, allowing one to describe the fate of inhaled drugs using top-down approaches. However, more progress needs to be made in improving physiologically based pharmacokinetic models and semi-mechanistic PK/PD models. These models should capture and predict the relevant pulmonary processes with more granularity.

ACKNOWLEDGEMENTS

We are thankful to our colleagues Manish Issar, Cary Mobley, and Patricia Khan for compiling the previous edition of this chapter.

REFERENCES

Agertoft, L., A. Andersen, E. Weibull, and S. Pedersen. 1999. "Systemic availability and pharmacokinetics of nebulised budesonide in preschool children." *Archives of Disease in Childhood* 80 (3): 241–247.

Agertoft, L., and S. Pedersen. 1993. "Importance of the inhalation device on the effect of budesonide." *Archives of Disease in Childhood* 69 (1): 130–133.

Amidon, G. L., H. Lennernäs, V. P. Shah, and J. R. Crison. 1995. "A theoretical basis for a biopharmaceutic drug classification: the correlation of in vitro drug product dissolution and in vivo bioavailability." *Pharmaceutical Research* 12 (3): 413–420.

Apiou-Sbirlea, G., S. Newman, J. Fleming, R. Siekmeier, S. Ehrmann, G. Scheuch, G. Hochhaus, and A. Hickey. 2013. "Bioequivalence of inhaled drugs: fundamentals, challenges and perspectives." *Therapeutic Delivery* 4 (3): 343–367. doi:10.4155/tde.12.161.

Argenti, D., B. Shah, and D. Heald. 1999. "A pharmacokinetic study to evaluate the absolute bioavailability of triamcinolone acetonide following inhalation administration." *Journal of Clinical Pharmacology* 39 (7): 695–702.

Arora, D., and M. Sakagami. 2007. "Kinetic assessment of aerosol particle dissolution and membrane permeation for testing commercial inhaler products." *The AAPS Journal* 9: W5241.

Arya, V., M. Issar, Y. Wang, G. Hochhaus, and J. D. Talton. 2005. "brain permeability of inhaled corticosteroids." *Journal of Pharmacy and Pharmacology* 57 (9): 1159–1167. doi:10.1211/jpp.57.9.0010.

Aswania, O. A., S. A. Corlett, and H. Chrystyn. 1997. "Development and validation of an ion-pair liquid chromatographic method for the quantitation of sodium cromoglycate in urine following inhalation." *Journal of Chromatography. B, Biomedical Sciences and Applications* 690 (1–2): 373–378.

Aswania, O. A., S. A. Corlett, and H. Chrystyn. 1998. "Determination of the relative bioavailability of nedocromil sodium to the lung following inhalation using urinary excretion." *European Journal of Clinical Pharmacology* 54 (6): 475–478.

Avram, M. J., D. A. Spyker, T. K. Henthorn, and J. V. Cassella. 2009. "The pharmacokinetics and bioavailability of prochlorperazine delivered as a thermally generated aerosol in a single breath to volunteers." *Clinical Pharmacology and Therapeutics* 85 (1): 71–77. doi:10.1038/clpt.2008.184.

Bäckman, P., S. Arora, W. Couet, B. Forbes, W. de Kruijf, and A. Paudel. 2017a. "Advances in experimental and mechanistic computational models to understand pulmonary exposure to inhaled drugs." *European Journal of Pharmaceutical Sciences.* doi:10.1016/j.ejps.2017.10.030.

Bäckman, P., U. Tehler, and B. Olsson. 2017b. "Predicting exposure after oral inhalation of the selective glucocorticoid receptor modulator, azd5423, based on dose, deposition pattern, and mechanistic modeling of pulmonary disposition." *Journal of Aerosol Medicine and Pulmonary Drug Delivery* 30 (2): 108–117. doi:10.1089/jamp.2016.1306.

Barnes, P. J., S. Pedersen, and W. W. Busse. 1998. "Efficacy and safety of inhaled corticosteroids. new developments." *American Journal of Respiratory and Critical Care Medicine* 157 (3 Pt 2): S1–S53. doi:10.1164/ajrccm.157.3.157315.

Bartels, C., M. Looby, R. Sechaud, and G. Kaiser. 2013. "determination of the pharmacokinetics of glycopyrronium in the lung using a population pharmacokinetic modelling approach." *British Journal of Clinical Pharmacology* 76 (6): 868–879. doi:10.1111/bcp.12118.

Beato, M., M. Kalimi, and P. Feigelson. 1972. "Correlation between glucocorticoid binding to specific liver cytosol receptors and enzyme induction in vivo." *Biochemical and Biophysical Research Communications* 47 (6): 1464–1472. doi:10.1016/0006-291X(72)90237-9.

Berge, M. van den, H. A. Kerstjens, R. J. Meijer, D. M. de Reus, G. H. Koëter, H. F. Kauffman, and D. S. Postma. 2001. "Corticosteroid-induced improvement in the PC20 of adenosine monophosphate is more closely associated with reduction in airway inflammation than improvement in the PC20 of methacholine." *American Journal of Respiratory and Critical Care Medicine* 164 (7): 1127–1132. doi:10.1164/ajrccm.164.7.2102135.

Berridge, M. S., D. L. Heald, G. J. Muswick, G. P. Leisure, K. W. Voelker, and F. Miraldi. 1998. "Biodistribution and kinetics of nasal carbon-11-triamcinolone acetonide." *Journal of Nuclear Medicine: Official Publication, Society of Nuclear Medicine* 39 (11): 1972–1977.

Bhagwat, S., U. Schilling, M.-J. Chen, X. Wei, R. Delvadia, M. Absar, B. Saluja, and G. Hochhaus. 2017. "predicting pulmonary pharmacokinetics from in vitro properties of dry powder inhalers." *Pharmaceutical Research* 34 (12): 2541–2556. doi:10.1007/s11095-017-2235-y.

Biggadike, K., R. M. Angell, C. M. Burgess, R. M. Farrell, A. P. Hancock, A. J. Harker, W. R. Irving et al. 2000. "Selective plasma hydrolysis of glucocorticoid gamma-lactones and cyclic carbonates by the enzyme paraoxonase: An ideal plasma inactivation mechanism." *Journal of Medicinal Chemistry* 43 (1): 19–21.

Bjermer, L., Y. G. Cai, B. Särnstrand, and R. Brattsand. 1994a. "Experimental Granulomatous Alveolitis in Rat. Effect of Antigen Manipulation, Smoke Exposure and Route of Administration." *Sarcoidosis* 11 (1): 52–57.

Bjermer, L., T. Sandström, B. Särnstrand, and R. Brattsand. 1994b. "Sephadex-induced granulomatous alveolitis in rat: effects of antigen manipulation." *American Journal of Industrial Medicine* 25 (1): 73–78.

Blake, K., R. Mehta, T. Spencer, R. L. Kunka, and L. Hendeles. 2012. "Bioavailability of inhaled fluticasone propionate via chambers/masks in young children." *The European Respiratory Journal* 39 (1): 97–103. doi:10.1183/09031936.00185510.

Boger, E., N. Evans, M. Chappell, A. Lundqvist, P. Ewing, A. Wigenborg, and M. Fridén. 2016. "Systems pharmacology approach for prediction of pulmonary and systemic pharmacokinetics and receptor occupancy of inhaled drugs." *CPT: Pharmacometrics & Systems Pharmacology* 5 (4): 201–210. doi:10.1002/psp4.12074.

Boger, E., P. Ewing, U. G. Eriksson, B.-M. Fihn, M. Chappell, N. Evans, and M. Fridén. 2015. "A novel in vivo receptor occupancy methodology for the glucocorticoid receptor: Toward an improved understanding of lung pharmacokinetic/pharmacodynamic relationships." *The Journal of Pharmacology and Experimental Therapeutics* 353 (2): 279–287. doi:10.1124/jpet.114.221226.

Borchard, G., M. L. Cassará, P. E. H. Roemelé, B. I. Florea, and H. E. Junginger. 2002. "Transport and local metabolism of budesonide and fluticasone propionate in a human bronchial epithelial cell line (Calu-3)." *Journal of Pharmaceutical Sciences* 91 (6): 1561–1567. doi:10.1002/jps.10151.

Borghardt, J. M., B. Weber, A. Staab, and C. Kloft. 2015. "Pharmacometric models for characterizing the pharmacokinetics of orally inhaled drugs." *The AAPS Journal* 17 (4): 853–870. doi:10.1208/s12248-015-9760-6.

Borghardt, J. M., B. Weber, A. Staab, C. Kunz, S. Formella, and C. Kloft. 2016a. "Investigating pulmonary and systemic pharmacokinetics of inhaled olodaterol in healthy volunteers using a population pharmacokinetic approach." *British Journal of Clinical Pharmacology* 81 (3): 538–552. doi:10.1111/bcp.12780.

Borghardt, J. M., B. Weber, A. Staab, C. Kunz, and C. Kloft. 2016b. "Model-based evaluation of pulmonary pharmacokinetics in asthmatic and COPD patients after oral olodaterol inhalation." *British Journal of Clinical Pharmacology* 82 (3): 739–753. doi:10.1111/bcp.12999.

Borgström, L. 1998. "Local versus total systemic bioavailability as a means to compare different inhaled formulations of the same substance." *Journal of Aerosol Medicine: The Official Journal of the International Society for Aerosols in Medicine* 11 (1): 55–63.

Borgström, L., and M. Nilsson. 1990. "A method for determination of the absolute pulmonary bioavailability of inhaled drugs: terbutaline." *Pharmaceutical Research* 7 (10): 1068–1070.

Bosquillon, C., M. Madlova, N. Patel, N. Clear, and B. Forbes. 2017. "A comparison of drug transport in pulmonary absorption models: isolated perfused rat lungs, respiratory epithelial cell lines and primary cell culture." *Pharmaceutical Research*, September, 1–9. doi:10.1007/s11095-017-2251-y.

Bot, A. I., T. E. Tarara, D. J. Smith, S. R. Bot, C. M. Woods, and J. G. Weers. 2000. "Novel lipid-based hollow-porous microparticles as a platform for immunoglobulin delivery to the respiratory tract." *Pharmaceutical Research* 17 (3): 275–283. doi:10.1023/A:1007544804864.

Boulet, L. P. 2002. "19. Markers of systemic actions of corticosteroids." In *Inhaled Steroids in Asthma: Optimizing Effects in the Airways*, R. P. Schleimer, P. M. O'Byrne, S. J. Szefler, and R. Brattsand, Eds., pp. 465–490. New York: Marcel Dekker.

Brattsand, R., and B. I. Axelsson. 1997. "Basis of airway selectivity of inhaled glucocoricoids." In *Inhaled Glucocoticoids in Asthma*, R. P. Schleimer, W. W. Busse, and P. M. O'Byrne, Eds., pp. 351–379. New York: Marcel Dekker.

Brindley, C., C. Falcoz, A. E. Mackie, and A. Bye. 2000. "Absorption kinetics after inhalation of fluticasone propionate via the diskhaler, diskus and metered-dose inhaler in healthy volunteers." *Clinical Pharmacokinetics* 39 Suppl 1: 1–8.

Burton, J. A., T. H. Gardiner, and L. S. Schanker. 1974. "Absorption of herbicides from the rat lung." *Archives of Environmental Health* 29 (1): 31–33.

Burton, J. A., and L. S. Schanker. 1974a. "Absorption of antibiotics from the rat lung." *Proceedings of the Society for Experimental Biology and Medicine. Society for Experimental Biology and Medicine (New York, N.Y.)* 145 (3): 752–756.

Burton, J. A., and L. S. Schanker. 1974b. "Absorption of corticosteroids from the rat lung." *Steroids* 23 (5): 617–624.

Burton, J. A., and L. S. Schanker. 1974c. "Absorption of sulphonamides and antitubercular drugs from the rat lung." *Xenobiotica; the Fate of Foreign Compounds in Biological Systems* 4 (5): 291–296. doi:10.3109/00498257409052057.

Byrnes, C. A., S. Dinarevic, E. A. Shinebourne, P. J. Barnes, and A. Bush. 1997. "exhaled nitric oxide measurements in normal and asthmatic children." *Pediatric Pulmonology* 24 (5): 312–318.

Byron, P. R., Z. Sun, H. Katayama, and F. Rypacek. 1994. "Solute absorption from the airways of the isolated rat lung. iv. Mechanisms of absorption of fluorophore-labeled poly-α,β-[*n* (2-hydroxyethyl)-DL-aspartamide]." *Pharmaceutical Research* 11 (2): 221–225. doi:10.1023/A:1018947122613.

Catley, M. 2007. "Dissociated steroids." *The Scientific World Journal* 7 (March): 421–430. doi:10.1100/tsw.2007.97.

Chaplin, M. D., W. Rooks, E. W. Swenson, W. C. Cooper, C. Nerenberg, and N. I. Chu. 1980. "Flunisolide metabolism and dynamics of a metabolite." *Clinical Pharmacology and Therapeutics* 27 (3): 402–413.

Chaudhuri, S. R., and V. Lukacova. 2010. "Simulating delivery of pulmonary (and intranasal) aerosolised drugs." *Orally Inhaled & Nasal Drug Products*, pp. 26–30.

Chege, J. K., and H. Chrystyn. 2000. "The relative bioavailability of salbutamol to the lung using urinary excretion following inhalation from a novel dry powder inhaler: The effect of inhalation rate and formulation." *Respiratory Medicine* 94 (1): 51–56. doi:10.1053/rmed.1999.0692.

Chen, D. L., and P. E. Kinahan. 2010. "Multimodality molecular imaging of the lung." *Journal of Magnetic Resonance Imaging: JMRI* 32 (6): 1409–1420. doi:10.1002/jmri.22385.

"Chronic Obstructive Pulmonary Disease: Developing Drugs for Treatment Guidance for Industry-Draft Guidance." Fda. Gov. n.d. Accessed February 26, 2018. https://www.fda.gov/downloads/drugs/guidances/ucm071575.pdf.

Dahlberg, E., A. Thalén, R. Brattsand, J. A. Gustafsson, U. Johansson, K. Roempke, and T. Saartok. 1984. "Correlation between chemical structure, receptor binding, and biological activity of some novel, highly active, 16 alpha, 17 alpha-acetal-substituted glucocorticoids." *Molecular Pharmacology* 25 (1): 70–78.

Daley-Yates, P. T., A. C. Price, J. R. Sisson, A. Pereira, and N. Dallow. 2001. "Beclomethasone dipropionate: Absolute bioavailability, pharmacokinetics and metabolism following intravenous, oral, intranasal and inhaled administration in man." *British Journal of Clinical Pharmacology* 51 (5): 400–409.

Daley-Yates, P. T., and D. H. Richards. 2004. "Relationship between systemic corticosteroid exposure and growth velocity: Development and validation of a pharmacokinetic/pharmacodynamic model." *Clinical Therapeutics* 26 (11): 1905–1919. doi:1.1016/j.clinthera.2004.11.017.

Daley-Yates, P. T., J. Tournant, and R. L. Kunka. 2000. "Comparison of the systemic availability of fluticasone propionate in healthy volunteers and patients with asthma." *Clinical Pharmacokinetics* 39 Suppl 1: 39–45.

Darquenne, C., J. S. Fleming, I. Katz, A. R. Martin, J. Schroeter, O. S. Usmani, J. Venegas, and O. Schmid. 2016. "Bridging the gap between science and clinical efficacy: physiology, imaging, and modeling of aerosols in the lung." *Journal of Aerosol Medicine and Pulmonary Drug Delivery* 29 (2): 107–126. doi:10.1089/jamp.2015.1270.

Davies, N., and M. R. Feddah. 2003. "A novel method for assessing dissolution of aerosol inhaler products." *International Journal of Pharmaceutics* 255 (May): 175–187. doi:10.1016/S0378-5173(03)00091-7.

Dellamary, L. A., T. E. Tarara, D. J. Smith, C. H. Woelk, A. Adractas, M. L. Costello, H. Gill, and J. G. Weers. 2000. "Hollow porous particles in metered dose inhalers." *Pharmaceutical Research* 17 (2): 168–174.

Delvadia, R., M. Hindle, P. W. Longest, and P. R. Byron. 2013. "In vitro tests for aerosol deposition ii: IVIVCS for different dry powder inhalers in normal adults." *Journal of Aerosol Medicine and Pulmonary Drug Delivery* 26 (3): 138–144. doi:10.1089/jamp.2012.0975.

Derendorf, H., G. Hochhaus, H. Möllmann, J. Barth, M. Krieg, S. Tunn, and C. Möllmann. 1993. "Receptor-based pharmacokinetic-pharmacodynamic analysis of corticosteroids." *Journal of Clinical Pharmacology* 33 (2): 115–123.

Derendorf, H., G. Hochhaus, S. Rohatagi, H. Möllmann, J. Barth, H. Sourgens, and M. Erdmann. 1995. "Pharmacokinetics of triamcinolone acetonide after intravenous, oral, and inhaled administration." *Journal of Clinical Pharmacology* 35 (3): 302–305.

Derendorf, H., and B. Meibohm. 1999. "Modeling of pharmacokinetic/pharmacodynamic (PK/PD) relationships: concepts and perspectives." *Pharmaceutical Research* 16 (2): 176–185.

Dershwitz, M., J. L. Walsh, R. J. Morishige, P. M. Connors, R. M. Rubsamen, S. L. Shafer, and C. E. Rosow. 2000. "Pharmacokinetics and pharmacodynamics of inhaled versus intravenous morphine in healthy volunteers." *Anesthesiology* 93 (3): 619–628.

Dickens, D., D. Wermeling, C. Matheney, W. John, W. Abramowitz, S. Sista, and T. Foster. 1999. "Flunisolide administered via metered dose inhaler with and without spacer and following oral administration." *Journal of Allergy and Clinical Immunology* 103: S132.

Diderichsen, P. M., E. Cox, S. W. Martin, A. Cleton, and J. Ribbing. 2013. "Characterizing systemic exposure of inhaled drugs: application to the long-acting B2-agonist PF-00610355." *Clinical Pharmacokinetics* 52 (6): 443–452. doi:10.1007/s40262-013-0048-7.

Digenis, G. A., E. P. Sandefer, R. C. Page, and W. J. Doll. 1998. "Gamma scintigraphy: An evolving technology in pharmaceutical formulation development-part 1." *Pharmaceutical Science & Technology Today* 1 (3): 100–108. doi:10.1016/S1461-5347(98)00032-7.

"Drug Administration Routes | Dermal Delivery | Inhaled Products | Injection." n.d. Accessed September 26, 2017. http://www.simulations-plus.com/software/gastroplus/additional-dosage/.

Druzgala, P., G. Hochhaus, and N. Bodor. 1991. "Soft drugs—10. blanching activity and receptor binding affinity of a new type of glucocorticoid: Loteprednol etabonate." *The Journal of Steroid Biochemistry and Molecular Biology* 38 (2): 149–154.

Edwards, C. D., C. Luscombe, P. Eddershaw, and E. M. Hessel. 2016. "Development of a novel quantitative structure-activity relationship model to accurately predict pulmonary absorption and replace routine use of the isolated perfused respiring rat lung model." *Pharmaceutical Research* 33 (11): 2604–2616. doi:10.1007/s11095-016-1983-4.

Edwards, D. A., A. Ben-Jebria, and R. Langer. 1998. "Recent advances in pulmonary drug delivery using large, porous inhaled particles." *Journal of Applied Physiology (Bethesda, Md.: 1985)* 85 (2): 379–385. doi:10.1152/jappl.1998.85.2.379.

Edwards, D. A., J. Hanes, G. Caponetti, J. Hrkach, A. Ben-Jebria, M. L. Eskew, J. Mintzes, D. Deaver, N. Lotan, and R. Langer. 1997. "Large porous particles for pulmonary drug delivery." *Science (New York, N.Y.)* 276 (5320): 1868–1871.

Ehrhardt, C., P. Bäckman, W. Couet, C. Edwards, B. Forbes, M. Fridén, M. Gumbleton et al. 2017. "Current progress toward a better understanding of drug disposition within the lungs: Summary proceedings of the first workshop on drug transporters in the lungs." *Journal of Pharmaceutical Sciences* 106 (9): 2234–2244. doi:10.1016/j.xphs.2017.04.011.

Ehrhardt, C., J. Fiegel, S. Fuchs, R. Abu-Dahab, U. F. Schaefer, J. Hanes, and C.-M. Lehr. 2002. "drug absorption by the respiratory mucosa: Cell culture models and particulate drug carriers." *Journal of Aerosol Medicine: The Official Journal of the International Society for Aerosols in Medicine* 15 (2): 131–139. doi:10.1089/089426802320282257.

Ehrhardt, C., and K.-J. Kim. 2008 *Drug Absorption Studies - In Situ, In Vitro and In Silico*. Springer. Accessed November 12, 2017. https://www.springer.com/us/book/9780387749006.

Enna, S. J., and L. S. Schanker. 1972. "Absorption of drugs from the rat lung." *The American Journal of Physiology* 223 (5): 1227–1231. doi:10.1152/ajplegacy.1972.223.5.1227.

Enna, S. J., and L. S. Schanker. 1973. "Phenol red absorption from the rat lung: Evidence of carrier transport." *Life Sciences* 12 (5, Part 1): 231–239. doi:10.1016/0024-3205(73)90357-3.

Ericsson, T., M. Fridén, C. Kärrman-Mårdh, I. Dainty, and K. Grime. 2017. "Benchmarking of human dose prediction for inhaled medicines from preclinical in vivo data." *Pharmaceutical Research* 34 (12): 2557–2567. doi:10.1007/s11095-017-2218-z.

Eriksson, J., E. Sjögren, H. Thörn, K. Rubin, P. Bäckman, and H. Lennernäs. 2018. "Pulmonary absorption – estimation of effective pulmonary permeability and tissue retention of ten drugs using an ex vivo rat model and computational analysis." *European Journal of Pharmaceutics and Biopharmaceutics* 124 (March): 1–12. doi:10.1016/j.ejpb.2017.11.013.

Esch, E. W., A. Bahinski, and D. Huh. 2015. "Organs-on-chips at the frontiers of drug discovery." *Nature Reviews Drug Discovery* 14 (4): nrd4539. doi:10.1038/nrd4539.

Esmailpour, N., P. Hogger, K. F. Rabe, U. Heitmann, M. Nakashima, and P. Rohdewald. 1997. "Distribution of inhaled fluticasone propionate between human lung tissue and serum in vivo." *European Respiratory Journal* 10 (7): 1496–1499.

Falcoz, C., A. E. Mackie, J. McDowall, J. McRae, L. Yogendran, G. P. Ventresca, and A. Bye. 1996. "Oral bioavailability of fluticasone propionate in healthy subjects." *British Journal of Clinical Pharmacology* 41: 459–460.

Falcoz, C., A. E. Mackie, J. Moss, J. Horton, G. P. Ventresca, A. Brown, E. Field, S. Harding, P. Wire, and A. Bye. n.d. "Pharmacokinetics of fluticasone propionate inhaled from the diskhaler and diskus after repeat doses in healthy subjects and asthmatic patients." *Journal of Allergy and Clinical Immunology* 1997 (99): S505.

Feng, Y., Z. Xu, and A. Haghnegahdar. 2016. "Computational fluid-particle dynamics modeling for unconventional inhaled aerosols in human respiratory systems." doi:10.5772/65361.

Feurstein, T., and M. Zeitlinger. 2011. "Microdialysis in lung tissue: monitoring of exogenous and endogenous compounds." In *Applications of Microdialysis in Pharmaceutical Science*, T.-H. Tsai, Ed., pp. 255–274. John Wiley & Sons, Inc. doi:10.1002/9781118011294.ch7.

Fiegel, J., C. Ehrhardt, U. F. Schaefer, C.-M. Lehr, and J. Hanes. 2003. "Large porous particle impingement on lung epithelial cell monolayers—toward improved particle characterization in the lung." *Pharmaceutical Research* 20 (5): 788–796.

Fielding, R. M., and R. M. Abra. 1992. "Factors affecting the release rate of terbutaline from liposome formulations after intratracheal instillation in the guinea pig." *Pharmaceutical Research* 9 (2): 220–223.

Forbes, B. 2000. "Human airway epithelial cell lines for in vitro drug transport and metabolism studies." *Pharmaceutical Science & Technology Today* 3 (1): 18–27. doi:10.1016/S1461-5347(99)00231-X.

Forbes, B., and C. Ehrhardt. 2005. "Human respiratory epithelial cell culture for drug delivery applications." *European Journal of Pharmaceutics and Biopharmaceutics: Official Journal of Arbeitsgemeinschaft Fur Pharmazeutische Verfahrenstechnik e. V* 60 (2): 193–205. doi:10.1016/j.ejpb.2005.02.010.

Fröhlich, E., A. Mercuri, S. Wu, and S. Salar-Behzadi. 2016. "Measurements of deposition, lung surface area and lung fluid for simulation of inhaled compounds." *Frontiers in Pharmacology* 7 (June). doi:10.3389/fphar.2016.00181.

Gabrielsson, J., and D. Weiner. 2012. "Non-compartmental analysis." *Methods in Molecular Biology (Clifton, N.J.)* 929: 377–389. doi:10.1007/978-1-62703-050-2_16.

Gaohua, L., J. Wedagedera, B. G. Small, L. Almond, K. Romero, D. Hermann, D. Hanna, M. Jamei, and I. Gardner. 2015. "Development of a multicompartment permeability-limited lung PBPK model and its application in predicting pulmonary pharmacokinetics of antituberculosis drugs." *CPT: Pharmacometrics & Systems Pharmacology* 4 (10): 605–613. doi:10.1002/psp4.12034.

Gardiner, T. H., and L. S. Schanker. 1974. "Absorption of disodium cromoglycate from the rat lung: evidence of carrier transport." *Xenobiotica* 4 (12): 725–731. doi:10.3109/00498257409052074.

Geller, D. A., A. K. Nussler, M. Di Silvio, C. J. Lowenstein, R. A. Shapiro, S. C. Wang, R. L. Simmons, and T. R. Billiar. 1993. "Cytokines, endotoxin, and glucocorticoids regulate the expression of inducible nitric oxide synthase in hepatocytes." *Proceedings of the National Academy of Sciences of the United States of America* 90 (2): 522–526.

Gerde, P., M. Malmlöf, L. Havsborn, C.-O. Sjöberg, P. Ewing, S. Eirefelt, and K. Ekelund. 2017. "DissolvIt: An in vitro method for simulating the dissolution and absorption of inhaled dry powder drugs in the lungs." *Assay and Drug Development Technologies* 15 (2): 77–88. doi:10.1089/adt.2017.779.

Ginsberg, G. L., B. Asgharian, J. S. Kimbell, J. S. Ultman, and A. M. Jarabek. 2008. "Modeling approaches for estimating the dosimetry of inhaled toxicants in children." *Journal of Toxicology and Environmental Health. Part A* 71 (3): 166–195. doi:10.1080/15287390701597889.

Goyal, N., and G. Hochhaus. 2010. "Demonstrating bioequivalence using pharmacokinetics: theoretical considerations across drug classes." *Respiratory Drug Delivery* 1: 261–272.

Green, S. A., A. P. Spasoff, R. A. Coleman, M. Johnson, and S. B. Liggett. 1996. "Sustained activation of a G protein-coupled receptor via 'anchored' agonist binding. molecular localization of the salmeterol exosite within the 2-adrenergic receptor." *The Journal of Biological Chemistry* 271 (39): 24029–24035.

Guillon, A., T. Sécher, L. A. Dailey, L. Vecellio, M. de Monte, M. Si-Tahar, P. Diot, C. P. Page, and N. Heuzé-Vourc'h. 2018. "Insights on animal models to investigate inhalation therapy: relevance for biotherapeutics." *International Journal of Pharmaceutics* 536 (1): 116–126. doi:10.1016/j.ijpharm.2017.11.049.

Guo, Z., Z. Gu, S. R. Howell, K. Chen, S. Rohatagi, L. Cai, J. Wu, and J. Stuhler. 2006. "Ciclesonide disposition and metabolism: Pharmacokinetics, metabolism, and excretion in the mouse, rat, rabbit, and dog." *American Journal of Therapeutics* 13 (6): 490–501. doi:10.1097/01.mjt.0000209688.52571.81.

Haddad, E.-B., S. L. Underwood, D. Dabrowski, M. A. Birrell, K. McCluskie, C. H. Battram, M. Pecoraro, M. L. Foster, and M. G. Belvisi. 2002. "Critical role for T cells in sephadex-induced airway inflammation: Pharmacological and immunological characterization and molecular biomarker identification." *The Journal of Immunology* 168 (6): 3004–3016. doi:10.4049/jimmunol.168.6.3004.

Hardy, J. G., and T. S. Chadwick. 2000. "Sustained release drug delivery to the lungs: an option for the future." *Clinical Pharmacokinetics* 39 (1): 1–4. doi:10.2165/00003088-200039010-00001.

Hastedt, J. E., P. Bäckman, A. R. Clark, W. Doub, A. Hickey, G. Hochhaus, P. J. Kuehl et al. 2016. "Scope and relevance of a pulmonary biopharmaceutical classification system AAPS/FDA/USP Workshop March 16-17th, 2015 in Baltimore, MD." *AAPS Open* 2 (1): 1. doi:10.1186/s41120-015-0002-x.

Hendeles, L., P. T. Daley-Yates, R. Hermann, J. De Backer, S. Dissanayake, and S. T. Horhota. 2015. "Pharmacodynamic studies to demonstrate bioequivalence of oral inhalation products." *The AAPS Journal* 17 (3): 758–768. doi:10.1208/s12248-015-9735-7.

Hendrickx, R., E. L. Bergström, D. L. I. Janzén, M. Fridén, U. Eriksson, K. Grime, and D. Ferguson. 2017. "Translational model to predict pulmonary pharmacokinetics and efficacy in man for inhaled bronchodilators." *CPT: Pharmacometrics & Systems Pharmacology*, December. doi:10.1002/psp4.12270.

Heyder, J., J. Gebhart, G. Rudolf, C. F. Schiller, and W. Stahlhofen. 1986. "Deposition of particles in the human respiratory tract in the size range 0.005–15 Mm." *Journal of Aerosol Science* 17 (5): 811–825. doi:10.1016/0021-8502(86)90035-2.

Hill, M., L. Vaughan, and M. Doovich. 1996. "Dose targeting for dry powder inhalers." In *Respiratory Drug Delivery*, Vol. V, R. N. Dalby, P. R. Byron, and S. Y. Farr, Eds., pp. 197–208. Buffalo Grove, IL: Interpharma Press Inc.

Hindle, M., and H. Chrystyn. 1992. "Determination of the relative bioavailability of salbutamol to the lung following inhalation." *British Journal of Clinical Pharmacology* 34 (4): 311–315.

Hindle, M., D. A. Newton, and H. Chrystyn. 1993. "Investigations of an optimal inhaler technique with the use of urinary salbutamol excretion as a measure of relative bioavailability to the lung." *Thorax* 48 (6): 607–610.

Hochhaus, G., L. S. Chen, A. Ratka, P. Druzgala, J. Howes, N. Bodor, and H. Derendorf. 1992a. "Pharmacokinetic characterization and tissue distribution of the new glucocorticoid soft drug loteprednol etabonate in rats and dogs." *Journal of Pharmaceutical Sciences* 81 (12): 1210–1215.

Hochhaus, G., H. Derendorf, H. Moellmann, and J. Talton. 2002. *Inhaled Steroids in Asthma: Optimizing Effects in the Airways*, pp. 283–307. New York: CRC Press.

Hochhaus, G., R. J. Gonzalez-Rothi, A. Lukyanov, H. Derendorf, H. Schreier, and T. Dalla Costa. 1995. "Assessment of glucocorticoid lung targeting by ex-vivo receptor binding studies in rats." *Pharmaceutical Research* 12 (1): 134–137.

Hochhaus, G., L. Hendeles, E. Harman, and H. Moellmann. 1993. "PK/PD analysis of albuterol action: Application to a comparative assessment of $\beta 2$-adrenergic drugs." *European Journal of Pharmaceutical Sciences* 1 (2): 73–80. doi:10.1016/0928-0987(93)90020-B.

Hochhaus, G., and H. Möllmann. 1992. "Pharmacokinetic/pharmacodynamic characteristics of the beta-2-agonists terbutaline, salbutamol and fenoterol." *International Journal of Clinical Pharmacology, Therapy, and Toxicology* 30 (9): 342–362.

Hochhaus, G., and H. Möllmann. 1995. "Beta-agonists: Terbutaline, albuterol, and fenoterol." In *Handbook of Pharmacokinetic/Pharmacodynamic Correlations*, H. Derendorf and G. Hochhaus, Eds., pp. 299–322. New York: CRC Press.

Hochhaus, G., H. Möllmann, H. Derendorf, and R. J. Gonzalez-Rothi. 1997. "Pharmacokinetic/pharmacodynamic aspects of aerosol therapy using glucocorticoids as a model." *The Journal of Clinical Pharmacology* 37 (10): 881–892. doi:10.1002/j.1552-4604.1997.tb04262.x.

Hochhaus, G., E. W. Schmidt, K. L. Rominger, and H. Möllmann. 1992b. "Pharmacokinetic/dynamic correlation of pulmonary and cardiac effects of fenoterol in asthmatic patients after different routes of administration." *Pharmaceutical Research* 9 (3): 291–297.

Hochhaus, G., S. Suarez, R. J. Gonzalez-Rothi, and H. Schreier. 1998. "Pulmonary targeting of inhaled glucocorticoids: How is it influenced by formulation." In *Respiratory Drug Delivery VI*, R. Dalby, P. Byron, and J. Farr (Eds.), pp. 45–52. Buffalo Grove, IL: Interpharm Press.

Hofmann, W. 2011. "Modelling inhaled particle deposition in the human lung—A review." *Journal of Aerosol Science* 42 (10): 693–724. doi:10.1016/j.jaerosci.2011.05.007.

Holford, N. H., and L. B. Sheiner. 1981. "Understanding the dose-effect relationship: clinical application of pharmacokinetic-pharmacodynamic models." *Clinical Pharmacokinetics* 6 (6): 429–453.

Huh, D. (Dan). 2015. "A human breathing lung-on-a-chip." *Annals of the American Thoracic Society* 12 (Supplement 1): S42–S44. doi:10.1513/AnnalsATS.201410-442MG.

Huh, D., B. D. Matthews, A. Mammoto, M. Montoya-Zavala, H. Y. Hsin, and D. E. Ingber. 2010. "Reconstituting organ-level lung functions on a chip." *Science* 328 (5986): 1662–1668. doi:10.1126/science.1188302.

Jacqmin, P., E. Snoeck, E. A. van Schaick, R. Gieschke, P. Pillai, J.-L. Steimer, and P. Girard. 2007. "Modelling response time profiles in the absence of drug concentrations: definition and performance evaluation of the K-PD model." *Journal of Pharmacokinetics and Pharmacodynamics* 34 (1): 57–85. doi:10.1007/s10928-006-9035-z.

Jones, H. M., and K. Rowland-Yeo. 2013. "Basic concepts in physiologically based pharmacokinetic modeling in drug discovery and development." *CPT: Pharmacometrics & Systems Pharmacology* 2 (August): e63. doi:10.1038/psp.2013.41.

Jonkers, R. E., M. C. Braat, R. P. Koopmans, and C. J. van Boxtel. 1995. "Pharmacodynamic modelling of the drug-induced downregulation of a beta 2-adrenoceptor mediated response and lack of restoration of receptor function after a single high dose of prednisone." *European Journal of Clinical Pharmacology* 49 (1–2): 37–44.

Kaellen, A., and L. Thorsson. 1999. In *ALA/ATS International Conference*, San Diego, CA.

Kandala, B., and G. Hochhaus. 2014. "Pharmacometrics in pulmonary diseases." In *Applied Pharmacometrics*, pp. 349–382. AAPS Advances in the Pharmaceutical Sciences Series. New York: Springer. doi:10.1007/978-1-4939-1304-6_12.

Kreyling, W. G., and G. Scheuch. 2000. "Clearance of particles deposited in the lungs." In *Particle-Lung Interactions*, pp. 323–376. Lung Biology in Health and Disease. CRC Press. doi:10.1201/b14423-11.

Krishnaswami, S., G. Hochhaus, and H. Derendorf. 2000. "An interactive algorithm for the assessment of cumulative cortisol suppression during inhaled corticosteroids therapy." *AAPS Pharmsci.*

Krishnaswami, S., G. Hochhaus, H. Möllmann, J. Barth, and H. Derendorf. 2005. "Interpretation of absorption rate data for inhaled fluticasone propionate obtained in compartmental pharmacokinetic modeling." *International Journal of Clinical Pharmacology and Therapeutics* 43 (3): 117–122.

Kumar, A., W. Terakosolphan, M. Hassoun, K.-K. Vandera, A. Novicky, R. Harvey, P. G. Royall et al. 2017. "A biocompatible synthetic lung fluid based on human respiratory tract lining fluid composition." *Pharmaceutical Research* 34 (12): 2454–2465. doi:10.1007/s11095-017-2169-4.

Labiris, N. R., and M. B. Dolovich. 2003a. "Pulmonary drug delivery. Part i: Physiological factors affecting therapeutic effectiveness of aerosolized medications." *British Journal of Clinical Pharmacology* 56 (6): 588–599. doi:10.1046/j.1365-2125.2003.01892.x.

Labiris, N. R., and M. B. Dolovich. 2003b. "Pulmonary drug delivery. Part ii: The role of inhalant delivery devices and drug formulations in therapeutic effectiveness of aerosolized medications." *British Journal of Clinical Pharmacology* 56 (6): 600–612. doi:10.1046/j.1365-2125.2003.01893.x.

Lanman, R. C., R. M. Gillilan, and L. S. Schanker. 1973. "Absorption of cardiac glycosides from the rat respiratory tract." *The Journal of Pharmacology and Experimental Therapeutics* 187 (1): 105–111.

Lee, S. L., B. Saluja, A. García-Arieta, G. M. L. Santos, Y. Li, S. Lu, S. Hou et al. 2015. "Regulatory considerations for approval of generic inhalation drug products in the US, EU, Brazil, China, and India." *The AAPS Journal* 17 (5): 1285–1304. doi:10.1208/s12248-015-9787-8.

Lin, L., and H. Wong. 2017. "Predicting oral drug absorption: mini review on physiologically-based pharmacokinetic models." *Pharmaceutics* 9 (4). doi:10.3390/pharmaceutics9040041.

Longest, P. W., M. Hindle, S. D. Choudhuri, and P. R. Byron. 2007. "Numerical simulations of capillary aerosol generation: CFD model development and comparisons with experimental data." *Aerosol Science and Technology* 41 (10): 952–973. doi:10.1080/02786820701607027.

Longest, P. W., and L. T. Holbrook. 2012. "In silico models of aerosol delivery to the respiratory tract – development and applications." *Advanced Drug Delivery Reviews* 64 (4): 296–311. doi:10.1016/j.addr.2011.05.009.

Longest, P. W., G. Tian, N. Khajeh-Hosseini-Dalasm, and M. Hindle. 2016. "Validating whole-airway CFD predictions of DPI aerosol deposition at multiple flow rates." *Journal of Aerosol Medicine and Pulmonary Drug Delivery* 29 (6): 461–481. doi:10.1089/jamp.2015.1281.

Lu, D., S. L. Lee, R. A. Lionberger, S. Choi, W. Adams, H. N. Caramenico, B. A. Chowdhury et al. 2015. "International guidelines for bioequivalence of locally acting orally inhaled drug products: Similarities and differences." *The AAPS Journal* 17 (3): 546–557. doi:10.1208/s12248-015-9733-9.

Lundin, P., T. Naber, M. Nilsson, and S. Edsbäcker. 2001. "Effect of food on the pharmacokinetics of budesonide controlled ileal release capsules in patients with active Crohn's disease." *Alimentary Pharmacology & Therapeutics* 15 (1): 45–51.

Mackie, A. E., G. P. Ventresca, R. W. Fuller, and A. Bye. 1996. "Pharmacokinetics of intravenous fluticasone propionate in healthy subjects." *British Journal of Clinical Pharmacology* 41 (6): 539–542.

Maier, G., C. Rubino, R. Hsu, T. Grasela, and R. A. Baumgartner. 2007. "Population pharmacokinetics of (R)-Albuterol and (S)-Albuterol in pediatric patients aged 4-11 years with asthma." *Pulmonary Pharmacology & Therapeutics* 20 (5): 534–542. doi:10.1016/j.pupt.2006.05.003.

Mathia, N. R., J. Timoszyk, P. I. Stetsko, J. R. Megill, R. L. Smith, and D. A. Wall. 2002. "Permeability characteristics of Calu-3 human bronchial epithelial cells: In vitro-in vivo correlation to predict lung absorption in rats." *Journal of Drug Targeting* 10 (1): 31–40. doi:10.1080/10611860290007504.

Matida, E. A., W. H. Finlay, M. Breuer, and C. F. Lange. 2006. "Improving prediction of aerosol deposition in an idealized mouth using large-eddy simulation." *Journal of Aerosol Medicine* 19 (3): 290–300. doi:10.1089/jam.2006.19.290.

May, S., B. Jensen, M. Wolkenhauer, M. Schneider, and C. M. Lehr. 2012. "Dissolution techniques for *in vitro* testing of dry powders for inhalation." *Pharmaceutical Research* 29 (8): 2157–2166. doi:10.1007/s11095-012-0744-2.

May, S., B. Jensen, M. Wolkenhauer, M. Schneider, and C.-M. Lehr. 2013. "Impact of deposition and the presence of surfactants on in vitro dissolution of inhalation powders." In *RDD Europe*, Berlin, Germany, pp. 343–348.

Meibohm, B., and H. Derendorf. 1997. "Basic concepts of pharmacokinetic/pharmacodynamic (PK/PD) modelling." *International Journal of Clinical Pharmacology and Therapeutics* 35 (10): 401–413.

Miller, R., S. Chaudhuri, V. Lukacova, V. Damian-Iordache, M. K. Bayliss, and W. S. Woltosz. 2010. "Development of a physiologically based pharmacokinetic (PBPK) model for predicting deposition and disposition following inhaled and intranasal administration." *Respiratory Drug Delivery* 2: 579–584.

Miller-Larsson, A., H. Mattsson, E. Hjertberg, M. Dahlbäck, A. Tunek, and R. Brattsand. 1998. "Reversible fatty acid conjugation of budesonide. Novel mechanism for prolonged retention of topically applied steroid in airway tissue." *Drug Metabolism and Disposition: The Biological Fate of Chemicals* 26 (7): 623–630.

Minto, C., B. Li, B. Tattam, K. Brown, J. P. Seale, and R. Donnelly. 2000. "Pharmacokinetics of epimeric budesonide and fluticasone propionate after repeat dose inhalation – intersubject variability in systemic absorption from the lung." *British Journal of Clinical Pharmacology* 50 (2): 116–124. doi:10.1046/j.1365-2125.2000.00218.x.

Mobley, C., and G. Hochhaus. 2001. "Methods used to assess pulmonary deposition and absorption of drugs." *Drug Discovery Today* 6 (7): 367–375.

Möllmann, H., H. Derendorf, J. Barth, B. Meibohm, M. Wagner, M. Krieg, H. Weisser, J. Knöller, A. Möllmann, and G. Hochhaus. 1997. "Pharmacokinetic/pharmacodynamic evaluation of systemic effects of flunisolide after inhalation." *The Journal of Clinical Pharmacology* 37 (10): 893–903. doi:10.1002/j.1552-4604.1997.tb04263.x.

Mortimer, K. J., T. W. Harrison, Y. Tang, K. Wu, S. Lewis, S. Sahasranaman, G. Hochhaus, and A. E. Tattersfield. 2006. "Plasma concentrations of inhaled corticosteroids in relation to airflow obstruction in asthma." *British Journal of Clinical Pharmacology* 62 (4): 412–419. doi:10.1111/j.1365-2125.2006.02712.x.

Mortimer, K. J., A. E. Tattersfield, Y. Tang, K. Wu, S. Lewis, G. Hochhaus, and T. W. Harrison. 2007. "Plasma concentrations of fluticasone propionate and budesonide following inhalation: effect of induced bronchoconstriction." *British Journal of Clinical Pharmacology* 64 (4): 439–444. doi:10.1111/j.1365-2125.2007.02856.x.

Nasr, H., and H. Chrystyn. 1997. "Relative bioavailability of gentamicin to the lungs following inhalation." *European Respiratory Journal* 10: 129s.

Newman, S. P., J. Brown, K. P. Steed, S. J. Reader, and H. Kladders. 1998. "Lung deposition of fenoterol and flunisolide delivered using a novel device for inhaled medicines: Comparison of respimat with conventional metered-dose inhalers with and without spacer devices." *Chest* 113 (4): 957–963.

Newman, S. P., and I. R. Wilding. 1999. "Imaging techniques for assessing drug delivery in man." *Pharmaceutical Science & Technology Today* 2 (5): 181–189.

Nilsson, F., P. Strandberg, R. Brattsand, and A. Miller-Larsson. 2001. "High airway selectivity of budesonide due to endogenous reversible esterification." *ATS*, San Francisco, CA.

Okusanya, O. O., S. M. Bhavnani, J. P. Hammel, A. Forrest, C. C. Bulik, P. G. Ambrose, and R. Gupta. 2014. "Evaluation of the pharmacokinetics and pharmacodynamics of liposomal amikacin for inhalation in cystic fibrosis patients with chronic pseudomonal infections using data from two phase 2 clinical studies." *Antimicrobial Agents and Chemotherapy* 58 (9): 5005–5015. doi:10.1128/AAC.02421-13.

Olsson, B. "Mimetikos Preludium Software – Emmace Consulting AB." n.d. Accessed February 27, 2018. http://www.emmace.se/mimetikos-preludium/.

Olsson, B., and P. Bäckman. 2014. "Mouth-throat models for realistic in vitro testing – a proposal for debate." *Respiratory Drug Delivery* 1: 287–294.

Olsson, B., E. Bondesson, L. Borgström, S. Edsbäcker, S. Eirefelt, K. Ekelund, L. Gustavsson, and T. Hegelund-Myrbäck. 2011. "Pulmonary drug metabolism, clearance, and absorption." In *Controlled Pulmonary Drug Delivery*, pp. 21–50. Advances in Delivery Science and Technology. Springer, New York. doi:10.1007/978-1-4419-9745-6_2.

Olsson, B., L. Borgström, H. Lundbäck, and M. Svensson. 2013. "Validation of a general in vitro approach for prediction of total lung deposition in healthy adults for pharmaceutical inhalation products." *Journal of Aerosol Medicine and Pulmonary Drug Delivery* 26 (6): 355–369. doi:10.1089/jamp.2012.0986.

Patel, J., D. Pal, V. Vangal, M. Gandhi, and A. L. Mitra. 2002. "Transport of HIV-protease inhibitors across 1 Alpha,25di-Hydroxy vitamin D3-treated Calu-3 cell monolayers: Modulation of P-glycoprotein activity." *Pharmaceutical Research* 19 (11): 1696–1703. doi:10.1023/A:1020761514471.

Patton, J. S. 1996. "Mechanisms of macromolecule absorption by the lungs." *Advanced Drug Delivery Reviews*, Pulmonary Polypeptide and Polynucleic Acid Delivery, 19 (1): 3–36. doi:10.1016/0169-409X(95)00113-L.

Pezron, I., R. Mitra, D. Pal, and A. K. Mitra. 2002. "Insulin aggregation and asymmetric transport across human bronchial epithelial cell monolayers (Calu-3)." *Journal of Pharmaceutical Sciences* 91 (4): 1135–1146.

Phillips, J. E. 2017. "Inhaled efficacious dose translation from rodent to human: A retrospective analysis of clinical standards for respiratory diseases." *Pharmacology & Therapeutics* 178 (October): 141–147. doi:10.1016/j.pharmthera.2017.04.003.

Price, O. "Multiple-Path Particle Dosimetry Model (MPPD v 3.04) | Www. Ara. Com." Accessed November 20, 2017. https://www.ara.com/products/multiple-path-particle-dosimetry-model-mppd-v-304.

Reddel, H. K., D. R. Taylor, E. D. Bateman, L.-P. Boulet, H. A. Boushey, W. W. Busse, T. B. Casale et al. 2009. "An official American Thoracic Society/European Respiratory Society statement: Asthma control and exacerbations: standardizing endpoints for clinical asthma trials and clinical practice." *American Journal of Respiratory and Critical Care Medicine* 180 (1): 59–99. doi:10.1164/rccm.200801-060ST.

Riley, T., D. Christopher, J. Arp, A. Casazza, A. Colombani, A. Cooper, M. Dey et al. 2012. "Challenges with developing in vitro dissolution tests for orally inhaled products (OIPs)." *AAPS PharmSciTech* 13 (3): 978–989. doi:10.1208/s12249-012-9822-3.

Rohatagi, S., V. Arya, K. Zech, R. Nave, G. Hochhaus, B. K. Jensen, and J. S. Barrett. 2003. "Population pharmacokinetics and pharmacodynamics of ciclesonide." *Journal of Clinical Pharmacology* 43 (4): 365–378.

Rohatagi, S., A. Bye, C. Falcoz, A. E. Mackie, B. Meibohm, H. Möllmann, and H. Derendorf. 1996. "Dynamic modeling of cortisol reduction after inhaled administration of fluticasone propionate." *Journal of Clinical Pharmacology* 36 (10): 938–941.

Rohatagi, S., G. Hochhaus, H. Möllmann, J. Barth, and H. Derendorf. 1995a. "Pharmacokinetic interaction between endogenous cortisol and exogenous corticosteroids." *Die Pharmazie* 50 (9): 610–613.

Rohatagi, S., G. Hochhaus, H. Mollmann, J. Barth, E. Galia, M. Erdmann, H. Sourgens, and H. Derendorf. 1995b. "Pharmacokinetic and pharmacodynamic evaluation of triamcinolone acetonide after intravenous, oral, and inhaled administration." *Journal of Clinical Pharmacology* 35 (12): 1187–1193.

Rohatagi, S., G. R. Rhodes, and P. Chaikin. 1999. "absolute oral versus inhaled bioavailability: Significance for inhaled drugs with special reference to inhaled glucocorticoids." *Journal of Clinical Pharmacology* 39 (7): 661–663.

Rohrschneider, M., S. Bhagwat, R. Krampe, V. Michler, J. Breitkreutz, and G. Hochhaus. 2015. "Evaluation of the Transwell system for characterization of dissolution behavior of inhalation drugs: Effects of membrane and surfactant." *Molecular Pharmaceutics* 12 (8): 2618–2624. doi:10.1021/acs.molpharmaceut.5b00221.

Rostami, A. A. 2009. "Computational modeling of aerosol deposition in respiratory tract: A review." *Inhalation Toxicology* 21 (4): 262–290. doi:10.1080/08958370802448987.

Rowland, M., C. Peck, and G. Tucker. 2011. "Physiologically-based pharmacokinetics in drug development and regulatory science." *Annual Review of Pharmacology and Toxicology* 51: 45–73. doi:10.1146/annurev-pharmtox-010510-100540.

Ryrfeldt, A., P. Andersson, S. Edsbäcker, M. Tönnesson, D. Davies, and R. Pauwels. 1982. "Pharmacokinetics and metabolism of budesonide, a selective glucocorticoid." *European Journal of Respiratory Diseases. Supplement* 122: 86–95.

Sadée, W., M. L. Richards, J. Grevel, and J. S. Rosenbaum. 1983. "In vivo characterization of four types of opioid binding sites in rat brain." *Life Sciences* 33 (January): 187–189. doi:10.1016/0024-3205(83)90474-5.

Sakagami, M. 2004. "Insulin disposition in the lung following oral inhalation in humans: A meta-analysis of its pharmacokinetics." *Clinical Pharmacokinetics* 43 (8): 539–552. doi:10.2165/00003088-200443080-00004.

Schanker, L. S., and J. A. Burton. 1976. "Absorption of heparin and cyanocobalamin from the rat lung." *Proceedings of the Society for Experimental Biology and Medicine* 152 (3): 377–380. doi:10.3181/00379727-152-39400.

Shek, P. N., Z. E. Suntres, and J. I. Brooks. 1994. "Liposomes in pulmonary applications: Physicochemical considerations, pulmonary distribution and antioxidant delivery." *Journal of Drug Targeting* 2 (5): 431–442. doi:10.3109/10611869408996819.

Siepmann, J., and F. Siepmann. 2013. "Mathematical modeling of drug dissolution." *International Journal of Pharmaceutics*, Poorly Soluble Drugs, 453 (1): 12–24. doi:10.1016/j.ijpharm.2013.04.044.

Son, Y.-J., and J. T. McConville. 2009. "Development of a standardized dissolution test method for inhaled pharmaceutical formulations." *International Journal of Pharmaceutics* 382 (1–2): 15–22. doi:10.1016/j.ijpharm.2009.07.034.

Stass, H., J. Nagelschmitz, S. Willmann, H. Delesen, A. Gupta, and S. Baumann. 2013. "Inhalation of a dry powder ciprofloxacin formulation in healthy subjects: A phase I study." *Clinical Drug Investigation* 33 (6): 419–427. doi:10.1007/s40261-013-0082-0.

Stefely, J. S., W. M. Hameister, P. B. Myrdal, and C. L. Leach. 1999. "Pulmonary sustained release of a novel steroid delivered by CFC-free metered dose inhaler in the dog." In *14th Annual Meeting of the American Association of Pharmaceutical Scientists*, New Orleans, LA.

Steimer, A., E. Haltner, and C.-M Lehr. 2005. "Cell culture models of the respiratory tract relevant to pulmonary drug delivery." *Journal of Aerosol Medicine* 18 (2): 137–182. doi:10.1089/jam.2005.18.137.

Stein, S. W., and C. G. Thiel. 2017. "The history of therapeutic aerosols: A chronological review." *Journal of Aerosol Medicine and Pulmonary Drug Delivery* 30 (1): 20–41. doi:10.1089/jamp.2016.1297.

Suarez, S., R. J. Gonzalez-Rothi, H. Schreier, and G. Hochhaus. 1998. "Effect of dose and release rate on pulmonary targeting of liposomal triamcinolone acetonide phosphate." *Pharmaceutical Research* 15 (3): 461–465. doi:10.1023/A:1011936617625.

Sykes, D. A., and S. J. Charlton. 2012. "Slow receptor dissociation is not a key factor in the duration of action of inhaled long-acting $\beta 2$-adrenoceptor agonists." *British Journal of Pharmacology* 165 (8): 2672–2683. doi:10.1111/j.1476-5381.2011.01639.x.

Szefler, S. J., and R. J. Martin. 2002. "16. Evaluation and comparison of inhaled steroids." In *Inhaled Steroids in Asthma: Optimizing Effects in the Airways*, R. P. Schleimer, P. M. O'Byrne, S. J. Szefler, and R. Brattsand, Eds., pp. 389–418. New York: Marcel Dekker.

Talton, J., J. Fitzgerald, R. Singh, and G. Hochhaus. 2000. "Nano-thin coatings for improved lung targeting of glucocorticoid dry powders. In vitro and in vivo characteristics." *Respiratory Drug Delivery VII* 1: 67–74.

Tayab, Z. R., and G. Hochhaus. 2005. "Pharmacokinetic/pharmacodynamic evaluation of inhalation drugs: Application to targeted pulmonary delivery systems." *Expert Opinion on Drug Delivery* 2 (3): 519–532. doi:10.1517/17425247.2.3.519.

Thorsson, L., S. Edsbäcker, and T. B. Conradson. 1994. "Lung deposition of budesonide from turbuhaler is twice that from a pressurized metered-dose inhaler P-MDI." *The European Respiratory Journal* 7 (10): 1839–1844.

Thorsson, L., S. Edsbäcker, A. Källén, and C. G. Löfdahl. 2001. "Pharmacokinetics and systemic activity of fluticasone via diskus and PMDI, and of budesonide via Turbuhaler." *British Journal of Clinical Pharmacology* 52 (5): 529–538.

Thorsson, L., F. Thunnisen, and S. Korn. 1998. "Formation of fatty acid conjugates of budesonide in human lung tissue in vivo." *American Journal of Respiratory and Critical Care Medicine* 157: A404.

Toogood, J. H. 1985. "An appraisal of the influence of dose frequency on the antiasthmatic activity of inhaled corticosteroids." *Annals of Allergy* 55 (1): 2–4.

Tronde, A., C. Bosquillon, and B. Forbes. 2008. "the isolated perfused lung for drug absorption studies." In *Drug Absorption Studies*, pp. 135–163. Biotechnology: Pharmaceutical Aspects. Boston, MA: Springer. doi:10.1007/978-0-387-74901-3_6.

Tronde, A., B. Nordén, A.-B. Jeppsson, P. Brunmark, E. Nilsson, H. Lennernäs, and U. H. Bengtsson. 2003. "Drug absorption from the isolated perfused rat lung—correlations with drug physicochemical properties and epithelial permeability." *Journal of Drug Targeting* 11 (1): 61–74. doi:10.1080/10611860 31000086117.

Tu, J. Y., K. Inthavong, and G. Ahmadi. 2013. "Fluid particle dynamics in the human respiratory system – a computational approach." doi:10.1007/978-94-007-4488-2.

Tunek, A., K. Sjödin, and G. Hallström. 1997. "Reversible formation of fatty acid esters of budesonide, an antiasthma glucocorticoid, in human lung and liver microsomes." *Drug Metabolism and Disposition: The Biological Fate of Chemicals* 25 (11): 1311–1317.

Van den Bosch, J. M., C. J. Westermann, J. Aumann, S. Edsbäcker, M. Tönnesson, and O. Selroos. 1993. "Relationship between lung tissue and blood plasma concentrations of inhaled budesonide." *Biopharmaceutics & Drug Disposition* 14 (5): 455–459.

Ventresca, G. P., A. E. Mackie, J. A. Moss, J. McDowall, and A. Bye. 1994. "Absorption of oral fluticasone propionate in healthy subjects." *American Journal of Respiratory and Critical Care Medicine* 149: A214.

Verma, R. K., M. Ibrahim, and L. Garcia-Contreras. 2015. "Lung anatomy and physiology and their implications for pulmonary drug delivery." In *Pulmonary Drug Delivery*, A. Nokhodchi and G. P. Martin, Eds., pp. 1–18. John Wiley & Sons, Ltd. http://onlinelibrary.wiley.com/doi/10.1002/9781118799536.ch1/summary.

Wan, H., H. L. Winton, C. Soeller, G. A. Stewart, P. J. Thompson, D. C. Gruenert, M. B. Cannell, D. R. Garrod, and C. Robinson. 2000. "Tight junction properties of the immortalized human bronchial epithelial cell lines Calu-3 and 16HBE14o-." *The European Respiratory Journal* 15 (6): 1058–1068.

Wang, C.-s., Ed. 2005. "Chapter 9 deposition models." In *Interface Science and Technology*, vol. 5, pp. 127–148. Inhaled Particles. Elsevier. doi:10.1016/S1573-4285(05)80013-4.

Wang, Y.-B., A. B. Watts, J. I. Peters, and R. O. Williams. 2014. "the impact of pulmonary diseases on the fate of inhaled medicines—A review." *International Journal of Pharmaceutics* 461 (1): 112–128. doi:10.1016/j.ijpharm.2013.11.042.

Weber, B., and G. Hochhaus. 2013. "A pharmacokinetic simulation tool for inhaled corticosteroids." *The AAPS Journal* 15 (1): 157–171. doi:10.1208/s12248-012-9420-z.

Weber, B., and G. Hochhaus. 2015. "A systematic analysis of the sensitivity of plasma pharmacokinetics to detect differences in the pulmonary performance of inhaled fluticasone propionate products using a model-based simulation approach." *The AAPS Journal* 17 (4): 999–1010. doi:10.1208/s12248-015-9768-y.

Wieslander, E., E. L. Delander, L. Järkelid, E. Hjertberg, A. Tunek, and R. Brattsand. 1998. "pharmacologic importance of the reversible fatty acid conjugation of budesonide studied in a rat cell line in vitro." *American Journal of Respiratory Cell and Molecular Biology* 19 (3): 477–484. doi:10.1165/ajrcmb.19.3.3195.

Wildhaber, J. H., S. G. Devadason, J. M. Wilson, C. Roller, T. Lagana, L. Borgström, and P. N. LeSouëf. 1998. "Lung deposition of budesonide from turbuhaler in asthmatic children." *European Journal of Pediatrics* 157 (12): 1017–1022.

Winton, H. L., H. Wan, M. B. Cannell, D. C. Gruenert, P. J. Thompson, D. R. Garrod, G. A. Stewart, and C. Robinson. 1998. "Cell lines of pulmonary and non-pulmonary origin as tools to study the effects of house dust mite proteinases on the regulation of epithelial permeability." *Clinical and Experimental Allergy: Journal of the British Society for Allergy and Clinical Immunology* 28 (10): 1273–1285.

Wu, K., A. L. Blomgren, K. Ekholm, B. Weber, S. Edsbaecker, and G. Hochhaus. 2009. "Budesonide and ciclesonide: Effect of tissue binding on pulmonary receptor binding." *Drug Metabolism and Disposition: The Biological Fate of Chemicals* 37 (7): 1421–1426. doi:10.1124/dmd.108.026039.

Wu, K., N. Goyal, J. G. Stark, and G. Hochhaus. 2008. "Evaluation of the administration time effect on the cumulative cortisol suppression and cumulative lymphocytes suppression for once-daily inhaled corticosteroids: A population modeling/simulation approach." *Journal of Clinical Pharmacology* 48 (9): 1069–1080. doi:10.1177/0091270008320607.

Wu, K., M. Looby, G. Pillai, G. Pinault, A. F. Drollman, and S. Pascoe. 2011. "Population pharmacodynamic model of the longitudinal fev1 response to an inhaled long-acting anti-muscarinic in COPD patients." *Journal of Pharmacokinetics and Pharmacodynamics* 38 (1): 105–119. doi:10.1007/s10928-010-9180-2.

Xu, J., R. Nave, G. Lahu, E. Derom, and H. Derendorf. 2010. "Population pharmacokinetics and pharmacodynamics of inhaled ciclesonide and fluticasone propionate in patients with persistent asthma." *Journal of Clinical Pharmacology* 50 (10): 1118–1127. doi:10.1177/0091270009354994.

Yang, S., L. Lee, and S. Pascoe. 2017. "Population pharmacokinetics modeling of inhaled umeclidinium for adult patients with asthma." *European Journal of Drug Metabolism and Pharmacokinetics* 42 (1): 79–88. doi:10.1007/s13318-016-0331-8.

Zhao, P., L. Zhang, J. A. Grillo, Q. Liu, J. M. Bullock, Y. J. Moon, P. Song et al. 2011. "Applications of physiologically based pharmacokinetic (PBPK) modeling and simulation during regulatory review." *Clinical Pharmacology & Therapeutics* 89 (2): 259–267. doi:10.1038/clpt.2010.298.

Section III

Active Pharmaceutical Ingredient/ Drug Product Manufacturing

7

Small Molecules: Process Intensification and Continuous Synthesis

Thomas D. Roper

CONTENTS

7.1 Introduction to Process Intensification

7.1.1 What Is Process Intensification

Process intensification is a term which encompasses both equipment-based and chemistry-based approaches to producing more chemical product in the same space or reducing the amount of space needed for a given process.[1] The concept has traditionally been used in the bulk chemical industry, but is now finding use in the fine chemical and pharmaceutical industry due to the increasing needs to control cost and avoid new capital investment in equipment and manufacturing sites. The initial definition was

Process Intensification Strategies for Active Pharmaceutical Ingredients	
Equipment Based	Process Based
Reactors	Increased yields
Separators	Increased Concentration
Crystallizers	Reaction Kinetics
Filters	Continuous Crystallization
Dryers	Drying Processes

FIGURE 7.1 Opportunity areas for process intensification.

proposed by imperial chemical industries (ICI) and generally related to the cost of capital plant equipment[2] and is now much more broadly defined. The concept is so often used and applied that the journal *Chemical Engineering and Processing: Process Intensification* (Elsevier) addresses the area from a chemical engineering perspective. In addition the RAPID Manufacturing Institute is a major research initiative sponsored by the United States Department of Energy. RAPID identified three areas of emphasis for application: (i) chemical commodity processing; (ii) natural gas upgrading, and (iii) renewable bio products. While production of pharmaceuticals is not directly addressed as an application by RAPID, the three areas of underpinning science and technology, namely: (i) module manufacturing; (ii) intensified process fundamentals; and (iii) modelling and simulation all find their uses within the realm of active pharmaceutical ingredient (API) manufacture.

With respect to the use of process intensification techniques within the context of pharmaceutical industry, there has been recognition that increased process efficiency is a competitive advantage and can directly affect the corporation bottom line. In addition, concepts of process intensification and resulting process control overlap significantly with FDA concepts of process analytical technology (PAT).[3] Implementation of PAT and process intensification are key components of a quality by design (QbD) file. The FDA has become interested in elements of process intensification, such as continuous processing and API particle generation which align with higher levels of process understanding and control. The FDA has taken firm action with respect to companies who do not have control of their manufacturing processes, thereby putting patients at risk. As a part of remediation and ensuring continuity of medicines supply, pharmaceutical suppliers are increasing their level of process understanding and control. The concepts of process intensification can serve as vehicles to increase understanding of chemical and pharmaceutical processes and aid in the support of PAT within the industry. A representation of the potential areas for process intensification as applied to API manufacture are given in Figure 7.1.

For the purposes of this chapter, process intensification will be dealt with on a broad basis, encompassing both chemical and engineering approaches which produce the same outcome, namely, the cost effective production of API from a minimized manufacturing footprint.

7.2 Methods of Measuring Process Intensification

In order to understand the baseline for existing and future processes, a set of pre-determined metrics is required in order to compare between previous, current, and proposed processes. These metrics can be understood in terms of chemistry-derived metrics and process-derived metrics. Chemistry metrics can be easily calculated by understanding the materials purpose, use, and fate in the process. Alternatively, process metrics comprise a much wider set of comparisons that range from energy utilization to cycle time among others. In this section, a selection of chemistry and process metrics will be reviewed including how they may be used in the context of API development and manufacture.

A starting point for metrics collection in API development would ideally be the original synthetic process utilized in the medicinal chemistry laboratories. However, often accurate data on workup volumes and isolation procedures are difficult to obtain and, in general, medicinal chemists' focus may not be primarily on ensuring the most efficient process. The initial delivery of API (albeit in medicinal or process labs) for toxicology can be on the order of 50 g for maximum tolerated dose studies. Preparation of this amount of API can serve as an appropriate baseline for measuring process improvement over time.

7.2.1 Chemistry Metrics

7.2.1.1 Metrics Used in the Context of Organic Chemistry

A fundamental metric of process efficiency is the number of transformations (chemical steps) in a process. This can be intuitively understood in that each synthetic transformation is comprised of unit operations, such as additions, reactions, separations, and crystallizations, which contribute to the overall metrics. Elimination of a single chemical transformation, therefore, eliminates a whole set of unit operations when compared to an initial synthesis. A group of process chemists from AstraZeneca and GlaxoSmithKline (GSK) have outlined the justification for changes in routes in a more comprehensive fashion.[4] A second fundamental measure of chemistry efficiency is percentage yield, which measures the efficiency of a specific reaction output against the theoretical output. This basic chemistry metric is useful in determining the molar efficiency of conversion of the limiting reagent only and does not take into consideration excess reagents or solvents and, hence, will not be explored further here.

The concept of *atom economy (AE)* has been developed by Trost[5] and is useful for understanding how atoms in the starting materials and reagents are incorporated into the desired product. Equation 7.1 provides a basic calculation for determining atom economy[6]:

$$\text{AE} = \frac{\text{MW}\left(\text{g} \cdot \text{mol}^{-1}\right) \text{ of product}}{\text{MW}\left(\text{g} \cdot \text{mol}^{-1}\right) \text{ of starting material and reagents}} \times 1000 \tag{7.1}$$

As can be observed from Equation 7.1, this method is useful in the context of organic chemistry in order to determine the percentage of the molecular weight of atoms from starting materials and reagents that are incorporated into the desired product. Higher atom economy is reflective of an efficient use of starting materials and reagents in synthesizing a molecule.

7.2.1.2 Holistic Green Chemistry Metrics

Academic and industrial groups have endeavored to find more complete ways of accounting for material use in the production of APIs. *Reaction mass efficiency* (RME) was developed by Curzons at GSK in order to more effectively account for yield and selectivity in green chemistry metrics.[6] RME (Equation 7.2) is defined in terms of weight and so accounts for excesses of materials used in order to produce the product.

$$\text{RME} = \frac{\text{mass of product}}{\text{mass of reactants}} \times 100 \tag{7.2}$$

The RME introduces the concept of metrics with respect to mass input rather than moles or molecular weights and therefore begins to more clearly define the total cost footprint of the process. In a further development of holistic chemistry metrics, Roger Sheldon developed the concept of E-factor in order to account for total material use in a process, with the exception of water.[7] Sheldon also identified the E-factor (Equation 7.3) associated with various industry groups, with particular notation that the pharmaceutical industry is the least efficient with respect to production of small molecules with E-factors in the area of 25–100, whereas the oil refining industry maintains E-factors of <0.1. Although many factors such as product history and volumes may be a reason for the inefficiency of the pharmaceuticals, the industry has taken on the challenge to become more efficient.

$$\text{E-Factor} = \frac{\text{mass of all input materials-mass of product}}{\text{mass of product}} \tag{7.3}$$

The metric of *process mass intensity* (PMI) has been agreed by the Green Chemistry Institute's Pharmaceutical Round Table as a standard for the industry and as a comparison across companies.[8] PMI

(Equation 7.4) is similar to E-factor in that all materials input are accounted for by mass with the exception of water and ideally will approach "1" as waste decreases.

$$PMI = \frac{\text{mass of all input materials}}{\text{mass of product}} \tag{7.4}$$

The use of PMI as a fundamental metric of efficiency is particularly easy to calculate as lab and pilot plant procedures require careful documentation of materials utilization. All chemistry metrics as defined above lack the inclusion of water as a waste product. While some aqueous phases may be discarded directly to waste, others contain varying amounts of metals or by-products which must be disposed of by costly means such as incineration, and, therefore, the inclusion of water as a part of the waste calculation is worthy of further debate.

The use of green chemistry metrics to produce a comparison among different routes of synthesis is a powerful way to demonstrate improvement over time or where justification is needed for the selection of one route over another. Chemists at DSM and Hoffmann-La Roche used this technique to compare three routes of synthesis and recommended the green chemistry metrics process as methodology to identify the most important areas of a synthesis for optimisation.[9]

7.2.2 Process Metrics

Process-based metrics cover a wide scope, and many have been outlined by Jimenez-Gonzalez and Constable.[10] The use of specific process metrics is defined by the needs of the scientist or organization based on the desirability of certain specific outcomes. For example, a scientist at a company which specializes in micronization will have important occupational safety metrics as a primary driver, whereas if the primary focus of the work is biocatalysis, then other considerations, such as catalyst stability or turnover number may be considered. For the purposes of API production, the emphasis will be on generally applicable metrics which can be compared across a process change history.

The *number and type of unit operations* is an important metric of process complexity. When using unit operations as a metric, initial definition of a series of high level and detailed operations are needed. Table 7.1 describes a set of standard unit operations which may be used to compare across different processes or routes.

Depending on the nature and length of the process, specific unit operations, both high level and detailed level may be selected as metrics to be tracked over time. Chemical process *cycle time* is another useful metric for consideration when evaluating the efficiency of a process, as it adds a time element to the chemistry and unit operations metrics. Chemistry metrics and unit operations may be minimized (for example), but if the remaining unit operations (such as reactions) are slow, then precious equipment time is being utilized, impacting personnel resource considerations, as well as creating an opportunity cost. In the case of *cycle time* evaluation, one is aiming for the lowest possible cycle time, while maintaining *product quality*.

TABLE 7.1

Examples of API Unit Operations

High Level Unit Operation (number)	Detailed Unit Operation (for example)
Chemical reactions	Additions
Separations	Heating or cooling
Mixing	Weighing operations
	Layer separations
	Crystallizations
	Chromatography operations
	Filtrations
	Drying operations
	Offloading of product

A final important metric of process intensification is the assurance of *product quality*. There are a number of ways to measure quality including calculation of process capability,[11] which is generally related to comparison against a single specification. Process capability (C_p) is defined in Equation 7.5, where the USL and LSL are the upper and lower specification limits, respectively, and σ is the process standard deviation. As can be observed, a higher process capability is more challenging when specifications are tight (i.e. USL and LSL are close to each other). It is therefore desirable, from a process capability point of view, to justify scientifically, the widest specification limits permissible, while still remaining well within patient safety and product performance expectations.

$$C_P = \frac{\text{USL} - \text{LSL}}{6\sigma} \tag{7.5}$$

Process capability can be useful when evaluating the effect of changes against a single critical specification, however, for the purposes of API production, we can simplify the metric since API batches produced must meet all the specifications before provision to a customer. Therefore, a simple measurement of the percentage of batches passed against the agreed API specification will suffice.

7.3 Process Intensification Strategies

7.3.1 Reduction of the Chemical Footprint

Limiting the amount and controlling the type of chemicals used throughout a synthetic scheme is a fundamental driver of process intensification in the pharmaceutical industry. Historically, process chemists have focused on developing plant and production ready processes, but without systematic driving principles which drive outcomes. In 1998, Anastas and Warner introduced the chemical and engineering community to the "12 principles of green chemistry,"[12] these 12 principles are an excellent starting point for a more systematic approach to API process development. Figure 7.2 outlines the general links between the 12 principles and a list of potential priorities of development chemists and engineers.

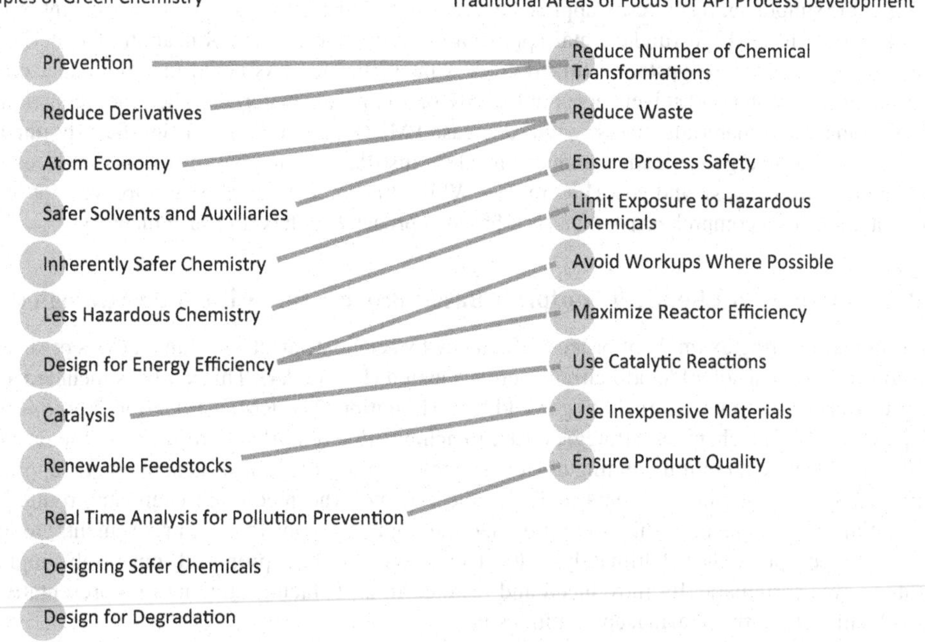

FIGURE 7.2 Alignment of the 12 principles of green chemistry with traditional API development challenges.

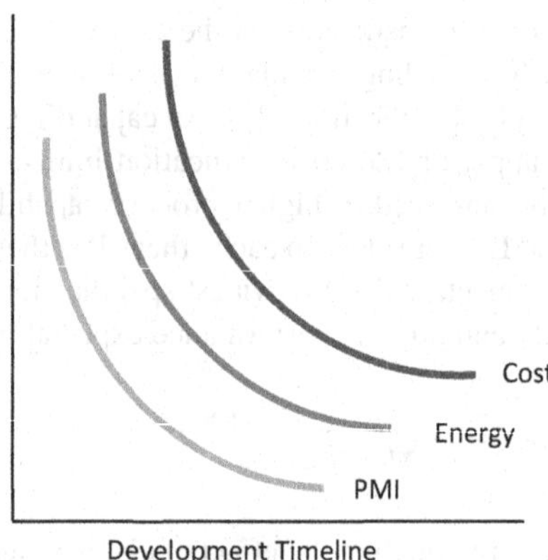

FIGURE 7.3 PMI tracks with energy consumption and cost.

The 12 principles of green chemistry, when combined with bespoke production requirements, comprise an excellent starting point with respect to optimization of chemical reactions. Tucker of Pfizer has made a similar analysis indicating how the principles align with an overall cost reduction strategy for pharmaceuticals.[13] These green chemistry concepts have now made their way to implementation further upstream in the API discovery and development process, as medicinal chemists now have begun to apply the principles of green chemistry. Initially, these approaches were based on replacement of solvents, but have now branched out into reagent selection,[14] and this example showed that medicinal chemists at Pfizer were able to implement greener oxidation reagents via use of a selection guide. A learning from this report is that chemists and engineers will utilize tools that facilitate green chemistry-based process intensification when they are available. This trend shows the utility of developing systematic approaches to green chemistry-based process intensification strategies at an early point in the discovery-development process, where previously medicinal chemists relied on traditional techniques which were familiar to them.

There are simplistic, yet effective approaches for chemistry-based approaches to process intensification. Chief among these is the fundamental approach of "reduction and simplification of material use" as methodology to drive downstream linked process intensification. As noted in a key paper on process mass intensity,[8] water and solvent account for 88% of all process materials. Therefore reduction of total reaction mass and materials diversity will decrease PMI (Equation 7.4) and significantly impact other metrics, such as energy utilization (reduced need for distillation), number of solvents (reduced need for put and take exchanges), and cost (Figure 7.3). While this approach can drive improvement of process intensity, it lacks a comprehensive materials-based approach to safety and sustainability.

7.3.2 Examples of Chemical Footprint-Based Process Intensification Strategies

In a standard setting example of process efficiency by scientists at Pfizer,[15] an analysis of several generations of synthesis of sildenafil citrate were evaluated (Figure 7.4). This analysis included a number of green chemistry metrics including, yield, AE (Equation 7.1), RME (Equation 7.2), *and* E-factor (Equation 7.3). The chemical strategies used to achieve this remarkable result were the development of highly selective and high yielding chemistry including use of a convergent synthetic approach that provided significant improvements to RME and AE over the medicinal chemistry route. Notably, the initial improvements in this route provided the highest proportion of improvements, followed by solvent-based approaches. Ultimately, solvent recovery, an often proposed, but rarely implemented strategy, was systematically introduced and resulted in an E-factor value more representative of the fine chemical than the pharmaceutical industry.

Chemists at Merck used a technology-based approach to process intensification in their development of sitagliptin and partnered with two external partners, Solviasis and Codexis, in achieving success.

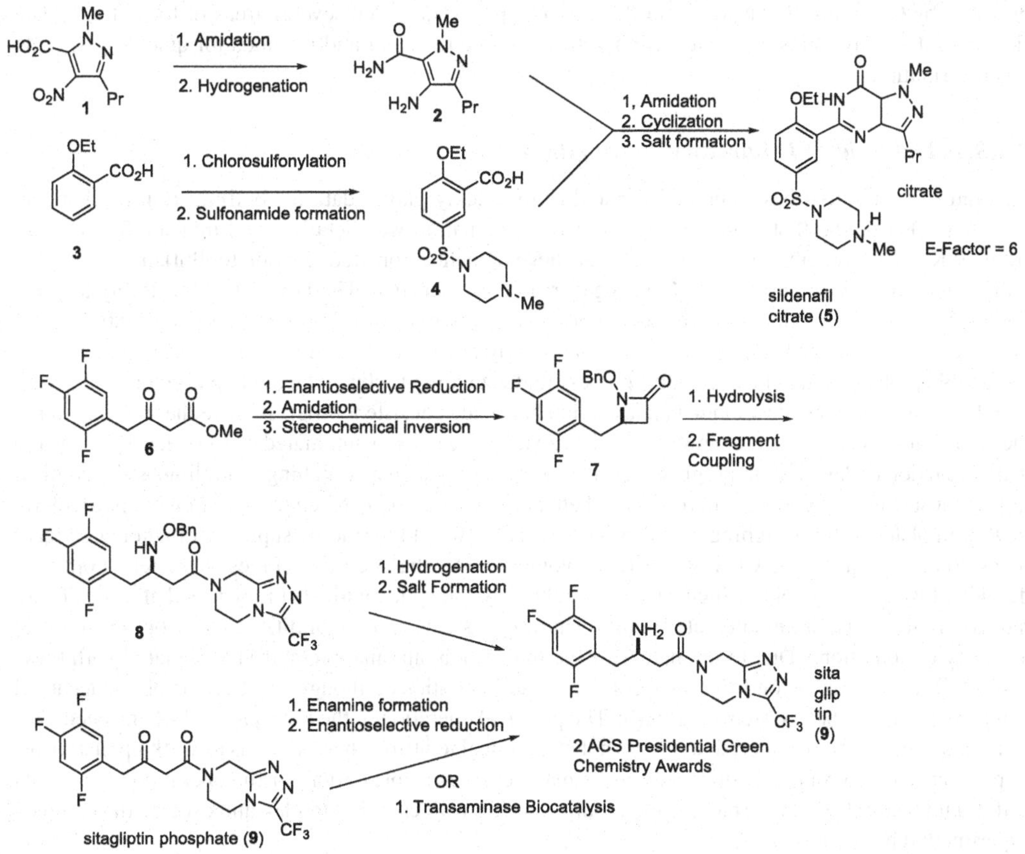

FIGURE 7.4 Synthetic schemes of sildenafil and sitagliptin.

The initial process chemistry introduced required chirality via a β-keto-ester reduction strategy, but then required the use of stereochemical inversion which results in poor AE. The second generation strategy relied on late stage introduction of chirality via a rhodium catalyzed asymmetric reduction. This much improved synthesis was awarded the ACS Presidential Green Chemistry Challenge Award. Chemists and engineers at Merck, however, were not satisfied and set to work to improve the process even further. Utilizing the emerging opportunities in biocatalysis, chemists at Merck partnered with Codexis to develop a bespoke transaminase enzyme which eliminated the need for the enantioselective reduction. So impressive was the result, that this third generation synthesis was also awarded the ACS Presidential Green Chemistry Challenge Award in a subsequent year.

7.3.3 The Importance of Process Understanding

Over time, pharmaceutical manufacturers have sought to improve the quality of their products through increased process understanding. The FDA, through its quality by design initiative, is now expecting a much higher level of product and process understanding than in the past.[16] Both patients (via the FDA) and industry benefit from the institutionalization of higher levels of process understanding which will result in lower rates of product failures, the reduced need for the FDA to take punitive actions, and the increased regulatory barriers to companies who are not able to demonstrate a science-based rationale for product development and control. In addition to the use of process understanding for the purposes of product quality, process understanding is a critical component needed in order to improve process intensity irrespective of whether a chemistry-based, and/or equipment-based strategies are used. A reflection of the history of process design and understanding in the pharmaceutical industry has been provided by Caron and Thomson from Pfizer.[17] The paper identified several areas of focus for "a data rich laboratory environment" which align with modern equipment and methods for quickly gathering this information.

7.3.3.1 The Role of Laboratory Automation

Laboratory automation has improved the ability to quickly gather data for optimization of chemical reactions. One of the first generations of process automation was detailed by Emiabata-Smith et al. from GSK.[18] This system, referred to as DART (development automated reaction toolkit), had integrated HPLC sampling which allowed the profiling of reactions over time. The DART had the ability to carry out ten reactions simultaneously which generated large amounts of reaction data. Prior to introduction of DART, collection of this amount of data would only been performed in order to solve a particularly intractable problem and not as a general process understanding tool which could be used on every reaction. Laboratory process development automation has made consistent progress since the introduction of the DART and recently been reviewed.[19] As the capacity to carry out automated process development and gather reaction understanding progresses, other technologies such as weighing, sampling, and analytical testing must continue to evolve. In the case where parallel small scale reactions are planned, particularly in 96 well plates, solids weighing becomes a bottleneck. Two of the leading suppliers of automated reaction automation equipment, Chemspeed Technologies and Unchained Labs, (Freeslate system) both have developed weighing systems which can accurately dispense solids with accuracy less that 1 mg. These modern systems also have automated liquid handling systems and the ability to carry out reactions at a variety of conditions. Due to the nature of the integration, automation, and IT associated with these systems, their cost is beyond that of most academic institutions although most major pharmaceutical companies employ these systems regularly. The practical operation of the Freeslate and Chemspeed platforms also need to be considered, as it may not be practical to utilize these systems as walk-up platforms. In practice, a core group of trained lead-users may be a reasonable option for the operation of the units and should be used as an internal service group, working with chemists to plan and execute the complex experimental protocols.

In one relevant example, chemists from Merck conducted a reaction optimization screening on a 1536 plastic microwell plate. They were able to optimize the room temperature cross-coupling of an aryl bromide with a cyclic amine while screening six bases and 16 phosphines. While the reactions were quenched after a short period of time, the analysis of the reaction mixture took place over the next 52 hours, and the products were analyzed by UPLC/MS. This rapid reaction optimization provided up to 98% conversion to product and set the stage for further scale-up.

In recent ground-breaking study from Pfizer, a continuous chemistry approach was used to screen optimized reaction conditions for a Suzuki-Miyaura coupling (Figure 7.5).

In this example of collection of data to support process understanding, 12 phosphine ligands, eight bases, and four solvents were screened against a substrate library of seven quinolines and four indazoles.[20] Notable aspects of this approach include the material sparing aspects of the experimental setup whereby only about 100 mg of each substrate was needed to complete the study. The process flow included the pre-mixing of the reactants prior to injection into the solvent flow. In this case, the reactants were allowed to diffuse into the surrounding solvent, rather than apply a segmented flow approach. This diffusion was managed by dividing the continuous reaction output into 96 well plate prior to analysis. In this way, each individual reaction could be sampled multiple times and analyzed with respect to

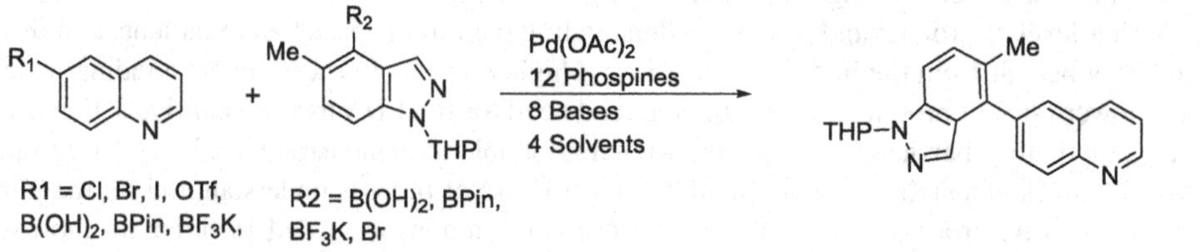

R1 = Cl, Br, I, OTf, $B(OH)_2$, BPin, BF_3K,

R2 = $B(OH)_2$, BPin, BF_3K, Br

$Pd(OAc)_2$
12 Phospines
8 Bases
4 Solvents

FIGURE 7.5 High throughput Suzuki-Miyaura coupling investigation and optimization in flow.

reference standards. The reactions could be run at a rate of 1500/day, which is a rate that challenges the ability to collect and visualize analytical data. To solve this challenge, the authors employed alternate sampling and injection processes using two UPLC/MS systems each running a 1.5 minute method. The work showed the practical potential of reaction optimization in continuous mode, along with the ability to screen reactions at a very rapid rate. Finally, this study successfully identified reaction conditions which were optimized across multiple substrates, an outcome which would have been impossible without such high-throughput reaction methodology.

7.3.3.2 Kinetic and Thermodynamic Data as Facilitators of Process Intensification

Process understanding of specific reaction data is important to understanding of scalability and safety of reactions, as well as using this information to understand the potential performance of chemistry across reactor sizes and types. An excellent background to safety and calorimetry is given by Dermaut in *Chemical Engineering in the Pharmaceutical Industry.*[21] Understanding reaction calorimetry and the relevant safety aspects are standard procedures when scaling into larger batch reactors or operating at increased concentrations. However, best practice for process intensification should include the collection of calorimetry data even when a change from batch to continuous chemistry is expected.[22] Collection of this type of data is standard practice for the chemical and pharmaceutical industry, however, laboratory reactors such as the Mettler Toledo EasyMax are capable of collecting this data and providing heat of reaction information.

Chemical reactions to produce pharmaceuticals have significant diversity in terms of reaction type and mechanism. In addition, many of the processes are scaled up very quickly to pilot plant reactors before full chemistry characterization can take place. Understanding of reaction kinetic data is an important mechanism for interpreting reaction scalability and interaction with mass transfer processes, and therefore chemists should strive for early collection of kinetic data whenever possible. Fortunately, modern equipment such as controlled reactors and in-situ FTIR are reducing the barrier to gathering such information. An excellent introduction to in-situ monitoring as an enabling technique for gathering of reaction progress data has been outlined by Donna Blackmond.[23] Blackmond has outlined that reaction progress kinetics can be conducted very simply if one has a method of in-situ analysis, as well as a curve-fitting software program. *In-situ* FTIR spectroscopy can be used to monitor the reaction concentration (or conversion) profile and converted to rate information via the integral method. The confidence of this data can be increased by using an orthogonal off-line analytical method such as HPCL or GC, which are routinely available during product development. In a follow-up paper, Blackmond outlined the use of both reaction calorimetry, as well as in-situ FTIR measurements to determine the mechanism of catalytic reactions, outlining how these two techniques can be used in a complementary fashion.[24]

As noted above, the use of *in-situ* monitoring techniques has become an important tool in understanding the profile of reactions which are being considered in the preparation of API. The benefit of in-situ monitoring is that it can be achieved with limited additional effort on the part of chemists by simply including the probe in the reaction vessel and having a software package capable of analyzing the output data. Figure 7.6 shows a typical reaction setup of a data-rich experiment which incorporates the potential for calorimetry and in-situ reaction monitoring. In-situ monitoring can be employed in a number of ways to facilitate process understanding and control in the context of process intensification.

In a continuous synthesis of a potent δ-opioid receptor, Ley used a ReactIR to analyse the reaction progression and time the addition.[25] The team had completed all the reactions in separate flow operations, however, when attempting to intensify the process by constructing an integrated flow system, the need arose to time the addition of the Burgess dehydrating reagent. ReactIR was used to monitor the appearance and dispersion of an intermediate and which provided the ability to both add the reagent with correct timing and concentration. In an example of the collection of kinetics in a flow mode, researchers at MIT[26] used ReactIR to measure the kinetics of a pyrrole formation under flow conditions by setting a gradual decrease in the resonance time in order to measure the change in conversion. By understanding the rate of decrease of the resonance time, the instantaneous resonance time could therefore be known and correlated to ReactIR data.

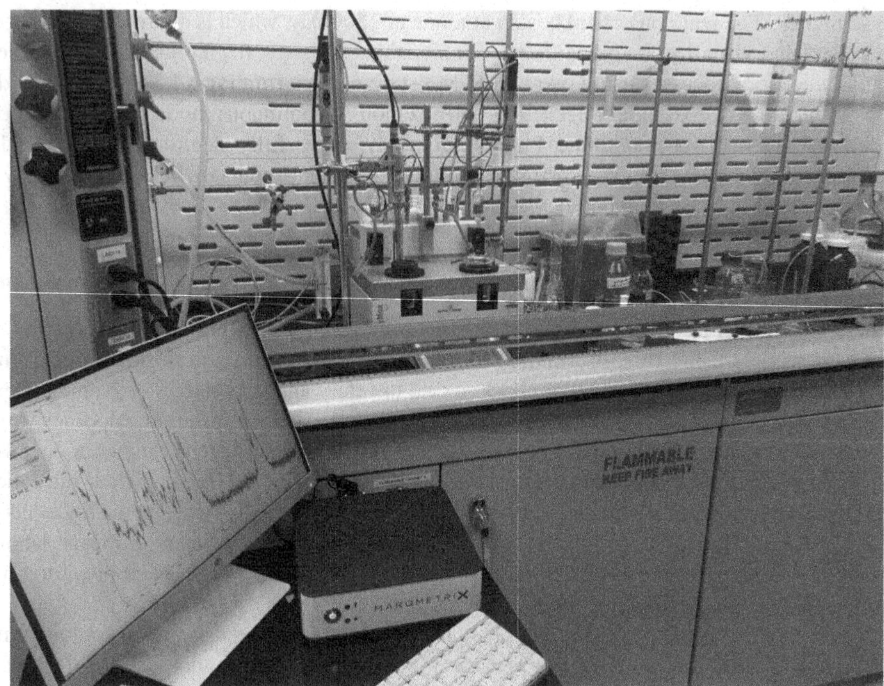

FIGURE 7.6 A data-rich experiment combining a reaction with in-situ spectroscopy and calorimetry.

The generation and control of API particles have attracted considerable study over recent years due to the importance of particle size and morphology to downstream formulation and ultimately pharmaceutical product performance. In an excellent example of data-rich experimentation in the field of API particle control, a batch crystallization of piroxicam was monitored using several in-situ techniques. Focused beam reflectance measurement (FBRM) was used to monitor particle counts of the crystallization nucleation process, and, subsequently, attenuated total reflectance-UV-vis spectrometry was used to monitor a supersaturated, seeded, cooled crystallisation.[27]

Process intensification techniques and knowledge generation continue to progress at a rapid pace, particularly with the focus on automation, data collection, and visualization techniques. Future trends in this area will be designed to maximize the amount of chemical experimentation conducted by the researcher as a function of time, while taking advantage of growing ability of chemists to design routes and experimental protocols by computer.

7.3.4 Equipment-Based Intensification Strategies for Continuous Chemistry

Scale-up of batch reactions from the laboratory to the pilot plant and the manufacturing site has been the historical mode of operation for the pharmaceutical industry. Many of the operations conducted on pilot or manufacturing scales are performed on well-engineered equipment which has its basis of design in laboratory glassware such as a round-bottom flask, reflux condenser, and Buchner funnel. The reason for this is likely due to an attempt to replicate laboratory result and quickly scale chemistry from the laboratory into equipment of similar operation in order to produce API for use in clinical trials. The advantage of this for the industry has been clear in the past, namely, that this type of equipment is largely multifunctional, meaning that a variety of chemistry can be run in a typical pilot plant reactor train, and the equipment can be turned over between products relatively easily, albeit with occasional extended cleaning times.

Chemists face severe constraints when scaling from the laboratory into multifunctional pilot plant equipment. These constraints restrict the available chemistry significantly and ultimately box the development chemist and engineer into a relatively small set of conditions out of the global set of potential

Reaction Type	Manufacturing Scale-Up Concern
Low temperature (<-30 °C)	Lack of equipment and cost
High temperature (>150 °C)	Lack of equipment and cost
Highly hazardous chemistry (e.g. nitrations)	Safety concerns
Organolithium chemistry	Need for cryogenic reactors
Photochemistry	Not practical due to limited light penetration into solvent
Highly exothermic chemistry	Reduced ability to control exotherm upon scale-up

FIGURE 7.7 Chemical transformations which are scale-challenged in the pharma industry.

methods to affect a chemical reaction. To mitigate against this, specialized batch reactors, such as cryogenic reactors, high temperature reactors, and pressure reactors have been developed to mitigate some of these deficiencies. Although many modern pharma pilot plants contain these types of specialized reactors, they may have only occasional use, and manufacturing plants are much less likely to invest in specialized technology. Hence, many types of specialized reactors, as well as chemistries, are often contracted to outside external contract manufacturing organizations (CMOs) who are able to provide services to the industry. Unfortunately, contracting specialized chemistry adds cost, and more importantly, significant time to an API campaign.

Figure 7.7 outlines some of the categories of chemical reactions which can be conducted on laboratory scale, but are generally discouraged in a multipurpose pilot plant facility (company dependent). Continuous flow chemistry has been widely used in the petroleum industry due to the large volumes, stable and well understood volume requirements, a cost constrained environment, and a liquid product output (i.e. pipe friendly). While the pharma industry has its own set of cost constraints, many of the volume and economic drivers present in the petroleum industry do not exist in the pharma industry, and therefore there has been little drive to implement continuous flow chemistry. Nevertheless, continuous chemistry offers scientific and engineering drivers (i.e. process intensification) which are common to both industries, such as control of product quality, ability to scale-out by building additional modules, ability to safely concentrate reactions, ability to conduct highly exothermic chemistry, and ability to access chemistries which are challenging to operate in batch (photochemistry, halogenation by molecular halides, nitrations, etc.). Traditionally, continuous flow chemistry has been the purview of chemical engineers in the petroleum industry, and therefore academic engineering curricula and research have developed to support the industry. However, both chemists and chemical engineers are now exploring the ability of flow chemistry to be used in the context of pharmaceutical production due to the scientific and regulatory opportunities outlined above.[28]

A refocus to continuous flow-based equipment both in the pharma process chemistry laboratory and in the pilot plant results in some significant differences when compared to batch processing. The performance of the pilot plant reactor as compared to a round-bottom flask drives a large amount of experimentation due to the constraints of the plant vessel including limitations on stirring, temperature ranges, addition times, and challenges in controlling exotherms. In contrast, a continuous flow device is simply a tube reactor in which heating or cooling elements are applied, and the pumps become the main actors as they control the stoichiometry or the reaction and rate of material production. In the case of microreactors, mixing occurs essentially instantaneously under laminar flow conditions. In the case where reactant mixing is determined to be critical, a static mixer can be used just prior to the reactor or inserted into the reactor itself. Continuous flow tube reactors present advantages in terms of material production and ease of scaling. For example a very typical laboratory flow rate through a 1 mm microreactor would be 1 mL/min, which at a 10% concentration of product would correspond to production of 144 g over the course of a day, which is a large amount for a laboratory and could be increased without any action by the scientist other than ensuring the feed tanks were sufficiently stocked. As reactor diameter increases beyond 1 mm id, the production of expected product increases significantly and will outstrip the ability of a general purpose laboratory to manage the waste, cost, and product output.

The following section presents a selection of reactors which are used to employ continuous processes in the API development or academic laboratory.

7.3.4.1 Microreactors

Microreactors are comprised of a simple tube through which reactants are pushed through via a pump. A selection of microreactors have previously been reviewed.[29] The simplest illustration of a flow chemistry setup is one or more HPLC pumps or syringe pumps which are connected to tubing which is temperature controlled by immersion in an oil bath (heating) or cooling bath (Figure 7.8). The tubing should be solvent and reagent compatible, and, as such, PTFE tubing presents an attractive material for use in the laboratory for screening experiments. These reactors have been used as screening reactors in a number of laboratories.[30] Coil microreactors are also available in a commercial form from Vapourtec (www.vapourtec.com), and these units are heated or cooled by airflow across the coils and include integrated diaphragm pumps which the company indicates will operate up to 10 barr. In an

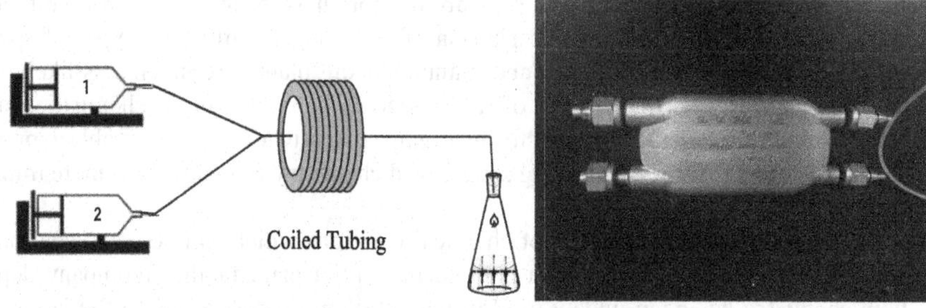

Schematic of a simple laboratory flow setup Chemtrix stainless-steel microreactor

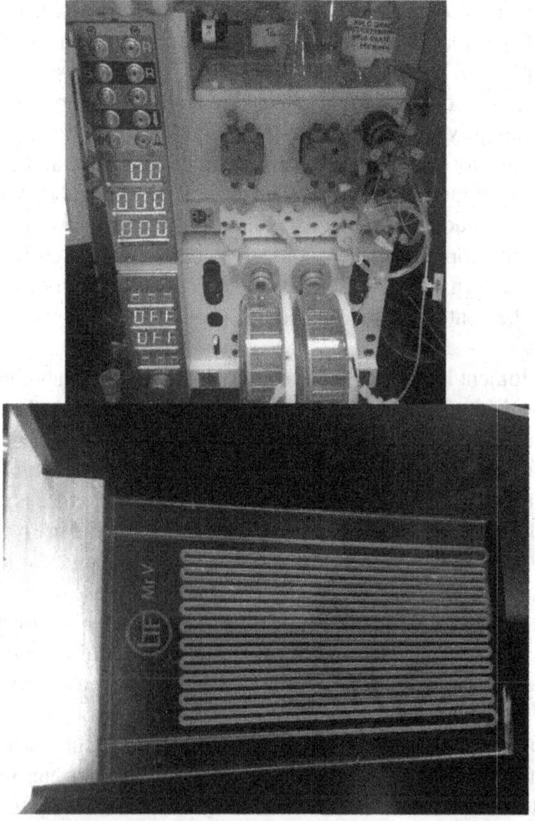

Vapourtec continuous reactor apparatus Little Things Factory (LTF) glass microreactor

FIGURE 7.8 Examples of microreactor systems.

example of selective and green chemistry, Jamison and co-workers conducted an N-monoalkylation of anlines with dimethyl carbonate at 250°C and 100 psi, conditions which would not have been possible in a typical batch reactor.[31]

Groups involved in materials engineering and chemistry continue to innovate on microreactors. In a recent publication of significance, a collaborative effort from MIT, Adamo and co-workers created bespoke coil reactors and used these reactors in a reconfigurable form to synthesize four different APIs.[32] This paper shows the significant potential for a reconfigurable system that has interchangeable and standardized components. For example, one of the APIs, diphenylhydramine hydrochloride, was prepared beginning with two starting materials that were delivered to the reactor without solvent and reacted at 180°C to and 1.7 MPa pressure to form a molten product within 15 minutes. Polyimide-based microreactors have been prepared by Kim et al., who have studied the mixing sensitive reduction of esters to aldehydes with DIBAL-H.[33] In addition, the polyimide-based flow system was also used to produce highly monodispersed PLGA particles via emulsification. Glass microfluidic reactors have found widespread applicability and have a very good breadth of operability in terms of chemistry variety, permitted temperature ranges, and ability to be operated above ambient pressure. Little Things Factory (www.ltf-gmbh.com) has developed a series of glass microreactors and the ability to fabricate microfluidic reactors based on customer specific requests. 3D printing techniques are now being used to develop bespoke microreactors from a wide variety of materials. This is particularly powerful methodology that allows the production of microreactors designed for a specific type of chemistry rather than assuming that every reactor must be able to accommodate a wide variety of chemistry.[34] In a particularly interesting commercial application, Chemtrix has produced 3D printed stainless steel reactors which are able to be externally heated or cooled (www.chemtrix.com). A growing number of laboratories are developing the capability to 3D print their own reactors. In one example, the Benaglia group from Milan created 3D printed microreactors from both polylactic acid (PLA) and high-impact polyethylene (HIPE). These reactors were used to conduct an enantioselective Henry reaction followed by a catalytic hydrogenation[35] (to afford products with good optical purity). These types of "homemade" 3D printed devices offer the opportunity for chemists and chemical engineers to work together to study the capabilities of different reactor configurations and their performance in chemical transformations.

7.3.4.2 Glass Plate Reactors for Process Intensification

Corning has developed a series of glass plate reactors (Advanced-Flow™ Reactors, www.corning.com/worldwide/en/innovation/corning-emerging-innovations/advanced-flow-reactors.html) with integrated heating and cooling capability which allow scalability to larger plates. The size and capacity of these reactors are only 60 mm × 72 mm and show the remarkable process intensification which can be achieved with continuous reactors when compared to a traditional chemical pilot or manufacturing plant. One of the smaller units, the *Low-Flow* system (Figure 7.9), accommodates flow rates from 2 mL/min–10 mL/min which translates to a potential capacity of 5 metric tons (MT) per annum. This reactor can be used for laboratory testing, and significant amounts of materials are needed for any systematic testing given the high flow rates of the system. The G1 glass plate reactors still retain a modest size of 155 mL × 125 mL while still being able to produce up to 50 MT per annum. It is worth considering that a full manufacturing building would normally be needed to produce this much material under traditional pharma production scenarios. Use of reactors of this size, along with robust chemical metering pumps are capable of producing large amounts of materials in a very small footprint, and therefore chemical material handling, both prior and subsequent to the reactor module, becomes one of the most critical aspects for production planning.

The Corning AF reactors have been used to produce diazomethane, a highly hazardous and explosive material which creates severe restrictions on its ability to be used at scale and even in a laboratory setting. Researchers at Corning and the University of Padova partnered to use both the *Low-Flow* and G1 versions of the reactors to produce diazomethane and subsequently methylate benzoic acid.[36] Initially, the reaction was optimized for solvent and conversion in the *Low-Flow* system, where a flow rate of 3.2 mL/min was found to be optimal. It was also reported that the reaction proceeded efficiently even

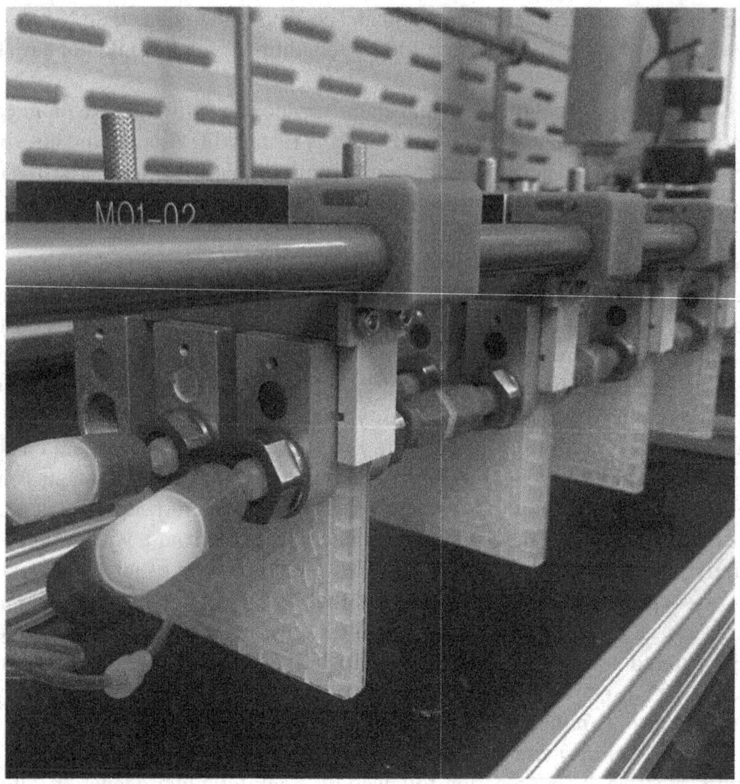

FIGURE 7.9 Corning low-flow glass plate reactor.

when a biphasic system was used due to the unique mixing capability of the heart-shaped glass channels. Upon direct scale-up to the G1 unit, and optimization, a quantitative yield of methyl benzoate was obtained at a resonance time of 28 seconds and a flow rate of 52.8 mL/min.

In another example of chemistry which can be carried out more conveniently in flow than in batch, the Corning *Low-Flow* reactor was used in the ozonolysis reaction of quinolines to form pyridine-dicarbolycic acids.[37] In this example, an ozone generator was positioned as a part of the system and gas flow was controlled by a mass-flow meter into a *Low-Flow* reactor, and excess ozone was diverted to waste. The quinoline was introduced into the reactor which contained eight low-flow plates (4.6 mL volume) and upon workup with H_2O_2, afforded a 73% yield of the desired dicarboxylic acid.

7.3.4.3 Spinning Disk Reactors

A spinning disk reactor (SDR) takes advantage of high rates of mass transfer, as well as extremely rapid micromixing times (0.01s–0.1s), which are produced as a result of the reactor disk spin rate which approaches 4500 rpm.[38] The reaction liquid is moved to the outside of the disk as a thin film and because of this, approaches the angular velocity of the disk. While a standard SDR reactor has a flat disk, other modifications have been made to facilitate catalytic or biocatalytic reactions. The SDRs (Figure 7.10) have exceptional mass transfer capabilities and perform very well where these processes dominate, including gas-liquid-solid-liquid and biphasic reactions. The reactors have found a number of uses including small molecule synthesis, polymer synthesis, and nanoparticle formation, and unlike microreactors, can accommodate the introduction or formation of particulates.[39]

The SDR has found several applications in small molecule synthesis. In one of the first applications applied to pharmaceuticals, researchers at SmithKline Beacham used the SDR to improve and optimize a biphasic Darzans reaction.[40] The same researchers identified that the SDR could be used to control

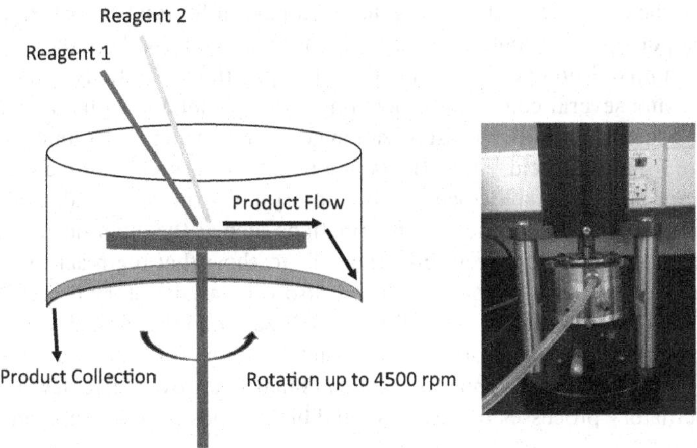

FIGURE 7.10 Basic schematic and photo of a lab SDR.

particle size in a crystallization by coating the spinning disk with PTFE.[40] In another example aimed at pharmaceutical manufacture, Gupton and co-workers took advantage of the mass transfer capabilities of the SDR in their synthesis of nevirapine by reacting a 3-amino pyridine with a suspension of sodium hydride. The deprotonated amine was then allowed to react with an ester to afford the transamination product, nevirapine.[41] The opportunities for this reactor remain open to investigation to increase both the scientific understanding and the practical application of such reactors.

7.3.4.4 Oscillatory Flow Reactor

The oscillatory flow reactor (OFR) offers a unique opportunity for process intensification based on a modification of a typical tube reactor. Unlike reactors with spinning parts or high flow rates, the tube-based apparatus creates mixing via use of a pump which creates oscillation within the reaction mixture. Because of this, a high rate of flow is not required to ensure mass transfer, material residence time can be significantly increased while still maintaining a continuous flow through the unit (Figure 7.11). The characteristics of the unit make it attractive for intensification of processes which may require longer resonance times (i.e. slower rates of reaction) and have solid-liquid transport requirements which may be challenging to operate in a typical tube type reactor. The design of the baffle, and baffle spacing, as well as other reactor system characteristics affect the performance of the reactor and can be optimized with respect to the application. An excellent review of parameters has been previously published.[42]

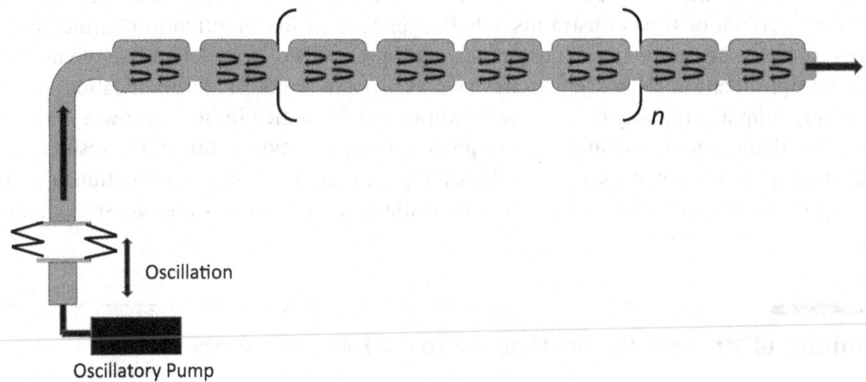

FIGURE 7.11 Diagram of an oscillatory flow reactor.

In their review of the OFR, researchers from the University of Strathclyde describe the capabilities with respect to the potential for continuous crystallization and outline how these reactors compare to mixed-suspension mixed-product removal (MSMPR) operations. Strathclyde has been a leader in the study of OFRs, and several compounds including paracetamol and *l*-glutamic acid (LGA) have been studied for producing controlled crystallization conditions using OFRs and similar reactor systems. In the case of *l*-glutamic acid,[43] the effects of a number of critical parameters such as mixing, seeding, temperature on meta-stable zone width, and crystal form were evaluated. The OFR type reactors have also been used for chemical transformations such as the biphasic alkylation reaction of phenylacetonitrile which was extensively investigated[44] to show that the reactors assisted in facilitating phase transfer conditions. Ni and co-workers also used a laboratory-based OFR to acetylate salicylic acid and subsequently conduct a cooling crystallization in the same device.[45] These reactors are effective as bioreactors as demonstrated in a batch mode by Vicente and co-workers,[46] where γ-decalactone was produced by *Yarrowia lipolytica*. Finally, an overall review of the merits and applications of oscillatory processes in chemistry and biology has been recently authored by Jensen and Abolhasani at MIT.[47]

7.3.4.5 Outlook for Process Intensification Strategies

The current state of process intensification can be arguably described as one where chemists and engineers undertake largely separate activities for intensification of processes. This occurs both in academics and industry and is therefore potentially self-affirming and self-replicating even with the most well intentioned teams, where chemists may lead a chemistry-based approach and, if time allows, alternative reactor-based intensification strategies may be employed. From many of the examples in Sections 7.3.4.2 through 7.3.4.5 (novel reactor types), the drivers of reports have been chemical engineers who have conducted impressive studies to characterize and use these systems, even coupling them with impressive PAT techniques. Despite this, the use of these types of reactors for pharmaceutical-based API synthetic processes have been relatively limited given their now well characterized abilities. Many of the uses for these reactors may currently lie outside the API synthesis space where they are employed in specialized circumstances, however, the opportunity exists for additional implementation in the production of pharmaceuticals.

The opportunity for organic chemists, analytical chemists, chemical engineers, and other engineering specialties to change overall pharmaceutical API process performance is significant. Academic institutions can play an important role by continuing to innovate on the variety of reactor types developed and finding innovative ways to reduce the cost of production. This has largely now happened with continuous chemistry, where many chemists now feel comfortable to convert their processes from batch to flow and many suppliers of simplified and user friendly microreactors exist. Despite the advantages, many companies have limited flow API manufacturing capabilities at scale, and despite the interest from the FDA, there are still relatively few registered continuous API synthetic steps. The reasons for this may be historical comfort with the round-bottom flask-glass-lined reactor scenario, organizational barriers, or time constraints. Challenges remain for adoption of continuous chemistry as a first intent strategy due to the current standard practices of parallel and automated reaction screening and optimization. However, as we have seen from some of the publications mentioned above, high throughput screening of reaction conditions and kinetics in flow is now a reality. When a cross-functional and intentional approach to process intensification is taken, the results are likely to be synergistic and far exceed the efforts of individual functions. In the next section, a number of examples of process intensification will be presented and several of the most impressive examples are from these collaborative efforts.

7.4 Examples of Process Intensification in API Manufacture

There are a number of examples of process intensification in the literature and some have been outlined above. In this section, additional examples of process intensification will be evaluated in more detail.

7.4.1 Process Intensification in a Hydrogenation of an API Intermediate

Ethyl 3-piperidine carboxylic acid (13) is derived from ethyl nicotinate (**11**) and is a potential intermediate used for the synthesis of (*R*)-tiagibine (**10**) which is marketed as an anti-convulsant (Figure 7.12). A collaborative group from the University of Cambridge, Takeda, and Pfizer worked together to develop technology and a process to address complexities in the synthesis of this compound.[48] Initially, the authors attempted to repeat the existing partial hydrogenation process (preparation of **12**) which was run in a small batch reactor, but required 100 psi of pressure and gave 85% conversion, but with a 7:1 mixture of products **12** and **13**, respectively. In order to increase the production rate a HEL FlowCAT reactor was evaluated which was potentially of the scale required to enable the throughput that the team was seeking. One of the important aspects of this paper is the description and supporting data which describe the detail of packing the catalyst column, an aspect that is sometimes omitted from studies where teams do not have the experience or equipment to pack their own columns. The authors were able to determine the optimal particle size (01. mm–0.8 mm) for packing in this particular setup and, in addition, demonstrated the ability to use smaller particle size in combination with glass beads, an aspect that might be important if commercial catalysts are of limited particle size options. Subsequently, the reaction was optimized to produce >80% conversion to 12 in a continuous process using a 5% Pd/Al_2O_3 catalyst with a controlled flow of hydrogen. Notably, in this reaction, the use of Pd/C, a widely used catalyst/support system, had limited ability to handle concentrations above 0.5 M. In one run, which proceeded for 22.5 hours, an 84:15 ratio of **12:13** was obtained, and the product could be isolated in 73% yield after separation from **13** by extraction.

The team then turned their attention to the complete hydrogenation of ethyl-nicotinate, which was previously conducted under conditions which would be challenging upon scale-up. Again, the superiority of Pd/Al_2O_3 was established in this particular reaction and the H-Cube reactor setup, which was used as a small scale screening apparatus. When the reaction was scaled to the HEL FlowCAT as a trickle-bed hydrogenation reactor, the desired product, **13**, was obtained with a throughput approaching 2 kg/day. The significance of the paper is due to its focus on the detail of column packing, careful evaluation of flow conditions, and demonstration of simple demonstrable scalability of continuous processes, an aspect which is often missing from traditional flow chemistry publications.

7.4.2 Process Intensification via Telescoping Reactions and Careful Measurements of Unit Operations

In Table 7.1 (Section 7.2.2), a list of unit operations were specified for potential use in evaluating the impact of process intensification activities. A team from Dow Chemical[49] used a careful analysis of unit operations to demonstrate required improvement in a chemical process over a short period of time (Figure 7.13). The process improvement required was a 50% decrease in cost to be achieved within 2 months. Given the constricted time allowed for improvements, the team focused on telescoping and removing unit operations rather than fundamentally changing the synthesis. The Dow team took a three prong approach to the process intensification activities which can serve as an example for this type of challenge: (i) telescope two of the reactions, which will remove some of the associated workup unit

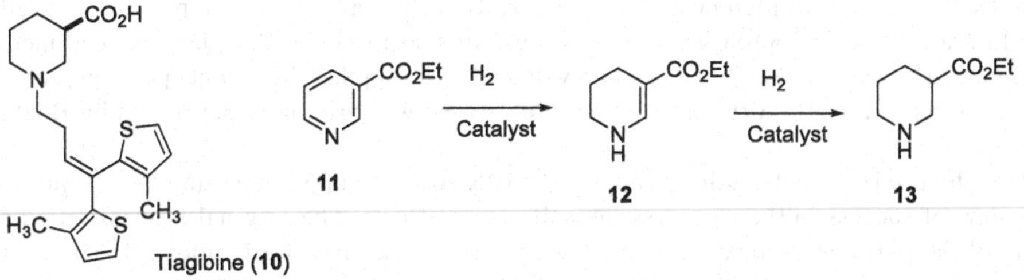

FIGURE 7.12 Pfizer's synthesis of ethyl piperidine-3-carboxylic acid.

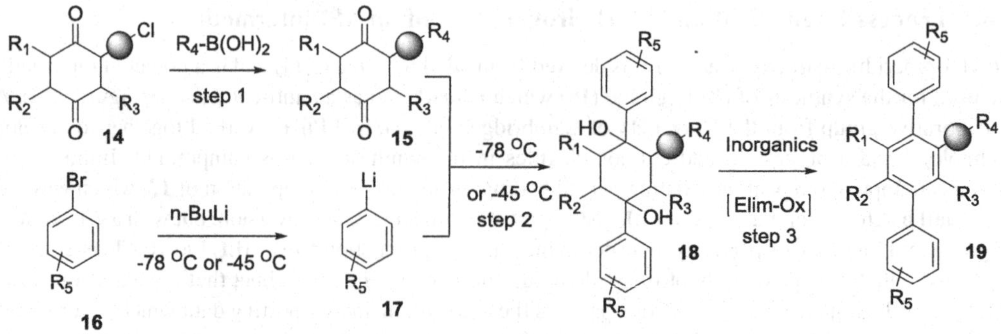

Metric	Original	Improved
Number of Isolation	2	1
Unit Operations	49	24
% Yield	36	48
Cycle Time	177	116
Cost	-	>50% reduction

FIGURE 7.13 Dow Chemical process intensification and metrics.

operations; (ii) replace numerous labor and material inefficient purification processes with crystallizations; and (iii) modify the cryogenic conditions from −78°C to a temperature which was more amenable to scale-up. The step 1 Suzuki coupling reaction yield was improved from 56% to 63% by improving the starting material quality and introducing a crystallization for Diketone **15** which eliminated multiple triturations and silica filtrations. The team was also able to demonstrate the feasibility of the lithium-halogen exchange at −45°C which facilitates scale-up. Finally, the group was able to telescope (remove a workup) stages 2 and 3 and directly crystallize Triphenyl **19** from the reaction mixture which successfully eliminated nine triturations and two silica gel filtrations.

The authors then undertook a systematic evaluation of materials, labor, and waste, as well as an analysis of unit operations, yield, and cycle times (Figure 7.13). This example of process intensification was chosen as excellent reference for a before-after analysis of processes in order to demonstrate overall improvement in a series of transformations where the chemistry was not changed, but significant waste and cost were removed.

7.4.3 Cost Reduction and Process Intensification of a Critical Medicine for the Treatment of AIDS

The cost of medicines continue to be a challenge for pharmaceutical innovators and generic firms, particularly with respect to those medicines associated with diseases which occur in nations with developing economies. In particular, drugs for the treatment of AIDS are generally complex molecules and have been introduced to the market with relatively short development timelines. As such, these molecules often have high costs which can restrict their availability to patients in need. The potential for a systematic approach (Figure 7.14) towards cost reduction on these critical medicines was recognized by Gupton, McQuade, and co-workers[50] who applied these concepts to process intensification efforts to the HIV drug nevirapine, (**20**), which was originally developed by Boehringer Ingelheim.

The team focused on a metrics driven approach using cost, unit operations, and *PMI* (Equation 7.4) as indicators of success in their process intensification efforts. The original process relied on the coupling of the pyridine-carboxylic acid **21** with CAPIC (**22**), to afford amide **23**. The cyclopropylamino moiety was introduced to afford CYCLOR (**26**) and, subsequently, cyclization produced neveripine (**20**). Overall, the original process demonstrated good efficiency with a 58% overall

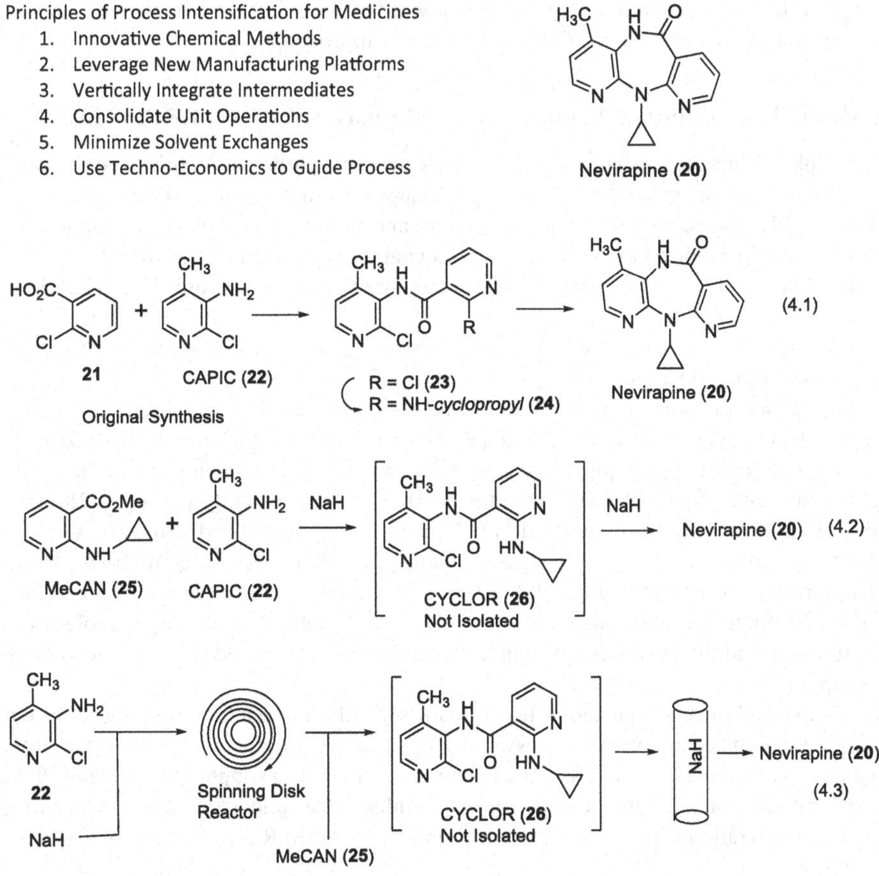

FIGURE 7.14 Gupton's synthesis of nevirapine.

yield, 15 unit operations, and a PMI of 67. The improved approach relied on a transamination of the 2-cyclopropylamino pyridine (MeCAN, **25**) with the 3-amino pyridine (CAPIC, **22**). The Gupton-McQuade group initially embarked on new syntheses of both of these materials in order to reduce costs. MeCAN (**25**) was synthesized in an overall yield of 86% and a PMI of 12 by a series of four transformations with only one isolated intermediate, beginning from 2-chloro-3-cyano-pyridine. More importantly, CAPIC (**22**), a 1,2,3 trisubstituted pyridine, was derived from the commodity chemicals acetone and malononitrie. The trisubstituted pyridine core was built up from these materials, using a dimethyl formamide equivalent, followed by cyclization to complete the pyridine ring preparation. Subsequently, several high-yielding transformations produced the desired CAPIC intermediate in an excellent 80% overall yield with a PMI of 18. To affect the transamination of **25** and **22**, both lithium hexamethyldisilazide (LiHMDS) and NaH were successful, with the latter being selected due to its atom economy. In the reaction, approximately two equivalents of NaH in diglyme at 65°C were used to produce the initial amide product CYCLOR (**26**), which was not isolated, but treated with another two equivalents of NaH in diglyme at 115 to produce nevirapine (**20**) in a single pot process. The authors were also able to demonstrate the conversion of this batch route into a continuous process. In the first step, CAPIC (**22**) was deprotonated with NaH with facilitation from a spinning disk reactor and transferred to a holding tank containing MeCAN (**25**), which was allowed to react to produced CYCLOR (**26**). This reaction is of particular note because it demonstrates the ability of the spinning disk reactor to process slurries such as NaH, without which this example of continuous chemistry may not have been achieved. The final cyclization to nevirapine was achieved by passing CYCLOR through a mixed packed bed of glass beads and NaH at 165°C. Overall, the modified process achieved a yield of 91%, four unit operations, and a PMI of 11, demonstrating the benefits of the Gupton-McQuade approach.

7.4.4 A Multikilo Continuous Manufacture of Prexasertib to cGMP Standards

Previous examples in this section have outlined a single step or multiple steps conducted in a continuous manner. There are also emerging methods and techniques for other important unit operations such as workups, solvent exchanges, crystallizations, filtrations, and drying. A multifunctional team of scientists from Eli Lilly recently reported the multifaceted and challenging production of over 24 kg of the chemotherapeutic kinase inhibitor prexasertib[41] by a fully continuous route (Figure 7.15). In addition to the standard elements of reaction engineering, the team also developed two continuous solvent exchanges and, more importantly, a fully automated MPMPR crystallization process along with subsequent filtration, washing, and drying operations.

The initial reaction of "Keto-nitrile **27**" to produce pyrazole **28** involved the use of hydrazine in a mixture of solvents, which in batch mode required a large excess of hazardous hydrazine. For this reaction, a bespoke stainless steel plug-flow reactor (tube reactor) was employed and the reaction run at higher pressure and employed a GC oven for heating and successfully produced **28** at a rate of >3.1 kg/day. As the reaction was conducted in flow, there was minimal hydrazine and starting material at use at any singe time point. This again demonstrates the ability of continuous chemistry to enable certain reactions which are difficult to carry out in batch owing to safety concerns. Following the reaction, a continuous extraction process was employed to purify the crude pyrazole and remove residual hydrazine, and then a solvent exchange to DMSO was conducted (in continuous mode) on a 20 L rotoevaporator.

Step 2 was a straightforward nucleophilic aromatic substitution reaction of chloride **29** with pyrazole **28**, which took place at normal processing temperatures to produce the penultimate intermediate **30**, at a rate of 2.8 kg/day. In this case, the Lilly team employed a simple PFR made of PFA tubing in order to limit the potential for degradation of stainless steel under the reaction conditions. At this point, a crystallization was needed to control quality. A MSSPR process employing two vessels

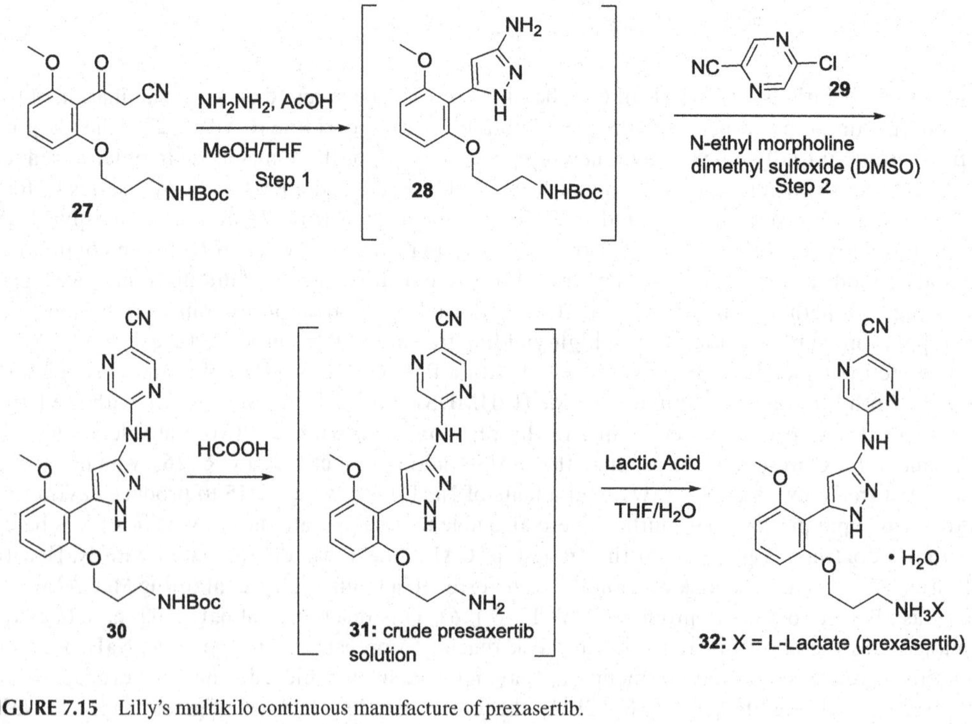

FIGURE 7.15 Lilly's multikilo continuous manufacture of prexasertib.

was used to crystallize the product upon addition of methanol. Subsequent to this, the slurries were transferred into two parallel filters which were automated so that while one filter was accepting a suspension of **30**, the other filter was conducing filtration, washing, drying, and redissolving actions. Outlined in detail in the *Science* publication, this series of actions is the result of an impressive level of planning and process control, which can enable intermediate purification in a longer series of unit operations, a critical enabler for control of API quality.

In step 3 of the process, the protecting group was removed from penultimate intermediate **30** by the use of another PFR created from simple PFA tubing, where the purity was facilitated by the removal of by-product gases via introduction of a nitrogen carrier gas to the formic acid-substrate mixture. Subsequent to the reaction, another solvent exchange operation removed the formic acid and lactic acid was added in excess, and tetrahydrofuran (THF) used as a diluent, prior to a standard batch type controlled crystallization. The significance of this paper is the discussion and demonstration of concepts of small-volume continuous manufacturing (SVC), which articulates the benefits of the use of continuous processing in the production of small scale pharmaceutical products. In this demonstration, the Lilly team integrated several reactions, parallel crystallization operations, and a final batch crystallization in an impressive synthesis of engineering and chemistry technologies.

7.5 The Outlook for Process Intensification of APIs

As this chapter has endeavored to illustrate, process intensification is a rapidly growing area of interest for both industry and academics, and a number of well-respected journals routinely publish work in the process intensification, continuous chemistry, and reactor technology areas of study. With more academic groups employing flow chemistry, reactor development, and associated analytical techniques, additional expertise is being introduced to industry-based challenges. An impressive example of this is the MIT-based Pharmacy on Demand platform,[32] where a series of four APIs were produced in a refrigerator-sized unit. These concepts have now been extended at MIT where a formulation module has now been added.[51] The pharmaceutical industry has recognized the potential value of process intensification both in terms of cost reduction and product quality, and many companies now have groups dedicated to the implementation of continuous flow chemistry. As the Lilly and MIT groups have demonstrated, the process intensification value stream does not stop at the end of a reaction, but continues on to downstream operations which also have a fundamental role in ensuring product quality.

There are significant opportunities for innovation in the area of process intensification as applied to small molecules. A key to achieving growth in the field is the partnership between chemistry, engineering, process control, and analytical functions. While this chapter has outlined several examples of flow chemistry conducted in a tube-based PFR, step changes in process intensification that the industry and FDA desire can only be attained through a team-based approach, with product quality as its driving force. Seven key areas for future focus in process intensification are listed below:

1. Advanced process control for automation
2. Integrated process analytical technologies including real-time release of products
3. Data collection and visualization techniques
4. Diversification of reactor type from plug-flow to more complex reactors
5. Integration of unit operations
6. Continued exploration of chemistry not suitable for traditional batch operations
7. Systematic approach to process intensification and green chemistry metrics

Taken as a whole, these seven areas of focus will drive overall improvements in process intensification within the pharmaceutical industry. Those academic and industrial groups dedicated to specific subspecialties of process intensification will increasingly need to collaborate in order to realize the potential for significant improvements API processes.

REFERENCES

1. Kim, Y. H., Park, L. K., Yiacoumi, S. & Tsouris, C. Modular chemical process intensification: A review. *Annu. Rev. Chem. Biomol. Eng.* **8**, 359–380 (2017).
2. Dautzenberg, F. & Mukherjee, M. Process intensification using multifunctional reactors. *Chem. Eng. Sci.* **56**, 251–267 (2001).
3. Hinz, D. C. Process analytical technologies in the pharmaceutical industry: The FDA's PAT initiative. *Anal. Bioanal. Chem.* **384**, 1036–1042 (2006).
4. Butters, M. et al. Critical assessment of pharmaceutical processes a rationale for changing the synthetic route. *Chem. Rev.* (2006). doi:10.1021/CR050982W.
5. Trost, B. M. The atom economy-a search for synthetic efficiency. *Source Sci. New Ser. Niqrot Zurim* **254**, 1471–1477 (1991).
6. Curzons, A. D., Mortimer, D. N., Constable, D. J. C. & Cunningham, V. L. So you think your process is green, how do you know? —Using principles of sustainability to determine what is green—a corporate perspective. *Green Chem.* **3**, 1–6 (2001).
7. Sheldon, R. A. The E factor: Fifteen years on. *Green Chem.* **9**, 1273 (2007).
8. Jimenez-Gonzalez, C., Ponder, C. S., Broxterman, Q. B. & Manley Glaxosmithkline, J. B. Using the right green yardstick: Why process mass intensity is used in the pharmaceutical industry to drive more sustainable processes. *Process Res. Dev.* **15**, 912–917 (2011).
9. Kuzemko, M. A., Van Arnum, S. D., & Niemczyk, H. J. A green chemistry comparative analysis of the syntheses of (E)-4-Cyclobutyl-2-[2-(3-nitrophenyl)ethenyl] Thiazole, Ro 24–5904. *Org. Process Res. Dev.* (2007). doi:10.1021/OP700008K.
10. Jimenez-Gonzalez, Concepcion, Constable, David. J. *Green Chemistry and Engineering: A Practical Design Approach* (John Wiley & Sons, Ltd., Hoboken, NJ, 2011).
11. Ryan, T. P. Process capability. In *Statistical Methods for Quality Improvement* (John Wiley & Sons, Ltd., Hoboken, NJ, 2011). doi:10.1002/9781118058114.
12. Anastas, P. & Eghbali, N. Green chemistry: Principles and practice. *Chem. Soc. Rev.* **39**, 301–312 (2010).
13. Tucker, J. L. Green chemistry, a pharmaceutical perspective. *Org. Process Res. Dev.* (2006). doi:10.1021/OP050227K.
14. Alfonsi, K. et al. Green chemistry tools to influence a medicinal chemistry and research chemistry based organisation. *Green Chem.* **10**, 31–36 (2008).
15. Dunn, P. J., Galvin, S. & Hettenbach, K. The development of an environmentally benign synthesis of sildenafil citrate (Viagra™) and its assessment by green chemistry metrics. *Green Chem.* **6**, 43–48 (2004).
16. Lawrence, X. Y. Pharmaceutical quality by design: Product and process development, understanding, and control. *Pharm. Res.* **25**, 781–791 (2008).
17. Caron, S. & Thomson, N. M. Pharmaceutical process chemistry: Evolution of a contemporary data-rich laboratory environment. *J. Org. Chem.* **80**, 2943–2958 (2015).
18. Emiabata-Smith, D. F., Crookes, D. L. & Owen, M. R. A practical approach to accelerated process screening and optimisation. *Org. Process Res. Dev.* (1999). doi:10.1021/OP990016D.
19. Chen, Q. & Grossmann, I. E. Recent developments and challenges in optimization-based process synthesis. *Annu. Rev. Chem. Biomol. Eng.* **8**, 249–283 (2017).
20. Perera, D. et al. A platform for automated nanomole-scale reaction screening and micromole-scale synthesis in flow. *Science* **359**, 429–434 (2018).
21. Dermaut, W. Process safety and reaction hazard assessment. In *Chemical Engineering in the Pharmaceutical Industry* (ed. D. J. am Ende) pp. 155–182 (John Wiley & Sons, Ltd., 2011).
22. Zhang, X., Stefanick, S. & Villani, F. J. Application of microreactor technology in process development. *Org. Process Res. Dev.* (2004). doi:10.1021/OP034193X.
23. Blackmond, D. G. Reaction progress kinetic analysis: A powerful methodology for mechanistic studies of complex catalytic reactions. *Angew. Chemie Int. Ed.* **44**, 4302–4320 (2005).
24. Blackmond, D. G. Kinetic profiling of catalytic organic reactions as a mechanistic tool. *J. Am. Chem. Soc.* **137**, 10852–10866 (2015).
25. Qian, Z., Baxendale, I. R. & Ley, S. V. A continuous flow process using a sequence of microreactors with in-line IR analysis for the preparation of N, N-Diethyl-4-(3-fluorophenylpiperidin-4-ylidenemethyl)benzamide as a potent and highly selective δ-Opioid receptor agonist. *Chem. A Eur. J.* **16**, 12342–12348 (2010).

26. Moore, J. S. & Jensen, K. F. "Batch" kinetics in flow: Online IR analysis and continuous control. *Angew. Chemie Int. Ed.* **53**, 470–473 (2014).
27. Hansen, T. B., Simone, E., Nagy, Z. & Qu, H. Process analytical tools to control polymorphism and particle size in batch crystallization processes. *Org. Process Res. Dev.* **21**, 855–865 (2017).
28. Baumann, M. & Baxendale, I. R. The synthesis of active pharmaceutical ingredients (APIs) using continuous flow chemistry. *Beilstein J. Org. Chem.* **11**, 1194–1219 (2015).
29. Jensen, K. F. Flow chemistry-microreaction technology comes of age. *AIChE J.* **63**, 858–869 (2017).
30. McQuade, D. T. & Seeberger, P. H. Applying flow chemistry: Methods, materials, and multistep synthesis. *J. Org. Chem.* **78**, 6384–6389 (2013).
31. Seo, H. et al. Selective N-monomethylation of primary anilines with dimethyl carbonate in continuous flow. *Tetrahedron* (2017). doi:10.1016/J.TET.2017.11.068.
32. Adamo, A. et al. On-demand continuous-flow production of pharmaceuticals in a compact, reconfigurable system. *Science* **352**, 61–67 (2016).
33. Min, K.-I., Lee, H.-J. & Kim, D.-P. Three-dimensional flash flow microreactor for scale-up production of monodisperse PEG–PLGA nanoparticles. *Lab Chip* **14**, 3987–3992 (2014).
34. Capel, A. J. et al. Design and additive manufacture for flow chemistry. *Lab Chip* **13**, 4583 (2013).
35. Rossi, S., Porta, R., Brenna, D., Puglisi, A. & Benaglia, M. Stereoselective catalytic synthesis of active pharmaceutical ingredients in homemade 3D-printed mesoreactors. *Angew. Chemie* **129**, 4354–4358 (2017).
36. Rossi, E., Woehl, P. & Maggini, M. Scalable in situ diazomethane generation in continuous-flow reactors. *Org. Process Res. Dev.* **16**, 1146–1149 (2012).
37. Lee, K., Lin, H. & Jensen, K. F. Ozonolysis of quinoline and quinoline derivatives in a Corning low flow reactor. *React. Chem. Eng.* **2**, 696–702 (2017).
38. Visscher, F., van der Schaaf, J., Nijhuis, T. A. & Schouten, J. C. Rotating reactors – A review. *Chem. Eng. Res. Des.* **91**, 1923–1940 (2013).
39. Pask, S. D., Nuyken, O. & Cai, Z. The spinning disk reactor: An example of a process intensification technology for polymers and particles. *Polym. Chem.* **3**, 2698 (2012).
40. Oxley, P., Brechtelsbauer, C., Ricard, F., Lewis, N. & Ramshaw, C. Evaluation of spinning disk reactor technology for the manufacture of pharmaceuticals. *Ind. Eng. Chem. Res.* (2000). doi:10.1021/IE990869U.
41. Verghese, J. et al. Increasing global access to the high-volume HIV drug nevirapine through process intensification. *Green Chem.* **19**, 2986–2991 (2017).
42. McGlone, T. et al. Oscillatory flow reactors (OFRs) for continuous manufacturing and crystallization. *Org. Process Res. Dev.* **19**, 1186–1202 (2015).
43. Ni, X. & Liao, A. Effects of mixing, seeding, material of baffles and final temperature on solution crystallization of l-glutamic acid in an oscillatory baffled crystallizer. *Chem. Eng. J.* **156**, 226–233 (2010).
44. Wilson, B., Sherrington, D. C. & Ni, X. Butylation of phenylacetonitrile in an oscillatory baffled reactor. *Ind. Eng. Chem. Res.* (2005). doi:10.1021/IE048855Y.
45. Ricardo, C. & Xiongwei, N. Evaluation and establishment of a cleaning protocol for the production of vanisal sodium and aspirin using a continuous oscillatory baffled reactor. *Org. Process Res. Dev.* **13**, 1080–1087 (2009).
46. Carr, R. et al. Directed evolution of an amine oxidase for the preparative deracemisation of cyclic secondary amines. *ChemBioChem* **6**, 637–639 (2005).
47. Abolhasani, M. & Jensen, K. F. Oscillatory multiphase flow strategy for chemistry and biology. *Lab Chip* **16**, 2775–2784 (2016).
48. Ouchi, T., Battilocchio, C., Hawkins, J. M. & Ley, S. V. Process intensification for the continuous flow hydrogenation of ethyl nicotinate. *Org. Process Res. Dev.* **18**, 1560–1566 (2014).
49. Desai, A. A., Molitor, E. J. & Anderson, J. E. Process intensification via reaction telescoping and a preliminary cost model to rapidly establish value. *Org. Process Res. Dev.* **16**, 160–165 (2012).
50. Cole, K. P. et al. Kilogram-scale prexasertib monolactate monohydrate synthesis under continuous-flow CGMP conditions. *Science* **356**, 1144–1150 (2017).
51. Azad, M. A. et al. A compact, portable, re-configurable, and automated system for on-demand pharmaceutical tablet manufacturing. *Int. J. Pharm.* **539**, 157–164 (2018).

8

Biologic Drug Substance and Drug Product Manufacture

Ajit S. Narang, Mary E. Krause, Shelly Pizarro, and Joon Chong Yee

CONTENTS

8.1 Introduction

Biologic drugs include proteins, peptides, and nucleic acids used in prophylactic or therapeutic applications. The use of insulin for type 1 diabetes mellitus is perhaps one of the oldest uses of protein therapeutics. The modern repertoire of protein drugs also includes monoclonal antibodies (mAbs) and antibody drug conjugates (ADCs) among others. Polypeptides with more than 30 amino acids are typically defined as large molecules or biologics. Nucleic acid drugs include anti-sense oligonucleotides (ODNs), RNA interference (RNAi) technologies such as small interfering RNA (siRNA), plasmid DNA, and virus-based gene therapy approaches, such as the use of recombinant adenoviruses and adeno-associated viruses. Anti-sense ODNs and siRNAs can reduce aberrant protein production, while gene therapy strategies increase the production of exogenous or endogenous therapeutic proteins in the patient's somatic cells.

Common characteristics of biologic drugs include large molecular weight, polymeric nature, and hydrophilicity. These drugs also tend to be structurally complex and fluid, i.e. having a primary, secondary, and tertiary structure that are sensitive to the environment. These drugs are usually produced in a biologic system. For example, antibodies are typically produced in cell culture or animals. These drugs exhibit at least some extent of compositional variability, i.e. the presence of structural variants within sub-populations that do not lead to substantial loss of activity or increased safety risk.

Biologic drugs also present unique challenges in their manufacture and use. For example, proteins and peptides have physical and chemical instabilities that can be difficult to control. These products also tend to have high manufacturing cost, instability in biological fluids, and rapid metabolism. Due to their poor membrane diffusivity and instability in the acidic gastric environment, most biologic drugs are not bioavailable orally and need to be administered parenterally by intravenous (IV) or subcutaneous (SC) injection. Sterility, therefore, is a key requirement in the manufacture of biologic drugs. Other parenteral routes of administration, such as intranasal, ocular, or lung delivery by inhalation, are also very attractive in that they bypass the issues that lead to poor oral bioavailability.

This chapter will focus predominantly on the cell culture-based manufacturing process of a typical mAb as a drug substance (DS) and a drug product (DP). A typical mAb DP manufactured by contemporary state-of-the-art recombinant DNA technology is produced in four clearly distinguishable steps:

1. Production of recombinant DNA, transfection of host cells, cell selection by screening for expression, cell expansion and characterization, and creation of a master cell bank (MCB) of a single clone.
2. Antibody production by microbial or cell culture technologies, commonly known as upstream production.
3. Antibody purification, typically using a series of column chromatography and buffer exchange techniques, commonly known as downstream purification.
4. Drug product formulation and development, which include identification of a stable buffer and excipient composition and the finished drug product modality (such as a lyophilized or a ready-to-use (RTU) solution product, and the use of vials, prefilled syringes, or novel delivery devices).

This chapter will describe these aspects of antibody DS and DP manufacturing, including the analytical techniques and quality attributes of biologic therapeutics that are applicable across the various stages of their manufacture. In addition, characteristics, manufacturing, and use of other biologic drugs, such as nucleic acids, and the intermediate molecular weight compounds will be described briefly.

8.2 Protein and Peptide Structure

Most proteins and peptides are folded three-dimensional (3D) assemblies of one or more polymeric chains of amino acids. Their structure is commonly described in terms of different levels of hierarchal complexity, as follows:

1. *Primary structure*: The primary structure consists of a chain of amino acids covalently linked to each other through peptide bonds—between the primary amine of one amino acid and the carboxylate carbon of the other. Depending upon the number of amino acids linked together, the peptide chain can be a dipeptide, tripeptide, oligopeptide, or a polypeptide. Polypeptides larger than ~30 amino acids are generally referred to as proteins.

   Twenty natural amino acids constitute the primary units of protein structure. Each amino acid consists of an alpha carbon connected to a primary amine group, a carboxylate group, and a unique side chain. The structural identity determines the properties of amino acids, such as acidity/basicity (with different ionization constants of their weakly acidic/basic functional groups) and hydrophilic/hydrophobic nature. The overall characteristic of a protein depends on the content, configuration, and surface exposure of the amino acid constituents.
2. *Secondary structure*: Spatial folding of a polypeptide chain, stabilized by non-covalent interactions (such as hydrogen bond) between amino acid side chains, forms the secondary structure of a protein. The secondary structure is fairly stable in the aqueous environment and often has patterns that repeat across naturally occurring proteins. These patterns can form domains of secondary structure within the larger three-dimensional structure of a protein. Two common patterns of secondary structural domains are α-helices and β-sheets.

   The α-helix is a right hand spiral conformation of a polypeptide chain where the backbone secondary nitrogen of an amino acid is connected through a hydrogen bond to the carboxyl carbon of the amino acid located three or four residues along the peptide chain. This recurring pattern leads to the burying of the hydrophilic, hydrogen bond forming residues of the peptide chain within the helix, while the hydrophobic regions are exposed on the surface. The α-helices are typically found in membrane proteins embedded in the hydrophobic regions of the lipid double layer.

   In β-sheets, the strands of amino acids in a peptide chain are laterally connected with hydrogen bonds, leading to the formation of a twisted, pleated sheet structure. These structures tend to be hydrophilic on the surface and present in secreted, water soluble proteins.
3. *Tertiary structure*: The surface of polypeptide chains, folded in their secondary structure, can further interact with the amino acid side chains of relatively distant amino acids, leading to stable folding into a tertiary structure. The spatial proximity of secondary structural elements determines the tertiary structure of a polypeptide—spatially close amino acids on the folded polypeptide chains can form attractive hydrogen bond, ionic, or hydrophobic interactions, resulting in stabilization of the tertiary structure (Mahato and Narang 2018). Under physiological conditions, proteins assume their distinctive tertiary structure of minimum free energy, which is a prerequisite for their biological function (Mahato and Narang 2018).
4. *Quaternary structure*: The quaternary structure of a protein typically consists of more than one polypeptide chain stably interacting with each other through non-covalent interactions. These associations of polypeptide chains can be in the form of dimers, trimers, or tetramers. Most proteins greater than 100 kDa have quaternary structure. Insulin, for example, is a hormone with a quaternary structure consisting of two polypeptide chains.

   Higher order structures of proteins are stabilized by multiple weak non-covalent interactions. This allows structural flexibility in the protein, which allows structural changes in response to the environment (e.g. change in pH) and upon interaction or binding with other proteins and small molecules.

8.3 Antibodies[1]

In the body, an antibody is a protein produced by β-lymphocytes in response to substances recognized as foreign ("antigens"). Antibodies recognize and bind to antigens, resulting in their inactivation or opsonization (binding of antibody to the membrane surface of invading pathogen, thus marking it for phagocytosis) or complement-mediated destruction. Antibodies are also known as immunoglobulins (abbreviated Ig) since they are immune-response proteins that are *globular* proteins (compact with higher orders of structure and hydrophilic surface making them soluble; as opposed to *fibrous* proteins, which have predominantly secondary structure and are insoluble). Of the five major types of antibodies (Table 8.1), immunoglobulin G (IgG) is preferred for therapeutic applications due to its wide distribution and function.

Structurally, Ig is commonly represented in a typical Y-arm structure (Figure 8.1) consisting of two large/heavy and two small/light polypeptide chains joined by disulfide bridges. Antibody fragments consist of a (mostly) constant region (designated, Fc) and an antigen-binding region (designated, Fab). Antibodies that recognize multiple sites of an antigen are termed *polyclonal*, whereas antibodies that target only a specific site are *monoclonal*. Identical immune cells make monoclonal antibodies, whereas polyclonal antibodies are produced by a mass of immune cells that may produce antibodies against

TABLE 8.1

Types of Antibodies

Antibody	Proportion of Total Antibodies	Where Found in the Body	Function	Size
IgA	10%–15%	Nose, breathing passages, digestive tract, ears, eyes, saliva, vagina, tears, and blood.	Protection on the mucosal surfaces of the body exposed to the outside environment.	
IgG	75%–80%	All body fluids. Smallest and the most common.	Fighting bacterial and viral infections. Only type of antibody that can cross placenta.	Smallest
IgM	5%–10%	Blood and lymph.	First type of antibody made in response to infection. Stimulate other immune cells.	Largest
IgE	Small amounts	Lungs, skin, mucous membranes.	React to pollen, fungal spores, and animal dander. May be involved in allergic reactions.	
IgD	Small amounts	Tissue that lines belly or chest	Not clear.	

Source: Mahato, R.I. and A.S. Narang, *Pharmaceutical Dosage Forms and Drug Delivery*, 3rd edn., CRC Press, Boca Raton, FL, 2018.

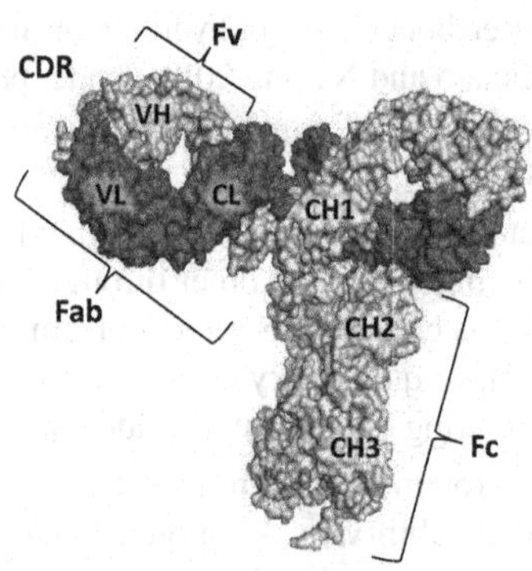

FIGURE 8.1 Typical structure of an antibody.

[1] This section reproduced with permission from Mahato and Narang (2018).

different regions of the antigen. In industrial applications, monoclonal antibodies are prepared using recombinant DNA technology in cultured cells. For human clinical applications, monoclonal antibodies are generally preferred. Polyclonal antibodies are utilized for diagnostic and lab use such as immunohistochemistry.

A number of IgG products have been developed for therapeutic use in various immune disorders (Table 8.2). Due to their specificity, there is a growing interest in the use of monoclonal antibodies and

TABLE 8.2
List of Some Commercial Products of Therapeutic Proteins

Protein Type	Protein Names	Description	Indication
Polyclonal antibodies (lyophilized)	Sandoglobulin	Human immune globulin for intravenous administration. It is a polyvalent antibody product that contains all IgG antibodies which regularly occur in the donor population in a concentrated form. It is prepared by fractionation of the plasma of volunteer donors. It is a lyophilised preparation.	Primary immune deficiencies such as severe combined immunodeficiency (SCID), common variable immunodeficiency, X-linked agammaglobulinemia; and immune thrombocytopenic purpura (ITP).
Polyclonal antibodies (solution)	Gammagard	Concentrated human IgG antibodies similar to that of normal plasma. It is manufactured from pooled human plasma from donors. It is available as a 10% ready-to-use sterile liquid formulation.	Primary immunodeficiencies.
Monoclonal antibodies	Rituximab	Monoclonal antibody that recognizes specific proteins on the surface of some lymphoma cells and triggers body's immune system.	Combination therapy for tumors such as non-Hodgkin's lymphoma (NHL) and chronic lymphocytic leukemia (CLL), and autoimmune diseases such as rheumatoid arthritis.
Radioactively tagged antibodies	Ibritumomab tiuxetan	Monoclonal antibody radioimmunotherapy. It is prepared from monoclonal mouse IgG1 antibody ibritumomab and uses the chelator tiuxetan, which has a radioactive isotope (yttrium-90 or indium-111).	B-cell non-Hodgkin's lymphoma.
Mose-antibodies	Tositumomab	IgG2 anti-CD20 monoclonal antibody of murine origin. Also available as radioactively labeled 131 I-tositumomab, which has covalently bound iodine-131.	Follicular lymphoma.
Chimeric antibodies	Infliximab	Monoclonal antibody against TNFα.	Psoriasis, Crohn's disease, ankylosing spondylitis, psoriatic arthritis, rheumatoid arthritis, and ulcerative colitis.
Humanized antibodies	Daclizumab	Monoclonal antibody against the α subunit of IL-2 receptor on T-cells.	To prevent the rejection in organ transplantation, especially in kidney transplantation.
Fusion proteins	Abatacept	Fusion protein that is composed of human Ig fused to the extracellular domain of cytotoxic T lymphocyte-associated antigen 4, a molecule involved in T-cell stimulation.	Rheumatoid arthritis.
Physiological proteins	Erythropoietin	Glycoprotein hormone that controls erythropoiesis (red blood cell production). It is available as a lyophilized preparation.	Kidney diseases, anemia, and cancer.
Antibody-drug conjugates	Kadcyla®	Human immunoglobulin conjugated to a small molecule anti-microtubule drug.	Breast cancer.

Source: Mahato, R.I. and A.S. Narang, *Pharmaceutical Dosage Forms and Drug Delivery*, 3rd edn., CRC Press, Boca Raton, FL, 2018.

their modifications as therapeutics. For example, a segment of a monomeric antibody Fab fragment that consists only of the smallest known antigen-binding segment of the variable domain is called a *domain antibody*. Antibodies that can bind two different antigens are called *bispecific antibodies*.

Early use of antibodies as therapeutics was restricted by the host immune response. This was especially the case for antibodies generated (by antigen injection) in foreign animal species, such as mouse. The antibodies generated in mouse were named with the suffix *~momab*. The use of humanized/human monoclonal antibodies produced using recombinant DNA technology, the predominant focus of this chapter, has helped to overcome these limitations.

Chimeric and Humanized antibodies are antibodies produced from non-human species whose protein sequences have been modified to increase their similarity to the antibody variants that are naturally found in humans. *Chimeric antibodies* consist of murine variable regions fused with human constant regions, resulting in ~65% human amino acid sequence. This reduces immunogenicity and increases plasma half-life. These antibodies are named with the suffix *~ximab*. For example, rituximab (Rituxan®) is a chimeric (mouse/human) antibody that targets B-cell surface CD20 receptors and is used for the treatment of autoimmune diseases and cancers of the white blood system, such as leukemia and lymphomas. *Humanized antibodies* are generated by grafting the murine variable amino acid domains (which determine antigen specificity) onto human antibodies, resulting in ~95% human amino acid sequence. These, however, have lower antigen binding affinity than murine antibodies. These antibodies are named with the suffix *~zumab*. For example, bevacizumab (Avastin®) is a humanized antibody that targets vascular endothelial growth factor (VEGF) and is recommended as first-line therapy in advanced colorectal cancer in combination with other drugs.

Human monoclonal antibodies can be produced using phage display or transgenic mice. Transferring the human Ig genes into the mouse genome can produce these antibodies. These antibodies are named with the suffix *~mumab*. For example, ipilimumab is a human mAb that inhibits the checkpoint receptor cytotoxic T lymphocyte-associated antigen 4 (CTLA-4) and is recommended for advanced-stage melanoma.

8.4 Physical and Chemical Instability of Biologic Drugs, Analytical Characterization Tools, and Stabilization Strategies

Biologic drug substance and drug product manufacturing processes must take into consideration the physicochemical characteristics of these molecules to ensure their stability throughout manufacture. Essential components of this strategy are the analytical characterization tools and techniques to quantify the physicochemical, biopharmaceutical, and biophysical properties of these compounds—which are applied throughout their manufacture, storage, and use. This section describes the common methods used for protein and antibody characterization.

8.4.1 Solubility

Most therapeutic proteins are administered as aqueous solutions. Therefore, achieving and maintaining solubility is a key requirement for the manufacture, storage, and use of these biologic drugs. High water solubility of these hydrophilic polymers is due to the hydrogen bonding and electrostatic interactions of the ionizable surface functional groups, which are typically weakly acidic or weakly basic. Since a protein contains many ionizable functional groups, each with a different ionization constant (pKa), the net charge on a protein can be negative (in the basic environment, pH > pI), positive (in the acidic pH environment, pH < pI), or zero (at a pH of the solution known as the isoelectric point, pI, where the proportion of positively charged functional groups are balanced by the negatively charged functional groups). At the pI, a protein does not migrate when placed in an electric field (such as during gel electrophoresis) and possesses the lowest solubility. Protein solubility increases as the solution pH migrates away from the pI. However, extremely acidic or basic pH environments are not physiologically compatible and can lead to chemical degradation of the protein. Hence, a balance of stability and solubility within the physiologically compatible range of pH values is sought in protein manufacturing and formulation.

8.4.2 Physical Instability

Changes in the higher order structure of a biomolecule, such as protein folding, usually without the involvement of formation or breakage of covalent bonds, is described as physical instability. Common forms of protein physical instability include the formation of dimers, trimers, or higher order structures in solution leading up to larger, sub-visible or visible aggregates/particles or precipitation, and adsorption (e.g. to container surfaces). Physical instability typically results from conformational changes that lead to surface exposure of hydrophobic residues in a protein.

The principles of colloidal stability, i.e. managing net electrostatic surface repulsion with the use of appropriate solution pH and salt concentration to shield surface charge, are at play in the physical instability of colloidal protein solutions. Thus, while stabilization of the native state of the protein by selection of the right pH and salt conditions in solution is key, it is also important to minimize exposure to various stresses that can lead to conformational perturbation. These stresses can include:

1. *Thermal*: For example, the rate of aggregation is usually higher with increasing temperature of processing and storage. In addition, the freezing/thawing process can also lead to localized environments with high excipient concentration and changes in pH that cause aggregation.
2. *Concentration*: Proteins tend to exhibit lower stability, i.e. higher rate of aggregation, at higher concentrations.
3. *Shear*: For example, high shear stress has the potential to increase the propensity for aggregation.
4. *Cavitation*: Sudden change in motion, such as dropping a container of a protein solution can lead to localized environments of very high pressure, where "seeding" of conformationally perturbed protein can take place.
5. *Interfacial stress*: Exposure to the air/water interface via agitation during shipping as also the exposure to the solid/liquid interface during freeze/thaw cycles can lead to protein aggregation.
6. *Ionic strength*: Increase in the salt concentration in solution can lead to decrease in surface polarity and electrostatic repulsion between protein molecules, promoting aggregation. Such local microenvironments can be present during freeze-thaw or lyophilization.
7. *pH*: For example, pH close to pI can lead to protein molecules with net neutral surface charges that tend to associate with other proteins, potentially causing agglomeration and aggregation.
8. *Water concentration*: For example, lyophilized protein must have some residual level of water—or stabilizing hydrophilic polymer—to keep the protein in the stable, native conformation and ensure rapid dissolution upon addition of water to the cake.

8.4.3 Chemical Instability

Chemical instability of proteins can include one or more of the following common reaction pathways:

1. Hydrolysis or proteolysis, i.e. breakage of the peptide bonds between amino acids can occur at extremes of pH and temperature. The most commonly observed proteolytic reactions in proteins and peptides involve the side chain amide groups of asparagine (Asn) and glutamine (Gln) and the peptide bond on the C-terminal side of an aspartic acid (Asp) or a proline (Pro) residue (Mahato and Narang 2018).
2. Deamidation of the side chain linkage in glutamine or asparagine residues to aspartate and glutamate, respectively, and isomerization (aspartate to iso-aspartate) can happen in particular sequences within a protein. These changes in amino acid side chains can lead to alterations in stabilizing interactions among amino acids within proteins, leading to conformational changes that can sometimes impact efficacy and safety of proteins.
3. *Oxidation*: Several amino acids have functional groups that can oxidize, leading to changes in protein structure, conformation, and function. These include sulfhydryl in cysteine, imidazole in histidine, thioether in methionine, phenol in tyrosine, and indole in tryptophan. Oxidation of proteins can occur due to atmospheric oxygen, presence of free radicals or peroxides in protein

solutions, or light—and may be catalyzed by the presence of metal contaminants in trace quantities. These may also be tied to changes in physical stability.

4. *Reduction*: Cleavage by reduction and rearrangement with oxidative coupling of cysteine disulfide bonds can change conformation of a protein. This phenomenon is commonly called disulfide exchange.
5. *Maillard reaction*: The presence of reducing sugars (e.g. glucose/dextrose) in the protein solution can lead to glycation of protein at the basic residues (such as the lysine amine). The reaction products can further rearrange and form coloured compounds through a series of reactions.

8.4.4 Analytical Characterization

In addition to the basic characterization for identification, appearance, potency, and water content, biomolecules are characterized for attributes that are specific to polymeric hydrophilic compounds that can possess a myriad of primary, secondary, and tertiary structures. For example, biophysical characterization of proteins includes the determination of *size, shape, and solution properties* of proteins through direct and indirect techniques that include (Mahato and Narang 2018):

- Hydrodynamic protein size measurement by analytical ultracentrifugation, gel filtration chromatography (also known as size exclusion chromatography), and gel electrophoresis.
- Binding affinity to the target protein by assays such as enzyme-linked immune sorbent assay (ELISA).
- Particulate formation by protein self-association or interaction with other components in solution by dynamic light scattering (DLS).
- Spectroscopic methods, such as circular dichroism (CD), intrinsic and extrinsic fluorescence, Fourier transform infrared (FTIR), and Raman, can help determine the stability of protein *conformation* in solution, in particular when paired with thermal melts.
- Identification of charge variants by isoelectric focusing. The different species elute at their pI, including the main peak. Thus, any acidic variants, that have additional acidic functional groups, elute differently than the main protein. Similarly, the basic variants have additional basic functional groups and elute differently than the main protein. For example, a protein that has undergone deamidation will appear as an acidic species due to the change from the neutral asparagine residue to an acidic aspartic acid residue. Changes in charge variants of proteins are also commonly analyzed by high-performance liquid chromatography (HPLC)-based ion exchange chromatography (IEX).
- Characterization of any molecular clippings by electrophoretic techniques such as reducing and non-reducing capillary electrophoresis. The difference between reducing and non-reducing conditions is the presence of agents (such as dithiothreitol and beta-mercaptoethanol) that can reduce the cystine disulfide bonds to cysteine sulfhydryls. Thus, these two methods provide very different information with respect to protein structure and constitution.
- Thermodynamic methods such as microcalorimetry and surface plasmon resonance can help delineate the state of protein association and interactions with other molecules in solution. These methodologies are not first-line or the most common methods of protein characterization.

8.5 Upstream Antibody Production by Mammalian Cells

mAb production by recombinant protein expression started with hybridoma and Chinese hamster ovary (CHO) cells. Several rodent- and human-derived cells are also used for therapeutic protein expression. These include 3T3, BHK, HeLa, and HepG2. However, CHO cells remain the most frequently used cell line for mAb production. CHO cells present several advantages such as resilience (can be grown in various media environments and scaled-up easily), fast generation times, easily adapted to suspension cell culture (as opposed to adherent cell cultures), and characteristics that make them amenable for genetic modification (e.g. low chromosome number and ease of transfection and selection of transgene-expressing cells). Early mutagenesis studies led to the isolation of certain auxotrophs—mutants that require particular nutrients for maintaining growth and viability over long culture periods.

The nutritional requirements of the auxotrophs form the basis of selection of cells post-transfection for those expressing exogenous proteins and has been utilized to also increase the transgene copy number and expression levels. Commonly used auxotrophs of CHO cells are the DG44 and DUKXB-11 host cell lines that are deficient in the dihydrofolate reductase (DHFR) enzyme. This enzyme reduces dihydrofolic acid to tetrahydrofolic acid, an essential cellular biochemical product for purine and thymidylate synthesis. Cells lacking the DHFR enzyme require glycine, hypoxanthine, and thymidine to grow (and are thus called triple auxotrophs). This property is utilized for the expression of a heterologous gene by co-transfection with a functional copy of the DHFR gene, such that the transfected cells do not require exogenously supplied glycine, hypoxanthine, and thymidine in the growth medium. Hence, cell culture in a deficient growth medium allows the selection of transfected cells. Another recombinant DNA expression strategy is the glutamine synthetase (GS) system utilized in GS deficient CHO cells. GS catalyzes the production of glutamine, an essential amino acid required for cellular metabolism, from glutamate and ammonia. Upon co-transfection of the recombinant gene and GS into host cells, the cells are cultivated in glutamine-free media to select for producing clones.

An additional selection marker commonly used is the addition of an antibiotic (e.g. hygromycin) to the cell culture medium, while the genetic sequence encoding for the antibiotic resistance gene is included in the gene transfer vector. Thus, during cell culture, only the cells that get transfected and actively transcribe and translate the exogenous DNA are able to survive.

These selected cells, however, are polyclonal since this is a collection of cells that have integrated the transgene at different locations on their expression systems and have other differences, such as post-translational modification (PTM), transgene expression. Selection of single clones, called clonal selection, is then performed by growth and isolation of single cells upon dilution and amplification in the deficient growth medium.

8.5.1 Cell Line Development

Cell line development typically involves:

1. Designing a vector that includes the transgene of interest along with the components required for gene expression in target cells (such as a promoter and an enhancer), target cell selection (e.g. DHFR gene and an optional secondary antibiotic selection gene), and elements that enhance transcriptional activity (such as polyA sequence and chromatin opening domains).
2. Transfection, i.e. introducing recombinant DNA into the host cells, using one of these technologies, such as lipid-based or polymer-based reagents, calcium phosphate precipitation, or electroporation.
3. Growth of transfected cells in an appropriate antibiotic-containing cell culture medium, which provides all nutrients except the one(s) that the auxotrophs rely on to survive.
4. An optional amplification step, which typically includes exposing the cells to increasing concentration of selective agent such as methotrexate (MTX). This enforces a stronger selection pressure on cell population such that the surviving cells have multiple copies of the recombinant DNA, with the exogenous DNA integrated at multiple transcription sites, and are able to express the DHFR gene (and the transgene of interest) at higher levels. In GS deficient CHO cells, methionine sulphoximine (MSX), an inhibitor of glutamine synthesis activity, is typically added to the cell culture media to amplify the copies of glutamine synthetase gene together with the transgene of interest.
5. Isolation of single cells from a diverse pool of cells by limiting-dilution cloning. In this method, cells are dispensed into each well of multiwell microtiter plates at very low cell density (<1 cell/well). Wells are monitored microscopically to ensure only those that are derived from a single

cell are used for subsequent selection. Supernatant from these individual wells can be assayed for productivity by methods such as enzyme-linked immunosorbent assay.

6. Isolation and growth of several cell clones that yield high product titer by expansion into larger microwell plates and subsequently into shaker flasks, which are monitored for growth and productivity profiles. Clones which deliver the highest protein titer may be selected for a second round of sub-cloning to further increase population homogeneity. This may not be necessary for clones derived from single cells, as evidenced by the imaging data during clone isolation and selection.
7. Selection and growth of a few candidate cell clones with the favorable characteristics of high protein titers, good growth characteristics (e.g. rate, viability, and metabolism), and acceptable protein quality. The research cell bank (RCB) is then prepared with an appropriate number of cells frozen in a dimethyl sulfoxide (DMSO) containing medium for future use. These few clones are further evaluated in production bioreactors and followed by more extensive characterization of the recombinant protein quality that is produced in larger scale. The most appropriate clone is then selected for further commercial process development.
8. Research cell banks are primarily used for research and development and can be used to produce material for toxicological assessment in animal species. For GMP-manufacturing and supply of drug substance in clinical trials and subsequent commercial production, a two-tiered cell banking system that includes MCBs and working cell banks (WCB) is created to ensure a continuous supply of cell banks for manufacturing use. Both MCBs and WCB undergo rigorous testing for genetic identity and biosafety.

The clone selection process is labor-extensive and time-consuming, typically employing high throughput screening methods and taking up approximately half a year. A majority of the surviving cell population shows only low or average level of protein production, whereas a small fraction of clones exhibit high protein productivity. Glycoforms, protein aggregates, and charge variants are also product quality attributes that are monitored in the clone selection process. Contemporary scientists seek to improve process efficiencies through technical and regulatory strategies such as increasing cellular growth rate, use of automation, and the use of monoclonal antibodies that are produced by a pool of cells (instead of single clone) and commonly referred to "antibodies produced by polyclonal cell population" in toxicology testing (Hu et al. 2017). Contemporary practices and aspects related to the generation of highly productive cell lines and the optimization of cell culture process conditions are outlined in a recent review (Li et al. 2010).

8.5.2 Increasing Transgene Expression Levels

A modification of the cell culture medium (i.e. addition of methotrexate) allows the selection of high transgene producing strain. Methotrexate blocks DHFR activity. Thus, surviving cells must upregulate the expression of the DHFR transgene to thrive in the deficient growth medium. By linking the expression of DHFR with the exogenous protein of interest, the selection process can increase the chances of obtaining a high production strain (Ng 2012).

Another strategy is designing vectors and selecting for high transcriptional activity at the site of integration of the exogenous DNA in the host cell genome. Preferential selection of clones where transgene integration has happened at the high transcriptional site of the host genome is attempted by increasing the selection pressure for DHFR clones through the use of mutant DHFR gene with reduced enzymatic activity or the use of a weak promoter for the DHFR gene (Chin et al. 2015). Design strategies include the use of chromatin opening elements in the exogenous DNA sequence. These include regions such as scaffold or matrix attachment regions and ubiquitous chromatin opening elements (Antoniou et al. 2013).

8.5.3 Productivity

Biopharmaceutical industry continuously strives to improve the volumetric productivity of high-quality therapeutic proteins. This has been approached through multiple strategies, such as cultivating high-density cultures in bioreactors with chemically defined cell culture medium, increasing the transgene expression levels, optimizing cell growth and productivity using pH and temperature, and improving protein capture and purification (downstream) techniques.

Taken together, these strategies have significantly increased achievable cell density (from <5 M cells/mL to >15 M cells/mL) and product titer (from <0.1 g/L to >5 g/L) in fed-batch cultures over the past few decades (Bareither et al. 2013; Huang et al. 2010; Padawer et al. 2013).

8.5.3.1 Scale of Manufacture and Nutrient Feeding in Bioreactors

CHO cells have been grown at high cell densities up to >30 × 10^6 cells/mL in large-scale production vessels (>15 kilo-liters). The upstream manufacturing process initiates with a vial thaw of a cell bank (Figure 8.2), and cells are expanded in progressively higher volumes in culture vessels such as shake flasks and/or wave bioreactors. Prior to inoculation of large production vessels, the cells are expanded through a series of inoculum train bioreactors. Depending on the scale of the production bioreactor, this upstream process may take 2 weeks–6 weeks from vial thaw.

Fed-batch process is the most common mode of operation for the production of recombinant protein in the biopharmaceutical industry. The operation of fed-batch does not typically involve complex control strategies, and the duration is short enough (approximately 2 weeks) to mitigate risks associated with contamination or equipment failure. Addition of concentrated culture medium throughout the culture helps replenish depleted nutrients, enabling longer culture times and higher viable cell densities. The optimization of cell culture medium is one of the key steps to prolonging cell longevity in the bioreactor and maximizing titer yields. Chemically defined and serum-free media used for the cultivation of CHO cells are highly complex. The media formulation can contain as many as 50 total components–70 total components, to provide the optimal balance of carbon source, amino acids, vitamins, growth factors, salts, and trace metals.

8.5.4 Glycosylation

Biological activity, including both pharmacokinetic and pharmacodynamic properties, of a protein requires proper folding and post-translational modification, such as glycosylation. This is the process where carbohydrate moieties are added to specific amino acid residues on a protein. Such proteins are called glycoproteins. Folding and post-translational modification also influence biophysical properties of protein therapeutics, such as solubility and conformational stability.

The molecular and conformational structure of the carbohydrate residues added to the protein are important to immune recognition as host versus foreign. Thus, glycosylation pattern on a protein that would be atypical of human glycosylation pattern can lead to immunogenic response. Hence, glycoproteins are

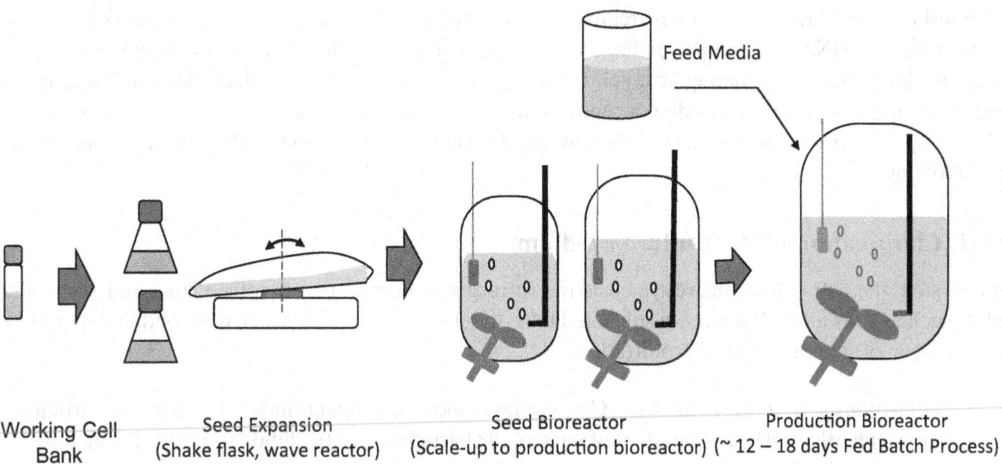

FIGURE 8.2 Schematic of cell culture steps in the manufacturing of recombinant mAb from CHO cells.

typically manufactured in mammalian cells. CHO cell glycoforms have proven to be both compatible and bioactive in humans. Cell culture environments in production bioreactor such as pH, temperature, or the presence of different carbon sources can have an impact on glycosylation profile (Hossler et al. 2009).

8.6 Downstream Purification

CHO-derived therapeutic proteins need to be extracted and purified from the components of the cell culture medium as well as cellular components and products—a large mixture of complex products, many of which are not well characterized. Chromatographic separation sciences constitute the mainstream product isolation and purification methodology for large molecule therapeutics. These operations fall under a broad category of steps that are collectively referred to as downstream purification or downstream processing. Chromatographic methods offer several advantages for target protein separation from complex mixtures such as high separation efficiencies (hundreds to thousands of theoretical plates) and the ability to separate small amounts of adsorbate from a large volume of solution, thus allowing concentration of the product and/or removal of the contaminants.

The steps involved in the downstream processing depend on whether the targeted protein is intracellular or secreted. Intracellular proteins can be cell membrane associated, present as an intracellular inclusion body, or as a soluble product in the cellular fluid. In any case, a specific extraction step precedes purification. For secreted proteins, harvest by centrifugation separates cells from the medium, where the desired protein can then be purified from the supernatant. Following extraction or clarification, typical downstream processing operations fall in the following three broad, sequential categories, each of which may be carried out in one or more unit operations to achieve the desired level of purity.

1. *Capture*: Protein capture involves isolation of the target protein from cell culture components and concentration in a stable (buffer) environment.
2. *Intermediate purification*: Intermediate purification involves the removal of bulk contaminants, such as host cell proteins and conformational variants of the target protein. This step may not be required, depending on the purity of the material obtained after the capture step and the desired application.
3. *Polishing*: The polishing step involves the removal of lower proportion and difficult to remove impurities, to achieve very high purity of the target protein.

Chromatographic purification is the mainstream technology for most of the protein purification steps. While improving purity, chromatographic steps applied in sequence tend to reduce the yield. A minimalistic approach that assures adequate product purity is, therefore, adopted on a case-by-case basis.

Important considerations for downstream purification processes include ensuring absence of contaminating host cell DNA and human pathogenic viruses. Current purification processes reach as low as picogram levels of contaminating host cell DNA per dose of the finished product. Also, a vast majority of the human pathogenic viruses do not replicate in CHO cells.

The steps involved in a typical downstream purification scheme of a recombinant mAb can include the following.

8.6.1 Clarification of the Culture Medium

In this step, the cell culture harvest, consisting of target protein in the dissolved state and suspended solids such as cells and cell debris, is subjected to sedimentation, centrifugation, deep bed or depth filtration, and one or more steps of microfiltration.

- *Sedimentation and centrifugation*: Gravitational and centrifugal rotational settling of particulate matter allows initial separation of most of the particles from the fluid for initial clarification.
- Depth filtration or deep bed filtration consists of a porous filtration medium that retains particles throughout the medium, rather than just on the surface. This process is particularly suitable

for fluids with high particle load since the filter can retain a large mass of particles before getting clogged. Depth filters provide high surface area and adsorptive surface. In addition to adsorbing impurities from cell culture supernatants, depth filters can also remove viruses (Yigzaw et al. 2006).

- Microfiltration involves passing the fluid through a specific pore size membrane to effect removal of microorganisms and suspended particles. Suspended particles are retained ("retentate") on the feed side of the membrane, while the dissolved liquids, including the protein of interest, passes through ("permeate"). A cross-flow filtration process, where the fluid is moved in a direction tangential to the membrane surface, is preferred compared to the dead-end filtration (where the fluid is forced through the membrane surface at a dead end to the direction of flow).

This step can be bypassed for low viscosity, dilute cell suspensions by the use of fluidized or expanded bed technique. In this method, the cell culture medium is made to flow upwards through a bed of dense adsorbent particles. As the particles fluidize, expand, and float, the cells and fluid can get through while the adsorbate (target protein) is adsorbed on the adsorbent. High density of the adsorbent allows resettling of the column after flushing and washing of the culture medium. This method, however, is only applicable to low viscosity, low density cell cultures—and, hence, is difficult to implement for most modern high-density cell cultures.

An alternative to expanded/fluidized bed capture without clarification is the use of packed bed of large size beads. In this case, the cell culture medium is made to pass down a packed bed of high-efficiency large diameter particles, so that both the cells and the liquid can pass through while the target protein is adsorbed on the adsorbent. This process is less sensitive to feed viscosity, but also less efficient due to the lower surface area of large size adsorbent particles.

8.6.2 Protein A Capture

Passage of the clarified medium containing the target mAb through a column consisting of staphylococcal protein A (called SPA, or simply protein A), or its smaller ligands, immobilized on porous beads, leads to selective binding and isolation of the antibody. This process is called *affinity chromatography*, since the separation is driven by the specific affinity of the stationary phase for the desired component of the mobile phase. SPA is a cell-wall associated protein domain on the surface of *S. aureus*. The porous beads are typically made of a resin that is acid and base resistant to allow for efficient column handling in different pH environments such as those commonly encountered for elution (low pH) and clean-in-place protocols (high pH).

Protein A binds all IgG sub-classes 1, 2, and 4 in a highly selective manner without interacting with the complementarity-determining region (CDR) of the antibody. Other ligands used for the protein capture affinity chromatography step include streptococcal protein G, a triazine-based ligand, or peptide-based ligands (Hober et al. 2007). The elution of captured antibody from protein A column is carried out using a low pH buffer, such as 0.1 M sodium citrate buffer at pH 3.0–3.5. SPA purification efficiently purifies the mAb from impurities such as host cell proteins and host DNA.

8.6.3 Low pH Viral Inactivation

A relatively short (<1 hour) incubation at low pH has been demonstrated to inactivate more than 4 $\log_{10}$ of large enveloped viruses such as X-MuLV. Viral inactivation requires incubation at a pH of 3.8 or below (Brorson et al. 2003). Since mAb elution from the protein A column is typically carried out using a low pH buffer, continued incubation of the antibody in the elution medium for a short period of time ensures inactivation of viruses. This low pH is achieved using low concentration of a strong acid, such as hydrochloric acid (HCl), or high concentration of a weak acid, such as acetic acid or citric acid. Higher concentrations of strong acids are avoided to minimize risk of localized high acid concentration that can be particularly damaging to the protein, resulting in issues such as aggregation and hydrolysis.

Low pH inactivation, of course, requires stability of the target protein under low pH conditions. This includes pumping the product intermediately into another vessel under low pH conditions to ensure complete exposure of the whole batch to the lower pH (and avoid the "hanging drop effect"). For products that cannot tolerate low pH incubation, chemical inactivation of enveloped retroviruses is sought by the use of a detergent (e.g. Triton X-100 or Tween 80 at 0.5%–1.0% concentration) or a detergent in combination with a solvent (e.g. tri-N-butyl phosphate) (Horowitz et al. 1992). If needed, the chemical inactivation step is preferably carried out earlier in the downstream purification scheme to allow complete removal of the inactivating agent from the finished product. It is also important to consider non-interference of the chemical inactivation step on downstream purification operations. For example, hydrophobic interaction chromatography can be significantly influenced by the presence of detergents, while protein A affinity chromatography and ion exchange chromatography are less likely to be impacted (Shukla and Aranha 2015).

8.6.4 Ion Exchange Chromatography

Ion exchange (IEX) chromatography is one of the most commonly used techniques for the purification of biomolecules including proteins, polypeptides, and polynucleotides. This charge-based separation technique is based on the difference in the charge between the target protein and the impurities or contaminants under specific elution conditions, such as pH and salt concentration. IEX utilizes the polyionic nature of these macromolecules and is based on the concepts of isoelectric point (pI) and ionic competition.

Isoelectric point is the pH at which a polyionic molecule carries no net electrostatic charge. At pH > pI, the net electrostatic charge is negative (a contribution, for example, from the unionized amines and the negatively charged carboxylate anions); while at pH < pI, the net electrostatic charge is positive (a contribution, for example, from the positively charged, ionized amines and the uncharged carboxylic acid groups). Utilizing these differences, IEX can be either cation exchange (CEX) or anion exchange (AEX) chromatography. CEX utilizes a negatively charged ion exchange resin, which has affinity for molecules with a net positive charge. CEX is run at a pH which is 0.5 units–1.5 units below the pI of the protein of interest. Conversely, AEX utilizes a positively charged ion exchange resin, which has affinity for molecules with a net negative charge. AEX is run at a pH which is 0.5 units–1.5 units above the pI of the protein of interest.

IEX resins are comprised of positively or negatively charged ionized groups attached to a solid matrix, such as cellulose, agarose, polymethacrylate, polystyrene, and polyacrylamide. Strong AEX resins bear a permanent positive charge and are based on quaternary ammonium ions, such as high Q (BioRad, Inc., Hercules, CA). Weak AEX resins could be tertiary amine based, such as diethylaminoethyl (DEAE). Weak CEX resins are weakly negatively charged and can be based on carboxylate groups, such as carboxymethyl; while strong CEX resins are strongly negatively charged and are based on, for example, sulfonate groups.

In a typical IEX experiment, an impure protein solution is loaded at a pH of the solution that facilitates the binding of the target protein to the resin (Figure 8.3). This is followed by a wash with the buffer alone to remove undesired proteins and impurities. The bound protein is then eluted from the column using either a salt gradient or a change in pH. Salt ions compete with the protein molecules for binding to the resin. Thus, weakly bound proteins with few charged groups elute at lower salt concentrations, while strongly bound proteins with many charged groups elute at high salt concentration. The use of pH gradient is based on steady change in the buffer pH towards the pI of the protein of interest. The protein elutes when the pH reaches the pI due to net charge neutralization. Salt gradient is more commonly used than pH changes to elute proteins from IEX columns due to complexities involved in pH adjustment and maintenance and the effect of pH on analytical methods. Sometimes, pH change is combined with salt-based elution.

In a typical protein purification scheme, both CEX and AEX are carried out sequentially. The use of salt gradient to elute the protein assumes stability of the protein in the presence of salt.

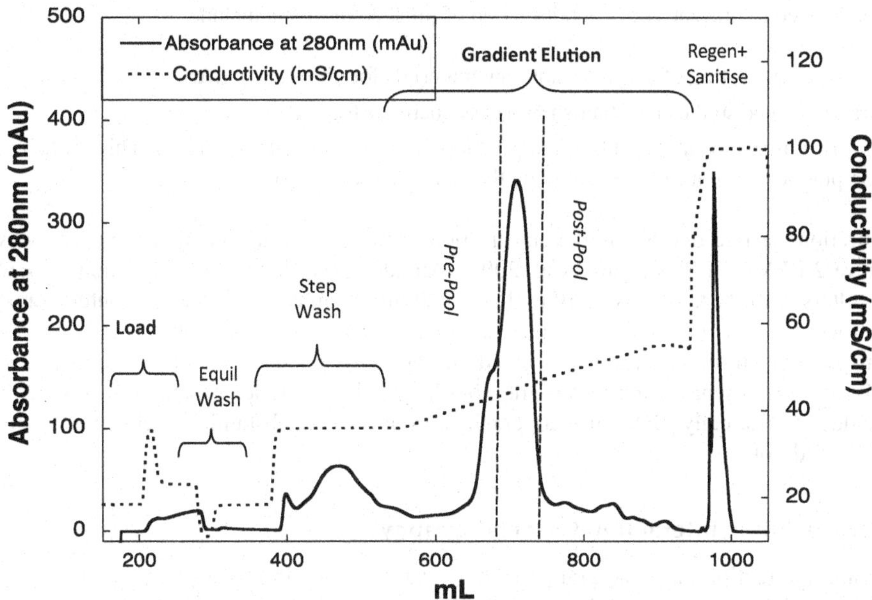

FIGURE 8.3 Cation exchange chromatogram showing a salt gradient elution and pooling criteria. Sulfopropyl (SP) high performance sepharose was loaded at 10 g/L density for the target protein and eluted in a 35%–85% gradient of 1.2 M sodium acetate in 25 mM HEPES pH 7.5. A 35% step wash is used to remove host cell proteins prior to elution. (Reproduced from Pizarro, S.A. et al., *Protein Expr. Purif.*, 72, 184–193, 2010. With permission.)

An analogous method is to apply IEX in a flow-through modality where the pH of the load solution is adjusted so that the target protein flows through the column and is readily recovered, while impurities are captured. This has an advantage in operational robustness and for yield. However, large volumes typically need to be managed for both load and elution pools.

In this case, for example, a negatively charged protein would simply flow through the cation exchange column, leaving behind positively charged proteins, then the flow through is loaded onto the anion exchange column, where it binds and undergoes gradient elution.

8.6.5 Viral Filtration

Iatrogenic transmission of pathogenic viruses is a key concern for cell culture-based products. In addition to the measures taken to reduce the risk of viral contamination of the final product, effective viral clearance during the downstream processing is a key requirement for clinical and commercial products. Viral clearance involves spiking studies for several downstream purification steps to demonstrate the removal and/or inactivation. Viral safety of cell culture-derived biotechnology products is also discussed in international council on harmonization (ICH) guidance Q5A(R1) and EMEA/CHMP/BWP/398498/2005.

The risk of viral contamination of cell culture-based biotechnology products can come from:

1. Contamination of cell line, raw materials, or adventitious viruses introduced during manufacturing.
2. The use of rodent cell lines that inherently express endogenous retroviral-like particles (RVLPs). Although the RVLPs are not infectious to humans, they can serve as a marker (baseline retroviral load) for the starting level to calculate the $\log_{10}$ (i.e. 10-fold) reduction value (LRV) of viral clearance required through the downstream processing.

Strategies adapted to prevent viral contamination of finished products include:

1. Selection and testing of cell lines and raw materials for absence of viruses.
2. Viral clearance studies to establish process capability for LRV.
3. Testing of intermediates and finished products to ensure absence of viruses. This is not a common practice since it requires knowing the exact viruses to test.

Depth filtration, carried out during the clarification of the cell culture medium, can remove viruses and achieve 2 LRVs–4 LRVs (Zhou et al. 2008). An additional downstream filtration through viral retentive filters, with pore size as small as 15 nm–20 nm, is an essential step in contemporary purification processes. This is a dedicated size exclusion chromatography step that aims for several log reductions (>5) of viral count (both enveloped and non-enveloped viruses) by filtration under pressure. This size-based separation seeks to filter out larger viral particles compared to smaller, soluble biomolecules. Additionally, IEX chromatography can provide a substantial level of LRV, depending on process conditions.

8.6.6 Hydrophobic Interaction Chromatography

Hydrophobic interaction chromatography (HIC) separates proteins based on their hydrophobicity. HIC utilizes an immobilized ligand, such as a straight chain alkane, on a hydrophilic carbohydrate matrix, such as cross-linked agarose. Protein with sufficient surface hydrophilicity gets adsorbed on the resin via interaction with the immobilized ligand. Hydrophobicity of the proteins and their interaction with the HIC column is influenced by the polarity of the solvent and salt concentration in solution.

Salts increase protein hydrophobicity by neutralizing and shielding the ionizable surface functional groups. In addition to salt, solution pH closer to the pI and the neutral pH range promotes protein surface hydrophobicity and adsorption with the HIC column. The relative propensity of salts for increasing the hydrophobicity and tendency for the salting out effect is indicated by the Hofmeister series, also known as the lyotropic series. The Hofmeister series is a rank ordering of the ability of ions to precipitate or crash out proteins from their solutions. At lower concentrations, these ions impact the stability of the secondary and tertiary structure of proteins, thus exposing hydrophobic groups that interact with the HIC column.

Differences in the hydrophobicity of different protein components in complex mixtures are utilized for protein separation and purification by HIC. The process conditions utilized in HIC are generally mild and tend to preserve the native state and activity of the protein. In particular, HIC is useful for removing protein aggregates—which have different hydrophobic properties compared to the native protein monomer. Ammonium sulfate and sodium chloride are two commonly used lyotropic salts used for HIC column purification.

8.6.7 Multimodal Chromatography

Recent advancements in synthesizing multifunctional ligands have led to a variety of commercially available resins developed with functional groups to target specific combinations of protein-ligand interactions (Johansson et al. 2003a, 2003b). These resins provide additional flexibility in designing effective purification processes and can be employed from capture to polishing steps because of the ligand's ability to interact with the target molecule through various intermolecular forces. However, the increased complexity of the protein-ligand interaction may pose additional challenges for method development of the desorption phases. The ligands have a blend of aromatic or non-aromatic groups coupled with the more traditional carboxylic acid- or amine-based ion exchange properties. Hydrogen acceptor groups close to the carboxylic or amine moiety also play a role in binding to the target molecule.

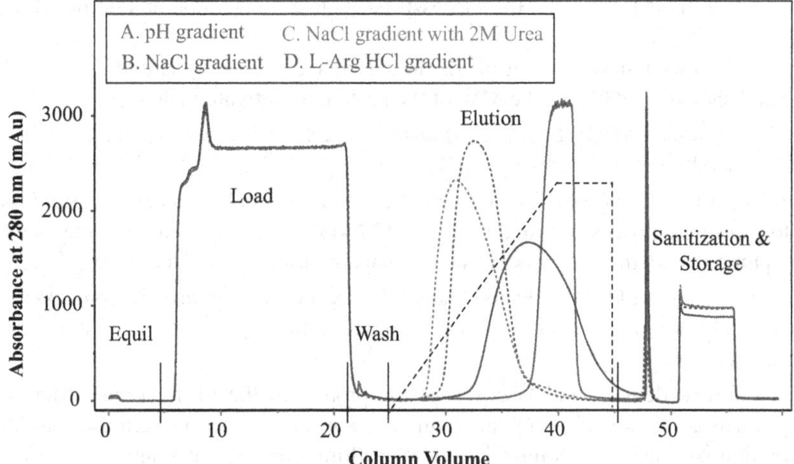

FIGURE 8.4 Capto MMC (mixed mode cation exchange) elution of a mAb using traditional elution gradient buffers and hydrogen disrupting agents. (Reproduced from Kaleas, K.A. et al., *J. Chromatogr. B Analyt. Technol. Biomed. Life Sci.*, 969, 256–263, 2014. With permission.)

In general, elution behaviors from mixed mode resins have been reported to be more challenging than traditional adsorption media, and the most successful buffers are pluripotent in nature so that they are able to simultaneously affect two or more kinds of interactions between a solute and a solid phase. Buffers such as 1 M sodium chloride or 20% ethanol were insufficient to elute the bound protein successfully from a mixed mode resin while buffers with urea or L-arginine HCl were effective (Arakawa et al. 2009; Girot et al. 2004). Several papers have also shown that desorption of the target protein from a mixed-mode ligand can be induced with electrostatic charge repulsion while accompanied by a shift in pH (Gao et al. 2007; Johansson et al. 2003a). Recent work to capture monoclonal antibodies using a mixed mode cation exchange resin CaptoMMC (Kaleas et al. 2014) showed diverse elution profiles when buffers of varying nature were used (Figure 8.4). Traditional pH or salt buffer gradients were enhanced to elute earlier by addition of urea or L-arginine to disrupt hydrogen bonding and hydrophobic moieties between the resin and the mAb.

8.6.8 Ultrafiltration and Diafiltration

Once proteins are purified through downstream chromatography steps, the next steps involve transitioning the protein into the formulation buffer (called buffer exchange or diafiltration, or DF) and increasing the protein concentration (called ultrafiltration, or UF). These steps are usually carried out together in a single unit operation, utilizing a process called tangential flow filtration (TFF). This unit operation involves continuous flow of the protein solution under high pressure in a direction tangential to the UFDF membrane. Buffer exchange happens by introduction of the target buffer into the protein solution. The semi-permeable membrane causes retention of the protein molecules in the circulation path (retentate), while certain amount of the buffer mixture is allowed to pass through the membrane (permeate). For buffer exchange, the retentate volume is held constant through pressure control mechanisms. Thus, over time, as more of the target buffer is introduced, the overall percentage of the target buffer increases and the levels of the initial buffer species remaining become minimal. To increase protein concentration, more permeate is pushed through the membrane than fresh buffer is introduced, so that the overall retentate volume is reduced and the concentration is increased.

Important considerations involved in the successful design and execution of TFF process involve:

- The nominal molecular weight cut-off of the UF membrane is typically between 5 kDa and 30 kDa and should be <30% of the MW of the protein to mitigate yield loss.
- Compatibility of the protein should be evaluated and established with the material of construction of the membrane.
- Protein's sensitivity to process shear should be evaluated, and, if necessary, steps should be taken to minimize process shear during the TFF operation. For example, the use of a diaphragm pump results in lower process shear compared to the peristaltic pump.
- Protein's stability should be evaluated and confirmed not only in both the process buffer and the formulation buffer, but also in the intermediate buffer conditions encountered during the TFF unit operation.
- Physical stability, density, and viscosity of the protein in the formulation buffer should be investigated as a function of both temperature and concentration of protein. Increase in protein concentration is typically accompanied by logarithmic increase in solution viscosity and the rate of protein aggregation, which are also functions of temperature.

8.7 Drug Product Formulation

Biologic drug products are marketed in several different configurations, including liquid (solution) filled vials or prefilled syringes, lyophilized powder in a vial, or concentrated solutions intended for either dilution in a parenteral fluid before administration or for direct subcutaneous injection using novel delivery devices. Proteins and peptides for parenteral administration are typically formulated as ready-to-use aqueous solutions or as a lyophilized solid mass that is reconstituted with water, isotonic dextrose solution, or isotonic sodium chloride solution immediately before administration; while proteins and peptides for inhalation and nasal routes of administration are typically formulated as dry powders (Mahato and Narang 2018). For stable molecules, nebulization of aqueous solutions is also a viable strategy. For example, Pulmozyme® (dornase alpha) is a solution which is aerosolized by a nebulizer during administration. It contains a CHO-produced recombinant human deoxyribonuclease I, an enzyme which cleaves the DNA present in the mucus of cystic fibrosis patients and reduces viscosity in the lungs, resulting in better clearance of secretions.

8.7.1 Solution Products

The inherent high solubility of proteins, peptides, and nucleic acids allows most biologic products to be manufactured as aqueous solutions. If the stability of the molecule allows, ready-to-use products are preferred from both a manufacturing standpoint and clinical administration standpoint. Formulation development is critical to enhance the stability of the molecule in solution. The development of a suitable pharmaceutical protein formulation usually involves the screening of a number of physiologically acceptable buffers, salts, chelators, anti-oxidants, surfactants, co-solvents, and preservatives (Table 8.3) (Mahato and Narang 2018). Formulation components are selected to address one or more requirements for protein formulations, such as the following (Mahato and Narang 2018):

- Increasing protein solubility by the use of surfactants and/or co-solvents and pH adjustment.
- Using and controlling pH of optimum stability by the use of buffering agents. Selection of an appropriate buffer type and strength is carried out to minimize specific/general-acid/base degradation of the protein.
- Physical stability improvement by the addition of polyhydric alcohols, carbohydrates, and amino acids. These components can hydrogen bond with the protein surface, stabilizing the native protein conformation.
- Stabilization of protein conformation by the addition of co-solvents such as glycerol or poly(ethylene glycol) (PEG), which may decrease the protein surface area in contact with the solvent.

TABLE 8.3

Typical Excipients in Protein Formulations

Category	Type	Functionality	Examples
Buffering agents	Non-amino acid buffers	Ensure optimal pH control	Acetate, citrate, carbonate, HEPES, maleate, phosphate, succinate, tartrate, TRIS
	Amino acids		Histidine
Tonic agents	Salts	Stabilization from aggregation, isotonicity	Sodium chloride, potassium chloride, calcium chloride, magnesium chloride, sodium gluconate, sodium sulfate, ammonium sulfate, magnesium sulfate, zinc chloride
Hydrophilic additives	Sugars	Conformation stabilizing agents, especially in lyophilized formulations, and isotonicity	Glucose, fructose, lactose, maltose, mannitol, sorbitol, sucrose, trehalose, inositol
	Other polyols		Glycerol, cyclodextrins
	Amino acids	Buffering action and non-specific interactions	Alanine, arginine, aspartic acid, lysine, proline, glycine
	Hydrophilic polymers	Polymer matrix in solution	Dextran, PEG
Solubilizers	Surfactants	Reduce surface tension, solubilization	Polysorbate, poloxamer, sodium lauryl sulfate
	Co-solvents	Increase protein solubility	Ethanol
Preservatives	Antioxidants	Preferentially oxidized over the protein substrate	Ascorbic acid, citric acid, glutathione, methionine, sodium sulfite
		Heavy metal binding	EDTA, DTPA, EGTA
	Antimicrobial preservation	Antimicrobial agents	Benzyl alcohol, benzoic acid, chlorobutanol, m-cresol, methyl paraben, propyl paraben

Source: Mahato, R.I. and A.S. Narang, *Pharmaceutical Dosage Forms and Drug Delivery*, 3rd edn., CRC Press, Boca Raton, FL, 2018.

Abbreviations: EDTA, ethylenediamine tetraacetic acid; DTPA, diethylene triamine pentaacetic acid; EGTA, ethylene glycol tetraacetic acid.

- Electrostatic interactions in proteins may be modulated by the alteration of the solvent polarity and dielectric constant, which may reduce the association tendency of a protein.
- Change in the ionic strength of the solution can alter protein surface charge density, impacting the association tendency of the protein molecules.
- Anti-microbial agents may be added to large volume parenteral solutions or multidose vials where repeated puncturing for dose withdrawal is expected, to preserve aqueous solutions of proteins against bacterial and fungal growth.
- Chelating agents and anti-oxidants may be added to prevent metal catalyzed oxidation or oxidation-induced chemical instability.
- Salts, buffers, and/or sugars are added to control osmolarity, which is required for parenteral formulations.

A typical manufacturing and administration process (Figure 8.5) of protein solution involves (Mahato and Narang 2018):

1. Thawing of the bulk drug substance (therapeutic protein).
2. Formulation (dilution and addition of excipients, if BDS is not fully formulated).
3. Filtration for removing any particulate matter and/or bioburden.
4. Filling of drug product in vials or syringes.
5. Visual inspection of filled vials or syringes for the presence of any particulate matter or critical defects in the primary components.
6. Labeling and packaging.
7. Storage and shipment of drug product.

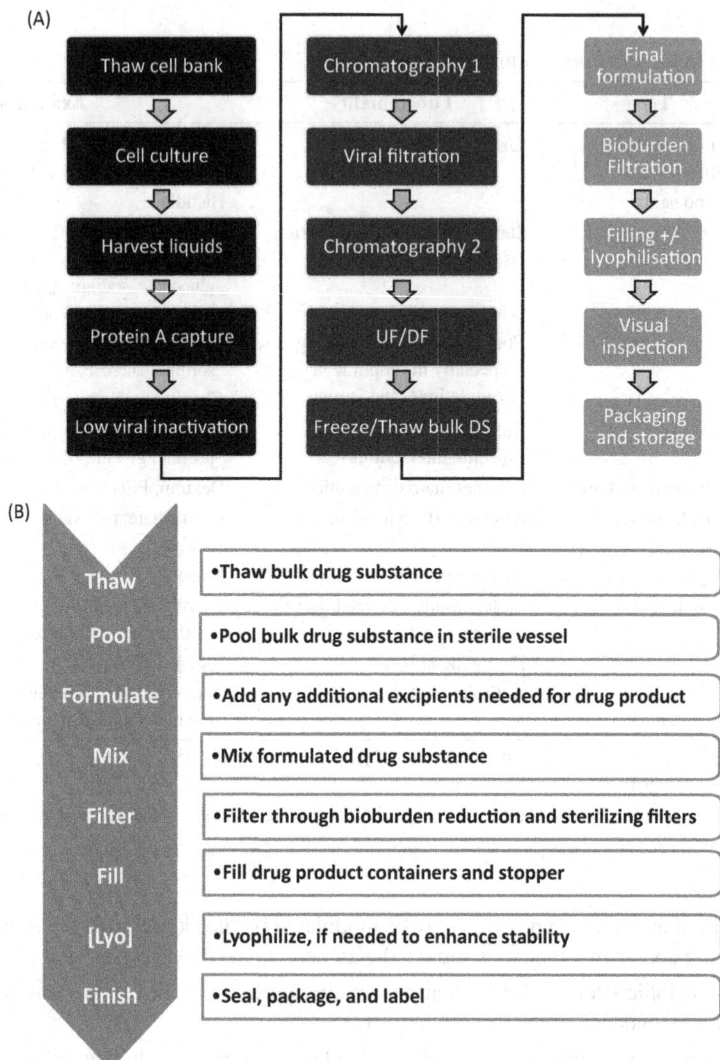

FIGURE 8.5 General schematic (A) for mAb drug substance and drug product process with (B) detailed process flow diagram for drug product manufacture.

Many of these processes may introduce sources of stress for the molecule (Figure 8.6) and affect stability, such as (Mahato and Narang 2018; Narang et al. 2016):

- Exposure to light during manufacturing, inspection, transportation, and storage may lead to oxidation of certain amino acid residues, potentially leading to aggregation.
- Shear and interfacial stress during pumping and filling operations.
- Cavitation during manufacturing and transportation can lead to the formation of microbubbles in the formulation, which can increase the propensity for aggregation and oxidation.
- Protein loss may occur due to adsorption to manufacturing equipment and filter membranes.
- When stainless steel tanks are employed, leaching of metal ions from manufacturing vessels into the protein formulation can lead to metal-catalyzed oxidation and protein instability. However, modern-day manufacturing practices utilize single-use plastic liners in process tanks to avoid the risk of metal leaching and also to eliminate cleaning verification needs and cross-contamination risk.

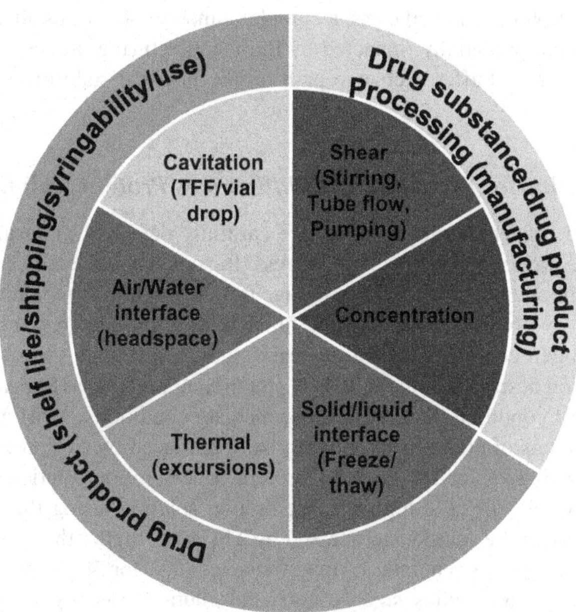

FIGURE 8.6 Types of stress that impact protein stability. (Reproduced from Narang, A.S. et al., *Biopharma Asia*, 5, 1, 2016. With permission.)

Special considerations of the role of formulation and packaging components on protein stability must be considered for long-term storage stability. For example, development of prefilled syringes of drug product solutions requires assessment of stability with the primary packaging components, such as small quantities of silicone oil present in syringes as a lubricant—which can promote protein aggregation and instability. Additionally, the secondary packaging must be able to prevent ambient light exposure that could promote protein oxidation and potential loss of activity.

8.7.2 High Concentration Protein Solution

Of the various injectable routes of parenteral administration of biologic drugs, SC injection is often preferred over intravenous administration since it can allow patient self-administration, reducing the need to visit clinic and the involvement of healthcare professionals in drug administration and improving the convenience for chronic therapies. Traditional SC administration, however, is limited by the amount of liquid that can be injected in a single injection (about 1 mL). This could be a problem for high dose drugs, as increases in protein concentration are often accompanied by significant increases in viscosity and physical instability. With increased viscosity, the force required to expel the drug solution from the syringe increases—reducing the syringeability (fill a syringe from the vial) and injectability (inject from the syringe into the patient) of a solution.

Enabling the SC injection of high dose drugs is an active area of research. Strategies that have been investigated include, for example, the following:

1. The use of slow injection pumps in clinical trials so that the rate of injection is matched to the rate of fluid absorption from the injection site—thus enabling larger injection volumes.
2. The use of autoinjector or semi-manual devices that enable application of high viscosity solutions with minimal force needed from the person administering the dose
3. The use of a recombinant human hyaluronidase enzyme in the drug product formulation (Halozyme's ENHANZE® technology). This enzyme catalyzes the degradation of hyaluronic acid, a constituent of the extracellular matrix, increasing tissue permeability.
4. The use of excipients, such as specific amino acids, to reduce the viscosity of high concentration biologics.

Physical stability of the protein is, nonetheless, a complex function of various attributes, such as conformational structure, that are potentially impacted by the manufacturing process. The case study below exemplifies the importance of buffer exchange path on the physical stability of a high concentration protein solution.

8.7.2.1 Case Study: Buffer Exchange Path Influences Protein Stability[2]

Protein purification and concentration processes are carefully designed to ensure maximum thermodynamic stability of the protein throughout the process. In some special cases, however, specific characteristics of the protein and sensitivity to particular buffer conditions (combination of pH and salt concentration) combined with requirements of the finished drug product (e.g. high concentration solution) can destabilize protein conformation. In this case study, a continuous buffer exchange process at high protein concentration destabilized an Fc fusion protein that is stable at low salt acidic pH condition and at high salt basic pH condition, but not the intermediate conditions of pH and salt concentration. High concentration solutions of an Fc fusion protein were produced by two processes: (a) TFF to high protein concentration or (b)TFF for DF to a low protein concentration solution followed by spin column concentration (SCC) for UF to a higher concentration solution, using the same upstream batch. Aggregation and viscosity of the solutions processed by TFF were higher than those processed by SCC upon storage at 25°C and 40°C for 3 months. After storage at 40°C for 3 months, clear differences were also evident in the hydrodynamic radius, size variants, and solution viscosity. To investigate whether the material produced by the two processes had any conformational differences, both samples were analyzed by DSF using a dye known to interact with hydrophobic residues as the protein unfolds gradually with temperature ramping. While DSC showed similar melting temperature (Tm) of the SCC and the TFF processed material, the interaction of hydrophobic dye with TFF-produced material started at a lower temperature as compared to the SCC-produced material. This suggested subtle conformational perturbation, greater hydrophobic surface exposure, and/or propensity for conformational changes in response to other stressors such as heat (e.g. in the DSF experiment) in the TFF-produced protein (Figure 8.7).

The process buffer (from the last step of downstream purification) and the formulation buffer are the two key players—the starting and the end point—of the buffer exchange process. These buffer systems are usually different due to certain practical constraints, such as the need for salt gradient purification from ion exchange columns. In either of these buffers, thermodynamic stability may

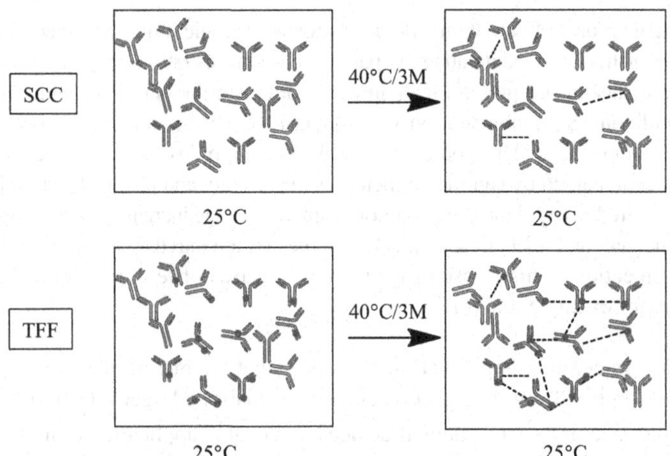

FIGURE 8.7 Schematic of the hypothetical impact of process shear and buffer milieu on viscosity comparing material produced by TFF and SCC processes. (Reproduced from Krause, M.E. et al., *Eur. J. Pharm. Biopharm.*, 131, 60–69, 2018. With permission.)

[2] This section reproduced with permission from Krause et al. (2018).

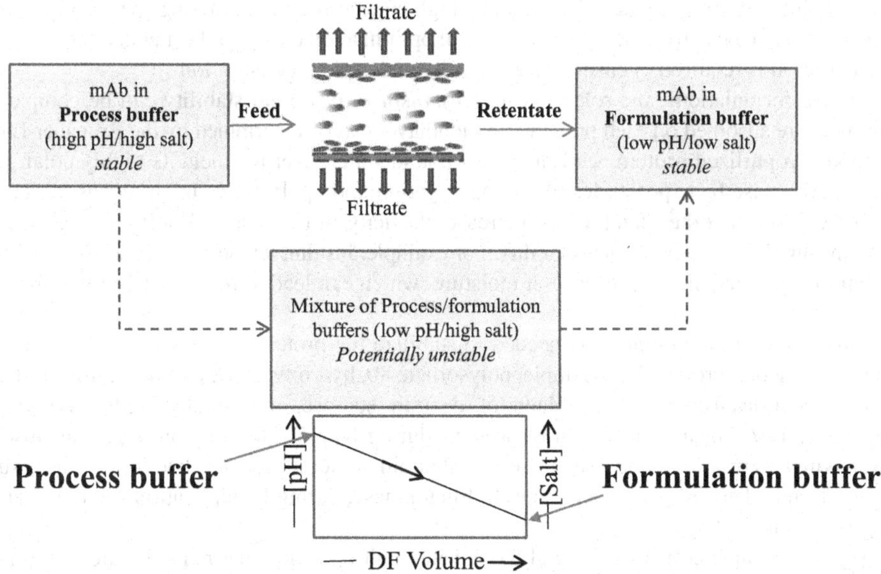

FIGURE 8.8 Schematic showing the TFF for the protein from stable conditions of the process buffer (higher in both pH and salt concentration) to those of the formulation buffer (lower in both pH and salt concentration) via a DF volume exchange that passes through intermediate conditions of lower protein stability. (Reproduced from Krause, M.E. et al., *Eur. J. Pharm. Biopharm.*, 131, 60–69, 2018. With permission.)

impact biochemical stability through solvent exposure of susceptible residues. To maximize protein stability during manufacture and ensure long-term stability, conditions which lead to the formation of partially unfolded intermediates are avoided, and consequently, conditions which stabilize the folded state are sought. Hence, the process buffer and the formulation buffer are selected to maximize protein stability. However, buffer exchange—from the purification buffer to the formulation buffer—can expose a protein to intermediate buffer states that can have differences in buffer type, pH, strength, and salt concentration (Figure 8.8). Unfavorable processing conditions can lead to the formation of partially unfolded intermediates. Retention of these intermediates in the final filtered drug product formulation can lead to differences in protein stability. This buffer exchange "path" can vary by the manufacturing process. The changes produced by the TFF process were attributable to the perturbation of protein conformation in intermediate buffer conditions combined with process shear.

This case study shows that the shearing of the protein can lead to almost indistinguishable immediate changes, but lasting changes that impact protein stability. These findings were further confirmed by applying shear stress to the protein in the formulation buffer at different rate and/or duration and quantifying protein aggregation. Taken together, these data indicated that the shearing of the protein can lead to subtle, yet lasting, differences in the protein conformation that impact protein stability over time.

It is important to emphasize that this case study highlights a special case of protein instability which is not commonly observed. In addition, this case study highlights the dependence of protein conformation and stability on processing and handling conditions during production.

8.7.3 Lyophilized Products[3]

Some proteins are unstable in solution and may not achieve an acceptable shelf-life, even under refrigerated (2°C–8°C) storage conditions. In such cases, freeze-drying or lyophilization is often employed to minimize the kinetics of degradation processes that occur in solutions. Many variables impact the

[3] This section reproduced with permission from Mahato and Narang (2018).

stability of lyophilized drug product. For example, high concentration of reacting species in the protein microenvironment can be detrimental. Further, careful optimization of residual water and protein-binding sugar concentration is required to ensure cake integrity and rapid reconstitution.

In lyophilized formulations, the role of *residual moisture* in protein stability can be complex. The amount of moisture adsorbed on each protein as a monolayer can be determined by the Brunauer-Emmett-Teller method. Lyophilized protein needs a closely bound water layer to shield its highly polar groups, which would otherwise be exposed, leading to aggregation and opalescence upon reconstitution. High moisture content, on the other hand, could increase plasticity in the system leading to high reactivity and compromising the physicochemical stability. For example, insulin, tetanus toxoid, somatotrophin, and human albumin aggregate in the presence of moisture, which can lead to reduced activity, stability, and diffusion.

The optimal formulation components needed to stabilize the protein during and after lyophilization depend on the particular protein. For example, polysorbate 80, hydroxypropyl β-cyclodextrin, and human serum albumin stabilized human IL-2. Mannitol, dextran, sucrose, and trehalose reduced aggregation in lyophilized TNF-α. Sugars stabilize most proteins during lyophilization by protecting against dehydration. Polyvinyl pyrrolidone and bovine serum albumin protect some tetrameric enzymes, such as asparaginase, lactate dehydrogenase, and phosphofructokinase, during lyophilization and rehydration by preventing protein unfolding.

Lyophilization is a high cost, long (several days), batch unit operation that requires careful formulation and process cycle development. The lyophilization process (Figure 8.9) involves freezing of a protein solution to a very low temperature (such as −50°C), followed by primary drying (sublimation of water from the frozen state) under vacuum at a higher temperature (such as −20°C), ensuring the temperature of each vial is maintained below the glass transition temperature in the frozen solution state (Tg') for the formulation. After a long primary drying period, secondary drying involves desorption of the remaining water under vacuum at higher temperature (usually 25°C). Sometimes an annealing step is inserted after initial freezing of solution and before primary drying. Annealing involves short-term increase of product temperature to allow reorientation of polymeric proteins and other components with excipients and provides better cake performance. Completion of each drying stage of lyophilization is ascertained through changes in the humidity in the lyophilization chamber (which indicates the rate of evaporation of water), change in the condensate weight or volume at the vacuum pump (which indicates amount of water removed), alignment of pressure readings from the Pirani gauge and the capacitance manometer, and/or change in product temperature through temperature

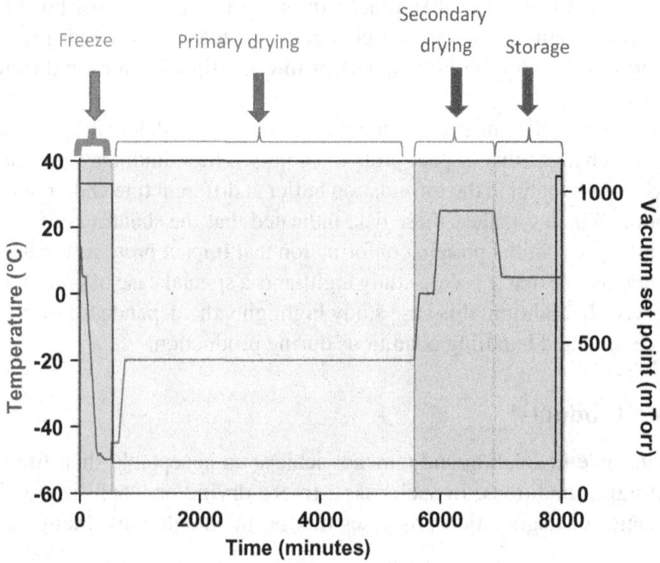

FIGURE 8.9 Schematic illustration of the steps of a conservative lyophilization cycle.

probes inserted in vials (which indicates changes in the heat of sublimation). When the pressure reading from a Pirani gauge matches that of the capacitance manometer, primary drying is complete. The Pirani gauge gives a high reading in the presence of water vapor, and when the gauges align, little water vapor is present.

8.7.4 Combination Products

Many parenteral protein therapeutics are used in life threatening and serious medical conditions, which often require more than one therapeutic agent. The parenteral administration of multiple therapeutic agents can seriously impact the quality of life of the patient, as extended chair time and/or multiple trips to the clinic may be required. Combination products that include, for example, two synergistic large molecules or one large and one small molecule in the same injection can have significant advantage over two separate injections or the need for infusion for drug delivery. However, in some cases, a combination product can increase the risk of physical and chemical instability of both the drugs.

The complexities involved in the development of combination products include analytical characterization, dose titration in clinical studies, and stability assessment. These challenges are being addressed through the development of improved analytical tools and novel technologies, and in the case of stability challenges, the potential use of devices that enable mixing of the two drug solutions immediately before injection—so that the duration of interaction between the two drugs is minimized.

8.8 Other Biologic Drugs

8.8.1 Intermediate Molecular Weight Compounds

A class of drugs that has recently grown in prominence in drug discovery research is that of compounds of molecular weight and properties that are intermediate between the traditional small and large molecular weight drugs. These intermediate molecular weight compounds share some characteristics of both the traditional small and large molecule drugs. For example:

1. Compared to traditional small molecule drugs, these compounds often lack a fixed three-dimensional molecular structure and do not crystallize. They, nonetheless, do possess a comparatively low number of ionizable functional groups and lend themselves to traditional biopharmaceutical assessment tools such as partition co-efficient and cell permeability assays. These compounds can often be prepared as pure, dry powders enabling ease of handling and have higher diffusivity than large molecule drugs.
2. Compared to traditional large molecule drugs, these compounds may not require cell culture for synthesis, can be manufactured using traditional chemical synthetic routes, and are small enough to exhibit diffusive cell membrane permeability, depending upon surface lipophilicity. Similar to large molecule compounds, they do have a three-dimensional conformation that can readily vary depending on the environment.

These drugs are exemplified by peptides, such as cyclosporin, and macrocyclic compounds, such as amphotericin B (Giordanetto and Kihlberg 2014). These compounds are typically synthetic or semi-synthetic in origin and are prepared as parenteral formulations, due to their low oral bioavailability. Considerations in the parenteral formulation of these compounds are fairly similar to those of small molecule and large molecule parenteral drugs, including factors such as pH, ionic strength, osmotic pressure, drug and salt concentration, pyrogenicity, and sterility.

8.8.2 Nucleic Acid Drugs

Nucleic acid drugs include anti-sense oligonucleotides (ODNs), RNA interference (RNAi) technologies such as small interfering RNA (siRNA), plasmid DNA, and virus-based gene therapy approaches, such as the use of recombinant adenoviruses and adeno-associated viruses. Anti-sense ODNs and siRNAs can reduce aberrant protein production, while gene therapy strategies increase the production of exogenous or endogenous therapeutic proteins in the patient's somatic cells.

The smaller nucleic acid drugs, such as siRNAs and ODNs, utilize a solid-phase synthesis process, where each nucleotide or deoxynucleotide derivative is conjugated to the previous nucleotide or deoxynucleotide in the 3′-5′ sequence (which is opposite of the natural process of 5′-3′ direction of polynucleotide synthesis). Each nucleotide addition is carried out with the intervening steps of protection and deprotection of the reactive functional groups. At the end of the desired length of nucleotide synthesis, the synthesized oligonucleotide is detached from the solid phase and brought into aqueous solution.

Larger nucleic acid drugs, such as plasmid DNA vectors and viral gene therapy vectors, such as adenoviruses and adeno-associated viruses, are modified within and isolated from their natural microorganisms of origin. For example, plasmids are isolated from bacteria. The transgene of interest, and other desired sequences, are inserted within the plasmid sequence in vitro using a combination of enzymes, by a process called recombinant DNA technology. The recombined plasmid is transfected into the cells that can replicate the plasmid. After the selection and growth of transfected cells, the plasmid with the transgene is isolated in larger quantities.

The manufactured plasmids or adenoviral vectors are formulated as parenteral solution drug products with considerations similar to the traditional small and large molecule drugs, such as pH, ionic strength, osmotic pressure, drug and salt concentration, pyrogenicity, and sterility.

8.9 Conclusions and Emerging Trends

Cell culture technologies for upstream production of biologics have made much progress over the years in terms of cell densities and product titers. Significant progress has also been made in the use of disposable technologies and process analytical technology that enables process efficiencies, trending, and control. Process improvements, combined with vector design, selection, and amplification approaches, promise greater production efficiencies. Other areas of continued research include the use of human cell lines and understanding the molecular biological basis of variability and cellular responses to environmental conditions using modern genomics and proteomics-based technologies.

For downstream operations, a number of technologies are available to suit the needs of the application (i.e. research, animal, or human studies) and desired level of purity. Protein stability and purity profiles are the key guiding principles during development to ensure consistent safety and activity of the therapeutic, and, as such, multiple molecular attributes are characterized during manufacturing at each stage of clinical development.

Drug product formulation and design continues to evolve with ever greater focus on the patient, emphasizing elements such as: (a) generating stable high concentration therapeutics that reduce the volume of injection and often enabling SC administration of high dose drugs, (b) lyophilization process improvements, (c) rapid developability assessment and high throughput stability screens for different types of stresses, and (d) the use of devices to make medicines more patient friendly.

Taken together, these advances continue to improve the range and scope of biologic drug products and their application to the prevention and treatment of human disease.

ABBREVIATIONS

AEX anion exchange (chromatography)
CDR complementarity-determining region
CEX cation exchange (chromatography)
CHO Chinese hamster ovary
DEAE diethylaminoethyl
DHFR dihydrofolate reductase
DP drug product
DS drug substance
HCP host cell proteins

IEX	ion exchange (chromatography)
IgG	immunoglobulin G
LRV	log10 (i.e., 10-fold) reduction value
mAb	monoclonal antibody
MCB	master cell bank
PAT	process analytical technology
pI	isoelectric point
RVLP	retroviral like particle

ACKNOWLEDGMENTS

Authors gratefully acknowledge the critical review and comments of our Genentech colleagues Inn Yuk, Michael Laird, and Chris Dowd.

REFERENCES

Antoniou, M. N., Skipper, K. A., & Anakok, O. (2013). Optimizing retroviral gene expression for effective therapies. *Hum Gene Ther, 24*(4), 363–374. doi:10.1089/hum.2013.062.

Arakawa, T., Kita, Y., Sato, H., & Ejima, D. (2009). MEP chromatography of antibody and Fc-fusion protein using aqueous arginine solution. *Protein Expr Purif, 63*(2), 158–163. doi:10.1016/j.pep.2008.09.011.

Bareither, R., Bargh, N., Oakeshott, R., Watts, K., & Pollard, D. (2013). Automated disposable small scale reactor for high throughput bioprocess development: A proof of concept study. *Biotechnol Bioeng, 110*(12), 3126–3138. doi:10.1002/bit.24978.

Brorson, K., Krejci, S., Lee, K., Hamilton, E., Stein, K., & Xu, Y. (2003). Bracketed generic inactivation of rodent retroviruses by low pH treatment for monoclonal antibodies and recombinant proteins. *Biotechnol Bioeng, 82*(3), 321–329. doi:10.1002/bit.10574.

Chin, C. L., Chin, H. K., Chin, C. S., Lai, E. T., & Ng, S. K. (2015). Engineering selection stringency on expression vector for the production of recombinant human alpha1-antitrypsin using Chinese Hamster ovary cells. *BMC Biotechnol, 15*, 44. doi:10.1186/s12896-015-0145-9.

Gao, D., Lin, D. Q., & Yao, S. J. (2007). Mechanistic analysis on the effects of salt concentration and pH on protein adsorption onto a mixed-mode adsorbent with cation ligand. *J Chromatogr B Analyt Technol Biomed Life Sci, 859*(1), 16–23. doi:10.1016/j.jchromb.2007.08.044.

Giordanetto, F., & Kihlberg, J. (2014). Macrocyclic drugs and clinical candidates: What can medicinal chemists learn from their properties? *J Med Chem, 57*(2), 278–295. doi:10.1021/jm400887j.

Girot, P., Averty, E., Flayeux, I., & Boschetti, E. (2004). 2-Mercapto-5-benzimidazolesulfonic acid: An effective multimodal ligand for the separation of antibodies. *J Chromatogr B Analyt Technol Biomed Life Sci, 808*(1), 25–33. doi:10.1016/j.jchromb.2004.04.034.

Hober, S., Nord, K., & Linhult, M. (2007). Protein A chromatography for antibody purification. *J Chromatogr B Analyt Technol Biomed Life Sci, 848*(1), 40–47. doi:10.1016/j.jchromb.2006.09.030.

Horowitz, B., Bonomo, R., Prince, A. M., Chin, S. N., Brotman, B., & Shulman, R. W. (1992). Solvent/detergent-treated plasma: A virus-inactivated substitute for fresh frozen plasma. *Blood, 79*(3), 826–831.

Hossler, P., Khattak, S. F., & Li, Z. J. (2009). Optimal and consistent protein glycosylation in mammalian cell culture. *Glycobiology, 19*(9), 936–949. doi:10.1093/glycob/cwp079.

Hu, Z., Hsu, W., Pynn, A., Ng, D., Quicho, D., Adem, Y. et al. (2017). A strategy to accelerate protein production from a pool of clones in Chinese hamster ovary cells for toxicology studies. *Biotechnol Prog, 33*(6), 1449–1455. doi:10.1002/btpr.2467.

Huang, Y. M., Hu, W., Rustandi, E., Chang, K., Yusuf-Makagiansar, H., & Ryll, T. (2010). Maximizing productivity of CHO cell-based fed-batch culture using chemically defined media conditions and typical manufacturing equipment. *Biotechnol Prog, 26*(5), 1400–1410. doi:10.1002/btpr.436.

Johansson, B. L., Belew, M., Eriksson, S., Glad, G., Lind, O., Maloisel, J. L., & Norrman, N. (2003a). Preparation and characterization of prototypes for multi-modal separation aimed for capture of positively charged biomolecules at high-salt conditions. *J Chromatogr A, 1016*(1), 35–49.

Johansson, B. L., Belew, M., Eriksson, S., Glad, G., Lind, O., Maloisel, J. L., & Norrman, N. (2003b). Preparation and characterization of prototypes for multi-modal separation media aimed for capture of negatively charged biomolecules at high salt conditions. *J Chromatogr A*, *1016*(1), 21–33.

Kaleas, K. A., Tripodi, M., Revelli, S., Sharma, V., & Pizarro, S. A. (2014). Evaluation of a multimodal resin for selective capture of CHO-derived monoclonal antibodies directly from harvested cell culture fluid. *J Chromatogr B Analyt Technol Biomed Life Sci*, *969*, 256–263. doi:10.1016/j.jchromb.2014.08.026.

Krause, M. E., Narang, S., Barker, G., Herzer, S., Deshmukh, S., Lan, W. et al. (2018). Buffer exchange path influences the stability and viscosity upon storage of a high concentration protein. *Eur J Pharm Biopharm*, 131, 60–69.

Li, F., Vijayasankaran, N., Shen, A., Kiss, R., & Amanullah, A. (2010). Cell culture processes for monoclonal antibody production. *MAbs*, *2*(5), 466–477.

Mahato, R. I. & Narang, A. S. (2018). *Pharmaceutical Dosage Forms and Drug Delivery* (3rd edn.). Boca Raton, FL: CRC Press.

Narang, A. S., Krause, M. E., & Puri, A. (2016). Formulation considerations for physical stability of high concentration biologics. *Biopharma Asia*, *5*(3), 1.

Ng, S. K. (2012). Generation of high-expressing cells by methotrexate amplification of destabilized dihydrofolate reductase selection marker. *Methods Mol Biol*, *801*, 161–172. doi:10.1007/978-1-61779-352-3_11.

Padawer, I., Ling, W. L., & Bai, Y. (2013). Case study: An accelerated 8-day monoclonal antibody production process based on high seeding densities. *Biotechnol Prog*, *29*(3), 829–832. doi:10.1002/btpr.1719.

Pizarro, S. A., Gunson, J., Field, M. J., Dinges, R., Khoo, S., Dalal, M. et al. (2010). High-yield expression of human vascular endothelial growth factor VEGF(165) in Escherichia coli and purification for therapeutic applications. *Protein Expr Purif*, *72*(2), 184–193. doi:10.1016/j.pep.2010.03.007.

Shukla, A. A. & Aranha, H. (2015). Viral clearance for biopharmaceutical downstream processes. *Pharm Bioprocess*, *3*(2), 127–138.

Yigzaw, Y., Piper, R., Tran, M., & Shukla, A. A. (2006). Exploitation of the adsorptive properties of depth filters for host cell protein removal during monoclonal antibody purification. *Biotechnol Prog*, *22*(1), 288–296. doi:10.1021/bp050274w.

Zhou, J. X., Solamo, F., Hong, T., Shearer, M., & Tressel, T. (2008). Viral clearance using disposable systems in monoclonal antibody commercial downstream processing. *Biotechnol Bioeng*, *100*(3), 488–496. doi:10.1002/bit.21781.

9

Scale-Up Considerations for Orally Inhaled Drug Products

Jeremy Clarke and S. van den Ban

CONTENTS

9.1 Introduction

Distinct to other pharmaceutical dose forms (U.S. Food and Drug Administration 1995, 1997a, 1997b), there is no existing Scale-Up and Post-Approval Changes guidance that details required in vitro and in vivo studies to support changes to manufacturing process, equipment, and scale for orally inhaled drug products (OIDPs). Over the last few years, the United States Food & Drug Administration (US FDA) has advanced recommendations for demonstration of bioequivalence for OIDPs through publication of draft product-specific guidance which details recommended in vitro and in vivo studies to establish bioequivalence (BE) of the test (T) and reference (R) dry powder inhalers (DPIs) (U.S. Food and Drug Administration 2013, 2015a, 2015b, 2016a, 2016b, 2016c, 2017a, 2017b, 2017c). A revised draft to the 1998 draft CDER guidance on "Metered Dose Inhaler (MDI) and Dry Powder Inhaler (DPI) Drug Products—Chemistry, Manufacturing, and Controls Documentation" is also planned for publication during the 2017 calendar year (U.S. Food and Drug Administration 2017d). However, scale-up considerations for OIDPs are not specifically addressed in these guidance documents. Conventionally, scale-up of pharmaceutical manufacturing processes has focused on scaling the component unit operations and generally has been based on empirical approaches. Evolving global regulatory expectations for improved understanding of manufacturing processes to improve product robustness and process capability challenge this scale-up template and highlight the need to develop mechanistic models that can predict drug product manufacturability, performance, and stability from first principles. Other emerging trends that challenge the current scale-up model include personalized medicine where customization of demand will call for manufacture of smaller, more frequent, "on demand" product batches (Gonce and Schrader 2012; Government Office for Science 2013) and technological innovations such as continuous manufacturing (Nasr et al. 2017), designed to facilitate improved consistency of product quality and where scale-up may become irrelevant or at least more modest compared to traditional batch processing.

A consequence of the current lack of a simple bioequivalence measure for OIDPs is a product/process "design freeze" earlier in development than for immediate release (IR) solid oral dosage forms; development of the commercial scale manufacturing process needing to be completed before initiating pivotal clinical studies. In comparison to IR solid oral dosage forms, absolute scale for OIDPs is typically smaller because of a low therapeutic dose (<1 mg) and formulation unit dose (<50 mg for powder-based systems). The use of a delivery device brings an added regulatory complexity as it brings OIDPs under the definition of combination products (U.S. Food and Drug Administration 2017e) and, from a technical standpoint, a manufacturing process for the delivery device also needs to be developed, transferred, and scaled.

In this chapter, scale considerations will be reviewed and exemplified for a dry powder inhaler process train and its constituent manufacturing unit operations. The aim is to demonstrate how scale effects can be anticipated and mitigated through appropriate risk assessment, better understanding of the fundamental science and identification of scale independent descriptors, and predictive tools.

9.2 Regulatory Context

Over 10 years ago, in its final report on "Pharmaceutical cGMPs for the 21st Century—A Risk-Based Approach," US FDA defined the goal of "[a] maximally efficient, agile, flexible manufacturing sector that reliably produces high-quality drug products without extensive regulatory oversight" (U.S. Food and Drug Administration 2004) and improving product quality to help reduce drug shortages and recalls was a key impetus for the launch of FDA's Office of Product Quality (Yu and Woodcock 2015). Interrogation of FDA Inspectional Observation Summaries ("483s") (U.S. Food and Drug Administration 2014a) gives an insight into factors that contribute to poor product quality, which include scale-related decisions such as "*equipment design, scale and location.*"

Guidance for industry on process validation (U.S. Food and Drug Administration 2011) details how product knowledge and process understanding should evolve through the process validation lifecycle and that "*...to understand the commercial process sufficiently, the manufacturer will need to consider the effects of scale...*" and "*...activities, such as experiments or demonstrations at laboratory or pilot scale, also assist in... prediction of performance of the commercial process....*" Scale is also identified as an important issue in the FDA Compliance Policy Guide (U.S. Food and Drug Administration 2016d) which advises agency staff on the standards and procedures to apply when determining compliance, "*...[readiness for manufacturing assessment includes] a review of the firm's scale-up studies...[and] firm may need to change the submitted proposed commercial process as scale-up studies are completed and knowledge is gained....*" From the EMA perspective (European Medicines Agency 2016), where a sponsor proposes a range of batch sizes, it must be justified that variations in batch size would not adversely alter the drug product critical quality attributes (CQAs). Process parameters that have not been shown to be scale independent will thus need to be revalidated once further scale-up is proposed post-authorization. Additionally, dry powder inhalers are considered "specialized dosage forms" for which the sponsor should provide production scale validation in the marketing authorization application dossier unless otherwise justified. However, it is noted that in its concept paper on revision of the guideline on the pharmaceutical quality of inhalation and nasal products, an item identified to address in the revision is "*complementary guidance how to justify that the manufacturing process may be considered as a standard process in accordance with the process validation guideline*" (European Medicines Agency 2017a). Finally, where a design space is presented in the dossier, any multivariate interactions between the design space parameters need to be studied, which should include a consideration of scale (European Medicines Agency 2017b). ICH Q12 Technical and Regulatory Considerations for Pharmaceutical Product Lifecycle Management (International Council for Harmonization of Technical Requirements for Pharmaceuticals for Human Use 2014) seeks to establish a framework for enhanced management of post-approval change, enabled by clear definition of the elements of the control strategy that would be subject to regulatory submission if changed, a risk-based categorization of reporting of change (notification, prior approval), and the use of post-approval change management protocols (PACMP) as a mechanism for prior agreement for future changes such as changes in scale.

Within the process validation lifecycle, Table 9.1. indicates where decisions related to scale can impact product quality:

TABLE 9.1

Product Validation Life Cycle—Impact of Scale on Product Quality

Process Validation Lifecycle Stage	Where Can It Go Wrong?
Process Design Define commercial manufacturing process based on knowledge gained through development and scale-up activities	• Choice/design of equipment and manufacturing process
Process Qualification Evaluate process design to determine if the process is capable of reproducible commercial manufacturing	• Effects of full scale not taken into consideration during design • Deviations from envisioned industrial process at pilot scale development, e.g. automation of manual processes, transport of pharmaceutical intermediates across manufacturing sites • Restrictions introduced by health, safety, and environmental legislation • Level and consistency of instrumentation to assess process performance similarity • Insufficient physicochemical characterization of output from each unit operation • Acceptance criteria not properly established as part of technology transfer
Continued Process Verification Routine production provides ongoing assurance that process remains in a state of control	• Effects of process changes not adequately studied or monitored

9.3 Developing Understanding of the Manufacturing Process

For the purposes of this chapter, scale considerations are restricted to typical unit operations of the manufacturing process for a dry powder inhaler which involve a number of consecutive operations of powder handling and powder transfer—particle size reduction (micronization), powder blending, and powder filling. As evidenced by several European public assessment reports (European Medicines Agency 2009, 2013, 2014), the "white space" between unit operations can also be impactful on product quality, and consideration of the impact of hold times of any process intermediates ("laagering") should also be considered during process development and scale-up.

A process flow can be created for each unit operation highlighting input attributes and process parameters that may impact the quality attributes of the output material. Criticality of each process parameter to product critical quality attributes is risk assessed based on scientific understanding and prior knowledge and, commensurate with the risk to product quality, the product control strategy can be established. Scale impact can be risk assessed under a failure mode effect analysis (FMEA) type scheme, the aim of this chapter being to provide the necessary scientific understanding to inform the knowledge base for such risk assessment.

For scale-up considerations related to drug substance and delivery device, the interested reader is directed towards, respectively, Chapters 7–8 and 18–21.

9.4 Particle Size Reduction

A representative process flow for micronization is provided in Figure 9.1.

The therapeutic effect of inhaled medicines depends on the dose deposited and its distribution within the lung, which in turn depend on the aerodynamic particle size distribution of the inhaled aerosol.

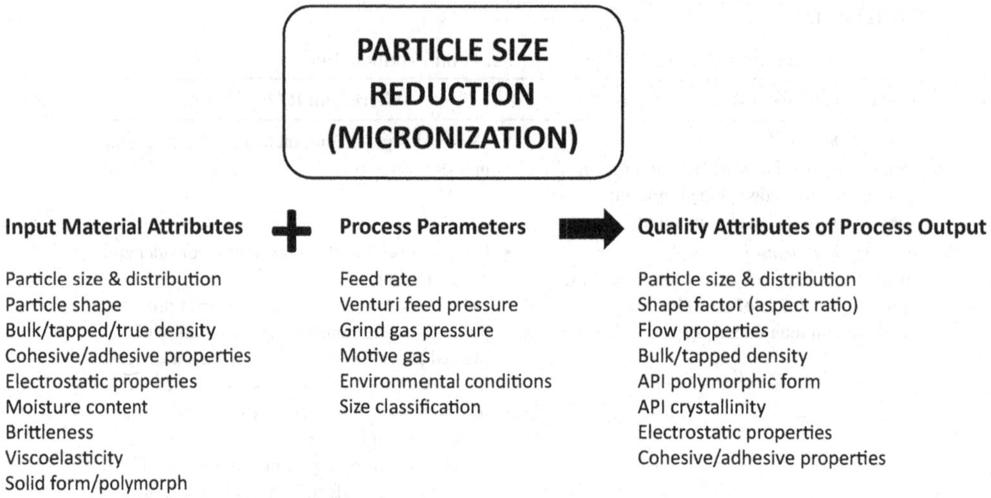

PARTICLE SIZE REDUCTION (MICRONIZATION)

Input Material Attributes		Process Parameters		Quality Attributes of Process Output
Particle size & distribution		Feed rate		Particle size & distribution
Particle shape		Venturi feed pressure		Shape factor (aspect ratio)
Bulk/tapped/true density		Grind gas pressure		Flow properties
Cohesive/adhesive properties		Motive gas		Bulk/tapped density
Electrostatic properties		Environmental conditions		API polymorphic form
Moisture content		Size classification		API crystallinity
Brittleness				Electrostatic properties
Viscoelasticity				Cohesive/adhesive properties
Solid form/polymorph				

FIGURE 9.1 Particle size reduction (micronization) process flow diagram.

For formulations containing particulate drug such as inhalation powders, it is thus critical to control particle size of the input active pharmaceutical ingredient (API), typically within the range 1–5 μm (cross reference Chapter 4?).

While a broad range of constructive bottom-up technologies have been described to engineer particles in the respirable range by first intent (Clarke 2006), most marketed dry powder inhalers are formulated using drug substance(s) particle size reduced using the spiral jet mill/micronizer. Effective size reduction in a spiral jet mill depends on geometry of the mill design (diameter of grinding chamber, shape, number, and angle of grinding nozzles), as well as operational parameters (solids feed rate, gas mass flow rate, and mechanical properties of material to be micronized). For a target particle size and throughput, control of the solids feed rate and gas mass flow rate assures a consistent output particle size distribution. The principle of operation of the spiral micronizer is based on acceleration of particles in a high velocity jet to promote particle-particle collisions with particles at relative low velocity present in the mill chamber although particle-wall collisions may occur. The micronized powder is separated from the gas flow, often via a cyclone. The cyclone design, diameter, and gas entry velocity impact particle-air separation efficiency and hence impact the final product particle size distribution obtained. Use of high efficiency cyclone designs permit an increased collection efficiency for particles less than approximately 5 μm.

In the mill chamber, powder is often introduced with a carrier or injector gas, typically nitrogen or compressed air. The Venturi effect and injector position create a relatively low pressure drop to introduce the powder from the feeder at a controlled rate into the carrier gas. The powder is then transported in its carrier gas and "injected" into the mill chamber. In the mill chamber, high velocity jets emanate from each nozzle; the velocity of the jet is sonic at the throat (choked flow, operation above the critical pressure ratio). Final expansion of the gas will take place beyond the nozzle throat. The Venturi effect results in particles being taken into the jet and accelerated to create high-intensity particle-particle collisions with particles moving at relatively low speed in the mill chamber (Zhao and Schurr 2002) have demonstrated the impact of different motive gases (helium, steam, compressed air, nitrogen, carbon dioxide) on the grinding limit (asymptote of the particle size distribution), lower molecular weight motive gases achieving a finer grinding limit due to higher sonic velocity and, therefore, kinetic energy.

The nozzles have a secondary function impacting the micronized particle size. The nozzles are equally spaced and directed or angled into the mill chamber such that the high velocity jets emanating the nozzles form a grinding zone and classification zone impacting maximum particle size or cut size; particles smaller than the cut size will exit the mill, while larger particles are retained until size reduced. The concentration of the product affects both the cut point and the separation efficiency of the classifier.

If the powder concentration in the micronizer is high, separation efficiency may deteriorate, resulting in coarser particles separated along with fine particles (Brodka-Pfeiffer et al. 2003). The mill chamber height and classifier height can impact residence time in the chamber and thereby size reduction. Equally, a wide slit width between the micronizing chamber and cyclone results in a lower suction effect and, consequently, additional comminution through increased micronizer residence time (Zuegner et al. 2006). Pressure drop over the cyclone is an important parameter to indirectly monitor separation performance (Dirgo and Leith 1985).

Visualization of micronization phenomena in spiral jet milling has been explored utilizing triboluminescent substances (manganese-activated zinc sulphide) (Kuerten and Rumpf 1966; Muschelknautz et al. 1970). The light intensity of manganese-activated zinc sulphide is proportional to newly created surface area is, hence, indicative of the micronization process. The impact of nozzle diameter, shape, angle, and arrangement were studied with particle size reduction observed to occur near the edge and back of the high velocity jet. The introduction position of the powder into the mill chamber and relative high injector pressure were found to distort the definition of the grinding zone and classification zone, resulting in a coarser product. Hence, geometrically, number of nozzles, size, and angle, as well as injection location is important to achieve requisite size reduction and operational performance.

The kinetic energy transferred from the high velocity gas jet to the particles is often taken as a measure of the intensity of collision. At choked flow (velocity at the nozzle throat is sonic), the kinetic energy of the gas is proportional to the mass gas flow rate, and dependent on the nozzle diameter, number of nozzles, pressure, and temperature of the gas. Often the temperature impact is considered negligible and mass (grinding) gas flow rate may then be approximated by grind gas pressure. The specific energy is the ratio of kinetic energy in the gas flow rate to the powder feed rate and is a macroscopic measure of the collision intensity and thus an important consideration in scale-up. However, specific energy may not be a suitable indicator of micronization performance because the effective acceleration distance may be limited, e.g. due to powder concentration in the mill and material specific breakage properties.

An increase in specific energy may result in a transition from particle breakage to particle attrition or fragmentation due to the stress required to initiate and propagate a crack on a particle surface (Rumpf 1973; Vogel and Peukert 2002). Operating above this transition may result in an increase in "fine" particulates (Midoux et al. 1999) or amorphous content (Ticehurst et al. 2000; Brodka-Pfeiffer 2003). Powder breakage behavior can result in a powder with heterogenous surface energetics due to preferential exposure of new crystal facets that can vary in facet specific surface energy (Shah et al. 2017). This can potentially modulate the balance of cohesive/adhesive particulate forces within the formulation and consequent impact on aerosolization performance.

For other products, e.g. due to material specific breakage properties, the specific energy may not be a performance differentiator and particle size distribution is limited by classification. Rodnianski et al. (2013) provide a derivation of cut size as a function of micronizer design, operating parameters, and particle sphericity, while MacDonald et al. (2016) describe a derivation for spiral jet mill cut size as a function of micronization settings, gas thermodynamic properties, and empirically derived constants for the material, corroborated by experimental evidence and prior knowledge from the scientific literature. A scale-up methodology is proposed for a high value material by using a small-scale mill to determine the material specific constants of the high value material and a cheaper surrogate material to determine mill specific constants at increased scale.

Rumpf 1960 reported on an analysis of mill chamber sizing for key geometrical parameters impacting performance. Geometrical similarity, impacting grinding, important in scale-up, may be based on machine mill chamber diameter, nozzle number, and nozzle diameter. For classification, classifier height, chamber height, and cyclone design are important to maintain performance at scale (Rodnianski et al. 2013; MacDonald et al. 2016).

Complementary to empirical experimentation described above is the use of computational simulation of the micronization process. Significant advances in computer technology and micronization modeling based on combining discrete element modeling (DEM) and computational fluid dynamics (CFD) to model particle motion and comminution provide capability to evaluate performance for equipment design, operating parameters, and mechanical breakage properties (Brosh et al. 2014).

Regulatory guidance on pharmaceutical quality of OIDPs highlights drug substance physicochemical properties which can influence product performance and thus necessitate evaluation during development and consideration in technology transfer and scale-up. For any product where drug substance is not in solution, the specification must include a control on particle size and particle size distribution. Consequently, the manufacturing process must be designed to provide precise control of particle size to deliver requisite product performance. Extant fundamental understanding of the micronization process reviewed above permits definition of clear principles to guide process scale-up and establishment of process controls to maintain a consistent particle size distribution across scales.

9.5 Powder Mixing

A representative process flow for the powder mixing unit operation is provided in Figure 9.2.

The formulation of inhalation powders typically contains particle size-reduced drug substance(s), a larger particle size excipient (carrier), and potentially additional components (e.g. magnesium stearate, leucine) to assure product performance and/or chemical/physical stability. Risk, cost, and time to qualify new excipients for lung delivery currently limit the choice of carrier to those materials with an established safety profile such as the sugars: lactose, glucose, and mannitol, with lactose monohydrate being predominant and well recognized as a safe excipient for inhalation formulations (Baldrick and Bamford 1997). Typically, formulation of an inhaled powder requires a balance of fine and coarse carrier particles to optimize both powder flow characteristics (Zeng et al. 1999) and powder aerosolization. While most products employ lactose monohydrate as a single excipient, the emergence of "dual excipient platform"-based products has been noted in a recent review (Shur et al. 2016).

The primary objective in powder mixing is to achieve uniformity of content. For oral solid dosage forms, technologies have been described that improve mix uniformity through various wet and dry coating processes, e.g. Huang et al. (2017) describe application of high intensity vibratory (acoustic) mixing as a dry coating approach to reduce cohesion of a model drug substance (micronized acetaminophen) using nano-silica powder which resulted in improved content uniformity of blends of processed acetaminophen powders with Avicel 102 compared to uncoated controls or those where silica was added during mixing. For dry powder inhalers, the choice of processing technologies is more restricted as, in addition to ensuring uniformity of content, close attention should also be given in formulation design to ensure resultant bulk powder properties (e.g. density, cohesion, shear properties, compressibility) and formulation microstructure are suitable for subsequent powder filling processes and product performance. The product is often

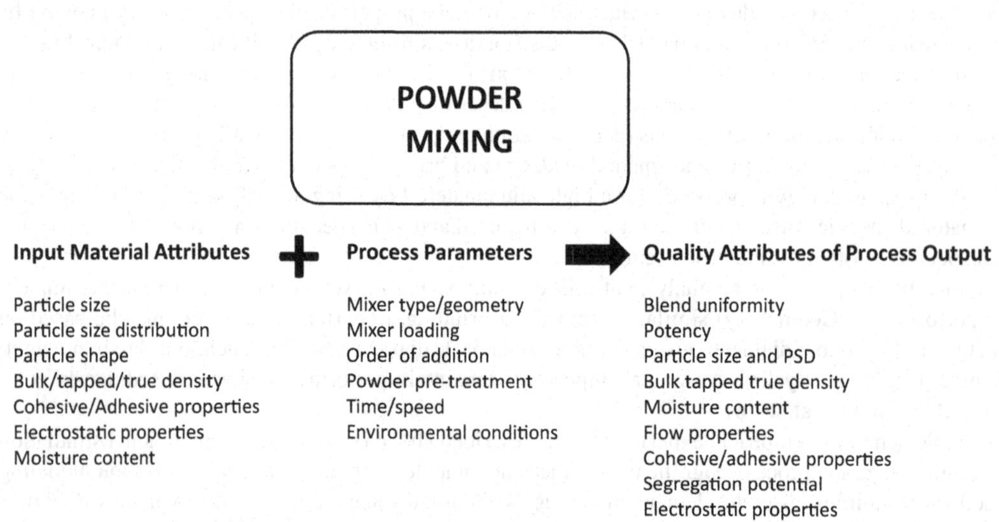

FIGURE 9.2 Powder mixing process flow diagram.

deliberately designed to be "metastable": at a macroscopic scale, the formulation must be sufficiently cohesive to facilitate precise/accurate filling and dose emission, while at a microscopic (particulate) scale, the balance of cohesive/adhesive forces must ensure reproducible aerosolization (Figure 9.3). As such, for dry powder inhalers, the product developer's dilemma is the need to assure short term formulation robustness (i.e. sufficient physical stability to survive the rigors of processing, transportation) and facilitate aerosolization when dosed to the patient. Practically, this often results in empirical optimization of the formulation and manufacturing process due to a paucity of knowledge on the influence of mixing processes on properties of the bulk formulation and downstream performance of the drug product (Shur et al. 2008). Shah et al. (2017) highlight the gap in mechanistic understanding of interaction of formulation and processing factors and the opportunity to use the understanding of how particle processing affects particle properties to optimize desired particle interactions and achieve optimal behavior of the powder bulk. Kaialy (2016) has reviewed interactions of variables in mixing (equipment, time, speed, order on addition) and physicochemical properties (particle size distribution, shape distribution, electrostatic charge, bulk, and surface properties) on content uniformity and aerosolization performance.

Nguyen et al. (2015) provide a detailed mixing mechanism map, identifying the following transformations:

1. **Mixing** between carrier particles and fine-particle agglomerates (random mixing)
2. **Deagglomeration** of fine (drug) particle agglomerates as a consequence of mechanical collision during mixing (drug-drug agglomerates with coarse carrier and/or walls of the mixing vessel and erosion/abrasion of agglomerates against coarse carrier particles
3. **Adhesion** of fine particles onto carrier surfaces by for, e.g. van der Waals forces
4. **Redistribution and exchange** of fine particles with carrier particles while press-on forces may cause compression of fine particles onto the carrier substance

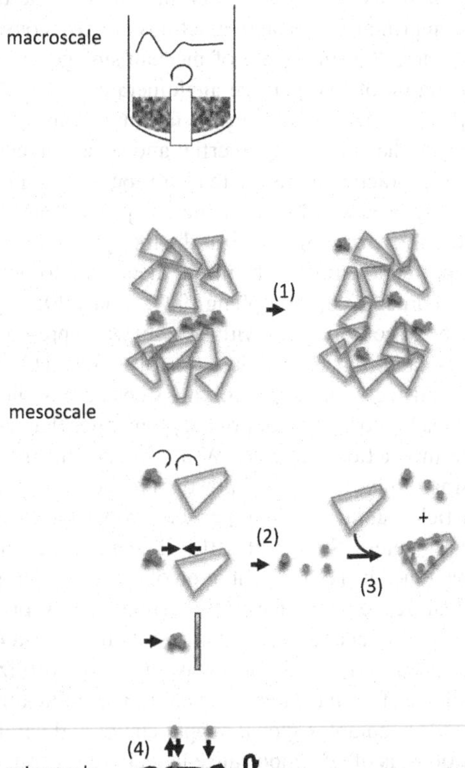

FIGURE 9.3 Illustration of mechanisms in mixing of inhalation powders across scales.

Grasmeijer et al. (2013) report an evaluation of the interactions between mixing time and other process variables (drug type, carrier size fraction, inhalation flow rate) on product performance (aerosolization efficiency) for several model dry powder formulations processed by low shear mixing. Observed interactions between mix quality (i.e. changes in drug particle morphology, particle size distribution, and mechanical stress-induced disorder) and product performance were consistent with a balance of the transformations described in the mixing mechanism map of Nguyen et al. (2015).

Literature reports describe the use of mixers based on different operating principles, which can be categorized as per Scale-Up and Post-Approval Changes equipment addendum (U.S. Food and Drug Administration 2014b) as low shear diffusion mixers and high shear convection mixers. Sarkar et al. (2017) describe a study of the mixing kinetics of a model binary system (fine lactose d50 < 5 µm as surrogate API with a coarse lactose carrier, d50 >> 100 µm) in low shear and high shear mixers, targeted at providing guidance on rational choice of blender. The study results confirm that irrespective of blender type, energy input is key to forming an adhesive mixture, but the significant process variables impacting mix quality differ between the mixer types (rotation speed and drug ratio for high shear mixer, speed alone for low shear mixer). Additionally, the advantage of short processing time within the manufacturing environment for high shear mixer needs to be balanced against potential abrasion of fine particles which could create amorphous material with attendant risk to physical stability for sensitive APIs. Hertel et al. (2017) report the influence of high shear mixing parameters (mixing time and rotation speed) and mixing order on the aerosolization performance of ternary component inhalation powders. Reduced aerosolization performance because of an increase in press-on forces at higher energy consumption of the mixer was observed on prolonged mixing time (linear correlation to press-on force) or higher rotation speed (quadratic relationship with press-on force).

Bridson et al. (2007) investigated and highlight the impact of the different mode of energy input into the high shear mixing of lactose monohydrate dependent on blade design; a knife edge-shaped blade was considered to induce frictional forces, while for a blunt-shaped blade, inertial forces dominated. In mixer design, this emphasizes the need to ensure powder is well-mixed on a macroscopic scale while ensuring that microscopic scale effects on primary particle interactions are also considered.

Nguyen at al. (2015) investigated the time scale of mechanisms governing the mixing process and reported the initial deagglomeration of fine-particle agglomerates as the rate limiting step to achieve blend uniformity based on particle size monitoring in mixing. Consequently, agglomerate size and strength are important, impacting the energy (e.g. inertial and shear forces) required to break-up cohesive API agglomerates. Industrial practice therefore tends to focus on application of high shear mixers in the commercial manufacturing process which provide adequate shear to overcome the agglomerate strength and disperse the API in the carrier and prevent the likelihood of drug-rich agglomerates.

Process design strategies reported to enhance the initial dispersion for low active content dry powder formulations include component order of addition (Zeng 1999; Kaialy 2016), geometric mixing (Venables and Wells 2001), and pre-mixing of cohesive API with lactose, while pre-coating inner walls of the mixing vessel with carrier powders can mitigate drug loss (Kaialy 2016). However, it should be noted that application of geometric mixing using multiple pre-mixing steps necessitates increased drug concentrations in initial blends that may lead to formation of drug agglomerates that are difficult to deagglomerate.

The importance of particle interactions (van der Waals forces, electrostatic force, capillary force, solid bridge force) to processing of pharmaceutical powders is the subject of a recent critical review of factors that can influence particle interactions, i.e. particle properties, environmental conditions, and powder processing methods/parameters (Shah et al. 2017). The metastable nature of the dry powder formulation will, in mixing, impact the level of redistribution of the active onto the carrier particle. Hence, carrier particle morphology features, e.g. crevices, large irregularities, or other deformations have an apparent increased adhesion ("highly active sites") that results in a greater stability and will in effect lead to a "sink," and the increased carrier adhesion may impact aerosolization performance (Kaialy 2016). Consistency of the carrier surface morphology is an important factor in a commercial process to meet the requirements of a modern complex global supply chain, and careful consideration to method of manufacture, storage conditions, is of key importance in technology transfer and scale-up from R&D to manufacturing. Note that industrial scale manufacturing processes may sometimes include a sieving or screening step of the API and carrier which can also impact their physicochemical properties and mixing performance. Formulation design strategies to minimize the impact of carrier surface morphology variation include the use of ternary excipients to control the adhesive force (e.g. laminar molecules such as magnesium stearate, Young et al. 2002) and addition of lactose fines in similar size range to micronized drug substance either during mixing process or as a pre-conditioning step (Zeng et al. 1999; Young et al. 2008; Kaialy 2016). Additionally, Young et al. (2008) report the potential of engineered carrier surfaces that are spatially uniform in adhesion of API to carrier with optimized API/carrier adhesion force to promote content uniformity and aerosolization performance. This offers opportunity to reduce sensitivity of product performance to the mixing process and scale-up thereof.

Moisture content and the environmental conditions (i.e. relative humidity and temperature) in mixing are important, as moisture may promote local dissolution and recrystallization leading to irreversible powder aggregation due to solid bridge formation (Hickey et al. 1990).

In liquid mixing, the concept of scale-up is well established and documented e.g. *Perry's Chemical Engineering Handbook* (Green 2007) and scale-up may be based on dimensionless power and Reynolds curves, specific power, as a function of impeller design. Conversely, powder mixing scale-up is relatively less well established, and there is a paucity of reported data in the literature. The rate limiting step of the mixing process as described by Nguyen et al. (2015) should inform the approach to scale-up and, dependent on the mechanism, scale-up may be based on mixing time or mixing speed or both. Scale-up rules for processing conditions are kinematic in nature, and often scale-up is based on maintaining a power relationship of impeller rpm (N) and diameter, D, e.g. ND^a, such as Froude number or tip speed of the impeller (Tardos 2004). In powder mixing, the impeller movement through the bulk results in shear, convection, dispersion, and the shear and normal forces generated introduce an overall motion of the powder inside the vessel and promotes deagglomeration of fine drug particulates. The stress transmission from the impeller to the powder is limited in range and insufficient in transmitting stresses very far into the powder bed. The resultant powder flow pattern is complex and varies with size and design of mixer; visual flow patterns of toroidal flow, roping, and bumping flow have been observed (Plank et al. 2003). The level of cohesion in the powder blend may impact the ability to impart shear and insertional forces on the bulk, for example, an increase in blender speed may aerate or levitate the bed, resulting in less effective transfer of momentum to the powder blend. This has been described as a powder bed that "bumps" up and down as the impeller moves underneath (Plank et al. 2003; Tardos 2004). Plank et al. (2003) have reported a temporary pause in powder movement consistent with the time delay required for the blade to move the powder bed. The use of a power-law for ND on scaling may hence shift the relative contribution of shear and impact to the powder mix and potentially impact product performance.

Tardos et al. (2004) investigated the magnitude of forces inside the granulator with calibrated particles to measure the shear-force distribution within the mixer as a basis for scale-up in high shear granulation. An index for the power-law-based scaling of ND, of 0.5 is based on Froude, while an index of 1 is equivalent to tip speed. To scale on constant shear stress, Tardos et al. (2004) empirically derived a value of 0.8 for a tangential impeller, while a coefficient of 0.85 was found for a radial impeller to scale from a 2.5 L to a 25 L high shear mixer. Constant shear stress across scale is likely important in the deagglomeration of fine particle agglomerates, and thus a power-law with an index of 0.8–0.85 is proposed as a reasonable starting point on which to base scale-up of dry powder inhaled mixtures in high shear mixers.

The importance of impeller design and geometrical similarity must be considered (Muzzio and Alexander 2005). Key geometric dimensions include powder bed height to diameter ratio, impeller geometry, and impeller design. For example, Tardos et al. (2004) reported the tangential-blade impeller transmitted more shear to the powder relative to the radial-blade impeller and bed height to diameter ratio impacted shear stress transmission. Commercially available mixing equipment is often designed with geometrically similar bowls sizes while various impellers designs may be available for each scale to optimize performance.

Additional insight into the powder mixing process has been gained through use of advanced techniques, such as positron emission particle tracking (PEPT), that track a radioactive labeled particle to permit the measurement of the flow pattern and shear force field to understand the impact of mechanical initiated motion into the powder (Bridgwater 2004). However, the size of the PEPT machine currently limits the size of the machine that can be investigated (Bridgwater 2004) and thus insight into process scale-up. For example, Hassanpour (2009) reports the flow field for a Cyclomix 1L and 5L and observed powder speed to be significantly less than the impeller speed (reflecting limited transmission of shear stress), significant differences in flow field at the two scales investigated, and the presence of high shear zones in the mixer rather than a uniform shear force distribution.

Shah et al. (2017) review the use of modeling approaches such as DEM to predict interparticle interactions, concluding that the ability to authentically simulate full scale commercial processes is limited by uncertainties over particle polydispersity (size and shape) and high demand on computational resources to model sufficient particles. Nevertheless, a recent study (Yang et al. 2015) has reported the use of DEM to evaluate effect of electrostatic force on particle mixing in a vibrating container and explored how different adhesive forces affect mixing behavior. Acknowledging the complexity of computational modeling of inter-particulate interactions during mixing to derive a mechanistic model, Barling et al. (2015) have proposed an iron oxide tracer method to assure equivalence of mixing conditions across mixer type, scale, and operating conditions and provide a more quantitative approach to blender scale-up. Dispersion of the iron oxide agglomerates and subsequent deagglomeration to primary particles during the mixing process is monitored by colorimetric measurement of hue and hue intensity, allowing construction of formulation deagglomeration/dispersion curves to predict equivalent mixing conditions and blend quality when moving to a new mixer.

Recognizing the multivariate influences of powder properties on product performance, Elia et al. (2016) describe the use of principal component analysis (PCA) to understand the correlation structure of the measured variables and partial least squares (PLS) regression to establish predictive models between powder characterization tests (rheology, density, particle size) and in vitro product performance (dose emission and aerosolization) as an aid to scale-up by providing a unit operation-by-unit operation insight into performance contribution rather than rely on end product testing. This places more emphasis on the use of powder characterization tests, for example, Yu et al. (2011) report prediction of powder flowability from particle size and shape distributions, while Wang et al. (2016) describe prediction of optimal flow for multicomponent mixtures based on shear cell measurements.

In conclusion, the complexity of the various interacting and competing mechanisms within the mixing operation is not fully understood and, consequentially, optimization is often empirical. Practically, optimal mixing conditions are established for every formulation; the understanding and prediction of interparticle forces in adhesive mixtures for inhalation require more research to enable in silico optimization. Efficiency of mixing is related to inertial, frictional, and shear force applied in mixing, and dependent on mixing equipment/conditions, physicochemical characteristics, carrier payload, and batch size (Kaialy 2016), and impacted by external factors, e.g. environmental conditions, handling protocols employed in an industrial set-up, e.g. screening and charging. The complex mechanisms involved in high shear powder mixing, the need to optimize various product attributes, the lack of established methods for scale-up, and absence of simple bioequivalence measure for OIDPs currently drive an approach where product is developed at the intended commercial manufacturing scale to avoid scale-up. However, clearly batch size selection at point of development may constrain future flexibility in the life cycle of the product.

9.6 Powder Filling

An illustrative inputs/process/outputs diagram for powder filling unit operation is presented in Figure 9.4.

Reproducible subdivision of inhalation powders at low dose into the inhalation powder primary pack (which may be a capsule, blister, reservoir, etc.) is challenging due to the typically low unit dose weight (Eskandar et al. 2011), which can range from <10 mg and up to 50 mg. Designing a robust manufacturing process requires a good understanding of the interaction between input material attributes and filling process parameters, and it is important that the selected dosing principle assures fill weight/content uniformity of unit doses as well as pharmaceutical performance (dose emission and aerosolization). Dosing principles are typically volumetric, e.g. dosator technologies used for encapsulation suitable for low dose necessitating challenging narrow dosator nozzle designs. Alternate dosing principles may be employed, but as evident from the patent literature, these tend to be proprietary in nature.

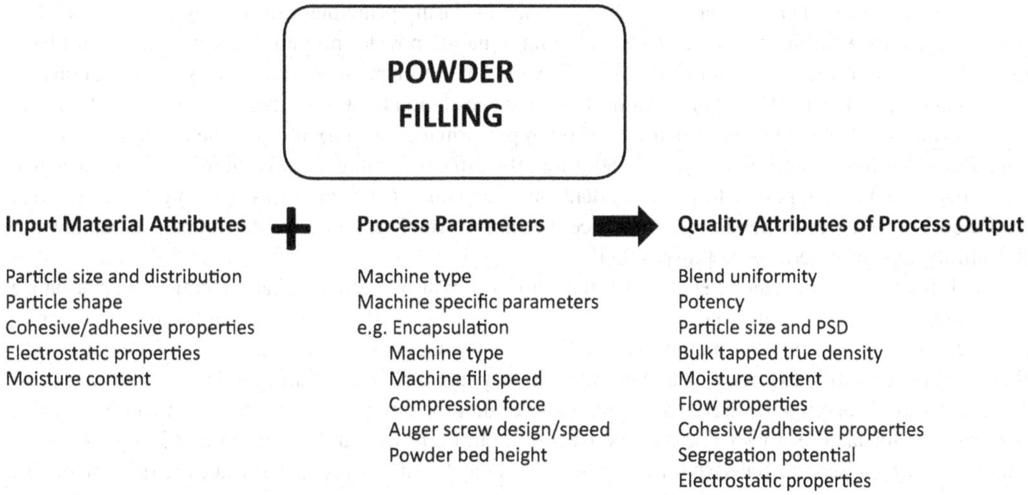

POWDER FILLING

Input Material Attributes + **Process Parameters** ➡ **Quality Attributes of Process Output**

Input Material Attributes

Particle size and distribution
Particle shape
Cohesive/adhesive properties
Electrostatic properties
Moisture content

Process Parameters

Machine type
Machine specific parameters
e.g. Encapsulation
Machine type
Machine fill speed
Compression force
Auger screw design/speed
Powder bed height

Quality Attributes of Process Output

Blend uniformity
Potency
Particle size and PSD
Bulk tapped true density
Moisture content
Flow properties
Cohesive/adhesive properties
Segregation potential
Electrostatic properties

FIGURE 9.4 Powder filling process flow diagram.

The typical filling cycle for a dosator-based system involves the following steps (Loidolt et al. 2017):

1. Dosator nozzle enters a conditioned powder bed.
2. Dosator nozzle progresses through powder bed until reaching a defined minimum distance from the bottom; compression of the powder occurs during this step controlled by the dosing height and powder bed height (compression may also result from mechanically controlled tamping).
3. Filled dosator nozzle is withdrawn from the powder bed and positioned over an empty capsule body.
4. Powder plug is ejected from dosator into the capsule body and the cap secured.

Powder flow characteristics of the inhalation powder must enable commercially viable manufacturing throughput. Powder cohesion must be balanced such that it is sufficient to form a stable plug for transfer without loss of the full or part of the unit dose, but also ensure requisite dose emission and aerosolization performance. The volumetric dosing principle is dependent on a constant density ("conditioned") powder bed, which must be reformed after a dose has been extracted. Cohesive powders may impact ability to reform the powder bed which can introduce unwanted effects such as powder arching, formation of air pockets. Over multiple cycles, there may also be time dependent changes in powder density (and thus dosed mass) which must be considered in technology transfer. Inevitably, achieving reproducible fill weight and fill weight uniformity thus depends on the close interaction of material attributes and process parameters. Hence, particularly in powder filling, the monitoring of key powder properties can be instructive for scale-up.

For example, a recent study (Stranzinger et al. 2017) evaluating two model powders with disparate bulk properties (large particles, good flowability, low cohesion and small particles, poor flowability and high cohesion) demonstrated the interplay between characteristics of materials to be filled (bulk powder properties) and the process parameters for the filling equipment.

Faulhammer et al. (2015a) describe development of a predictive statistical model for fill weight and fill weight variability for an encapsulation process based on filling parameters (e.g. dosator diameter, dosing chamber length, powder layer depth) and material attributes (e.g. wall friction angle, bulk density, basic flowability energy). The model was reported to successfully predict fill weight, but not fill weight uniformity. Podczeck and Jones (2004) provide a guideline for powder suitability for encapsulation based on Carr's index as a measure of powder density. Powders with a Carr index between 15–35 are deemed suitable for capsule filling, lower values impacting plug formation, while higher values are detrimental to powder bed reformation.

Seyfang et al. (2014) have demonstrated for a range of dosing principles how dosing performance (fill weight variability) can be predicted from static and dynamic powder properties. Sim et al. (2014) have taken the concept further by establishing a predictive link between powder permeability and drug delivery performance. Lu et al. (2017) report a similarly strong correlation between a dynamic measure of powder flow (normalized basic flow energy) and dispersion performance for mixtures of fine and coarse lactose containing varying proportion of fines. In addition, the effect of storage at high humidity (85% Relative Humidity [RH]) was reported to be dependent on fines content, i.e. mixtures with high fines content exhibited sensitivity to dispersion performance, but not flowability, while for the coarse lactose powder flowability was impacted, but not dispersion.

The influence of the characteristics of the carrier on drug product pharmaceutical performance (aerosolization efficiency) and manufacturability (dosator capsule filling) has been studied by Faulhammer et al. (2015b) in a model system employing salbutamol sulfate with lactose and mannitol carriers modified by wet decantation to remove fine particles. The impact on blending, capsule filling, and in vitro performance was observed to be carrier specific, with decantation having a greater impact on aerosolization performance for lactose (lower fine particle fraction), but on processability for mannitol (higher weight variability) which was attributed to differences in formulation microstructure (surface distribution of API on the carrier surface).

As a first step in DEM simulation of the capsule filling process to determine material attributes and process parameters that achieve a robust process with low variation in dosed mass, Loidolt et al. (2017) report a DEM investigation of the first step of the filling cycle (filling of the dosator nozzle) to compare behavior of coarse/fine and cohesive/non-cohesive powders. Two factors were observed to influence the dosed mass—the ratio of particle to dosator diameter which impacts particle packing within the dosator chamber and powder flow which impacts filling and compression behavior. Different filling mechanisms were revealed for non-cohesive and cohesive powders, providing a mechanistic explanation for the relative importance of powder bed height on fill weight in experimental studies on cohesive and non-cohesive powders.

In conclusion, the strong interaction between powder properties and dosing performance drives the maintenance of the same filling principle on scale-up, limited only by capacity of the hopper from which powder feeds the filling process. Practically, this typically results in a scale-out rather than scale-up approach, i.e. assurance of translation of dosing performance across scales is achieved by expanding the number of filling stations.

9.7 Concluding Remarks

In this chapter, the key unit process operations in the manufacture of an inhaled powder—particle size reduction (micronization), powder mixing, and powder filling—have been reviewed with the aim of providing guidance on approaches to process scale-up. Approaches have been defined for scale-up, where possible, based on mechanistic understanding of underlying principles, although their (im)maturity constrains the ability to define clear rules for process scale-up and establish the necessary process controls to maintain a robust, consistent process output across scales. Promising alternative approaches are described where characteristics of process intermediates are used as surrogate product performance indicators to inform and direct scale-up. Advances in computational simulation are providing additional insight complementing the knowledge gained from traditional experimentation, but while improved understanding has removed the empirical nature of scale-up, significant gaps in understanding remain. It is desirable that modern regulatory mechanisms exist to provide a clear path for risk-based, post-approval changes for OIDPs such as manufacturing process scale that reflect current knowledge, such that industry can deliver innovation to achieve efficient pharmaceutical manufacturing as originally highlighted in US FDA's original PAT Framework (U.S. Food and Drug Administration 2004) and further developed in ICH Q12 (ICH 2014).

REFERENCES

Baldrick, P., and D. G. Bamford. 1997. A toxicological review of lactose to support clinical administration by inhalation. *Food Chem Toxicol* 35(7): 719–733.

Barling, D., D. Morton, and K. Hapgood. 2015. Pharmaceutical dry powder blending and scale-up: Maintaining equivalent mixing conditions using a colored tracer powder. *Powder Technol* 270(B): 461–469.

Bridgwater, J., S. Forrest, and D. J. Parker. 2004. PEPT for agglomeration? *Powder Technol* 140(3): 187–193.

Bridson, R. H., P. T. Robbins, Y. Chen et al. 2007. The effects of high shear blending on α-lactose monohydrate. *Int J Pharm* 339(1–2): 84–90.

Brodka-Pfeiffer, K., P. Langguth, P. Graβ, and H. Häusler. 2003. Influence of mechanical activation on the physical stability of salbutamol sulphate, *Eur J Pharm Biopharm* 56(3): 393–400.

Brosh, T., H. Kalman, A. Levy, I. Peyron, and F. Ricard. 2014. DEM–CFD simulation of particle comminution in jet-mill. *Powder Technol* 257: 104–112.

Clarke, J. G. 2006. Inspired by design: Evaluating novel particle production technologies. *Abstracts of Respiratory Drug Delivery 2006* 1: 287–296.

Dirgo, J., and D. Leith. 1985. Cyclone collection efficiency: comparison of experimental results with theoretical predictions. *Pharm Dev Technol* 4(4): 401–415.

Elia, A., M. Cocchi, C. Cottini et al. 2016. Multivariate data analysis to assess dry powder inhalers performance from powder properties. *Powder Technol* 301: 830–838.

Eskandar, F., M. Lejeune, and S. Edge. 2011. Low powder mass filling of dry powder inhalation formulations. *Drug Dev Ind Pharm* 37(1): 24–32.

European Medicines Agency. 2009. Assessment report for Onbrez Breezhaler. EMA/659981/2009.

European Medicines Agency. 2013. CHMP Assessment report for Ultibro Breezhaler. EMA/CHMP/296722/2013.

European Medicines Agency. 2014. CHMP Assessment report for BiResp Spiromax. EMA/CHMP/175684/2014.

European Medicines Agency. 2016. Guideline on process validation for finished products – Information and data to be provided in regulatory submissions. EMA/CHMP/CVMP/QWP/BWP/70278/2012-Rev1, Corr.1, 21 November 2016.

European Medicines Agency. 2017a. Concept paper on revision of the guideline on the pharmaceutical quality of inhalation and nasal products – Draft. EMA/CHMP/QWP/115777/2017.

European Medicines Agency. 2017b. Questions and answers: Improving the understanding of NORs, PARs, DSp and normal variability of process parameters. EMA/CHMP/CVMP/QWP/354895/2017.

Faulhammer, E., M. Llusa, P. R. Wahl et al. 2015a. Development of a design space and predictive statistical model for capsule filling of low-fill-weight inhalation products. *Drug Dev Ind Pharm, Early Online*: 1–10.

Faulhammer, E., V. Wahl, S. Zellnitz, J. G. Khinast, and A. Paudel. 2015b. Carrier-based dry powder inhalation: Impact of carrier modification on capsule filling processability and in vitro aerodynamic performance. *Int J Pharm* 491(1–2): 231–242.

Gonce, A., and U. Schrader. 2012. Plantopia? A mandate for innovation in pharma manufacturing. http://www.mckinsey.com/~/media/mckinsey/industries/pharmaceuticals%20and%20medical%20products/our%20insights/pharma%20manufacturing%20for%20a%20new%20era/plantopia.ashx.

Government Office for Science. 2013. Future of manufacturing project: Evidence Paper 29. https://www.gov.uk/government/uploads/system/uploads/attachment_data/file/283903/ep29-factory-of-the-future.pdf.

Grasmeijer, F., P. Hagedoorn, H. W. Frijlink, and H. A. de Boer. 2013. Mixing time effects on the dispersion performance of adhesive mixtures for inhalation. *PLoS One* 8(7): 1–18.

Green, D. W. 2007. *Perry's Chemical Engineering Handbook*. New York: McGraw-Hill.

Hassanpour, A., C.C. Kwan, B.H. Ng et al. 2009. Effect of granulation scale-up on the strength of granules. *Powder Technol* 189(2): 304–312.

Hertel, M., E. Schwarz, M. Kobler, S. Hauptstein, H. Steckel, and R. Scherließ. 2017. The influence of high shear mixing on ternary dry powder inhaler formulations. *Int J Pharm* 534(1–2): 242–250.

Hickey, A.J., I. Gonda, W.J. Irwin et al. 1990. Effect of hydrophobic coating on the behavior of a hygroscopic aerosol powder in an environment of controlled temperature and relative humidity. *J Pharm Sci* 79(11): 1009–1014.

Huang, Z., W. Xiong, K. Kunnath, S. Bhaumik, and R. N. Davé. 2017. Improving blend content uniformity via dry particle coating of micronized drug powders. *Eur J Pharm Sci* 104: 344–355.

International Council for Harmonisation of Technical Requirements for Pharmaceuticals for Human Use (ICH). 2014. *Technical and Regulatory Considerations for Pharmaceutical Product Lifecycle Management Final Concept Paper.* http://www.ich.org/fileadmin/Public_Web_Site/ICH_Products/Guidelines/Quality/Q12/Q12_Final_Concept_Paper_July_2014.pdf.

Kaialy, W. 2016. On the effects of blending, physicochemical properties, and their interactions on the performance of carrier-based dry powders for inhalation – A review. *Adv Colloid Interface Sci* 235: 70–89.

Kuerten, H., and H. Rumpf. 1966. Zerkleinerungsuntersuchungen mit triboluminescierenden Stoffen. *Chemie-Ing Technik* 38(3): 331–341.

Loidolt, P., S. Madlmeir, and J. G. Khinast. 2017. Mechanistic modeling of a capsule filling process. *Int J Pharm* 532(1): 47–54.

Lu, X. Y., L. Chen, C. Y. Wu, H. K. Chan, and T. Freeman. 2017. The effects of relative humidity on the flowability and dispersion performance of lactose mixtures. *Materials* 10(592): 1–9.

MacDonald, R., D. Rowe, E. Martin, and L. Gorringe. 2016. The spiral jet mill cut size equation. *Powder Technol* 299: 26–40.

Midoux, N., P. Hošek, L. Pailleres, and J. R. Authelin. 1999. Micronization of pharmaceutical substances in a spiral jet mill. *Powder Technol* 104: 113–120.

Muschelknautz, E., G. Giersiepen, and N. Rink. 1970. Strömungsvorgänge bei der Zerkleinerung in Strahlmühlen. Chemie Ingenieur Technik 42(1): 6–15.

Muzzio, F. J., and A. W. Alexander. 2005. Scale-up of powder blending operations. *Pharmaceutical Technology, Scaling Up Manufacturing* s34–s44.

Nasr, M. M., M. Krumme, Y. Matsuda et al. 2017. Regulatory perspectives on continuous pharmaceutical manufacturing: Moving from theory to practice: September 26–27, 2016, International symposium on the continuous manufacturing of pharmaceuticals, *J Pharm Sci* 106(11): 3199–3206.

Nguyen, D., A. Rasmuson, I. N. Björn, and K. Thalberg. 2015. Mechanistic time scales in adhesive mixing investigated by dry particle sizing. *Eur J Pharm Sci* 69: 19–25.

Plank, R., B. Diehl, H. Grinstead et al. 2003. Quantifying liquid coverage and powder flux in high-shear granulators. *Powder Technol* 134: 223–234.

Podczeck, F., and B. Jones. 2004. *Pharmaceutical Capsules* (Second Edition). London, UK: Pharmaceutical Press.

Rodnianski, V., N. Krakauer, K. Darwesh et al. 2013. Aerodynamic classification in a spiral jet mill. *Powder Technol* 243: 10–119.

Rumpf, H. 1973. Physical aspects of comminution and new formulation of a law of comminution. *Powder Technol* 7(3): 145–159.

Rumpf, H. 1960. Prinzipien der Prallzerkleinerung und ihre Anwendung bei der Strahlmahlung. *Chemie-Ing Technik* 32(3): 129–135.

Sarkar S., B. Minatovicz, K. Thalberg, and B. Chaudhuri. 2017. Development of a rational design space for optimizing mixing conditions for formation of adhesive mixtures for dry-powder inhaler formulations. *J Pharm Sci* 106(1): 129–139.

Seyfang, K., E. M. Littringer, M. Lober, and E. Schwarz. 2014. Correlation between properties of dry powder inhaler model formulations and their filling performance: Comparison of different dosing methods. *Abstracts of Respiratory Drug Delivery 2014 Volume* 2: 427–431.

Shah, U. V., V. Karde, C. Ghoroi, and J. Y. Heng. 2017. Influence of particle properties on powder bulk behaviour and processability. *Int J Pharm* 518(1–2): 138–154.

Shur, J., R. Price, D. Lewis et al. 2016. From single excipients to dual excipient platforms in dry powder inhaler products. *Int J Pharm* 514(2): 374–383.

Shur, J., H. Harris, M. D. Jones et al. 2008. The role of fines in the modification of the fluidization and dispersion mechanism within dry powder inhaler formulations. *Pharm Res* 25(7): 1931–1940.

Sim, S., K. Margo, J. Parks et al. 2014. An insight into powder entrainment and drug delivery mechanisms from a modified Rotahaler®. *Int J Pharm* 477(1–2): 351–360.

Stranzinger, S., E. Faulhammer, V. Calzolari et al. 2017. The effect of material attributes and process parameters on the powder bed uniformity during a low-dose dosator capsule filling process. *Int J Pharm* 516(1–2): 9–20.

Tardos, G.I., K.P. Hapgood, O.O. Ipadeola et al. 2004. Stress measurements in high-shear granulators using calibrated "test" particles: Application to scale-up. *Powder Technol* 140(3): 217–227.

Ticehurst, M. D., P. A. Basford, C. I. Dallman et al. 2000. Characterisation of the influence of micronisation on the crystallinity and physical stability of revatropate hydrobromide. *Int J Pharm* 193(2): 247–259.

U.S. Food and Drug Administration. 1995. Guidance for industry: Scale up considerations immediate release solid oral dosage forms Scale-Up and Postapproval Changes: Chemistry, manufacturing, and controls, in vitro dissolution testing, and in vivo bioequivalence documentation. https://www.fda.gov/downloads/Drugs/GuidanceComplianceRegulatoryInformation/Guidances/UCM070237.pdf.

U.S. Food and Drug Administration. 1997a. Guidance for industry: SUPAC-MR: Modified release solid oral dosage forms Scale-Up and Postapproval Changes: Chemistry, manufacturing, and controls; in vitro dissolution testing and in vivo bioequivalence documentation. https://www.fda.gov/downloads/Drugs/GuidanceComplianceRegulatoryInformation/Guidances/UCM070640.pdf.

U.S. Food and Drug Administration. 1997b. Guidance for Industry: Nonsterile semisolid dosage forms Scale-Up and Postapproval Changes: Chemistry, manufacturing, and controls; in vitro release testing and in vivo bioequivalence documentation. https://www.fda.gov/downloads/Drugs/GuidanceComplianceRegulatoryInformation/Guidances/UCM070930.pdf.

U.S. Food and Drug Administration. 2004. Final report on pharmaceutical cGMPs for the 21st century – A risk-based approach. https://www.fda.gov/downloads/Drugs/DevelopmentApprovalProcess/Manufacturing/QuestionsandAnswersonCurrentGoodManufacturingPracticescGMPforDrugs/UCM176374.pdf.

U.S. Food and Drug Administration. 2011. Guidance for industry, process validation: General principles and practices. https://www.fda.gov/ucm/groups/fdagov-public/@fdagov-afda-orgs/documents/document/ucm334560.pdf (accessed 31 August 2017).

U.S. Food and Drug Administration. 2013. Draft guidance on fluticasone propionate; salmeterol Xinafoate. https://www.fda.gov/downloads/Drugs/GuidanceComplianceRegulatoryInformation/Guidances/UCM367643.pdf.

U.S. Food and Drug Administration. 2014a. FDA inspectional observation summaries FY 2014. http://www.fda.gov/ICECI/Inspections/ucm424098.htm (accessed 31 August 2017).

U.S. Food and Drug Administration. 2014b. Guidance for industry: SUPAC: Manufacturing equipment addendum. https://www.fda.gov/downloads/Drugs/GuidanceComplianceRegulatoryInformation/Guidances/UCM346049.pdf.

U.S. Food and Drug Administration. 2015a. Draft guidance on aclidinium bromide. https://www.fda.gov/downloads/Drugs/GuidanceComplianceRegulatoryInformation/Guidances/UCM460918.pdf.

U.S. Food and Drug Administration. 2015b. Draft guidance on formoterol fumarate. https://www.fda.gov/downloads/Drugs/GuidanceComplianceRegulatoryInformation/Guidances/UCM461064.pdf.

U.S. Food and Drug Administration. 2016a. Draft guidance on indacaterol maleate. https://www.fda.gov/downloads/Drugs/GuidanceComplianceRegulatoryInformation/Guidances/UCM495054.pdf.

U.S. Food and Drug Administration. 2016b. Draft guidance on fluticasone furoate. https://www.fda.gov/downloads/Drugs/GuidanceComplianceRegulatoryInformation/Guidances/UCM495024.pdf.

U.S. Food and Drug Administration. 2016c. Draft guidance on fluticasone furoate; vilanterol trifenatate. https://www.fda.gov/downloads/Drugs/GuidanceComplianceRegulatoryInformation/Guidances/UCM495023.pdf.

U.S. Food and Drug Administration. 2017a. Draft guidance on salmeterol xinafoate. https://www.fda.gov/downloads/Drugs/GuidanceComplianceRegulatoryInformation/Guidances/UCM581189.pdf.

U.S. Food and Drug Administration. 2017b. Draft guidance on fluticasone propionate. https://www.fda.gov/downloads/Drugs/GuidanceComplianceRegulatoryInformation/Guidances/UCM581179.pdf.

U.S. Food and Drug Administration. 2017c. Draft guidance on tiotropium bromide. https://www.fda.gov/downloads/Drugs/GuidanceComplianceRegulatoryInformation/Guidances/UCM581192.pdf.

U.S. Food and Drug Administration. 2017d. Guidance agenda: New & revised draft guidances CDER is planning to publish during calendar year 2017. https://www.fda.gov/downloads/Drugs/GuidanceComplianceRegulatoryInformation/Guidances/UCM417290.pdf.

U.S. Food and Drug Administration. 2016d. Compliance policy guides, Chapter 4 – human drugs. http://www.fda.gov/ICECI/ComplianceManuals/CompliancePolicyGuidanceManual/ucm116271.htm (accessed 31 August 2017).

U.S. Food and Drug Administration. 2017e. Guidance for industry and FDA staff: Current good manufacturing practice requirements for combination products. https://www.fda.gov/downloads/RegulatoryInformation/Guidances/UCM429304.pdf.

Venables, H. J., and J. I. Wells. 2001. Powder mixing. *Drug Dev Ind Pharm* 27(7): 599–612.

Vogel, L., and W. Peukert. 2002. Characterisation of grinding-relevant particle properties by inverting a population balance model. *Part Syst Char* 19(3): 149–157.

Wang, Y., R. D. Snee, W. Meng, and F. J. Muzzio. 2016. Predicting flow behavior of pharmaceutical blends using shear cell methodology: A quality by design approach. *Powder Technol* 294: 22–29.

Yang, J., C. Y. Wu, and M. Adams. 2015. DEM analysis of the effect of electrostatic interaction on particle mixing for carrier-based dry powder inhaler formulations. *Particuology* 23: 25–30.

Young, P.M., D. Cocconi, P. Colombo et al. 2002. Characterization of a surface modified dry powder inhalation carrier prepared by particle smoothing. *J Pharm Pharmacol* 54(10): 1339–1344.

Young, P.M., D. Roberts, H. Chiou et al. 2008. Composite carriers improve the aerosolisation efficiency of drugs for respiratory delivery. *J Aerosol Sci* 39(1): 82–93.

Yu, L. X., and J. Woodcock. 2015. FDA pharmaceutical quality oversight. *Int J Pharm* 491(1–2): 2–7.

Yu, W., K. Muteki, L. Zhang, and G. Kim. 2011. Prediction of bulk powder flow performance using comprehensive particle size and particle shape distributions. *J Pharm Sci* 100(1): 284–293.

Zhao, Q. Q., and G. Schurr. 2002. Effect of motive gases on fine grinding in a fluid energy mill. *Powder Technol* 122(2–3): 129–135.

Zeng, X. M., G. P. Martin, S. K. Tee et al. 1999. Effects of particle size and adding sequence of fine lactose on the deposition of salbutamol sulphate from a dry powder formulation. *Int J Pharm* 182: 133–144.

Zuegner, S., K. Marquardt, and K. Zimmerman. 2006. Influence of nanomechanical crystal properties of the comminution process of particulate solids in spiral jet mills. *Eur J Pharm Biopharm* 56(3): 393–400.

10

Quality by Control

Helen N. Strickland and Beth Morgan

CONTENTS

10.1 Introduction

This chapter addresses statistical considerations in implementing a framework for the assessment of quality for inhalation aerosol products, such as, metered dose inhaler (MDI) and dry powder inhaler (DPI) drug products intended for commercial distribution. Although this framework focuses on the statistical quality control aspects of MDI and DPI drug products developed using traditional product development approaches, it is also a component of the quality assessment for products developed using a risk- and science-based approach, where the intent could be to utilize advanced statistical process control procedures. The International Council for Harmonization (ICH) defines quality as "the degree to which a set of inherent properties of a product, system or process fulfills requirements" (ICH Q6A 1999). For most MDI and DPI products developed traditionally, pharmaceutical quality is regarded as the suitability of a drug substance or drug product for intended use, which is operationally achieved by demonstrating that a product has been manufactured in accordance with Current Good Manufacturing Practice (CGMP) regulations and the inherent properties conform to regulatory specifications (Woodcock 2004). For MDIs and DPIs developed using a risk- and science-based approach, good pharmaceutical quality is: (1) producing product that has an acceptable minimal risk of not clinically performing as labeled,

(2) producing product absent of contamination, and (3) supplying product that is readily available to the patient (Yu and Woodcock 2015). Regardless of the development approach, controlling the quality of any drug product is a statutory requirement. The degree of success a firm achieves, in controlling the pharmaceutical quality of its MDI and DPI drug products, is related to the proper application of statistical quality control and/or statistical process control methods throughout the product's lifecycle.

10.2 Regulatory and Statutory Requirements for Pharmaceutical Quality

In the United States, GMPs for drugs (finished pharmaceuticals and components) are legally enforceable requirements under statutory CGMP requirements of section 501(a)(2)(B) of the Federal Food, Drug, and Cosmetic Act (the Act) (21 U.S.C. 351(a)(2)(B)). GMPs and CGMPs are regulations that specify the scientific and engineering controls required for drug manufacture. GMPs and CGMPs are based on the same principles, but CGMP emphasizes the use of the most current technology and standards; GMPs are more widely used than CGMPs (Kungu 2018). For the United States, CGMP regulations for finished pharmaceuticals are provided in 21 CFR (Code of Federal Regulation) parts 210 and 211. The following CGMP regulations in CFR Title 21 Section 211 for finished pharmaceuticals pertain to the application of quality assurance and quality control statistics:

- *21 CFR 211.165 (c)*: Any sampling and testing plans shall be described in written procedures that shall include the method of sampling and the number of units per batch to be tested; such written procedure shall be followed.
- *21 CFR 211.165 (d)*: Acceptance criteria for the sampling and testing conducted by the quality control unit shall be adequate to assure that batches of drug products meet each appropriate specification and appropriate statistical quality control criteria as a condition for their approval and release. The statistical quality control criteria shall include appropriate acceptance levels and/or appropriate rejection levels.
- *21 CFR 211.166 (a) (1)*: Sample size and test intervals based on statistical criteria for each attribute examined to assure valid estimates of stability.
- *21 CFR 211.110 (b)*: Valid in-process specifications for such characteristics shall be consistent with drug product final specifications and shall be derived from previous acceptable process average and process variability estimates where possible and determined by the application of suitable statistical procedures where appropriate.
- *21 CFR 211.180 (e)*: Written records required by this part shall be maintained so that data therein can be used for evaluating, at least annually, the quality standards of each drug product to determine the need for changes in drug product specifications or manufacturing or control procedures.

In addition to general CGMP finished pharmaceutical requirements, inhaled drug products are further differentiated in the US as they are defined as combination products under 21 CFR Part 4. Combination products are defined as products composed of any combination of a drug and a device; a biological product and a device; a drug and a biological product; or a drug, device, and a biological product. Therefore, quality for a combination product is a function of not only the quality of the formulated drug product and device separately, but ultimately, a function of how these components perform together.

10.3 Quality Lifecycle Guidelines

The product lifecycle for drug products as presented in ICH Q10 consists of four lifecycle stages: pharmaceutical development, technology transfer, commercial manufacture, and product discontinuation. ICH Q10 describes a pharmaceutical quality system model based on International Organization for

Standardization (ISO) quality system concepts as applied to the product lifecycle. If implemented, the ICH Q10 model facilitates the manufacture, control, and supply of good pharmaceutical quality drug product to patients while complementing or enhancing regional GMP requirements (ICH Q10 2008).

Process validation (PV) is required by CGMP regulations. PV is described as a set of activities "taking place over the lifecycle of the product and process" (FDA 2011). These activities comprise "the collection and evaluation of data, from the process design stage through commercial production, which establishes scientific evidence that a process is capable of consistently delivering quality product" (FDA 2011). The process validation lifecycle activities begin in the latter part of the pharmaceutical development phase and stop at the end of the commercial phase. Process design (stage 1) is carried out during the early development phase with the goal to define the commercial manufacturing process and to develop the process control strategy. Process qualification (stage 2) contains two elements: design of the facility and qualification of the equipment and utilities, and process performance qualification (PPQ). The goal of PPQ is to evaluate if the process is capable of reproducibly manufacturing product of good pharmaceutical quality. Continued process verification (stage 3), although not formally referenced in the guideline, should be treated as a minimum of two substages, pre-routine commercial and routine commercial to align with the recommendations in the guidance that "continued monitoring and sampling of process parameters and quality attributes at the level established during the process qualification stage until sufficient data are available to generate significant variability estimates" (FDA 2011). These estimates "provide the basis for establishing levels and frequency of routine sampling and monitoring" (FDA 2011). This substage concept facilitates obtaining ongoing assurance that the validated process remains in a state of control with the ability to detect undesired process variability or unexpected changes in the process as required by CGMP regulations to control drug product quality.

A meaningful and systematic process validation plan integrates science, risk management, and statistics to collect and evaluate appropriate data throughout the product lifecycle. The goals of the process validation plan are to document evidence that sources of variation that impact the manufacturing process' ability to consistently produce finished drug product of appropriate quality can be identified, detected, and controlled.

The quality measures reflecting identity, strength, quality, and purity of a drug product are often called critical quality attributes (CQAs) and include, for example, delivered dose or aerodynamic particle size distribution (APSD) stage groupings. These are attributes that should be derived from the quality target product profile (QTPP) requirements as well as the process control strategy and specifications. The QTPP requirements are the characteristics of a drug product that would ideally be achieved to ensure the desired quality (FDA 2018). The QTPP may include route of administration, dosage form, delivery, dosage strength, container closure, and drug product quality criteria (e.g. sterility, purity, stability, and drug release) (ICH Q8(R2) 2009). The quality target product profile links to the target product profile (TPP). A *TPP* is a format for a summary of a drug development program described in terms of labeling concepts (FDA 2007). The intent is to define what is required of the product for the patient and market (TPP), that then is translated into requirements for the quality of the product to reliably deliver that to the patient (QTPP), that is then translated into measurements that can be monitored and controlled to reliably deliver that quality and reduce process variability. In this way, the industry is moving from being reactive and addressing corrective actions downstream to being proactive in defining quality upstream (ICH Q10: 2008).

10.4 Quality Standards: Registered and Pharmacopeial

Regulatory specifications consist of a list of tests and appropriate acceptance criteria which a drug substance or drug product (when tested in accordance with the referenced analytical procedures) should meet to be deemed as "conforming to specification" from batch release to expiry (ICH Q6A 1999). Table 10.1 contains a list of the general product quality tests and performance quality tests (a.k.a. end-product tests) that are included in the United States Pharmacopeia (USP 40-NF 33 2018). These tests are associated with important quality attributes defined by the United States Food and Drug Administration for MDI and DPI drug product (FDA 2018). Typically, specification limits are either: (1) empirically derived from the *in vitro* test results observed on the batches from which *in vivo* response data have been obtained or (2) taken from the specification limits provided in

TABLE 10.1
USP General Product Quality and Product Performance Test

Inhalation Aerosol	Inhalation Powder
Identification	Identification
Assay	Assay
Impurities and degradation products	Impurities and degradation products
Water content	Content uniformity (pre-metered)
Foreign particulate matter	Water content
Leachables	Foreign particulate matter
Spray pattern	Microbial limit
Microbial limit	Net content (device-metered)
Alcohol content (if present)	Osmolality
Net fill weight	Leachables
Leak rate	Net fill weight
	Plume geometry
Delivered dose	Residual solvents
APSD	Volatile and semi-volatile leachables
	Emitted dose
	APSD

regional pharmacopeias (i.e., European Pharmacopoeia, United States Pharmacopeia, and Japanese Pharmacopoeia). In either case, the intent is to make an inference regarding the quality of the untested units in the batch.

The United States CGMP regulations mandate that appropriate statistical practices are to be employed for determining the acceptance criteria utilized by the quality control unit for the sampling and testing of drug product batches as a condition for approval and release (i.e. batch release). In the November 2012 issue of Pharmacopeial Forum, a stimulus article entitled *Methods for Measuring Uniformity in USP* was published, and although not the primary intent, the USP acknowledged: (1) the result of any testing applied, for compendial purposes, only to the sample, (2) compendial assessments were not intended "to support an inference to a larger number of units, e.g. a batch, from which the sample is drawn," and (3) compendial standards applied "at all times in the life of the article from production to expiration" even though USP does not require any testing to be done (USP 2012). Therefore, as stated in the article and implied in the General Notices, "USP tests are not intended for determining whether a batch is suitable for release and it is the responsibility of the manufacturer to determine batch release (or process monitoring) criteria" such that "potential samples have a sufficiently high probability of meeting USP standards when tested" (USP 2012).

MDI and DPI drug products developed via a traditional product development approach rely on in-process testing and end-product testing of lagging indicators of quality to demonstrate conformance to specification, often applying USP tests and compendial standards as the specifications, despite recent publications. For these situations, acceptance sampling and control charting are common statistical quality control (SQC) methods. Drug products developed using a quality by design approach would demonstrate conformance to specification through a combination of implemented statistical process control (SPC) methods on leading indicators of quality and implementing SQC methods on lagging indicators of quality.

10.5 Statistical Process Control and Statistical Quality Control

SPC and SQC utilize similar statistical methodologies, however, distinct differences exist between the two applications. SPC is the application of statistical techniques and/or statistical or "stochastic control algorithms" to analyze process inputs (independent variables) with the intent of one or more of the following: (1) "to increase knowledge about a process;" (2) "to steer a process to behave in the desired way" and (3) to characterize variation of final-product parameters to guide improvements in process performance

(ISO/TR 11462-1:2001). The basic tool for SPC is the control chart. Lagging indicator (product based) control charts instead of leading indicator (process based) control charts are most common within the pharmaceutical industry currently. Product-based control is also referred to as "after the event statistical product control" (ISO/TR 18532:2009). Lagging indicator control charts are used more frequently within the pharmaceutical industry because the technical linkages between process inputs and process parameters (i.e. critical material attributes [CMAs] and critical process parameters [CPPs]) and product characteristics (i.e. CQAs) are generally not identified through prior knowledge, scientific understanding based on first principles, or empirical understanding based on design of experiments (DoE).

SQC is the application of statistical tools, primarily control charting and acceptance sampling methodologies, to analyze the quality characteristics of the process outputs (i.e. dependent variables) with the intent to demonstrate product quality stability and/or product quality acceptability. In addition to acceptance sampling, ISO recommends what is referred to as the "guarantee system" for demonstrating conformance to specifications (ISO/TR 18532:2009). Acceptance sampling, by itself, is the least efficient approach because as a decision-making procedure, it is completely determined by the information from the sample that was chosen. In contrast, the guarantee system for assuring conformance to specification relies on all the knowledge that was established during process design linking CMAs and CPPs to CQAs. It builds in the necessary assurance of continued suitability and capability of the process.

The ICH Quality Implementation Working Group discussed four important data elements, similar in principle to the ISO "guarantee system," for assessing if a batch may be released to market. These ISO elements for batch release consist of: (1) regulatory compliance data, (2) system data related to environmental, facility, utilities, and equipment for the current batch, (3) product-related data based on the manufacturing process, and (4) product-related data from quality control. ICH Quality Implementation Working Group emphasized the use of an enhanced control strategy, allowing conformance to specification to be demonstrated through increased process monitoring of all system related data such that all deviation or atypical events are identified and corrected, increased use of SPC for process inputs and CPPs, and an increase in the control charting in-process and final drug quality characteristics (CQAs) with less reliance on SQC acceptance sampling data (ICH Q&A 2010).

The data collection and data evaluation options provided in this chapter focus on demonstrating process stability and product acceptability while leveraging all relevant product and process specific knowledge. Demonstrating process stability corresponds to assessing how effective the proposed process control strategy is in allowing the process to operate as expected, and then demonstrating that the process continues to operate as expected. Demonstrating product acceptability corresponds to assessing how well the process output (product) conforms to product requirements defined in terms of product specifications, and then demonstrating that the output quality is consistent.

The data collection and data evaluation plans presented in this chapter acknowledge the difference between sampling for quality verification, sampling for monitoring process performance, and sampling for process control. In general, manufacturing processes consist of leading measurements and lagging measurements. Leading measurements are made on process inputs and are independent variables. Some leading measurements are process parameters such as speed, force, flow volume, and temperature. Other leading measurements can be the actual output of an upstream process, such as loss on drying, drug concentration, drug substance purity, excipient particle size distribution, or drug-related impurities. Lagging measurements are made on the process output and are typically measurements of the inherent characteristics of the product. If the inherent characteristics are related to product requirements, then those are referred to as quality characteristics (ISO 3534-1, 2006).

Process-based inferences imply SPC is utilized for leading indicators that impact product quality. This assumes that appropriate technical linkages between process inputs and processing parameters (CMAs and CPPs—the leading indicators) and product characteristics (CQAs—the lagging indicators) have been identified through prior knowledge, scientific first principles, or design of experiments. The intent of enhanced data collection (sampling) and data evaluation for CPPs during PPQ is not for prospective process control purposes. The objective is to show, via monitoring, that the control strategy used for the leading indicators works as intended.

If the technical linkages between CPPs and CQAs have not been identified, as is the case for most legacy products, then enhanced data collection and evaluation of the CPPs should be performed with the intent to characterize the CPPs and establish control charts for process monitoring. This could be accomplished by following recommendations for implementation of effective statistical process control. If the control strategy incorporates product-based lagging indicators, additional data collection and data evaluation activities are required during PPQ. The product-based lagging indicators may be intermediate process outputs or final process outputs linked to final product quality characteristics. In either case, these process outputs may be deemed CQAs, depending on the results of a quality risk assessment. It is very important to realize that if the "variation is not under statistical control, then it is foolhardy to attempt to predict the characteristics of the population from a sample chosen at random" (ISO 18532).

For example, delivered dose uniformity (DDU) and APSD are deemed major performance measures related to dose delivery to the patient (USP 40-NF 33 2018). Dose delivery to the patient is considered an inherent property indicative of MDI and DPI drug product suitability and as such, these are two of the critical quality attributes considered for inclusion in the regulatory specification (FDA 2018). These critical quality attributes are defined as continuous measurements or continuous data. A different type of CQA would be defect data or categorical data. An example of this type of CQA might be function testing to ensure a device indexes correctly. Either a sampled device indexes properly or it does not, but this functionality is also critical for ensuring the correct delivery of the dose of drug product to the patient, and, therefore, both attributes would be considered CQAs.

Two case studies have been developed to show the application of SQC tools to both attribute and continuous data within a product lifecycle management framework. Both case studies present a scenario for validating a process from PPQ into routine commercial production in which the sample size, acceptance sampling plan, data evaluation, and process monitoring utilize SQC tools. Case study 1 presents the issues to consider when developing the framework for a product defect designated as major, and case study 2 presents a scenario for delivered dose data, considered a continuous measurement.

10.6 Case Study 1: Attribute Sampling Plan from PPQ to Routine Release

In this example, an acceptance sampling plan is needed for a defect following the process validation lifecycle principles as described above. A guiding principle in this case study and the following one is that, within each lifecycle phase, a series of activities occur for data collection and data evaluation that then influence the decisions and data collection of the subsequent phase. The data collection phase includes activities related to both determining sample sizes, but also ensuring that the sample is representative of material throughout the batch. Through discussions with both development and the quality organizations, the consumer risk quality for this defect was defined to be 0.5%. This means that the company needs to ensure with high degree of confidence that a process producing as many as 5000 defective units per one million units would be readily detected, which may or may not lead to batch rejection. This defect rate is, often, referred to as the limiting quality or rejectable quality level. Ideally, this defect level should be established based on understanding impact to the patient for drug product delivery.

The primary focus for PPQ is to ensure that the process is in a state of statistical control, and to demonstrate that the process does not produce batches whose quality is worse than the stated CRQ. An additional focus for the producer is to understand the risk or probability of passing PPQ for the number of batches defined.

10.6.1 Data Collection of PPQ

Regardless of details of the acceptance sampling plan, enhanced sampling of the critical process parameters and material attributes should also be implemented. The next step is to define the acceptance sampling plan to apply through PPQ. It is also helpful to consider natural segments throughout the batch from which the units can be sampled. For example, there may be 10 kegs or larger units that comprise the batch for the filling process, and these provide natural segments from which the units can be sampled.

There are many options for an acceptance sampling plan. The purpose of this case study is to present some of those options along with the rationale for the final decision. The final decision for a sampling plan and number of PPQ batches should not be based, solely, on the statistical properties of the sampling plan. The statistical properties should be considered along with knowledge of the product and process and the technical risk assessment for the product. The statistical considerations follow this general approach:

1. Define different sampling plans, for one batch, with a focus on consumer risk
2. Understand, across one batch, the percent defective for which the process needs to be operating to minimize producer risk for those plans
3. Quantify the consumer risk along with the percent defective to minimize producer risk for the *entire* validation across multiple batches, and use this information along with the technical risk assessment to make a final decision for the acceptance sampling plan and the total number of batches to produce in PPQ

The first step within PPQ is to develop options focusing on consumer risk. One plan is to choose an isolated lot acceptance sampling plan indexed on a limiting quality value of 0.5% from ISO 2859-2 (1985). This plan requires sampling 800 units in total (80 per segment across ten segments). The plan will pass (i.e. the batch will be released to market) if the number of defective units from the sample of 800 is less than or equal to 1. This sampling plan has a 9.1% chance of passing at the limiting quality value of 0.5%. This means that the consumer risk for this plan is 9.1%; i.e. there is a 9.1% chance that a batch that contains 0.5% defective would be released to the market. Another option is to choose an acceptance sampling plan that allows zero defects and controls the consumer risk to be 5% as opposed to, approximately, 9%. This is a user defined acceptance sampling plan. This plan would sample 600 units (60 per segment), and the batch would be released if the number of defects observed was zero. A final option would be a user-defined plan that allowed one defective unit, but still controlled the consumer risk to be 5% at the limiting quality value of 0.5%. This acceptance sampling plan would sample 950 units (95 per segment), and the batch would be released to market if the number of defective units was less than or equal to 1. This highlights that there are three possible sampling plan options, but they do not provide the same level of consumer risk protection.

The second step is to determine the quality level (i.e. the percent defective in the batch) in which the producer would have at least a 95% probability of passing this acceptance sampling plan for one batch. This is often referred to as the producer risk quality. Different sampling plans will require the process to be operating at different defect levels to assure a producer risk of 5%; i.e. to pass 95% of the time. Table 10.2 summarizes this information across the three sampling plans. Figure 10.1 provides the operating characteristic (OC) curves for these three plans. The sample sizes for user defined plans can be calculated from the binomial distribution, assuming the probability of selecting a defective unit is not altered or changed by selecting the sample itself. This is a reasonable assumption if the sample size is 10% or less of the batch size. If this is not a reasonable assumption, the OC curve should be based on the hypergeometric distribution (Hahn and Meeker 1991). Table 10.2 highlights two points to consider. The first point is that the consumer risk coverage is not the same across all three plans. The ISO standard acceptance plan approximately doubles the consumer risk compared to the other two plans, which would need to be justified. The second point to consider is that, between the two plans that control the consumer risk to be 5%, the plan requiring zero defects to pass also requires the process defect level to be, approximately, 1/5 the defect level of the plan allowing one defective unit. In general, zero defect plans have a very different shape to the OC curve compared to plans that allow one defect to be observed. Even for small values of the percent

TABLE 10.2

Comparison of Possible Acceptance Sampling Plans for Consumer Risk and Defect Rate to Pass 95% of the Time for $n = 1$ Batch for PPQ

Sampling Plan	Total Number Sampled	Allowable Number of Defects	Consumer Risk (%)	Process Defect Rate (%) Corresponding to 95% Chance of Passing Sampling Plan
A	800	1	9.1	0.0444
B	600	0	4.9	0.0085
C	950	1	4.9	0.0374

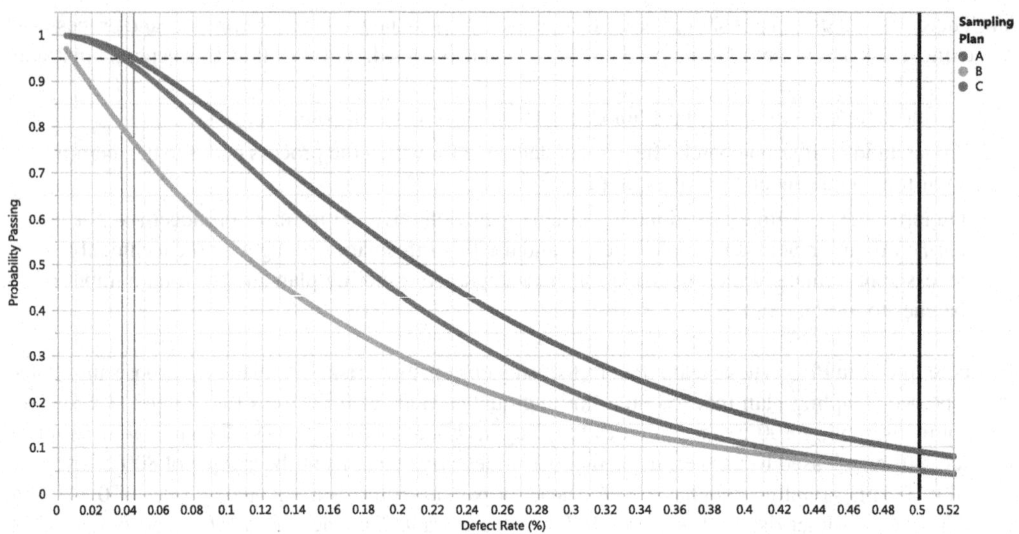

FIGURE 10.1 Operating characteristic curves for sampling plans A, B, and C with vertical line at limiting quality level of 0.5% and vertical lines at process defect rate to pass sampling plan 95% of the time.

defective, the probability of acceptance drops rapidly (ISO/TR 8550-1:2007). This should be well understood by the producer before implementation of such a plan. At this point, since both user-defined acceptance sample plans have the same consumer risk, the decision becomes more focused on what information the producer has for the expected defect rate. If historical data show that the defect rate of this process is expected to consistently stay as low as 0.0085%, then the company could choose plan B (0 defect) and still have high probability of passing and save resources. However, if a defect rate of 0.0085% is not assured, then the company puts itself at risk for choosing this plan and not passing PPQ.

The overall PPQ validation effort will not require just one batch to be produced. Several batches need to be manufactured. From the technical risk assessment, three batches or five batches are being considered. Figure 10.2 shows the operating characteristic curves for acceptance (i.e. passing the validation) for three consecutive batches and five consecutive batches. Notice each time that the curve from the ISO standard plan is the most liberal of the three with a higher consumer risk and a higher proportion defective to pass 95% of the time. The user-defined plan with zero defects is the steepest curve, and the user-defined plan allowing one defective unit is between the other two, but closer to the ISO standard plan. Like the table above, the consumer risk and the producer risk quality values for passing PPQ based on n = 3 or n = 5 batches are reported in Table 10.3. These consumer

TABLE 10.3

Comparison of Possible Acceptance Sampling Plans for Consumer Risk and Defect Rate to Pass 95% of the Time for n = 3 Batches or n = 5 Batches for PPQ

Number of Batches for PPQ	Sampling Plan	Total Number Sampled	Allowable Number of Defects	Consumer Risk (%)	Process Defect Rate (%) Corresponding to 95% Chance of Passing Sampling Plan
3	A	800	1	9.1	0.044
	B	600	0	4.9	0.009
	C	950	1	4.9	0.037
5	A	800	1	9.1	0.044
	B	600	0	4.9	0.009
	C	950	1	4.9	0.037

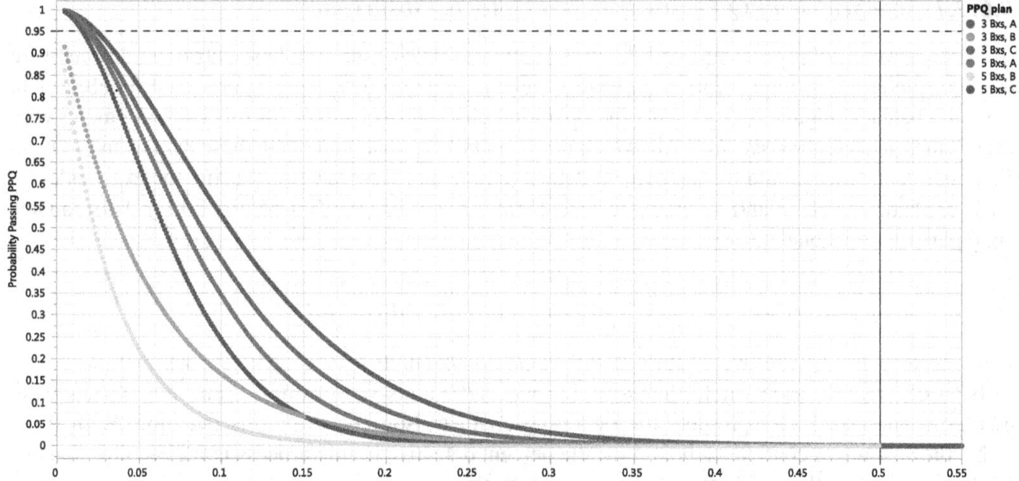

FIGURE 10.2 Operating characteristic curves for sampling plans A, B, and C for $n = 3$ batches and $n = 5$ batches.

risks and producer risks are calculated based on passing the individual acceptance sampling plans a total of three times or five times. Based on both sets of OC curves, accounting for consumer risk for one batch, producer risk quality for one batch, the producer risk quality for the entire validation effort, and the technical risk assessment, the decision was made to conduct PPQ on five batches, implementing the user-defined acceptance sampling plan allowing one defective unit to be observed per batch (PPQ = 5 batches, sampling plan = C, sample $n = 950$ per batch, accept if zero or one defect observed). This will define the sampling plan for PPQ.

10.6.2 Data Evaluation of PPQ

Two scenarios are described here to contrast how the results from one stage should influence the decisions of the next stage in the product lifecycle. In the first scenario, PPQ passed with no defects, and, in the second scenario, PPQ passed with defects observed. Again, regardless of the different scenarios, the general steps being followed for data evaluation of PPQ are:

1. Analysis of CPPs data collected through PPQ to demonstrate within batch state of control; the statistical tools used here are standard Shewhart Xbar-S charts, boxplots and scatter plots, and analysis of variance techniques for demonstrating no significant differences across stratum or segments. See Montgomery (2013) for a discussion of these methods.
2. Estimation of the true percent defective in the process and determination of an upper confidence bound on that true percent defective.

Step 1 above will not be detailed here as the analysis of process data for demonstrating statistical control using control charts and Analysis of variance (ANOVA) techniques are well documented when significant differences do not exist across the stratum. This is a critical step because this analysis gives assurance, through the data collected, that the batches were processed similarly and are consistent in performance. It is this assurance of consistency that individual batches can be treated as coming from an overall process that allows us to pool the data for estimating the true percent defective from data collected through PPQ and to consider the batches as representative as a series of batches and not isolated lots. If the processing of the batches cannot be considered consistent and the batches cannot be pooled, then the validation team would need to discuss impacts of that outcome on the broader validation effort. It is assumed for both scenarios below that the data can be pooled across batches.

10.6.2.1 Scenario 1: PPQ Passes with No Defects Observed

Five batches were sampled, sampling 950 units from each batch, and, in this scenario, no defects were observed; therefore, in total, 4750 units were sampled, and zero defects were observed, pooling data across the batches. Figure 10.3 presents the operating characteristic curve for this outcome along with the OC curve representing scenario 2 in which five defects were observed. With these data from PPQ, the 95% upper confidence bound for the percent defective in this process is 0.063% using the exact calculation as explained in Hahn and Meeker's text, *Statistical Intervals* (ISO/TR 8550-2:2007). This equates to 630 parts per million defective.

10.6.2.2 Scenario 2: PPQ Passes with Five Defects Observed

In this scenario, five batches were sampled with sampling 950 units from each batch, but now, one defect had been observed in each batch; therefore, in total, 4750 units were sampled, and five defects were observed. Figure 10.3 also presents the operating characteristic curve for this outcome. With these results, the 95% upper confidence bound for the percent defective in this process is 0.22%. This equates to 2200 parts per million defective. These data show that the process could be operating with almost 4 times the defect rate compared to scenario 1, and therefore, the decisions and outcomes in stage 3A should not look the same between these scenarios, given the information that PPQ has provided on the performance of the process is not the same.

10.6.3 Data Collection of Stage 3A Continued Process Verification

In stage 3A, the goal is to ensure, through sampling and monitoring, that the process remains in a validated state consistent with performance from PPQ, and that the sampling and monitoring will detect unplanned or undesirable changes in variation. Statistically, the balance of goals during this stage becomes more complex. First, there is the desire to be sampling in such a way that allows a natural progression to stage 3B if stage 3A is passed. Secondly, there is the desire, from the producer, to be able to pass each batch to the market on its own merits, and, thus, assurance of consumer risk at the individual

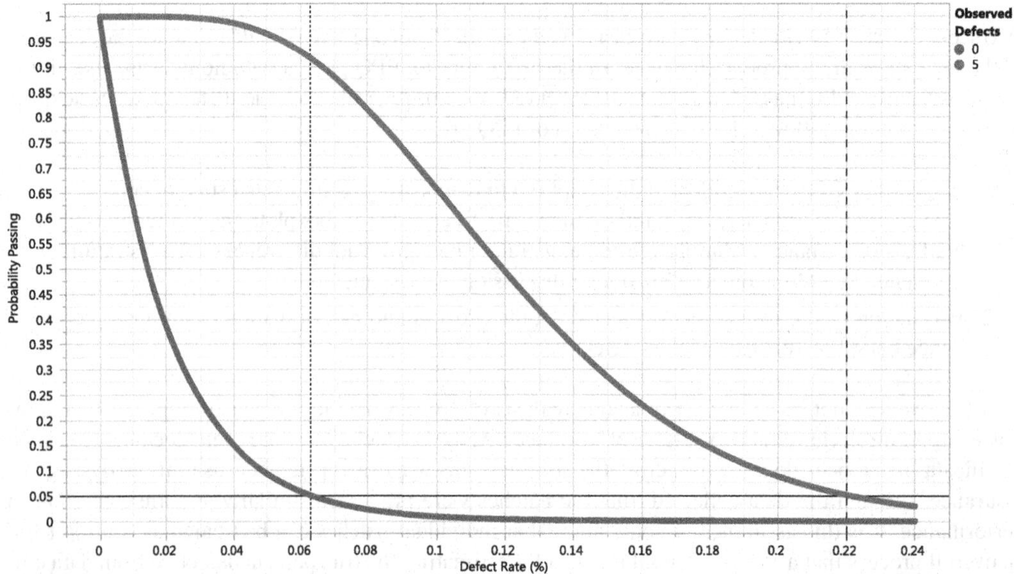

FIGURE 10.3 Operating characteristic curves for sampling plan B in which zero defects were observed across five batches and five defects were observed across five batches. For each outcome, the 95% upper confidence bound for the true defect rate is indicated with the vertical line.

batch level needs to be maintained at levels reasonably close to PPQ. Thirdly, there is the desire to be able to detect if the defect rate in the process increased compared to PPQ. Finally, the plan needs to be acceptable from the producer risk vantage point. To contrast these considerations, given the different scenarios from PPQ with different outcomes, this section will discuss determining the stage 3A sampling protocol for both scenarios above. Recall, in scenario 2, the data from PPQ reflect a higher average proportion defective in the process compared to scenario 1, and, therefore, considerations of how to proceed in stage 3A should not be the same between these scenarios. As an overall approach, balancing the considerations above, the steps followed in this section are:

1. Given the calculated upper confidence bound from the data assessment phase of PPQ, consider different sampling plans, such that, if the defect rate equals the calculated upper confidence bound on the percent defective, the batch would pass 95% of the time. This could be viewed as aligning the upper confidence bound from PPQ with an acceptance quality limit (AQL) sampling plan to be used, eventually, for routine release testing (stage 3B). These plans could be user defined or standards. The relationship between the limiting quality level (in this case, 0.5%) and the AQL also needs to be considered in that a working principle is that the LQ value should be a minimum of 3 times greater than the AQL (ISO 2859-2:1985). These AQL level plans represent the acceptance sampling plan for stage 3B, routine release testing. Statistically, we are now using the data from PPQ to provide information on an upper bound of the average defect rate and defining the sampling such that batches should pass 95% of the time if the process stayed at that average defect rate or "acceptable quality level." This step ensures that the average percent defective (or upper bound) observed from PPQ is aligned with the final plan for routine release.
2. Choose a sample size that is a multiple of the AQL acceptance sampling plans outlined in step 1 that will ensure that if the true percent defective significantly changed (doubled) compared to PPQ, that the plan would detect that. Also, the heightened testing should ensure that the consumer risk continues to be appropriately controlled at an individual batch level. This step ensures that there will be a natural transition between stage 3A to 3B, that the plan can respond to an undesirable increase in the percent defective, and that the consumer risk is controlled for an individual batch.
3. Choose or establish the number of batches for stage 3A. This is often determined by factors that are not directly statistical in that the number should represent what the company expects for different sources of variation. If this is not possible, statistically, the number could be determined based on the number such that the variation in the process average stabilizes (i.e. the change in the half width of the confidence interval stabilizes). This would ensure that the number of batches was sufficient such that additional sampling did not substantially improve the estimate of the overall process average.
4. Based on the possible sampling plans defined for each batch and the number of batches in stage 3A (steps 2 and 3 above), determine the total number of units sampled across stage 3A and the total number of defects allowed with those possible sampling plans. Construct an operating characteristic curve for these plans, assuming that data can be pooled because at this stage in the product lifecycle, the batches should represent units that are being sampled from one overall process.
5. Choose, as the final plan, the acceptance sampling plan in which the percent defective to pass 95% of the time from the operating characteristic curve above aligns with the upper confidence bound from PPQ. This ensures that the chosen plan would have a high likelihood of being observed at the end of stage 3A, pooling data, if the process continues at its current (upper bound) defect rate and that the producer and consumer risks are minimized. Given the defect rate observed in PPQ, if there is no testing plan that shows high likelihood of being observed at the end of stage 3A, treating batches as coming from a series, then the company must maintain PPQ level testing and continue to assess the data periodically. If the defect rate drops as more batches are collected, then the decision to move forward into stage 3A can be re-assessed and steps 1–5 can be repeated.

10.6.3.1 Scenario 1: Data Collection for Stage 3A, PPQ = 0/4750 Defects Observed

In scenario 1, the upper 95% confidence bound on the percent defective was 0.063%. Following step 1 above, acceptance sampling plans are needed for stage 3B such that the probability of passing is 95% if the true percent defective is either 0.065% or 0.10%, depending on the nature of the defect. These values were chosen to align outcomes from PPQ with established defect rates in ISO 2859-1. These sampling plans could be user defined or could be based on a standard AQL sampling plan. Table 10.4 shows different options for stage 3B for the final sampling plan in terms of sample size, accept/reject number, whether the plan is user defined or not, and the probability of passing at that defect (acceptable quality) level. This table shows directly that the standard acceptance sampling plans may not always be the best options for every case. One of the hidden costs that producers accept implementing the standards without understanding the background behind development of the standards is increased testing and resources. Also, this table shows that allowing a defect to be observed is possible, but at the cost of increased sampling. Based on this, the decision is taken to consider only user-defined plans. The sample size for the user-defined plan for AQL = 0.10% and accept on zero is increased to 60 for convenience reasons in sampling the batch. The same principle was applied for $n = 380$. Therefore, at this point, there will be four sampling plans to consider: ($n = 60$, accept = 0), ($n = 380$, accept = 1), ($n = 80$, accept = 0), and ($n = 550$, accept = 1).

Next, multiples of these sampling plans are reviewed to determine the sample size needed to detect, with reasonable assurance, an increase in the defect rate with the constraint of testing no more than the number sampled and tested during PPQ. In other words, statistically, the question becomes what sample size is required such that if the true percent defective increased to 0.15% (approximately double the bound of 0.063%), that this plan would then have a reduced chance of passing, and, therefore, detect the increased defect rate?

Table 10.5 shows the sample size in multiples of sampling plans for stage 3A such that each plan has approximately a 50% chance of passing if the defect rate increased to 0.15%. Sampling plans such that the level exceeded the number tested during PPQ were not considered as these do not represent a savings in resources. Recall, a defect rate of 0.15% would be considerably higher than even a worst case from PPQ and would, therefore, represent a significant shift in product quality compared to what has been observed. The sample size of 480 represents an 8-fold increase if using the stage 3B plan of $n = 60$ and a 6-fold increase if using the stage 3B plan of $n = 80$. The sample size of 760 represents a doubling of the stage 3B plan for testing 380 units; the stage 3B plan for 550 cannot even be doubled without testing more than PPQ. Therefore, there are, realistically, two different options to consider.

To decide between these options, we now need to consider how many units will be sampled across the entire stage 3A process, and this will depend on the number of batches to test. As mentioned, often the number of batches to test should be decided based on practical considerations of the volume of product manufactured and the turnover for inventory such that the breadth of natural variation in the process should be experienced during stage 3A. In this case, it was determined that it would take 3 months of production to experience multiple input lots. Demand for the product was such that five lots or batches were produced each month. Therefore, a total of 15 batches will comprise stage 3A. This will mean a total tested of either 7200 units or 11,400 units, depending on whether 480 units or 760 units are sampled for each batch. To determine the final sampling plan, the probability of passing a sampling plan of 7200 or

TABLE 10.4
Options for Stage 3B

Acceptable Quality Level (%)	Sample Size	Accept/Reject	Type of Plan	Probability of Passing This Plan at Acceptable Quality Level
0.065	80	0/1		0.95
	550	1/2		0.95
	800	1/2		0.90
0.10	60	0/1		0.94
	380	1/2		0.94
	800	2/3		0.95

TABLE 10.5

Options for Stage 3A, Individual Batches, Scenario 1

Sample Size	Accept/Reject	Probability of Passing If Defect Rate = 0.15%
80	0/1	0.89
60	0/1	0.91
380	1/2	0.89
240	0/1	0.70
360	0/1	0.58
480	0/1	0.49
760	1/2	0.68

TABLE 10.6

Options for Stage 3A in Total, Scenario 1

Sample Size	Accept/Reject Across Entire Stage 3A	Probability of Passing If Defect Rate = 0.063% (1—Producer Risk) (%)	Probability of Passing If Defect Rate = 0.5% (Consumer Risk) (%)
7200 = 15 × 480	0/1	1.1	0.0
11,400 = 15 × 760	15/16	99.6	0.0

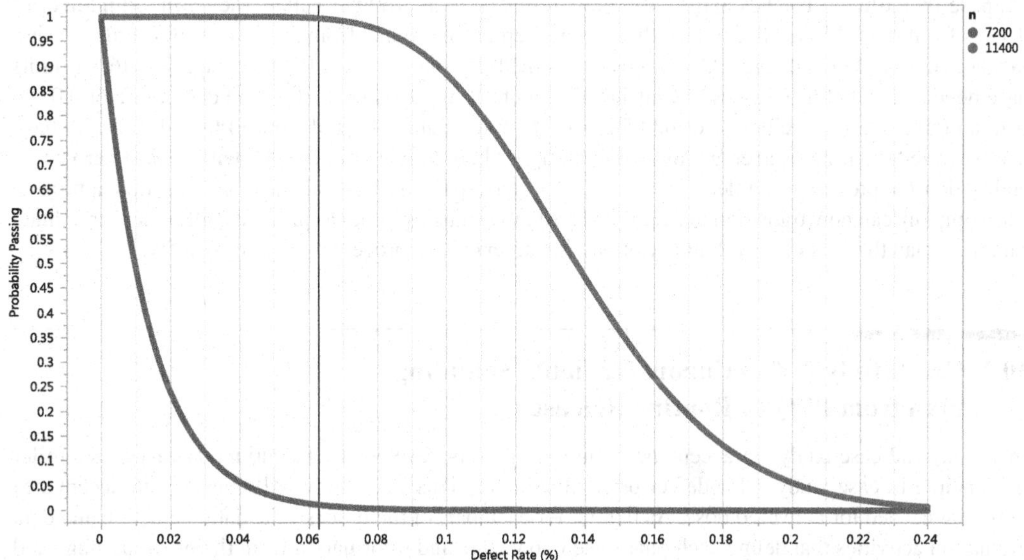

FIGURE 10.4 Operating characteristic curves comparing different sampling plans for case study for stage 3A.

11,400 with corresponding accept/reject numbers is compared for a true percent defective of 0.063% and 0.5%. These points represent the percent defective for where the process could be operating (worst case) and the percent defective that is unacceptable for release to the market. Table 10.6 gives these probabilities. This table clearly shows the significantly increased risk of failing stage 3A if the company chooses a zero defect plan for 15 batches if the defect level is as high as 0.063%. This is also shown in the OC curves comparing these plans in Figure 10.4. For interest, the comparison is also made to the ISO standard plan for the same number of batches. The company decides to implement a PPQ protocol plan in which 15 batches will be produced, and the sampling plan per batch will be to sample 760 units within each batch and allow one defect per batch to be observed. This plan has a considerably lower producer risk compared to the zero defect plan for stage 3A and saves approximately 1000 units that can be sold to the market compared to the standard plan.

10.6.3.2 Scenario 2: Data Collection for Stage 3A, PPQ = 5/4750 Defects Observed

In this scenario, the 95% upper confidence bound for the percent defective in this process is 0.22%. There are AQL sampling plans at 0.25%; however, this would mean that the limiting quality level of 0.5% is only twice the estimated upper bound for the process average. This is one immediate indication that the process has not demonstrated a low enough defect rate to reduce sampling and proceed into stage 3A. Also, if the defect rate were to increase above 0.22% and, for example, double, the defect rate would then be almost equal to the limiting quality level of 0.5% for which there can be at most a 5% chance of passing the batch if the defect rate increased to that level. Therefore, with the data collected from PPQ, there is no evidence that sampling can be reduced immediately. The company must maintain a sampling plan of sampling 950 and accept the batch if one defect is observed. Since this will be maintaining PPQ levels of sampling, the recommendation would be to re-assess the results after five more batches, meaning PPQ sampling would have occurred for a total of ten batches to determine if the upper bound for the percent defective has decreased. If it has, then the steps could be implemented as above in scenario 1 with a lower upper confidence bound on the percent defective. In this scenario, the company cannot immediately reap the benefits of reducing sampling until lower defect levels have been observed.

10.6.4 Data Assessment for Stage 3A

Suppose that after 15 batches and 11,400 units tested in total (760 per batch), the observed number of defects from stage 3A was five. Given that batches represent product from a series or an overall process, the data across PPQ and stage 3A can now be pooled. In total, across PPQ and stage 3A, 16,150 units have been tested and five defective units have been observed. This is an observed defect rate of 0.031% with an upper confidence bound of 0.065%. At this point, data collected from PPQ and stage 3A have demonstrated the process average, including an upper bound, is within 0.065% with almost zero probability that the process has a defect rate of 0.5% to have passed PPQ and stage 3A with this approach. The company can now transition to routine release testing, using either a standard AQL or a user defined sampling plan that has high probability of passing at an overall process average of 0.065%.

10.7 Case Study 2: Continuous Variable Sampling Plan from PPQ to Routine Release

In this second case study, an acceptance sampling plan is developed for continuous variables similar in principle to case study 1 for defect or attribute data. This case study will consider an acceptance sampling needed for delivered dose. As before, for each part of the process, the data collection and data evaluation activities that define each phase use knowledge and information from the previous stage and inform actions to be taken for the subsequent stage.

In this example, the quality standard for delivered dose is defined such that the process should be producing product in which no more than 6.25% of units are above 120% label claim and no more than 6.25% of units are below 80% label claim. Statistically, this means that if the process were producing units such that 6.25% of the units were at or above 120% label claim or at or below 80% label claim, there should be little chance that those units would be released for commercial distribution. Therefore, unacceptable performance for the *process* would be one in which $p_{\text{Lower}} > 0.0625$ OR $p_{\text{Upper}} > 0.0625$, where p_{Lower} is the true proportion of the units in the batch with dose below 80% label claim, and p_{Upper} is the true proportion of the units in the batch with dose above 120% label claim. Product considered acceptable would be product in which $p_{\text{Lower}} <= 0.0625$ AND $p_{\text{Upper}} <= 0.0625$. This is analogous to the limiting quality level of 0.5% in case study 1 in which the quality standard is defined, and the consumer risk well controlled for

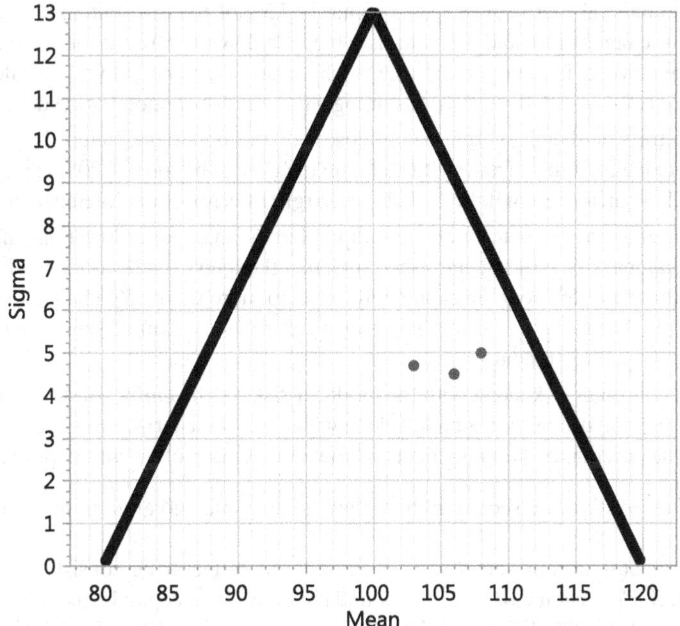

FIGURE 10.5 Limiting quality region defined where the true proportion of units less than 80 % LC and/or greater than 120 % LC is less than or equal to 0.0625.

each individual batch through PPQ, but stage 3B release acceptance sampling does not need to demonstrate that quality standard with the same level of consumer risk as PPQ. Visually, this quality standard can be represented in Figure 10.5 that shows combinations of true process means and standard deviations for which no more than 6.25% of units are outside 80%–120% label claim. Combinations within the triangle represent product that meets the quality standard and combinations outside the triangle represent product that would not meet the quality standard. Statistically, this is a framework similar in approach to equivalence testing for mean differences (Owen 1964), but based on proportions of a population. The approach is called the parametric tolerance interval two one-sided t-test (PTI-TOST) and has been discussed in literature as well as directly included in the updated guidance.

As before, the primary focus for PPQ is to ensure that the process is in a state of statistical control and that the process is producing, with high probability or confidence, no more than the stated number of allowable defects based on the quality standard defined above. From a producer perspective, another primary objective in planning for PPQ is to assess the probability of passing with a defined number of batches, given the previous history of data collected.

10.7.1 Data Collection for PPQ

Different demonstration tests and acceptance criterion (i.e. statistical methodology approaches) can be developed to address the same quality standard. However, all options presented here, even if specific numbers change, follow this general approach for establishing the sampling and testing plan for PPQ:

1. Determine batches from development or previous history that would be considered typical of the large-scale manufacturing process. Determine from this set of batches the batch closest to the boundary between acceptable product and unacceptable product. That would be the batch closest to the boundary of the triangle region in Figure 10.5. This batch represents a case in which heightened testing would be required to demonstrate that the quality standard has been met, but this batch is also typical of what could be observed through PPQ. Therefore, the sampling plan is developed to ensure that such a batch with these characteristics would pass the demonstration test and meet the stated quality standard. Using the mean and standard deviation for this batch,

determine the interval that is expected to contain 87.5% of the distribution with no more than 6.25% above the upper limit and no more than 6.25% below the lower limit, assuming the batch mean and standard deviation represent true batch values. This interval will be calculated as the intersection of two one-sided intervals assuming a normal distribution for the data.
2. Once limits are calculated for this batch closest to the boundary, determine the difference between the calculated limit from that batch and the closest bound of 120% label claim or 80% label claim. This difference will be called the margin of error of the tolerance bound.
3. Use that margin of error to determine the sample size for an upper or lower one-sided tolerance bound. This sample size will be established such that the interval will contain at least 93.75% of the distribution with 95% confidence and will have no more than a 5% chance to contain more than 93.75% plus the margin of error. This step establishes the sample size for each PPQ batch and ensures the quality standard.
4. Quantify the consumer risk along with the producer risk for the *entire* validation activity across multiple batches, and use this information along with the technical risk assessment to make a final decision for the acceptance sampling plan and the total number of batches to produce in PPQ.

Implementation of these steps are shown in the following example and align in principle to the steps in case study 1.

Suppose development data representative of large-scale manufacturing consists of the three batches shown in Figure 10.5. The batch closest to the boundary between acceptable and unacceptable product has a batch mean equal to 108% LC (label claim) and a standard deviation of 5%. If these were the true batch parameter values, then the interval to contain at least 93.75% below and 93.75% above is calculated as: 108% ± (1.534 * 5%) which equals [100.33%, 115.67%]. The value of 1.534 is the quantile from a standard normal distribution such that 93.75% of the distribution is below that value. The difference between 120% and 115.67% is 4.33%; this is the margin of error to use in the calculation of the sample size for tolerance intervals. This margin of error ensures that the interval will cover at least 93.75% of the batch distribution 95% of the time, and that the interval will contain no more than 98.08% (93.75% + 4.33%) 5% of the time. This approach for sample sizing is to ensure that the sample size increases as a batch comes closer to the boundary between acceptable and unacceptable quality. The methodology is based on the paper by Faulkenberry and Weeks (1968). Assuming a normal distribution for the data and defining the coverage to be 93.75% for a one-sided tolerance interval, the confidence to be 95%, and the margin of error to be 4.33% with a 5% probability of containing more than the margin of error, a sample size of $n = 100$ is needed for each batch. This establishes that $n = 100$ units are needed to test for each PPQ batch. Just as in case study 1, we now need to determine how many batches will define PPQ.

Based on this assessment and through the technical risk assessment process, the decision is made to conduct PPQ with three batches and testing 100 units per batch.

10.7.2 Data Evaluation of PPQ

Similar in principle to case study 1, the general steps being followed for data evaluation of PPQ are outlined here:

1. Critical process parameter data collected through PPQ are analyzed to demonstrate within batch state of control from data collected; the statistical tools used here are standard Shewhart Xbar-S charts, boxplots and scatter plots, and analysis of variance techniques for detecting if significant differences exist across stratum or segments.
2. Estimation of the true bounds of the process to contain 87.5% of the distribution with 95% confidence with no more than 6.25% above 120% LC or below 80% LC, assuming batches are representative of a series of batches from an overall process.

As before, even though step 1 will not be detailed, this analysis is critical because it provides assurance that batches were processed similarly and are consistent and can be considered as a "series." Consistency across the batches supports pooling the data as representative of one overall process.

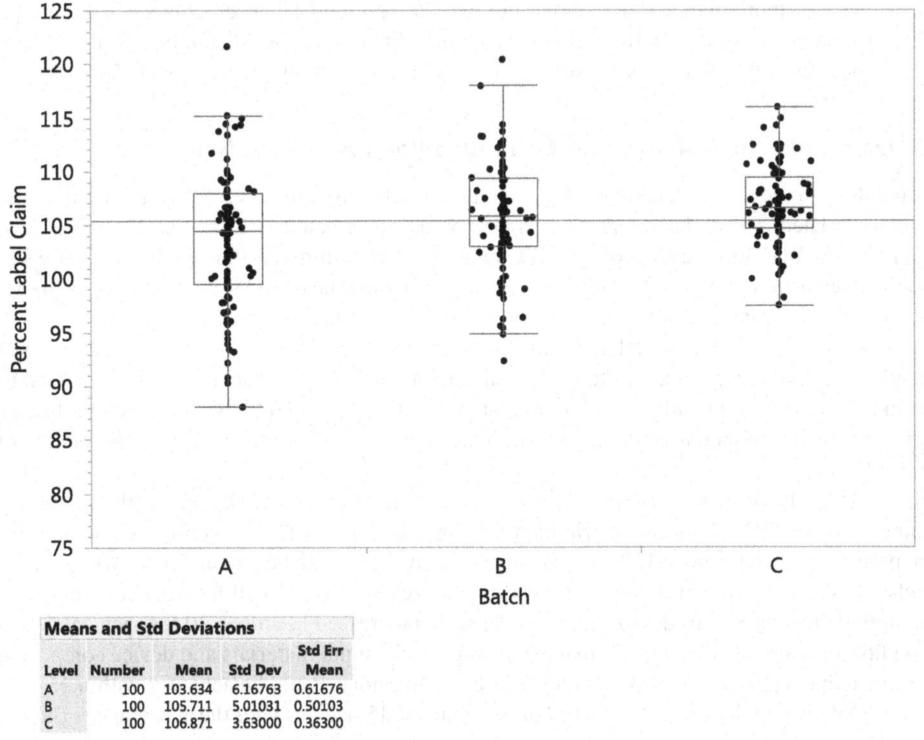

Means and Std Deviations

Level	Number	Mean	Std Dev	Std Err Mean
A	100	103.634	6.16763	0.61676
B	100	105.711	5.01031	0.50103
C	100	106.871	3.63000	0.36300

FIGURE 10.6 Case study 2 boxplots of delivered dose results for each PPQ batch.

Figure 10.6 shows the delivered dose results generated from the three batches, along with summary statistics for each batch. The intersection of the two one-sided tolerance intervals (i.e. the PTI-TOST interval) to contain no more than 6.25% above 120% LC or below 80% LC with 95% confidence for each batch is contained within 80% LC–120% LC so the assurance of the quality standard is met for each individual batch controlling the consumer risk at an individual batch level. The calculated intervals were [92.51%, 114.76%], [96.67%, 114.75%], and [100.32%, 113.42%] for batch A, batch B, and batch C, respectively. The data are comparable and are pooled to represent results from one overall process to decide the sampling strategy for stage 3A.

Figure 10.7 shows the distribution of all results pooled. The overall mean of the process is 105.4% LC with a standard deviation of 5.2%. A PTI-TOST interval to contain 87.5% of the distribution with 95%

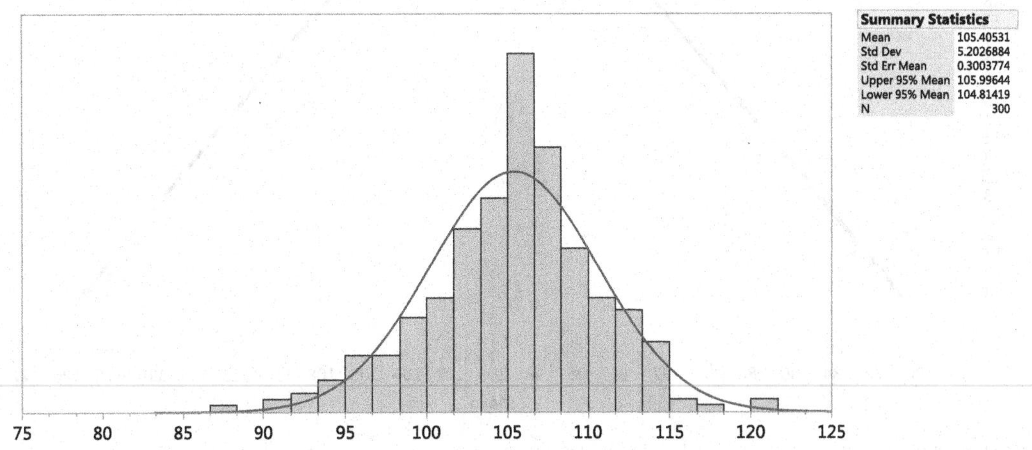

Summary Statistics

Mean	105.40531
Std Dev	5.2026884
Std Err Mean	0.3003774
Upper 95% Mean	105.99644
Lower 95% Mean	104.81419
N	300

FIGURE 10.7 Case study 2 histogram of delivered dose results for PPQ batches combined.

confidence with no more than 6.25% in either tail based on pooling all observations is calculated to be [96.65%, 114.16% LC]. Therefore, the process, given the PPQ data alone, should be producing no more than 6.25% of delivered dose results above 114.16% label claim or below 96.65% label claim.

10.7.3 Data Collection of Stage 3A Continued Process Verification

At this point, from the larger sample of PPQ data, the estimated margin of error for sample size calculations can be updated. The updated margin of error would be calculated as 120% LC–114.16% LC, which is equal to 5.84%. With sample sizes of $n = 300$, there would be minimal difference in a PTI-TOST interval and the intersection of two one-sided intervals, assuming the mean and standard deviation to be true values, and, therefore, the margin of error will be estimated as the difference between the goalpost and the closest value from the PTI-TOST interval. The goals for stage 3A have not changed: (1) the sample size should practically align in a way to easily transition to 3B, (2) each batch should be released to the market independent of the results of any other batch, (3) the plan should have increased probability to detect if the defect rate increased significantly, and, finally, (4) the producer risk should be quantified and understood.

At this point in the process, with the margin of error estimate updated to be 5.84%, the sample size is determined such that 93.75% of the distribution is below 120% LC with 95% confidence, which ensures that the proportion of data above 120% LC is no more than 6.25% with 95% confidence. This sample size is calculated as $n = 29$. However, since the final test for release testing will follow a counting test procedure, initially testing $n = 10$ devices, the sample size is increased to an $n = 30$ for each batch. Again, based on flow of materials through the manufacturing site for input materials and device components, it is determined that a reasonable coverage or turnover of inventory would be achieved within 15 batches. Therefore, 30 delivered dose results will be collected across 15 batches with the acceptance criterion for release testing applied.

To detect significant deviations of the process, the batches will be monitored with tightened limits applied to the triangle plot. These tightened limits were determined based on a k critical value for the tolerance interval analysis equal to 2.084259 for an $n = 30$ and are shown in Figure 10.8 compared to the

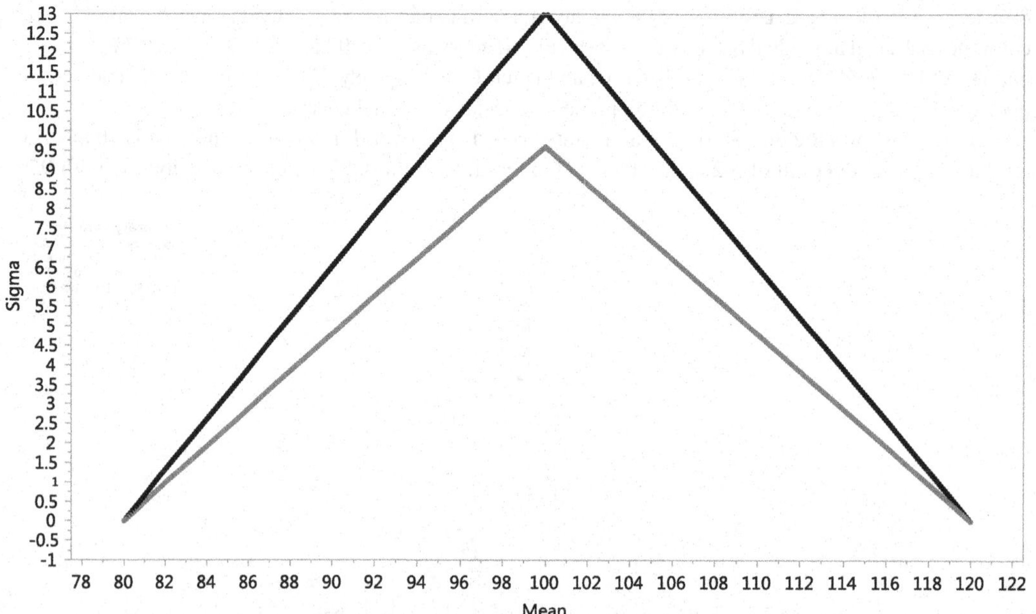

FIGURE 10.8 True limiting quality region (black) defined where the true proportion of units less than 80% LC and/or greater than 120% LC is less than or equal to 0.0625 versus 95% confidence operating region based on sample size of 30 units.

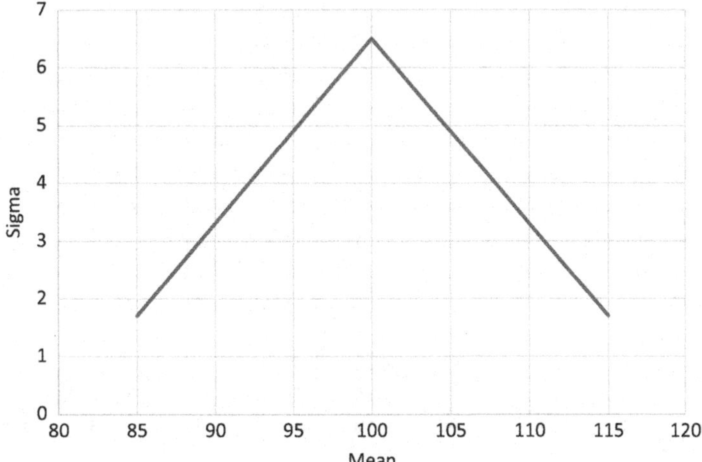

FIGURE 10.9 Minimum operation region (gray) for 95% passing rate of 15 consecutive batches for sample size of 30 units.

limits that represent true batch means and standard deviations to ensure no more than 6.25% outside 80% LC or 120% LC. In this plot, the boundary in black represents the region in which the quality standard is met for true values of batch means and standard deviations. The boundary in red represents the region in which the quality standard is assured with 95% confidence based on a sample size of n = 30. Batch means and standard deviations will be plotted through stage 3A on this plot, and if a batch falls outside the smaller triangular region, but within the larger triangular region, that batch will be investigated prior to release to the market. In this way, detection of a significant change is assured.

Alternatively, X-bar/S charts can be implemented as another option to the triangle plot. However, the X-bar charts need to account for batch to batch variation as well as the within batch variation, which is not the standard approach for X-bar charts in most software packages. Also, the limits need to be based on averages based on a sample size of n = 30. An S chart could be implemented from the PPQ data, but, again, ensuring the limits are based on a sample size of n = 30. The advantage of the triangle plot over the standard X-bar/S charts is that the risk of false alarms is minimized; that is, the X-bar/S charts will have an increased probability that a batch that truly meets the quality standard will be investigated erroneously.

As before, the overall operating characteristic curve for testing n = 30 units across 15 batches is determined to assess the probability of passing stage 3A validation from a consumer risk perspective and producer risk and is shown in Figure 10.9. This shows that there is almost no chance that product that does not meet the quality standard will be released to the market passing a stage 3A sampling plan based on 15 batches and 30 units per batch.

10.7.3.1 Data Assessment for Stage 3A

Once all batches are produced from stage 3A and PPQ and have met the acceptance criterion, we now have 750 delivered dose measurements across 18 batches. These data are plotted in Figure 10.10. Once again, an upper one-sided 95% confidence bound to contain 93.75% of the distribution above and below is calculated from these 750 delivered dose measurements and is within 80% LC to 120% LC as the lower bound is 96.62% LC and the upper bound is 113.38% LC. We now have strong evidence that batches produced from this process meet the quality standard. We are now ready to reduce testing for stage 3B and perform ongoing monitoring.

At this point, it is important to highlight that the specifications for stage 3B and routine release testing should not be the same as the acceptance criterion and sampling plan implemented during PPQ and stage 3A, regardless of the type of data collected. As shown in the example for defects, acceptance sampling plans for routine release are based on or aligned with AQL principles in which a

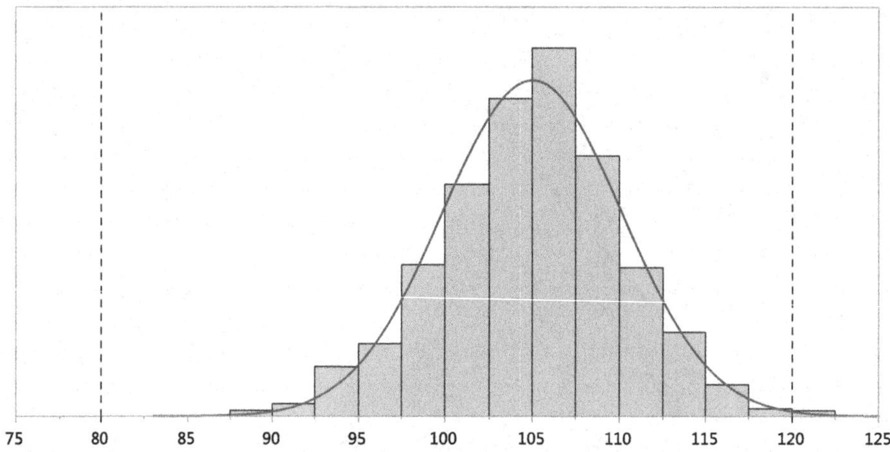

FIGURE 10.10 Plot of all results from PPQ and stage 3A.

process average is established through PPQ and stage 3A, and the sampling plan for stage 3B (routine release testing) is then to ensure that, if the process stays at that average, there is high probability of batch acceptance. Sampling during PPQ was done to ensure the quality standard for individual batches, and sampling during stage 3A was performed to transition between evaluating the data from individual batches to evaluating the data as coming from a series of batches or overall process. A different standard should not be introduced for continuous data; the same overall principle should be applied to align with established international standards. Therefore, application of the PTI-TOST approach as batch release criterion with the same characteristics as PPQ should not continue past PPQ as that would mean, in essence, implementing a limiting quality plan into stage 3A and stage 3B. The batch release criterion could be developed applying PTI-TOST with lower confidence, or a counting procedure could be implemented along with a program to continually monitor and trend the data to detect if process characteristics significantly changed.

Given the above, the batch release criterion will be based on a counting test, but ongoing monitoring will be performed in one of two ways, similar in approach to the recommendations through stage 3A:

1. A triangle plot could be constructed, similar to the one in Figure 10.8 and used for routine monitoring, using either the limits from stage 3A or limits updated with the sample size for release testing, which would be less than the amount sampled during stage 3A and thus would narrow the operating range.
2. Xbar-S charts could be implemented for the appropriate sample size and constructed accounting for batch variation.

The case studies presented previously have outlined the statistical principles and the statistical thinking for developing sampling plans and acceptance criterion for attribute data and continuous data. However, neither of the case studies are amenable for testing from PPQ to routine release for attributes that are extremely time consuming to obtain and measure. An example of this type of attribute for inhaled products is, potentially, APSD (aerodynamic particle size distribution) data. Often this type of data is obtained manually via twin impinger, Andersen cascade impactor, or Next Generation Impactor. Collecting 20 replicates–30 replicates for APSD data per batch for application of the tolerance interval approach is not, typically, feasible to do unless automation has been implemented. Even testing enough to make claims on the within batch variation with high statistical confidence for each batch is often challenging; therefore, what should be done for this attribute since it is a critical attribute for product development and release?

There are several possibilities, but currently, no consensus standard routinely used across the industry exists for these situations. One possibility is to establish direct relationships between in-process testing and APSD and apply the approach above to the in-process data. However, the industry has not been able to routinely establish these relationships, particularly for legacy products. Another possibility is to collect additional samples through PPQ and stage 3A (typically a multiple of release testing) and show multivariately that the data are not significantly different than representative data generated from development. This would be similar to the approach outlined in *Good Cascade Impactor Practices, AIM and EDA for Orally Inhaled Products* (Tougas et al. 2013). For this approach, a tolerance interval could still be applied, treating the data as coming from an overall process, to show that the data from this *process* (rather than individual batches) were contained within specification with high probability prior to going to routine batch release. Finally, a statistical approach could be used to test enough to detect departures (or significant differences) from what was, typically, observed from representative development data in terms of behavior of batch mean or variation.

Another option for this CQA would be to consider implementation of abbreviated impactor methods (AIM) or techniques of efficient data analysis (EDA). A quality standard could be defined from the abbreviated distribution that would maintain the producer and consumer risk compared to the quality standard from the full impaction data. This means defining a quality standard for the abbreviated impactor data that would not pass if the quality standard was not passed from the full distribution. In this way, understanding the characteristics of the batch would be maintained, but in a less resource intensive way, and the tolerance interval approach outlined here could be considered, in full implementation. And, finally, if a company invested significantly in an automation program to automate APSD testing such that the resource burden was alleviated, then, again, the tolerance interval approach as outlined above could be considered.

10.8 Conclusion

This chapter summarized the regulatory and compendial framework and statistical tools and statistical thinking that can be considered in demonstrating a process is suitable to be routinely releasing drug product to the market and is under a state of statistical control. We have presented case studies, both for attribute data and continuous data, that show the statistical thinking, rationale, and approaches that could be used to justify a holistic sampling approach as the product transitions from development through PPQ and into continued process verification and routine release. This framework, approach, and thinking can be implemented now, even while recognizing that many of the quality attributes that reflect the manufacturing process may or may not be directly related to patient impact. As the industry continues to struggle to learn more of the relationship between *in vitro* characteristics and *in vivo* outcomes (true quality by design), the approaches outlined here can be implemented to ensure that the current state of manufacturing processes continue to consistently deliver product to patients.

References

Hahn, G. J. and W. Q. Meeker. 1991. *Statistical Intervals—A Guide for Practitioners*. New York: Wiley, p. 412.

ISO/TR 11462-1:2001. *Guidelines for Implementation of Statistical Process Control (SPC) - Part 1: Elements orf SPC*. Geneva, Switzerland: International Organization for Standardization.

ISO/TR 18532:2009. *Guidance on the Application of Statistical Method to Quality and to Industrial Standardization*. Geneva, Switzerland: International Organization for Standardization.

ISO/TR 8550-1:2007. *Guidance on the Selection and Usage of Acceptance Sampling Systems for Inspectio of Discrete Items in Lots – Part 1: Acceptance Sampling*. Geneva, Switzerland: International Organization for Standardization.

ISO/TR 8550-2:2007. *Guidance on the Selection and Usage of Acceptance Sampling Systems for Inspectio of Discrete Items in Lots – Part 2: Sampling by Attributes*. Geneva, Switzerland: International Organization for Standardization.

ISO 2859-2:1985. *Samplig Procedures for Inspection by Attributes—Part 2: Sampling Plans Indexed by Limiting Quality (LQ) for Isolated Lot Inspection*. Geneva, Switzerland: International Organization for Standardization.

Montgomery, D. C. 2013. *Introduction to Statistical Quality Control*. Hoboken, NJ: Wiley.

Owen, D. B. 1964. Control of percentages in both tails of the normal distribution. *Technometrics*, 6(4), 377–387. doi:10.1080/00401706.1964.10490202.

Tougas, T. P., J. P. Mitchell, and S. A. Lyapustina. 2013. *Good Cascade Impactor Practices, AIM and EDA for Orally Inhaled Products*. Springer US. doi:10.1007/978-1-4614-6296-5.

Section IV

Particle Engineering/Processing

11

Milling and Blending: Producing the Right Particles and Blend Characteristics for Dry Powder Inhalation

Bernice Mei Jin Tan, Lai Wah Chan, and Paul Wan Sia Heng

CONTENTS

11.1 Introduction

Milling and blending are fundamental unit operations required in the preparation of dry powder inhalation (DPI) products. There are two basic reasons for this: (1) only respirable particles within the aerodynamic size range of 1 µm–5 µm can be deposited in the lung and (2) the inhalation performance and manufacturability of DPI products are greatly improved by the addition of inert coarse carrier particles to the respirable drug particles. Micronization of drug and blending with a carrier are therefore the most basic processes to produce inhalable mixtures. Many commercial DPI products are designed as lactose-based interactive mixtures. Lactose carriers improve both the aerosolization of drug particles and the content and dosing uniformity of the product. Drug-only formulations were introduced when inhalable particles could be accurately dosed from reservoir systems and readily aerosolized upon inhalation. In these formulation systems, milling and blending operations are replaced by complex particle engineering techniques. The specially designed inhalable particles, usually by spray-drying, are often larger-sized, spherical, and porous. Coupled with various improvements in device design (Healy et al. 2014), these single component formulations are able to maintain or improve on the respirable fraction produced by carrier-based formulations (de Boer et al. 2017).

In recent years, at least six DPI formulations based on binary excipient mixtures of lactose monohydrate and magnesium stearate have been clinically approved (Shur et al. 2016; Lau et al. 2017). While this is not an entirely new concept, the launch of these commercial products represents a new interest in carrier-based formulations containing even a ternary excipient. Magnesium stearate may impart the following benefits to the DPI product: lubrication of powder particles, modulation of drug-carrier physical interactions, reduction in moisture uptake, and inhibition of chemical reactions between the drug and lactose (Lau et al. 2017). There is limited information in the public domain regarding the methods by which the ternary excipient is incorporated into the formulations. Some possibilities include simple blending with the excipient or the pre-treatment of drug particles with the excipient by high intensity blending, mechanofusion, or co-milling (Jetzer et al. 2018). The inclusion of ternary excipients in carrier-based mixtures allows for more diverse possibilities in DPI formulation designs. However, particle design of components by milling and blending of the formulations remain central to the preparation of these three-component systems.

This chapter comprises two sections. The first focuses on fundamental concepts in particle design by comminution, in particular by the micronization process, such as the energy requirements in size reduction and the target particle size. The different milling techniques are also discussed with reference to their propensity for milling-induced amorphization of drug. The second section reviews the blending mechanisms involved in the formation of interactive mixtures and the attainment of blend uniformity. Lastly, the influence of blending on the cohesive-adhesive balance (CAB) is discussed as it is the CAB which ultimately determines the aerosolization performance of a DPI product.

11.2 Preparation of Inhalable Particles by Milling

Milling is a critical unit operation to prepare drug particles for delivery by inhalation. It is described as a process where mechanical energy is applied to physically break down coarse particles into finer particles (Loh et al. 2015). In the typical production of an inhalable drug, bulk active pharmaceutical ingredient (API) crystals obtained from a crystallization process are filtered, dried, and micronised to the desired particle size (Telko and Hickey 2005). The micronized particles may then be conditioned for a suitable duration to promote controlled recrystallization (Ward and Schultz 1995; Jones et al. 2008; Moura et al. 2016) so that predictable stability and release profiles of the final product can be obtained. The milling equipment required for micronization is different from those that are commonly used for routine comminution, which generally produce particles larger than 10 μm and of relatively wide size distributions. Compared to powders used for other solid dosage forms, the critical physicochemical attributes of inhalable particles are substantially different. For example, the aerodynamic diameter and surface morphology of drug particles may influence the DPI performance greatly. On the other hand, flowability of inhalable particles meant for a carrier-based formulation is not as critical compared to that of powders used in direct compression of tablets. This section will highlight the key considerations in milling operations to produce drug particles for inhalation. The fluid energy mill and mechanical impact mills are most frequently cited for this purpose. These mills are largely differentiated based on their size reduction capability, containment system, and product throughput. Besides size and shape considerations, milling-induced amorphization is also a critical attribute of milled drug particles. The latter attribute may be undesirable, but is inevitable in high energy milling. In attempts to circumvent this problem, wet milling has been explored. It should be noted that respirable particles do not necessarily have to be within the commonly mentioned geometric size range of 1 μm–5 μm, especially for specially engineered particles using techniques such as spray-drying or controlled crystallization. Nevertheless, milling has much wider commercial applications than crystallization because it is universally applicable to all pharmaceutically relevant materials (Loh et al. 2015). Techniques which involve particle growth, rather than size reduction, will not be discussed here in detail.

11.2.1 Fundamentals of Milling—Energy Requirements and Target Particle Size

The three main theories of milling by Rittinger (1867), Kick (1885), and Bond (1952) describe the relationships between the energy required for comminution and the degree of size reduction (O'Connor et al. 2006). These models were obtained from the fitting of empirical data from different types of materials and mills and are well described in literature (Ghadiri et al. 2007; Baláž 2008). Walker et al.

considered the three models as integrals of the same differential equation and simplified them into a general equation as shown below (Mann 1937):

$$\frac{dE}{dx} = -\frac{c}{x^n} \tag{11.1}$$

where *dE* is the amount of energy required to cause a reduction in size of *dx* per unit mass of material, and both *n* and *c* are constants. The value of *n* may be taken to represent the degree of resistance to fracture, and this value increases as particles become smaller (Parrott 1974). When *n* values of 2, 1, and 1.5 are substituted into Equation 11.1, the resulting equations express the models of Rittinger, Kick, and Bond, respectively. Of the three models, the Rittinger model describes most accurately cases where the increase in surface area per unit mass of original material is large. The model proposes that the comminution energy is directly proportional to the new surface area created. It is widely accepted that the Rittinger model is most applicable to fine grinding, such as micronization of powders. Therefore, the energy requirements in micronization increase exponentially as the particle size is reduced. On the other hand, the Kick model describes the crushing of very large particles, while the Bond model is broadly suitable for milling of material to an intermediate size range. The actual energy requirements in milling are expected to be significantly higher than those predicted by the models. This is because much of the milling energy will be dissipated as kinetic, heat, and/or sound energy in the mill. The predicted energy requirement also does not account for the energy absorbed during elastic deformation of particles, which has been noted to be several times greater than that required to create new surfaces (Ghadiri et al. 2007; Baláž 2008). It has been estimated that less than 1% of the total energy input during milling is used for actual size reduction (O'Connor et al. 2006). Hence, these models can at most provide qualitative information about the milling process. More detailed analyses of milling processes from a modeling perspective can be found elsewhere in the literature (Tanaka 1966; Parrott 1974; Baláž 2008; Naik and Chaudhuri 2015).

The target particle size and size distribution are two critical properties of milled drug for inhalation. It is more of the aerodynamic diameter, rather than the geometric diameter, of inhalable particles that governs their potential deposition profiles in the lung. The aerodynamic diameter is defined as the diameter of a hypothetical spherical particle with unit density having the same motion characteristics (i.e. settling velocity) as the particle in question (Flagan and Seinfeld 1988). The relationship between the aerodynamic and geometric diameters of a particle may be described as follows (Chen and Fryrear 2001; Telko and Hickey 2005):

$$d_A = d_G\sqrt{\frac{\rho}{X}} \tag{11.2}$$

where d_A is the aerodynamic diameter, d_G is the geometric diameter, ρ is the density of the particle, and *X* is the dynamic shape factor. The shape factor equals to unity for a perfect sphere and less as it deviates from sphericity. Clearly, the shape factor cannot be accurately determined for three-dimensional particles and has to be estimated by common shape parameters such as sphericity or aspect ratio. Nevertheless, the inclusion of the shape factor in the equation helps to account for the deviation in aerodynamic behavior of irregularly shaped particles. It can be seen that the geometric diameter, density, and shape are the critical attributes influencing the magnitude of the aerodynamic size of a respirable drug. The true density of particles are expected to be unchanged after milling, while there is very limited information on the control of particle shapes using mill parameters (Chan et al. 2002). For a milled drug, particle size and size distribution are therefore the only two important characteristics of particles that can be practically altered by milling. It is also evident from Equation 11.2 that the geometric size is not likely to be equal to the aerodynamic size as milled particles will never be spherical. A consequential question then arises: how should the geometric size specifications of an inhalable drug be defined? Aerodynamic particle size is not only dependent on the properties of the drug particles, but also the formulation, device and *in vitro* test parameters. While the geometric particle size is still a good approximation, the ideal size of the milled drug should be selected based on the *in vitro* deposition data and only with reference to the actual DPI formulation.

11.2.2 Milling Techniques

11.2.2.1 Jet Milling

Fluid energy mills (also known as jet mills) are the mills of choice based on comparisons of the energy efficiency, control of particle size, product throughput, containment, contamination risk, and heat generation (Dobson and Rothwell 1969; Murnane et al. 2009; Yu-Wei et al. 2015). Jet mills are advantageous for highly potent and low volume APIs, typical of DPI drugs, as the milling chamber can be fully contained and kept free from contamination. In addition, the lack of rotating elements in the mill results in much lower heat generation compared to mechanical impact mills. Jet mills are capable of producing particles within the range of about 0.5 μm–50 μm. There are various designs of the jet mill, but their basic size reduction mechanisms are largely similar (Chamayou and Dodds 2007). The energy for milling is delivered by propelling particles in high velocity air jets to cause collisions, and the micronization process takes place by impact grinding. As a result of extensive fragmentation, particles tend to be irregular in shape which contributes to greater inter-particulate friction, interlocking, and poorer flow properties. Nitrogen gas, rather than atmospheric air, can be used in conditions that necessitate the avoidance of oxygen due to the chemical reactivity of the drug. Rapid volume expansion of the compressed gas also results in a cooling effect which is beneficial for thermolabile drugs. The higher the grinding gas pressure used, the finer will be the particle size of milled product. As fragmentation is the main mechanism of size reduction, the size distribution of particles in the milling chamber is generally wide. Classifying systems are therefore integrated into jet mills to separate the fines below a certain cut-off size from the larger particles. As gas is continuously delivered into the milling chamber, fine milled particles are conveyed through the classifier system with the exiting gas while coarser particles remain in the milling chamber. After passage through the classifier, fines are collected in the cyclone while ultra-fine sub-micron particles entrained in the exhaust gas are removed by the dust collector system with an exhaust filter. Very narrow size distributions of milled product can be produced by the jet mill. The rate of material feed into the mill was found to affect the size distribution of milled particles. Both high and low feed rates led to a greater spread in the size distributions in a spiral jet mill (Dobson and Rothwell 1969). The limit of size reduction in the jet mill was reported at a grinding pressure of 6 bar for salbutamol sulphate (Ward and Schultz 1995). A further increase in the grinding pressure only contributed to an increase in the amorphous content of milled product, but not size reduction.

The two common designs of jet mills for the pharmaceutical industry are the spiral jet mill and the fluidized bed opposed jet mill. In a spiral jet mill, a high speed spiral vortex is created when high pressure gas jets enter through numerous nozzles positioned tangential to the milling chamber (Müller et al. 1996). The feed material enters the milling chamber by an injector gas stream. The spiral gas column will cause the coarser particles to experience higher centripetal forces and are flung with orbits of larger circumferences while finely milled particles are less affected and are entrained with the portion of the gas stream leaving via the classification centre of the chamber. Coarser particles remaining will be conveyed back to the active milling site for further grinding. In a fluidized bed opposed jet mill, the feed material is conveyed into the mill by screw feeder and falls into the milling chamber by gravity. Opposing jets of gas are directed towards a central point in space where particles collide at high velocities and fragment. Unlike the static air classifier in the spiral jet mill, a wheel classifier in the fluidized bed opposed jet mill is located above the grinding zone (Alpine 2016). Fine milled particles entrained in the exiting gas will leave through the rotating wheel classifier spun at a high rotation speed which determines the upper cut-off limit for the milled particles to leave while coarser particles are retained in the chamber for further milling.

In addition to the milling of a pure API in a jet mill, milling of co-crystals and co-milling strategies have been investigated for improving the physical and/or pharmacokinetic properties of the DPI formulation. Micronized co-crystals of itraconazole were found to be superior to both the amorphous spray-dried and micronized crystalline itraconazole in rat pulmonary absorption studies (Karashima et al. 2017). Jet-milled co-crystals did not show evidence of co-crystal dissociation or losses in crystallinity. They simultaneously maintained formulation advantages of both amorphous and crystalline forms of the drug; greater physical/chemical stability over the amorphous form and higher intrinsic dissolution rates compared to the crystalline form. Co-milling in a jet mill has been investigated for direct preparation of inhalable mixtures, eliminating the need for a subsequent blending step. In this process, a mixture of drug and excipient (carrier and/or force control agent) is fed into the jet mill, and the product is a micronized uniform mixture. Since jet milling is a high energy process, very few agglomerates can be formed during milling and the components are more uniformly mixed compared to mechanical blending. Due to the inherent characteristics (e.g. particle size, crystal hardness, fragmentation mechanism) of each component, their respective size distributions in the co-milled product were found to be different with the same mill setting (Lau et al. 2017). The size of drug particles and excipient particles in a co-milled product cannot be individually determined by microscopy or laser diffraction. By assuming that the size distribution of each component is similar regardless of whether it is milled alone or in combination, rough estimations of the drug particle size can then be made. The inclusion of magnesium stearate during the co-milling of lactose and beclomethasone dipropionate led to less deterioration in the aerosol performance during storage at 75% relative humidity (RH). It was suggested that magnesium stearate could either form a protective coating on the amorphous regions of milled lactose or directly limit the formation of amorphous regions on lactose. In another study, co-milling of fusafungine and lactose in a jet mill was reported to be an essential step to create intimate mixtures of drug and fine excipient before blending with the coarse carrier (Giry et al. 2006). Physical blending of micronized drug, fine lactose, and coarse carrier could not achieve the same blend microstructure. The fine particle fraction (FPF) of formulations produced involving the co-milling step improved significantly to over 20% compared to less than 10% in the formulations without co-milling.

11.2.2.2 Other Mechanical Mills

Ball mills are more commonly used for micronization in academic research. Size reduction occurs by impact and attrition (Parrott 1974), and the size reduction limit is approximately 1 μm. Material is placed in the milling chamber with the grinding medium which usually consists of hard ceramic or steel balls. As the milling chamber is rotated, the balls slide in a cascading motion and cause attrition to particles located between the balls. Particles may also fragment when they collide with sufficient impact with balls falling from a height. Variables such as the size of balls, speed of rotation, and milling duration influence the size of milled product. Rapid centrifugal or vibratory movements to the mill can provide greater intensity to ball milling. The feed load in the milling chamber affects the efficiency of milling. An optimum fill of grinding medium is approximately 30%–50% of the milling chamber volume. The material should be added to fill the void spaces between the balls and just cover the grinding medium. Large amounts of heat are produced in the ball mill due to friction between the balls and may result in chemical/solid-state instability of the feed material. In one study, significant particle size reduction occurred in a ball-mill before any detectable increase in the amorphous content of salbutamol sulphate (Gaisford et al. 2010). With a milling time of 5 minutes, the median particle size of drug was reduced from 13 μm to 4 μm while amorphous content increased to 5%. After 20 minutes, the median particle size reduced slightly to 2.5 μm, but the amorphous content increased significantly to 17%. Approaching the limit of size reduction, it can be seen that additional milling energy contributes greatly to the solid-state instability rather than size reduction. Gradual wear of the balls also poses a contamination risk for the milled material. Compared to other micron-level milling techniques, the ball milling process is relatively easy to use and comparatively inexpensive, but results may be variable and the process is difficult to scale up. Thus, ball milling has limited applications in the commercial manufacture of inhalable drugs (Telko and Hickey 2005).

Size reduction in a pin mill occurs mainly by impact grinding. Material enters from the centre of the mill and falls onto a rotating platform. The rapid rotating motion causes the particles to be thrown outwards and through the grinding zone of rotating pins. The particles collide with pins that are concentrically mounted, both on a spinning rotor and a stationary plate. The rotation speed and number of pins determine the frequency of impact collisions and, therefore, the size of milled product. Milled particles continue to travel out of the grinding zone and are collected at the bottom of the mill. Like the ball mill, the size reduction limit of pin-milled particles is approximately 1 μm (Telko and Hickey 2005).

11.2.2.3 Wet Milling

Wet milling methods have been developed as alternatives to jet mills or mechanical impact mills to avoid both amorphization of milled product and electrostatic charging. Literature suggests that wet milling may reduce, but not entirely eliminate amorphous content in milled drug (Ostrander et al. 1999; Date and Patravale 2004). Recrystallization of amorphous regions on drug particles during storage may affect their size distribution, morphology, and surface properties (Malamatari et al. 2016). No commercial inhalable products have been produced by wet milling to date (Zhang et al. 2011), although it remains popular in academic research. Micron-sized particles can be produced either by micronization in wet media (Moura et al. 2016) or controlled crystallization by the addition of an anti-solvent in the presence of a stabilizer (Steckel et al. 2003a, 2003b; Murnane et al. 2009). Particles are then obtained after spray-drying of the dispersion.

The bead mill is commonly used for wet milling of drugs into nanoparticles, to less than 1 μm, in a time-consuming process that may extend from hours to days (Zhang et al. 2011). The operation of the bead mill is similar to the ball mill; grinding media is required and the rotation of an agitator/vessel results in size reduction by attrition and impaction. In order to prevent crystallinity changes (such as hydrate formation or amorphization), a suitable solvent in which the drug can be dispersed, but not dissolved (preferably having solubility lower than 5 mg/mL) is used as the wet media (Malamatari et al. 2016). A survey in literature suggests that nanoparticles for inhalation can be produced using wet milling (the other popular method being high pressure homogenization). Drugs which have been investigated include budesonide (Shrewsbury et al. 2009), beclomethasone dipropionate (Ostrander et al. 1999), itraconzole (Yang et al. 2010), fluticasone dipropionate (Chiang et al. 2009), and ciclesonide (Chiang et al. 2010). The nanoparticles typically range from 100 nm to 400 nm (Zhang et al. 2011). Almost all drugs were formulated as nebulizer solutions, suggesting that wet milling has limited applicability for dry formulations. Milling adjuvants such as surfactants or polymers are often required as stabilizers or to reduce aggregation (Loh et al. 2015). The lack of toxicological information for inhalation delivery of such adjuvants is a major barrier for the commercial adoption of such formulations. With proper control of milling parameters, dry inhalable particles can also be produced by wet milling. Dry particles of theophylline were produced in a bead mill using isopropyl alcohol as the wet media, followed by spray-drying of the suspension (Malamatari et al. 2016). It was necessary to include mannitol as a milling adjuvant to enhance size reduction. Spray-dried particles containing theophylline:mannitol and theophylline alone had median diameters of 2.2 μm and 4.6 μm, respectively. There was no loss of crystallinity of theophylline after milling, suggesting that the wet media promoted rapid recrystallization of amorphous regions formed on particle surfaces (Kayaert and Van den Mooter 2012). Alternatively, wet media may limit heat generation during milling and inhibit the amorphization process (Monteiro et al. 2013). In one study, pure budesonide nanoparticles were produced by bead milling for 10 hours followed by lyophilization (El-Gendy et al. 2012). Although these nanoparticles had a primary particle size of about 300 nm, they existed as dry agglomerates of 1 μm–3 μm. The FPF of the nanoparticle formulation was 66% and almost double that of a commercial budesonide DPI product (34%; Pulmicort®).

Particles produced using the wet and dry methods can exhibit significantly different physical properties, in particular, their surface morphology. The gross morphologies of wet-milled salmeterol xinafoate and fluticasone propionate particles appeared different from the corresponding particles micronized in the jet mill (Murnane et al. 2009). In another study, smoother particles of fluticasone propionate, mometasone furoate, and salmeterol xinafoate (with much reduced surface area) were attributed to the presence of liquid media which helped to remove surface defects (Moura et al. 2016). Most notably, the amorphous contents of particles produced using wet processes were lower than those produced by jet milling. This may be explained by the lower direct energy input to particles during micronization in wet media compared to jet milling.

11.2.3 Milling-Induced Amorphization

Conventional micronization techniques produce particles with suitable geometric and aerodynamic size distributions, but these particles have poor flow. One well-known disadvantage of milling is the increase in amorphous content of crystalline particles. A high energy method, such as ball, pin, or jet milling, induces many surface dislocations which result in amorphous regions on crystalline particles. These regions can increase the surface energy and cohesiveness of the powder (Brodka-Pfeiffer et al. 2003). It has been reported that amorphous regions due to milling can only be induced on particle surfaces. Direct physical evidence of milling-induced surface damage to a lactose crystal, corresponding to disorder of a few molecular layers (Andreou et al. 2009), was observed using the atomic force microscope (Price and Young 2005). A similar observation was reported for micronized budesonide particles (Jones et al. 2008). Milled crystalline material with low amorphous content (<1%) may therefore exhibit adhesive behavior that is similar to highly amorphous material (Newell et al. 2001; Gaisford et al. 2010). While spray-drying can directly produce inhalable particles with favorable aerodynamic properties, spray-dried products may be almost fully amorphous (Steckel et al. 2003b; Thi et al. 2008; Karashima et al. 2017). Re-crystallization will occur upon the sorption of water. Thus, changes in storage humidity and temperature may alter particle size (typically by particle growth) (Ward and Schultz 1995) and adhesion characteristics of the drug. These factors have the potential to cause gradual drifts in the *in vitro* drug deposition profiles throughout the shelf-life of the product. In addition to milled drug, the contribution of amorphous content in lactose carrier to product instability has also been noted (Das et al. 2009; Vollenbroek et al. 2010).

The amorphous content of drug or carrier may be investigated using spectroscopic, thermal, and gravimetric methods; powder X-ray diffraction (PXRD), inverse phase gas chromatography, differential scanning calorimetry (Ward and Schultz 1995), isothermal calorimetry (Ward and Schultz 1995; Newell et al. 2001; Gaisford et al. 2010; Alam et al. 2014), solution calorimetry (Newell et al. 2001), and dynamic vapor sorption (DVS) (Ward and Schultz 1995; Vollenbroek et al. 2010; Müller et al. 2015). A detailed comparison of thermal, spectroscopic, and vapor sorption methods for the quantification of amorphous content in salbutamol sulphate has been published (Grisedale et al. 2011). There are generally more literature reports on lactose compared to inhalation drugs, but the concepts described below are similar. Thermal methods measuring the heat change upon moisture sorption and re-crystallization are useful for estimating surface amorphous content. PXRD and solution calorimetry are more useful to estimate amorphous content in the bulk material. It has been reported that spectroscopic methods are not sufficiently sensitive to detect low amorphous contents in lactose carriers for inhalation (Shrewsbury et al. 2009). In one study, the limit of quantification of amorphous content using PXRD was reported as 1% (Chen et al. 2001). Gravimetric methods such as DVS exhibited a level of quantification of 0.5% (Vollenbroek et al. 2010). The relationship between amorphous content and surface energy is not as straightforward as expected (i.e. higher amorphous content results in higher surface energy). Researchers have argued that an "amorphous nature" cannot be exactly defined or characterized, and it is theoretically possible that different amorphous (and energy) states could be induced by different processing methods. This was aptly demonstrated by the discrepancies observed between amorphous content and surface energies of lactose powders prepared using different methods (Newell et al. 2001). Amorphous content of lactose was measured using solution calorimetry as the method accounts for the entire bulk and not only the crystal surfaces. A physical mixture of 99% crystalline and 1% amorphous lactose had very similar surface energy to 100% crystalline lactose. Spray-dried lactose (100% amorphous content) exhibited lower surface energies than milled lactose (0.7% amorphous content). One possible explanation for the discrepancy was that the surface disorder of milled lactose particles had higher energies than that of the spray-dried powder. A similar observation was reported in another study; spray-dried and freeze-dried lactose exhibited significantly different moisture sorption properties although both samples were fully amorphous (Vollenbroek et al. 2010). Hence, there is probably no true reference standard for fully amorphous lactose. This poses a problem as the majority of measurement methods require the use of "calibration standards" (Grisedale et al. 2011), which are pre-determined mixtures of fully amorphous and fully crystalline material. A method which does not require the use of calibration standards was proposed as follows: amorphous content can be calculated from the ratio of the enthalpy of crystallization at the melting temperature for the amorphous fraction to the heat of fusion of fully crystalline material (Phillips 1997). This method was demonstrated for micronized methylprednisolone.

11.3 Blending of Powders for Inhalation

Blending is both an essential and a critical process in solid dosage form manufacture. The primary purpose of blending, in the manufacture of tablets or capsules, is to achieve uniform and ideally, also non-segregating mixtures of drug and excipients. During the process, there should be minimal alterations to the physicochemical properties and/or size distributions of the constituent powders. Similar to milling operation, the nature of inhalable particles signifies that blending requirements differ greatly compared to mixtures of free-flowing powders. For interactive mixtures in DPIs, the blending process serves an additional functional purpose; to create the desired blend organization with an optimal cohesive-adhesive balance (CAB). This is because the blend organization, which refers to the physical arrangement and interactions between the active drug and excipient particles, has a direct influence on the aerosolization performance of a DPI formulation.

11.3.1 Characteristics of an Interactive Mixture

Materials of similar size and size distributions form random mixtures while those with highly dissimilar size characteristics, micronized and coarse particles, form interactive mixtures (Yeung and Hersey 1979). In an ideal random mixture, all samples of the mixture are identical in composition. There are equal, but negligible, forces of interaction between the individual particles (Poux et al. 1991). Gravity is the main force acting on particles in a free-flowing random mixture while motion or vibration may bring about segregation. Irregular particle shapes and high moisture contents are conditions which increase inter-particle interactions and reduce flowability. Ideal interactive mixtures, however, consist of non-random "ordered" units which are randomly distributed in the mixture. Each ordered unit is comprised of a coarse particle with many fine particles adhering to its surface. The adhesive forces between the fine and coarse particles are much greater than the gravitational forces acting on fine particles. This limited freedom of movement of fine particles (relative to coarse particles) imparts some "order" to the mixture and counteracts the effect of gravity on segregation (Yip and Hersey 1977). At the same time, coarse particles remain free-flowing and act as physical carriers of fine particles.

11.3.2 Mechanisms of Blending—Interactive Mixtures

Blending can occur by three main mechanisms: convective, shear, and diffusive blending (Poux et al. 1991; Twitchell 2007; Kaialy 2016). Convective (or macro-) blending occurs when large fractions of powder move randomly in the blender aided by a rotating blade or tumbling action. Diffusive (or micro-) blending occurs when individual particles move randomly to create a statistically uniform mixture at the scale of several particles. Shear blending results from the forced movement of one layer of powder over another due to velocity gradients. For example, the rotating impeller of a high shear blender creates transient shear planes which collapse as it cuts through the powder bed. In mixtures containing free-flowing powders of similar particle size and density, convective and diffusive blending in a low shear blender can produce a sufficiently blended mixture. In drug-carrier mixtures for inhalation, a certain degree of blend uniformity can be quickly achieved by low to medium shear blending; where drug in agglomerated form are uniformly blended with large carrier particles. Due to the limited energy input, this blend organization will be maintained regardless of mixing time. An even higher energy input (such as that from a high shear blender) is necessary for effective shearing and de-agglomeration of micronized drug powders (Clarke et al. 2001; Sebti et al. 2007; Le et al. 2012) and the redistribution of individual drug particles on carrier surfaces. De-agglomeration has been shown to be the rate-limiting step (Nguyen et al. 2015, 2016) and hence determines the total blending time required. Experimental evidence showed that the reduction in drug agglomerate size followed first-order kinetics, at the initial stages of blending, in both the Turbula® blender and V-Mixer (de Villiers 1997). The drug agglomerate size then remained relatively constant, indicating the transition from random to interactive blending. The time taken to reach this transition stage ranged from 40 minutes to 90 minutes. Blend uniformity of inhalation mixtures is thus better defined by attainment of the blend organization found in an ideal interactive mixture (i.e. uniformity at the level of individual carrier particles). At the same time, convective blending is also necessary to ensure uniform distribution of carrier particles within the powder.

Blending equipment may be classified based on their input of blending energy as low shear, medium shear, or high shear blenders. The power input to a stationary blender, equipped with an internal agitator, can be calculated from the torque of the rotating agitator and its rotational speed (Kaialy 2016). Examples of low shear blenders include the tumbling, planetary, double cone, conical screw, and ribbon types of blenders. The blender fill ratio, rotation speed, and blending time are critical parameters of rotating blenders (de Boer et al. 2012). High shear blenders are normally equipped with variable-speed agitators which rotate in the powder bed and the critical parameters include blender fill ratio, agitator speed, and blend time. An extensive review of the different blender types and their characteristics such as the blender design, applications, ease of cleaning, power, and volume capacity is available in the literature (Poux et al. 1991). Each blender has its own predominant blending mechanism and should be selected based on factors such as processing time, degree of blend uniformity achievable, and aerosolization performance after blending. Colored tracers have been successfully employed to study blending mechanisms as well as to categorize blenders based on their blending intensities. In one study, fine Rhodamine B particles (dark pink in color) were used with mannitol pellets and micronized lactose to study the redistribution of fines in adhesive mixtures in a high shear mixer (Nguyen et al. 2016). The lightness of color, using the CIELCh color space values, was used to monitor the migration of lactose fines to carrier particles. It was reported that a state of equilibrium for both redistribution of adhered fines and random mixing was established over very short timescales, in the order of a few minutes. As the model carrier used was spherical pellets, the effect of irregular particle shapes and surface roughness on mixing mechanisms could not be elucidated. Sub-micronized iron oxide, representing the micronized drug, was blended with lactose carriers in another study (Barling et al. 2015). The sequential phases of blending, namely, the dispersion of agglomerates, de-agglomeration, and finally particle breakage, could be differentiated based on the measured color space values. The Turbula® blender only enabled the dispersion of agglomerates regardless of mixing time while the high shear blender resulted in deagglomeration. Mechanofusion at speeds above 2000 rpm resulted in breakage of lactose particles. Thus, the analysis of color values was proposed as a method to define blend quality and the end-point of blending.

In addition to blending by physical agitation, newer mechanisms of blending have also been investigated for research applications. Resonant acoustic mixing (RAM), which uses low frequency and high intensity acoustic energy to fluidize and disperse powders uniformly at the micro-scale (~50 μm), has been utilized for interactive mixtures in DPI (Tanaka et al. 2018). The process is reported to be gentler and energy-efficient due to direct energy transfer to the mixing load with minimal losses due to friction. Small-scale blending of salmeterol xinafoate and fluticasone propionate with lactose carrier by RAM for about 150 seconds resulted in comparable drug content uniformity and *in vitro* deposition profiles to commercial reference products (Tanaka et al. 2018).

11.3.3 Blend Uniformity and Segregation

The content of micronized drug in a DPI formulation is typically low, less than 2%, weight by weight (w/w). It has been reported that an increase in the proportion of fine component to 5%, w/w in an interactive mixture greatly increased the blending time required to achieve blend uniformity (Staniforth et al. 1981). When considering blend uniformity of DPI mixtures, it is important to match the scale of scrutiny with the dosage unit of the DPI product. The United States Pharmacopeia criteria for content uniformity for DPI is 85%–115% of the label claim while the relative standard deviation (RSD) of 10 dosage units should be less than or equal to 6%. The industry standard is usually more stringent and is often set at 90%–110%. Long duration of blending in a low shear blender, such as a tumbling or V-shaped blender, is normally required to achieve an acceptable variation in drug content (Tanaka et al. 2018). A pre-blending step which involves geometric dilution of the drug might reduce blending time (Carstensen and Rhodes 1984). High shear blenders are therefore often preferred in production due to their higher energy input/efficiency and shorter blending time.

High shear blenders specifically designed for DPI formulation, such as the Turbo Rapid Variable (TRV) blender from Gesellschaft für Entstaubungsanlagen (GEA) and the Cyclomix® from Hosokawa Micron, are equipped with agitators of large surface areas to efficiently impart the blending energy to the powder mass.

Blending and segregation may be considered as processes in dynamic equilibrium. While segregation mechanisms in powders are widely reported (Williams 1976; Hogg 2009), few studies investigated the segregation of interactive mixtures in detail. Due to the relative simplicity of the chemical and physical compositions of DPI mixtures (typically binary/ternary mixtures) and the restricted mobility of adhesive particles, only a few mechanisms are directly relevant. The differences in particle size and density are the two main contributing factors to segregation. Segregation of interactive mixtures may occur under the following scenarios (Poux et al. 1991); during blending (referred as de-mixing) or in downstream handling/processing. De-mixing is characterized by an increase in the RSD of drug content beyond a critical blending time. Prolonged blending times in a Turbula® blender were shown to result in de-mixing (Poux et al. 1991). This was attributed to excessive inertial or shear forces which resulted in the disruption of adhesive forces between drug and carrier particles. It has been reported that interactive mixtures which require long blending times also have higher segregation potential (Staniforth et al. 1981). The coarse and fine components in these systems are thought to have lower "affinities" (adhesion strength) for each other and are thus easier to be separated by external forces such as vibration. Segregation due to differences in particle size occurs as fine agglomerates move through the inter-particulate voids of the powder bed more readily than carrier particles (Hogg 2009). This process is encouraged by vibration which causes a transient dilation of the bed and an increase in particle mobility. Carrier particles themselves may also segregate due to differences in particle size or shape. In this case, however, the non-uniform distribution of drug particles on carrier particles often precedes the segregation of carrier particles themselves. A gradual decrease in drug content with increased blending time may be observed and attributed to segregation (Kaialy 2016). Fine drug particles may be lost due to adhesion to the walls of the blender as the van der Waals and electrostatic forces greatly exceed the gravitational forces on particles with small masses.

11.3.4 Achieving the Cohesive-Adhesive Balance through Blending

The relationships between blending parameters (blender type, blending time, and speed) and DPI performance (drug adhesion/FPF) are rarely straightforward. These disparities in literature reports could probably be related to the differing criteria which researchers use to define the "optimal" blending time along with other variables in experimental conditions and procedures. The optimal blending time should be defined as the time required to achieve the optimal state of CAB. The CAB refers to the fine balance between cohesion (drug-drug) and adhesion (drug-carrier) forces that will dictate the achievable best *in vitro* performance of the DPI. Hence, the optimal blending time can be broadly defined as the blending time which ensures that: (i) de-agglomeration and uniform distribution of drug particles over carrier surfaces have occurred, (ii) blend uniformity at the scale of a unit dose has been achieved, (iii) adhesion strength between drug and carrier is sufficient to withstand segregation forces, and (iv) adhesion strength is sufficiently weak to permit easy detachment of drug during aerosolization by the air shear forces. The third and fourth points may be considered as competing outcomes. It is therefore quite apparent that the "optimal" blending time for any particular formulation/blender cannot be easily defined without extensive experimental validation work. Besides the control by blending time, force control agents can also be used to modulate the cohesive-adhesive balance of interactive mixtures. The inclusion of magnesium stearate in the drug-lactose powder of the Fostair® NEXThaler (beclomethasone dipropionate and formoterol fumarate) has been thought to reduce the association between the two APIs and their adhesion to the carrier. Experimental evidence showed that the FPF of both drugs were increased while their mass median aerodynamic diameters (MMAD) were decreased in the presence of magnesium stearate (Jetzer et al. 2018). Magnesium stearate was strongly co-associated with drug particles up to the point of deposition.

For any given type of blender, the increase of blending speed and time generally promotes blend uniformity up to a certain limit. The negative impacts of prolonged blending time or high blending speed have been widely reported. There was a clear negative relationship between the energy input of the Picomix® and the FPF of DPI formulations (Hertel et al. 2017). Longer blending times in high shear blenders promote stronger drug-carrier adhesion (de Villiers 1997; Podczeck 1997; Kaialy 2016). This is because the impeller blades tend to exert compressive forces on the powder. The compaction of powder was visually observed when excessive impeller speeds were used in one study (Sebti et al. 2007), suggesting the press-on forces were significant too. A quadratic relationship between the mixing energy and press-on forces has been proposed (Selvam and Smyth 2011). At the particulate level, press-on forces can increase drug adhesion to smooth surfaces while forcing drug particles into large crevices. Drug particles residing in crevices occupy positions of greatest stability (Kulvanich and Stewart 1987) and thus are significantly more difficult to displace. It was reported that the degree of drug adhesion, as measured by a centrifugation method, increased with blending time (Podczeck 1997), but eventually reached a point of saturation (Kulvanich and Stewart 1987). It was recommended that the optimal blending time should be defined at this point, where the interactive mixture would be reasonably stable to segregation and yet not too adhesive. Mixing speed does not influence the adhesion force or MMAD in a linear fashion (Podczeck 1997). The minimum adhesion value (corresponding to minimum MMAD) of a salmeterol xinafoate-lactose formulation was obtained at a medium, but not higher or lower, blending speed in a Turbula® mixer. An increase in the mixing speed led to more rapid de-agglomeration of drug at early stages of blending (de Villiers 1997). However, an excessive amount of blending energy may result in the milling and attrition of powders even when the duration is short (Hertel et al. 2017). A large amount of fines was generated, accompanied by a 3-fold increase in the specific surface area, after a batch of lactose (63 μm–90 μm) was blended for 1 minute at 500 rpm in a high shear blender (Shur et al. 2008). In comparison, no such changes were observed in the Turbula® T2F or Vortex mixer. When powders with low moisture contents are blended at high speeds, development of electrostatic charges may exert a negative influence on blend uniformity. This is because the degree of charging is related to the number of contacts/collisions between particles while charge dissipation is improved in the presence of moisture. This could be mitigated by introducing intermittent "rest" periods during blending for charges to dissipate (Le et al. 2012).

The influence of blending order of ingredients in a ternary mixture has been investigated due to the reported benefits of fine excipient on the FPF (Zeng et al. 1999, 2000). Fine excipient particles can modulate the physical interactions between drug and carrier particles (Tan et al. 2015). It is usually recommended that the fine excipient be blended with the coarse carrier first (before blending with the drug), although other studies have suggested no such benefit due to a redistribution mechanism at play (Lucas et al. 1998; Louey and Stewart 2002). Saturation of the high energy "active sites" by fine excipient particles prevents strong adhesion of micronized drug on these active sites (Kulvanich and Stewart 1987; El-Sabawi et al. 2006; Pilcer et al. 2012). This will ease their detachment from carrier surfaces during aerosolization. While this is theoretically plausible, the negative impact of this blending order on content uniformity has to be considered. In one study, coarse lactose was blended with beclomethasone dipropionate first (before fine lactose), and the RSD of drug content was 3.0% after 15 minutes (Zeng et al. 2000). However, a total of 60 minutes of blending was necessary to achieve the RSD of 4.1% when coarse lactose was first blended with fine lactose followed by the drug. In other studies, it was found that blending order had no influence on FPF when the drug content was above the range of 0.9% to 1.5%, w/w (Jones et al. 2010). It appears that blending order studies may be significantly more complex and the final blend organization determined the influence of blending order on FPF. In cases where the drug was predominantly adhered to carrier surfaces in the final mixture, blending order was of importance. When the drug was extensively redistributed or formed mixed agglomerates with fine excipient particles, blending order had less impact on the FPF. Thus, formulation factors such as the particle size of the fine excipient and content ratios of drug to fine excipient to coarse carrier are other important considerations in blending.

11.4 Conclusion

Milling and blending can be viewed as complementary techniques for the preparation of inhalable particles for DPI. Due to the inherent physicochemical and solid-state properties of micronized particles, such irregular morphologies, high surface energy and poor flow, it is almost always necessary to formulate them with a carrier. Jet milling remains as the micronization technique of choice for commercial applications due to its milling efficiency, low temperature environment, high throughput, and containment systems. While milling-induced amorphization is a true concern in any size reduction process, proper optimization of milling parameters or conditioning of drug may reduce its effect on product stability. Compared to milling of drug, blending of interactive mixtures is significantly more complex. In addition to blend uniformity, blending may be used to control the CAB in the interactive mixtures. Various options in formulation and blending techniques include: blending with force-control agents, modification of blending order, selection of blender design, and optimization of the speed and time of blending. Researchers have not reached a consensus on the impact of the above-mentioned variables on DPI performance. This is because the blending outcomes are also highly dependent on formulation variables, such as carrier particle size, surface properties, drug cohesiveness and adhesiveness, drug load, carrier to drug ratio, amorphous content, and many more. The inclusion of a ternary excipient adds further complexity to formulation design. Continued experimentation and optimization of milling and blending processes will allow for more efficient yet simplified ways to improve manufacturing and product performance.

LIST OF ABBREVIATIONS

3D three-dimensional
API active pharmaceutical ingredient
CAB cohesive-adhesive balance
CIE Commission international de l'éclairage (International Commission on Illumination)
DPI dry powder inhalation
DVS dynamic vapor sorption
FPF fine particle fraction
MMAD mass median aerodynamic diameter
PXRD powder X-ray diffraction
RAM resonant acoustic mixing
RSD relative standard deviation
TRV turbo rapid variable

REFERENCES

Alam, Shamsul, Mahmoud Omar, and Simon Gaisford. 2014. "Use of heat of adsorption to quantify amorphous content in milled pharmaceutical powders." *International Journal of Pharmaceutics* 459 (1):19–22. doi:10.1016/j.ijpharm.2013.11.052.

Alpine, Hosokawa. 2018. *Fluidised Bed Opposed Jet Mill AFG.* Hosowaka Alpine 2016 [cited 10 February 2018].

Andreou, J. G., P. J. Stewart, and D. A. V. Morton. 2009. "Short-term changes in drug agglomeration within interactive mixtures following blending." *International Journal of Pharmaceutics* 372 (1):1–11. doi:10.1016/j.ijpharm.2008.12.042.

Baláž, Peter. 2008. "High-energy milling." In *Mechanochemistry in Nanoscience and Minerals Engineering*, edited by Peter Baláž, pp. 103–132. Berlin, Germany: Springer.

Barling, David, David A. V. Morton, and Karen Hapgood. 2015. "Pharmaceutical dry powder blending and scale-up: Maintaining equivalent mixing conditions using a coloured tracer powder." *Powder Technology* 270:461–469. doi:10.1016/j.powtec.2014.04.069.

Bond, Fred Chester. 1952. "The third theory of comminution." *Transactions of the American Institute of Mining, Metallurgical and Petroleum Engineers* 193:484–494.

Brodka-Pfeiffer, Katharina, Peter Langguth, Peter Graβ, and Heribert Häusler. 2003. "Influence of mechanical activation on the physical stability of salbutamol sulphate." *European Journal of Pharmaceutics and Biopharmaceutics* 56 (3):393–400. doi:10.1016/S0939-6411(03)00134-6.

Carstensen, Jens Thurø, and Christopher T. Rhodes. 1984. "Optimization of preblending in random mixing." *Drug Development and Industrial Pharmacy* 10 (7):1017–1023. doi:10.3109/03639048409038302.

Chamayou, Alain, and John A. Dodds. 2007. "Chapter 8: Air jet milling." In *Handbook of Powder Technology*, edited by Agba D. Salman, Mojtaba Ghadiri and Michael J. Hounslow, pp. 421–435. Amsterdam, the Netherlands: Elsevier Science B.V.

Chan, Lai Wah, Cameron C. Lee, and Paul Wan Sia Heng. 2002. "Ultrafine grinding using a fluidized bed opposed jet mill: Effects of feed load and rotational speed of classifier wheel on particle shape." *Drug Development and Industrial Pharmacy* 28 (8):939–947. doi:10.1081/DDC-120006426.

Chen, Weinan, and Donald W. Fryrear. 2001. "Aerodynamic and geometric diameters of airborne particles." *Journal of Sedimentary Research* 71 (3):365–371. doi:10.1306/2DC4094A-0E47-11D7-8643000102C1865D.

Chen, Xiaoming, Simon Bates, and Kenneth R. Morris. 2001. "Quantifying amorphous content of lactose using parallel beam X-ray powder diffraction and whole pattern fitting." *Journal of Pharmaceutical and Biomedical Analysis* 26 (1):63–72. doi:10.1016/S0731-7085(01)00346-6.

Chiang, Po-Chang, Jason W. Alsup, Yurong Lai, Yiding Hu, Bruce R. Heyde, and David Tung. 2009. "Evaluation of aerosol delivery of nanosuspension for pre-clinical pulmonary drug delivery." *Nanoscale Research Letters* 4 (3):254–261. doi:10.1007/s11671-008-9234-1.

Chiang, Po-Chang, Yiding Hu, Jason D. Blom, and David C. Thompson. 2010. "Evaluating the suitability of using rat models for preclinical efficacy and side effects with inhaled corticosteroids nanosuspension formulations." *Nanoscale Research Letters* 5 (6):1010–1019. doi:10.1007/s11671-010-9597-y.

Clarke, Martyn J., Michael J. Tobyn, and John N. Staniforth. 2001. "The formulation of powder inhalation systems containing a high mass of nedocromil sodium trihydrate." *Journal of Pharmaceutical Sciences* 90 (2):213–223. doi:10.1002/1520-6017(200102)90:2<213::AID-JPS12>3.0.CO;2-7.

Das, Shyamal, Ian Larson, Paul Young, and Peter Stewart. 2009. "Influence of storage relative humidity on the dispersion of salmeterol xinafoate powders for inhalation." *Journal of Pharmaceutical Sciences* 98 (3):1015–1027. doi:10.1002/jps.21500.

Date, Abhijit A., and V. B. Patravale. 2004. "Current strategies for engineering drug nanoparticles." *Current Opinion in Colloid & Interface Science* 9 (3):222–235. doi:10.1016/j.cocis.2004.06.009.

de Boer, Anne H., Chan Ha-Kim, and Robert Price. 2012. "A critical view on lactose-based drug formulation and device studies for dry powder inhalation: Which are relevant and what interactions to expect?" *Advanced Drug Delivery Reviews* 64 (3):257–274. doi:10.1016/j.addr.2011.04.004.

de Boer, Anne H., Paul Hagedoorn, Marcel Hoppentocht, Francesca Buttini, Floris Grasmeijer, and Henderik W. Frijlink. 2017. "Dry powder inhalation: Past, present and future." *Expert Opinion on Drug Delivery* 14 (4):499–512. doi:10.1080/17425247.2016.1224846.

de Villiers, Melgardt M. 1997. "Description of the kinetics of the deagglomeration of drug particle agglomerates during powder mixing." *International Journal of Pharmaceutics* 151 (1):1–6. doi:10.1016/S0378-5173(97)04893-X.

Dobson, B., and Eric Rothwell. 1969. "Particle size reduction in a fluid energy mill." *Powder Technology* 3 (1):213–217. doi:10.1016/0032-5910(69)80080-X.

El-Gendy, Nashwa, Parthiban Selvam, Pravin Soni, and Cory Berkland. 2012. "Development of budesonide nanocluster dry powder aerosols: Processing." *Journal of Pharmaceutical Sciences* 101 (9):3425–3433. doi:10.1002/jps.23168.

El-Sabawi, Dina, Stephen Edge, Robert Price, and Paul M. Young. 2006. "Continued investigation into the influence of loaded dose on the performance of dry powder inhalers: Surface smoothing effects." *Drug Development and Industrial Pharmacy* 32 (10):1135–1138. doi:10.1080/03639040600712920.

Flagan, Richard C., and John H. Seinfeld. 1988. "Aerosols." In *Fundamentals of Air Pollution Engineering*, pp. 290–357. Englewood Cliffs, NJ: Prentice-Hall.

Gaisford, Simon, Mansa Dennison, Mahmoud Tawfik, and Matthew D. Jones. 2010. "Following mechanical activation of salbutamol sulphate during ball-milling with isothermal calorimetry." *International Journal of Pharmaceutics* 393 (1):75–79. doi:10.1016/j.ijpharm.2010.04.004.

Ghadiri, Mojtaba, Chih Chi Kwan, and Yulong Ding. 2007. "Chapter 14: Analysis of milling and the role of feed properties." In *Handbook of Powder Technology*, edited by Agba D. Salman, Mojtaba Ghadiri and Michael J. Hounslow, pp. 605–634. Amsterdam, the Netherlands: Elsevier Science B.V.

Giry, Karine, Jean Manuel Péan, L. Giraud, S. Marsas, Hervé Rolland, and Patrick Wüthrich. 2006. "Drug/lactose co-micronization by jet milling to improve aerosolization properties of a powder for inhalation." *International Journal of Pharmaceutics* 321 (1):162–166. doi:10.1016/j.ijpharm.2006.05.009.

Grisedale, Louise C., Matthew J. Jamieson, Peter S. Belton, Susan A. Barker, and Duncan Q. M. Craig. 2011. "Characterization and quantification of amorphous material in milled and spray-dried salbutamol sulfate: a comparison of thermal, spectroscopic, and water vapor sorption approaches." *Journal of Pharmaceutical Sciences* 100 (8):3114–3129. doi:10.1002/jps.22484.

Healy, Anne Marie, Maria Inês Amaro, Krzysztof J. Paluch, and Lidia Tajber. 2014. "Dry powders for oral inhalation free of lactose carrier particles." *Advanced Drug Delivery Reviews* 75:32–52. doi:10.1016/j.addr.2014.04.005.

Hertel, Mats, Eugen Schwarz, Mirjam Kobler, Sabine Hauptstein, Hartwig Steckel, and Regina Scherließ. 2017. "The influence of high shear mixing on ternary dry powder inhaler formulations." *International Journal of Pharmaceutics* 534 (1):242–250. doi:10.1016/j.ijpharm.2017.10.033.

Hogg, Richard. 2009. "Mixing and segregation in powders: Evaluation, mechanisms and processes." *KONA Powder and Particle Journal* 27:3–17. doi:10.14356/kona.2009005.

Jetzer, Martin W., Bradley D. Morrical, Marcel Schneider, Stephen Edge, and Georgios Imanidis. 2018. "Probing the particulate microstructure of the aerodynamic particle size distribution of dry powder inhaler combination products." *International Journal of Pharmaceutics* 538 (1):30–39. doi:10.1016/j.ijpharm.2017.12.046.

Jones, Matthew D., João G. F. Santo, Bilal Yakub, Mansa Dennison, Husein Master, and Graham Buckton. 2010. "The relationship between drug concentration, mixing time, blending order and ternary dry powder inhalation performance." *International Journal of Pharmaceutics* 391 (1–2):137–147. doi:10.1016/j.ijpharm.2010.02.031.

Jones, Matthew D., Paul M. Young, Daniela Traini, Jagdeep Shur, Stephen Edge, and Robert Price. 2008. "The use of atomic force microscopy to study the conditioning of micronised budesonide." *International Journal of Pharmaceutics* 357 (1–2):314–317. doi:10.1016/j.ijpharm.2008.01.042.

Kaialy, Waseem. 2016. "On the effects of blending, physicochemical properties, and their interactions on the performance of carrier-based dry powders for inhalation—A review." *Advances in Colloid and Interface Science* 235:70–89. doi:10.1016/j.cis.2016.05.014.

Karashima, Masatoshi, Noriyasu Sano, Syunsuke Yamamoto, Yuta Arai, Katsuhiko Yamamoto, Nobuyuki Amano, and Yukihiro Ikeda. 2017. "Enhanced pulmonary absorption of poorly soluble itraconazole by micronized cocrystal dry powder formulations." *European Journal of Pharmaceutics and Biopharmaceutics* 115:65–72. doi:10.1016/j.ejpb.2017.02.013.

Kayaert, Pieterjan, and Guy Van den Mooter. 2012. "Is the amorphous fraction of a dried nanosuspension caused by milling or by drying? A case study with Naproxen and Cinnarizine." *European Journal of Pharmaceutics and Biopharmaceutics* 81 (3):650–656. doi:10.1016/j.ejpb.2012.04.020.

Kick, Friedrich. 1885. *Das Gesetz der proportionalen Widerstande und seine anwendung*. Leipzig, Germany: Arthur Felix.

Kulvanich, Poj, and Peter J. Stewart. 1987. "The effect of blending time on particle adhesion in a model interactive system." *Journal of Pharmacy and Pharmacology* 39 (9):732–733.

Lau, Michael, Paul M. Young, and Daniela Traini. 2017. "Co-milled API-lactose systems for inhalation therapy: Impact of magnesium stearate on physico-chemical stability and aerosolization performance." *Drug Development and Industrial Pharmacy* 43 (6):980–988. doi:10.1080/03639045.2017.1287719.

Le, V. N. P., Thanh Huong Hoang Thi, E. Robins, and Marie Pierre Flament. 2012. "Dry powder inhalers: Study of the parameters influencing adhesion and dispersion of fluticasone propionate." *AAPS PharmSciTech* 13 (2):477–484. doi:10.1208/s12249-012-9765-8.

Loh, Zhi Hui, Asim Kumar Samanta, and Paul Wan Sia Heng. 2015. "Overview of milling techniques for improving the solubility of poorly water-soluble drugs." *Asian Journal of Pharmaceutical Sciences* 10 (4):255–274. doi:10.1016/j.ajps.2014.12.006.

Louey, Margaret D., and Peter J. Stewart. 2002. "Particle interactions involved in aerosol dispersion of ternary interactive mixtures." *Pharmaceutical Research* 19 (10):1524–1531.

Lucas, Paul, Kerry Anderson, and John N. Staniforth. 1998. "Protein deposition from dry powder inhalers: fine particle multiplets as performance modifiers." *Pharmaceutical Research* 15 (4):562–569.

Malamatari, Maria, Satyanarayana Somavarapu, Kyriakos Kachrimanis, Mark Bloxham, Kevin M. G. Taylor, and Graham Buckton. 2016. "Preparation of theophylline inhalable microcomposite particles by wet milling and spray drying: The influence of mannitol as a co-milling agent." *International Journal of Pharmaceutics* 514 (1):200–211. doi:10.1016/j.ijpharm.2016.06.032.

Mann, Charles A. 1937. "Principles of chemical engineering. By W. H. Walker, W. K. Lewis, W. H. McAdams, and E. R. Gilliland." *The Journal of Physical Chemistry* 41 (9):1231. doi:10.1021/j150387a017.

Monteiro, Alexandre, Afolawemi Afolabi, and Ecevit Bilgili. 2013. "Continuous production of drug nanoparticle suspensions via wet stirred media milling: A fresh look at the Rehbinder effect." *Drug Development and Industrial Pharmacy* 39 (2):266–283. doi:10.3109/03639045.2012.676048.

Moura, Cláudia, Filipe Neves, and Eunice Costa. 2016. "Impact of jet-milling and wet-polishing size reduction technologies on inhalation API particle properties." *Powder Technology* 298:90–98. doi:10.1016/j.powtec.2016.05.008.

Müller, Frank, Reinhard F. Polke, and G. Schädel. 1996. "Spiral jet mills: Hold up and scale up." *International Journal of Mineral Processing* 44–45:315–326. doi:10.1016/0301-7516(95)00042-9.

Müller, Thorsten, Regina Krehl, Jörg Schiewe, Claudius Weiler, and Hartwig Steckel. 2015. "Influence of small amorphous amounts in hydrophilic and hydrophobic APIs on storage stability of dry powder inhalation products." *European Journal of Pharmaceutics and Biopharmaceutics* 92:130–138. doi:10.1016/j.ejpb.2015.03.006.

Murnane, Darragh, Gary P. Martin, and Christopher Marriott. 2009. "Dry powder formulations for inhalation of fluticasone propionate and salmeterol xinafoate microcrystals." *Journal of Pharmaceutical Sciences* 98 (2):503–515. doi:10.1002/jps.21450.

Naik, Shivangi, and Bodhisattwa Chaudhuri. 2015. "Quantifying dry milling in pharmaceutical processing: A review on experimental and modeling approaches." *Journal of Pharmaceutical Sciences* 104 (8):2401–2413. doi:10.1002/jps.24512.

Newell, Helen E., Graham Buckton, David A. Butler, Frank Thielmann, and Daryl R. Williams. 2001. "The use of inverse phase gas chromatography to measure the surface energy of crystalline, amorphous, and recently milled lactose." *Pharmaceutical Research* 18 (5):662–666. doi:10.1023/A:1011089511959.

Nguyen, Duy, Anders Rasmuson, Ingela Niklasson Björn, and Kyrre Thalberg. 2015. "Mechanistic time scales in adhesive mixing investigated by dry particle sizing." *European Journal of Pharmaceutical Sciences* 69:19–25. doi:10.1016/j.ejps.2014.12.016.

Nguyen, Duy, Anders Rasmuson, Kyrre Thalberg, and Ingela Niklasson Björn. 2016. "A study of the redistribution of fines between carriers in adhesive particle mixing using image analysis with coloured tracers." *Powder Technology* 299:71–76. doi:10.1016/j.powtec.2016.05.030.

O'Connor, Robert E., Joseph B. Schwartz, and Linda A. Felton. 2006. "Powders." In *Remington: The Science and Practice of Pharmacy*, edited by David B. Troy and Paul Beringer. Baltimore, MD: Lippincott Williams & Wilkins.

Ostrander, Kevin D., H. William Bosch, and Donna M. Bondanza. 1999. "An in-vitro assessment of a NanoCrystal™ beclomethasone dipropionate colloidal dispersion via ultrasonic nebulization." *European Journal of Pharmaceutics and Biopharmaceutics* 48 (3):207–215. doi:10.1016/S0939-6411(99)00049-1.

Parrott, Eugene L. 1974. "Milling of pharmaceutical solids." *Journal of Pharmaceutical Sciences* 63 (6):813–829. doi:10.1002/jps.2600630603.

Phillips, Elaine M. 1997. "An approach to estimate the amorphous content of pharmaceutical powders using calorimetry with no calibration standards." *International Journal of Pharmaceutics* 149 (2):267–271. doi:10.1016/S0378-5173(96)04812-0.

Pilcer, Gabrielle, Nathalie Wauthoz, and Karim Amighi. 2012. "Lactose characteristics and the generation of the aerosol." *Advanced Drug Delivery Reviews* 64 (3):233–256. doi:10.1016/j.addr.2011.05.003.

Podczeck, Fridrun. 1997. "The development of a cascade impactor simulator based on adhesion force measurements to aid the development of dry powder inhalations." *Chemical and Pharmaceutical Bulletin (Tokyo)* 45 (5):911–917.

Poux, Martine, P. Fayolle, Joël Bertrand, D. Bridoux, and Jacques Louis Bousquet. 1991. "Powder mixing: Some practical rules applied to agitated systems." *Powder Technology* 68 (3):213–234. doi:10.1016/0032-5910(91)80047-M.

Price, Robert, and Paul M. Young. 2005. "On the physical transformations of processed pharmaceutical solids." *Micron* 36 (6):519–524. doi:10.1016/j.micron.2005.04.003.

Sebti, Thambi, Francis Vanderbist, and Karim Amighi. 2007. "Evaluation of the content homogeneity and dispersion properties of fluticasone DPI compositions." *Journal of Drug Delivery Science and Technology* 17 (3):223–229. doi:10.1016/S1773-2247(07)50040-7.

Selvam, Parthiban, and Hugh D. C. Smyth. 2011. "Effect of press-on forces on drug adhesion in dry powder inhaler formulations." *Journal of Adhesion Science and Technology* 25 (14):1659–1670. doi:10.1163/016942410X533390.

Shrewsbury, Stephen B., Andrew P. Bosco, and Paul S. Uster. 2009. "Pharmacokinetics of a novel submicron budesonide dispersion for nebulized delivery in asthma." *International Journal of Pharmaceutics* 365 (1):12–17. doi:10.1016/j.ijpharm.2008.08.012.

Shur, Jagdeep, Haggis Harris, Matthew D. Jones, J. Sebastian Kaerger, and Robert Price. 2008. "The role of fines in the modification of the fluidization and dispersion mechanism within dry powder inhaler formulations." *Pharmaceutical Research* 25 (7):1631–1640. doi:10.1007/s11095-008-9538-y.

Shur, Jagdeep, Robert Price, David Lewis, Paul M. Young, Grahame Woollam, Dilraj Singh, and Stephen Edge. 2016. "From single excipients to dual excipient platforms in dry powder inhaler products." *International Journal of Pharmaceutics* 514 (2):374–383. doi:10.1016/j.ijpharm.2016.05.057.

Staniforth, John N., John E. Rees, and John B. Kayes. 1981. "Relation between mixing time and segregation of ordered mixes." *Journal of Pharmacy and Pharmacology* 33 (1):175–176. doi:10.1111/j.2042-7158.1981.tb13745.x.

Steckel, Hartwig, Norbert Rasenack, and Bernd W. Müller. 2003a. "In-situ-micronization of disodium cromoglycate for pulmonary delivery." *European Journal of Pharmaceutics and Biopharmaceutics* 55 (2):173–180. doi:10.1016/S0939-6411(02)00168-6.

Steckel, Hartwig, Norbert Rasenack, Peter Villax, and Bernd W. Müller. 2003b. "In vitro characterization of jet-milled and in-situ-micronized fluticasone-17-propionate." *International Journal of Pharmaceutics* 258 (1):65–75. doi:10.1016/S0378-5173(03)00153-4.

Tan, Bernice Mei Jin, Celine Valeria Liew, Lai Wah Chan, and Paul Wan Sia Heng. 2015. "Particle surface roughness – Its characterisation and impact on dry powder inhaler performance." In *Pulmonary Drug Delivery*, pp. 199–222. Chichester, UK: John Wiley & Sons.

Tanaka, Ryoma, Naoyuki Takahashi, Yasuaki Nakamura, Yusuke Hattori, Kazuhide Ashizawa, and Makoto Otsuka. 2018. "Performance of an acoustically mixed pharmaceutical dry powder delivered from a novel inhaler." *International Journal of Pharmaceutics* 538 (1):130–138. doi:10.1016/j.ijpharm.2018.01.001.

Tanaka, Tatsuo. 1966. "Comminution laws. Several probabilities." *Industrial & Engineering Chemistry Process Design and Development* 5 (4):353–358. doi:10.1021/i260020a001.

Telko, Martin J., and Anthony J. Hickey. 2005. "Dry powder inhaler formulation." *Respir Care* 50 (9):1209–1227.

Thi, Thanh Huong Hoang, Florence Danède, Marc Descamps, and Marie-Pierre Flament. 2008. "Comparison of physical and inhalation properties of spray-dried and micronized terbutaline sulphate." *European Journal of Pharmaceutics and Biopharmaceutics* 70 (1):380–388. doi:10.1016/j.ejpb.2008.04.002.

Twitchell, M. Andrew. 2007. "Mixing." In *Aulton's Pharmaceutics: The Design and Manufacture of Medicines*, edited by Michael E. Aulton, pp. 152–167. New York: Churchill Livingstone.

Vollenbroek, Jasper, Gerald A. Hebbink, Susanne Ziffels, and Hartwig Steckel. 2010. "Determination of low levels of amorphous content in inhalation grade lactose by moisture sorption isotherms." *International Journal of Pharmaceutics* 395 (1–2):62–70. doi:10.1016/j.ijpharm.2010.04.035.

von Rittinger, Peter Ritter. 1867. *Lehrbuch der Aufbereitungskunde*. Berlin, Germany: Ernst and Korn.

Ward, Gary H., and Robert K. Schultz. 1995. "Process-induced crystallinity changes in albuterol sulfate and its effect on powder physical stability." *Pharmaceutical Research* 12 (5):773–779. doi:10.1023/a:1016232230638.

Williams, James C. 1976. "The segregation of particulate materials. A review." *Powder Technology* 15 (2):245–251. doi:10.1016/0032-5910(76)80053-8.

Yang, Wei, Keith P. Johnston, and Robert O. Williams. 2010. "Comparison of bioavailability of amorphous versus crystalline itraconazole nanoparticles via pulmonary administration in rats." *European Journal of Pharmaceutics and Biopharmaceutics* 75 (1):33–41. doi:10.1016/j.ejpb.2010.01.011.

Yeung, Charles C., and John A. Hersey. 1979. "Ordered powder mixing of coarse and fine particulate systems." *Powder Technology* 22 (1):127–131. doi:10.1016/0032-5910(79)85015-9.

Yip, Chee Wai, and J. A. Hersey. 1977. "Ordered or random mixing: Choice of system and mixer." *Drug Development and Industrial Pharmacy* 3 (5):429–438. doi:10.3109/03639047709055622.

Yu-Wei, Lin, Wong Jennifer, Qu Li, Chan Hak-Kim, and Zhou Qi. 2015. "Powder production and particle engineering for dry powder inhaler formulations." *Current Pharmaceutical Design* 21 (27):3902–3916. doi:10.2174/1381612821666150820111134.

Zeng, Xian Ming, Gary Peter Martin, Seah-Kee Tee, Abeer Abu Ghoush, and Christopher Marriott. 1999. "Effects of particle size and adding sequence of fine lactose on the deposition of salbutamol sulphate from a dry powder formulation." *International Journal of Pharmaceutics* 182 (2):133–144. doi:10.1016/S0378-5173(99)00021-6.

Zeng, Xian Ming, Kiranpal H. Pandhal, and Gary P. Martin. 2000. "The influence of lactose carrier on the content homogeneity and dispersibility of beclomethasone dipropionate from dry powder aerosols." *International Journal of Pharmaceutics* 197 (1):41–52. doi:10.1016/S0378-5173(99)00400-7.

Zhang, Jian, Libo Wu, Hak-Kim Chan, and Wiwik Watanabe. 2011. "Formation, characterization, and fate of inhaled drug nanoparticles." *Advanced Drug Delivery Reviews* 63 (6):441–455. doi:10.1016/j.addr.2010.11.002.

12

Engineering Stable Spray-Dried Biologic Powder for Inhalation

Nicholas Carrigy and Reinhard Vehring

CONTENTS

12.1 Introduction

In 1865, Charles A. La Mont of New York claimed invention of a method of desiccating egg-batter into fine particles, whereby the egg-batter is forced into a spray using a "powerful blast of air" and made to "fall through a current of heated air" [1]. A similar patent regarding drying and concentration of liquid and solid substances in general was granted in 1872 [2]. These patents appear to be the first descriptions of the process now known as spray drying, which can be defined as the atomization of feed formulation (either solution or suspension) into a hot drying gas to evaporate the solvent, thereby creating dry particles from the solute materials.

The schematic of a typical laboratory-scale spray dryer, given in Figure 12.1, shows some details of the process. In this setup, the feed is pumped to a twin-fluid atomizer which generates droplets that are dried in a drying chamber and collected in a collection bottle using a cyclone. The applications and advantages of spray drying are discussed in the following paragraphs.

Spray drying is the most commonly used technique for microencapsulation in the food industry [3,4] and for dehydration of dairy products [5]. Indeed, a milk spray dryer in New Zealand can generate nearly 10 tons of milk powder per hour [6]. Spray drying is also widely used for producing dry and stable food additives and flavors [3,4,7,8], fruit and vegetable juices [4,9,10], coffee and tea [11], probiotic bacteria [12–18], and nutraceuticals [19]. Spray drying to produce particles with thick shells can be used for prolonged scent release and volatile retention [8], as well as for protecting oil from oxidation [3,20]. Other industries that use spray drying include, but are not limited to, the pharmaceutical, ceramic, polymer,

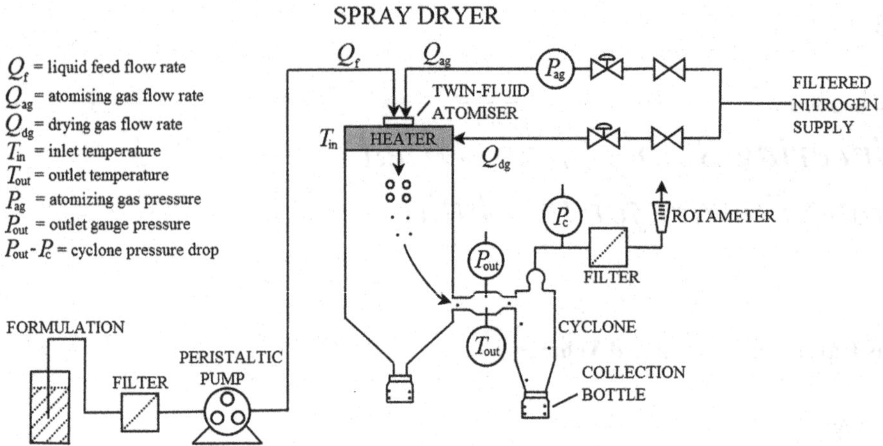

FIGURE 12.1 Schematic showing an example setup for a laboratory-scale open-loop spray dryer.

detergent, pesticide, mining, and chemical industries [4,11,21]. Spray drying is even being considered for water recovery on the International Space Station [22,23].

The success and widespread use of spray drying is due largely to it being a continuous, fast, scalable, bottom-up approach that allows for particle properties such as particle size and distribution, surface composition, roughness, and particle density to be controlled [24], with comparatively low cost [3,4,14,25–30]. By contrast, lyophilization does not allow for the level of control over particle properties that spray drying provides, as generally, secondary milling or sieving is required [31,32]. Additionally, lyophilization is a lengthy batch process and requires infrastructure for freezing and generating sub-atmospheric pressures.

The removal of water associated with drying reduces weight and volume, which can reduce transportation costs and make handling and storage easier [33]. Additionally, many studies have demonstrated superior thermal stability of biologics in dry dosage forms as compared to liquid dosage forms [34–39], which is associated with decreased water-mediated degradation. An improved shelf-life could eliminate the need for cold-chain infrastructure, which can fail and lead to vaccine wastage, and is not available everywhere in developing countries [36,37,39–49]. There is also a risk of transmitting blood-borne diseases when needles are used, and this can be addressed by instead using inhaled vaccine delivery, which has the additional benefits of eliminating needle pain, needle-stick injuries, and needle disposal issues [36,40,44–46,50]. The potential for dry dosage forms to have long-term ambient temperature storage stability may also allow for easier stockpiling and distribution during pandemics [31,48,49,51].

Spray dried vaccines intended for inhalation include influenza vaccines [34,35,52–54], a pneumonia vaccine [55], a measles vaccine [56], Newcastle disease vaccines for poultry [57,58], a listeria vaccine [59], a hepatitis B vaccine [60], and various tuberculosis vaccines [61–67]. By offering immediate protection at the exposure site for diseases transmitted by aerosol, inhaled vaccine powder affords comparable or greater mucosal immunity than does liquid subcutaneous or intramuscular vaccine delivery, and may even result in systemic immunity [35,40,53,54,60,61]. Indeed, large trials with measles vaccine delivered by nebulizer have demonstrated higher antibody titers with the inhalation route as compared to injection [68–71]. However, there is a general concern about adverse reaction to foreign material depositing in the lung [72–75]. This is particularly the case for the delivery of lipid-based vectors [61,75] and delivery to asthmatics [45,50] or immunocompromised patients [45]. Smokers may also be at risk [76]. The adjuvant-like response generated by inhaled powder may eliminate the need for an adjuvant in the formulation [54,60,64], which is important as little is known about the safety of adjuvants in the lung [40]. There are also safety and toxicity concerns with inhaling residual organic solvents sometimes used in spray dried formulations [77]. While spray dried vaccines can be resuspended for injection rather than direct inhalation [37,39,48,78,79], enhancements to stability can be lost upon reconstitution as can the advantages of needle-free delivery; moreover, reconstitution creates a need for a sterile rehydration medium, which can complicate preparation and transportation [80].

Biologics are gaining market share relative to small molecules, with 52% of the top 100 product sales expected to be biologics by the year 2022 [81], and it is thus expected that there will be many applications other than vaccines where spray drying biologics can prove beneficial. Research has shown that monoclonal antibodies (mABs), which have been the most frequently approved biologics recently [82], can be successfully spray dried [83–87], and work has been done to scale-up the spray drying process for bulk mAB storage applications [38,86]. Currently, commercially available inhalable biologics include colistin methosulfonate, bovine pulmonary surfactants, Pulmozyme® (recombinant human DNase), and AFREZZA® (fast-acting insulin) [31,88]. Spray drying has been used for generating materials in regulatory-approved inhaled products such as for EXUBERA® inhaled insulin [89], Tobramycin Inhalation Powder [90], BEVESPI AEROSPHERE® [91,92], and the topically applied biologic RAPLIXA® [26]. Further details are available in the literature regarding spray drying insulin [89,93–95] and tobramycin [90,96], which have been rendered room-temperature stable for years by glass stabilization, a process discussed later in this chapter. The most common application of spray drying in the pharmaceutical industry, however, is the generation of an amorphous form of the excipient lactose to improve compaction properties of tablets [21]. There is also much interest in using spray drying to generate amorphous solid dispersions to deliver poorly water-soluble drugs [97–101].

Another application of spray drying in the pharmaceutical industry is for controlled release of a drug or biologic substance in the lungs. The morphology of the spray dried particles, for example, thickness and surface area, can affect the dissolution and diffusion of material through the outer layer of the particle [24]. Due to the small size of spray dried particles for inhalation, release is rapid unless the solubility and diffusion are very low; hence, slowly biodegradable polymers with high molecular weight are typically used [24]. Of the many materials available, poly(lactic-*co*-glycolic acid) (PLGA) is the most commonly used [24]. Nano-PLGA particles (that can be delivered to the lungs within lactose microparticles) are too small to be efficiently phagocytosed by alveolar macrophages and have been used for controlled release of an antibody [102]. Other biologics for which PLGA has been used to provide controlled release include spray dried antigen [64,103] and interleukin [104]. A review of the use of PLGA for inhalation applications is available elsewhere [105].

Spray dried biologics may be able to address the rise in antibiotic resistance and the slow development of new antibiotics. Examples of such biologics include bacteriophage [106–121], anti-microbial peptides [122,123], and bacterial cell wall hydrolases [122]. Pulmonary delivery of bacteriophage to mice [118,124] and humans [108,125] has generally produced positive results with few if any side effects. Spray dried bacteriophage powder has been produced with high titer [126–129] and has demonstrated long-term stability with refrigerated [128] and room temperature storage [126].

Successful development of stable spray dried biologic products can be a challenging task. In the following sections, the main stages in engineering spray dried biologics for inhalation are discussed, with a focus on the development of dispersible powders with long-term stability. This discussion includes detailed descriptions of: (1) purification and formulation, (2) atomization, (3) solvent evaporation and particle formation, (4) particle collection and analysis, (5) aerosolization, and (6) lung deposition. Then, theoretical and practical aspects of glass stabilization and stability testing are discussed. Finally, the development of a spray dryer process model and non-equilibrium supplemented phase diagram is demonstrated.

12.2 Purification and Formulation

After isolation and initial characterization, biologics are typically purified and formulated with stabilizers before spray drying. The degree of purification and formulation is typically much less in the laboratory than in the development of commercial products, and it should be considered that impurities can affect stability and particle formation. The purification process will also vary between biologics. For mABs, the purification process may involve clarification with disk-stack centrifuge, multiple filtration steps, low-pH virus inactivation, and multiple chromatographic steps including protein A capture [130–132]. Purification can come at a substantial cost, due in part to the high price of the resin used in chromatography [132]; thus, alternatives such as high performance tangential flow filtration and aqueous two-phase processing have been suggested [133,134]. However, cost analysis has indicated that alternatives may not be warranted [131]. The interested reader is directed elsewhere for more information regarding biologic purification [130–138].

Purified biologics usually cannot be spray dried on their own without substantial inactivation and hence require stabilizing excipients. Ideally, the excipients would not involve materials from animals as these could be contaminated with viruses [139]. The function and concentration of each excipient in the formulation as well as the selection and control of the manufacturing process must be justified to regulatory agencies [140], and, hence, a mechanistic understanding of what each excipient in the formulation does and how the process parameters affect the final product is clearly of interest. Additionally, a mechanistic approach allows the number of experiments required to develop a product with target characteristics to be reduced [31,97,141]. However, rather than mechanistic modeling, past experience and statistical design of experiments (DoE) are often used for determining formulation and process parameters for spray drying [12,34,51,93,95,142–146]. Unfortunately, DoE has limited ability to translate the results across scales and formulations and may require many experiments [97].

Factors that can inactivate biologics during formulation and processing include shear [15,31,147–151], osmotic stress or ionic strength [31,121,152,153], electric fields [154,155], UV light [106,156–159], heat [15,31,41,121,153,159,160], desiccation (which can be related to osmotic stress and ionic strength) [15,31,41,159,161], pH [31,41,106,121,153], and pressure [31,160]. Minimizing these stresses during formulation and spray drying can be crucial to developing an effective biologic product.

Pre-adapting bacteria to environmental stresses such as heat, osmotic pressure, and starvation may help to increase their stress resistance and survival during spray drying [14,15]. Bacteria harvested during the stationary phase may be more resistant to drying [14]. Damage or strain history may be important to consider. Viruses have been adapted for use at different temperatures [162,163].

Increasing the stress resistance at the interior of large biologics such as viruses, bacteria, or red blood cells, may require getting stabilizers into the biologic [24,48,164]. Placing the biologic in a hyperosmotic solution containing the stabilizer may be useful in this regard, but this depends on the permeability of the membrane and whether or not the biologic possesses active transport mechanisms to bring in or expel substances [48,164,165]. Adding compounds to increase membrane fluidity and to take advantage of phase transitions at elevated temperatures may also be helpful for getting stabilizers into the biologic [48,164].

Usually, a major stress on biologics during spray drying is desiccation, which can be addressed by adding a suitable glass stabilizer to the formulation. While many sugars can be used for glass stabilization, those that participate in the Maillard reaction (such as lactose) should be avoided [36]. Trehalose is an excellent glass former and stabilizer and does not participate in the Maillard reaction, although it is not yet approved for inhalation. For reconstitution purposes, it may be important to consider that solution viscosity increases with dissolved trehalose concentration [166], and that high viscosity would result in the need for larger needles which are more painful [38]. Generally, better stabilization is achieved with trehalose than with sucrose [166]. Glass stabilization with trehalose is discussed further later in this chapter.

Spray drying amorphous disaccharide glass stabilizers on their own tends to result in cohesive, solid particles, which are not very flowable or dispersible, typically exhibiting low collection yields in spray dryers. A crystalline shell former, such as leucine, can be used to decrease particle cohesiveness and to lower particle density, thereby improving flowability and dispersibility [24]. The combination of trehalose and leucine has commonly been used in the literature [52,126,128,129,167,168] and has been shown to provide the best stabilization of certain biologics out of different formulations tested, while producing a dispersible powder [126,128,129,167].

The pH of aqueous leucine solution is ~5.98, near the isoelectric point, where formally there is no surface charge [169]. The surface activity, solubility, and particle morphology will depend on pH, which should be considered when adding a buffer to the formulation.

For leucine to increase dispersibility, it should be present in high concentration on the surface of the spray dried particles. A high concentration on the surface requires high initial saturation of the leucine relative to the other materials, which may be undesirable if the particles need to consist of a high mass fraction of the active (biologic) [24]. Trileucine has therefore been considered as an alternative, as it reaches a high concentration at the surface at lower feed concentrations, due to a lower solubility in water and higher surface activity [24,170]. The wrinkled structure of trileucine particles, which may be associated with the shell being too thin to maintain a spherical shape [171], is expected to result in a high emitted dose from carrier-free dry powder inhalers [170,171] and potentially less flow dependence [172].

The solvent used for preparing biologic formulations for spray drying is typically water. Spray drying with propellant [173] and ethanol [173–175] as solvents, among others [100], can be performed using a closed-loop (drying gas recycling) configuration, allowing for the spray drying of substances with low aqueous solubility as well as potentially for improved thermal efficiency and particle morphology. However, it is crucial to check that the biologic is stable or can be stabilized in the chosen solvent [176] and inhaled toxicity of residual solvent in the particles must be considered in non-aqueous systems [77]. Emulsion formulation preparation may involve the use of a high-shear mixer and a high-pressure homogenizer before spray drying [91], and the effect of the preparation method on the biologic activity should be tested. The formulation of biologics is discussed further in Chapter 15.

Prior to entering the atomizer, the formulation, which is termed the feed, should be well-mixed to ensure that the biologic material is evenly distributed in the solvent. Some larger biologics may entangle or settle if not properly mixed. On a laboratory-scale, mixing can be performed using a magnetic stirrer [12]. The effect of the container and the feed lines on biologic activity should also be tested, as it is known, for example, that proteins, because of their amphipathic nature, can adsorb to surfaces such as on plastic and glassware, in a protein- and surface material-dependent manner [177–185]. The feed can be cooled prior to drying if required for biologic stability; however, this may affect particle size, as discussed in the next section.

12.3 Atomization

In a spray dryer, an atomizer is used to generate droplets from the liquid feed formulation. The droplets subsequently dry to produce solid particles. This section reviews characteristics of commonly used atomizers, the generated shear stress and air-liquid interfacial stress on biologics, and the use of surfactants and other excipients to displace biologics from the surface of atomized droplets. The interested reader is directed to textbooks for background information regarding the atomization process [11,186,187].

Commercial spray dryers commonly use rotary or twin-fluid atomizers [33,188]. Rotary atomizers impinge a liquid jet onto the centre of a rotating disk, which discharges the liquid radially by its rotational motion [186]. The particle size can be controlled by the rate of rotation, but wider drying chambers are needed for higher rotation rates [189]. The disk is typically rotated using a gas-driven turbine for a smaller disk or an electric motor for a larger disk [188]. Very high production rates are possible in production-scale rotary atomizers (up to 40 kg s^{-1}) [186], with little risk of clogging [187]. While rotary atomizers tend to produce more uniform droplets than twin-fluid atomizers, the latter are preferable for developing particles for delivery to the lungs due to the smaller size of the droplets produced [188].

Twin-fluid atomizers use the energy from a high-pressure atomizing gas to break the liquid feed into a spray of droplets. The droplet diameter is related to the ratio of the mass flow rates of atomizing gas and liquid feed [141,188]. An increase in feed viscosity, for example, when using a higher dissolved solids content or reducing feed temperature, will tend to produce larger droplets [11,186,188]. Production-scale twin-fluid atomizers are available, such as the Schlick-05 [190]. Large amounts of compressed gas may be required in open-loop configurations and so on scale-up closed-loop configurations, where the atomizing and drying gas are recycled, may be desirable [189].

The wide distribution of droplet sizes produced by twin-fluid atomizers may not be desirable in some pharmaceutical inhalation applications. To address this concern, as well as to study the particle formation process and to generate plenty of uniform particles for analytical work, the use of monodisperse atomizers in research spray dryers has become increasingly common [171,173,191]. While further work is required to scale-up these monodisperse atomizers to accommodate higher throughput rates, they can be useful in applications where only small quantities of biologic powder need to be developed.

Shear stress can be present in the pressurized liquid flow through the liquid channel of twin-fluid atomizers [31], as well as past the exit of the orifice [18]. Shear stress during atomization is typically considered low enough not to cause biologic inactivation [31,192]. However, in one study, less inactivation was observed using a pilot scale rotary atomizer as compared to a pilot scale twin-fluid atomizer, which was hypothesized to be related to a characteristic shear rate that was three orders of magnitude higher for the twin-fluid atomizer [18]. Another study found that using higher atomizing gas pressure with a twin-fluid nozzle led to more biologic inactivation [193]. While these studies point towards shear stress as being a cause of inactivation, this has not been proven because the biologic was assayed from the produced powder rather than from the droplets generated by the atomizer. A filter could be attached to the atomizer to capture and assay atomized droplets [194].

It has been suggested that using larger initial droplet sizes will result in less stress on the biologic, since less energy is needed to break up the liquid jet into larger droplets [41]. Another consideration is that with decreasing droplet size, the surface area to volume ratio increases. Proteins will tend concentrate at the air-liquid interface during drying due to their large size, which prevents quick diffusion away from the receding interface (this is discussed further in the next section). The accumulation and adsorption at the air-liquid interface can lead to the unfolding and exposure of the hydrophobic interior of the protein to the air-phase, which can further lead to hydrophobic aggregation and inactivation by the irreversible loss of the native structure of the protein [31,148,149,195,196]. The surface accumulation effect may be enhanced by the fact that proteins are typically amphiphilic and hence essentially surface active macromolecules [179,184,185,197].

It is widely accepted that surfactants can displace proteins at the surface and decrease aggregation and inactivation during processing [185,195–202]. The accumulation of surfactants on the droplet surface is a process that occurs transiently during droplet evaporation. In addition to transport from the bulk to the surface and adsorption onto the surface, high molecular weight surfactants will take time to orient at the surface [203]. Some surfactants can accumulate on the surface and decrease surface tension in the millisecond time scale (within the droplet lifetime typically encountered in laboratory-scale spray drying), although most surfactants will not reach an equilibrium surface tension within this time scale [203,204]. Addition of even small amounts of surfactant can lead to smooth, spherical particles [24,198,202–205]. A concern with using surfactants is that they may solubilize some membrane components for certain biologics [56].

Leucine and trileucine, discussed previously, are potential alternatives for displacing the biologic at the surface. Trileucine decreases surface activity in solution in a concentration-dependent manner and competes with protein on the air-liquid interface, which can decrease denaturation and aggregation of protein [170]. Further details regarding surface enrichment are given in the following section.

12.4 Solvent Evaporation and Particle Formation

This section reviews the basic particle engineering concepts needed to understand the particle formation process, including solvent evaporation, surface enrichment, time available for crystallization, and aerodynamic diameter. Crystallization and shell deformation processes are discussed, as is the development of more complex particles.

The low humidity and high temperature of the drying gas drive evaporation of the solvent from the atomized droplets. The evaporation process involves coupled heat and mass transfer [11,171]. The drying droplet surface stays near the wet bulb temperature of the drying gas (which is much lower than the nominal drying gas temperature) for most of the evaporation process [11]. Evaporative cooling results in the outlet drying gas temperature decreasing with increasing feed flow rates. Computational fluid dynamics (CFDs) can be used to model spatial distributions of temperature [206] and evaporation rate in spray dryers [188]. CFD has shown that particles caught up in eddies may be exposed to the high inlet temperature without evaporative cooling to provide protection [188]. For small droplets, solvent evaporation and particle formation commonly take place in co-current drying chambers, in which atomized droplets and drying gas flow in the same direction. For large droplets, a counter-current configuration can be used to increase the time for solvent evaporation; however, in this configuration, the hottest air contacts the driest particles [11], which may not be suitable for heat-sensitive biologics.

The radial recession of the droplet surface due to evaporation causes solute to increase in concentration near the surface, unless the solute can diffuse quickly to the interior of the droplet. A commonly used particle formation model for this process is the Vehring-Foss-Lechuga (VFL) model [171], which is based upon assumptions of one-dimensional spherical symmetry and no convection except Stefan flow. The VFL model does not account for surface activity, shell deformation, or non-constant evaporation rates during initial temperature equilibration and the falling rate period [171]. In reality, the evaporation rate depends upon the local temperature and relative humidity, solute concentration according to Raoult's law, and the diameter according to the Kelvin effect, among other factors [207].

The ratio of surface concentration to mean concentration of the solute in the droplet is termed surface enrichment [24]. The surface enrichment can be considered a function of the Péclet number, Pe_i, which is proportional to the ratio of evaporation rate, κ, to the diffusion coefficient, D_i, of the solute (i) in the solvent [171]:

$$Pe_i = \frac{\kappa}{(8D_i)} \tag{12.1}$$

The steady state evaporation rate can be predicted using hygroscopic theory [171,207] if tabulated data are not available. The diffusion coefficient can be predicted from the Stokes-Einstein equation [208]:

$$D_i = \frac{kT}{(3\pi\mu d_{\text{mol},i})} \tag{12.2}$$

where k is the Boltzmann's constant, T is the temperature of the droplet, μ is the dynamic viscosity of the droplet, and the molecular diameter $d_{\text{mol},i}$ can be estimated from the bond length and structure of the solute molecule.

The evaporation rate and diffusion coefficient may need to be modeled as functions of time. In co-solvent systems, one solvent may evaporate faster than the other, resulting in a transient evaporation rate [24]. Near the end of the droplet lifetime, the solute concentration increases, which increases the viscosity of the droplet and decreases the diffusion coefficient, and, hence, a model has incorporated a time-dependent viscosity in Equation (12.2) [208].

The droplet surface recedes faster than the dissolved or suspended components with a Péclet number greater than 1 diffuse, resulting in surface enrichment of those components [24]. Components with Péclet numbers less than 1 remain relatively evenly distributed [24]. If phase transition (crystal nucleation) occurs, the local dissolved solute concentration is lowered, which can be modeled as a sink condition [209]. The mobility of the nucleated material is drastically reduced resulting in negligible diffusion and a very large Péclet number [24].

Small solute molecules, for example disaccharide sugars such as trehalose, have lower Péclet numbers than large solute molecules such as proteins or most other biologics. Thus, the biologic will tend to reside on the surface of the particle (exhibit high surface enrichment), and be exposed to surface stresses at the air-liquid interface, unless there is an excipient that will out-compete the biologic to reside on the surface.

In Figure 12.2, the surface enrichment, E_i, defined as the ratio of surface concentration, $C_{s,i}$, to mean concentration, $C_{m,i}$, in the droplet, is shown to increase with Péclet number. This figure, which is useful for a first estimate of the radial distribution of components in the particle, shows the constant surface enrichment that would result at the end of the droplet lifetime, were there no precipitation event, and is a good approximation within the range shown [210]. To model the change in surface enrichment over time, more complex analytical models have been developed, which extend the VFL model to larger Péclet numbers, and which can be used to estimate the shell thickness at the time of saturation [210].

In spray drying, nucleation and crystallization or precipitation generally occur first at the surface, where the local concentration is high enough to overcome the local saturation concentration. By performing a

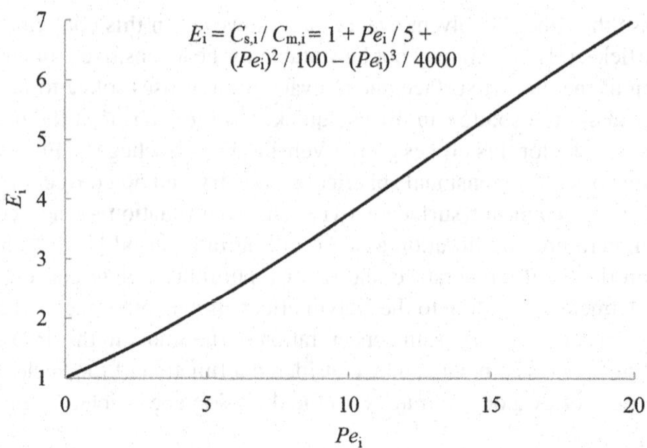

FIGURE 12.2 Surface enrichment, E_i, versus Péclet number, Pe_i, according to the steady state VFL model, given by Vehring et al. [171]. Large molecules such as polymers and biologics have large Péclet numbers and hence high surface enrichment, while amino acids and disaccharide sugars typically have low Péclet numbers and hence low surface enrichment.

mass balance on the solute and assuming a constant evaporation rate, it can be shown that the time for the solute to reach saturation at the surface, $\tau_{sat,i}$, is given by [24]:

$$\tau_{sat,i} = \tau_D\left[1-\left(S_{0,i}E_i\right)^{2/3}\right] \tag{12.3}$$

where the droplet lifetime, τ_D, is given by [24]:

$$\tau_D = \frac{(d_0)^2}{\kappa} \tag{12.4}$$

where d_0 is the initial diameter of the droplets emitted by the atomizer. As most atomizers emit polydisperse sprays, a range of these characteristic times will be present. The droplet lifetime can be used to predict whether the drying chamber of a given spray dryer provides enough residence time for droplets of a particular diameter to complete the drying process.

Also required in Equation (12.3) is the initial saturation ratio, $S_{0,i}$, which is given by [24]:

$$S_{0,i} = \frac{C_{0,i}}{C_{sat,i}} \tag{12.5}$$

where $C_{0,i}$ is the initial concentration of dissolved solute in the solvent, and $C_{sat,i}$ is the saturation concentration of the dissolved solute in the solvent.

The difference between the droplet lifetime and the time to reach saturation is termed the time available for crystallization, also known as the precipitation window, $\tau_{p,i}$, and is given by [24]:

$$\tau_{p,i} = \tau_D - \tau_{sat,i} = \frac{\left(S_{0,i}E_i\right)^{2/3}(d_0)^2}{\kappa} \tag{12.6}$$

Whether the solute forms crystals that grow within this time available for crystallization depends on many factors. Time is required for crystal nucleation, growth, and polymorph transitions, which proceed according to the Ostwald step rule [24]. Many factors can affect the times required, including droplet temperature, which tends to increase the rate of nucleation [209]. Studies have suggested a critical supersaturation (in the range of 1–10), which depends on material properties, must be reached for spontaneous nucleation to occur [211,212].

If the time available for crystallization is not long enough for the crystals to reach equilibrium, a mixture of different polymorphs will result [24]. The presence of the most stable form increases the rate that the less stable polymorphs convert to the most stable form [24]; such a system would likely be unstable on storage. Additionally, if the time available for crystallization is too short, some or all of the solute may not grow crystals and instead will precipitate in a disordered, higher energy state, termed amorphous [141]. A mixture of amorphous and crystalline states of the same material may also not be stable on storage. Once the amorphous phase starts to crystallize, expelled water can enter the remaining amorphous matrix and speed up the rate of conversion to crystalline form, which could cause rapid product failure [24]. Physically unstable systems like these are difficult to scale-up, as residence times may be different in large spray dryers [24]. As the time available for crystallization is shorter for smaller droplets, leading to crystals not having the same time to grow [24], production of potentially unstable systems like these may be a particular concern for polydisperse sprays. Additionally, at the centre of a droplet, water evaporation is slower and crystals may have more time to grow [213]. Studies have quantified the growth of larger and broader crystals with increased time available for crystallization [173,208,212] and have demonstrated the formation of larger crystals growing from smaller crystals on microparticles in a high humidity environment [213]. Controlling crystal size is important since it affects rugosity and hence particle cohesiveness and dispersibility [214].

Certain materials can be used to inhibit or delay the onset of crystallization [84,213,215,216]. Inhibiting crystallization can lead to glass stabilization with materials that normally crystallize quickly like mannitol [84], although decreased yield may be present without a crystalline shell [215]. Delaying crystallization can lead to smaller crystals and a smoother surface [213].

Buffer, ions, and impurities will increase in concentration during the evaporation process and may be enriched on the surface. Any changes in pH could affect the biologic and will affect protein solubility [217] and hence particle formation. Increases in ionic concentration during evaporation can exert osmotic stresses on the biologics. Small amounts of impurities can substantially decrease crystal growth rates [218].

Trehalose and leucine have been studied extensively as excipients for particles containing biologics. In trehalose and leucine systems, it is desirable to dissolve the trehalose in the liquid feed with a low initial saturation ratio so that it will precipitate near the end of the drying process into an amorphous solid suitable for stabilization of biologics. By contrast, leucine should be dissolved in the liquid feed with a high initial saturation ratio, leading to a long time available for crystallization, which allows crystals to grow at the surface of the drying droplet and form a shell that decreases particle cohesiveness. The shell is typically not exclusively composed of leucine, but can nevertheless lead to acceptable dispersibility [126]. As the leucine shell forms early in the evaporation process, while the droplets are relatively large, hollow particles, with low particle density, ρ_p, result; it has been shown that more void space and lower particle density result with increasing time available for crystallization [208,212]. The particle density can be predicted from measurements of volume equivalent diameter, d_v, (e.g. by estimating the hydrodynamic diameter using scanning electron microscopy for a sufficiently large number of particles) and aerodynamic diameter, d_a, (e.g. using aerodynamic particle sizing techniques such as impactors), using the relationship obtained by equating the settling velocities [24,219]:

$$d_a = d_v\left(\rho_p/\rho*\right)^{1/2} \tag{12.7}$$

where ρ^* is a reference density equal to 1000 kg/m^3.

The aerodynamic diameter of the dry particles can be predicted via a mass balance [24,141]:

$$d_a = d_0\left(C_0/\rho*\right)^{1/3}\left(\rho_p/\rho*\right)^{1/6} \tag{12.8}$$

where C_0 is the concentration of the solute in the feed and d_0 is the initial droplet diameter emitted from the atomizer. These equations assume spherical droplets and particles and neglect the Cunningham slip correction factor [141]. These equations are useful during scale-up to ensure particle size is not greatly affected by changing feed concentrations and initial droplet diameters [24]. The aerodynamic diameter is an important factor for estimating the lung dose of the emitted aerosol using extrathoracic deposition models, as discussed later in this chapter.

Models are available to predict the shell thickness and particle density of spray dried particles, which operate on the assumption that the shell forms immediately upon the saturation concentration being reached on the surface, and that the shell density is the mass-averaged true density of the materials [210]. Further work is required to develop more exact models not requiring these simplifying assumptions.

Leucine shells may deform substantially [168], provided impurities do not interfere with this process [194]. Experimental and theoretical studies of shell deformation processes are available in the literature [220–230]. One prevailing theory argues that elastic shell deformation occurs when capillary forces in menisci that form between nanoparticles (which could perhaps apply to small crystals of leucine) overcome stabilizing electrostatic forces between nanoparticles [220].

Another related important aspect of particle formation that has yet to be incorporated into particle engineering models for spray drying applications is the role of surface activity in surface enrichment, which may be relevant for trileucine shell formation.

Trileucine forms a non-crystalline thin shell or coating that cannot support a spherical shape and deforms substantially. Like trileucine, polymers and other large molecular weight compounds have restricted molecular motions and hence tend to not crystallize or crystallize much slower than low molecular weight compounds [218].

More complex approaches can be used to produce low density particles by spray drying. Volatile salts or other templating agents can be sublimated to form voids, typically by incorporating a secondary drying step [24,90,174,231]. Templating has been used to produce PulmoSphere™ particles [232], which are part of the commercial Tobramycin Inhalation Powder, administered with the TOBI® Podhaler™ [90]. These particles are stable for 3 years at 30°C and 75% relative humidity (stored in a blister pack), result in less variable dosing, and require only low inspiratory efforts [90,96,232]; however, further excipients are needed for glass stabilization. PulmoSphere™ particles incorporate distearoylphosphatidylcholine (which is endogenous to the lungs) as a shell former and can be suspended for use with pressurised metered-dose inhalers, nebulizers, or liquid instillation [96,232]. Advanced particle engineering is discussed further in Chapter 14.

12.5 Particle Collection

Cyclones are the most commonly used equipment in industry for collecting spray dried microparticles [33,195]. A cyclone is typically situated just downstream of the drying chamber, its use allowing for the capture of the particles in a collection bottle (see Figure 12.1).

The low yield typically encountered in laboratory-scale spray dryers with small batch sizes is generally improved upon scale-up [80]. Losses due to wall deposition upstream of the cyclone typically occur for large or highly surface-charged particles, while losses of small particles typically occur at the exit of the cyclone [188]. A dual cyclone design has been implemented for accommodating the increased drying gas flow rate during scale-up [38].

Use of pure spray dried trehalose typically results in a low yield due to its cohesive nature. Particles can also agglomerate in cyclones [233]. CFD has been used to model particle trajectories as a means of evaluating spray dryer designs that may minimize wall deposition and agglomeration [206,234–236]. Fragile particles may fracture or deform when impacting the cyclone wall (termed attrition), which has been related to the inlet velocity of the cyclone [233]. Attrition may damage biologics residing on the surface of microparticles, but such damage has not been quantified.

Conditions in the collector should be controlled to ensure consistent powder properties. External surface thermometers have been used to estimate the temperature in the collection bottle [95]. The collector can be thermostated using a water bath [237], which can also be used to control the relative humidity in the collection bottle and hence the moisture content in the powder.

In standard laboratory-scale spray dryers, the collection bottle is typically quickly removed and capped after the run is completed to minimize thermal degradation and entry of moisture into the bottle from the surroundings. There may be time-dependent degradation in the collection bottle for large batch sizes without bottle replacement [95]. In these instances, collectors can be changed intermittently. For aseptic systems, a valve can shut off flow to the collection bottle, allowing for replacement of the collection bottle in a clean room at set time intervals during continuous operation.

After collection, a secondary drying step (for example, in a vacuum desiccator, convection-tray dryer, or fluidized bed system) may be used to lower the moisture content of the powder or to remove residual organic solvent [100,188,238]. Decreasing moisture content by using a secondary drying step may be more suitable than using a higher drying gas temperature for heat-sensitive biologics [238]. A secondary moisture-equilibration step, for example, using a humidity-controlled chamber or saturated salt solution, can be used to target a desired moisture content. Moisture equilibration is discussed further later in this chapter.

12.6 Particle Analysis

While mechanistic models can be used to predict the properties of the freshly spray dried particles, the analysis discussed in this section should be performed to verify the predicted results. Analysis can also be performed at different time points during stability studies. Many analytical techniques are available and not all can be discussed here.

Techniques available for quantifying the amount of amorphous and crystalline material present in spray dried powder are reviewed in the literature [239]. Such analysis is important since, as discussed previously, partially crystalline excipients should be avoided, as these can act as a template to increase the rate of crystallization. One method for quantitative crystallinity measurement is Raman spectroscopy, in which an infrared laser is directed at the powder, and the intensity of the portion of light that is inelastically scattered to a different wavelength is measured [126,168,240–242]. Crystalline material results in narrow spectral lines, while amorphous material results in a broader scattering pattern. Since small masses of powder are typically used for analysis, relative humidity control is important during Raman spectroscopy to prevent water uptake and solid-state change. Although interfering fluorescence may not be a large concern for high purity small molecule drug powders [241], biologics may not be highly purified during preliminary development, and, hence, it may be more difficult to perform quantitative Raman spectroscopy, due to residual fluorescence. Still, Raman spectroscopy has been used to screen excipients for providing long-term stability to spray dried mABs [83]. Powder X-ray diffraction is an alternative to Raman spectroscopy for solid phase analysis, but it is more difficult to quantify small masses of amorphous material in a primarily crystalline powder [241].

Modulated differential scanning calorimetry (MDSC) can be used to determine the glass transition temperature of the powder [128,243]. Enthalpic relaxation heat flow measured by MDSC can be used to assess the amorphous content in a partially crystalline sample [244]. Dynamic vapor sorption can be used to determine the moisture uptake behavior of the powder [126–128]. These techniques are discussed in more detail later in this chapter.

X-ray photoelectron spectroscopy, also known as electron spectroscopy for chemical analysis, can be used to measure the elemental surface composition of spray dried powders [87,126,170,171,174,196,199,200,202,204,212,245–248]. The elemental surface composition can be useful for determining the ratios of excipients on the surface and for comparison to theoretical surface enrichment described previously. This is, however, strictly speaking, a near-surface method, and, hence, the measurements may not be able to accurately measure a coating thinner than the penetration depth of the instrument [24]. Alternatively, time-of-flight secondary ion mass spectroscopy can provide qualitative near-surface composition measurements [246].

Scanning electron microscopy is commonly used to examine particle morphology, which is then compared to expectations from particle formation theory. Scanning electron microscopy can also be used for estimating crystal size [212]. If the interior of the particle is of interest, particles can be cut with ion-beam milling and then the cross section can be viewed using scanning electron microscopy [93,141,173,208,212,249,250]. This method also yields shell thickness [208,250]. X-ray photoelectron spectroscopy on ion-beam milled particles can potentially determine if the radial internal distributions of materials match particle formation theory [212]. Milling, when performed at multiple locations [141], can also verify predications of void space from particle formation models. For example, it has been shown using ion-beam milling that for polydisperse powders, large particles may contain void space, whereas smaller particles do not [141], in agreement with theoretical predictions. Compressed bulk density can also be used to predict if there are internal voids or porous materials [141]. Porosity may decrease with increasing surface corrugation [249].

A unique feature of spray dried biologics is that it is generally necessary to quantify the level of biological activity in the collected powder. This can be done with bioassays, which are often more variable and costly than chemical assays, such as, those used for small-molecule antibiotics [31]. Additionally, bioassays are generally performed in the liquid state and hence a method of rehydration is necessary. Therefore, any possible inactivation due to spray drying may not be able to be separated from inactivation due to rehydration. The activity of biologics after rehydration has been shown to be affected by temperature [14,15,251–256], rate or duration of rehydration [15,251,253,256–258] (likely related to osmotic stress), resuspension medium composition [15,156,251,256,258], exposure to UV radiation [156], and powder composition [258]. Biologics can leak if rehydration causes phase change [252,259–262].

A generalized method for resuspending spray dried biologics for bioassay is not available. It can be assumed that the rehydration method resulting in the lowest overall spray drying and rehydration inactivation most closely represents the inactivation due to spray drying, provided there is no increase in biologic activity in the resuspension media, for example, due to cell division. For dry powders meant for inhalation, however, it may be most relevant to resuspend in a medium representative of the fluid in the lungs, provided one can perform an accurate bioassay in such a medium. Reconstitution may occur in mucus in the upper respiratory tract and surfactant in the lower respiratory tract, both of which contain anti-microbial molecules [263]. *In vitro* studies in mucus or surfactant may therefore be useful for testing biologic reconstitution survival in a realistic medium [263].

12.7 Aerosolization

This section reviews considerations regarding the use of various inhalation devices for delivering biologics. Spray dried powder is usually intended for delivery with a dry powder inhaler (DPI), but powder can also be suspended for delivery from nebulizers, pressurized metered-dose inhalers (pMDIs), or soft mist inhalers (SMIs). Device selection depends on the intended use of the biologic and the dose to be delivered.

Not surprisingly, the most common method for aerosolizing dry powder is to use a DPI. Loading the powder may require filling into a capsule, which is a well-established technique in industry [25,89] and should be done in a temperature- and humidity-controlled environment. Triboelectric charging can be an issue for powder filling, and, hence, it may be beneficial to retain some moisture in the powder and filling environment. Cohesive powders can also be difficult to fill. Advantages of using DPIs include the obviation of any need for on-site reconstitution, which might otherwise require the transport of sterile liquid (not desirable for use in developing countries, as discussed previously), less administration time than with nebulizers [96], and the possible elimination of any need for adjuvants in vaccine preparation (as discussed previously).

Nebulizers are commonly used for aerosol delivery as they allow for the delivery of large doses without the need for breath coordination and refilling is simple; however, nebulizers can be bulky, comparatively expensive, and require electricity. Biologics have been shown to sustain acceptable losses of activity after aerosolization from nebulizers [264,265]. However, this is not always the case, as use of certain biologic and nebulizer combinations can result in substantial inactivation [264,266]. The use of jet nebulizers can be particularly damaging to biologics, a problem that may be due to the hydrodynamic shear stress during droplet production and the repeated baffle impaction and recirculation that the biologic is exposed to in the device [264,266]. With nebulizers, the inhaled volume of aerosol may vary between patients, leading to variability in the dose reaching the lungs. Accordingly, it is suspected that the administration of measles vaccine to children in Mexico using nebulizers with disposable paper cups led to variable dosing. Nevertheless, this means of measles aerosol vaccine delivery has proven successful [68–71,267].

Nebulizers can also be used to deliver aerosol vaccines to people in a tent or other enclosure [268,269]; this practice is also expected to result in dose variability.

Biologics have been spray dried and resuspended in pMDIs [270,271], which may be particularly useful for administration in developing countries [31]. Bacteriophage can sustain acceptable losses of activity after aerosolization from a pMDI [31]. To minimize extrathoracic deposition, and to allow for the same pMDI to be used with multiple patients, which may be useful for vaccine delivery in developing countries, face masks and valved holding chambers can be used. However, it has been demonstrated that the fraction of air inhaled through the holding chamber rather than the environment determines the dose, and that this fraction is related to potential face mask leaks [272]. Therefore, if face masks are not held tightly onto the face, for example, because the same face mask or holding chamber is used for multiple patients and cross-contamination needs to be avoided, then a low and variable lung dose may be expected [272].

SMIs may also be useful for administering biologics; indeed, an SMI insulin product is being developed [273]. It has been demonstrated that inactivation of anti-tuberculosis bacteriophage D29 with an SMI was relatively small, comparable to that with a vibrating mesh nebulizer, and much less than with a jet nebulizer [264].

The use of CFD and analytical models can help to determine the strain rates encountered in commercial aerosolization devices [274] and hence to predict if biologic inactivation will result. Transmission electron micrographs taken after aerosolization and powder resuspension may be compared to images taken of the initial formulation to determine if visible damage is present and related to inactivation of the biologic [275], but it is difficult to find the biologic when imaging if the biologic is not in high number [193]. Inactivation due to aerosolization should be considered when selecting the inhalation device and the loaded dose. The loss of aerosol due to extrathoracic deposition and the inactivation after deposition in the lungs also plays a role when determining dose, as discussed in the following section.

12.8 Lung Deposition

This section reviews the use of deposition modeling and idealized *in vitro* models for predicting the lung dose of inhaled aerosol, and loss of biologic activity upon deposition in the lungs, both of which are useful for determining the nominal dose to deliver.

Aerosol must pass through the extrathoracic region prior to entering the lungs [207]. It logically follows that extrathoracic deposition models are particularly useful for estimating the lung dose of inhaled aerosol [207,276,277]. Different extrathoracic deposition profiles are expected for different patient age groups [207,276,277]. Much less data are available on extrathoracic deposition in pediatrics than in adults [277], a paucity that can have implications for vaccine delivery to children in developing countries. Furthermore, different particle sizes for children than for adults may be required for optimal lung deposition, because of differences in extrathoracic dimensions (including smaller airways in children) and inhalation flow patterns [276]. In some cases lung dose per unit body surface area may be a better parameter than total lung dose for predicting whether or not the intended effect will be achieved [276,278]. Infants are nasal breathers and hence a pMDI with attached valved holding chamber and face mask is sometimes used for aerosol delivery, but again a proper face mask seal is crucial for delivering a high dose [272].

In vitro extrathoracic deposition models typically neglect aerosol exhalation and neither consider hygroscopic particles nor the effect of disease on airway dimensions or the effect of coughing on deposition [276]. CFD can be useful for modeling local deposition patterns and may include effects of hygroscopic growth and condensation of the aerosol in the airways [277].

Among many other parameters, the particle size of the aerosol emitted from inhalation devices is important for predicting lung deposition. The size of individual dried particles can be predicted from particle formation theory. However, for DPI delivery, the particle size distribution of the aerosol is affected by incomplete process yield, size selective retention in the filling process and inhalation device, and incomplete dispersion of the powder. The particle size emitted from different aerosolization devices, and the biological activity within certain size ranges, can be measured using an impactor or multistage liquid impinger [126–128]. Idealized geometries, which are available for infants [272,279], children [280,281], and adults [282–284], can be included upstream of the impactor or a filter to quantify extra-thoracic deposition and to better estimate the dose and particle size distribution that enters the lungs. Ideally, environmental chambers are used to maintain representative temperature and relative humidity when performing these *in vitro* measurements [141]. Airway surface liquid concentration models can then be used to extend the particle size specific information to predict deposition and biologic concentration in different lung generations [265].

Upon deposition in the lungs, biologics are subject to degradation mechanisms, which are discussed in more detail elsewhere [285]. Some biologics may be able to evade lung defense mechanisms for long enough to produce the desired effect. For example, bacteriophage D29 can infect tuberculosis inside macrophage before being inactivated [286].

Once the biologic aerosol is likely to achieve the desired effect in the lungs, the product development process can proceed. It is in most cases necessary to stabilize the biologic so that the aerosolization device and biologic combination has a reasonable shelf-life. Glass stabilisation, discussed in the next section, is the preferred method for stabilizing labile biologics.

12.9 Glass Stabilization

This section discusses an important aspect of ensuring the stability of desiccated biologics during storage, glass stabilization. Other physical and chemical degradation pathways such as deamidation and oxidation can occur in the solid state and these are discussed in detail elsewhere [177,287].

As discussed previously, the fast evaporation process in spray drying can result in precipitation of dissolved material into a high energy, disordered, glassy state if the time available for crystallization is too short or the material does not have a natural tendency to crystallize. Glasses, amorphous materials that exhibit a glass transition at the temperature where the time for relaxation to a lower viscosity equals the typical time scale of an experiment (usually ~100 seconds), are essentially very high viscosity liquids (10 orders–12 orders of magnitude higher after vitrification than in the initial liquid state) [288]. The solid-like behavior of glasses is due to reduction in molecular motions and long relaxation times [288]. Amorphous solids are more soluble (with quicker dissolution) than their lower energy state more structured crystalline counterparts and have a higher thermal expansion coefficient [289,290]. Amorphous solids may have some short-range molecular order, but do not have the long-range order present in crystalline solids [289,290]. Water molecules may freely diffuse through the solid phase of glassy solids [288]. Unlike small molecules, which are generally more stable in crystalline form, amorphous excipients provide better stabilization of biologics [36].

Some organisms can survive severe dehydration by accumulating disaccharides such as trehalose and sucrose [291]. This characteristic is thought to be related to the ability of these disaccharides to form glasses. The most common mechanisms hypothesized to explain the stabilization upon desiccation by glass stabilisers have been water (hydrogen bond) replacement and vitrification [31,35,47,195,260,291–293].

Water replacement stabilization theory has been suggested on the grounds that lysozyme or bovine serum albumin lyophilized with trehalose produces a similar infrared spectrum to hydrated trehalose (but different than trehalose lyophilized on its own), and this "hydration" by trehalose correlates with stabilization [292,294]. Essentially, the effect of the protein on the sugar structure is hypothesized to have the same effect as water [292]. More specifically, this is believed to mean that hydrogen bonds between polar amino acids and water are replaced by hydrogen bonds between the amino acids and the stabilizing sugar, preventing denaturation of the protein (associated with exposure of inner hydrophobic structure) due to drying [31,47,291,292].

Vitrification stabilization primarily considers immobilization of the biologic in the glassy matrix. Reduced molecular mobility decreases denaturation, and physical separation may decrease aggregation [31,47,291]. These two theories are not mutually exclusive as glass formation is thought to be a necessary condition for hydrogen bond replacement [294]. However, vitrification on its own may be insufficient for glass stabilization. For example, it has been shown that even though dextran forms a glassy matrix, it is not very good at providing glass stabilization [291]. In fact, the larger the molecular weight of dextran, the less it stabilizes, despite an increasing glass transition temperature, from which it has been hypothesized that steric hindrance in large molecular weight dextran interfered with hydrogen bond replacement [291]. Furthermore, studies have shown that small molecular weight glass formers stabilize better than large molecular weight glass formers (even though glass transition temperature increases almost linearly with molecular weight), a difference thought to be related to the greater ability of small glass formers to directly interact by hydrogen bond replacement because of their lower free volume [17,291,293]. While physical stability requires that the glassy matrix not undergo a glass transition and become less viscous or crystallize, the above argument clearly demonstrates that storage well below the glass transition temperature is not all that is required for stability. If a glass transition and subsequent excipient crystallization event occurs, biological inactivation may result [295], because crystallization would lead to a loss of hydrogen bonds with the biologic.

From the above arguments, the reason trehalose is a good glass stabilizer and preserver of biologics may in part be due to it being small enough to effectively provide hydrogen bond replacement, while being large enough that it has a sufficient glass transition temperature to ensure it remains amorphous when stored at ambient temperature, low humidity conditions. Moreover, trehalose molecules have many locations available for hydrogen bonding [166]. It has been suggested that the sugar-protein ratio in a formulation should be designed based on the number of bonding sites on the protein that need to be replaced [243].

Despite its relatively small size, trehalose may not be able to replace all hydrogen bonds with the protein; hence, adding a small amount of even lower molecular weight compound, such as sorbitol, may fill some of the remaining excess free volume and allow for additional hydrogen bonding to the protein to improve stability. The use of small amounts of plasticizers such as glycerol may improve stability despite lowering the glass transition temperature [185,296,297]. This effect is thought to be related to the slowing down of the fast dynamics of short-range relaxations, which appear to be more important for long-term biological stability than long-range relaxation occurring at glass transition, as short-range relaxations occur well below the glass transition temperature [185,298,299]. The use of incoherent neutron scattering and isothermal microcalorimetry may be useful for modeling these relaxations in screening studies [87,299]. Isothermal microcalorimetry instruments can be used to measure heat flow from many powders simultaneously and with great sensitivity, a feature that may prove useful for screening, and for indicating the rate of reactions within the powder, including those between components, as part of excipient compatibility testing.

Isothermal microcalorimetry can be adapted to perform relative humidity (RH)-perfusion microcalorimetry in order to assess suitable storage conditions by predicting long-term chemical and physical stability [300–302]. Heat flow is measured upon exposure of the powder to different relative humidity streams. This measurement can be performed at several temperatures so that the effect of both temperature and relative humidity can be determined [302]. Using RH-perfusion microcalorimetry, it has been observed that at an increase in energy of interaction (not associated with phase or morphology change) between water vapor and glass occurs at a threshold relative humidity (hydration limit), which is thought to relate to water vapor saturating binding sites within the amorphous phase, as the water content at this relative humidity is near the monolayer value from Brunauer-Emmett-Teller theory [237]. The hydration limit is thought to represent the amorphous analogue of the deliquescence point of crystalline material [237]. Below the hydration limit, the water vapor, which may freely diffuse in the amorphous solid matrix, is soluble in the solid, and above the hydration limit additional absorbed water vapor acts as solvent on the amorphous solid, since the heat of water sorption approaches the enthalpy of condensation of water [237]. If so, the supersaturated solution above the hydration limit may initiate crystal growth [300].

A minimum in oxidation rate is expected at the (monolayer) hydration level [288]. Essentially, the monolayer of water may block reaction sites [288]. Other studies have suggested that retaining some residual moisture in the powder may improve stability. Decreased aggregation with 2%–3% moisture relative to 1% moisture has been demonstrated for lyophilized mAB powder [243], and better stability without secondary drying in a lyophilizer from 3% moisture to 1% or less moisture has been demonstrated for spray dried measles vaccine [56].

It has been suggested that the hydration limit may relate to a zero mobility temperature [300], and that a system specific mobility temperature may eventually replace the empirical T_g–50 rule of thumb [288], which assumes long-term physical stability is present when the powder is stored 50°C below the wet glass transition temperature [303]. Indeed, some materials such as amorphous indomethacin crystallize relatively quickly well below the glass transition temperature, which is thought to be due to the large molecular mobility and the quick relaxation of amorphous phases [304,305]. Ultimately, the chemical nature of the formulation determines the stability in a glassy matrix [288]. Stability testing, discussed in the next section, can experimentally demonstrate whether glass stabilization is successful.

12.10 Stability Testing

Stability testing is essentially stress testing required by regulatory agencies to determine the storage conditions and shelf-life of spray dried biologic products. The stability testing requirements are not well defined for all biologic products. One should speak with regulators early in the development process as different procedures may apply for different biologics [139,306].

The analytical techniques described in the Particle Analysis section, in particular bioassays, should be performed at each time point in the stability tests. Performing different analytical measurements at the same time can be important for determining causes of instability. For example, if biologic inactivation is found to occur at a specific time point, moisture content measurement by Karl Fischer titration may indicate increased moisture content (which could be due to a leak in the packaging), solid state analysis may indicate crystallization has occurred (because of an increased moisture content), and scanning electron microscopy may indicate that the morphology of the dried particles has changed (through moisture-induced crystallization events).

There are many different types of stability tests that can be performed to determine when the product fails. Typically, regulatory agencies require long-term and accelerated stability testing, the methods and protocols for which can be found elsewhere [307–311].

Long-term, or real-time, stability measurements are used to determine the shelf-life of the product and should be performed until degradation is seen or the target shelf-life is passed [309–312]. Using multiple samples is particularly important for biologics, as there can be large variability [313]. Long-term stability tests are typically conducted monthly for the first 3 months and then at 3-month intervals thereafter until the end of the first year, every 6 months until the end of the second year, and annually thereafter [309]. For climate zones I and II, 25°C is the long-term stability temperature for room temperature storage, while for climate zones III and IV, it is 30°C [310]. There are no general recommendations for acceptable loss of biological activity [309]. In many instances, a biphasic loss on storage is observed [41,51,56] that may be related to damage from the spray drying process [14].

In accelerated stability tests, the product is stressed at higher temperature, typically for shorter periods of time, to increase degradation rates [311]. The theory of accelerated degradation kinetics is discussed elsewhere [313]. Since the loss of biologic activity and other changes to the powder such as solid phase changes may be non-linear functions of temperature and time, extrapolation of accelerated to long-term stability may not be simple. For example, the time until physical instability is observed for a given difference between wet glass transition temperature and storage temperature is expected to have a non-linear relationship, but the exact relationship is material dependent and usually not known *a priori*.

Cyclic temperature stress testing provides evidence of instability not seen in isothermal long-term and accelerated stability tests and is useful in development and troubleshooting [310,312]. Quicker degradation may result during cyclic stress testing than isothermal testing.

Small chambers can be used for accelerated and cyclic stability studies, whereas long-term stability studies may be performed in walk-in chambers engineered to provide a uniform temperature exposure; these may be fitted with temperature readouts and alarms [310]. In preliminary laboratory work, spray dried powder can be stored over saturated salt solution in a desiccator to control relative humidity and the desiccator placed in the stability chamber at a set temperature [237]. Relative humidity ranges for saturated salt solutions are available in the literature [314,315]. However, this method can require much storage space and does not test the effect of interactions of the powder with the container, for example, those associated with leachables and extractables, which should be tested [41,309]. Additionally, the ability of the proposed packaging to protect against humidity should be tested [309].

In preliminary stability testing, representative simulated packaging may be used. It is often overlooked that bottles, vials, and bags are semipermeable to water vapor [311] and should not be used on their own to package spray dried biologics, as high relative humidity storage can inactivate biologics in spray dried powder [128]. Thus, for preliminary stability measurements, spray dried powder can be packaged with desiccant, which is designed to act like a moisture buffer that slows down the effects of moisture ingress; this is due to the large internal surface area of the desiccant to which water can adsorb [316]. Molecular sieve desiccant possesses a high moisture sorption capacity at low relative humidity, whereas silica gel desiccant is useful for protection from higher relative humidity because of a more linear relationship between moisture sorption capacity and relative humidity [317]. Larger quantities of dry desiccant or powder will lower the relative humidity in the container through larger moisture sorption capacity [317].

The change in relative humidity within packaging over the time of a stability test can be estimated from moisture sorption isotherms and the moisture vapor transmission rate of the packaging system, along with ambient conditions [317]. In practice, it is typical for moisture to transfer quickly from the dosage form to the desiccant until the relative humidity is equilibrated; thereafter, external moisture will slowly enter the packaging and increase the water content of the powder and desiccant over time [317].

It may be of interest to store the powder at a low, but optimized non-zero moisture content since very dry powder may lead to increased degradation and electrostatic charging can make filling and handling difficult [33,47,188]. The simplest method for equilibrating moisture for passive relative humidity control is to place the materials in an environmental chamber that is set to the desired relative humidity and temperature [316]. The moisture adsorbed to the packaging material and desiccant and in the headspace of the packaging material should be equilibrated to the desired level prior to packaging. The desiccant is most crucial to equilibrate, as it generally has the highest moisture capacity. Equilibration can be verified by placing the desiccant in a sealed container (such as a bottle) within the environmental chamber and measuring the relative humidity in the bottle with a hygrometer [316]. A supplemented phase diagram can be used to choose moisture equilibration parameters, as discussed later in this chapter.

Biologic powders have been packaged to protect against moisture using heat-sealed aluminum foil bags containing desiccant [49,52]. It is crucial that there are no humidity excursions during the stability testing period, which can last on the order of years; hence, double packaging and double heat sealing are recommended. In addition to desiccant, for some biologics, it may be useful to add antioxidant and perform a nitrogen purge when packaging [59,255]. Instead of an external antioxidant pack, excipients such as ascorbic acid can be added to the spray drying formulation to work as an oxygen scavenger [18].

12.11 Process Modeling

In this section, thermodynamic modeling of a spray drying process is used to predict the outlet temperature and relative humidity for different inlet conditions. This is important since the outlet temperature and relative humidity are key factors in determining the biological and physical stability of the developed particles. The process model presented here is similar to those presented in the literature [97,318]. It is developed by applying a mass and energy balance on the spray dryer under steady state conditions. The following paragraphs contain a brief derivation of the process model.

For incompressible liquids and ideal gases at constant pressure, the relation between enthalpy, h, and temperature, T, at two locations (here, "in" and "out") is given by:

$$h_{\text{out}} - h_{\text{in}} = c_p\left(T_{\text{out}} - T_{\text{in}}\right) \tag{12.9}$$

where c_p is the specific heat capacity. For this equation to be valid, c_p must be constant, and, thus, this equation alone does not adequately describe the enthalpy change when phase change is present, such as when there is evaporation, in which case, latent heat must also be considered.

The steady state conservation of energy equation developed considering a control volume around the spray dryer, neglecting energy changes associated with kinetic energy and elevation, is given by:

$$\dot{m}_{ag}h_{ag,in} + \dot{m}_{dg}h_{dg,in} + \dot{m}_w h_{w,in} = \dot{Q}_{loss} + \dot{m}_{ag}h_{ag,out} + \dot{m}_{dg}h_{dg,out} + \dot{m}_w h_{w,out} \tag{12.10}$$

where $\dot{m}$ refers to mass flow rate, the subscript "ag" represents atomizing gas, "dg" drying gas, and "w" liquid feed solvent (considered as water here). Unless sufficient insulation is used, the spray dryer cannot be considered adiabatic and the heat loss, $\dot{Q}_{loss}$, is non-zero. Using the enthalpy relation in Equation (12.9) and considering latent heat of evaporation, $\Delta h_{w,evap}$, Equation (12.10) can be rearranged as:

$$\dot{Q}_{loss} = \dot{m}_{dg}c_{p,dg}\left(T_{in} - T_{out}\right) - \dot{m}_w \Delta h_{w,evap} \tag{12.11}$$

where the sensible heat associated with the liquid feed and atomizing gas have been omitted for the sake of simplicity. It is assumed that the drying gas is at 0% relative humidity, the effect of dissolved solids can be neglected, c_p of the drying gas is constant over the ranges tested, and the gas is incompressible and ideal as stated previously. For closed-cycle systems, which are often used after scale-up, the model may differ, particularly if the inlet drying gas has a non-zero relative humidity [97].

The dryer heat loss decreases the temperature the droplet or particle is exposed to and increases the relative humidity and hence moisture content of the produced powder [31]. The heat loss can be most easily modeled empirically; here, the case where the heat loss can be approximated as a linear function of the outlet temperature is considered:

$$\dot{Q}_{loss} = \alpha T_{out} + \beta \tag{12.12}$$

where α and β are experimentally determined constants.

Combining Equations (12.11) and (12.12) gives:

$$\alpha T_{out} + \beta = \dot{m}_{dg}c_{p,dg}\left(T_{in} - T_{out}\right) - \dot{m}_w \Delta h_{w,evap} \tag{12.13}$$

which can be rearranged to:

$$T_{out} = \frac{\left(\dot{m}_{dg}c_{p,dg}T_{in} - \dot{m}_w \Delta h_{w,evap} - \beta\right)}{\left(\dot{m}_{dg}c_{p,dg} + \alpha\right)} \tag{12.14}$$

The outlet relative humidity, RH_{out}, can be calculated according to:

$$RH_{out} = \left(P_w / P_{w,sat}\right) \times 100\% \tag{12.15}$$

where the water vapor partial pressure, P_w, is given by:

$$P_w = P_{out} \times (\dot{m}_{w,feed}/M_w)/[(\dot{m}_{w,feed}/M_w) + (\dot{m}_{dg}/M_{dg}) + (\dot{m}_{ag}/M_{ag})] \tag{12.16}$$

where P_{out} is the pressure at the outlet which can be measured (see Figure 12.1) and predicted empirically for different process conditions, the powder moisture content is neglected, and M refers to molecular weight. The saturation vapor pressure, $P_{w,sat}$, can be determined as a function of T_{out}, for example, according to the Antoine equation for water vapor pressure [319]:

$$P_{w,sat} = 10 \wedge \left\{7.113 - \left[1685.6/\left(T_{out} - 43.154\right)\right]\right\} \tag{12.17}$$

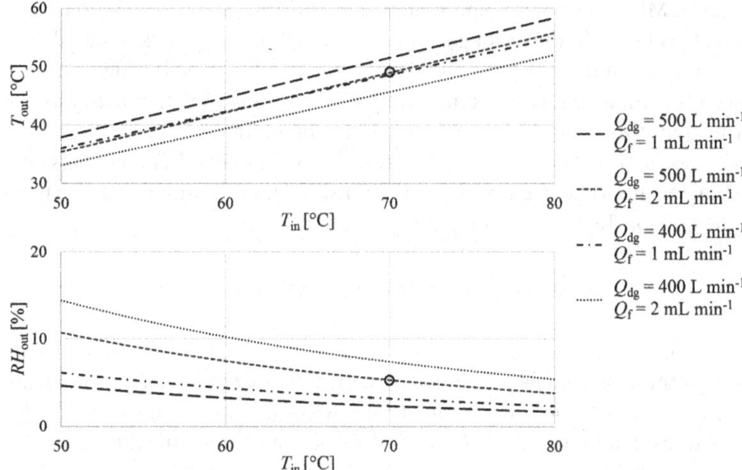

FIGURE 12.3 Outlet temperature and outlet relative humidity for different inlet temperatures, drying gas flow rates, and liquid feed flow rates based on a spray dryer process model developed for the laboratory-scale spray dryer in Figure 12.1. Chosen process parameters used in Figures 12.4 and 12.5 are indicated by circles.

where T_{out} is in units of Kelvin and $P_{w,sat}$ is in units of kilopascals.

The relative humidity calculated using Equation (12.15) can be verified by replacing the outlet temperature probe used in typical commercial laboratory-scale spray dryers with a combined temperature and relative humidity probe. Note that the outlet temperature and relative humidity may differ from the temperature and relative humidity in the collection bottle. External surface thermometers can be used to measure the temperature of the collection bottle [95]. A common method for controlling the temperature and hence relative humidity in the collection bottle is to use a water bath [237].

From Equations (12.14) and (12.15), the outlet temperature and outlet relative humidity can be modeled for various inlet temperatures and gas flow rates. The process model plots in Figure 12.3 illustrate this relationship. As expected, higher drying gas flow rate and higher inlet temperature lead to higher outlet temperature and lower outlet relative humidity, while higher liquid feed flow rate leads to lower outlet temperature (due to evaporative cooling) and higher outlet relative humidity.

The necessary use of lower process temperatures with biologics leads to higher relative humidity for the same drying gas and feed flow rates, which corresponds to greater moisture uptake in the powder. Process modeling is useful for predicting how scenarios like this will affect the properties of the powder. This is possible by using the outlet relative humidity to predict the moisture content in the powder, and to relate this to stability, as discussed further in the next section.

12.12 Supplemented Phase Diagram

A supplemented phase diagram can be used to predict the physical and possibly the biological stability of powder for different storage conditions. The first step in developing the supplemented phase diagram is to determine the moisture uptake of the powder for different relative humidity levels. The relationship between equilibrium moisture content and relative humidity can be obtained experimentally, for example, using dynamic vapor sorption and Karl Fischer (KF) instruments. Equilibrium moisture uptake for amorphous trehalose can also be estimated from the literature [320–323], but more data at low relative humidity levels are desirable.

The glass transition temperature of an amorphous powder decreases with increasing moisture content, an effect known as plasticization [288]. The glass transition temperature can be determined using MDSC. The use of a sinusoidal heating rate overlaid on a ramp heating rate in MDSC allows for the distinction between reversible and non-reversible heat flow for easier detection of glass transitions [243].

Lower heating rates in MDSC are more representative of real-time stability and give lower glass transition temperature values [324], but take longer to perform and provide weaker signals that may be difficult to detect. It is important that the pan and lid are hermetically sealed during MSDC measurements, otherwise, the dry glass transition temperature (only relevant to 0% relative humidity storage) will be measured; unfortunately, this mistake is often made in the literature.

When the glass transition temperature is known only for individual components within a powder containing a well-mixed amorphous glass, the glass transition temperature of the mixture, $T_{g,\text{mix}}$, can be estimated using the Gordon-Taylor equation [325]:

$$T_{g,\text{mix}} = \left(w_1 T_{g,1} + K w_2 T_{g,2}\right) / \left(w_1 + K w_2\right) \tag{12.18}$$

where $1 = w_1 + w_2$, with w referring to mass fraction. Equation (12.18) can also be used to predict the glass transition temperature of a single amorphous excipient for different moisture contents. An estimate for the constant K is 7.5 for trehalose (subscript 1) and water (subscript 2), when trehalose is assumed to have a dry glass transition temperature $T_{g,1} = 387$ K and water is assumed to have a glass transition temperature $T_{g,2} = 138$ K [326].

Summaries of the wet glass transition temperature of trehalose for different moisture contents are given in the literature [323,327]. Figure 12.4 gives the wet glass transition temperature of trehalose for different relative humidity levels predicted by the Gordon-Taylor equation using the constants given previously, along with the corresponding moisture content. The predictions are more accurate at higher relative humidity levels. Note that the glass transition temperature here is only for the moist trehalose component of a particle. For a mixture of amorphous components or partially ordered shell or coating, the glass transition temperature may vary with the radial dimension of the particle [24]. At the same moisture content, sucrose has a much lower glass transition temperature than trehalose, and therefore may not be as suitable of a glass stabilizer for storage at room temperature [323,326].

A non-equilibrium supplemented phase diagram conveniently combines the previously discussed factors of temperature, moisture, and time into a single graph, enabling predictions of physical stability for an amorphous powder [31]. With this approach, the stability of the biologic in the amorphous matrix formulation can be estimated prior to any experiments, saving development time and resources. Figure 12.5 shows a supplemented phase diagram for the spray drying of trehalose with the process conditions presented in Figure 12.3, plasticization data from Figure 12.4, and a storage condition of 5% relative humidity and 30°C.

The drying occurs very quickly, as the droplet lifetime predicted from Equation (12.4) is very small, on the order of milliseconds for the spray dryer in Figure 12.1, and, thus, the dried particles form early

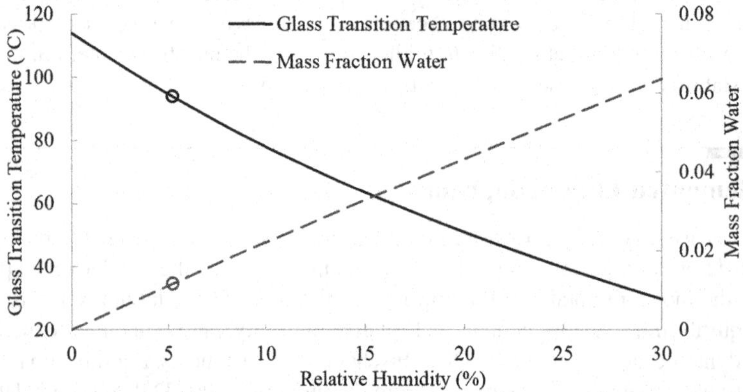

FIGURE 12.4 Glass transition temperature and mass fraction of water in amorphous trehalose equilibrated at different relative humidity levels. Glass transition temperature was predicted using the Gordon-Taylor equation (12.18) for a trehalose-water system using $K = 7.5$ [326], while the mass fraction of water is determined from Roe et al. The values expected at the spray dryer outlet for the process parameters chosen in Figure 12.3 are indicated by circles. (From Roe, K.D. and Labuza, T.P., *Int. J. Food Prop.*, 8, 559–574, 2005.)

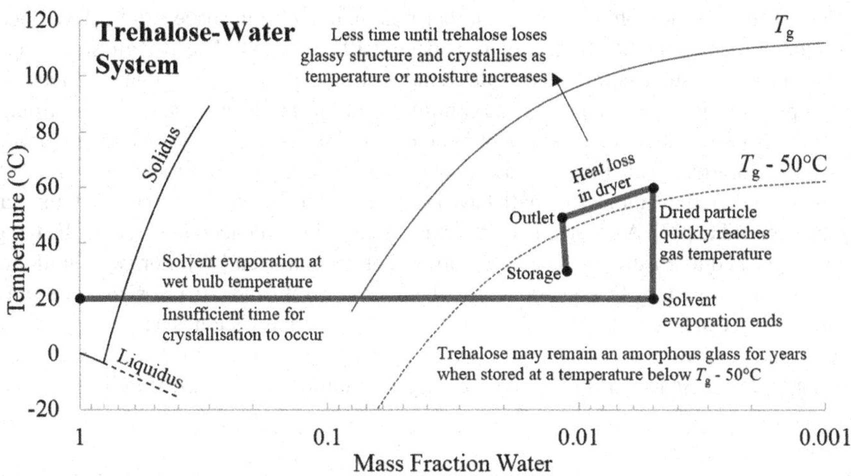

FIGURE 12.5 Non-equilibrium supplemented phase diagram for a trehalose-water system. The solidus and liquidus were approximated from data available in Chen et al. and Roe et al. The thick line represents an approximation of the spray drying process from atomization to storage for the parameters chosen in Figure 12.3. The plasticization curve (glass transition temperature for different mass fractions of water) was developed using values from the Gordon-Taylor equation as per Figure 12.4. The storage condition is 5% relative humidity and 30°C. (From Chen, T. et al., *Cryobiology*, 40, 277–282, 2000; Roe, K.D. and Labuza, T.P., *Int. J. Food Prop.*, 8, 559–574, 2005.)

in the dryer. The quick evaporation occurs at a temperature much lower than the drying gas temperature due to evaporative cooling and can be approximated by the wet bulb temperature [31]. It is assumed that after evaporation ends, the particle temperature quickly increases to the surrounding gas temperature [31]. Further modeling would be required to determine the surrounding gas temperature at the location in the dryer where the particles are at the end of the droplet lifetime (only an estimate is given in Figure 12.5). As further heat loss occurs during the drying process, the relative humidity will increase accordingly, as cooler air has a lower saturated vapor pressure according to Equation (12.17). This increase in relative humidity may lead to more moisture in the powder near the outlet and in the collection bottle than further upstream. The collector temperature is usually assumed to be the same as the outlet temperature [31], but it is likely lower without external control. The collector temperature can be raised to decrease relative humidity in the collector and hence decrease the moisture content in the powder, as explained previously.

The storage temperature is typically lower than the outlet temperature. A rule of thumb is that the wet glass transition temperature of the biologic powder should be 50°C above the storage temperature for long-term stability to be expected [303]. The relative humidity of the powder and packaging material should be designed as per Figures 12.4 and 12.5, to ensure the correct moisture content is achieved to meet this requirement. It can be seen that leaks that raise the moisture content of the powder (move the storage condition to the left in the supplemented phase diagram) can detrimentally affect long-term physical stability. Additionally, following different process paths on this diagram may lead to different levels of biologic inactivation. As explained previously, the use of a system-specific mobility transition temperature may eventually replace the T_g– 50 rule of thumb [288].

Long-term room temperature stability of bacteriophage in a leucine and trehalose powder stored under dry conditions has been demonstrated [126]. Stability without refrigeration is a particularly useful attribute with respect to distribution of biologics to developing countries. While dry storage is simple and practical in many applications, it may not be optimal for all biologics, as previously explained. When a powder is required to have stability at comparatively high relative humidity, the use of a high glass transition temperature polymeric excipient such as pullulan can prevent trehalose from crystallizing at high relative humidity and temperature, improving the storage stability in those conditions [320]. Excellent chemical and aggregation stability of salmon calcitonin and human growth hormone stored at high relative humidity has been demonstrated with trileucine [170].

Further to the supplemented phase diagram, a thermodynamic design space can be developed within which good stability and manufacturability is expected [97,140,328]. The design space consists of constraints to parameters such as inlet and outlet temperature, drying gas flow rate, and feed flow rate. The outlet temperature is constrained to a maximum based on degradation and to a minimum based on relative humidity considerations [97]. Hot-bench experiments, whereby visible observations for cohesiveness, discoloration, or melting are made on a small amount of powder spread over a metal strip with a known thermal gradient along its length have been suggested to define a maximum temperature the powder can be exposed to [97]. A constraint on the minimum ratio of the feed flow rate to drying gas flow rate has been suggested to ensure an acceptable throughput is achieved [97]. For twin-fluid atomizers, the atomizing gas flow rate may be constrained by the feed flow rate and particle size considerations.

Physical instability can lead to biological instability [295], and many studies have demonstrated more loss of biologic activity with increasing drying gas temperature [12,14,95,146,193,255,329]. Developing a thermodynamic design space for biological stability in addition to physical stability is a subject for future work.

12.13 Conclusions

Applying engineering principles to the spray drying process expedites the development of stable spray dried biologic powder for inhalation that may eliminate the need for cold chain infrastructure and thus increase market access in developing countries. Formulation using leucine or trileucine as shell-forming excipients and trehalose as a glass stabilizer are promising combinations for the development of dispersible and stable spray dried biologic powders.

Scale-up and aseptic spray drying have proven feasible with some spray dried biologics produced at a manufacturing scale having already reached the market.

Twin-fluid atomizers can produce particles with sizes suitable for inhalation and typically result in an acceptable level of shear stress on the biologic. Inactivation of biologics at the air-liquid interface may occur in the drying process, and can be decreased through the use of suitable excipients.

The droplet evaporation and particle formation processes are relatively well understood. Particle engineering models are available to predict the characteristics of spray dried particles, including the surface enrichment and radial distributions of different excipients, solid state, and particle size. Once dried, the particles are typically collected into a collection bottle using a cyclone, from which samples can be taken and analyzed using various particle analysis techniques to verify the predictions from particle engineering models.

The separation of biologic inactivation due to spray drying and rehydration of the powder for bioassay is difficult, and the use of rehydration media representative of lung fluid can be informative. Aerosolization of spray dried biologic powder can be performed with DPIs, and suspension of spray dried biologic powder in a suitable liquid medium allows for aerosolization with nebulizers, pMDIs, and SMIs. Since biologic inactivation due to aerosolization is variable between strains and inhalation devices, it needs to be tested on a case-by-case basis. A comprehensive analysis of losses, including extrathoracic deposition and device losses such as face mask leaks or device retention, should be undertaken when designing the dosage form and choosing the dose.

Trehalose is often a suitable excipient for glass stabilization of biologics. The reason trehalose is a good glass stabilizer appears to be related to its high glass transition temperature, high hydration number, and small size, which allows for direct replacement of hydrogen bonds lost by the biologic during desiccation. The RH-perfusion microcalorimetry technique may be particularly useful for predicting long-term physical stability of spray dried powder and may eventually replace the use of the $T_g - 50$ rule of thumb for predicting long-term physical stability. When performing long-term stability studies, it is crucial to ensure the packaging maintains a suitable relative humidity for the duration of the study. The use of moisture equilibrated desiccant for passive relative humidity control may be useful in this regard.

The conditions that powder is exposed to at the outlet of a spray dryer can be predicted using a process model derived from a mass and energy balance on the spray dryer. The temperature and relative humidity to which the droplets and particles are exposed throughout the spray drying process can be overlaid on a supplemented phase diagram, which is developed from plasticization data for the glass stabilizer. Use of this diagram allows for prediction of long-term stability and manufacturability early in product development.

Suggested directions for future work include determining material properties and characterizing the inhalation toxicology of alternative excipients, characterizing the mechanisms of biologic inactivation in response to selected stresses, and characterizing the use of excipients to stabilize against these specific stresses. Additionally, investments in aseptic spray drying, clinical trials, and the development of straightforward regulatory guidelines will contribute to the engineering and commercialization of more spray dried biologic products for inhalation.

REFERENCES

1. La Mont, C.A. 1865. Improvement in preserving eggs. Patent US51263A.
2. Peroy, S.R. 1872. Improvement in drying and concentrating liquid substances by atomizing. Patent US125406A.
3. Desai, K.G.H., Park, H.J. 2005. Recent developments in microencapsulation of food ingredients. *Drying Technol* 23:1361–1394.
4. Anandharamakrishnan, C., Padma Ishwarya, S. 2015. *Spray Drying Techniques for Food Ingredient Encapsulation*. Chichester, UK: John Wiley & Sons.
5. Schuck, P., Jeantet, R., Bhandari, B. et al. 2016. Recent advances in spray drying relevant to the dairy industry: A comprehensive critical review. *Drying Technol* 34:1773–1790.
6. Masters, K. 1994. Scale-up of spray dryers. *Drying Technol* 12:235–257.
7. Gharsallaoui, A., Roudaut, G., Chambin, O., Voilley, A., Saurel, R. 2007. Applications of spray-drying in microencapsulation of food ingredients: An overview. *Food Res Int* 40:1107–1121.
8. Ré, M.I. 1998. Microencapsulation by spray drying. *Drying Technol* 16:1195–1236.
9. Shishir, M.R.I., Chen, W. 2017. Trends of spray drying: A critical review on drying of fruit and vegetable juices. *Trends Food Sci Technol* 65:49–67.
10. Verma, A., Singh, S.V. 2015. Spray drying of fruit and vegetable juices-A review. *Crit Rev Food Sci Nutr* 55:701–719.
11. Masters, K. 1972. *Spray Drying: An Introduction to Principles, Operational Practice and Applications*. London, UK: Leonard Hill Books.
12. Behboudi-Jobbehdar, S., Soukoulis, C., Yonekura, L., Fisk, I. 2013. Optimization of spray-drying process conditions for the production of maximally viable microencapsulated *L. acidophilus* NCIMB 701748. *Drying Technol* 31:1274–1283.
13. Dianawati, D., Mishra, V., Shah, N.P. 2016. Survival of microencapsulated probiotic bacteria after processing and during storage: A review. *Crit Rev Food Sci Nutr* 56:1685–1716.
14. Huang, S., Vignolles, M.L., Chen, X.D. et al. 2017. Spray drying of probiotics and other food-grade bacteria: A review. *Trends Food Sci Technol* 63:1–17.
15. Broeckx, G., Vandenheuvel, D., Claes, I.J.J., Lebeer, S., Kiekens, F. 2016. Drying techniques of probiotic bacteria as an important step towards the development of novel pharmabiotics. *Int J Pharm* 505:303–313.
16. Perdana, J., Bereschenko, L., Fox, M.B. et al. 2013. Dehydration and thermal inactivation of *Lactobacillus plantarum* WCFS1: Comparing single droplet during drying to spray and freeze drying. *Food Res Int* 54:1351–1359.
17. Perdana, J., Fox, M.B., Siwei, C., Boom, R.M., Schutyser, M.A.I. 2014. Interactions between formulation and spray drying conditions related to survival of *Lactobacillus plantarum* WCFS1. *Food Res Int* 56:9–17.
18. Ghandi, A., Powell, I.B., Broome, M., Adhikari, B. 2013. Survival, fermentation activity and storage stability of spray dried *Lactococcus lactis* produced via different atomization regimes. *J Food Eng* 115:83–90.
19. Murugesan, R., Orsat, V. 2012. Spray drying for the production of nutraceutical ingredients – A review. *Food Bioprocess Tech* 5:3–14.
20. Carneiro, H.C.F., Tonon, R.V., Grosso, C.R.F., Hubinger, M.D. 2013. Encapsulation efficiency and oxidative stability of flaxseed oil microencapsulated by spray drying using different combinations of wall materials. *J Food Eng* 115:443–451.

21. Broadhead, J., Edmond Rouan, S.K., Rhodes, C.T. 1992. The spray drying of pharmaceuticals. *Drug Dev Ind Pharm* 18:1169–1206.
22. Wisniewski, R. 2015. Spray drying technology review. *45th International Conference on Environmental Systems*, Bellevue, WA.
23. Jones, H.W., Wisniewski, R., Flynn, M. 2014. Space and industrial brine drying technologies. *44th International Conference on Environmental Systems*, Tuscon, Arizona.
24. Vehring, R. 2008. Pharmaceutical particle engineering via spray drying. *Pharm Res* 25:999–1022.
25. Schwartzbach, H. 2011. Achieving aseptic drying with spray drying technologies. *Pharm Technol Eur* 23(9):90–92. http://www.pharmtech.com/achieving-aseptic-drying-spray-drying-technologies.
26. Siew, A. 2016. Exploring the use of aseptic spray drying in the manufacture of biopharmaceutical injectables. *Pharm Technol* 40(7):24–27. http://www.pharmtech.com/exploring-use-aseptic-spray-drying-manufacture-biopharmaceutical-injectables.
27. Quinn, J.J. 1965. The economics of spray drying. *Ind Eng Chem* 57:35–37.
28. Holsinger, V.H., McAloon, A.J., Onwulata, C.I., Smith, P.W. 2000. A cost analysis of encapsulated spray-dried milk fat. *J Dairy Sci* 83:2361–2365.
29. Pharmaceutical Technology Editors. 2010. The possibilities and challenges of spray drying. *Pharm Technol Eur* 22(5):22–24. http://www.pharmtech.com/possibilities-and-challenges-spray-drying.
30. Roser, B. 1991. Trehalose, a new approach to premium dried foods. *Trends Food Sci Technol* 2:166–169.
31. Hoe, S., Boraey, M.A., Ivey, J.W., Finlay, W.H., Vehring, R. 2014. Manufacturing and device options for the delivery of biotherapeutics. *J Aerosol Med Pulm Drug Deliv* 27:315–328.
32. Ledet, G.A., Graves, R.A., Bostanian, L.A., Mandal, T.K. 2015. Spray-drying of biopharmaceuticals. In *Lyophilized Biologics and Vaccines: Modality-based Approaches*, ed. D. Varshney, M. Singh, 273–297. New York: Springer Science+Business Media.
33. Walters, R.H., Bhatnagar, B., Tchessalov, S., Izutsu, K.I., Tsumoto, K., Ohtake, S. 2014. Next generation drying technologies for pharmaceutical applications. *J Pharm Sci* 103:2673–2695.
34. Kanojia, G., Willems, G.J., Frijlink, H.W., Kersten, G.F.A., Soema, P.C., Amorij, J.P. 2016. A design of experiment approach to predict product and process parameters for a spray dried influenza vaccine. *Int J Pharm* 511:1098–1111.
35. Saluja, V., Amorij, J.P., Kapteyn, J.C., de Boer, A.H., Frijlink, H.W., Hinrichs, W.L.J. 2010. A comparison between spray drying and spray freeze drying to produce an influenza subunit vaccine powder for inhalation. *J Control Release* 144:127–133.
36. Weers, J.G., Tarara, T.E., Clark, A.R. 2007. Design of fine particles for pulmonary drug delivery. *Expert Opin Drug Deliv* 4:297–313.
37. Afkhami, S., LeClair, D.A., Haddadi, S. et al. 2017. Spray dried human and chimpanzee adenoviral-vectored vaccines are thermally stable and immunogenic *in vivo*. *Vaccine* 35:2916–2924.
38. Gikanga, B., Turok, R., Hui, A., Bowen, M., Stauch, O.B., Maa, Y.F. 2015. Manufacturing of high-concentration monoclonal antibody formulations via spray drying-the road to manufacturing scale. *PDA J Pharm Sci Technol* 69:59–73.
39. Chen, D., Kapre, S., Goel, A. et al. 2010. Thermostable formulations of a hepatitis B vaccine and a meningitis A polysaccharide conjugate vaccine produced by a spray drying method. *Vaccine* 28:5093–5099.
40. Sou, T., Meeusen, E.N., de Veer, M., Morton, D.A.V., Kaminskas, L.M., McIntosh, M.P. 2011. New developments in dry powder pulmonary vaccine delivery. *Trends Biotechnol* 29:191–198.
41. Tlaxca, J.L., Ellis, S., Remmele Jr., R.L. 2015. Live attenuated and inactivated viral vaccine formulation and nasal delivery: Potential and challenges. *Adv Drug Deliv Rev* 93:56–78.
42. World Health Organization. 2005. *Monitoring Vaccine Wastage at Country Level: Guideline for Programme Managers*. Geneva, Switzerland: World Health Organization. http://apps.who.int/iris/handle/10665/68463 (accessed March 12, 2018).
43. Huang, J., Garmise, R.J., Crowder, T.M. et al. 2004. A novel dry powder influenza vaccine and intranasal delivery technology: Induction of systemic and mucosal immune responses in rats. *Vaccine* 23:794–801.
44. LiCalsi, C., Christensen, T., Bennett, J.V., Phillips, E., Witham, C. 1999. Dry powder inhalation as a potential delivery method for vaccines. *Vaccine* 17:1796–1803.
45. Lu, D., Hickey, A.J. 2007. Pulmonary vaccine delivery. *Expert Rev Vaccines* 6:213–226.
46. Wang, S.H., Thompson, A.L., Hickey, A.J., Staats, H.F. 2012. Dry powder vaccines for mucosal administration: Critical factors in manufacture and delivery. In *Mucosal Vaccines: Modern Concepts, Strategies, and Challenges*, ed. P.A. Kozlowski, 121–156. Berlin, Germany: Springer-Verlag.

47. Ohtake, S., Lechuga-Ballesteros, D., Truong-Le, V., Patzer, E.J. 2015. Strategies for heat-stable vaccines. In *Vaccine Development and Manufacturing*, eds. E.P. Wang, R. Ellis, N.S. Pujar, 287–318. Hoboken, NJ: John Wiley & Sons.
48. Amorij, J.P., Huckriede, A., Wilschut, J., Frijlink, H.W., Hinrichs, W.L.J. 2008. Development of stable influenza vaccine powder formulations: Challenges and possibilities. *Pharm Res* 25:1256–1273.
49. Zhu, C., Shoji, Y., McCray, S. et al. 2014. Stabilization of HAC1 influenza vaccine by spray drying: Formulation development and process scale-up. *Pharm Res* 31:3006–3018.
50. Laube, B.L. 2005. The expanding role of aerosols in systemic drug delivery, gene therapy, and vaccination. *Respir Care* 50:1161–1176.
51. Lovalenti, P.M., Anderl, J., Yee, L. et al. 2016. Stabilization of live attenuated influenza vaccines by freeze drying, spray drying, and foam drying. *Pharm Res* 33:1144–1160.
52. Sou, T., Morton, D.A.V., Williamson, M., Meeusen, E.N., Kaminskas, L.M., McIntosh, M.P. 2015. Spray-dried influenza antigen with trehalose and leucine produces an aerosolizable powder vaccine formulation that induces strong systemic and mucosal immunity after pulmonary administration. *J Aerosol Med Pulm Drug Deliv* 28:361–371.
53. Smith, D.J., Bot, S., Dellamary, L., Bot, A. 2003. Evaluation of novel aerosol formulations designed for mucosal vaccination against influenza virus. *Vaccine* 21:2805–2812.
54. Amorij, J.P., Saluja, V., Petersen, A.H., Hinrichs, W.L.J., Huckriede, A., Frijlink, H.W. 2007. Pulmonary delivery of an inulin-stabilized influenza subunit vaccine prepared by spray-freeze drying induces systemic, mucosal humoral as well as cell-mediated responses in BALB/c mice. *Vaccine* 25:8707–8717.
55. Kunda, N.K., Alfagih, I.M., Miyaji, E.N. et al. 2015. Pulmonary dry powder vaccine of pneumococcal antigen loaded nanoparticles. *Int J Pharm* 495:903–912.
56. Ohtake, S., Martin, R.A., Yee, L. et al. 2010. Heat-stable measles vaccine produced by spray drying. *Vaccine* 28:1275–1284.
57. Corbanie, E.A., Remon, J.P., van Reeth, K., Landman, W.J.M., van Eck, J.H.H., Vervaet, C. 2007. Spray drying of an attenuated live Newcastle disease vaccine virus intended for respiratory mass vaccination of poultry. *Vaccine* 25:8306–8317.
58. Huyge, K., van Reeth, K., de Beer, T. et al. 2012. Suitability of differently formulated dry powder Newcastle disease vaccines for mass vaccination of poultry. *Eur J Pharm Biopharm* 80:649–656.
59. Kunda, N.K., Wafula, D., Tram, M., Wu, T.H., Muttil, P. 2016. A stable live bacterial vaccine. *Eur J Pharm Biopharm* 103:109–117.
60. Muttil, P., Prego, C., Garcia-Contreras, L. et al. 2010. Immunization of guinea pigs with novel hepatitis B antigen as nanoparticle aggregate powders administered by the pulmonary route. *AAPS J* 12:330–337.
61. Garcia Contreras, L., Awashthi, S., Hanif, S.N.M., Hickey, A.J. 2012. Inhaled vaccines for the prevention of tuberculosis. *J Mycobac Dis* S1:002.
62. Tyne, A.S., Chan, J.G.Y., Shanahan, E.R. et al. 2013. TLR2-targeted secreted proteins from *Mycobacterium tuberculosis* are protective as powdered pulmonary vaccines. *Vaccine* 31:4322–4329.
63. Lu, D., Garcia-Contreras, L., Muttil, P. et al. 2010. Pulmonary immunization using antigen 85-B polymeric microparticles to boost tuberculosis immunity. *AAPS J* 12:338–347.
64. Lu, D., Garcia-Contreras, L., Xu, D. et al. 2010. Poly (lactide-co-glycolide) microspheres in respirable sizes enhance an *in vitro* T cell response to recombinant *Mycobacterium tuberculosis* antigen 85B. *Pharm Res* 24:1834–1843.
65. Jin, T.H., Tsao, E., Goudsmit, J., Dheenadhayalan, V., Sadoff, J. 2010. Stabilizing formulations for inhalable powders of an adenovirus 35-vectored tuberculosis (TB) vaccine (AERAS-402). *Vaccine* 28:4369–4375.
66. Garcia-Contreras, L., Wong, Y.L., Muttil, P. et al. 2008. Immunization by bacterial aerosol. *Proc Natl Acad Sci USA* 105:4656–4660.
67. Wong, Y.L., Sampson, S., Germishuizen, W.A. et al. 2007. Drying a tuberculosis vaccine without freezing. *Proc Natl Acad Sci USA* 104:2591–2595.
68. Bennett, J.V., de Castro, J.F., Valdespino-Gomez, J.L. et al. 2002. Aerosolized measles and measles-rubella vaccines induce better antibody booster responses than injected vaccines: randomized trials in Mexican schoolchildren. *Bull World Health Organ* 80:806–812.
69. de Castro, J.F., Bennett, J.V., Gallardo Rincon, H., Alvarez y Munoz, M.T., Partida Sanchez, L.A.E., Santos, J.I. 2005. Evaluation of immunogenicity and side effects of triple viral vaccine (MMR) in adults, given by two routes: Subcutaneous and respiratory (aerosol). *Vaccine* 23:1079–1084.

70. Dilraj, A., Cutts, F.T., de Castro, J.F. et al. 2000. Response to different measles vaccine strains given by aerosol and subcutaneous routes to schoolchildren: A randomised trial. *Lancet* 355:798–803.
71. Dilraj, A., Sukhoo, R., Cutts, F.T., Bennett, J.V. 2007. Aerosol and subcutaneous measles vaccine: Measles antibody responses 6 years after re-vaccination. *Vaccine* 25:4170–4174.
72. Patton, J.S., Platz, R.M. 1992. (D) Routes of delivery: case studies: (2) Pulmonary delivery of peptides and proteins for systemic action. *Adv Drug Deliv Rev* 8:179–196.
73. Wolff, R.K. 1998. Safety of inhaled proteins for therapeutic use. *J Aerosol Med Pulm Drug Deliv* 11:197–219.
74. Hyde, S.C., Pringle, I.A., Abdullah, S. et al. 2008. CpG-free plasmids confer reduced inflammation and sustained pulmonary gene expressions. *Nat Biotechnol* 26:549–551.
75. Ruiz, F.E., Clancy, J.P., Perricone, M.A. et al. 2001. A clinical inflammation syndrome attributable to aerosolized lipid-DNA administration in cystic fibrosis. *Hum Gene Ther* 12:751–761.
76. Heinemann, L. 2008. The failure of exubera: Are we beating a dead horse? *J Diabetes Sci Technol* 2:518–529.
77. Chow, A.H.L., Tong, H.H.Y., Chattopadhyay, P., Shekunov, B.Y. 2007. Particle engineering for pulmonary drug delivery. *Pharm Res* 24:411–437.
78. Peyre, M., Audran, R., Estevez, F. et al. 2004. Childhood and malaria vaccines combined in biodegradable microspheres produce immunity with synergistic interactions. *J Control Release* 99:345–355.
79. Boehm, G., Peyre, M., Sesardic, D. et al. 2002. On technological and immunological benefits of multivalent single-injection microsphere vaccines. *Pharm Res* 19:1330–1336.
80. McAdams, D., Chen, D., Kristensen, D. 2012. Spray drying and vaccine stabilization. *Expert Rev Vaccines* 11:1211–1219.
81. Evaluate Ltd. 2017. EvaluatePharma® World Preview 2017, Outlook to 2022. http://www.evaluategroup.com/public/Reports/EvaluatePharma-World-Preview-2017.aspx (accessed March 9, 2018).
82. Walsh, G. 2014. Biopharmaceutical benchmarks 2014. *Nat Biotechnol* 32:992–1000.
83. Sane, S.U., Wong, R., Hsu, C.C. 2004. Raman spectroscopic characterization of drying-induced structural changes in a therapeutic antibody: Correlating structural changes with long-term stability. *J Pharm Sci* 93:1005–1018.
84. Costantino, H.R., Andya, J.D., Nguyen, P.H. et al. 1998. Effect of mannitol crystallization on the stability and aerosol performance of a spray-dried pharmaceutical protein, recombinant humanized anti-IgE monoclonal antibody. *J Pharm Sci* 87:1406–1411.
85. Schüle, S., Schulz-Fademrecht, T., Garidel, P., Bechtold-Peters, K., Frieß, W. 2008. Stabilization of IgG1 in spray-dried powders for inhalation. *Eur J Pharm Biopharm* 69:793–807.
86. Bowen, M., Turok, R., Maa, Y.F. 2013. Spray drying of monoclonal antibodies: Investigating powder-based biologic drug substance bulk storage. *Drying Technol* 31:1441–1450.
87. Abdul-Fattah, A.M., Truong-Le, V., Yee, L. et al. 2007. Drying-induced variations in physico-chemical properties of amorphous pharmaceuticals and their impact on stability (I): Stability of a monoclonal antibody. *J Pharm Sci* 96:1983–2008.
88. Mohanty, R.R., Das, S. 2017. Inhaled insulin – current direction of insulin research. *J Clin Diagn Res* 11:OE01–OE02.
89. White, S., Bennett, D.B., Cheu, S. et al. 2005. EXUBERA®: Pharmaceutical development of a novel product for pulmonary delivery of insulin. *Diabetes Technol Ther* 7:896–906.
90. Miller, D.P., Tan, T., Nakamura, J., Malcolmson, R.J., Tarara, T.E., Weers, J.G. 2017. Physical characterization of tobramycin inhalation powder: II. State diagram of an amorphous engineered particle formulation. *Mol Pharm* 14:1950–1960.
91. Vehring, R., Lechuga-Ballesteros, D., Joshi, V., Noga, B., Dwivedi, S.K. 2012. Cosuspensions of microcrystals and engineered microparticles for uniform and efficient delivery of respiratory therapeutics from pressurized metered dose inhalers. *Langmuir* 28:15015–15023.
92. Doty, A., Schroeder, J., Vang, K. et al. 2018. Drug delivery from an innovative LAMA/LABA co-suspension delivery technology fixed-dose combination MDI: Evidence of consistency, robustness, and reliability. *AAPS PharmSciTech* 19:837–844.
93. Maltesen, M.J., Bjerregaard, S., Hovgaard, L., Havelund, S., van de Weert, M. 2008. Quality by design – Spray drying of insulin intended for inhalation. *Eur J Pharm Biopharm* 70:828–838.
94. Sadrzadeh, N., Miller, D.P., Lechuga-Ballesteros, D., Harper, N.J., Stevenson, C.L., Bennett, D.B. 2010. Solid-state stability of spray-dried insulin powder for inhalation: Chemical kinetics and structural relaxation modeling of Exubera above and below the glass transition temperature. *J Pharm Sci* 99:3698–3710.

95. Ståhl, K., Claesson, M., Lilliehorn, P., Lindén, H., Bäckström, K. 2002. The effect of process variables on the degradation and physical properties of spray dried insulin intended for inhalation. *Int J Pharm* 233:227–237.
96. Geller, D.E., Weers, J., Heuerding, S. 2011. Development of an inhaled dry-powder formulation of Tobramycin using PulmoSphere™ technology. *J Aerosol Med Pulm Drug Deliv* 24:175–182.
97. Dobry, D.E., Settell, D.M., Baumann, J.M., Ray, R.J., Graham, L.J., Beyerinck, R.A. 2009. A model-based methodology for spray-drying process development. *J Pharm Innov* 4:133–142.
98. Baghel, S., Cathcart, H., O'Reilly, N.J. 2016. Polymeric amorphous solid dispersions: A review of amorphization, crystallization, stabilization, solid-state characterization, and aqueous solubilization of biopharmaceutical classification system class II drugs. *J Pharm Sci* 105:2527–2544.
99. Paudel, A., Worku, Z.A., Meeus, J., Guns, S., van den Mooter, G. 2013. Manufacturing of solid dispersions of poorly water soluble drugs by spray drying: Formulation and process considerations. *Int J Pharm* 453:253–284.
100. Singh, A., van den Mooter, G. 2016. Spray drying formulation of amorphous solid dispersions. *Adv Drug Deliv Rev* 100:27–50.
101. Vasconcelos, T., Marques, S., das Neves, J., Sarmento, B. 2016. Amorphous solid dispersions: Rational selection of a manufacturing process. *Adv Drug Deliv Rev* 100:85–101.
102. Kaye, R.S., Purewal, T.S., Oya Alpar, H. 2009. Simultaneously manufactured nano-in-micro (SIMANIM) particles for dry-powder modified-release delivery of antibodies. *J Pharm Sci* 98:4055–4068.
103. Lee, H.K., Park, J.H., Kwon, K.C. 1997. Double-walled microparticles for single shot vaccine. *J Control Release* 44:283–293.
104. Thomas, T.T., Kohane, D.S., Wang, A., Langer, R. 2004. Microparticulate formulations for the controlled release of interleukin-2. *J Pharm Sci* 93:1100–1109.
105. Ungaro, F., d'Angelo, I., Miro, A., La Rotonda, M.I., Quaglia, F. 2012. Engineered PLGA nano- and micro-carriers for pulmonary delivery: Challenges and promises. *J Pharm Pharmacol* 64:1217–1235.
106. Kutter, E., Sulakvelidze, A. 2005. *Bacteriophages: Biology and Applications*. Boca Raton, FL: CRC Press.
107. Huff, W.E., Huff, G.R., Rath, N.C., Balog, J.M., Donoghue, A.M. 2002. Prevention of *Escherichia coli* infection in broiler chickens with a bacteriophage aerosol spray. *Poult Sci* 81:1486–1491.
108. Abedon, S.T. 2015. Phage therapy of pulmonary infections. *Bacteriophage* 5:e1020260.
109. Abedon, S.T., Kuhl, S.J., Blasdel, B.G., Kutter, E.M. 2011. Phage treatment of human infections. *Bacteriophage* 1:66–85.
110. Chan, B.K., Abedon, S.T., Loc-Carrillo, C. 2013. Phage cocktails and the future of phage therapy. *Future Microbiol* 8:769–783.
111. Haq, I.U., Chaudhry, W.N., Akhtar, M.N., Andleeb, S., Qadri, I. 2012. Bacteriophages and their implications on future biotechnology: A review. *Virol J* 9:9.
112. Hatfull, G.F., Vehring R. 2016. Respirable bacteriophage aerosols for the prevention and treatment of tuberculosis. In *Drug Delivery Systems for Tuberculosis Prevention and Treatment*, ed. A.J. Hickey, A. Misra, P.B. Fourie, 277–292. Chichester, UK: John Wiley & Sons.
113. Kutter, E., de Vos, D., Gvasalia, G. et al. 2010. Phage therapy in clinical practice: Treatment of human infections. *Curr Pharm Biotechnol* 11:69–86.
114. Loc-Carrillo, C., Abedon, S.T. 2011. Pros and cons of phage therapy. *Bacteriophage* 1:111–114.
115. Merabishvili, M., Pirnay, J.P., Verbeken, G. et al. 2009. Quality-controlled small-scale production of a well-defined bacteriophage cocktail for use in human clinical trials. *PLoS ONE* 4:e4944.
116. Międzybrodzki, R., Borysowski, J., Weber-Dąbrowska, B. et al. 2012. Chapter 3 – Clinical aspects of phage therapy. *Adv Virus Res* 83:73–121.
117. Parracho, H.M.R.T., Burrowes, B.H., Enright, M.C., McConville, M.L., Harper, D.R. 2012. The role of regulated clinical trials in the development of bacteriophage therapeutics. *J Mol Genet Med* 6:279–286.
118. Semler, D.D., Goudie, A.D., Finlay, W.H., Dennis, J.J. 2014. Aerosol phage therapy efficacy in *Burkholderia cepacia* complex respiratory infections. *Antimicrob Agents Chemother* 58:4005–4013.
119. Ślopek, S., Weber-Dąbrowska, B., Dąbrowski, M., Kucharewicz-Krukowska, K. 1987. Results of bacteriophage treatment of suppurative bacterial infections in the years 1981–1986. *Arch Immunol Ther Exp (Warsz)* 35:569–583.
120. Malik, D.J., Sokolov, I.J., Vinner, G.K. et al. 2017. Formulation, stabilisation and encapsulation of bacteriophage for phage therapy. *Adv Colloid Interface Sci* 249:100–133.

121. Hoe, S., Semler, D.D., Goudie, A.D. et al. 2013. Respirable bacteriophages for the treatment of bacterial lung infections. *J Aerosol Med Pulm Drug Deliv* 26:317–335.
122. Parisien, A., Allain, B., Zhang, J., Mandeville, R., Lan, C.Q. 2008. Novel alternatives to antbiotics: Bacteriophages, bacterial cell wall hydrolases, and antimicrobial peptides. *J Appl Microbiol* 104:1–13.
123. Kwok, P.C.L., Grabarek, A., Chow, M.Y.T. et al. 2015. Inhalable spray-dried formulation of D-LAK antimicrobial peptides targeting tuberculosis. *Int J Pharm* 491:367–374.
124. Chang, R.Y.K., Chen, K., Wang, J. et al. 2018. Proof-of-principle study in a murine lung infection model of antipseudomonal activity of phage PEV20 in a dry-powder formulation. *Antimicrob Agents Chemother* 62:e01714–e01717.
125. Sulakvelidze, A., Alavidze, Z., Glenn Morris, Jr., J., 2001. Bacteriophage therapy. *Antimicrob Agents Chemother* 45:649–659.
126. Leung, S.S.Y., Parumasivam, T., Nguyen, A. et al. 2018. Effect of storage temperature on the stability of spray dried bacteriophage powders. *Eur J Pharm Biopharm* 127:213–222.
127. Leung, S.S.Y., Parumasivam, T., Gao, F.G. et al. 2016. Production of inhalation phage powders using spray freeze drying and spray drying techniques for treatment of respiratory infections. *Pharm Res* 33:1486–1496.
128. Leung, S.S.Y., Parumasivam, T., Gao, F.G. et al. 2017. Effect of storage conditions on the stability of spray dried, inhalable bacteriophage powders. *Int J Pharm* 521:141–149.
129. Matinkhoo, S., Lynch, K.H., Dennis, J.J., Finlay, W.H., Vehring, R. 2011. Spray-dried respirable powders containing bacteriophages for the treatment of pulmonary infections. *J Pharm Sci* 100:5197–5205.
130. Liu, H.F., Ma, J., Winter, C., Bayer, R. 2010. Recovery and purification process development for monoclonal antibody production. *mAbs* 2:480–499.
131. Kelley, B. 2007. Very large scale monoclonal antibody purification: The case for conventional unit operations. *Biotechnol Prog* 23:995–1008.
132. Gottschalk, U. 2017. *Process Scale Purification of Antibodies*, 2nd edition. Hoboken, NJ: John Wiley & Sons.
133. Gagnon, P. 2012. Technology trends in antibody purification. *J Chromatogr A* 1221:57–70.
134. Azevedo, A.M., Rosa, P.A.J., Filipa Ferreira, I., Raquel Aires-Barros, M. 2009. Chromatography-free recovery of biopharmaceuticals through aqueous two-phase processing. *Trends Biotechnol* 27:240–247.
135. Janson, J.C. 2011. *Protein Purification: Principles, High Resolution Methods, and Applications*, 3rd edition. Hoboken, NJ: John Wiley & Sons.
136. GE Healthcare. 2010. Strategies for protein purification: Handbook. https://www.gelifesciences.com/en/bs/solutions/protein-research/knowledge-center/protein-handbooks (accessed June 21, 2017).
137. Grzenia, D.L., Carlson, J.O., Ranil Wickramasinghe, S. 2008. Tangential flow filtration for virus purification. *J Membr Sci* 321:373–380.
138. van Reis, R., Brake, J.M., Charkoudian, J., Burns, D.B., Zydney, A.L. 1999. High-performance tangential flow filtration using charged membranes. *J Membr Sci* 159:133–142.
139. Withington, R. 2001. Regulatory issues for phage-based clinical products. *J Chem Technol Biotechnol* 76:673–676.
140. European Medicines Agency. 2017. ICH guideline Q8 (R2) on pharmaceutical development. http://www.ema.europa.eu/docs/en_GB/document_library/Scientific_guideline/2009/09/WC500002872.pdf (accessed April 20, 2018).
141. Hoe, S., Ivey, J.W., Boraey, M.A. et al. 2014. Use of a fundamental approach to spray-drying formulation design to facilitate the development of multi-component dry powder aerosols for respiratory drug delivery. *Pharm Res* 31:449–465.
142. Chaul, L.T., Conceição, E.C., Bara, M.T.F., Paula, J.R., Couto, R.O. 2017. Engineering spray-dried rosemary extracts with improved physicomechanical properties: A design of experiments issue. *Rev Bras Farmacogn* 27:236–244.
143. Faghihi, H., Najafabadi, A.R., Vatanara, A. 2017. Optimization and characterization of spray-dried IgG formulations: A design of experiments approach. *DARU J Pharm Sci* 25:22.
144. Prinn, K.B., Costantino, H.R., Tracy, M. 2002. Statistical modeling of protein spray drying at the lab scale. *AAPS PharmSciTech* 3:E4.
145. Saboo, S., Tumban, E., Peabody, J. et al. 2016. Optimized formulation of a thermostable spray-dried virus-like particle vaccine against human papillomavirus. *Mol Pharm* 13:1646–1655.
146. de Jesus, S.S., Filho, R.M. 2014. Drying of α-amylase by spray drying and freeze-drying – A comparative study. *Braz J Chem Eng* 31:625–631.

147. Branston, S., Stanley, E., Ward, J., Keshavarz-Moore, E. 2011. Study of robustness of filamentous bacteriophages for industrial applications. *Biotechnol Bioeng* 108:1468–1472.
148. Maa, Y.F., Hsu, C.C. 1997. Protein denaturation by combined effect of shear and air-liquid interface. *Biotechnol Bioeng* 54:503–512.
149. Levy, M.S., Collins, I.J., Yim, S.S. et al. 1999. Effect of shear on plasmid DNA in solution. *Bioprocess Biosyst Eng* 20:7–13.
150. Beckard, I.B., Asimakis, P., Bertolini, J., Dunstan, D.E. 2011. The effect of shear flow on protein structure and function. *Biopolymers* 95:733–745.
151. Biddlecombe, J.G., Craig, A.V., Zhang, H. et al. 2007. Determining antibody stability: Creation of solid-liquid interfacial effects within a high shear environment. *Biotechnol Prog* 23:1218–1222.
152. Cordova, A., Deserno, M., Gelbart, W.M., Ben-Shaul, A. 2003. Osmotic shock and the strength of viral capsids. *Biophys J* 85:70–74.
153. Jończyk, E., Kłak, M., Międzybrodzki, R., Górski, A. 2011. The influence of external factors on bacteriophages-review. *Folia Microbiol (Praha)* 56:191–200.
154. Drees, K.P., Abbaszadegan, M., Maier, R.M. 2003. Comparative electrochemical inactivation of bacteria and bacteriophage. *Water Res* 37:2291–2300.
155. Nanjiao, Y., Rong, F., Juan, Z. Yong, Y. 2013. Inactivation of *Escherichia coli* phage by pulsed electric field treatment. *J Chem Pharm Res* 5:210–214.
156. Plowright, W., Herniman, K.A.J., Rampton, C.S. 1971. Studies on rinderpest culture vaccine. IV. The stability of the reconstituted product. *Res Vet Sci* 12:40–46.
157. Greene, G.I., Babel, F.J. 1948. Effect of ultraviolet irradiation on bacteriophage active against *Streptococcus lactis*. *J Dairy Sci* 31:509–515.
158. Iriarte, F.B., Balogh, B., Momol, M.T., Smith, L.M., Wilson, M., Jones, J.B. 2007. Factors affecting survival of bacteriophage on tomato leaf surfaces. *Appl Environ Microbiol* 73:1704–1711.
159. Iwasawa, Y., Ishihara, K. 1967. Resistance of *Staphylococcus aureus* to desiccation, heat and ultraviolet rays in relation to phage pattern. *Jpn J Microbiol* 11:305–309.
160. Müller-Merbach, M., Rauscher, T., Hinrichs, J. 2005. Inactivation of bacteriophages by thermal and high-pressure treatment. *Int Dairy J* 15:777–784.
161. Cambell-Renton, M.L. 1941. Experiments on drying and on freezing bacteriophage. *J Pathol* 53:371–384.
162. Arribas, M., Kubota, K., Cabanillas, L., Lázaro, E. 2014. Adaptation to fluctuating temperatures in an RNA virus is driven by the most stringent selective pressure. *PLoS ONE* 9:e100940.
163. Maassab, H.F., DeBorde, D.C. 1985. Development and characterization of cold-adapted viruses for use as live virus vaccines. *Vaccine* 3:355–369.
164. Satpathy, G.R., Török, Z., Bali, R. et al. 2004. Loading red blood cells with trehalose: A steps towards biostabilization. *Cryobiology* 49:123–136.
165. Santivarangkna, C., Higl, B., Foerst, P. 2008. Protection mechanisms of sugars during different stages of preparation process of dried lactic acid starter cultures. *Food Microbiol* 25:429–441.
166. Ohtake, S., Wang, Y.J. 2011. Trehalose: Current use and future applications. *J Pharm Sci* 100:2020–2053.
167. Chang, R.Y., Wong, J., Mathai, A. et al. 2017. Production of highly stable spray dried phage formulations for the treatment of *Pseudomonas aeruginosa* lung infection. *Eur J Pharm Biopharm* 121:1–13.
168. Feng, A.L., Boraey, M.A., Gwin, M.A., Finlay, P.R., Kuehl, P.J., Vehring, R. 2011. Mechanistic models facilitate efficient development of leucine containing microparticles for pulmonary drug delivery. *Int J Pharm* 409:156–163.
169. Gliński, J., Chavepeyer, G., Platten, J.K. 2000. Surface properties of aqueous solutions of L-leucine. *Biophys Chem* 84:99–103.
170. Lechuga-Ballesteros, D., Charan, C., Stults, C.L.M. et al. 2008. Trileucine improves aerosol performance and stability of spray-dried powders for inhalation. *J Pharm Sci* 97:287–302.
171. Vehring, R., Foss, W.R., Lechuga-Ballesteros, D. 2007. Particle formation in spray drying. *J Aerosol Sci* 38:728–746.
172. Chew, N.Y.K., Chan, H.K. 2001. Use of solid corrugated particles to enhance powder aerosol performance. *Pharm Res* 18:1570–1577.
173. Ivey, J.W., Bhambri, P., Church, T.K., Lewis, D.A., Vehring, R. 2018. Experimental investigations of particle formation from propellant and solvent droplets using a monodisperse spray dryer. *Aerosol Sci Technol* 52:702–716.

174. Boraey, M.A., Hoe, S., Sharif, H., Miller, D.P., Lechuga-Ballesteros, D., Vehring, R. 2013. Improvement of the dispersibility of spray-dried budesonide powders using leucine in an ethanol-water cosolvent system. *Powder Technol* 236:171–178.
175. Ji, S., Thulstrup, P.W., Mu, H. et al. 2016. Effect of ethanol as a co-solvent on the aerosol performance and stability of spray-dried lysozyme. *Int J Pharm* 513:175–182.
176. Ibrahim, B.M., Jun, S.W., Lee, M.Y., Kang, S.H., Yeo, Y. 2010. Development of inhalable dry powder formulation of basic fibroblast growth factor. *Int J Pharm* 385:66–72.
177. Manning, M.C., Chou, D.K., Murphy, B.M., Payne, R.W., Katayama, D.S. 2010. Stability of protein pharmaceuticals: An update. *Pharm Res* 27:544–575.
178. Goebel-Stengel, M., Stengel, A., Taché, Y., Reeve Jr., J.R. 2011. The importance of using the optimal plastic and glassware in studies involving peptides. *Anal Biochem* 414:38–46.
179. Hlady, V., Buijs, J. 1996. Protein adsorption on solid surfaces. *Curr Opin Biotechnol* 7:72–77.
180. Höger, K., Mathes, J., Frieß, W. 2015. IgG1 adsorption to siliconized glass vials-influence of pH, ionic strength, and nonionic surfactants. *J Pharm Sci* 104:34–43.
181. Mathes, J.M. 2010. Protein adsorption to vial surfaces – Quantification, structural and mechanistic studies. PhD Diss., Ludwig-Maximilians-Universität München.
182. Nakanishi, K., Sakiyama, T., Imamura, K. 2001. On the adsorption of proteins on solid surfaces, a common but very complicated phenomenon. *J Biosci Bioeng* 91:233–244.
183. Rabe, M., Verdes, D., Seeger, S. 2011. Understanding protein adsorption at solid surfaces. *Adv Colloid Interface Sci* 162:87–106.
184. MacRitchie, F. 1978. Proteins at interfaces. *Adv Protein Chem* 32:283–326.
185. Abdul-Fattah, A.M., Kalonia, D.S., Pikal, M.J. 2007. The challenge of drying method selection for protein pharmaceuticals: Product quality implications. *J Pharm Sci* 96:1886–1916.
186. Lefebvre, A.H., McDonell, V.G. 2017. *Atomization and Sprays*, 2nd edition. Boca Raton, FL: CRC Press.
187. Ashgriz, N. 2011. *Handbook of Atomization and Sprays: Theory and Applications.* New York: Springer Science+Business Media, LLC.
188. Snyder, H.E., Lechuga-Ballesteros, D. 2008. Spray drying: Theory and pharmaceutical applications. In *Pharmaceutical Dosage forms – Tablets: Unit operations and Mechanical Properties, 3rd edition*, eds. L.L. Augsburger, S.W. Hoag, 227–260. Boca Raton, FL: CRC Press.
189. Cal, K., Sollohub, K. 2010. Spray drying technique. I: Hardware and process parameters. *J Pharm Sci* 99:575–586.
190. Thybo, P., Hovgaard, L., Andersen, S.K., Sæderup Lindeløv, J. 2008. Droplet size measurements for spray dryer scale-up. *Pharm Dev Technol* 13:93–104.
191. Liu, W., Chen, X.D., Selomulya, C. 2015. On the spray drying of uniform functional microparticles. *Particuology* 22:1–12.
192. Ameri, M., Maa, Y.F. 2006. Spray drying of biopharmaceuticals: Stability and process considerations. *Drying Technol* 24:763–768.
193. Vandenheuvel, D., Singh, A., Vandersteegen, K., Klumpp, J., Lavigne, R., van den Mooter, G. 2013. Feasibility of spray drying bacteriophages into respirable powders to combat pulmonary bacterial infections. *Eur J Pharm Biopharm* 84:578–582.
194. Carrigy, N.B., Liang, L., Wang, H. et al. 2018. Mechanistic modeling expedites the development of spray dried biologics. *In Proceedings of 21st International Drying Symposium*, eds. J.A. Cárcel, G. Clemente, J.V. García-Pérez, A. Mulet, C. Rosselló, 1551–1558. València, Spain: Editorial Universitat Politècnica de València.
195. Abdul-Fattah, A.M., Truong, V.L. 2010. Drying process methods for biopharmaceutical products: An overview. In *Formulation and Process Development Strategies for Manufacturing Biopharmaceuticals*, eds. F. Jameel, S. Hershenson, 705–738. Hoboken, NJ: John Wiley & Sons.
196. Millqvist-Fureby, A., Malmsten, M., Bergenståhl, B. 1999. Spray-drying of trypsin – Surface characterisation and activity preservation. *Int J Pharm* 188:243–253.
197. Maa, Y.F., Prestrelski, S.J. 2000. Biopharmaceutical powders: Particle formation and formulation considerations. *Curr Pharm Biotechnol* 1:283–302.
198. Lee, G. 2002. Spray-drying of proteins. In *Rational Design of Stable Protein Formulations: Theory and Practice,* eds. J.F. Carpenter, M.C. Manning, 135–158. New York: Kluwer Academic/Plenum Publishers.

199. Adler, M., Lee, G. 1999. Stability and surface activity of lactate dehydrogenase in spray-dried trehalose. *J Pharm Sci* 88:199–208.
200. Adler, M., Unger, M., Lee, G. 2000. Surface composition of spray-dried particles of bovine serum albumin/trehalose/surfactant. *Pharm Res* 17:863–870.
201. Mumenthaler, M., Hsu, C.C., Pearlman, R. 1994. Feasibility study on spray-drying protein pharmaceuticals: Recombinant human growth hormone and tissue-type plasminogen activator. *Pharm Res* 11:12–20.
202. Abdul-Fattah, A.M., Lechuga-Ballesteros, D., Kalonia, D.S., Pikal, M.J. 2008. The impact of drying method and formulation on the physical properties and stability of methionyl human growth hormone in the amorphous solid state. *J Pharm Sci* 97:163–184.
203. Kawakami, K., Sumitani, C., Toshihashi, Y., Yonemochi, E., Terada, K. 2010. Investigation of the dynamic process during spray-drying to improve aerodynamic performance of inhalation particles. *Int J Pharm* 390:250–259.
204. Nuzzo, M., Millqvist-Fureby, A., Sloth, J., Bergenstahl, B. 2015. Surface composition and morphology of particles dried individually and by spray drying. *Drying Technol* 33:757–767.
205. Maa, Y.F., Costantino, H.R., Nguyen, P.A., Hsu, C.C. 1997. The effect of operating and formulation variables on the morphology of spray-dried protein particles. *Pharm Dev Technol* 2:213–223.
206. Jaskulski, M., Wawrzyniak, P., Zbiciński, I. 2015. CFD model of particle agglomeration in spray drying. *Drying Technol* 33:1971–1980.
207. Finlay, W.H. 2001. *The Mechanics of Inhaled Pharmaceutical Aerosol: An Introduction*. London, UK: Academic Press.
208. Baldelli, A., Power, R.M., Miles, R.E.H., Reid, J.P., Vehring, R. 2016. Effect of crystallization kinetics on the properties of spray dried microparticles. *Aerosol Sci Technol* 50:693–704.
209. Leong, K.H. 1987. Morphological control of particles generated from the evaporation of solution droplets: Theoretical considerations. *J Aerosol Sci* 18:511–524.
210. Boraey, M.A., Vehring, R. 2014. Diffusion controlled formation of microparticles. *J Aerosol Sci* 67:131–143.
211. He, G., Bhamidi, V., Tan, R.B.H., Kenis, P.J.A., Zukoski, C.F. 2006. Determination of critical supersaturation from microdroplet evaporation experiments. *Cryst Growth Des* 6:1175–1180.
212. Baldelli, A., Vehring, R. 2016. Control of the radial distribution of chemical components in spray-dried crystalline microparticles. *Aerosol Sci Technol* 50:1130–1142.
213. Lin, R., Woo, M.W., Wu, Z. et al. 2017. Spray drying of mixed amino acids: The effect of crystallization inhibition and humidity treatment on the particle formation. *Chem Eng Sci* 167:161–171.
214. Baldelli, A., Vehring, R. 2016. Analysis of cohesion forces between monodisperse microparticles with rough surfaces. *Coll Surf A* 506:179–189.
215. Sou, T., Forbes, R., Gray, J. et al. 2016. Designing a multi-component spray-dried formulation platform for pulmonary delivery of biopharmaceuticals: The use of polyol, disaccharide, polysaccharide and synthetic polymer to modify solid-state properties for glass stabilization. *Powder Technol* 287:248–255.
216. Yu, L., Mishra, D.S., Rigsbee, D.R. 1998. Determination of the glass properties of D-mannitol using sorbitol as an impurity. *J Pharm Sci* 87:774–777.
217. Bergfors, T.M. 2001. *Protein Crystallization: Techniques, Strategies, and Tips: A Laboratory Manual*. La Jolla, CA: International University Line.
218. Roos, Y.H., Drusch, S. 2016. *Phase Transition in Foods*, 2nd edition. Kidlington, UK: Academic Press.
219. Hinds, W.C. 1999. *Aerosol Technology: Properties, Behavior, and Measurement of Airborne Particles*, 2nd edition. New York: John Wiley & Sons.
220. Lintingre, E., Lequeux, F., Talini, L., Tsapis, N. 2016. Control of particle morphology in the spray drying of colloidal suspensions. *Soft Matter* 12:7435–7444.
221. Biswas, P., Sen, D., Mazumder, S., Basak, C.B., Doshi, P. 2016. Temperature mediated morphological transition during drying of spray colloidal droplets. *Langmuir* 32:2464–2473.
222. Boulogne, F., Giorgiutti-Dauphiné, F., Pauchard, L. 2013. The buckling and invagination process during consolidation of colloidal droplets. *Soft Matter* 9:750–757.
223. Pathak, B., Basu, S. 2015. Phenomenology and control of buckling dynamics in multicomponent colloidal droplets. *J Appl Phys* 117:244901.

224. Sadek, C., Pauchard, L., Schuck, P. et al. 2015. Mechanical properties of milk protein skin layers after drying: Understanding the mechanisms of particle formation from whey protein isolate and native phosphocaseinate. *Food Hydrocoll* 48:8–16.
225. Sen, D., Mazumder, S., Melo, J.S., Khan, A., Bhattyacharya, S., D'Souza, S.F. 2009. Evaporation driven self-assembly of a colloidal dispersion using spray drying: Volume fraction dependent morphological transition. *Langmuir* 25:6690–6695.
226. Sen, D., Melo, J.S., Bahadur, J. et al. 2010. Buckling-driven morphological transformation of droplets of a mixed colloidal suspension during evaporation-induced self-assembly by spray drying. *Eur Phys J E* 31:393–402.
227. Tsapis, N., Dufresne, E.R., Sinha, S.S. et al. 2005. Onset of buckling in drying droplets of colloidal suspensions. *Phys Rev Lett* 94:018302.
228. Bahadur, J., Sen, D., Mazumder, S., Bhattacharya, S., Frielinghaus, H., Goerigk, G. 2011. Origin of buckling phenomenon during drying of micrometer-sized colloidal droplets. *Langmuir* 27:8404–8414.
229. Carlson, R.L., Sendelbeck, R.L., Hoff, N.J. 1967. Experimental studies of the buckling of complete spherical shells. *Exp Mech* 7:281–288.
230. Sloth, J., Jørgensen, K., Bach, P., Jensen, A.D., Kiil, S., Dam-Johansen, K. 2009. Drying of suspensions for pharma and bio products: Drying kinetics and morphology. *Ind Eng Chem Res* 48:3657–3664.
231. Nandiyanto, A.B.D., Okuyama, K. 2011. Progress in developing spray-drying methods for the production of controlled morphology particles: From the nanometer to submicrometer size ranges. *Adv Powder Technol* 22:1–19.
232. Weers, J., Tarara, T. 2014. The PulmoSphere™ platform for pulmonary drug delivery. *Ther Deliv* 5:277–295.
233. Haig, C.W., Hursthouse, A., McIlwain, S., Skyes, D. 2014. The effect of particle agglomeration and attrition on the separation efficiency of a Stairmand cyclone. *Powder Technol* 258:110–124.
234. Fletcher, D.F., Guo, B., Harvie, D.J.E., Langrish, T.A.G., Nijdam, J.J., Williams, J. 2006. What is important in the simulation of spray dryer performance and how do current CFD models performs? *Appl Math Model* 30:1281–1292.
235. Keshani, S., Ramli Wan Daud, W., Nourouzi, M.M., Namvar, F., Ghasemi, M. 2015. Spray drying: An overview on wall deposition, process and modeling. *J Food Eng* 146:152–162.
236. Langrish, T.A.G. 2007. New engineered particles from spray dryers: Research needs in spray drying. *Drying Technol* 25:981–993.
237. Lechuga-Ballesteros, D., Bakri, A., Miller, D.P. 2003. Microcalorimetric measurement of the interactions between water vapor and amorphous pharmaceutical solids. *Pharm Res* 20:308–318.
238. Wong, J., Ricci, M., Chan, H.K. 2016. Spray drying strategies to stop tuberculosis. In *Drug Delivery Systems for Tuberculosis Prevention and Treatment*, eds. A.J. Hickey, A. Misra, P.B. Fourie, 161–196. Chichester, UK: John Wiley & Sons.
239. Shah, B., Kakumanu, V.K., Bansal, A.K. 2006. Analytical techniques for quantification of amorphous/crystalline phases in pharmaceutical solids. *J Pharm Sci* 95:1641–1665.
240. Wang, H., Boraey, M.A., Williams, L., Lechuga-Ballesteros, D., Vehring, R. 2014. Low-frequency shift dispersive Raman spectroscopy for the analysis of respirable dosage forms. *Int J Pharm* 469:197–205.
241. Vehring, R. 2005. Red-excitation dispersive Raman spectroscopy is a suitable technique for solid-state analysis of respirable pharmaceutical powders. *Appl Spectrosc* 59:286–292.
242. Strachan, C.J., Rades, T., Gordon, K.C., Rantanen, J. 2007. Raman spectroscopy for quantitative analysis of pharmaceutical solids. *J Pharm Pharmacol* 59:179–192.
243. Breen, E.D., Curley, J.G., Overcashier, D.E., Hsu, C.C., Shire, S.J. 2001. Effect of moisture on the stability of a lyophilized humanized monoclonal antibody formulation. *Pharm Res* 18:1345–1353.
244. Mahlin, D., Bergström, C.A.S. 2013. Early drug development predictions of glass-forming ability and physical stability of drugs. *Eur J Pharm Sci* 49:323–332.
245. Shur, J., Nevell, T.G., Ewen, R.J. et al. 2008. Cospray-dried unfractionated heparin with L-leucine as a dry powder inhaler mucolytic for cystic fibrosis therapy. *J Pharm Sci* 97:4857–4868.
246. Li, L., Sun, S., Parumasivam, T. et al. 2016. L-leucine as an excipient against moisture on *in vitro* aerosolization performances of highly hygroscopic spray-dried powders. *Eur J Pharm Biopharm* 102:132–141.
247. Fäldt, P., Bergenståhl, B., Carlsson, G. 1993. The surface coverage of fat on food powders analyzed by ESCA (electron spectroscopy for chemical analysis). *Food Struct* 12:225–234.

248. Kim, E.H.J., Chen, X.D., Pearce, D. 2003. On the mechanisms of surface formation and the surface compositions of industrial milk powders. *Drying Technol* 21:265–278.
249. Heng, D., Tang, P., Cairney, J.M. et al. 2007. Focused-ion-beam milling: A novel approach to probing the interior of particles used for inhalation aerosols. *Pharm Res* 24:1608–1617.
250. Baldelli, A., Boraey, M.A., Nobes, D.S., Vehring, R. 2015. Analysis of the particle formation process of structured microparticles. *Mol Pharm* 12:2562–2573.
251. Beker, M.J., Rapoport, A.I. 1987. Conservation of yeasts by dehydration. In *Advances in Biochemical Engineering/Biotechnology*, ed. A. Fiechter, 127–171. Berlin, Germany: Springer-Verlag.
252. Crowe, J.H., Hoekstra, F.A., Crowe, L.M. 1989. Membrane phase transitions are responsible for imbibitional damage in dry pollen. *Proc Natl Acad Sci USA* 86:520–523.
253. Poirier, I., Maréchal, P.A., Richard, S., Gervais, P. 1999. *Saccharomyces cerevisiae* viability is strongly dependant on rehydration kinetics and the temperature of dried cells. *J Appl Microbiol* 86:87–92.
254. Speck, M.L., Myers, R.P. 1946. The viability of dried skim-milk cultures of *Lactobacillus bulgaricus* as affected by the temperature of reconstitution. *J Bacteriol* 52:657–663.
255. Wang, Y.C., Yu, R.C., Chou, C.C. 2004. Viability of lactic acid bacteria and bifidobacteria in fermented soymilk after drying, subsequent rehydration and storage. *Int J Food Microbiol* 93:209–217.
256. Morgan, C.A., Herman, N., White, P.A., Vesey, G. 2006. Preservation of micro-organisms by drying; A review. *J Microbiol Methods* 66:183–193.
257. Leach, R.H., Scott, W.J. 1959. The influence of rehydration on the viability of dried micro-organisms. *J Gen Microbiol* 21:295–307.
258. Muller, J.A., Stanton, C., Sybesma, W., Fitzgerald, G.F., Ross, R.P. 2010. Reconstitution conditions for dried probiotic powders represent a critical step in determining cell viability. *J Appl Microbiol* 108:1369–1379.
259. Hoekstra, F.A., Golovina, E.A., van Aelst, A.C., Hemminga, M.A. 1999. Imbibitional leakage from anhydrobiotes revisited. *Plant Cell Environ* 22:1121–1131.
260. Ingvarsson, P.T., Yang, M., Nielsen, H.M., Rantanen, J., Foged, C. 2011. Stabilization of liposomes during drying. *Expert Opin Drug Deliv* 8:375–388.
261. Crowe, L.M., Crowe, J.H., Rudolph, A., Womersley, C., Appel, L. 1985. Preservation of freeze-dried liposomes by trehalose. *Arch Biochem Biophys* 242:240–247.
262. Marsh, D., Watts, A., Knowles, P.F. 1976. Evidence for phase boundary lipid. Permeability of Tempo-choline into dimyristoylphosphatidylcholine vesicles at the phase transition. *Biochemistry* 15:3570–3578.
263. de Swart, R.L., LiCalsi, C., Quirk, A.V. et al. 2007. Measles vaccination of macaques by dry powder inhalation. *Vaccine* 25:1183–1190.
264. Carrigy, N.B., Chang, R.Y., Leung, S.S.Y. et al. 2017. Anti-tuberculosis bacteriophage D29 delivery with a vibrating mesh nebulizer, jet nebulizer, and soft mist inhaler. *Pharm Res* 34:2084–2096.
265. Golshahi, L., Seed, K.D., Dennis, J.J., Finlay, W.H. 2008. Toward modern inhalational bacteriophage therapy: Nebulization of bacteriophages of *Burkholderia cepacia* complex. *J Aerosol Med Pulm Drug Deliv* 21:351–359.
266. Lentz, Y.K., Worden, L.R., Anchordoquy, T.J., Lengsfeld, C.S. 2005. Effect of jet nebulization on DNA: Identifying the dominant degradation mechanism and mitigation methods. *J Aerosol Sci* 36:973–990.
267. Cutts, F.T., Clements, C.J., Bennett, J.V. 1997. Alternative routes of measles immunization: A review. *Biologicals* 25:323–338.
268. Roth, Y., Chapnik, J.S., Cole, P. 2003. Feasibility of aerosol vaccination in humans. *Ann Otol Rhinol Laryngol* 112:264–270.
269. Sabin, A.B. 1983. Immunization against measles by aerosol. *Rev Infect Dis* 5:514–523.
270. Jones, S.A., Martin, G.P., Brown, M.B. 2006. Stabilisation of deoxyribonuclease in hydrofluoroalkanes using miscible vinyl polymers. *J Control Release* 115:1–8.
271. Liao, Y.H., Brown, M.B., Jones, S.A., Nazir, T., Martin, G.P. 2005. The effects of polyvinyl alcohol on the in vitro stability and delivery of spray-dried protein particles from surfactant-free HFA 134a-based pressurised metered dose inhalers. *Int J Pharm* 304:29–39.
272. Carrigy, N.B., O'Reilly, C., Schmitt, J., Noga, M., Finlay, W.H. 2014. Effect of facial material softness and applied force on face mask dead volume, face mask seal, and inhaled corticosteroid delivery through an idealized infant replica. *J Aerosol Med Pulm Drug Deliv* 27:290–298.
273. Dance Biopharm Inc. 2017. Dance Biopharm and Phillips-Medisize enter into joint development agreement for advanced inhaled insulin delivery. https://www.dancebiopharm.com/news-and-events/press-releases/detail/8/dance-biopharm-and-phillips-medisize-enter-into-joint (accessed April 20, 2018).

274. Arulmuthu, E.R., Williams, D.J., Baldascini, H., Versteeg, H.K., Hoare, M. 2007. Studies on aerosol delivery of plasmid DNA using a mesh nebulizer. *Biotechnol Bioeng* 98:939–955.
275. Astudillo, A., Leung, S.S.Y., Kutter, E., Morales, S., Chan, H.K. 2018. Nebulization effects on structural stability of bacteriophage PEV 44. *Eur J Pharm Biopharm* 125:124–130.
276. Carrigy, N.B., Ruzycki, C.A., Golshahi, L., Finlay, W.H. 2014. Pediatric *in vitro* and *in silico* models of deposition via oral and nasal inhalation. *J Aerosol Med Pulm Drug Deliv* 27:149–169.
277. Carrigy, N.B., Martin, A.R., Finlay, W.H. 2015. Use of extrathoracic deposition models for patient-specific dose estimation during inhaler design. *Curr Pharm Des* 21:3984–3992.
278. Finlay, W.H., Golshahi, L., Noga, M. 2012. New validated extrathoracic and pulmonary deposition models for infants and children. In *Respiratory Drug Delivery 2012*, eds. R.N. Dalby, P.R. Byron, J.P. Peart, J.D. Suman, S.J. Farr, P.M. Young, 325–336. River Grove, IL: Davis Healthcare International Publishing, LLC.
279. Javaheri, E., Golshahi, L., Finlay, W.H. 2013. An idealized geometry that mimics average infant nasal airway deposition. *J Aerosol Sci* 55:137–148.
280. Golshahi, L., Finlay, W.H. 2012. An idealized child throat that mimics average pediatric oropharyngeal deposition. *Aerosol Sci Technol* 46:i–iv.
281. Ruzycki, C.A., Golshahi, L., Vehring, R., Finlay, W.H. 2014. Comparison of *in vitro* deposition of pharmaceutical aerosols in an idealized child throat with *in vivo* deposition in the upper respiratory tract of children. *Pharm Res* 31:1525–1535.
282. Stapleton, K.W., Guentsch, E., Hoskinson, M.K., Finlay, W.H. 2000. On the suitability of κ-ε turbulence modeling for aerosol deposition in the mouth and throat: A comparison with experiment. *J Aerosol Sci* 31:739–749.
283. Matida, E.A, Finlay, W.H., Lange, C.F., Grgic, B. 2004. Improved numerical simulation of aerosol deposition in an idealized mouth-throat. *J Aerosol Sci* 35:1–19.
284. Copley Scientific. 2018. Alberta Idealised Throat (AIT). http://www.copleyscientific.com/home/inhaler-testing/aerodynamic-particle-size/improved-in-vitro-in-vivo-correlation-ivivc/alberta-idealised-throat-ait (accessed April 26, 2018).
285. Depreter, F., Pilcer, G., Amighi, K. 2013. Inhaled proteins: Challenges and perspectives. *Int J Pharm* 447:251–280.
286. Xiong, X., Zhang, H.M., Wu, T.T. et al. 2014. Titer dynamic analysis of D29 within MTB-infected macrophages and effect on immune function of macrophages. *Exp Lung Res* 40:86–98.
287. Lai, M.C., Topp, E.M. 1999. Solid-state chemical stability of proteins and peptides. *J Pharm Sci* 88:489–500.
288. Lechuga-Ballesteros, D., Miller, D.P., Zhang, J. Residual water in amorphous solids: Measurement and effects on stability. In *Amorphous Food and Pharmaceutical Systems*, ed. H. Levine, 275–316. Cambridge, UK: Royal Society of Chemistry Publishing.
289. Zallen, R. 1983. *The Physics of Amorphous Solids*. Weinheim, Germany: Wiley-VCH Verlag GmbH & Co. KGaA.
290. Yu, L. 2001. Amorphous pharmaceutical solids: Preparation, characterization and stabilization. *Adv Drug Deliv Rev* 48:27–42.
291. Crowe, J.H., Carpenter, J.F., Crowe, L.M. 1998. The role of vitrification in anhydrobiosis. *Annu Rev Physiol* 60:73–103.
292. Carpenter, J.F., Crowe, J.H. 1989. An infrared spectroscopic study of the interactions of carbohydrates with dried proteins. *Biochemistry* 28:3916–3922.
293. Mensink, M.A., Frijlink, H.W., van der Voort Maarschalk, K., Hinrichs, W.L.J. 2017. How sugars protect proteins in the solid state and during drying (review): Mechanisms of stabilization in relation to stress conditions. *Eur J Pharm Biopharm* 114:288–295.
294. Arakawa, T., Prestrelski, S.J., Kenney, W.C., Carpenter, J.F. 2001. Factors affecting short-term and long-term stabilities of proteins. *Adv Drug Deliv Rev* 46:307–326.
295. Vandenheuvel, D., Meeus, J., Lavigne, R., van den Mooter, G. 2014. Instability of bacteriophage in spray-dried trehalose powders is caused by crystallization of the matrix. *Int J Pharm* 472:202–205.
296. Averett, D., Cicerone, M.T., Douglas, J.F., de Pablo, J.J. 2012. Fast relaxation and elasticity-related properties of trehalose-glycerol mixtures. *Soft Matter* 8:4936–4945.
297. Weng, L., Elliott, G.D. 2015. Local minimum in fragility for trehalose/glycerol mixtures: Implications for biopharmaceutical stabilization. *J Phys Chem B* 119:6820–6827.

298. Laitinen, R., Löbmann, K., Strachan, C.J., Grohganz, H., Rades, T. 2013. Emerging trends in the stabilization of amorphous drugs. *Int J Pharm* 453:65–79.
299. Cicerone, M.T., Soles, C.L. 2004. Fast dynamics and stabilization of proteins: Binary glasses of trehalose and glycerol. *Biophys J* 86:3836–3845.
300. Lechuga-Ballesteros, D., Miller, D.P. 2006. The hydration limit of amorphous solids and long-term stability. In *Water Properties of Food, Pharmaceutical, and Biological Materials*, eds. M. del Pilar Buera, J. Welti-Chanes, P.J. Lillford, H.R. Corti, 303–308. Boca Raton, FL: CRC Press.
301. Chan, H.K., Clark, A.R., Feeley, J.C. et al. 2004. Physical stability of salmon calcitonin spray-dried powders for inhalation. *J Pharm Sci* 93:792–804.
302. Miller, D.P., Lechuga-Ballesteros, D. 2006. Rapid assessment of the structural relaxation behavior of amorphous pharmaceutical solids: Effect of residual water on molecular mobility. *Pharm Res* 23:2291–2305.
303. Hancock, B.C., Shamblin, S.L., Zografi, G. 1995. Molecular mobility of amorphous pharmaceutical solids below their glass transition temperatures. *Pharm Res* 12:799–806.
304. Andronis, V., Zografi, G. 1998. The molecular mobility of supercooled amorphous indomethacin as a function of temperature and relative humidity. *Pharm Res* 15:835–842.
305. Yoshioka, M., Hancock, B.C., Zografi, G. 1994. Crystallization of indomethacin from the amorphous state below and above its glass transition temperature. *J Pharm Sci* 83:1700–1705.
306. Verbeken, G., Pirnay, J.P., de Vos, D. et al. 2012. Optimizing the European regulatory framework for sustainable bacteriophage therapy in human medicine. *Arch Immunol Ther Exp (Warsz)* 60:161–172.
307. World Health Organization. 2009. Stability testing of active pharmaceutical ingredients and finished pharmaceutical products. WHO Technical Report Series, No. 953, 2009 – Annex 2. http://apps.who.int/medicinedocs/en/d/Js19133en/ (accessed March 13, 2018).
308. Mazzeo, A., Carpenter, P. 2009. Stability studies for biologics. In *Handbook of Stability Testing in Pharmaceutical Development: Regulations, Methodologies, and Best Practices*, ed. K. Huynh-Ba, 353–369. New York, NY: Springer Science+Business Media, LLC.
309. International Conference on Harmonisation. 1995. Stability testing of biotechnological/biological products: Q5C. http://www.ich.org/products/guidelines/quality/article/quality-guidelines.html (accessed April 20, 2018).
310. Bajaj, S., Singla, D., Sakhuja, N. 2012. Stability testing of pharmaceutical products. *J Appl Pharm Sci* 02:129–138.
311. U.S. Food & Drug Administration. 2003. Guidance for industry: Q1A(R2) stability testing of new drug substances and products. http://academy.gmp-compliance.org/guidemgr/files/Q1A(R2).PDF (accessed April 20, 2018).
312. Kommanaboyina, B., Rhodes, C.T. 1999. Trends in stability testing, with emphasis on stability during distribution and storage. *Drug Dev Ind Pharm* 25:857–868.
313. Allison, L.M.C., Mann, G.F., Perkins, F.T., Zuckerman, A.J. 1981. An accelerated stability test procedure for lyophilized measles vaccines. *J Biol Stand* 9:185–194.
314. Greenspan, L. 1977. Humidity fixed points of binary saturated aqueous solutions. *J Res Natl Stand Sec A* 81A:89–96.
315. Young, J.F. 1967. Humidity control in the laboratory using salt solutions–A review. *J Chem Technol Biotechnol.* 17:241–245.
316. Weintraub, S. 2002. Demystifying silica gel. *Proceedings of the Objects Specialty Group Session 30th AIC Annual Meeting*, Miami, FL, pp. 169–194.
317. Waterman, K.C., MacDonald, B.C. 2010. Package selection for moisture protection for solid, oral drug products. *J Pharm Sci* 99:4437–4452.
318. Ivey, J.W., Vehring, R. 2010. The use of modeling in spray drying of emulsions and suspensions accelerates formulation and process development. *Comput Chem Eng* 34:1036–1040.
319. Rumble, J.R. 2018. *CRC Handbook of Chemistry and Physics*, 98th edition. Boca Raton, FL: CRC Press.
320. Teekamp, N., Tian, Y., Visser, J.C. et al. 2017. Addition of pullulan to trehalose glasses improves the stability of β-galactosidase at high moisture conditions. *Carbohydr Polym* 176:374–380.
321. Iglesias, H.A., Chirife, J., Buera, M.P. 1997. Adsorption isotherm of amorphous trehalose. *J Sci Food Agric* 75:183–186.

322. Fan, F., Roos, Y.H. 2016. Crystallization and structural relaxation times in structural strength analysis of amorphous sugar/whey protein systems. *Food Hydrocoll* 60:85–97.
323. Roe, K.D., Labuza, T.P. 2005. Glass transition and crystallization of amorphous trehalose-sucrose mixtures. *Int J Food Prop* 8:559–574.
324. Moynihan, C.T., Easteal, A.J., Wilder, J. Dependence of the glass transition temperature on heating and cooling rate. *J Phys Chem* 78:2673–2677.
325. Gordon, M., Taylor, J.S. 1952. Ideal copolymers and the second-order transitions of synthetic rubbers. I. Non-crystalline copolymers. *J Chem Technol Biotechnol* 2:493–500.
326. Crowe, L.M., Reid, D.S., Crowe, J.H. 1996. Is trehalose special for preserving dry biomaterials? *Biophys J* 71:2087–2093.
327. Chen, T., Fowler, A., Toner, M. 2000. Literature review: Supplemented phase diagram of the trehalose-water binary mixture. *Cryobiology* 40:277–282.
328. Gaspar, F., Vicente, J., Neves, F., Authelin, J.R. 2014. Spray drying: Scale-up and manufacturing. In *Amorphous Solid dispersions: Theory and Practice*, eds. N. Shah, H. Sandhu, D.S. Choi, H. Chokshi, A.W. Malick, 261–302. New York: Springer.
329. Ananta, E., Volkert, M., Knorr, D. 2005. Cellular injuries and storage stability of spray-dried *Lactobacillus rhamnosus* GG. *Int Dairy J* 15:399–409.

13

Supercritical Fluid Manufacture

Ana Aguiar-Ricardo and Eunice Costa

CONTENTS

13.1 Background

A supercritical fluid (SCF) process for particles production was first reported in Hannay and Hogarth (1879). In spite of this fact, it was only within the last four decades that supercritical fluid techniques were systematically investigated for micronization of pharmaceuticals, natural substances, pigments, (bio)polymers, superconductor precursors, among others (Tong et al. 2001, Shariati and Peters 2003, Reverchon 1999). Different SCF techniques have been proposed taking advantage of the peculiar properties of the supercritical solvent, particularly supercritical carbon dioxide ($scCO_2$) (Brunner 2004). The SCF is defined as a fluid that is above its critical temperature (T_C) and pressure (p_C), being CO_2 the most common one due to its relatively low critical temperature (31.18°C) and mild critical pressure (7.4 MPa). Feature properties of a SCF are the liquid-like densities, the gas-like transport properties, and the continuous adjustable solvent power by fine tuning the temperature and pressure. Taking advantage of these properties, several SCF-based techniques have been developed for particle generation overcoming technical and environmental problems associated to the conventional ones (Türk 2014).

The micronization of pharmaceuticals using SCF-assisted processes presents many advantages, namely, the high purity of nano/submicron or microparticles generated and the ability of precisely controlling size distribution(s). The rapid expansion of supercritical solutions (RESS), the simplest supercritical micronization technique, can be used to produce pure or encapsulated drug particles, but a variety of composite drug delivery systems can be produced using other SCF-assisted techniques. The SCF processes may be broadly classified in three groups depending on the $scCO_2$ role in the processing: (i) SCF as solvent and the precipitation occurs from supercritical solutions; (ii) as anti-solvent with precipitation occurring from saturated solutions; and (iii) as co-solute with precipitation occurring from gas saturated solutions (Martin and Cocero 2008, Palakodaty and York 1999). The RESS process as well as the rapid expansion from supercritical to aqueous solution (RESAS) process have been included in the first group. The process supercritical anti-solvent (SAS) was subsequently developed into many other processes such as gas anti-solvent (GAS), aerosol solvent extraction system (ASES), the supercritical fluid extraction of emulsion (SFEE), and solution enhanced dispersion by supercritical fluids (SEDS). The third group includes the particles from gas saturated solutions (PGSS) process and several other derived processes, as the carbon dioxide-assisted nebulization (CAN-BD) process, the supercritical enhanced atomization (SEA), the supercritical-assisted atomization (SAA), also designated as supercritical-assisted spray drying (SASD), the PGSS drying and the depressurization of an expanded liquid organic solution (DELOS), among others.

With the advent of nanoparticle formulations and controlled release systems of small molecule therapeutics and biopharmaceuticals, increased interest in the development of SCF-based processes for particle formation emerged. Particularly, with supreme importance for the development of inhalation formulations, in which the ability to fine-tune particle properties and the flexibility in processing different active principles are requirements mostly for metered dose inhalers (MDIs) and dry powder inhalers (DPIs). The pipeline of drugs under development for the treatment of respiratory diseases include a range of molecules spanning from high-dosage anti-infectives to complex and/or labile peptides and proteins (Depreter et al. 2013). For these particular classes of molecules, the traditional adhesive mixtures with lactose for DPI (also known as carrier-based formulations) cannot be applied since they only enable the delivery of drugs in the order micrograms and also do not allow the stabilization of sensitive molecules. Hence, alternative drug-alone or composite particle formulations, in which the active pharmaceutical ingredient is embedded in an excipient matrix, are becoming more predominant (Pilcer and Amighi 2010). These engineered particles are typically more efficient and less flow-dependent than traditional DPI formulations, ultimately benefiting patients (Weers and Miller 2015).

This chapter describes the SCF-based techniques that have been exploited to produce particles fine enough to be appropriately transported to the lungs (i.e. for inhalation product development). The basic concepts and technologies are introduced, with emphasis on formulation issues considering the pulmonary route of administration, for example, control of particle size and distribution, physical stability, solid state, powder characterization, and effects on bioavailability. A thorough understanding of fluid phase equilibria near the critical conditions and their possible influence on the particle formation mechanisms are essential when manipulating the experimental conditions to achieve changes in the solid state and particle properties in a controlled manner.

13.2 Fundamentals of Particle Formation in Supercritical Fluid

13.2.1 Solubility and Supersaturation

The application of SCFs for micronization of pharmaceuticals involve solutions containing solutes in very diluted concentrations (molar solubilities less than 10^{-5}). In order to design and optimize the processes for particle formation, it is necessary to have data on the solubility of compounds on the supercritical fluid media (Kumar and Johnston 1988). The measurement of drug solubility in $scCO_2$ is highly time-consuming and costly. Thus, several theoretical and empirical models have been developed to predict the solubility of drugs in supercritical solvents. Models based on equations of state (EoS) (Huang et al. 2001, Yazdizadeh et al. 2011), empirical models based on association models (Ch and Madras 2010, Mendez-Santiago and Teja 1999), on solvate complex models (Chrastil 1982), and on density-based models (Si-Moussa et al. 2017) were proposed.

As already mentioned, the driving force for a precipitation process is the supersaturation of the solution. The supersaturation, S, is the ratio between the composition of the fluid and the composition at equilibrium. It measures the departure of composition from the equilibrium state and is calculated through Equation (13.1):

$$S = S = \frac{f_i\ (T,p)}{f_{ieq}(T,p)} = \frac{y_i\ (T,p)\ \phi_i\left(T,\ p, y_i\right)}{y_{ieq}\ (T,p)\ \phi_i^{eq}\left(T,\ p, y_{ieq}\right)} \tag{13.1}$$

where y_i is the mole fraction of solute i at the temperature and pressure of the fluid, y_{ieq} is the saturation composition at the temperature and pressure in the expansion vessel, $\phi_i\ (T, p,\ y_i)$ is the solute fugacity coefficient in the real mixture, and $\phi_i^{eq}\ (T, p,\ y_{ieq})$ is the equilibrium solute fugacity coefficient in the mixture.

To calculate the supersaturation of a solute in $scCO_2$, a good method must be available. Since the solutions of drug compounds in SCF are diluted, the conditions of phase equilibria in the solid compound-SCF system can be described in terms of the equality of fugacities of the solute in the solid and fluid phases:

$$f_i^S(T,p) = f_i^{SCF}(Y,p,y_i) \tag{13.2}$$

where superscripts S and SCF refer to the solid phase and supercritical fluid phase, respectively. The fugacity for each component can be described as follows:

$$f_i^{SCF} = \phi_i^{SCF}\ y_i\, p \tag{13.3}$$

where y_i is the mole fraction of the solid compound in the SCF phase, ϕ_i^{SCF} is the fugacity coefficient in the SCF phase, p is the pressure in the system, and f_i^{SCF} is the fugacity of the solid compound (which has the dimensions of pressure). If we have a multicomponent system, the fugacity coefficients for each i component can be calculated as following:

$$\ln \phi_i^{SCF} = \frac{1}{RT}\int_V^{\infty}\left[\left(\frac{\partial p}{\partial n}\right)_{T,V,n_i} - \frac{RT}{V}\right]dV - lnZ \tag{13.4}$$

where V is the total volume of the system, Z is the compressibility coefficient, and n_i is the number of moles of component i. To determine the fugacity coefficient using the mixing rule in Equation (13.4), the cubic equation of state is applied. Since the solvent ($scCO_2$) is not dissolved in a solid, fugacity is defined as:

$$f_i^S(T,p) = p_i^{sub}(T)\phi_i^{sub}(T,p_i^{sub})\exp\left[\int_{p_i^{sub}}^{p}\frac{\vartheta_i^S}{RT}\,dp\right] \tag{13.5}$$

where p_i^{sub} is the sublimation pressure (the vapor pressure of the pure solid compound) at a specified temperature; ϑ_i^S is the molar volume of the pure solid compound, which is not pressure dependent; and $\phi_i^{sub}\left(T,\ p_i^{sub}\right)$ is the fugacity coefficient at T and p_i^{sub}. By combining Equations (13.4) and (13.5) the solubility is described as:

$$y_i = \frac{p_i^{sub}(T)\exp\left[\dfrac{\vartheta_i^S\left(p - p_i^{sub}\right)}{RT}\right]}{p\ \phi_i^{SCF}} = \frac{p_i^{sub}(T)}{p}E \tag{13.6}$$

$$E = \frac{\exp\left[\vartheta_i^S\left(p - p_i^{\text{sub}}\right)/RT\right]}{\phi_i^{\text{SC}}} p \quad (13.7)$$

The fugacity coefficient in Equation (13.7) is calculated using an equation of state and the convenient mixing rules and interaction parameters. The most commonly used EoS to correlate solubilities of solids in $scCO_2$ are the Peng-Robinson with quadratic mixing rules (van der Waals 1873) and the Perturbed-Chain Statistical Associating Fluid Theory (Gross 2005, Spyriouni et al. 2011).

The mole fraction of dissolved solid compound in the $scCO_2$ is given by:

$$y_i = \frac{p_i^S(T)\exp\left[\frac{V_i^S p}{RT}\right]}{\phi_i^S p} \quad (13.8)$$

where $p_i^S(T)$ is the vapor pressure of the dissolved compound at a given temperature, V_i^S is the molar volume of the dissolved compound, and ϕ_i^S is the fugacity coefficient. The vapor pressure might be calculated according to the Antoine equation.

13.2.2 Modeling of the Solubility of Solid Active Entities in $scCO_2$ with and without Co-solvents

In general, the determination of solubility in $scCO_2$ using the activity coefficient models and equations of state are very time consuming, requiring efficient and robust computational methods, and the access to many properties, such as critical parameters of pure components, sublimation vapor pressure, and molecular parameters, which are very often not available. To overcome these problems, semi-empirical methods as the Chrastil equation have been applied. Chrastil described the first-density model, which is grounded on the formation of a solvato-complex at equilibrium, i.e. it is considered the assembling of an aggregate between the solute and the solvent molecules. The Chrastil model has three parameters (*A*, *B*, and *k*) which are determined by fitting the experimental solubility data of solute *i* in the SCF as described in Equation (13.9), where ρ_{SCF} (in kg m^{-3}) is the density of the pure SCF (Chrastil 1982):

$$y_{\text{ieq}} = \rho_{\text{SCF}}{}^{\kappa} \cdot \exp\left(\frac{A}{T} + B\right) \Leftrightarrow \ln y_{\text{ieq}} = k \cdot \ln \rho_{\text{SCF}} + \frac{\alpha}{T} + \beta \quad (13.9)$$

In Equation (13.9), the parameter *A* is correlated with the enthalpy of solvation and enthalpy of vaporization, *B* is a function of the molecular weight of the solute, *k* denotes the number of molecules of the *SCF* solvating the molecule of solute *i*. The exponential term comes from the Boltzmann weight argument in the form of "exp (–*E*/*RT*)," and *T* is the absolute temperature. It should be remarked that Chrastil's equation is not valid for a solubility higher than 100 kg m^{-3} –200 kg m^{-3} and is only applicable in a narrow range of temperatures (Sparks et al. 2008).

Several attempts were made to extend the density-model proposed by Chrastil to systems including co-solvents. Sauceau et al. proposed another equation (Equation 13.10) where the parameter k_s is the total number of molecules forming the solvato-complex $AB_{k1}C_{k3}$ (Sauceau et al. 2003). The number of molecules surrounding one solute molecule is given by the sum of the number of molecules of the solvent *B*, k_1, plus the number of molecules of co-solvent *C*, k_3, and ρ is the density of the mixture (*SCF* + co-solvent), and the calculated solubility must be fitted to experimental data obtained from ternary systems.

$$T\, ln\left(\frac{y_{\text{ieq}} p}{p^{\text{std}}}\right) = A + B\,\rho_{\text{SCF}} + C\,\text{x}T + \sum_{\text{cos}} D\text{x}\, y_3^{\text{cos}} \quad (13.10)$$

y_3 is the co-solvent mole fraction and Equation (13.10) is applicable for fixed concentration of co-solvent. González et al. (2001) developed another modified Chrastil's equation to calculate the solute solubility in the SCF with a co-solvent. A modified term correlated to the co-solvent concentration in the mixture was added, as expressed in the González equation (13.11):

$$y_{ieq} = \rho_{SCF}^{k} . m^{\gamma} . \exp\left(\frac{A}{T} + B\right) \tag{13.11}$$

where ρ_{SCF} denotes the density of the pure SCF, k describes the associated number of the SCF molecules in the solvato-complex, m is the co-solvent molar fraction in the binary mixture SCF-co-solvent, and the number of co-solvent molecules associated with the solute molecules is γ. With the González model, there is no need to calculate the fluid density, but four parameters need to be fitted: A, B, k, and γ.

The González equation was modified using the q-exponential function and the variables and the adjustable parameters with the meaning as defined above (Tabernero et al. 2014):

$$y_{ieq} = \rho_{SCF}^{k} \cdot m^{\gamma} \cdot \exp_q\left(\frac{A_q}{T}\right) \tag{13.12}$$

Many semi-empirical equations following the Chrastil approach were developed to estimate the solubility of pharmaceutical entities in $scCO_2$ as well as in SCF-co-solvent systems. The density-based models described by different authors (Adachi and Lu 1983, Bartle et al. 1991, Kumar and Johnston 1988, Mendez-Santiago and Teja 1999, Sparks et al. 2008, Valle and Aguilera 1988) gave reasonable solubility predictions although requiring the determination of many parameters for each solute under study. It is not possible to establish the best equation to predict more accurately the solubility of pharmaceutics in SCFs (Tabernero et al. 2010). Many other semi-empirical models for correlating the solubilities of solids in $scCO_2$ with co-solvents and co-solutes were proposed (Reddy and Madras 2011, 2012, Sovova 2001, Tang et al. 2010). Comparing the data reported in literature, these equations were accurate to predict the solubility of pharmaceutical compounds, with different polarities and in a wide range of molecular weight, in SCFs. In general, in spite of the vast number of parameters that must be determined for each system, the predictions from semi-empirical equations give better approximations to experimental data than the cubic equations of state.

13.2.3 Fluid Mechanics and Expansion Path of Supercritical Solution Through a Nozzle Device

When a supercritical solution expands rapidly through a nozzle device, the fluid transits from supercritical to a two-phase state or to a low-pressure gas. In very rapid expansions, homogeneous nucleation is expected to occur. The nucleation rate depends on the properties of the solvents being expanded, the cooling effect due to depressurization, and the resulting high supersaturation. Many supercritical CO_2-assisted precipitation processes involve the expansion through a nozzle into a low-pressure gas. The process is usually described considering four regions, as schematically shown in Figure 13.1a: (i) the inlet region of the nozzle, (ii) the capillary nozzle design, (iii) the supersonic free jet, and (iv) the subsonic free jet. In the inlet region (part I), the flow area reduces suddenly from the inlet tube to the nozzle diameter. In part II, a turbulent flow occurs inside the capillary nozzle, followed by the flow expansion at the outlet of the capillary nozzle into a supersonic free jet with the largest pressure drop. Here is where the flux acquires maximum velocity. At lower p_{exp}, and T_{exp}, and pre-expansion values, spontaneous solvent condenzation might occur. The condenzation starts in the Wilson point (Figure 13.1b). At the end of supersonic free jet, a Mach shock occurs which is a pressure wave travelling with the speed of sound caused by a slight change of pressure added to a compressible flow. The temperature and pressure rise suddenly over the Mach disk and the density increases. The velocity decreases from supersonic to subsonic values, close to an ideal gas state, and the formed droplets evaporate almost instantaneously in the expansion vessel. The solubility y_2 depends on the pressure and temperature. Before the Mach disk,

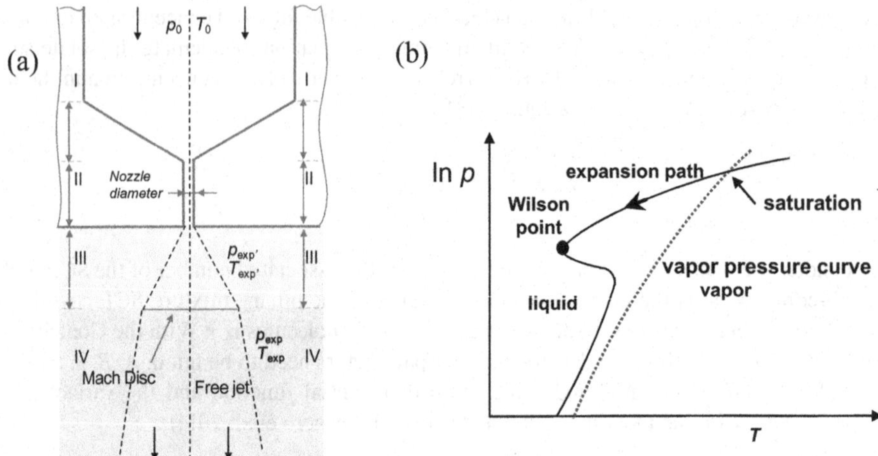

FIGURE 13.1 (a) Scheme of the expansion device showing the considered parts: inlet region (I), capillary nozzle (II), supersonic free jet (III), and subsonic free jet (IV); (b) schematic expansion path showing the saturation point and the Wilson point, whereas the condenzation starts. (Adapted from Helfgen, B. et al., *J. Supercrit. Fluids* 26, 225–242, 2003.)

the rapid decrease in pressure and temperature leads to the rapid decrease of solubility and, consequently, a sudden increase in supersaturation with consequent formation of solid particles (Liu et al. 2014).

The mechanism for particle generation in the rapid expansion process in SCFs was investigated by 2D simulation (Liu et al. 2014). The results from the simulation indicated that the greatest nucleation rate is found near the nozzle exit and that particle precipitation inside the nozzle might occur. In part III, after the nozzle exit, but before the Mach disk, the solute mole fraction in equilibrium, y_{2eq}, at rather smaller temperature and pressure than the values for expansion vessel, $p_{exp'}$ and $T_{exp'}$, decreases to as low as 10^{-15} while the supersaturation increases to as high as 10^{12}. After the Mach disk, the temperature T_{exp} is achieved, leading to an increase in solubility and, thus, a decrease in supersaturation *S*. However, the solution is still saturated, and the particles will continue to grow progressively in the expansion vessel.

To understand the evolution of supersaturation along the expansion path, and how its variation profile is interrelated (Figure 13.1a) with the size, shape, and density of particles formed, mathematical models of nucleation and growth were developed (Debenedetti et al. 1993). The number of critical nuclei formed by unit time and unit volume is designated as the nucleation rate, *J*, and can then be calculated by Equation (13.13) (Debenedetti 1990):

$$J = 2N_{tot}\,\beta\sqrt{\frac{\sigma\, v_2^{\frac{2}{3}}}{kT}}\;.\exp\left\{-\frac{16\pi}{3}\left(\frac{\sigma\, v_2^{\frac{2}{3}}}{kT}\right)^3\left[\frac{1}{lnS - K\,y_2^e\,(S-1)}\right]^2\right\} \tag{13.13}$$

where β is the thermal flux of solute molecules ($\beta = P\,y_2/\,(2\pi mkT)^{1/2}$) for ideal gas behavior, N_{tot} is the solute's concentration in the supercritical fluid, and σ is the interfacial tension between the supercritical fluid and the solid solute. There is no experimental data on interfacial tension available for most of the mixtures of interest for RESS experiments, thus, an estimate of 0.02 Nm^{-1} is often used in modeling calculations (Liu et al. 2014). The critical radius of the nuclei, assuming spherical shape, is then given by:

$$r^* = 2\frac{\sigma\, v_2}{kT}\left[\frac{1}{lnS - K\,y_2^e\,(S-1)}\right] \tag{13.14}$$

This critical radius gives the threshold size of the nuclei from which irreversible condenzation will occur regardless the supersaturation.

13.3 Micronization with $scCO_2$ as Solvent: Rapid Expansion of Supercritical Solutions (RESS)

The RESS process was firstly reported in 1987, and it consists of two main steps: first, the dissolution (or extraction) of the solid product in the high-pressure SCF and, secondly, the expansion of the SCF stream through a nozzle with precipitation of the solute (Matson et al. 1987). Upon the expansion step, the density of the solvent decreases suddenly, reducing its solvent power, and the solute is no longer soluble at the gas-like solvent density. Consequently, instantaneous nucleation occurs, and the crystals grow at very high supersaturation. After the expansion, the solvent becomes a gas, delivering dry and solvent free products. In this process, no further washing and drying steps are needed.

As explained in Section 13.2.1, the driving force for particle formation is the supersaturation associated to the rapid reduction of solvent density upon expansion with the consequent decrease of solute solubility. The rates of nucleation and particle growth are dictated by the rapid change of the saturation ratio. Starting the process with low concentrations of solute in the SCF leads to smaller changes of supersaturation ratio, decreasing the number of nuclei formed. Expanding solutions with lower concentration of the solute in $scCO_2$ leads to smaller particles and a narrower particle size distribution (PSD). This is clearly demonstrated by the micronization of beclomethasone-17,21-dipropionate (BDP) (Charpentier et al. 2008). With increasing concentration, less spherical particles are formed by the RESS process. This experimental evidence is contrary to the classical theory of nucleation (Matson et al. 1987), where higher concentrations are associated to higher supersaturation ratio and thus higher nucleation rates, reducing the particle size due to the greater number of produced nuclei. This apparent contradiction is explained because, regardless of the supersaturation ratio, and according to the theory of Lele and Mawson (Mawson et al. 1995), the particle size and shape of the particles formed are determined also by the location of the initial solute condenzation along the expansion path. The expansion occurs in less than 10^{-5} s, thus, if the particles start to nucleate from the solution in the end of the capillary nozzle, they will have no time to grow and small spherical particles are formed. However, if the particles start to nucleate in the nozzle entrance, then there will be enough time to grow and larger particles can be formed. According to Charpentier et al. (2008) fiber formation can occur if the cloud point is achieved upstream of the nozzle entrance and the solute starts to precipitate there. The same rationale can explain the experimental evidence that with increasing nozzle diameter, particles change from spheres to elongated shapes. Overall, the controlled growth of particles formed by RESS can be achieved by selecting experimental conditions such as: the temperature and pressure in the extraction chamber; the concentration of the solutes in the fluid streams; the solvent and co-solvent composition in the SCF; the size and geometry of the nozzle; the temperature at the expansion chamber; and the distance of collector from the nozzle (depending on the precipitation vessels design) (Figure 13.2).

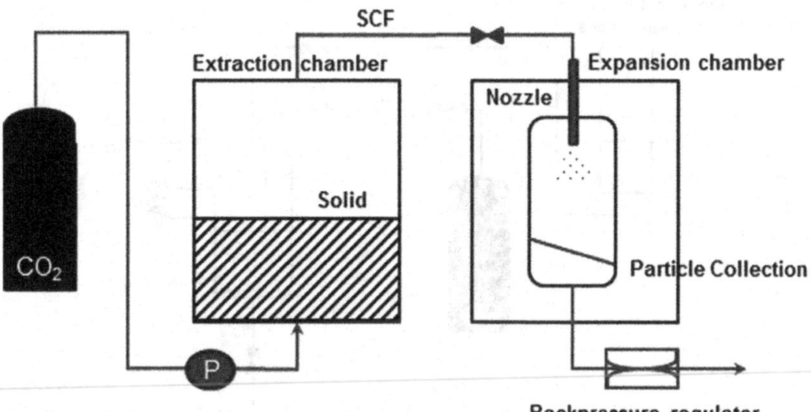

FIGURE 13.2 Schematic representation of RESS experimental apparatus.

The RESS process has two main limitations: (i) the poor solubility of medicines in $scCO_2$, and (ii) the recovery of the particles formed. The main strategy to increase the drugs' solubility involves using an entrainer: a small amount of organic solvent acting as a co-solvent (Mishima et al. 1999).

One method that is described in literature as derived from RESS is the adsorptive precipitation of drugs from supercritical mixtures, a method which is recognized as being able to improve the overall loading, in a porous matrix, of a poorly soluble drug in $scCO_2$. The loading might be improved if the matrix swells in the presence of $scCO_2$ and a controlled depressurization is then performed, or by adding an entrainer or modifier, and also by precipitation within a porous material upon fast depressurization leaving the drug in the pores confinement (Garcia-Gonzalez et al. 2015, Miura et al. 2010). Another strategy to improve the drug loading might be accomplished if specific stronger interactions can be established between the solid matrix and the drug (da Silva et al. 2011a, 2011b). The methodology was demonstrated for the development of oral drug delivery systems, but could be easily extended for inhalation aerosols.

The spraying of $scCO_2$ into an aqueous solvent led to another micronization process, known as RESAS (Pathak et al. 2004).

13.4 Micronization with $scCO_2$ as Anti-solvent

13.4.1 Gas Anti-solvent (GAS) or Supercritical Fluid Anti-solvent (SAS)

Gas anti solvent (GAS) or supercritical fluid anti solvent (SAS) precipitation refers to the expansion of a solute-containing solvent by a SCF. Pivotal studies in GAS processing of guanidine were performed by Gallagher and co-workers (1989) on which it was shown that properties such as particle size, morphology, and particle size distribution of the solute could be varied by fine-tuning the gas anti-solvent addition rate. The SCF anti-solvent addition rate will both influence the interaction between nucleation rate and the growth rate of the crystals as well as the solute supersaturation.

The application of supercritical anti-solvent techniques require that the compound is practically insoluble in SCF, which is the case of most drugs. These techniques are based on the same mechanism: SCF is added to a solution of the target substrate, thus decreasing the solvent power of the solvent in which the substrate is dissolved, leading to supersaturation, and ultimately precipitation or recrystallization of the component, depending on whether it is a recrystallizing solid (Jung and Perrut 2001). The solvent and the SCF need to be miscible, and, hence, organic solvents are typically used for preparing the target substance solution. As shown in Figure 13.3, the high-pressure precipitator is partially filled with the solution of the target substance, and the SCF is pumped until the target pressure/fraction is reached as defined by the equilibrium solubility considerations of the organic solvent in the SCF discussed in

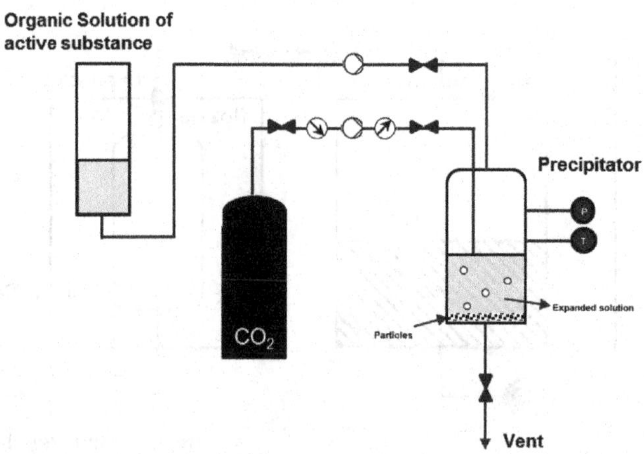

FIGURE 13.3 Gas anti-solvent simplified experimental apparatus.

Section 13.2. The expanded solution is then vented and the particles collected and potentially washed with fresh SCF. The main challenge of this technique might be the control over the solute saturation, hence, the final particle properties, throughout the process, particularly in batch operating conditions. As a consequence, there are little references on the direct application of GAS/SAS for drugs relevant to inhalation applications. However, there were several techniques based on the use of SCF as anti-solvent that have been successfully used on the processing of a vast array of molecules suitable for inhalation, as detailed in the next sections.

13.4.2 Aerosol Solvent Extraction System Technique (ASES)

The ASES technique comprises feeding an organic solution of the compound of interest through a nozzle as fine aerosol into a high-pressure precipitator containing compressed CO_2 (Figure 13.4). The feed solution is fed at a pressure higher than the operating pressure of the precipitator. The dissolution of the SCF into the droplet leads to the liquid expansion and reduction of its solvent power, causing a sudden supersaturation and precipitation into small and uniform particles. The particles are collected on a filter at the bottom of the precipitator and the SCF-expanded solvent vented. The secondary stripping of the collected particles from residual solvents can then be performed through feeding fresh CO_2. The concept is similar to the GAS/SAS technique, but occurs at the droplet level, maximizing the SCF to solvent ratio and mass transfer and thus accelerating the drying process. Overall, the particle properties can be controlled by manipulating the following process parameters: the organic solution solvent, the solute concentration, the solution feed rate into the precipitator, the spray droplet size distribution, the spray velocity, and the SCF temperature and pressure in the high-pressure vessel. ASES has been applied for processing both small molecules and biopharmaceuticals for inhalation, enabling a narrow particle size distribution, uniform shape, and control over the final physical-chemical properties. Examples include ipratropium bromide (Kim and Shing 2008), several steroids (Steckel et al. 1997), and biopharmaceuticals (Shoyele and Cawthome 2006).

13.4.3 Solution Enhanced Dispersion with Supercritical Fluid Technique (SEDS)

Solution enhanced dispersion with supercritical fluid technique (SEDS) is another variation of SCF anti-solvent technique initially developed by the University of Bradford in 1994—Figure 13.4 (Hanna and York 1995). Herein, the apparatus comprises a co-axial nozzle that allows simultaneous feeding of the organic solution of the target active in the inner capillary and the SCF in the outer ring, enabling intense mixing of

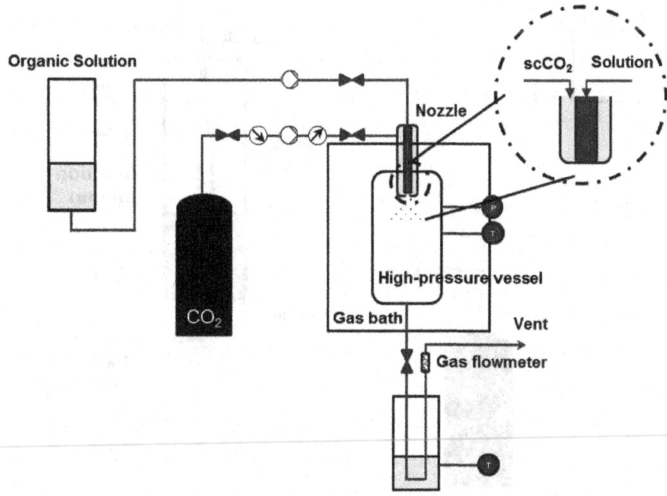

FIGURE 13.4 SEDS technique simplified experimental apparatus.

the SCF with the solvent and higher transfer rates at the nozzle tip. A mixing length can be introduced at the end of the nozzle to intensify the pre-mixing. In addition, expansion of the SCF also enhances atomization and generates a very fine aerosol inside the high-pressure precipitator. The pressure inside the vessel is controlled using a back-pressure regulator; coupled with temperature control, appropriate conditions for solvent extraction, as discussed in Section 13.2, are ensured. In order to micronize water-soluble compounds such as sugars or proteins while circumventing the limited solubility of $scCO_2$ in water, a three-fluid nozzle can be employed in which an organic solvent is introduced in the second co-axial passage.

This technique has been extensively optimized by several research groups since then with particular emphasis on respiratory delivery applications. Several molecules such as budesonide and salmeterol were successfully engineered via SEDS and formulated for pulmonary delivery (Amani et al. 2009). For salmeterol xinafoate, SEDS enabled the preparation of pure polymorphs with controlled particle size through fine-tuning of the recrystallization conditions, which is particularly relevant considering that a mixture of polymorphs is typically obtained through conventional crystallization processes (Beach et al. 1999). Another example is Semprana® (previously branded as Levadex®), which comprises a MDI formulation of dihydroergotamine crystallized by SEDS for the treatment of severe migraine and was the first new drug application submitted to the FDA on SCF-engineered drug (Cipolla and Gonda 2011).

13.4.4 Supercritical Fluid Extraction of Emulsions (SFEE)

The SFEE process enables the continuous production of solid lipid nanoparticles (Chattopadhyay et al. 2007). Basically, the process consists in adding a $scCO_2$ stream at the bottom of a counter current column and an oil-in-water emulsion containing the drug and the lipid in the top of the column (Figure 13.5). As the $scCO_2$ extracts the oily solvent, the nanoparticles precipitate out of the solution. Due to CO_2-lipid interactions, plasticization might occur during extraction, decreasing significantly the glass transition temperature, T_g, and the melting temperature of the lipid. The precipitation process is fast, facilitating a steady operation and enabling the production of particles with uniform particle distribution.

Ketoprofen- and indomethacin-loaded solid lipid nanoparticle formulations for inhalation were successfully manufactured by SFEE (Schuster et al. 1997). The oil-in-water emulsion is prepared by dissolving the drug in an organic solvent, e.g. chloroform for dissolving ketoprofen or indomethacin, with

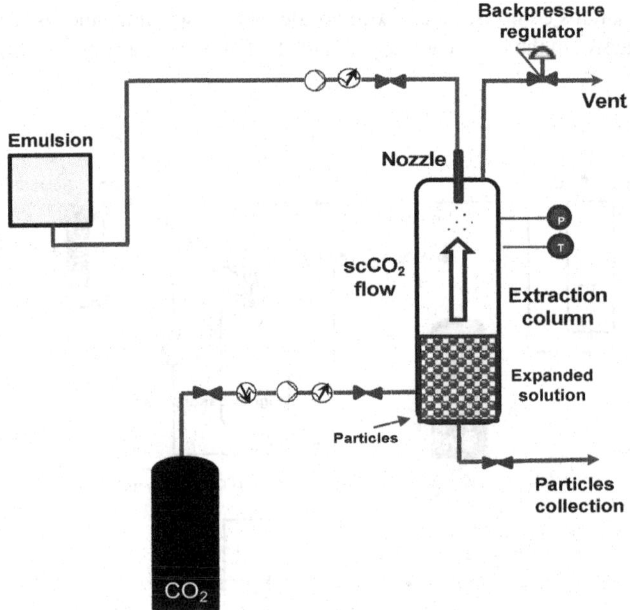

FIGURE 13.5 SFEEs simplified experimental apparatus.

the addition of a surfactant. Then, the organic solution is dispersed into an aqueous phase which passes throughout a high-pressure homogenizer. The steady emulsion is pumped, pre-heated, and then introduced to the top of the extracting unit for the organic solvent removal. The operating pressure and temperature conditions are chosen in order to minimize lipid and drug losses by venting through the CO_2 stream. The aqueous lipid nanosuspensions are collected continuously through the bottom of the extraction unit. The partial CO_2 dissolution in the organic phase of the emulsion causes its expansion while acting as anti-solvent leading to the precipitation of the lipid nanoparticle formation. CO_2 is highly efficient in removing impurities with low molecular weight leading to highly pure solid lipid nanoparticle (SLN) suspensions. The size and the drug loading efficiency of the SLN were essentially dependent on the droplet size of the emulsion and the nature of the oil-in-water emulsion.

The aerosol platforms prepared via SFEE showed large reduction of crystallinity, but kept high drug loadings in stable conditions within the solid lipid nanoparticles. The aerosolization studies of the SLN suspensions as a fine mist using the AERx pulmonary delivery system demonstrated good aerodynamic properties as determined via Andersen cascade impactor measurements.

13.4.5 Combinational Supercritical CO_2 Techniques

The increasing number of poorly water-soluble drugs have driven researchers to develop combined supercritical methods to overcome the low bioavailability of poorly absorbed drugs. One example of this approach is the production of submicron-sized particles of essentially meta-stable indomethacin polymorphs using both SAS and RESAS processes (Tozuka et al. 2010). In this process, the liquid CO_2 is first pumped into a high-pressure vessel to mix with the drug solution at a certain pressure and controlled temperature, and then the multicomponent supercritical solution is co-sprayed, rapidly expanding via a co-axial orifice device into an aqueous media, instead of a gas phase, via a back-pressure regulator (Figure 13.6). This system enables the production of nanoparticles which are stabilized through sonication of the solution, but for the preparation of a powder, further freeze-drying is required. The $scCO_2$ processed powders presented enhanced drug dissolution profiles as a result of the reduced particle and consequent surface area together with the formation of more soluble drug polymorphs.

Another example of combinatorial approaches is the supercritical fluid drying of aqueous solution, following similar principles as described in SEDS (Tozuka et al. 2010). Herein, the $scCO_2$ is fed through a co-axial nozzle in order to atomize the solution into a high-pressure precipitator where extraction with $scCO_2$ at a given pressure and temperature condition is performed. Modifiers such as ethanol or acetone in the $scCO_2$ stream can be added to enhance water extraction and, hence, minimize the residual moisture of the dried powder (Bouchard et al. 2008). In addition, further stripping of the particles collected

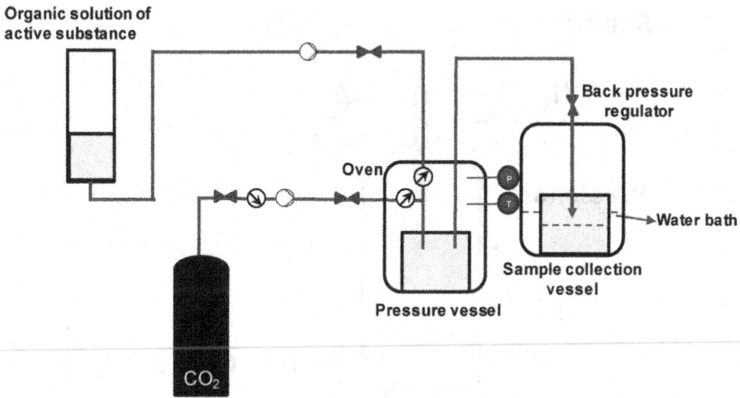

FIGURE 13.6 Simplified processing apparatus combining SAS and RESAS processes.

in the high-pressure precipitator with fresh $scCO_2$ can also be performed as a secondary drying step. This process has been applied for preparing protein and trehalose formulations with potentially inhalable particle size (Nuchuchua et al. 2014).

13.5 Micronization with $scCO_2$ as Co-solute

13.5.1 Supercritical Fluid-Assisted Atomization Methods

In 1991, Masters defined clearly that "Spray drying is the transformation of feed from a fluid state into a dried particulate form by spraying the feed into a hot drying medium" (Masters 1991). By analogy, the SAA methods also transform the feed from a fluid state into a dried particulate form by spraying the feed into a hot drying medium. Thus, SAA is indeed a spray drying process, this is the reason why SAA was later coined as SASD by Aguiar-Ricardo and co-workers (Aguiar-Ricardo 2017, Cabral et al. 2016).

SAA methods benefit of using $scCO_2$ as an atomization aid. CAN-BD was firstly introduced in 1997 for processing aqueous solutions (Sievers and Karst 1997), circumventing the challenge of processing hydrophilic compounds using CO_2. Herein, the aqueous solution and the near critical or $scCO_2$ are put in contact for a short period of time in a low-dead volume tee. The resulting emulsion is atomized into a very fine aerosol through a capillary flow restrictor into a precipitator at near ambient pressure, where a co-current stream of hot air or nitrogen leads to the evaporation of water and the precipitation of the solids, similar to conventional spray drying. The final particle properties can be controlled via the feed composition, temperature, and pressure as well as restrictor size. There are several examples on the application of CAN-BD for processing a diverse range of molecules with a particle size suitable for respiratory delivery (Cape et al. 2008).

Reverchon (2002) introduced the SAA in which the near-zero volume tee was replaced by a packed saturator to ensure close contact and solubilization of the CO_2 in the aqueous or organic solution at high pressure and temperature, hence, avoiding the large pressure drop in the tee observed via CAN-BD and sprayed through a thin injection nozzle into the precipitation and drying vessel. The micronized particles are captured in a stainless-steel filter at the bottom of the precipitator (Figure 13.7). In the saturator, a quasi-equilibrium $scCO_2$-expanded solution is formed, characterized by a lower viscosity and surface tension when compared with the solution at ambient conditions. The reduction in viscosity and surface tension enables a more efficient primary atomization at the nozzle tip, which together with the secondary atomization that occurs with the release of CO_2 leads to a very fine spray. SAA or SASD becomes a very effective micronization method, commonly considered as an improved method derived from CAN-BD and from PGSS (Costa et al. 2018). Several examples can be found in the literature on the processing of a diverse array of materials via SAA, ranging from polymers, protein, and pharmaceuticals with properties that can enable their delivery to the lungs. Similar to spray drying, typically the drying kinetics are faster than the recrystallization kinetics of crystalline solutes, leading to the formation of amorphous spherical

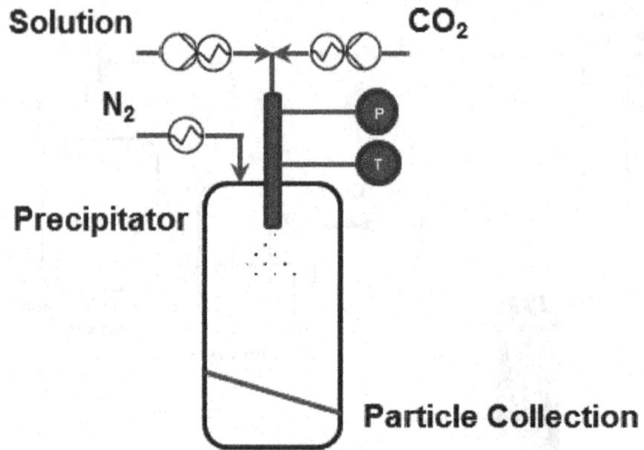

FIGURE 13.7 Supercritical CO_2-assisted atomization simplified experimental apparatus.

materials by SAA. However, beclomethasone dipropionate was successfully isolated as crystalline materials through rational manipulation of feed properties and process conditions (Reverchon et al. 2010).

As with other SCF techniques, knowledge on the vapor-liquid equilibria allows the design of the experimental conditions to ensure a fine control over the particle size and morphology of the final powders. Typically, input factors such as feed solution concentration, pre-expansion pressure, and temperature, as well as gas-to-liquid ratio can be used to control powder attributes. However, the interplay of complex phenomena, namely, the role of CO_2 as both a co-solute that enhances atomization and as an antisolvent that contributes to supersaturation inside the atomized droplets, together with the contribution of co-current gas in drying and particle formation, makes the process hard to model. Aguiar-Ricardo and co-workers have applied lean tools such as statistical modeling for the benefit of process optimization (Aguiar-Ricardo 2017, Cabral et al. 2016), as further detailed below.

13.5.2 Supercritical-Assisted Atomization/Supercritical CO_2-Assisted Spray Drying

SAA or SASD technology has been thoroughly explored as an efficient, versatile, potentially continuous, and scalable technique for the preparation of micro and nanoparticle formulations of a diverse range of molecules with properties suitable for pulmonary delivery, including thermolabile compounds (Adami et al. 2011, Della Porta et al. 2006, Hong et al. 2018, Reverchon 2002). Several research groups pursued an intense research in further optimizing this technique for more challenging target substances and for pulmonary delivery applications.

Zhu and co-workers introduced a hydrodynamic cavitation mixer to the standard SAA apparatus with the benefit of improving the mass transfer between the $scCO_2$ and the liquid solution and, hence, the atomization and applied it to the micronization of levofloxacin (Hong et al. 2018), lysozyme (as a model protein) (Du et al. 2011), and parathyroid hormone (Cai et al. 2008) for an inhalation application. This process enables small particle sizes with well-defined size distribution, while maintaining the activity and secondary structure for the biomolecules studied. In the particular case of parathyroid hormone (a polypeptide), chitosan oligosaccharides were used in the formulation to potentially maximize absorption while stabilizing the biomolecule through hydrogen bonding. The final composite formulations were successfully aerosolized using a capsule-based DPI (HandiHaler) and enabled appropriate fine particle fractions (FPF), as determined by cascade impaction.

Reverchon and co-workers also kept developing the SAA technique and in 2011 introduced a new configuration operated at reduced pressure to micronize thermo-labile target substances (Adami et al. 2011). In this apparatus, the precipitator is under a slight vacuum, which leads to the solvent boiling point depression and, hence, a reduced precipitation temperature. This configuration was successfully employed in the preparation of well-defined and spherical microparticles (with ~1 μm–4 μm) of biocompatible polymers with low glass transition temperature (T_g), such as polyL-lactide (Adami et al. 2011), polyethylene glycol (PEG) (Liparoti et al. 2012), and poly (D, L-lactide) (PDLLA) (Labuschagne et al. 2014) while avoiding polymer coalescence or aggregation as the precipitator temperature was below the polymers T_g. The process with PEG and PDLLA was employed for encapsulating a pesticide, rotenone, and an antibiotic for tuberculosis treatment, rifampicin (Martin et al. 2013). Bovine serum albumin (BSA) was also micronized through this configuration without any modification on the protein secondary structure (Adami et al. 2011).

The SASD technique was further optimized by Aguiar-Ricardo and co-workers via the introduction of a high efficiency cyclone and/or filter bag downstream of the precipitator and drying chamber, similarly to a conventional spray drying apparatus, that allows the continuous collection of the micronized powders throughout processing—Figure 13.8 (Cabral et al. 2016). Research conducted had a clear aim of engineering drug delivery systems that can accommodate a diverse range of active pharmaceutical ingredient for lung delivery, hence, expanding the range of applications for SASD. An initial work was performed on engineering chitosan microparticles, a biodegradable and mucoadhesive polymer, following a DoE approach in order to understand the impact of the several input process parameters in the microparticles properties and aerodynamic performance in a capsule-based DPI device (Cabral et al. 2016). This knowledge was applied to the formulation of chitosan microparticles loaded with oxazoline-grafted polyurea dendrimers (Restani et al. 2016) and with oxazoline-grafted

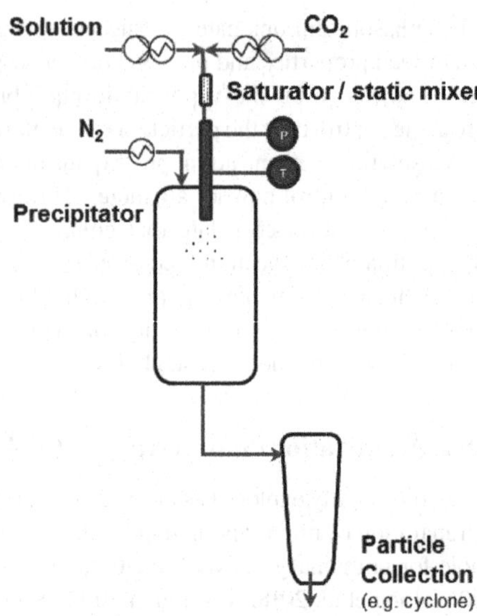

FIGURE 13.8 Supercritical CO_2-assisted spray drying simplified experimental apparatus.

gold-coated magnetite nanoparticles (Silva et al. 2017). In these examples, drug delivery was modulated via nano-in-micro formulation of ibuprofen in dendrimers and of magnetite nanoparticles inside chitosan microparticles towards minimizing its toxicity, maximizing stability while ensuring that it is suitable for lung delivery, with fine particle fractions up to 55% in capsule-based DPIs. Another study considered the micronization of a low T_g polymer, poly (D-L-lactide-co-glycolide) (PLGA), loaded with a model biomolecule, in which it was shown that the addition of L-leucine as a dispersibility enhancer can be added to improve PLGA performance, as reflected in an increased aerodynamic performance (up to 43% FPF) (Tavares et al. 2017). Temtem and co-workers (2017) also reported another study involving the optimization of the SASD process and its benchmarking with conventional spray drying for the manufacturing of trehalose and L-leucine composite particles for inhalation, an excipient matrix that can accommodate both small active ingredients and biomacromolecules. Well-defined composite particles with FPF as high as 86% under good process yields were successfully generated through manipulation of the input parameters, showing that SASD, like conventional spray drying, is a well behaved process in which the final product properties can be predicted based on local statistical models (Temtem et al. 2017).

Overall, the advances described above may lead to a wider use of SASD in the processing of pharmaceuticals and also underline the relative importance of SASD, amongst other supercritical fluid techniques, for engineering advanced composite particles particularly for pulmonary delivery.

13.5.3 Particles from Gas Saturated Solutions and Depressurization of an Expanded Liquid Organic Solution Techniques

Particles from Gas Saturated Solutions (PGSS) process takes advantage of the plasticizing effect of $scCO_2$ in several solids and was initially patented by Weidner et al. (2000). The target substance is melted and saturated with the dense CO_2 either in a high-pressure vessel for a batch process or in a static mixer for a continuous process and pumped through a high-pressure nozzle into a precipitator under ambient pressure, as shown in Figure 13.9. Mixing with CO_2 leads to a melting point depression

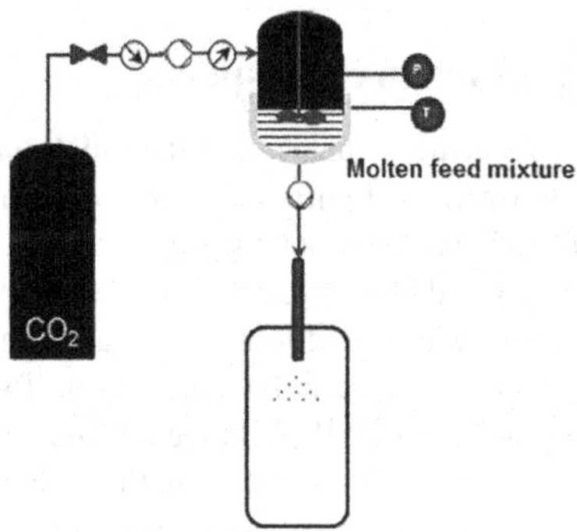

FIGURE 13.9 Precipitation from gas saturated solutions simplified experimental apparatus.

and viscosity reduction, enabling the micronization of the target substance at relatively mild conditions of temperature and pressure. At the nozzle and upon depressurization, the molten feed is atomized into droplets, which solidify into particles as a consequence of the gas expansion Joule-Thomson cooling effect. In the continuous configuration, the PGSS apparatus can also include a cyclone to collect the fine particles, whereas the main fraction is collected at the precipitator. Polyethylene glycol (PEG) was used as model to demonstrate that the particle size distribution, morphology, and density of the final powders can be fine-tuned via the feed composition, namely, ratio of $scCO_2$, to the target substance, feed temperature, and pre-expansion pressure (Lack et al. 2005). The design of the final powder can, hence, leverage from upfront knowledge solid-liquid-gas equilibrium between CO_2 and the target substance.

The particle sizes typically obtained through this technique are above the inhalable range (>20 μm in size). Furthermore, PGSS application is limited to polymers, fat, oils, and only a few pharmaceutical compounds, in which CO_2 is highly soluble. PGSS-drying process was developed to expand the applicability to processing aqueous solutions of polar compounds. In this process, an aqueous solution of the target substance and $scCO_2$ are simultaneously and continuously fed to a high-pressure static mixer, reaching a quasi-equilibrium (being different from SAA technique since the solution is saturated in CO_2). Upon atomization, a fine spray is formed due to the rapid gas expansion and water is extracted by the CO_2, leading to the formation of particles. The process can be designed taking into account the vapor-liquid equilibrium data of water and CO_2 to ensure successful drying. Given the relatively low solubility of CO_2 in water, high ratios of CO_2 to water are typically required, although may be significantly reduced by adding co-solvents, e.g. ethanol. This technique enables the micronization of powders to lower particles sizes than PGSS and additional levels of control in fine-tuning the particle properties (Martin et al. 2010). The main advantages of these techniques when compared with other techniques are their relative simplicity and scalability and have already been applied commercially.

Depressurization of an expanded liquid organic solution technique was introduced by Ventosa and co-workers (2001) and Ventosa et al. (2003). Herein, after the solubilization of a compressed gas such as CO_2 in an organic solution of the target substance, the solution is expanded into a precipitator at ambient pressure, leading to a sudden decrease in temperature as a consequence of the Joule-Thomson effect, followed by supersaturation and precipitation of the target substance. Similarly to anti-solvent techniques, it has been applied to crystallization, but unlike GAS, the temperature and pressure parameters are set so that the compressed CO_2 acts as a co-solvent to the organic solution of the target substance (Ventosa et al. 2003). There are only a few examples on the application of DELOS that are not particularly relevant for inhalation applications, given the low particle sizes.

13.6 Conclusion Remarks and Future Prospects

ScCO_2 technologies for particle engineering of pharmaceutical materials or drug delivery systems are very promising especially in the manufacture of pulmonary drug delivery systems, taking into consideration the tight requirements in terms of final aerosol properties.

The 2018 FDA draft guidance on Metered Dose Inhaler (MDI) and Dry Powder Inhaler (DPI) Products Quality Considerations refers to supercritical fluid technology as an alternative pharmaceutical engineering approach in micronizing drug substances and in ensuring uniform final formulations (FDA and CDER 2018). This is a clear acknowledgement of the relative advantages of supercritical fluid processes for inhalation applications and of all the research conducted in this field that led to clear understanding of the impact of the process and material inputs on the final product properties that enables the development of inhalation products through quality by design principles.

There are several studies, even beyond those that were mentioned beforehand, in which powders with properties suitable for respiratory delivery in terms of particle size, size distribution, and morphology were micronized. However, some of those studies have not assessed the resulting aerodynamic performance with an inhaler device, nor insights in terms of clinical superiority of these particulate formulations and, hence, the full potential of the technology remains to be realized.

13.6.1 Application of scCO_2 Techniques for the Preparation of Neat Drug Particles

The advent of scCO_2-based micronization techniques aimed at preparing crystalline active pharmaceutical ingredient (API), with high purity and a fine control over polymorphism and particle size distribution, amongst other properties, for satisfying the requirements of the pharmaceutical industry. Successful examples of the application of RESS and SEDS for the preparation of MDI and DPI formulations of RESS- and SEDS-engineered have been presented herein.

It should also be emphasized that with RESS, no organic solvent waste is generated, addressing major economic and environmental issues, since not only do organic solvents typically account for 80%–90% of the mass balance of a pharmaceutical batch operation (Constable et al. 2007), but their use is also under the scope of increasing regulatory restrictions (De Soete et al. 2017, Jessop et al. 2015).

13.6.2 Application of scCO_2 Techniques for the Preparation of Composite Drug Particles

The implementation of amorphous solid dispersions, as a solubilizing strategy for the increasing number of poorly water-soluble drugs in the industry pipeline and as a stabilizing approach for peptides and proteins, fostered the development of the scCO_2-assisted particle formation techniques. These techniques have expanded to advanced drug delivery systems, such as microencapsulation for controlled release or for optimizing aerodynamic performance in the case of inhalation applications or nanoparticles for maximizing drug uptake. The application of scCO_2 techniques such as SASD, that can successfully process a wide range of feedstocks and that allow a fine control over the particle properties, is particularly relevant for engineering particles for DPI in which there is a demand for more efficient and patient-focused formulations that are less susceptible to dose variability arising from inhalation flow and maneuver and device handling patient-to-patient differences. Formulation robustness can be introduced a priori via thoughtful particle design and understanding of the particle formation processes through environmentally "greener" approaches.

13.6.3 Scale-Up Issues

One major concern for the wide application of SCF techniques is their scalability. Considering the high potency of most molecules delivered to the lungs, most formulations comprise only a few micrograms of drug and, hence, scalability might not be an issue for the preparation of neat API particles. However, for composite systems in which the drug is engineered in an excipient matrix, concerns over the high-pressure footprint on a safety and economic standpoint, as well as over the process scalability, namely, in ensuring that the particle properties are maintained from early clinical phases to commercial stage, are relevant. In that perspective, processes such as SEDS, PGSS-drying, and SASD have the highest potential in terms of scalability for inhalation applications, considering that only a limited portion of the whole apparatus is high-pressure rated and leveraging from the fact that clinical and commercial products have been enabled by these techniques.

On the other hand, from all the SCF techniques, RESS is the one that is more fully understood. Additional mechanistical insight on the $scCO_2$ anti-solvent and co-solute techniques, including studies in terms of droplet and particle formation mechanisms, in correlation with the final outcome in terms of particle size, size distribution, density, and morphology would be key in ensuring a wider implementation of these technologies in the pharmaceutical industry.

REFERENCES

Adachi, Y., and B. C. Y. Lu. 1983. "Supercritical fluid extraction with carbon-dioxide and ethylene." *Fluid Phase Equilibria* 14:147–156. doi:10.1016/0378-3812(83)80120-4.

Adami, R., S. Liparoti, and E. Reverchon. 2011. "A new supercritical assisted atomization configuration, for the micronization of thermolabile compounds." *Chemical Engineering Journal* 173 (1):55–61. doi:10.1016/j.cej.2011.07.036.

Aguiar-Ricardo, A. 2017. "Building dry powder formulations using supercritical CO2 spray drying." *Current Opinion in Green and Sustainable Chemistry* 5:12–16. doi:10.1016/j.cogsc.2017.03.005.

Amani, A., H. Chrystyn, B. J. Clark, M. E. Abdelrahim, and P. York. 2009. "Evaluation of supercritical fluid engineered budesonide powder for respiratory delivery using nebulisers." *Journal of Pharmacy and Pharmacology* 61(12):1625–1630. doi:10.1211/jpp/61.12.0006.

Bartle, K. D., A. A. Clifford, S. A. Jafar, and G. F. Shilstone. 1991. "Solubilities of solids and liquids of low volatility in supercritical carbon-dioxide." *Journal of Physical and Chemical Reference Data* 20 (4):713–756. doi:10.1063/1.555893.

Beach, S., D. Latham, C. Sidgwick, M. Hanna, and P. York. 1999. "Control of the physical form of salmeterol xinafoate." *Organic Process Research & Development* 3 (5):370–376. doi:10.1021/op990160z.

Bouchard, A., N. Jovanovic, A. Martin, G. W. Hofland, D. J. A. Crommelin, W. Jiskoot, and G. J. Witkamp. 2008. "Effect of the modifier on the particle formation and crystallization behaviour during precipitation from aqueous solutions." *Journal of Supercritical Fluids* 44 (3):409–421. doi:10.1016/j.supflu.2007.09.015.

Brunner, G. 2004. *Supercritical Fluids as Solvents and Reaction Media*. Amstredam, the Netherlands: Elsevier.

Cabral, R. P., A. M. L. Sousa, A. S. Silva, A. I. Paninho, M. Temtem, E. Costa, T. Casimiro, and A. Aguiar-Ricardo. 2016. "Design of experiments approach on the preparation of dry inhaler chitosan composite formulations by supercritical CO2-assisted spray-drying." *Journal of Supercritical Fluids* 116:26–35. doi:10.1016/j.supflu.2016.04.001.

Cai, M. Q., Y. X. Guan, S. J. Yao, and Z. Q. Zhu. 2008. "Supercritical fluid assisted atomization introduced by hydrodynamic cavitation mixer (SAA-HCM) for micronization of levofloxacin hydrochloride." *Journal of Supercritical Fluids* 43 (3):524–534. doi:10.1016/j.supflu.2007.07.008.

Cape, S. P., J. A. Villa, E. T. S. Huang, T. H. Yang, J. F. Carpenter, and R. E. Sievers. 2008. "Preparation of active proteins, vaccines and pharmaceuticals as fine powders using supercritical or near-critical fluids." *Pharmaceutical Research* 25 (9):1967–1990. doi:10.1007/s11095-008-9575-6.

Ch, R., and G. Madras. 2010. "An association model for the solubilities of pharmaceuticals in supercritical carbon dioxide." *Thermochimica Acta* 507–508:99–105. doi:10.1016/j.tca.2010.05.006.

Charpentier, P. A., M. Jia, and R. A. Lucky. 2008. "Study of the RESS process for producing beclomethasone-17,21-dipropionate particles suitable for pulmonary delivery." *Aaps Pharmscitech* 9 (1):39–46. doi:10.1208/s12249-007-9004-x.

Chattopadhyay, P., B. Y. Shekunov, D. Yim, D. Cipolla, B. Boyd, and S. Farr. 2007. "Production of solid lipid nanoparticle suspensions using supercritical fluid extraction of emulsions (SFEE) for pulmonary delivery using the AERx system." *Advanced Drug Delivery Reviews* 59 (6):444–453. doi:10.1016/j.addr.2007.04.010.

Chrastil, J. 1982. "Solubility of solids and liquids in supercritical gases." *Journal of Physical Chemistry* 86 (15):3016–3021. doi:10.1021/j100212a041.

Cipolla, D. C., and I. Gonda. 2011. "Formulation technology to repurpose drugs for inhalation delivery." *Drug Discovery Today: Therapeutic Strategies* 8 (3):123–130. doi:10.1016/j.ddstr.2011.07.001.

Constable, D. J. C., C. Jimenez-Gonzalez, and R. K. Henderson. 2007. "Perspective on solvent use in the pharmaceutical industry." *Organic Process Research & Development* 11 (1):133–137. doi:10.1021/op060170h.

Costa, C., T. Casimiro, and A. Aguiar-Ricardo. 2018. "Optimization of supercritical CO2-assisted atomization: Phase behavior and design of experiments." *Journal of Chemical and Engineering Data* 63 (4):885–896. doi:10.1021/acs.jced.7b00820.

da Silva, M. S., F. L. Nobrega, A. Aguiar-Ricardo, E. J. Cabrita, and T. Casimiro. 2011a. "Development of molecularly imprinted co-polymeric devices for controlled delivery of flufenamic acid using supercritical fluid technology." *Journal of Supercritical Fluids* 58 (1):150–157. doi:10.1016/j.supflu.2011.05.010.

da Silva, M. S., R. Viveiros, P. I. Morgado, A. Aguiar-Ricardo, I. J. Correia, and T. Casimiro. 2011b. "Development of 2-(dimethylamino)ethyl methacrylate-based molecular recognition devices for controlled drug delivery using supercritical fluid technology." *International Journal of Pharmaceutics* 416 (1):61–68. doi:10.1016/j.ijpharm.2011.06.004.

De Soete, W., C. Jimenez-Gonzalez, P. Dahlin, and J. Dewulf. 2017. "Challenges and recommendations for environmental sustainability assessments of pharmaceutical products in the healthcare sector." *Green Chemistry* 19 (15):3493–3509. doi:10.1039/c7gc00833c.

Debenedetti, P. G. 1990. "Homogeneous nucleation in supercritical fluids." *AIChE Journal* 36 (9):1289–1298. doi:10.1002/aic.690360902.

Debenedetti, P. G., J. W. Tom, X. Kwauk, and S. D. Yeo. 1993. "Rapid expansion of supercritical solutions (RESS)—Fundamentals and applications." *Fluid Phase Equilibria* 82:311–321. doi:10.1016/0378-3812(93)87155-t.

Della Porta, G., S. F. Ercolino, L. Parente, and E. Reverchon. 2006. "Corticosteroid microparticles produced by supercritical-assisted atomization: Process optimization, product characterization, and "in vitro" performance." *Journal of Pharmaceutical Sciences* 95 (9):2062–2076. doi:10.1002/jps.20703.

Depreter, F., G. Pilcer, and K. Amighi. 2013. "Inhaled proteins: Challenges and perspectives." *International Journal of Pharmaceutics* 447 (1–2):251–280. doi:10.1016/j.ijpharm.2013.02.031.

Du, Z., Y. X. Guan, S. J. Yao, and Z. Q. Zhu. 2011. "Supercritical fluid assisted atomization introduced by an enhanced mixer for micronization of lysozyme: Particle morphology, size and protein stability." *International Journal of Pharmaceutics* 421 (2):258–268. doi:10.1016/j.ijpharm.2011.10.002.

FDA, and CDER. 2018. Metered Dose Inhaler (MDI) and Dry Powder Inhaler (DPI) Products–Quality Considerations: Guidance for industry. USA: U.S. Department of Health and Human Services; Food and Drug Administration; Center for Drug Evaluation and Research.

Gallagher, P. M., M. P. Coffey, V. J. Krukonis, and N. Klasutis. 1989. "Gas antisolvent recrystallization: New process to recrystallize compounds insoluble in supercritical fluids." In *Supercritical Fluid Science and Technology*, edited by K. P. Johnston and J. M. L. Penninger, pp. 334–354. Washington, DC: American Chemical Society.

Garcia-Gonzalez, C. A., M. Jin, J. Gerth, C. Alvarez-Lorenzo, and I. Smirnova. 2015. "Polysaccharide-based aerogel microspheres for oral drug delivery." *Carbohydrate Polymers* 117:797–806. doi:10.1016/j.carbpol.2014.10.045.

Gonzalez, J. C., M. R. Vieytes, A. M. Botana, J. M. Vieites, and L. M. Botana. 2001. "Modified mass action law-based model to correlate the solubility of solids and liquids in entrained supercritical carbon dioxide." *Journal of Chromatography A* 910 (1):119–125. doi:10.1016/s0021-9673(00)01120-1.

Gross, J. 2005. "An equation-of-state contribution for polar components: Quadrupolar molecules." *AIChE Journal* 51 (9):2556–2568. doi:10.1002/aic.10502.

Hanna, M., and P. York. 1995. Method and apparatus for the formation of particles. WO Patent 95/01221, filed June 30, 1994, and issued January 12, 1995.

Hannay, J. B., and J. Hogarth. 1879. "Solubility of solids in gases" *Proceedings of the Royal Society of London* 29:324–326.

Helfgen, B., M. Turk, and K. Schaber. 2003. "Hydrodynamic and aerosol modelling of the rapid expansion of supercritical solutions (RESS-process)." *Journal of Supercritical Fluids* 26 (3):225–242. doi:10.1016/s0896-8446(02)00159-6.

Hong, D. X., Y. L. Yun, Y. X. Guan, and S. J. Yao. 2018. "Preparation of micrometric powders of parathyroid hormone (PTH1-34)-loaded chitosan oligosaccharide by supercritical fluid assisted atomization." *International Journal of Pharmaceutics* 545 (1–2):389–394. doi:10.1016/j.ijpharm.2018.05.022.

Huang, C. C., M. O. Tang, W. H. Tao, and Y. P. Chen. 2001. "Calculation of the solid solubilities in supercritical carbon dioxide using a modified mixing model." *Fluid Phase Equilibria* 179 (1–2):67–84. doi:10.1016/s0378-3812(00)00483-0.

Jessop, P. G., F. Ahmadpour, M. A. Buczynski, T. J. Burns, N. B. Green, R. Korwin, D. Long et al. 2015. "Opportunities for greener alternatives in chemical formulations." *Green Chemistry* 17 (5):2664–2678. doi:10.1039/c4gc02261k.

Jung, J., and M. Perrut. 2001. "Particle design using supercritical fluids: Literature and patent survey." *Journal of Supercritical Fluids* 20 (3):179–219. doi:10.1016/s0896-8446(01)00064-x.

Kim, Y. H., and K. S. Shing. 2008. "Supercritical fluid-micronized ipratropium bromide for pulmonary drug delivery." *Powder Technology* 182 (1):25–32. doi:10.1016/j.powtec.2007.04.009.

Kumar, S. K., and K. P. Johnston. 1988. "Modelling the solubility of solids in supercritical fluids with density as the independent variable." *Journal of Supercritical Fluids* 1 (1):15–22. doi:10.1016/0896-8446(88)90005-8.

Labuschagne, P. W., R. Adami, S. Liparoti, S. Naidoo, H. Swai, and E. Reverchon. 2014. "Preparation of rifampicin/poly(D, L-lactice) nanoparticles for sustained release by supercritical assisted atomization technique." *Journal of Supercritical Fluids* 95:106–117. doi:10.1016/j.supflu.2014.08.004.

Lack, E., E. Weidner, Z. Knez, S. Gruner, B. Weinreich, and H. Seidlitz. 2005. "Particle generation with supercritical CO_2." *Proceedings of the Vienna International Conference on Micro- and Nano-Technology* 1:141–147.

Liparoti, S., R. Adami, and E. Reverchon. 2012. "PEG micronization by supercritical assisted atomization, operated under reduced pressure." *Journal of Supercritical Fluids* 72:46–51. doi:10.1016/j.supflu.2012.08.009.

Liu, J. W., G. Amberg, and M. Do-Quang. 2014. "Numerical simulation of particle formation in the rapid expansion of supercritical solution process." *Journal of Supercritical Fluids* 95:572–587. doi:10.1016/j.supflu.2014.08.033.

Martin, A., and M. J. Cocero. 2008. "Micronization processes with supercritical fluids: Fundamentals and mechanisms." *Advanced Drug Delivery Reviews* 60 (3):339–350. doi:10.1016/j.addr.2007.06.019.

Martin, A., M. P. Huu, A. Kilzer, S. Kareth, and E. Weidner. 2010. "Micronization of polyethylene glycol by PGSS (Particles from Gas Saturated Solutions)-drying of aqueous solutions." *Chemical Engineering and Processing* 49 (12):1259–1266. doi:10.1016/j.cep.2010.09.014.

Martin, L., S. Liparoti, G. Della Porta, R. Adami, J. L. Marques, J. S. Urieta, A. M. Mainar, and E. Reverchon. 2013. "Rotenone coprecipitation with biodegradable polymers by supercritical assisted atomization." *Journal of Supercritical Fluids* 81:48–54. doi:10.1016/j.supflu.2013.03.032.

Masters, K. 1991. "Applications in the food industry." In *Spray Drying Handbook*, edited by K. Masters, pp. 587–638. New York: Longman Scientific & Technical.

Matson, D. W., J. L. Fulton, R. C. Petersen, and R. D. Smith. 1987. "Rapid expansion of supercritical fluid solutions: Solute formation of powders, thin-films, and fibers." *Industrial & Engineering Chemistry Research* 26 (11):2298–2306. doi:10.1021/ie00071a021.

Mawson, S., K. P. Johnston, J. R. Combes, and J. M. Desimone. 1995. "Formation of poly(1,1,2,2-tetrahydroperfluorodecyl acrylate) submicron fibers and particles from supercritical carbon-dioxide solutions." *Macromolecules* 28 (9):3182–3191. doi:10.1021/ma00113a021.

Mendez-Santiago, J., and A. S. Teja. 1999. "The solubility of solids in supercritical fluids." *Fluid Phase Equilibria* 158:501–510. doi:10.1016/s0378-3812(99)00154-5.

Mishima, K., K. Matsuyama, and M. Nagatani. 1999. "Solubilities of poly(ethylene glycol)s in the mixtures of supercritical carbon dioxide and cosolvent." *Fluid Phase Equilibria* 161 (2):315–324. doi:10.1016/s0378-3812(99)00211-3.

Miura, H., M. Kanebako, H. Shirai, H. Nakao, T. Inagi, and K. Terada. 2010. "Enhancement of dissolution rate and oral absorption of a poorly water-soluble drug, K-832, by adsorption onto porous silica using supercritical carbon dioxide." *European Journal of Pharmaceutics and Biopharmaceutics* 76 (2):215–221. doi:10.1016/j.ejpb.2010.06.016.

Nuchuchua, O., H. A. Every, G. W. Hofland, and W. Jiskoot. 2014. "Scalable organic solvent free supercritical fluid spray drying process for producing dry protein formulations." *European Journal of Pharmaceutics and Biopharmaceutics* 88 (3):919–930. doi:10.1016/j.ejpb.2014.09.004.

Palakodaty, S., and P. York. 1999. "Phase behavioral effects on particle formation processes using supercritical fluids." *Pharmaceutical Research* 16 (7):976–985. doi:10.1023/a:1011957512347.

Pathak, P., M. J. Meziani, T. Desai, and Y. P. Sun. 2004. "Nanosizing drug particles in supercritical fluid processing." *Journal of the American Chemical Society* 126 (35):10842–10843. doi:10.1021/ja046914t.

Pilcer, G., and K. Amighi. 2010. "Formulation strategy and use of excipients in pulmonary drug delivery." *International Journal of Pharmaceutics* 392 (1–2):1–19. doi:10.1016/j.ijpharm.2010.03.017.

Reddy, S. N., and G. Madras. 2011. "A new semi-empirical model for correlating the solubilities of solids in supercritical carbon dioxide with cosolvents." *Fluid Phase Equilibria* 310 (1–2):207–212. doi:10.1016/j.fluid.2011.08.021.

Reddy, S. N., and G. Madras. 2012. "Modeling of ternary solubilities of solids in supercritical carbon dioxide in the presence of cosolvents or cosolutes." *Journal of Supercritical Fluids* 63:105–114. doi:10.1016/j.supflu.2011.11.016.

Restani, R. B., A. S. Silva, R. F. Pires, R. Cabral, I. J. Correia, T. Casimiro, V. D. B. Bonifacio, and A. Aguiar-Ricardo. 2016. "Nano-in-micro poxylated polyurea dendrimers and chitosan dry powder formulations for pulmonary delivery." *Particle & Particle Systems Characterization* 33 (11):851–858. doi:10.1002/ppsc.201600123.

Reverchon, E. 1999. "Supercritical antisolvent precipitation of micro- and nano-particles." *Journal of Supercritical Fluids* 15 (1):1–21. doi:10.1016/s0896-8446(98)00129-6.

Reverchon, E. 2002. "Supercritical-assisted atomization to produce micro- and/or nanoparticles of controlled size and distribution." *Industrial & Engineering Chemistry Research* 41 (10):2405–2411. doi:10.1021/ie010943k.

Reverchon, E., R. Adami, M. Scognamiglio, G. Fortunato, and G. Della Porta. 2010. "Beclomethasone microparticles for wet inhalation, produced by supercritical assisted atomization." *Industrial & Engineering Chemistry Research* 49 (24):12747–12755. doi:10.1021/ie101574z.

Sauceau, M., J. J. Letourneau, D. Richon, and J. Fages. 2003. "Enhanced density-based models for solid compound solubilities in supercritical carbon dioxide with cosolvents." *Fluid Phase Equilibria* 208 (1–2):99–113. doi:10.1016/s0378-3812(03)00005-0.

Schuster, J., R. Rubsamen, P. Lloyd, and J. Lloyd. 1997. "The AERX™ aerosol delivery system." *Pharmaceutical Research* 14 (3):354–357. doi:10.1023/a:1012058323754.

Shariati, A., and C. J. Peters. 2003. "Recent developments in particle design using supercritical fluids." *Current Opinion in Solid State & Materials Science* 7 (4–5):371–383. doi:10.1016/j.cossms.2003.12.001.

Shoyele, S. A., and S. Cawthome. 2006. "Particle engineering techniques for inhaled biopharmaceuticals." *Advanced Drug Delivery Reviews* 58 (9–10):1009–1029. doi:10.1016/j.addr.2006.07.010.

Si-Moussa, C., A. Belghait, L. Khaouane, S. Hanini, and A. Halilali. 2017. "Novel density-based model for the correlation of solid drugs solubility in supercritical carbon dioxide." *Comptes Rendus Chimie* 20 (5):559–572. doi:10.1016/j.crci.2016.09.009.

Sievers, R. E., and U. Karst. 1997. Methods for fine particle formation. US Patent 5,639,441, filled April 8, 1994, and issued June 17, 1997: Board of Regents of University of Colorado, Boulder, CO.

Silva, M. C., A. S. Silva, J. Fernandez-Lodeiro, T. Casimiro, C. Lodeiro, and A. Aguiar-Ricardo. 2017. "Supercritical CO2-assisted spray drying of strawberry-like gold-coated magnetite nanocomposites in chitosan powders for inhalation." *Materials* 10 (1):74. doi:10.3390/ma10010074.

Sovova, H. 2001. "Solubility of ferulic acid in supercritical carbon dioxide with ethanol as cosolvent." *Journal of Chemical and Engineering Data* 46 (5):1255–1257. doi:10.1021/je0101146.

Sparks, D. L., R. Hernandez, and L. A. Estevez. 2008. "Evaluation of density-based models for the solubility of solids in supercritical carbon dioxide and formulation of a new model." *Chemical Engineering Science* 63 (17):4292–4301. doi:10.1016/j.ces.2008.05.031.

Spyriouni, T., X. Krokidis, and I. G. Economou. 2011. "Thermodynamics of pharmaceuticals: Prediction of solubility in pure and mixed solvents with PC-SAFT." *Fluid Phase Equilibria* 302 (1–2):331–337. doi:10.1016/j.fluid.2010.08.029.

Steckel, H., J. Thies, and B. W. Muller. 1997. "Micronizing of steroids for pulmonary delivery by supercritical carbon dioxide." *International Journal of Pharmaceutics* 152 (1):99–110. doi:10.1016/s0378-5173(97)00071-9.

Tabernero, A., S. V. de Melo, R. Mammucari, E. M. M. del Valle, and N. R. Foster. 2014. "Modelling solubility of solid active principle ingredients in sc-CO2 with and without cosolvents: A comparative assessment of semiempirical models based on Chrastil's equation and its modifications." *Journal of Supercritical Fluids* 93:91–102. doi:10.1016/j.supflu.2013.11.017.

Tabernero, A., E. M. M. del Valle, and M. Á. Galán. 2010. "A comparison between semiempirical equations to predict the solubility of pharmaceutical compounds in supercritical carbon dioxide." *Journal of Supercritical Fluids* 52 (2):161–174. doi:10.1016/j.supflu.2010.01.009.

Tang, Z., J. S. Jin, Z. T. Zhang, X. Y. Yu, and J. N. Xu. 2010. "Solubility of 3,5-dinitrobenzoic acid in supercritical carbon dioxide with cosolvent at temperatures from (308 to 328) K and pressures from (10.0 to 21.0) MPa." *Journal of Chemical and Engineering Data* 55 (9):3834–3841. doi:10.1021/je100331h.

Tavares, M., R. P. Cabral, C. Costa, P. Martins, A. R. Fernandes, T. Casimiro, and A. Aguiar-Ricardo. 2017. "Development of PLGA dry powder microparticles by supercritical CO2-assisted spray-drying for potential vaccine delivery to the lungs." *Journal of Supercritical Fluids* 128:235–243. doi:10.1016/j.supflu.2017.06.004.

Temtem, M., C. Moura, T. Casimiro, E. Costa, and A. Aguiar-Ricardo. 2017. "Benchmarking supercritical CO2-assisted spray drying with conventional spray drying for the manufacture of inhalation formulations." *Respiratory Drug Delivery* 1:153–166.

Tong, H. H. Y., B. Y. Shekunov, P. York, and A. H. L. Chow. 2001. "Characterization of two polymorphs of salmeterol xinafoate crystallized from supercritical fluids." *Pharmaceutical Research* 18 (6):852–858. doi:10.1023/a:1011000915769.

Tozuka, Y., Y. Miyazaki, and H. Takeuchi. 2010. "A combinational supercritical CO2 system for nanoparticle preparation of indomethacin." *International Journal of Pharmaceutics* 386 (1–2):243–248. doi:10.1016/j.ijpharm.2009.10.044.

Türk, M. 2014. *Particle Formation with Supercritical Fluids: Challenges and Limitations*. Amsterdam, the Netherlands: Elsevier.

Valle, J. M. del, and J. M. Aguilera. 1988. "An improved equation for predicting the solubility of vegetable-oils in supercritical CO2." *Industrial & Engineering Chemistry Research* 27 (8):1551–1553. doi:10.1021/ie00080a036.

van der Waals, J. D. 1873. "On the continuity of the gaseous and liquid states." PhD, Physics, University of Leiden, Leiden, the Netherlands.

Ventosa, N., S. Sala, and J. Veciana. 2003. "DELOS process: A crystallization technique using compressed fluids: 1. Comparison to the GAS crystallization method." *Journal of Supercritical Fluids* 26 (1):33–45. doi:10.1016/s0896-8446(02)00189-4.

Ventosa, N., S. Sala, J. Veciana, J. Torres, and J. Llibre. 2001. "Depressurization of an expanded liquid organic solution (DELOS): A new procedure for obtaining submicron- or micron-sized crystalline particles." *Crystal Growth & Design* 1 (4):299–303. doi:10.1021/cg0155090.

Weers, J. G., and D. P. Miller. 2015. "Formulation design of dry powders for inhalation." *Journal of Pharmaceutical Sciences* 104 (10):3259–3288. doi:10.1002/jps.24574.

Weidner, E., Z. Knez, and Z. Novak. 2000. Process for the production of particles or powders. US Patent 6,056,791, filed November 7, 1997, and issued May 2, 2000.

Yazdizadeh, M., A. Eslamimanesh, and F. Esmaeilzadeh. 2011. "Thermodynamic modeling of solubilities of various solid compounds in supercritical carbon dioxide: Effects of equations of state and mixing rules." *Journal of Supercritical Fluids* 55 (3):861–875. doi:10.1016/j.supflu.2010.10.019.

14

Particle Engineering Technology for Inhaled Therapies

David Lechuga-Ballesteros, Susan Hoe, and Benjamin W. Maynor

CONTENTS

14.1 Introduction

Examples of engineered particles for pulmonary delivery are shown in Figure 14.1. All particles shown display a mass median aerodynamic diameter (MMAD) of less than five micrometers and can be efficiently delivered to the lung using a passive dry powder inhaler (driven by patient inhalation), with aerosol performance being largely independent of the flow rate within a clinically relevant range. These engineered particles also represent examples of the new generation of dry powder inhalers that do not require the use of large lactose crystals as "carriers" to aid in flowability and dispersion.

Engineered particles shown in Figure 14.1 are manufactured via spray drying and have been successfully scaled up to support phase 3 clinical trials or commercial manufacturing. The composition of the engineered particles shown in Figure 14.1 is representative of classes of excipients that have been successfully used to manufacture non-cohesive, dispersible particles which are also able to efficiently perform in high relative humidity environments (Li et al. 2016), which are a subsection of all excipients used in inhalation formulations outlined in Table 14.1.

Phospholipids such as dipalmitoyl phosphatidylcholine (DPPC) and distearoyl phosphatidylcholine (DSPC), amino acids such as iso-leucine and leucine, oligopeptides such as di-leucine and tri-leucine, as well as fumaryl diketopiperazine (FDKP) on a class on its own, can be defined as "functional excipients" used to engineer particles with low particle density and low surface energy, both properties that can be desirable for a successful dry powder aerosol. Other useful excipients that are used as bulking agents and stabilizer for proteins or peptides are sugars like trehalose, sucrose, and raffinose, sugar alcohols such as mannitol, and buffers such as sodium citrate.

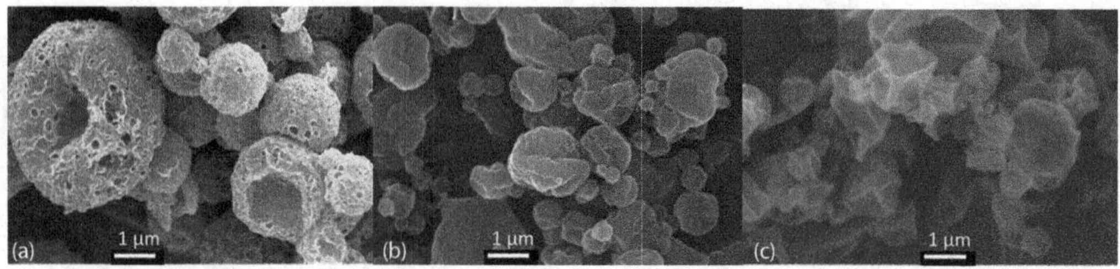

FIGURE 14.1 (a) Spray drying from an emulsion of water, PFOB, DSPC, and $CaCl_2$; (b) spray dried leucine particle; and (c) spray dried trileucine particle.

TABLE 14.1

List of Known Excipients Used in the Formulation of Inhaled Products. Where Blank, the Excipient is Strictly Used as an Additive with No Further Processing

Excipient	Use in Formulation	Formulation Technique
Approved		
DPPC	Surfactant	Aqueous dispersion
DSPC	Microcarrier	Spray drying
DSPC	Dispersibility bulking agent	Spray drying
FDKP	Carrier	Lyophilization
Mannitol	Osmolality	Spray drying
Lactose	Carrier	Micronization/blending
Buffer salts (e.g. citrate, sulfate)	Buffer, glass stabilizer	Spray drying
Polyvinyl pyrrolidone (PVP) K12	Suspension stabilizer	
Polyethylene glycol (PEG) 1000	Lubricant	
Magnesium stearate	Lubricant	
Glycerol	Particle size modification	
Ethanol	Co-solvent	
Disodium cromoglycate	Dessicant	
In clinical development		
Leucine	Dispersibility	Spray drying
Trileucine	Dispersibility	Spray drying
Trehalose	Glass stabilizer, bulking agent	Spray drying
Fumaryl diketopiperazine (FDKP)	Carrier	Spray drying
Liposomal components (e.g. PEGylated lipids, conjugated lipids)	Controlled-release agent	Liposome
Dipalmitoylphosphatidylcholine (DPPC)	Dispersibility, bulking agent	Liposome
Literature only		
PLA, PLGA	Controlled-release agent	Spray drying
Polysaccharides (inulin, hydroxyether starch, other starches)	Dispersibility, bulking agent	Spray drying
Cyclodextrins	Dispersibility, bulking agent	Spray drying

For engineered particles made via spray drying, the particle formation process is greatly dependent on excipient physicochemical properties. In the case of phospholipid-based particles, because of their aqueous insolubility, phospholipids require use of an ethanolic solution (Vanbever et al. 1999) or an emulsion-based feedstock (Ivey and Vehring 2010). Water-soluble excipients like leucine and trileucine can be spray dried from an aqueous-based feedstock (Lechuga-Ballesteros et al. 2008). Selection of sugar, sugar alcohols, and buffers is also driven by the feedstock composition and liquid state (i.e. solution, emulsion, suspension). The particle formation for the FDKP particles depends on FDKP solubility as a function of pH. In the case of sugars, spray drying and other drying techniques, including molding promote the formation of the amorphous solid state which is advantageous to stabilize biotherapeutics. In the following sections, we highlight relevant properties of excipients commonly used to engineer particles for inhalation.

14.2 Sugars, Polyols, and Plasticizers for Glass Stabilization

The active molecular structure of a biotherapeutic is fully hydrated. Biostabilization during dehydration is dependent on the replacement of water hydrogen bonding with hydrogen bonding between biotherapeutic and excipient, thus molecules able to hydrogen bond with an elevated glass transition temperature are preferred. Glass transition increases with molecular weight, hence, sucrose (dry T_g ~ 73°C) is preferred to fructose or glucose (T_g ~ 38°C), for instance (Weers et al. 2007). However, higher molecular weight molecules with the ability to hydrogen bond are not very effective stabilizers as they form amorphous solids with a larger fraction of free volume that allows for local molecular mobility. Low molecular weight polyols, referred to as "plasticizers" because their addition decreases the glass transition of the formulated amorphous solid, are often used as they have been shown to reduce molecular mobility.

The term *glass state stabilization* refers to the use of an inert substance such as sugar molecules (e.g. glucose, fructose, sucrose, trehalose, raffinose, etc.) or polyols (e.g. mannitol or sorbitol) that are rich in hydroxyl groups (R-OH), which effectively replace the hydrogen bonds that water forms with the protein in solution as it is removed during the drying process. Sugars have a water-like ability to hydrogen bond and can replace water-protein interactions. Disaccharides such as trehalose (dry T_g ~ 117°C), raffinose (T_g ~ 113°C), and sucrose (dry T_g ~ 73°C) are preferred due to their high glass transition when dried into an amorphous solid.

In addition to forming hydrogen bonds with the protein, sugars dry into amorphous solids, also referred to as *supercooled liquid* or *glass*, some with a sufficiently high glass transition temperature to decrease molecular mobility enough to provide room temperature stability. Protection of labile biological products during desiccation is achieved by the presence of sugar molecules. Preservation is achieved through specific interactions via hydrogen bonding and immobilization of the protein in a highly viscous liquid. Free volume between protein molecules can be minimized by addition of small molecule plasticizers that hydrogen bond to the sugar glass network to improve stability by further reducing non-translational molecular mobility (Cicerone and Soles 2004).

Commonly used excipients to form stable organic glasses are lactose, sucrose, raffinose, trehalose, and sodium citrate. Glass stabilization technology was successfully used to engineer spray dried inhalable insulin (Exubera® by Pfizer) using citrate, mannitol, and glycine, providing a superior long-term stability compared to insulin in solution (Sadrzadeh et al. 2010). Glycine acts as a buffer for the protein during manufacturing, mannitol is used as the plasticizer, and sodium citrate both provides the ionic strength required to dissolve insulin in the spray dryer feedstock and acts as a glass former (high glass transition). In addition to its superior solid-state stability, spray dried insulin powders displayed excellent aerosol properties in both dry and wet environments. Spray dried amorphous sugars tend to render cohesive powders with poor aerosol performance. However, in the case of Exubera®, insulin is surface active and possesses a high glass transition; as a result, during particle formation, it enriches the droplet surface and dominates the particle surface properties, negating the need for additional excipients to decrease cohesion. This is not always the case, as some peptides, such as spray dried salmon calcitonin, present poor aerosol performance and addition of excipients to modify surface properties to decrease cohesion is often needed (Chan et al. 2004).

14.3 Hydrophobic Amino Acids and Oligopeptides

Hydrophobic amino acids, such as leucine and iso-leucine, as well as hydrophobic oligopeptides such as di- and tri-leucine, have been successfully used as functional excipients in spray drying, (Yamashita et al. 1998, Lechuga-Ballesteros et al. 2008) and leucine has been used in PRINT® technology particles

(Garcia et al. 2012). These excipients share physicochemical properties such as low aqueous solubility and surface activity which define particle density and surface energy, respectively (Vehring 2007, Lechuga-Ballesteros et al. 2008).

For non-surface active, water-soluble molecules, engineering a spray dried particle with acceptable aerosol performance requires control of particle cohesion. Powder cohesiveness is inversely correlated to both: (a) particle rugosity, which controls interparticle contact; and (b) surface energy, which reduces overall particle cohesivity (Lechuga-Ballesteros et al. 2008). Like sugars, water-soluble small molecule drugs form cohesive powders with poor aerosol performance when spray dried (Lechuga-Ballesteros et al. 2008). The use of surface-active excipients can achieve a wrinkled particle morphology (particle rugosity) and decreased surface energy (Lechuga-Ballesteros et al. 2008). In addition, adequate *in vitro* aerosol performance must be achieved under humid conditions to ensure proper dosing in realistic environmental scenarios (Yamashita et al. 1998, Li et al. 2016).

Spray dried powders for inhalation formulated with isoleucine (Yamashita et al. 1998), leucine (Vehring 2007, Kuo et al. 2014, Li et al. 2016), and trileucine (Lechuga-Ballesteros et al. 2008) display excellent aerosol performance and physical stability. Improvement in the aerosol properties of water-soluble molecules (>20 mg/mL) such as antibiotics or cromolyn has been demonstrated with the use of trileucine (Lechuga-Ballesteros et al. 2008).

Both leucine and trileucine have been shown to increase the emitted dose (ED) of small hydrophilic molecules. For example, the ED of nano-spray dried powder containing gentamicin improved from 35% to more than 75% and the Fine Particle Mass (FPM) < 3.3 μm increased from 28% to 48% upon the addition of as little as 2% wt. trileucine. Addition of 25% Percentage Mass fraction (% w/w) trileucine to gentamicin produced a nano-spray dried powder with an ED > 90% (Kuo and Lechuga-Ballesteros 2013). In a study involving co-spray dried trileucine and netilmicin, an improvement in dispersibility correlated with increased trileucine surface concentration, decrease in surface energy, and with corrugated morphology, which decreases contact points and further decreases interparticle cohesion (Kuo and Lechuga-Ballesteros 2003).

For spray dried powders containing low water solubility drugs, and using leucine to enhance aerosolization properties, cosolvents have been used to successfully control the solubility of the drug with respect to the excipient. For example, the relative solubility of budesonide and leucine is inverted depending on the cosolvent ratio (Boraey et al. 2013), and a cosolvent composition must be chosen where budesonide solubility is higher than that of leucine, knowing that the component with the lower solubility will enrich the particle surface (Vehring et al. 2007). The technique successfully "encapsulates" budesonide and improves its dispersibility, due to the precipitation of leucine early in the particle formation process, resulting in lower density particles with a less cohesive surface.

Some hydrophobic molecules, like cyclosporine, and water-soluble surface-active molecules, like insulin, present intrinsically good dispersibility properties; however, they may still require an excipient depending on their dose requirements.

In addition to improving the physical stability and aerosol performance of peptide- and protein-containing spray dried powders for inhalation, trileucine also helps to conserve their chemical stability during processing and storage. Results from dynamic surface tension measurements suggest that the protective effect is due to trileucine's surface activity properties. Trileucine effectively competes for the air/liquid interface, thus preventing degradation of surface-active proteins (Lechuga-Ballesteros et al. 2008).

14.4 Phospholipids

The use of phospholipids is widespread in the formulation of intravenous oncology therapies (e.g. Doxil®), where the composition of liposomes is designed to encapsulate the cytotoxic drug, modify absorption, distribution, metabolism, and excretion (ADME) characteristics, and thus improve the safety and efficacy of the drug. Given the proliferation of saturated and unsaturated phospholipids in mammalian lung surfactant (see Table 14.2), phospholipids are also an excipient option for inhalation. Phospholipids have successfully been used to manufacture liposomal dispersions for pulmonary delivery. Inhaled dipalmitoyl phosphatidylcholine (DPPC) is used as a lung surfactant in a formulation (Survanta®) for prevention and treatment of respiratory distress syndrome in premature newborns. Linhaliq® and Lipoquin®

TABLE 14.2
Major Components in Mammalian Lung Surfactant

Component	Composition in Bovine Surfactant (%)	Composition in Porcine Surfactant (%)
DPPC (16:0/16:0)	40	60
1-palmitoyl-2-oleoyl-sn-glycero-3-phosphocholine (POPC) (16:0/18:1)	20	12
Surfactant proteins (SP-A, SP-B, SP-C, SP-D)	10	10
Palmitoylmyristoyl-PC (PMPC) (16:0/14:0)	7	10
Palmitoylpalmitoleoyl-PC (16:0/16:1)	10	8
Phosphatidylglycerol (PG)	10	–
Cholesterol	2.5	–

Source: Bernhard, W. et al., *Am. J. Respir. Crit. Care Med.*, 162, 1524–1533, 2000; Zasadzinski, J.A. et al., *Curr. Opin. Colloid Interface Sci.*, 6, 506–513, 2001; Zuo, Y.Y. et al., *Biochim. Biophys. Acta*, 1778, 1947–1977, 2008.

liposomal ciprofloxacin for nebulization (HSPC:Chol) and Insmed's ALIS (Amikacin liposomal inhalation solution) (DPPC:Chol 2:1 neutrally charged) are two other examples of inhaled phospholipid formulations. Liposomal dispersions have been proven ideal to increase the residence time of the drug in the lung and thereby frequency of administration and increase local effect, properties advantageous for inhaled antibiotics for lung infections (Cipolla et al. 2014).

During spray drying, phospholipids are expected to precipitate and form a variety of phases in the solid particle (such as monolayers, bilayers, gel phase, ripple phase, liquid crystalline phase). To ensure that these particles remain physicochemically stable during the spray drying process and during storage, phospholipids with a higher melting point are selected in order to formulate lipid particles with major phase transition temperatures above spray dryer outlet/collector temperature, and above ambient storage temperature. Two phospholipids stand out as the most used for spray dried powders for inhalation, DPPC and distearoyl phosphatidylcholine (DSPC), which although not endogenous have been shown to be safe for inhalation.

14.4.1 Dipalmitoylphosphatidylcholine (DPPC)

DPPC has been used extensively as a dispersibility agent in many spray dried formulations. Inhaled insulin was developed in the late 1990s by Alkermes/Eli Lilly (AIR® Advanced Inhalation Research) in large low-density lactose/albumin/DPPC particles that entered phase III clinical trials (Muchmore et al. 2007, Onoue et al. 2008). Due to the water insolubility of DPPC (<1 μg/mL at 25°C), it requires the use of ethanolic aqueous solutions at low solids content to manufacture APIs into low-density particles. The investigational inhaled L-dopa formulation in CVT-301 (Acorda Therapeutics), containing 90% w/w L-dopa, 8% w/w DPPC, and 2% NaCl has been developed for the treatment of Parkinson's disease, another example of the inhalation route being used for systemic drug delivery (LeWitt et al. 2017).

14.4.2 Distearyoylphosphatidylcholine (DPSC)

One of the most successfully used phospholipids in particle engineering is spray dried DSPC in combination with calcium chloride, creating porous and low-density particles (Weers et al. 2007). Engineered particles based on DSPC are found in two commercial products: TOBI® Podhaler (inhaled tobramycin DPI) and Bevespi® (Long-acting b_2-agonist (LABA)/LAMA inhaled combination in a Pressurized metered dose inhaler (pMDI) cosuspension) and several products in clinical trials. The TOBI® Podhaler DPI is based on the PulmoSphere™ technology where the drug is dissolved or suspended in an emulsion feedstock containing perfluorooctylbromide (PFOB) as the organic phase and DSPC and calcium chloride in the aqueous phase. Due to its liquid crystalline nature in the spray dried particle, DSPC bilayers stabilized with calcium chloride are able to interact with moderately high relative humidity long enough to consistently produce an efficient aerosol when actuated from a passive DPI device (Geller et al. 2011).

Bevespi® pMDI is based on the Aerosphere™ technology where spray dried porous particles made of DSPC and calcium chloride act both as a suspending agent of micronized crystalline API particles in a fluoroalkane suspension and as an aerosol performance aid (Vehring et al. 2012). The hallmark of the Aerosphere™ technology is the ability to formulate combination products containing two or more APIs, which are delivered with the same aerodynamic properties. Several products utilizing DSPC are in late phase clinical trials (AstraZeneca's PT010, a LABA/LAMA/Inhaled corticosteroid (ICS) combination, and Bayer's ciprofloxacin DPI, both currently in phase III clinical trials).

14.5 Mannitol

The only commercial products which contain mannitol are Exubera® (recombinant human insulin) and Bronchitol® (mannitol for diagnostic purposes), both of which are spray dried formulations. Mannitol has several factors in its favor as an inhaled excipient: (1) it is a non-reducing sugar; (2) it can act as a low hygroscopicity bulking agent when spray dried; and (3) it can be used as an amorphous glass matrix to stabilize proteins.

14.5.1 Crystalline Mannitol Polymorphs

Polymorph selection and purity is an important consideration in the selection of crystalline mannitol for formulation development. The crystalline anhydrous form of mannitol exists in three known polymorphs: α (metastable), β (stable), and δ (metastable) (Chan et al. 2004). While commercial mannitol is usually in the β form, spray dried formulations have tended to produce a combination of α and β forms immediately after processing and converted to the β form over time. Higher spray drying outlet temperatures have been associated with greater α-mannitol content (Al-Khattawi et al. 2015), suggesting that this polymorph is formed preferentially in droplet drying conditions where a short crystallization time is promoted. The metastable δ form has been occasionally identified in spray dried protein formulations, which will be discussed further below.

With respect to physical powder properties, spray dried crystalline mannitol has been reported as having <1% w/w moisture sorption at 25°C, between 0% and 94% Relative Humidity (RH) (Burger et al. 2000, Young et al. 2014), regardless of polymorph, conferring the desired powder property of low hygroscopicity to the formulation. In contrast, Yoshinari et al. (2002) reports the δ form as having a greater sorption (7.2% w/w) than the stable β form (3.2% w/w) after 20 hours at 25°C/97% RH—and the increased presence of moisture may impact stability of the coformulated active. In addition, solvent interaction with water triggers conversion of the δ form back into the β form (Yoshinari et al. 2002), impairing product storage stability. However, if not exposed to excessive moisture (i.e. coformulated with a moisture-protecting shell former such as leucine), the δ form may be maintained long-term (Burger et al. 2000), if it is difficult to eliminate this polymorph from the powder formulation. For example, a study of spray dried 1:1 (w/w) mannitol/trypsin identified the presence of both β and δ forms immediately after production; however, after 1 month storage of powder at 40°C/75% RH, the moisture content of the powder did not increase from 3.0% w/w at initial timepoint, and the δ form was retained in the powder (Hulse et al. 2009). Burger et al. (2000) also claim >5 year stability of the δ form at 25°C if kept dry, but does not specify the moisture content criteria.

14.5.2 Amorphous Mannitol

The use of mannitol as a glass stabilizer in an inhalation product is challenging, due to its low dry T_g of 11°C. Unless the intent is to lyophilize the powder formulation for long-term refrigerated storage, and immediate powder reconstitution prior to inhalation, a room-temperature stable inhaled formulation using mannitol requires the presence of additional excipients and strict moisture control to arrest physicochemical instability. An early study by Costantino et al. (1998) looking at spray dried monoclonal antibody with amorphous mannitol observed crystallization occurring during 1 year of powder storage at 5°C/38% RH and 30°C/23% RH, corresponding to a significant drop in FPF, when mannitol mass fraction was at 30% w/w and above. However, an investigation into degradation kinetics of the Exubera® spray dried insulin formulation found that the combination of mannitol, glycine, and sodium citrate conferred a high composite T_g (81°C) once co-spray dried with insulin. As a result, temperature-dependent insulin degradation was mitigated, where monomer purity was maintained at above 98% for the 40°C storage condition after 6 months (Sadrzadeh et al. 2010). In the absence of a protein in the formulation, as in the case of the Exubera formulation, the presence of glycine in amounts from 11% to 50% w/w did not appear to hinder mannitol crystallization in spray dried composites (Sou et al. 2013), suggesting mannitol interacts with the protein acting as a plasticizer stabilizer.

14.6 Fumaryl Diketopiperazine (FDKP)

Examples described in patents filed by, and granted to, Mannkind Corporation (the developer of AFREZZA® inhaled insulin) provide some insight into particle engineering with this excipient. The process described for the production of FDKP microparticles is as follows: FDKP is initially dissolved into ammonium hydroxide solution at basic pH, then combined with an acetic acid solution to crash FDKP out of solution. The suspension is then subjected to high shear mixing, while the FDKP crystals self-assemble, to produce precipitated microparticles which are recovered by a washing and concentration step with deionized water and tangential flow filtration. In order to use these particles as a formulation platform, an annex solution of protein is added to the microsphere suspension, and then adjusted for pH once again, before cryogranulation into pellets, and then lyophilization of the frozen pellets into the final bulk powder. This method of protein adsorption onto FDKP microparticles is referred to as, "Technosphere®" technology by MannKind (Grant et al. 2017).

Interestingly, this technology represents an instance where lyophilization is directly applicable to inhalation drug delivery of dry powders. The control of powder dispersibility is guided by specific surface area (SSA) of the microparticles, which is itself an indirect parameter for the size of individual FDKP crystals in the assembly. The microparticle size is controlled by the rate of FDKP crystal growth, through adjustments to acid/base titration and FDKP content in solution. Generally speaking, promotion of nucleation and faster crystallization (by increased acid or FDKP content) leads to smaller crystals within the process step timeframe, and a higher SSA. An ideal SSA range of 35 m^2/g–60 m^2/g was identified for optimal aerosol performance of the Technosphere® insulin formulation. Below the range indicated the presence of insulin bridging, while above the range, the high rugosity may lead to particle interlocking and reduced powder dispersibility (Grant et al. 2017).

Another Mannkind patent describes spray drying of the FDKP/insulin suspension to produce highly rugose and folded particles (Leone-Bay et al. 2017), a morphology consistent with particle formation models from atomized droplets. Given the lower molecular mobility of peptides and proteins compared to small molecules, and the increased aqueous solubility of FDKP salts, during the droplet lifetime, insulin could be expected to enrich the rapidly receding droplet surface while FDKP would remain distributed throughout solution. As a result, insulin reaches supersaturation and precipitates at the droplet surface, leading to the formation of a void in the dried particle. The particle then collapses or folds, creating a particle morphology commonly observed with other spray dried formulations containing shell formers such as leucine or trileucine.

The spray dried FDKP/insulin formulation is amorphous (Leone-Bay et al. 2010). Insulin stability in the powder after exposure to accelerated conditions (40°C/75% RH for up to 17 days), in terms of percent degradation and percent formation of the A_{21}-desamidoinsulin degradant, was improved relative to the lyophilized formulation, which contains crystalline FDKP (Leone-Bay et al. 2017). The contribution of amorphous FDKP to protein stability may be via glass stabilization, but it does not impart moisture robustness to the spray dried particle (such as with trileucine and higher mass fractions of leucine). Another patent outlining several spray dried oxytocin formulations reports improved stability over 32 weeks at 40°C/75% RH when a 10% isoleucine/89% trehalose formulation platform was replaced by 10% isoleucine/59% trehalose/30% disodium FDKP; however, a formulation containing 10% trileucine/87% trehalose outperformed both (Fabio et al. 2018).

14.6.1 Safety and Pharmacokinetics (PK)

The selection of FDKP as an inhaled excipient is of note as it is a derivative of cyclic dipeptide diketopiperazine; cyclic peptides have been identified as a class of "penetration enhancer" excipient for transdermal delivery (Namjoshi and Benson 2010). In the context of inhalation drug delivery, the function of FDKP is to rapidly dissolve in the epithelial lining fluid (which it can do rapidly at neutral pH) and free insulin protein to be absorbed across the lung epithelia and into the systemic circulation. However, given that penetration enhancers as a class include mechanisms such as plasma membrane disruption or expansion of tight cell junctions, FDKP has been especially subject to questions of safety and toxicology.

The absolute systemic bioavailability of FDKP after inhalation of Technosphere® powder by diabetic and non-diabetic patients in two phase I PK studies was reported to be 22%–25%, comparable to urinary excretion data (20%–23% of dose collected), confirming the relatively high systemic distribution of FDKP (Potocka et al. 2010). Both insulin and FDKP were cleared from the lung in a similarly rapid fashion in a phase I proof of mechanism study, with bronchioalveolar lavage sample concentrations below limit of quantification by 12 hours and terminal $t_{1/2}$ of ~1 hour (Cassidy et al. 2011). A recent review article by Heinemann et al. (2016) provides a comprehensive summary of PK and PD studies conducted to date with Technosphere® insulin.

In phase II and III clinical trials summarized by Kugler et al. (2015), Technosphere® insulin powder was generally well tolerated, with the most common adverse effect being cough and throat irritation.

14.7 PRINT® Technology

PRINT® technology (Liquidia Technologies, Research Triangle Park, NC) is a unique particle engineering approach that allows for the design and scalable manufacturing of particles for pharmaceutical products. The technology uses a proprietary micromolding approach to produce particles of controlled size, shape, and compositional parameters that maximize deagglomeration and aerosol performance (Mack et al. 2012).

A PRINT particle is formed by filling the cavities of the mold with API or formulated drug product, shown in Figure 14.2. Initially, the desired drug product (API and excipient) is dissolved and is cast into a uniform film onto a secondary substrate (typically a polymeric sheet). The drug product film is then laminated to the mold and passed through heated rollers. This transiently heats the drug product and applies conformal pressure to the mold, assisting material flow of the drug product film into the mold cavities. After molding, the particle laminate quickly cools (within 1 second–2 seconds) and solid particles are produced. At this point the PRINT particles are typically amorphous or semicrystalline, but if other morphologies are desired, crystalline, shape-specific particles can be produced. Once the desired particle morphology is achieved, the mold is then removed from the particles, leaving behind an array of monodisperse, shape-specific PRINT particles. These particles are dislodged from the array using a proprietary "harvester" and collected as a bulk powder that is suitable for secondary operations such as bulk drying, capsuling, or blistering.

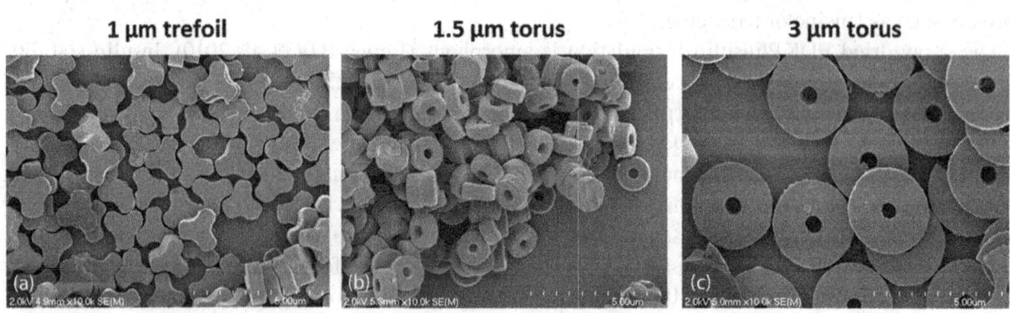

FIGURE 14.2 (a–c) Engineered particles manufactured with PRINT technology. (Courtesy of Ben Maynor.)

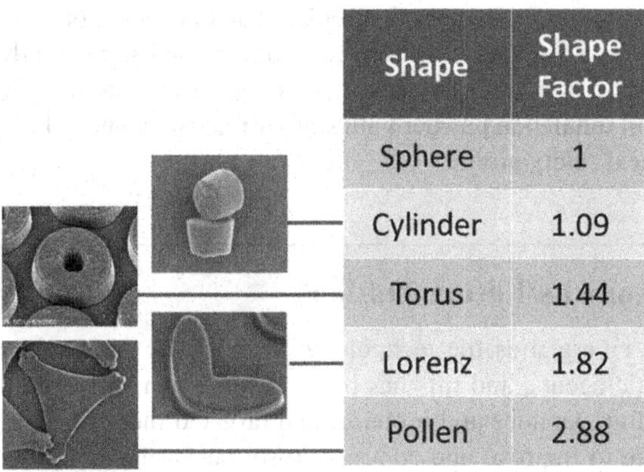

Shape	Shape Factor
Sphere	1
Cylinder	1.09
Torus	1.44
Lorenz	1.82
Pollen	2.88

FIGURE 14.3 PRINT particles manufactured with different shape factors. (Courtesy of Benjamin Maynor.)

For spray dried powders, the polydispersity and complexity of particle morphology have left shape factor largely ignored in analytical modeling and prediction of aerosol properties, even though it is a parameter in the commonly used equation for aerodynamic diameter:

$$d_a = \sqrt{\frac{\rho_p}{\rho^*}\frac{C_c(d_v)}{C_c(d_a)}\frac{1}{\lambda}}d_v \tag{14.1}$$

where λ is the dynamic shape factor, ρ_p is particle density, and C_c is the Cunningham slip factor (Boraey and Vehring 2014). The control over particle geometry, and therefore shape factor, afforded by the PRINT micromolding method shown in Figure 14.3 enables a closer investigation of the impact of particle engineering on regional aerosol deposition in the lung (Garcia et al. 2012, Fromen et al. 2013). The ability to predictably influence the deposition of drug through aerodynamic particle size control of the aerosol could have important clinical ramifications (Usmani et al. 2005).

As with spray dried amorphous materials, coformulation with leucine has been used to provide moisture robustness to the PRINT particles manufactured with lactose, trehalose, and other sugars. For formulations where a crystalline stolid state is desired (i.e. small molecules), an "in-mold" annealing step consisting of holding the particles in the mold for a specified period under controlled ambient conditions can be employed to allow crystallization to occur. PRINT technology has been used to formulate a variety of proteins from small peptides to full-length monoclonal antibodies with good control over particle size/shape, preservation of protein activity and stability, high respirable dose, high fine particle fraction, and preservation of protein stability (Garcia et al. 2012, Rahhal et al. 2016).

14.7.1 Particle Engineering Impact on PK and Toxicology

Due to their monodispersity and unique geometries, the responses of macrophages and other cell types in the lung to PRINT particles is of significant interest. The rate of macrophage uptake of PRINT particles has shown dependence on particle geometry; broader, flatter shapes were phagocytosed at a slower rate than shapes with higher aspect ratios (Champion and Mitragotri 2006, Shen 2014). PRINT particles delivered to mice, ranging from 80 nm to 6 microns, were internalized by macrophages and observed in the lungs after 7 days, without triggering of host immunity (Roberts et al. 2013). A dry powder formulation of PRINT treprostinil/trehalose/L-leucine particles was developed to enable single-breath administration of treprostinil from a capsule-based dry powder inhaler. Single-dose PK studies in rats and dogs and 14-day repeat-dose studies in rats demonstrated similar PK profile of this formulation to nebulized treprostinil solution (Anderson et al. 2017). A 14-day, repeat-dose toxicity evaluation of the dry powder PRINT-treprostinil particles found drug-related toxicological findings were broadly similar between the trepostinil dry powder and nebulized solution. In this 14-day study, placebo PRINT particles and

PRINT-treprostinil powder groups, increased alveolar macrophages, not associated with inflammation, were seen in all rats, and findings had resolved or diminished significantly at the end of recovery (Dillberger et al. 2017). These non-clinical studies indicate that Liquidia was able to successfully formulate and deliver treprostinil inhalation powder with similar relative bioavailability to nebulized solution, with acceptable non-clinical safety profile.

14.8 Concluding Remarks/Future Outlook

Particle engineering has emerged as the technology of choice to enable the pulmonary delivery of non-crystalline therapeutic agents, and this has been driven by an increased industry focus on large molecule delivery, including peptides and proteins, and targeted therapies using monoclonal antibodies. In addition, the desire to improve and control aerosol performance in the product has motivated the inhalation field to find ways to fine-tune particle properties, exemplified by the particle engineering approaches described in this chapter. A considerable challenge has been the limited availability of functional excipients, which in one sense has also encouraged development of particle engineering techniques to fully exploit what excipients are already generally regarded as safe (GRAS) for inhalation. However, as more products are approved the number of GRAS excipients for pulmonary applications is expected to increase.

With this comes an increased complexity in formulation design, and a strong understanding of solid-state properties of the actives and excipients *in toto* will enhance in-use and long-term stability of drug products made with this technology. Through an improved understanding of how excipients and actives interact in these engineered formulations, there are also opportunities to strengthen development of formulations with modified release dosing profiles, which in the clinical literature has been limited so far to liposomal formulations.

Complexities of the particle engineering process, be it spray drying or molding, requires further understanding to control key particle qualities such as particle size, particle density, surface energy, moisture content, and solid-state stability. Moreover, development of manufacturing technology is a key aspect of ensuring scale up to support large clinical trials and eventual commercial distribution.

In spite all the technical challenges, particle engineering has revealed opportunities to formulate and deliver small and large molecules previously thought too difficult to develop for inhalation and further innovation in the area can only be expected in the years to come as the technology becomes widely adopted.

REFERENCES

Al-Khattawi, Ali, Jasdip Koner, Peter Rue, Dan Kirby, Yvonne Perrie, Ali Rajabi-Siahboomi, and Afzal R. Mohammed. 2015. "A pragmatic approach for engineering porous mannitol and mechanistic evaluation of particle performance." *European Journal of Pharmaceutics and Biopharmaceutics* 94 (August): 1–10. doi:10.1016/j.ejpb.2015.04.011.

Anderson, Stephanie, Patrick Normand, Manal Hantash, John Dillberger, Robert Roscigno, and William Wargin. 2017. "Pharmacokinetics (PK) of inhaled treprostinil are similar when delivered as LIQ861 dry powder or nebulized solution." In: *The Toxicologist: Supplement to Toxicological Sciences*, Society of Toxicology, 2017. Abstract no. 1681.

Bernhard, Wolfgang, Jasmin Mottaghian, Andreas Gebert, Gunnar A. Rau, Horst Von Der Hardt, and Christian F. Poets. 2000. "Commercial versus native surfactants." *American Journal of Respiratory and Critical Care Medicine* 162 (4): 1524–1533. doi:10.1164/ajrccm.162.4.9908104.

Boraey, Mohammed A., Susan Hoe, Hajar Sharif, Danforth P. Miller, David Lechuga-Ballesteros, and Reinhard Vehring. 2013. "Improvement of the dispersibility of spray-dried budesonide powders using leucine in an ethanol–water cosolvent system." *Powder Technology* 236 (February): 171–178. doi:10.1016/j.powtec.2012.02.047.

Boraey, Mohammed A., and Reinhard Vehring. 2014. "Diffusion controlled formation of microparticles." *Journal of Aerosol Science* 67 (January): 131–143. doi:10.1016/j.jaerosci.2013.10.002.

Burger, Artur, Jan-Olav Henck, Silvia Hetz, Judith M. Rollinger, Andrea A. Weissnicht, and Hemma Stöttner. 2000. "Energy/temperature diagram and compression behavior of the polymorphs of D-mannitol." *Journal of Pharmaceutical Sciences* 89 (4): 457–468. doi:10.1002/(sici)1520-6017(200004)89:4<457::aid-jps3>3.0.co;2-g.

Cassidy, James P., Nikhil Amin, Mark Marino, Mark Gotfried, Thomas Meyer, Knut Sommerer, and Robert A. Baughman. 2011. "Insulin lung deposition and clearance following Technosphere® insulin inhalation powder administration." *Pharmaceutical Research* 28 (9): 2157–2164. doi:10.1007/s11095-011-0443-4.

Champion, Julie A., and Samir Mitragotri. 2006. "Role of target geometry in phagocytosis." *Proceedings of the National Academy of Sciences* 103 (13): 4930–4934. doi:10.1073/pnas.0600997103.

Chan, Hak-Kim, Andrew R. Clark, Jane C. Feeley, Mei-Chang Kuo, S. Russ Lehrman, Katherine Pikal-Cleland, Danforth P. Miller, Reinhard Vehring, and David Lechuga-Ballesteros. 2004. "Physical stability of salmon calcitonin spray-dried powders for inhalation." *Journal of Pharmaceutical Sciences* 93 (3): 792–804. doi:10.1002/jps.10594.

Cicerone, Marcus T. and Christopher L. Soles. 2004. "Fast dynamics and stabilization of proteins: binary glasses of trehalose and glycerol." *Biophysics Journal*, 86 (6): 3836–3845. doi:10.1529/biophysj.103.035519.

Cipolla, David, Boris Shekunov, Jim Blanchard, Anthony Hickey. 2014. "Lipid-based carriers for pulmonary products: Preclinical development and case studies in humans." *Advanced Drug Delivery Reviews*, 75: 53–80. doi:10.1016/j.addr.2014.05.001.

Costantino, Henry R., James D. Andya, Phuong-Anh Nguyen, Nancy Dasovich, Theresa D. Sweeney, Steven J. Shire, Chung C. Hsu, and Yuh-Fun Maa. 1998. "Effect of mannitol crystallization on the stability and aerosol performance of a spray-dried pharmaceutical protein, recombinant humanized anti-IgE monoclonal antibody." *Journal of Pharmaceutical Sciences* 87 (11): 1406–1411. doi:10.1021/js9800679.

Dillberger, John, Patrick Normand, Robert Roscigno, and Stephanie Anderson. 2017. "Inhaled treprostinil toxicity profile is similar administered as LIQ861 dry powder or nebulized solution." In: *The Toxicologist: Supplement to Toxicological Sciences*, Society of Toxicology, 2017. Abstract no. 1683.

Fabio, Karine, Joseph J. Guarneri, Kieran Curley, Marshall L. Grant, and Andrea Leone-Bay. "Heat-stable dry powder pharmaceutical compositions and methods." U.S. Patent 9,925,144 B2 filed July 18, 2014 and issued March 27, 2018.

Fromen, Catherine A., Tammy W. Shen, Abigail E. Larus, Peter Mack, Benjamin W. Maynor, J. Christopher Luft, and Joseph M. DeSimone. 2013. "Synthesis and characterization of monodisperse uniformly shaped respirable aerosols." *AIChE Journal* 59 (9): 3184–3194. doi:10.1002/aic.14157.

Garcia, Andres, Peter Mack, Stuart Williams, Catherine Fromen, Tammy Shen, Janet Tully, Jonathan Pillai et al. 2012. "Microfabricated engineered particle systems for respiratory drug delivery and other pharmaceutical applications." *Journal of Drug Delivery* 2012: 1–10. doi:10.1155/2012/941243.

Geller, David E., Jeffry G. Weers, and Silvia Heuerding. 2011. "Development of an inhaled dry-powder formulation of tobramycin using PulmoSphere™ technology." *Journal of Aerosol Medicine and Pulmonary Drug Delivery* 24 (4): 175–182.

Grant, Marshall L., Grayson W. Stowell, and Paul Menkin. "Diketopiperazine microparticles with defined specific surface areas." U.S. Patent 9,630,930 B2 filed April 11, 2014, and issued April 25, 2017.

Heinemann, Lutz, Robert Baughman, Anders Boss, and Marcus Hompesch. 2016. "Pharmacokinetic and pharmacodynamic properties of a novel inhaled insulin." *Journal of Diabetes Science and Technology* 11 (1): 148–156. doi:10.1177/1932296816658055.

Hulse, Wendy L., Robert T. Forbes, Michael C. Bonner, and Matthias Getrost. 2009. "Influence of protein on mannitol polymorphic form produced during co-spray drying." *International Journal of Pharmaceutics* 382 (1–2): 67–72. doi:10.1016/j.ijpharm.2009.08.007.

Ivey, James W., and Reinhard Vehring. 2010. "The use of modeling in spray drying of emulsions and suspensions accelerates formulation and process development." *Computers & Chemical Engineering* 34 (7): 1036–1040. doi:10.1016/j.compchemeng.2010.02.031.

Kugler, Anne J., Kristin L. Fabbio, David Q. Pham, and Daniel A. Nadeau. 2015. "Inhaled technosphere insulin: A novel delivery system and formulation for the treatment of types 1 and 2 diabetes mellitus." *Pharmacotherapy: The Journal of Human Pharmacology and Drug Therapy* 35 (3): 298–314. doi:10.1002/phar.1555.

Kuo, Mei-Chang, and David Lechuga-Ballesteros. "Compositions comprising an active agent." U.S. Patent 8,501,240 B2 filed May 7, 2009 and issued August 6, 2013.

Kuo, Mei-Chang, and David Lechuga-Ballesteros. "Dry powder compositions having improved dispersivity." U.S. Patent 6,518,239 B1 filed April 13, 2000 and issued February 11, 2003.

Kuo, Mei-Chang, Michael Eldon, and Yiqiong Yuan. "Insulin derivative formulations for pulmonary delivery." U.S. Patent 8,900,555 B2 filed July 27, 2007 and issued December 2, 2014.

Lechuga-Ballesteros, David, Chatan Charan, Cheryl L.M. Stults, Cynthia L. Stevenson, Danforth P. Miller, Reinhard Vehring, Vathana Tep, and Mei-Chang Kuo. 2008. "Trileucine improves aerosol performance and stability of spray-dried powders for inhalation." *Journal of Pharmaceutical Sciences* 97 (1): 287–302. doi:10.1002/jps.21078.

Leone-Bay, Andrea, Robert Baughman, Chad Smutney, and Joseph Kocinsky. 2010. "Innovation in drug delivery by inhalation." *ONdrugDelivery Magazine*, November. http://ondrugdelivery.com/publications/OINDP%20November%202010/Mannkind.pdf.

Leone-Bay, Andrea, Destardi Moye-Sherman, and Bryan R. Wilson. "Diketopiperazine salts for drug delivery and related methods." U.S. Patent 9,675,674 B2 filed January 8, 2016 and issued June 13, 2017.

LeWitt, Peter A., Rajesh Pahwa, Alexander Sedkov, Ann Corbin, Richard Batycky, and Harald Murck. 2017. "Pulmonary safety and tolerability of inhaled levodopa (CVT-301) administered to patients with Parkinson's disease." *Journal of Aerosol Medicine and Pulmonary Drug Delivery*, November. doi:10.1089/jamp.2016.1354.

Li, Liang, Siping Sun, Thaigarajan Parumasivam, John A. Denman, Thomas Gengenbach, Patricia Tang, Shirui Mao, and Hak-Kim Chan. 2016. "L-Leucine as an excipient against moisture on in vitro aerosolization performances of highly hygroscopic spray-dried powders." *European Journal of Pharmaceutics and Biopharmaceutics* 102 (May): 132–141. doi:10.1016/j.ejpb.2016.02.010.

Mack, Peter, Katie Horvath, Andres Garcia, Janet Tully, and Benjamin Maynor. 2012. "Particle engineering for inhalation formulation and delivery of biotherapeutics." *Inhalation*, August. http://liquidia.com/publications/Liquidia_Inhalation_Magazine_August_2012.pdf.

Muchmore, Douglas B., Bernard Silverman, Amparo De La Peña, and Janet Tobian. 2007. "The AIR® inhaled insulin system: System components and pharmacokinetic/glucodynamic data." *Diabetes Technology & Therapeutics* 9 (s1): S-41–S-47. doi:10.1089/dia.2007.0218.

Namjoshi, Sarika, and Heather A. E. Benson. 2010. "Cyclic peptides as potential therapeutic agents for skin disorders." *Biopolymers* 94 (5): 673–680. doi:10.1002/bip.21476.

Onoue, Satomi, Naofumi Hashimoto, and Shizuo Yamada. 2008. "Dry powder inhalation systems for pulmonary delivery of therapeutic peptides and proteins." *Expert Opinion on Therapeutic Patents* 18 (4): 429–442. doi:10.1517/13543776.18.4.429.

Potocka, Elizabeth, James P. Cassidy, Pamela Haworth, Douglas Heuman, Sjoerd van Marle, and Robert A. Baughman Jr. 2010. "Pharmacokinetic characterization of the novel pulmonary delivery excipient fumaryl diketopiperazine." *Journal of Diabetes Science and Technology* 4 (5): 1164–1173. doi:10.1177/193229681000400515.

Rahhal, Tojan B., Catherine A. Fromen, Erin M. Wilson, Marc P. Kai, Tammy W. Shen, J. Christopher Luft, and Joseph M. DeSimone. 2016. "Pulmonary delivery of butyrylcholinesterase as a model protein to the lung." *Molecular Pharmaceutics* 13 (5): 1626–1635. doi:10.1021/acs.molpharmaceut.6b00066.

Roberts, Reid A., Tammy Shen, Irving C. Allen, Warefta Hasan, Joseph M. DeSimone, and Jenny P. Y. Ting. 2013. "Analysis of the murine immune response to pulmonary delivery of precisely fabricated nano- and microscale particles." *PLoS ONE* 8 (4): e62115. doi:10.1371/journal.pone.0062115.

Sadrzadeh, Negar, Danforth P. Miller, David Lechuga-Ballesteros, Nancy J. Harper, Cynthia L. Stevenson, and David B. Bennett. 2010. "Solid-state stability of spray-dried insulin powder for inhalation: chemical kinetics and structural relaxation modeling of exubera above and below the glass transition temperature." *Journal of Pharmaceutical Sciences* 99 (9): 3698–3710. doi:10.1002/jps.21936.

Shen, Tammy W. 2014. "Development and characterization of print particles as drug delivery vehicles in the lung." Doctoral diss., University of North Carolina at Chapel Hill.

Sou, Tomás, Lisa M. Kaminskas, Tri-Hung Nguyen, Renée Carlberg, Michelle P. McIntosh, and David A.V. Morton. 2013. "the effect of amino acid excipients on morphology and solid-state properties of multi-component spray-dried formulations for pulmonary delivery of biomacromolecules." *European Journal of Pharmaceutics and Biopharmaceutics* 83 (2): 234–243. doi:10.1016/j.ejpb.2012.10.015.

Usmani, Omar S., Martyn F. Biddiscombe, and Peter J. Barnes. 2005. "Regional lung deposition and bronchodilator response as a function of β2-agonist particle size." *American Journal of Respiratory and Critical Care Medicine* 172 (12): 1497–1504. doi:10.1164/rccm.200410-1414oc.

Vanbever, Rita, Jeffrey D. Mintzes, Jue Wang, Jacquelyn Nice, Donghao Chen, Richard Batycky, Robert Langer, and David A. Edwards. 1999. "Formulation and physical characterization of large porous particles for inhalation." *Pharmaceutical Research*, 16 (11): 1735–1742. doi:10.1023/a:1018910200420.

Vehring, Reinhard, David Lechuga-Ballesteros, Vidya Joshi, Brian Noga, and Sarvajna K. Dwivedi. 2012. "Cosuspensions of microcrystals and engineered microparticles for uniform and efficient delivery of respiratory therapeutics from pressurized metered dose inhalers." *Langmuir* 28 (42): 15015–15023. doi:10.1021/la302281n.

Vehring, Reinhard, Willard R. Foss, and David Lechuga-Ballesteros. 2007. "Particle formation in spray drying." *Journal of Aerosol Science* 38 (7): 728–746. doi:10.1016/j.jaerosci.2007.04.005.

Vehring, Reinhard. 2007. "Pharmaceutical particle engineering via spray drying." *Pharmaceutical Research* 25 (5): 999–1022. doi:10.1007/s11095-007-9475-1.

Weers, Jeffry G., Thomas E. Tarara, and Andrew R. Clark. 2007. "Design of fine particles for pulmonary drug delivery." *Expert Opinion on Drug Delivery* 4 (3): 297–313. doi:10.1517/17425247.4.3.297.

Yamashita, Chikamasa, Toru Nishibayashi, Susumu Akashi, Hajime Toguchi, and Masaaki Odomi. 1998. "A novel formulation of dry powder for inhalation of peptides and proteins." In: *Respiratory Drug Delivery VI*, edited by Richard Dalby, Stephen J. Farr, and Peter Byron, pp. 483–485. Buffalo Grove, IL: Interpharm Press.

Yoshinari, Tomohiro, Robert T. Forbes, Peter York, and Yoshiaki Kawashima. 2002. "Moisture induced polymorphic transition of mannitol and its morphological transformation." *International Journal of Pharmaceutics* 247 (1–2): 69–77. doi:10.1016/s0378-5173(02)00380-0.

Young, Paul M., Rania O. Salama, Bing Zhu, Gary Phillips, John Crapper, Hak-Kim Chan, and Daniela Traini. 2014. "Multi-breath dry powder inhaler for delivery of cohesive powders in the treatment of bronchiectasis." *Drug Development and Industrial Pharmacy* 41 (5): 859–865. doi:10.3109/03639045.2014.909841.

Zasadzinski, Joseph A., Junqi Ding, Heidi E. Warriner, Frank Bringezu, and Alan J Waring. 2001. "The physics and physiology of lung surfactants." *Current Opinion in Colloid & Interface Science* 6 (5–6): 506–513. doi:10.1016/s1359-0294(01)00124-8.

Zuo, Yi Y., Ruud A.W. Veldhuizen, A. Wilhelm Neumann, Nils O. Petersen, and Fred Possmayer. 2008. "Current perspectives in pulmonary surfactant—Inhibition, enhancement and evaluation." *Biochimica et Biophysica Acta (BBA) - Biomembranes* 1778 (10): 1947–1977. doi:10.1016/j.bbamem.2008.03.021.

Section V

Drug Product Formulation

15

Emerging Pulmonary Delivery Strategies in Gene Therapy: State of the Art and Future Considerations

Gabriella Costabile and Olivia M. Merkel

CONTENTS

15.1 Introduction

Since the first studies that have shown the potential of using DNA anti-sense oligonucleotides (AON) to modulate target gene expression in the 1970s, the administration of nucleic acids has moved from the concept of a tool for possible drug target identification to an effective therapeutic class (Seguin and Ferrari 2009). In general, there are two main approaches to affect the genetics of targeted cells: (i) gene therapy, where DNA is delivered with the aim of providing a functional copy of a defective gene in the patient, such as double stranded DNA (dsDNA), single stranded (ssDNA), and plasmid DNA or (ii) the delivery of therapeutic nucleic acids which include microRNA (miRNA), short hairpin RNA (shRNA), antisense oligonucleotides (AONs) and small interfering RNA (siRNA). In the case of miRNA, shRNA, and siRNA, the RNA species are processed via the Dicer complex, and loaded into the RNA-induced silencing complex (RISC), which then binds to messenger RNA (mRNA) molecules to either degrade them or modulate their expression. In contrast, AONs are delivered as a single-stranded species and must find their complementary mRNA sequences without the aid of an auxiliary protein (such as Argonaute in the RISC complex). This approach is typically used to target tumors, but can also be used when a genetic disorder results in elevated levels of gene expression (Oliveira et al. 2016).

Regardless the possible approaches to affect the genetics of targeted cells, to be effectively used, gene therapy molecules have to be properly delivered: nowadays, it is well known that there is no one vector that is suited for all applications, but the gene transfer agent (GTA) has to be carefully chosen depending on the cell type to be targeted, the number of treatments (one versus repeated administration) required, and the size and nature of the nucleic acid to be delivered. In this regard, several studies have shown that local delivery displayed better bioavailability in target tissues, therefore, in this sense, the opportunity to selectively target the lungs is a fascinating option to treat severe pulmonary diseases.

Nowadays, the lungs, that are perhaps the most ancient route of drug delivery, are considered as a port of entry to systemic circulation for a broad range of therapies (Stein and Thiel 2017). As early as 1,500 BCE, the ancient Egyptians inhaled vapors to treat a variety of diseases. Unfortunately, the lungs were soon forgotten as a major route of drug delivery, and only in the 1950s, serious consideration of the lungs was resurrected with the invention of the first metered dose inhaler (MDI) (Newman 2005, Rubin and Fink 2005). The introduction of MDI in 1956 was the major breakthrough in the treatment of respiratory diseases, particularly asthma, and has since been followed by a period of unprecedented innovation marked by the introduction of DPI available on the market and the monumental efforts to develop insulin inhalers for non-invasive treatment of diabetes.

Based on this consideration, in recent years, gene therapy applied to the lung has been the target of intense research and development by the pharmaceutical and biotechnology industry for a wide range of acute and chronic lung diseases such as asthma, chronic obstructive pulmonary disease (COPD), cancer, and cystic fibrosis (CF). Gene therapy is particularly attractive for those diseases that currently do not have satisfactory treatment options (Griesenbach and Alton 2009, Seguin and Ferrari 2009, Alamgeer et al. 2013, Villaflor and Salgia 2013, Yeh and Horwitz 2017). Asthma affects an estimated 300 million people worldwide and is expected to rise up to 400 million over the next 15 years–20 years (Nunes et al. 2017). In spite of all the therapies available today, asthma remains uncontrolled in many patients. In fact, moderate to severe patients often fail to completely respond to conventional therapy, and these patients account for >50% of the total healthcare costs associated with asthma (Seguin and Ferrari 2009). In contrast to asthma, COPD is a collective term used to describe a chronic lung disease usually induced by tobacco smoking or chronic exposure to irritants, that is characterized by progressive obstruction of airflow, increased shortness of breath with chronic cough, and phlegm production in most patients. COPD is projected to be the third leading cause of death worldwide by 2030 by the WHO (Ferrari et al. 2007). Pharmacological treatments aim to improve quality of life, control symptoms, and reduce exacerbation risk, but no medications have been conclusively shown to modify long-term decline or to improve survival in COPD (Seguin and Ferrari 2009, Yeh and Horwitz 2017). As a third important lung disease, lung cancer is very heterogeneous and involves several molecular targets (Alamgeer et al. 2013, Villaflor and Salgia 2013). Despite a decrease in mortality due to both the reduction of tobacco consumption and great advances achieved in therapies, there is still a significant lack of treatment success, especially because of drug resistance. Thus, lung and bronchial cancer are still the major cause of cancer-related death for both genders, in many geographic regions (Siegel et al. 2013). Cancer development and progression is the addition of genetic events, such as activation of dominant oncogenes and inactivation of tumor suppressor genes; therefore, an effective cancer treatment can have these genetic events as target involving therapeutic nucleic acids specifically targeted in order to regulate the abnormal genetic expressions in cancer cells with consequent higher efficiency and reduction of systemic cytotoxicity. New and improved treatments are urgent and nucleic acid-based delivery may be an important strategy for tumor suppression (Patil et al. 2010). On the other hand, gene therapy is expected to be more successful to treat monogenic disorders such as cystic fibrosis compared to more complex genetic diseases (Griesenbach and Alton 2009). CF is the most common lethal autosomal recessive disease in the Caucasian population and, even if several organs are affected, the lung implication is the main cause of morbidity and mortality in CF individuals. The most commonly mutated gene in CF, the cystic fibrosis transmembrane conductance regulator (CFTR), is a chloride channel located in the apical membrane of epithelial cells and was cloned in 1989 (Riordan et al. 1989). Cystic fibrosis has been one of the first diseases considered as potential target for gene therapy. In fact, as above mentioned, the GTA has to be carefully chosen depending on the cell type to be targeted, but also because, additionally, extracellular barriers such as mucus/sputum and the degree of inflammation may depend both on disease type and severity within a given disease. In this sense, CF serves as a "proof-of-principle" to evaluate the efficacy of pulmonary gene therapy for a chronic, life-long disease, which would require gene expression for the individual's whole life-time.

15.2 Therapeutic Nucleic Acids: Characteristics, Stability and Administration

Over the last decades, therapeutic nucleic acids have witnessed an explosion of interest in academia and industry for the treatment of various diseases due to their ability to express or inhibit specific genes. Genetic therapeutics offer the possibility to knock down gene expression, to alter mRNA splicing, to target trinucleotide repeat disorders, to target non-coding RNAs involved in transcriptional and epigenetic regulation in order to upregulate target genes, to express genes, and to edit the genome. Those are all forms of therapeutics intervention that we never could even dream of achieving with small-molecules or antibodies (Dowdy 2017).

Despite all the therapeutic potential associated with them, nucleic acids have physicochemical characteristics that affect their pharmacokinetics and pharmacodynamics, resulting in limited therapeutic applications. The delivery of nucleic acids across the phospholipid bilayer which constitutes the cell and nuclear membranes remains the biggest hurdle to overcome in order to obtain effective therapeutics. It is not an exaggeration to say that the attempt to successfully deliver nucleic acid-based therapeutics is the attempt to tackle a billion year's worth of evolutionary defenses. We should consider that life started on this planet ~4 billion years ago when the primordial DNA/RNA and macromolecular soup became encapsulated by a lipid bilayer that allowed chemical reactions to take place inside without interference from RNAs and macromolecules on the outside. Lipid bilayers allow small neutral, slightly hydrophobic molecules <1,000 Daltons (Da) to passively diffuse across them, at the same time preventing that large, charged molecules, such as DNA/RNAs, can cross them. Furthermore, these macromolecules are easily taken up by endocytosis, remaining trapped inside of the endosome and behind the lipid bilayer, which leaves them separated from the cytoplasm and nucleus. Thus, delivery of nucleic acids across the lipid bilayers out of the endosome and into the cytoplasm in a non-toxic manner remains the biggest hurdle to developing effective therapeutics and is the key technological problem to solve before we can tap into the full potential of genetic therapeutics.

To this concern, specifically related to nucleic acids characteristics, we should also add all the other limitations directly imposed by the administration route chosen for the delivery. Usually, nucleic acids are administered through the parenteral route. This administration route is one of the most commonly used for macromolecular drugs, but in the nucleic acids case, the main problem is their elevated instability in the bloodstream. Owing to their structure, nucleic acids undergo degradation by nucleases and are rapidly cleared from the bloodstream by the kidneys and scavenger receptors on liver hepatocytes, thus having reduced systemic half-life. Additionally, their excretion is very fast. Furthermore, systemic administration is an invasive route which can lead to reduced compliance by patients and, consequently, increased costs of therapy, especially when prolonged or chronic treatment is required (Patton et al. 2004).

In order to overcome the problems associated with parenteral administration, the pharmaceutical industry has been channeling efforts on developing systems for the delivery of nucleic acids without resorting to injections. In general, oral administration is considered the most attractive route for drug delivery because of its convenience and high acceptance by patients. However, this route is not very straightforward for nucleic acids delivery because of a number of anatomical and physiological barriers resulting in very low bioavailability. In fact, nucleic acids are highly instable in the gastrointestinal tract; they undergo rapid degradation at low gastric pH, experience enzymatic degradation by endonuclease and exonuclease in the small and large intestines, and get clearance by phagocytes such as macrophages. Additionally, the physical barrier of epithelial tight junctions and negatively charged mucus along with negative charge on the cell surface prevent uptake of nucleic acids, which are also negatively charged. As a result of all of the above barriers, only a very small percentage of the delivered dose becomes available at the cellular sites for uptake, where additional challenges are encountered (Moroz et al. 2016, Attarwala et al. 2017, Morales et al. 2017).

Parallel to the oral route, inhalation has been thoroughly studied and seems to be the most effective alternative to parenteral administration, especially for macromolecules. Inhalation is a desirable route of administration to deliver therapeutic nucleic acids not only for its non-invasive nature and lower endonuclease activity in the airways compared to the bloodstream, but it is a route of choice for drug administration because of several additional advantages, such as the large surface area for absorption (~75 m^2) and thin (0.1 µm–0.5 µm) alveolar epithelium, permitting rapid absorption, absence of first-pass metabolism, rapid onset of action, and high bioavailability. Furthermore, if it is generally true that locally targeted delivery of drugs acting in the lungs can improve efficacy and decrease unwanted systemic side effects over small molecules, this is especially true for the use of therapeutic nucleic acids where a specific activity is strictly required. In fact, the direct administration to the site of action by inhalation allows the nucleic acids to reach and enter target cells, preventing the intra-pulmonary degradation of nucleic acids and, at the same time, avoiding systemic toxicity; moreover, a long half-life of nucleic acids in the lungs would lead to daily or even longer chronic dosing and improved patient compliance. However, despite the theoretical ease of non-invasive access to the lung, it is perhaps unsurprising that gene transfer into the airway epithelium is a difficult issue to overcome. The lung has evolved to keep foreign particles out (see above), including gene transfer agents. The deposition of particles at the lower respiratory tract is a complex phenomenon, and its efficiency depends on several aspects including physiological factors such as humidity and geometry of the airways, respiratory capacity (inspiratory flow rate, breathing frequency, and tidal volume), and the inhalation technique used by the patient, as well as factors inherent to the particles, such as the mean diameter, surface and shape, density, and their aerodynamic properties. Finally, it also depends on the type of formulation, delivery device used, and its capacity to produce the aerosol. The combination of all these aspects causes for the drug to undergo consecutive losses between delivery and absorption steps. Thus, the absorbed dose is usually below the dose initially present in the delivery device and, in the worst case, the final result leads to a non-reproducible pharmacokinetic and pharmacodynamic response.

Taking all these considerations together, it can be brought to conclusion that gene therapy is only theoretically a simple therapeutic method. Replacing a distorted gene with a healthy one, or complementing a missing gene in order to express the required protein, in practice are complex operations due to several obstacles that must be overcome.

Hence, for ensuring the arrival of DNA/RNA molecules via inhalation route in the nucleus/cell without degradation, it is necessary to use a gene delivery system able not only to protect the DNA/RNA molecules from degradation, but able to pass through the extracellular and cellular barriers imposed by the lung.

15.3 Overcoming Barriers in Pulmonary Gene Delivery

The delivery of therapeutic DNA/RNA molecules to their target tissue is a challenging task.

As explained above, despite all the therapeutic potential, nucleic acid-based therapeutics have physiochemical characteristics which strongly affect their pharmacokinetics and pharmacodynamics, resulting in a significant challenge for clinical applications. Furthermore, because of their negative charge, the DNA/RNA molecules lack the ability to penetrate the cell membrane, arrive in the cytoplasm, and, eventually, enter the nucleus. Thus, in order to achieve effective gene therapy via inhalation, conducive delivery strategies have to be developed.

The ideal transfer carrier, capable of ensuring the success of gene therapy, must satisfy the following criteria:

1. It must be capable of transporting nucleic acids whatever their size;
2. The vector must deliver the genetic cargo only to certain types of cells, especially when the target cells are scattered throughout the body or when they are part of a heterogeneous population;
3. It must not trigger a strong immune response;
4. It must lead to the sustained and regular expression of its genetic cargo;
5. It must be able to infect both dividing and non-dividing cell;
6. It must be easy to prepare, inexpensive, and commercially available at high concentrations;
7. When integration into the genome is required, the vector has to be able to integrate the gene into a specific region (Ibraheem et al. 2014).

It is easy to understand how the possibility to produce specifically engineered carriers could not only promote cellular uptake and give back a selective activity, but at the same time it could also guarantee protection to the genetic cargo. An optimized carrier is also expected to allow a reduction in the administered drug dose or in the number of administrations, or it may further help to combine two or more therapeutic molecules into one drug product and have broader specific targeted effects.

The technology currently in use for aerosol delivery was originally developed for small molecule drugs and not for the administration of macromolecules such as DNA or RNA, thus, the reengineering of inhalers for nucleic acids delivery is mandatory in order to achieve a therapeutic effect. In the past decades, with the progression of nanotechnology, several kinds of carriers composed of various materials have been widely applied in the field of gene delivery. The delivery systems can be broadly categorized into viral and non-viral vectors, according to their nature.

15.4 Viral Vectors

A virus is a biological entity that can penetrate into the cell nucleus of the host and exploit the cellular machinery to express its own genetic material and replace it, then spread to other cells. Viral vectors refer to the use of viruses to deliver genetic materials to the cell. They are extremely attractive because of their ability to enter the cells and their nucleus, but also to induce high transduction efficiency and, depending on the type of viruses employed, e.g. retroviruses, provide also transient or long-term gene expression which is currently difficult to accomplish with non-viral methods (Ibraheem et al. 2014). Several kinds of modified "non-aggressive" viruses have been studied to be used as potential vectors Table 15.1.

In fact, the pathogenic part of their genome has to be removed, while the non-pathogenic part, which allows it to infect the cell, has to be retained. However, clinical application of viral vectors is limited by their toxicity, insertional mutagenesis (e.g. retroviruses), and immunogenicity (e.g. adenoviruses). In fact, viral vectors may cause a very strong immune response that can be fatal for the patient. Other important limitations to the application of viral vectors are: (i) the limited size of genetic material that can be delivered by the virus and (ii) the elevated cost for the production of a large number of viral vectors. Despite all these disadvantages that still remain to be overcome, at the moment, viral vectors are the most often used to transfer nucleic acids due to their high *in vivo* transduction efficacy. Furthermore, gene therapy products that have been commercialized until now are all based on viral vectors.

TABLE 15.1

Viral Gene Vectors for Lung Diseases

Viral Vector	Advantages	Disadvantages	Ref.
Adenovirus	Large nucleic acid packaging capacity (36 Kb); non-integrating; no insertional mutagenesis.	Requires basolaterally expressed receptors for cell entry; no integration into host genome with transient gene expression; repeated administration inefficient because of immune response.	[Moroz et al. (2016), Rawlins et al. (2008), Toietta et al. (2003)]
Adeno-associated virus	Infect dividing and non-dividing cells; broad cellular tropism; non-pathogenic; low immunogenicity; more stable gene expression compared to AdV.	Limited packaging capacity (4.7 Kb); the best-suited serotypes for lung administration still need to be individualized.	[Newman (2005), Koehler et al. (2005), Tosi et al. (2004)]
Negative strand RNA virus	Not able to enter the nucleus, no risk of insertional mutagenesis.	Transient gene expression; repeated administration inefficient.	[Ostedgaard et al. (2005), Fischer (2007), Duan et al. (2001)]
Lentivirus	Insert capacity 10 Kb; infect dividing and non-dividing cells; stable gene expression.	Potential insertional mutagenesis; limited tissue tropism.	[Ferrari et al. (2007)]

15.4.1 Adenovirus

Adenoviruses (AdV) have been one of the first viral gene vectors tested in inhaled gene therapy clinical trials. They are non-enveloped DNA viruses, icosahedral capsid virions with diameters ranging from 70 nm to 100 nm. AdV has a genome capacity (36 kb) that is much larger than typical viruses. This allows relatively large therapeutic nucleic acids to be packaged, such as sequences encoding CFTR and alpha1-antitrypsin deficiency (AATD), respectively, the main genetic factors related to the onset of CF and COPD. Adenovirus vectors have a broad cell tropism and can infect non-dividing cells. This is an important advantage considering the slow turnover rate of airway epithelium (Rawlins and Hogan 2008). The disadvantage of these vectors is their episomal status in the host cell allowing only transient expression of the therapeutic gene. However, this aspect could also be considered as an advantage from a safety point of view, considering that, up to now, insertional mutagenesis without the integration into the genome has been not observed. Apart from this aspect, their main limitation is that they can induce inflammatory responses in the host organism, which can be also amplified by repeated administration as most likely required for inhaled gene therapy applications. To address this problem, several approaches have been investigated: (i) administration of immunosuppressors and corticosteroids, (ii) the development of helper-dependent ("gutted") adenoviral vectors, which are depleted of all viral genes, becoming in this way less immuno-stimulatory and safer compared to first generation viruses, which have only a subset of viral genes deleted, and (iii) the generation of a "stealth virus," which is invisible to the immune system, by coating the virus capsid with polyethylene glycol (PEG). PEGylation of the virus capsid reduced cytotoxic T cells and antibody production and significantly prolonged transgene expression from 4 days to 42 days. But still, repeated administration of the AdV modified with the same PEG was not successful (Croyle et al. 2001, Toietta et al. 2003, Tosi et al. 2004, Koehler et al. 2005).

Lastly, the coxsackievirus-adenovirus receptor (CAR) that is responsible for AdV entry into airway epithelial cells, resides on the basolateral side of the epithelium, resulting in a limitation of the potential efficacy *in vivo*. Related to this limitation, some studies have already shown how in absence of epithelial damage adenovirus-mediated gene transfer is inefficient in CF patients, despite encouraging results in nasal and pulmonary tissues of pre-clinical models and being well-tolerated at low to intermediate doses in humans (Walters et al. 1999, Griesenbach and Alton 2009).

15.4.2 Adeno-Associated Virus

Recent viral gene therapy trials have shifted to the use of adeno-associated virus (AAV), as it overcomes many limitations of adenoviruses. The AAV is a single stranded DNA virus and belongs to the family of parvoviruses. Its capsid contains two types of genes: *rep* and *cap*, respectively, encoding for polypeptides essential for replication and encapsidation. As vectors for gene delivery purposes, AAV has attracted much interest due to several desirable characteristics, such as the ability to infect a broad number of cells types, superior escape from immune system surveillance compared with other viruses, broad tissue tropism, high transduction efficiency, long duration of episomal expression, and, above all, a very good safety profile has been shown in various clinical trials (Duan et al. 1998, Daya and Berns 2008). Nevertheless, there are also some drawbacks that need to be overcome, for instance, the limited packaging capacity of the virus, that can only barely hold the CFTR gene (4.7 kb). Furthermore, the infection of target cells is mediated by cell surface-associated glycans depending on the AAV serotypes, and the individualization of the best-suited AAV serotypes for lung administration still needs to be addressed (Griesenbach and Alton 2009). The serotype AAV2 was the first one tested in clinical trials of inhaled gene therapy on CF patients (Wagner et al. 2002, Flotte et al. 2003, Moss et al. 2007). The results show that even if efficient gene transfer was demonstrated for nasal application, the lung function of CF patients was not improved (Wagner et al. 2002, Flotte et al. 2003, Moss et al. 2007). The possible explanations may be both: (i) the limited capacity of AAV2 to transduce airway epithelial cells via the apical membrane. In fact, as already seen for AdV, also AAV2 needs a receptor that is primarily expressed on the basolateral side of the airway epithelium in order to introduce nucleic acids into the cells (Wagner et al. 2002, Flotte et al. 2003). And (ii) repeated administrations may lead to the development of an anti-viral immune response (Summerford and Samulski 1998, Wagner et al. 2002, Flotte et al. 2003, Wu et al. 2006, Moss et al. 2007).

Attempting to overcome the limitation of AAV2, alternative AAV serotypes have been taken into consideration including AAV1, AAV5, AAV6, and AAV9 (Halbert et al. 2001, Gao et al. 2004, Limberis and Wilson 2006). In particular, AAV5 mediated 50-fold greater gene transfer efficiency than AAV2 in air-liquid interface (ALI) culture of primary human airway epithelium *in vitro* (Zabner et al. 2000, Sirninger et al. 2004, Virella-Lowell et al. 2005). The better transduction in airway epithelial cells can be explained because of a different receptor involved: the α2,3 N-linked receptor is expressed on the apical side (Liu et al. 2007). On the other hand, a higher gene transfer efficiency after intra-tracheal administration of AAV1 in the airway of chimpanzees has been seen in comparison with AAV5, motivating their development for inhaled gene therapy. However, it is important to keep in mind that chimpanzees are genetically different from humans, and, thus, this tropism needs to be tested in human cultures prior to being used in clinical trials (Liu et al. 2007, Flotte et al. 2010).

Referring to the small packaging capacity of the AVV capsid, several methods have been evaluated to achieve a higher encapsulation. So far, all the CF gene therapy trials have used the full-length wild-type CFTR gene to produce functional CFTR proteins, limiting the selection of other important elements such as the promoter and enhancer components and, thus, resulting in low expression caused by a weak promoter. In this regard, Ostedgaard et al. have shown that a CFTR cDNA, in which a portion of the R-domain has been deleted, leads to a partial correction of chloride transport *in vitro* (Ostedgaard et al. 2005). Fischer et al. established proof-of-principle that AAV2/5 carrying a truncated CFTR cDNA leads to vector-specific mRNA and protein expression in non-human primates (Fischer et al. 2007), indicating that the full-length wild-type CFTR gene is not necessary to produce functional CFTR proteins. As further alternative approach, splitting of the therapeutic cDNA has also been taken in consideration. It required promoter elements in two different viruses, which after the transfection in the same cell may recombine and generate a full-length therapeutic gene. This approach has been applied by Duan and co-workers using AAV2 (Duan et al. 2001). Their results show that the dual vector efficiency never matches the efficiency of the single vector, but refinements of these approaches may ultimately enhance efficiencies to their theoretical maximums. For example, defining the optimal length of the overlapping sequence would likely increase the efficiency of intermolecular recombination approaches. Additionally, as both dual vector approaches require co-infection of the same cell with two viral genomes, improvements in infectivity using alternative serotypes and higher titer virus would likely also increase the efficiencies. On the other hand, Halbert et al. have shown that upon intra-nasal administration of two AAV6 carrying overlapping fragments, the production of the encoded protein is comparable to the administration of a single AAV6 carrying the whole genome, suggesting that this recombination step may not significantly affect the transgene expression (Halbert et al. 2002).

15.4.3 Negative Strand RNA Virus

The murine parainfluenza virus type 1 (or Sendai virus (SeV)), the human respiratory syncytial virus (RSV), and the human parainfluenza virus type 3 (PIV3) are all efficiently able to transfect airway epithelial cells via the apical membrane using sialic acid and cholesterol, which are abundantly present on the apical surface of airway epithelial cells (Ferrari et al. 2004, Zhang et al. 2005). These viruses have a negative strand RNA genome and replicate in the cytoplasm. These viruses do not enter the nucleus and do not carry a risk of insertional mutagenesis because of the fact that there is not a DNA intermediate. Only SeV has been assessed in animal models *in vivo*, and it is very efficient in transducing airway epithelial cells. First-generation recombinant SeV carrying the CFTR cDNA has been shown to be able in the production of a functional CFTR chloride channels *in vitro* and after transfection of the nasal epithelium in CF knockout mice *in vivo* (Ferrari et al. 2007). The second generation of SeV vectors has been obtained by deleting the F-protein from the viral backbone (ΔF), making in this way the viruses transmission-incompetent while the transduction efficiency was not affected (Ferrari et al. 2004).

Inoue et al. have further improved the ΔF/SeV vector by introducing mutations into the matrix (M) and hemagglutinin-neuraminidase (HN) proteins, which reduced the amount of virus-like particles that are produced after transfection, thereby improving the safety profile (Inoue et al. 2003). SeV-mediated gene expression is transient (lasting for about 7 days) and currently repeated administration is inefficient. Immuno-modulatory strategies such as astolerization of mice to SeV immunodominant epitopes have so far not improved gene expression after repeated administration (Griesenbach et al. 2006). Although SeV may be useful for acute diseases that require only transient gene expression, in the context of CF, the use of SeV will be, as for adenovirus, restricted to pre-clinical proof-of-principle studies, until repeated administration problems can be solved.

15.4.4 Lentivirus

Retroviruses have been also investigated as potential viral vectors in gene therapy. A peculiar characteristic of these viruses is that they can retro-transcribe RNA to DNA using the cells' environments. Compared to AdV and AVV, they are able to integrate their whole nucleic acids into the host genome, and this of course can be an advantage if we consider the consequent long and stable transduction, but, on the other hand, it may also open the way for insertional mutations (Perricone et al. 2001). Furthermore, these kinds of viruses are not able to infect non-replicating cells, and this is certainly an important disadvantage for lung administration, considering the slow turnover of epithelial cells. In contrast to retroviruses, lentiviruses are able to transfect non-dividing cells, including post-mitotic cells such as parenchymal lung cells. Thus, recombinant human (HIV), feline (FIV), or equine (EIAV) immunodeficiency viruses can be suitable vectors for pulmonary gene therapy and have been already reported in literature. Lentiviral vectors have a packaging capacity large enough to accommodate full-length genes such as CFTR (Sakuma et al. 2012). However, they have a limited tissue tropism, and, thus, capsid engineering is required to enable their use in gene therapy applications. Initial inhaled gene transfer studies with lentiviruses focused on vectors pseudo types with vesicular stomatitis virus G glycoprotein (VSV-G), and this approach was used to generally improve the lentivirus' tropism. However, to achieve efficient transfection in mouse nose, pre-treatments with a compound able to disrupt tight junctions were necessary, suggesting that the transduction was achieved through the basolateral surface (Farrow et al. 2013, Cmielewski et al. 2014).

To bypass the need of adjuvant treatments, hybrid lentiviruses vectors were engineered by incorporating envelope proteins from SeV or baculo-virus. In fact, as mentioned above, members of the paramyxovirus family such as SeV and RSV transfect airway epithelial cells very efficiently due to their rapid interaction between the envelope glycoproteins and the cholesterol and sialic acid residues on the cell surface, respectively, demonstrating high tropism for the apical surface in the airway epithelium (Griesenbach and Alton 2013). Mitomo et al. (2010) were able to apically transduce polarized primary Cystic Fibrosis Human Airway Epithelium (CF HAE) cultures *in vitro* and CF mouse nasal epithelium *in vivo* using SeV-pseudotyped SIV (Mitomo et al. 2010). The transgene expression in mouse nasal epithelium lasted up to 1 year after a single administration with no sign of immune responses (Griesenbach et al. 2012). Even if this approach has significantly advanced the use of lentiviral vectors for inhaled gene therapy applications, lentiviruses would still likely need to be re-administrated, and therefore may face the same immune response problems as other viral vectors. This problem needs to be properly addressed and, until now, encouraging results have been published (Sinn et al. 2008).

15.5 Non-Viral Vectors

The majority of inhaled therapy clinical trials especially for obstructive lung diseases to date have evaluated virus-based gene vectors. However, intrinsic limitations to their use over the lifetime of a patient, including therapy-inactivating immunogenicity and insufficient gene transfer in human airways to elicit clinical benefits have spurred interest in the development of synthetic systems (Wang et al. 2012). Non-viral carriers have the potential to overcome many of the limitations of viral vectors and have emerged as a safer, cheaper, and "easier to be produced" alternative, especially counting on the continuous advance in the field of material science and nano-engineering. Along with the diversity of available materials, the synthesis, characterization, and functionalization of biocompatible nanomaterials for gene delivery purposes have been prompt and many researches are focused on the improvement of these non-viral synthetic systems. Non-viral vectors offer, at least theoretically, a number of advantages: easy preparation with low cost and large quantities (Zhang et al. 2008), low immune response, and lower risks in multiple administrations compared to viral vectors (Griesenbach et al. 2002). Moreover, these materials are supposed to be biocompatible and able to facilitate cellular internalization, escaping from the endosome and able to release the nucleic acids into the cytoplasm (Bergen et al. 2008). In addition, they can transfer large, multiple, and/or diverse nucleic acid payloads (Yin et al. 2014), and they can be stored for long periods due to their stability (Li and Huang 2000, Kircheis et al. 2001, Munier et al. 2005). The major drawback to their use in large scale is the low transfection efficiency (Putnam 2006). In fact, many cellular and intra-cellular barriers, that viruses overcome naturally, need to be considered during the engineering of these systems. Nevertheless, the major benefit of synthetic non-viral delivery systems is that they can be easily manipulated. Thus, to address this important issue, several strategies are available mostly using surface modifications, for instance, coating with PEG in order to enhance mucus penetration (Boylan et al. 2012) or target specific cell types and enhance intra-cellular delivery (Son et al. 2012). In general, non-viral deliveries include lipid-based vectors, polymer-based vectors, and inorganic material-based vectors Figure 15.1.

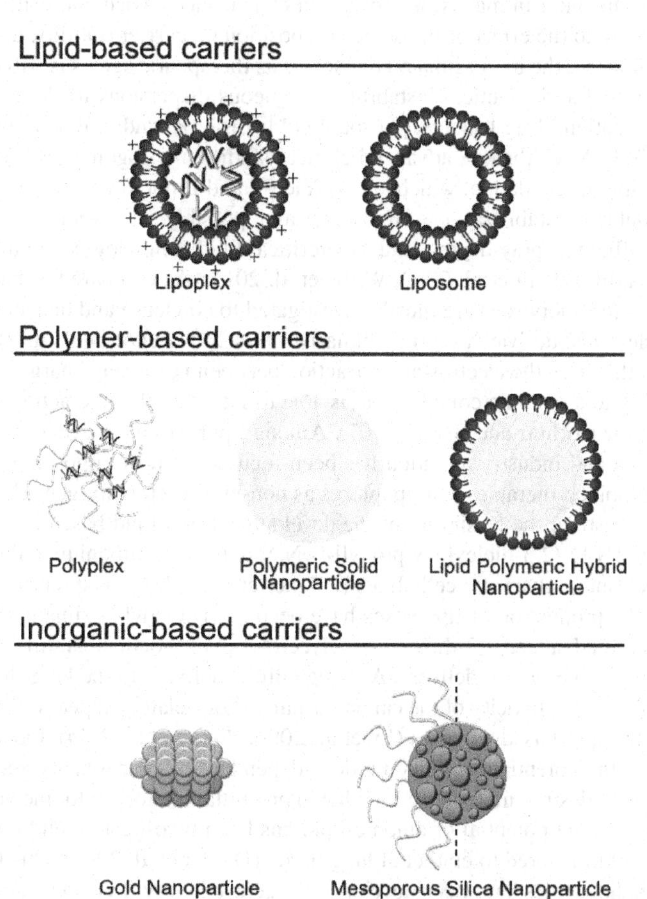

FIGURE 15.1 Summary of non-viral delivery approaches including lipid-based vectors, polymer-based vectors, and inorganic material-based vectors.

15.5.1 Lipid-Based Carriers

Lipids are a class of biological molecules defined by their hydrophobic and/or amphiphilic nature and, due to their high transfection efficiency as well as high drug loading capacity of both hydrophilic and hydrophobic drugs, are very attractive for the development of delivery systems. Moreover, one of the major advantages of lipid-based carriers is the possibility to reaching liposomal systems that can be easily engineered to yield a desired size, surface charge, composition, and morphology by just modifying the phospholipid composition (Foged 2012, Markman et al. 2013, Colombo et al. 2015). The most commonly employed lipid materials in drug carriers development, such as phospholipids and cholesterol, are well tolerated since they constitute a significant portion of the naturally occurring pulmonary surfactant pool (Jaafar-Maalej et al. 2012, Cipolla et al. 2013). Furthermore, the hydrophobic nature of lipids, especially of neutral lipids, reduces the absorption of ubiquitous vapor onto particles during inhalation, limiting aggregation, and adhesion phenomena (Pilcer and Amighi 2010). Lipid-based gene delivery systems include lipoplexes that electrostatically self-assemble with negatively charged nucleic acids, liposomes (neutral, anionic, and cationic) composed of phospholipids bilayer, and solid-lipid nanoparticles with a solid lipid core matrix enclosed in a lipid monolayer. Liposome-encapsulated drugs represent very promising drug delivery systems for lung targeting (Jaafar-Maalej et al. 2012, Allen and Cullis 2013, Cipolla et al. 2013). From a technological standpoint, liposomes have a great design versatility since single lipid blocks can be assembled, resulting in tuned physicochemical properties and, consequently, adequate interactions with mucus, biofilm matrix, and bacterial cell surface (Allen and Cullis 2013). Of course, attention should be paid to the effect of liposome composition on carrier stability, drug entrapment efficiency, and release. Indeed, the use of inhaled liposomes as therapeutic agents is still challenged by their well-established physical and chemical instability in aqueous dispersions for long-term storage, often causing vesicle aggregation, drug leakage, phospholipid hydrolysis, and/or oxidation (Chen et al. 2010, Allen and Cullis 2013). Nevertheless, advanced clinical studies are ongoing on two neutral liposomal formulations for antibiotic inhalation, which are Arikace™ and Lipoquin™ (ARD-3100). Furthermore, many methods available for stabilization of liposomes and, possibly, achievement of DPI liposomal formulations (e.g. lyophilizing, spray-drying, and supercritical fluid technology) are currently being investigated (Chen et al. 2010, Misra et al. 2009, Willis et al. 2012). As compared to bare liposomes, lipid cationic nanocarriers (or lipoplexes) are mostly investigated to condense and deliver negatively charged DNA and short nucleic acid derivatives intra-cellularly (Dass 2004, Alton et al. 2013). In fact, a lipoplex is a delivery system that uses the electrostatic attraction between negatively charged nucleic acids and a cationic lipid, leading to a cationic complex that is able to facilitate the interaction with the negatively charged cell membrane (Akhtar and Benter 2007). Among lipid-based carriers of interest in inhalation therapy, both research and industry attention has been focused on novel liposome-based formulations for antibiotic and combined therapies and lipoplexes as non-viral vectors for gene therapy. Felgner et al. were the first to demonstrate the feasibility of the development of a lipid-based carrier by using a non-natural cationic lipid [N-[1-(2,3-dioleyloxy)propyl]-N,N,N-trimethylammonium chloride (DOTMA)] to deliver plasmid DNA into eukaryotic cells lines (Felgner et al. 1987). Since then, other cationic lipids commonly used in the production of lipoplexes have been 1,2-Dioleoyl-3-trimethylammoniumpropane (DOTAP), or the more advanced 1,2-dioleoyl-sn-glycerol-3-phosphoethanolamine (DOPE), especially used in order to improve the *in vivo* delivery. Although direct delivery to the lung should limit systemic side effects of lipoplexes, the toxicity of the carrier, usually dose-related, appears still critical for *in vivo* translation of cationic lipid-based particles (Lv et al. 2006, Weber et al. 2014). Indeed, the major issue related to their use is the potential for inducing dose-dependent cellular toxicity and, when complexed with DNA, triggering undesired macrophage-mediated pro-inflammatory cytokine production. As alternative to cationic lipids, the potential of anionic lipid has been investigated, and their safety has been demonstrated when administered to epithelial lung tissue (Dokka et al. 2000). Due to their high safety and stability, anionic liposomes have been developed for gene delivery (Lee and Huang 1996, Patil et al. 2004, Kapoor and Burgess 2012). However, these vectors have limited applications, mainly because of the poor association between nucleic acid molecules and anionic lipids caused by electrostatic repulsion that leads to a low encapsulation efficacy; furthermore, the electrostatic repulsion also affects the transfection efficacy. In order to overcome this issue, some authors propose the use of cationic helper molecules such as calcium chloride, poly (amino acid), or some arginine rich oligomers in order to form an initial complex with nucleic acids which is then encapsulated in or among anionic liposomes to form the lipoplex. Still, the potential cytotoxicity of these helper molecules needs to be addressed. Solid lipid nanoparticles (SLNs) are also being explored as a viable alternative to liposomes for drug and gene delivery to the lung. SLNs constitute of a solid lipid core matrix that is enclosed and stabilized by a lipid monolayer on the surface. Compared with liposomes, the chemical and physical stability in biological environments are both higher. SLNs have evolved into particles known as nanostructured lipid carriers (NLCs), made of a blend of a solid lipid and an oil consisting in a semi-crystal structure with more flexibility and are able to better accommodate drugs (Weber et al. 2014). NLCs have the same advantages as SLNs, that is controlled drug release, improved chemical stability of encapsulated drug molecules, and simple and inexpensive production, also on a large scale. Especially the production aspect is a great advantage compared to liposomes.

15.5.2 Polymer-Based Carriers

Although it can be dated back to the 1990s (Edwards et al. 1997), the concept of using polymer particles for pulmonary delivery has evolved over time and is experiencing a growing research interest in recent years. A fundamental feature of polymer systems, which is only partly shared by liposomal carriers, relies on their ability to exert a prolonged drug release. This is crucial to reduce the number of administrations and increase patient adherence to complex therapeutic regimens required by chronic lung diseases, such as CF (Geller and Madge 2011). Polymer particles also have the potential: (i) to increase *drug stability in vivo* and its shelf life; (ii) to co-deliver different molecules with complementary functionalities; and (iii) to promote cell uptake of delivered drug cargos. Indeed, various systemic and cellular barriers imposed to nucleic acid-based therapeutics, including nucleases, the cell membrane, endosomal compartment, and nuclear membrane may be successfully circumvented by adequately designed polymer carriers. Nevertheless, to be successful, design of inhalable Nanoparticles (NPs) should take into account well-defined rules to overcome limitations associated with the pulmonary route of administration, providing adequate composition, size, and surface modification along with respirability. Furthermore, polymeric NPs have to be able to escape the endosome and prevent their subsequent degradation after fusion with a lysosome. Still, more generally, the fate of nanomaterials under physiological conditions must be determined and eventual undesired interactions with protein or other components, that can result in aggregation, have to be considered. In general, this class of vectors can be further subdivided into polycations that electrostatically self-assemble with negatively charged nucleic acids to form so-called polyplexes and polymeric solid nanoparticles which encapsulate their load. Poly(ethylenimine) (PEI), is used as non-viral gene transfer agent since the 1990s, and today it is still one of the most popular polymers in lung delivery of nucleic acids, especially siRNA. It has been extensively explored as a state of the art gene carrier for *in vitro* and *in vivo* applications. PEI readily forms polyplexes with nucleic acids via electrostatic self-assembly. Despite the high transfection efficiency and the possibility to be used as multifunctional excipient, for instance, in the inhaled therapy of CF due to its confirmed synergic anti-microbial properties against *P. aeruginosa* (Khalil et al. 2008), several drawbacks have to be taken into account. Most importantly, PEI is not a degradable polymer and can aggregate in the lung and bloodstream, resulting in high toxicity. To overcome this limitation, PEI with low molecular weight has been shown to be less toxic *in vivo*, but also exhibits lower transfection ability (Kasper et al. 2013). Based upon these results, derivatives of PEI obtained from PEI with low molecular weight and a variety of modifications have been studied (Beyerle et al. 2011). Even if some promising results regarding transfection efficacy have been achieved, the potential of PEI-based gene carriers needs to be improved. Among polymers currently under investigation, synthetic biodegradable polymers represent the most promising class of materials for pulmonary delivery, as evidenced by increasing literature data, fulfilling also important safety concerns. Chitosan is a natural polysaccharide that is generally accepted as biocompatible and biodegradable (Mao et al. 2010). It can form stable complexes with DNA, has low cytotoxicity, and is suitable for gene delivery to the lung because of its mucoadhesive characteristics (Koping-Hoggard et al. 2004). Some studies have already demonstrated the efficacy of inhalable chitosan siRNA dry powders composed of unmodified chitosan mediating effective induction of gene silencing *in vitro* in lung models (Okuda et al. 2013, Ihara et al. 2015). The major drawbacks are: (i) poor water solubility and (ii) low transfection efficiency. In order to improve these limitations, several polymer modifications have been tested, producing, for instance, a guanidinylated chitosan (GCS) (Luo et al. 2012) or an O-carboxymethylchitosan-*graft*-branched polyethylenimine (OCMPEI) (Park et al. 2013). The polyplexes were injected intravenous (i.v.) and mediated excellent green fluorescent protein (GFP) expression in the lung, supporting the idea that this delivery system may as well be successful for nucleic acids delivery in the lung after i.v. or even local administration. Another promising biodegradable co-polymer is poly(lactic-co-glycolic acid) (PLGA) which has generated tremendous research interest due to its excellent biocompatibility as well as the possibility to tailor its biodegradability by varying monomer composition (lactide/glycolide ratio), molecular weight, and chemical structure (i.e. capped and uncapped end-groups) (Ungaro et al. 2012a). PLGAs characterized by very different *in vivo* life-times, ranging from 3 weeks to over a year, are available and approved for human use. Among all commercially available PLGA types, those characterized by a rapid *in vitro* degradation are undoubtedly preferred for inhalation and have shown improved toxicity profile compared to other synthetic polymers on both healthy (Coowanitwong et al. 2008, Jensen et al. 2012) and CF human airway epithelial cells (De Stefano et al. 2011, Ungaro et al. 2012b).

Drug encapsulation within PLGA co-polymers is regarded also as a powerful means to achieve its sustained release for long time frames and, in case of labile drugs, to effectively protect the molecule from *in vivo* degradation occurring at the administration site. To increase the availability of the delivered drug at the lung target, engineered inhalable PLGA particles have been developed through the addition of specific excipients (Ungaro et al. 2012a). On the nanosized level, particle surface modification with helper hydrophilic polymers (e.g. PEG, poloxamer, chitosan, polyvinyl alcohol) have been found useful to modulate carrier interactions with lung cellular and extracellular barriers (Mura et al. 2011, Ensign et al. 2012). To tune NP interaction with the lung microenvironment, hydrophilic polymers, both mucoadhesive (e.g. chitosan, hyaluronic acid) and mucoinert (PEG), have been employed to impart the desired surface properties (Tang et al. 2009). Despite promising results, the effect of hydrophilic polymers in modulating PLGA NP/mucus interactions is still unclear and debated. It has recently been observed that PLGA NPs of 200 nm–500 nm modified at surface with non-adhesive PEG, so-called mucus penetrating particles, may deeply penetrate human mucus secretions (Tang et al. 2009). Nevertheless, surface modifications of PLGA NPs may have also a significant impact on their interaction with the target cell. For example, the uptake of PLGA NPs into macrophages may be significantly reduced upon PEGylation. Overcoming the cell membrane to reach intra-cellular targets is especially mandatory, in case of emerging nucleic-acid therapeutics (Lam et al. 2012, Patel et al. 2015). Lastly, since PLGA nanoparticles exhibit a negative surface charge, they can be modified with hydrophilic and cationic polymers, such as PEI and chitosan, for electrostatic adsorption of nucleic acids. To adsorb siRNA, negatively charged PLGA nanoparticles are often modified with a strong cationic polymer, such as PEI. In a typical study, PEI-modified nanoparticles were used for co-delivery of paclitaxel and an siRNA therapeutic for cancer therapy. Paclitaxel, the hydrophobic anti-cancer drug, was encapsulated in PLGA nanoparticles, and stat3 siRNA was adsorbed onto the PLGA-PEI nanoparticles through electrostatic interaction. The researchers used fluorescence measurements to confirm that stat3 siRNA and Paclitaxel (PTX) were delivered simultaneously to A549 lung cancer cells via PLGA-PEI nanoparticles. Stat3 is activated in lung cancer cells (A549 and A549/T12), and siRNA-based silencing of the stat3 gene using PLGAPEI-TAX-S3SI nanoparticles rendered cancer cells more sensitive to PTX and produced more cellular apoptosis than PLGA-PEI-TAX did (Su et al. 2012). Lastly, Lipid-PLGA hybrid nanoparticles with core-shell morphology have been especially designed for siRNA delivery (Raemdonck et al. 2014, d'Angelo et al. 2018). In particular, recent progresses in nanotechnologies and emerging knowledge on the properties of the nano-bio interface have paved the way towards core-shell lipid-polymer hybrid NPs, where the synthetic polymeric core is surrounded with a phospholipid bilayer of natural origin (De Backer et al. 2015).

15.5.3 Inorganic-Based Carriers

Most delivery systems in clinical use for drug delivery are based on liposomal or polymer carrier. However, also inorganic nanoparticles are widely studied, and inorganic materials are used for a variety of applications devised for diagnostic and therapeutic purposes. Some of the inorganic materials used in drug delivery are calcium phosphate, gold, iron oxide, and silica. It is clear how, in the attempt to achieve effective delivery systems, physical properties, such as size, shape, charge density, elasticity, and colloidal stability are important attributes that determine the suitability of inorganic materials for a specific function. In fact, many inorganic materials offer ease of functionalization, unique electrical and optical properties, biocompatibility, as well as low cytotoxicity, and, because of all these advantages, they are so highly sought after in the drug delivery field (Qiu et al. 2016). Lipid/calcium/phosphate (LCP) nanoparticles, composed, respectively, of lipid calcium and phosphate, have been proposed to deliver siRNA in the treatment of lung cancer and its metastases and exhibited a remarkable ability to improve the transfection efficacy of nucleic acid drugs (Li et al. 2010, Zhang et al. 2013b). LCPs have been evaluated after administration *via* intravenous injection in a lung cancer xenograft model. In particular, Li et al. developed LCP modified on the surface by PEG conjugation in order to actively target the sigma receptor in lung cancer cells, and siRNA labeled with Cy5.5 was loaded in the LCPs (Li et al. 2010). On the other hand, Zhang et al. proposed the LCPs as co-delivery system for siRNA and gemcitabine monophosphate as chemotherapeutic drug (Zhang et al. 2013a, 2013b). Li et al. showed that siRNA is efficiently able to reach the primary H460 xenograft, and about 50% luciferase knockdown was reported in the luciferase expressing primary tumor. On the other hand, the combined therapy mediates not only the induction of the apoptosis in the tumor cells, but also a dramatic inhibition of tumour growth. At the same time, very low toxicity *in vivo* was observed (Zhang et al. 2013a). However, it needs to be noted that the xenografts model does not necessarily reflect the accumulation and uptake into the lung or a lung tumor. Therefore, further studies are required in order to evaluate if LCPs are effectively able to reach the lung upon aerosolization and, subsequently, to evaluate also their activity when locally applied.

Additionally, metal-based nanoparticles have been widely studied for applications in imaging and drug delivery, and gold nanomaterials are so far the most widely investigated type. Gold offers a surface characterized by high flexibility which assists its functionalization and enables gold nanoparticles to be ideal for application as gene delivery system (Giljohann et al. 2009). On the other hand, one of the biggest challenges preventing gold nanoparticles (AuNPs) from entering the clinic is tuning and optimizing surface and physical properties to ensure maximum functionality without inducing toxic effects at the biological level. To this regard, Conde et al. have prepared AuNPs by first modifying the surface with PEG and later adding the targeting peptide arginine-glycine-aspartate (RGD). Lastly, on the surface c-myc siRNA was conjugated and carried by the system. The AuNPs produced were intratracheally administrated through instillation in mice CMT/167 bearing lung carcinoma tumors. The results obtained clearly show an efficient c-myc oncogene down-regulation with a reduction in tumor growth. Nevertheless, further studies are required considering that also a strong inflammatory reaction has been observed suggesting the idea that immune responses might enhance the effectiveness of the anti-tumor treatment (Conde et al. 2013). In another study, Guo et al. produced a pH-dependent gene delivery system. AuNPs were chemically modified with carboxylic acid chains and then coated with PEI as pH-dependent charge-reversal polyelectrolyte for controlled release of siRNA and plasmid DNA after pH change in the endosome (Guo et al. 2010). Mesoporous silica-based nanoparticles (MSNs) are novel drug carriers with unique properties, such as high loading capability with tunable pore sizes and volumes for transport of a wide variety of cargo molecules (Trewyn et al. 2007). MSNs are chemically stable, safe, and biodegradable which makes them a promising gene delivery system, especially for the application in the therapy of complex diseases such as cancer. In fact, thanks to their particular structure, MSNs can be functionalized to effectively deliver two or more therapeutics agents at the same time, and this possibility appears particularly helpful against multiple drug resistance (MDR) phenomena. In order to overcome this MDR issue, a co-delivery strategy that utilizes an siRNA to silence the expression of P-glycoprotein and MDR protein family, together with an appropriate anti-cancer drug is regarded with great interest and early *in vitro* studies have already shown successful results. For instance, Meng and co-workers reported that MSNs can be functionalized to effectively deliver the chemotherapeutic agent doxorubicin as well as Pgp siRNA to a drug-resistant cancer cell line (KB-V1 cells) to accomplish cell killing in an additive or synergistic fashion. Consistent with this hypothesis, the results demonstrate the effectiveness of MSNs as a platform to deliver a siRNA that knocks down gene expression of a drug exporter that can be used to improve drug sensitivity to a chemotherapeutic agent (Meng et al. 2010).

In light of these results, MSNs have been investigated also as lung delivery systems in lung cancer therapy. van Rijt and co-workers showed that tight surface modification on MSNs can induce an optimal release of the drug, not only *in vitro* in a human lung tissue model, but also in an advanced mouse model (Kras mutant mice) that closely reflects the human pathophysiology (van Rijt et al. 2015). Furthermore, the same MSNs were evaluated *in vivo* upon direct (intratracheal) instillation in the lungs of mice. Specifically looking at the pulmonary distribution, clearance rate, cell specific uptake, and induction of inflammatory response, the results obtained, such as low surface specific toxicity, wide distribution, and slow clearance rate, make this drug delivery system promising not only for the treatment of lung cancer, but, in perspective, for the treatments of other severe lung diseases.

15.6 Clinical Translation

In 2012, the European Medicines Agency (EMA) approved Glybera (alipogene tiparvovec) as the first gene therapy treatment for sale in the European Union. Even if Glybera has been withdrawn in October 2017 due to lack of demand, its approval still represents the culmination of many years of research on DNA delivery with the help of viruses. In fact, Glybera is an adeno-associated virus (AAV)-mediated delivery of DNA for the treatment of the inherited metabolic disorder lipoprotein lipase deficiency (Yla-Herttuala 2012, Schuster, 2013, 2014, Ferreira et al. 2014, Watanabe et al. 2015, Mullard 2016).

For the record, Glybera was not the first approved viral vector for gene therapy worldwide: in 2003, China approved the first gene therapy product, Gendicine™, based on an AdV vector and indicated for the treatment of head and neck squamous cell carcinoma (Li et al. 2015). Later, China approved the second gene therapy product, Oncorine™, in 2005, which is also based on an AdV vector and is indicated for the treatment of late stage refractory nasopharyngeal cancer (Liang 2012); in 2015, the gene therapy product IMLYGIC™ was approved in the United States, which is based on a herpes simplex virus (HSV) vector and is indicated for local treatment of unresectable cutaneous, subcutaneous, and nodal lesions in patients with melanoma recurrent after initial surgery (Pol et al. 2016). Despite the fact that none of these products are intended for pulmonary administration, it is clear how viral-vectors are in advantage compared to non-viral vectors. Despite all the promise about the use of non-viral carriers, there is no gene therapy that involves a non-viral vector on the market. Additionally, clinical trials of inhaled gene therapies employ more viral-based delivery systems than non-viral carriers (Griesenbach and Alton 2009, Mueller and Flotte 2013).

Gene vectors tested for inhaled therapy to date have failed to demonstrate a clear clinical benefit despite encouraging results obtained in animal models Table 15.2.

The leading material of non-viral vectors for lung cancer and metastasis treatment in the clinics is based on a lipid vector: in 2012, Lu and co-workers (2012) used lipid-based NP comprising of DOTAP carrying pDNA encoding tumor suppressing candidate 2 (TUSC2), a tumor suppressor that is commonly inactivated in lung cancer. These NPs were administered intravenously and tested in a phase I clinical trial. TUSC2 is supposed to mediate apoptosis in rapidly dividing, but not in healthy cells. The reduced tumor metabolic activity observed in general and the comparison of pre- and post-treatment scans of a single patient support the efficacy of this NP system, nevertheless, a range of toxic effects were seen in treated patients. Even if it was unclear whether these effects were due to off-target effects of gene expression or non-specificity of the NP, these studies underline how NP systems can be safely administered in lung cancer patients, but at the same time a direct action supported by the use of a targeted system and the direct administration is strictly required (Lu et al. 2012).

In this sense, siRNA has been the first to make significant progress in the treatment of respiratory diseases with a couple of clinical studies investigating its efficacy *via* pulmonary delivery. In the ALS-RSV01 study conducted by Alnylam Pharmaceuticals, their cholesterol-modified siRNA to treat respiratory syncytial virus (RSV) infection in lung transplant patients was evaluated upon nebulization in a phase II completed clinical study (Zamora et al. 2011, Gottlieb et al. 2016). Another inhaled siRNA-based therapeutic that passed the phase I safety trial and entered the phase II efficacy trial is Excellair™.

TABLE 15.2
Summary of Clinical Trials of NPs used for Gene Delivery in Respiratory Diseases

Company or University	Condition	Nucleic Acid	System	Delivery	Status	Year	Ref.
Alnylam Pharmaceuticals	RSV infection in lung transplant patients	N protein siRNA (ALN_RSV01)	Naked siRNA	Inhalation	Phase II completed	2011	Liang (2012), Pol et al. (2016)
University of Texas MD Anderson Cancer Center	Lung cancer	pDNA encoding tumor suppressing candidate 2	1,2-Dioleoyl-3-trimethylammoniumpropane, cholesterol liposome	Intravenous	Phase I	2012	Li et al. (2015)
ZaBeCor Pharmaceuticals	Asthma	Syk siRNA (Excellair®)	Naked siRNA	Inhalation	Phase I completed Phase II	2012	Mueller et al. (2013), Lu et al. (2012)
Imperial College of London	Cystic fibrosis	pDNA encoding CFTR	Cationic liposome	Inhalation	Phase II completed	2015	Gottlieb et al. (2016)

This study was aimed to treat asthma and was conducted by the ZaBeCor Pharmaceuticals Company. Although the results from Excellair™ I trial looked very promising, to date there is not information about the current state (Watts and Corey 2010, Burnett et al. 2011). Lastly, Alton et al. have recently completed a phase IIb clinical trial demonstrating that nebulization of a cationic liposome used as gene vectors, carrying a pDNA encoding the CFTR gene, was safely inhaled by CF patients also providing a modest, but significant beneficial effect (Alton et al. 2015). Taken together, these are all promising and encouraging results. Nevertheless, the research journey still seems to be long before an efficient non-viral carrier for gene therapy will be approved on the market.

In August 2018, the Food and Drug Administration "https://www.fda.gov/NewsEvents/Newsroom/PressAnnouncements/ucm616518.htm" approved the first-ever small interfering RNA (siRNA) product, and Alnylam secured approval and Orphan Drug Designation for its siRNA product Onpattro (patisiran), marking a significant milestone in the history of siRNA therapy and opening the path to other possible therapies.

15.7 Future Prospective

Nowadays, gene therapy is considered one of the most attractive therapeutic strategies to treat pulmonary diseases, especially considering that numerous genetic targets and the monogenic nature of pathologies as CF have been identified. Nevertheless, the therapeutic potential of nucleic acids in the treatment of lung diseases has yet to be fully explored, partially due to the physicochemical characteristics that affect their pharmacokinetics and pharmacodynamics and partially because of the challenging administration route. Extensive research has been conducted in order to develop suitable delivery strategies and to date, these strategies can be grouped in two big families, viral and non-viral delivery systems, which can be further subdivided in other small families. Each of these families have several advantages, but still several drawbacks. Viral vectors offer high transfection efficacy due to their origin, but, at the same time, they are often not able to encapsidate all the genetic material required and too often they induce high immune responses. In order to overcome these limitations, research attention has been focused on the development of non-viral vectors that seem to be able to protect the payload, which can be carried in high amounts without inducing immune responses, but, at the same time, are characterized by a low transfection efficacy. What today seems to be the best approach in order to overcome the limitations imposed by the characteristics of single strategies is to merge the different characteristics in order to develop a strengthened delivery system (i.e. stealth virus with PEGylated capsid or hybrid lipid/polymer nanoparticles). However, what is important to underline is that, in order to avoid failure in clinical trials, independent of the approach applied, relevant pre-clinical models are needed to better predict the performance in clinical trials. For instance, an *in vitro* improved transfection or transgene expression often does not correlate with the results obtained after *in vivo* administration. *In vitro* and *in vivo* experiments need to be designed carefully, taking in consideration complex cellular models which can better mimic the human physiology or physiopathology. Three-dimensional tumor spheroids and air-liquid interface airway cultures based on human primary cancer and airway epithelial cells, respectively, are a few examples of system that can better represent the barriers to *in vivo* delivery (de Souza Carvalho et al. 2014). Also, considering the importance of mucus as barrier in inhaled therapy, especially in case of obstructive diseases such as COPD and CF, the use of *ex vivo* models may be helpful to evaluate the real ability to penetrate through the human airway mucus barrier (Schuster et al. 2013, 2014). Moreover, most pre-clinical studies have been conducted in short-term mice models for their low cost. But murine lungs are different from human lungs and are not able to reproduce the human pathologies. There is a lack of data from animal models where the profiles of nanoparticles distribution, deposition, uptake, as well as the risk-benefit ratios and cost-benefit ratios may differ in significant ways from that in the mouse lung. Finally, even if an ideal *in vitro/in vivo* model satisfactory to individualize the best drug delivery system was developed, only information about the transport in lung lining fluid, uptake, and gene expression could be assessed. This information is not enough to predict the aerosolization profile of the formulation, which is essential not only to reach the cellular targets in the deep lung, but also to arrive at the right dose in order to produce a pharmacological benefit. In conclusion, a global knowledge about the dosage form, the organism, the cells involved, and molecular biology process supported by relevant pre-clinical settings is crucial to success with gene therapy against lung diseases.

REFERENCES

Akhtar, S., and I. F. Benter. 2007. "Nonviral delivery of synthetic siRNAs in vivo." *J Clin Invest* 117 (12):3623–3632. doi:10.1172/jci33494.

Alamgeer, M., V. Ganju, and D. N. Watkins. 2013. "Novel therapeutic targets in non-small cell lung cancer." *Curr Opin Pharmacol* 13 (3):394–401. doi:10.1016/j.coph.2013.03.010.

Allen, T. M., and P. R. Cullis. 2013. "Liposomal drug delivery systems: From concept to clinical applications." *Adv Drug Deliv Rev* 65 (1):36–48. doi:10.1016/j.addr.2012.09.037.

Alton, E. W., A. C. Boyd, S. H. Cheng, S. Cunningham, J. C. Davies, D. R. Gill, U. Griesenbach et al. 2013. "A randomised, double-blind, placebo-controlled phase IIB clinical trial of repeated application of gene therapy in patients with cystic fibrosis." *Thorax* 68 (11):1075–1077. doi:10.1136/thoraxjnl-2013-203309.

Alton, E. W. F. W., D. K. Armstrong, D. Ashby, K. J. Bayfield, D. Bilton, E. V. Bloomfield, A. C. Boyd et al. 2015. "Repeated nebulisation of non-viral CFTR gene therapy in patients with cystic fibrosis: A randomised, double-blind, placebo-controlled, phase 2b trial." *Lancet Respir Med* 3 (9):684–691. doi:10.1016/s2213-2600(15)00245-3.

Attarwala, H., M. Han, J. Kim, and M. Amiji. 2017. "Oral nucleic acid therapy using multicompartmental delivery systems." *Wiley Interdiscip Rev Nanomed Nanobiotechnol.* doi:10.1002/wnan.1478.

Bergen, J. M., I. K. Park, P. J. Horner, and S. H. Pun. 2008. "Nonviral approaches for neuronal delivery of nucleic acids." *Pharm Res* 25 (5):983–998. doi:10.1007/s11095-007-9439-5.

Beyerle, A., A. Braun, O. Merkel, F. Koch, T. Kissel, and T. Stoeger. 2011. "Comparative in vivo study of poly(ethylene imine)/siRNA complexes for pulmonary delivery in mice." *J Control Release* 151 (1):51–56. doi:10.1016/j.jconrel.2010.12.017.

Boylan, N. J., J. S. Suk, S. K. Lai, R. Jelinek, M. P. Boyle, M. J. Cooper, and J. Hanes. 2012. "Highly compacted DNA nanoparticles with low MW PEG coatings: In vitro, ex vivo and in vivo evaluation." *J Control Release* 157 (1):72–79. doi:10.1016/j.jconrel.2011.08.031.

Burnett, J. C., J. J. Rossi, and K. Tiemann. 2011. "Current progress of siRNA/shRNA therapeutics in clinical trials." *Biotechnol J* 6 (9):1130-1146. doi:10.1002/biot.201100054.

Chen, C., D. Han, C. Cai, and X. Tang. 2010. "An overview of liposome lyophilization and its future potential." *J Control Release* 142 (3):299–311. doi:10.1016/j.jconrel.2009.10.024.

Cipolla, D., I. Gonda, and H. K. Chan. 2013. "Liposomal formulations for inhalation." *Ther Deliv* 4 (8):1047–1072. doi:10.4155/tde.13.71.

Cmielewski, P., N. Farrow, M. Donnelley, C. McIntyre, J. Penny-Dimri, T. Kuchel, and D. Parsons. 2014. "Transduction of ferret airway epithelia using a pre-treatment and lentiviral gene vector." *BMC Pulm Med* 14:183. doi:10.1186/1471-2466-14-183.

Colombo, S., D. Cun, K. Remaut, M. Bunker, J. Zhang, B. Martin-Bertelsen, A. Yaghmur, K. Braeckmans, H. M. Nielsen, and C. Foged. 2015. "Mechanistic profiling of the siRNA delivery dynamics of lipid-polymer hybrid nanoparticles." *J Control Release* 201:22–31. doi:10.1016/j.jconrel.2014.12.026.

Conde, J., F. Tian, Y. Hernandez, C. Bao, D. Cui, K. P. Janssen, M. R. Ibarra, P. V. Baptista, T. Stoeger, and J. M. de la Fuente. 2013. "In vivo tumor targeting via nanoparticle-mediated therapeutic siRNA coupled to inflammatory response in lung cancer mouse models." *Biomaterials* 34 (31):7744–7753. doi:10.1016/j.biomaterials.2013.06.041.

Coowanitwong, I., V. Arya, P. Kulvanich, and G. Hochhaus. 2008. "Slow release formulations of inhaled rifampin." *AAPS J* 10 (2):342–348. doi:10.1208/s12248-008-9044-5.

Croyle, M. A., N. Chirmule, Y. Zhang, and J. M. Wilson. 2001. "'Stealth' adenoviruses blunt cell-mediated and humoral immune responses against the virus and allow for significant gene expression upon readministration in the lung." *J Virol* 75 (10):4792–4801. doi:10.1128/jvi.75.10.4792-4801.2001.

d'Angelo, I., G. Costabile, E. Durantie, P. Brocca, V. Rondelli, A. Russo, G. Russo et al. 2018. "Hybrid lipid/polymer nanoparticles for pulmonary delivery of siRNA: Development and fate upon in vitro deposition on the human epithelial airway barrier." *J Aerosol Med Pulm Drug Deliv.* doi:10.1089/jamp.2017.1364.

Dass, C. R. 2004. "Lipoplex-mediated delivery of nucleic acids: Factors affecting in vivo transfection." *J Mol Med (Berl)* 82 (9):579–591. doi:10.1007/s00109-004-0558-8.

Daya, S., and K. I. Berns. 2008. "Gene therapy using adeno-associated virus vectors." *Clin Microbiol Rev* 21 (4):583–593. doi:10.1128/cmr.00008-08.

De Backer, L., K. Braeckmans, M. C. Stuart, J. Demeester, S. C. De Smedt, and K. Raemdonck. 2015. "Bio-inspired pulmonary surfactant-modified nanogels: A promising siRNA delivery system." *J Control Release* 206:177–186. doi:10.1016/j.jconrel.2015.03.015.

de Souza Carvalho, C., N. Daum, and C. M. Lehr. 2014. "Carrier interactions with the biological barriers of the lung: Advanced in vitro models and challenges for pulmonary drug delivery." *Adv Drug Deliv Rev* 75:129–140. doi:10.1016/j.addr.2014.05.014.

De Stefano, D., F. Ungaro, C. Giovino, A. Polimeno, F. Quaglia, and R. Carnuccio. 2011. "Sustained inhibition of IL-6 and IL-8 expression by decoy ODN to NF-kappaB delivered through respirable large porous particles in LPS-stimulated cystic fibrosis bronchial cells." *J Gene Med* 13 (4):200–208. doi:10.1002/jgm.1546.

Dokka, S., D. Toledo, X. Shi, V. Castranova, and Y. Rojanasakul. 2000. "Oxygen radical-mediated pulmonary toxicity induced by some cationic liposomes." *Pharm Res* 17 (5):521–525.

Dowdy, S. F. 2017. "Overcoming cellular barriers for RNA therapeutics." *Nat Biotechnol* 35 (3):222–229. doi:10.1038/nbt.3802.

Duan, D., P. Sharma, J. Yang, Y. Yue, L. Dudus, Y. Zhang, K. J. Fisher, and J. F. Engelhardt. 1998. "Circular intermediates of recombinant adeno-associated virus have defined structural characteristics responsible for long-term episomal persistence in muscle tissue." *J Virol* 72 (11):8568–8577.

Duan, D., Y. Yue, and J. F. Engelhardt. 2001. "Expanding AAV packaging capacity with trans-splicing or overlapping vectors: A quantitative comparison." *Mol Ther* 4 (4):383–391. doi:10.1006/mthe.2001.0456.

Edwards, D. A., J. Hanes, G. Caponetti, J. Hrkach, A. Ben-Jebria, M. L. Eskew, J. Mintzes, D. Deaver, N. Lotan, and R. Langer. 1997. "Large porous particles for pulmonary drug delivery." *Science* 276 (5320):1868–1871.

Ensign, L. M., C. Schneider, J. S. Suk, R. Cone, and J. Hanes. 2012. "Mucus penetrating nanoparticles: Biophysical tool and method of drug and gene delivery." *Adv Mater* 24 (28):3887–3894.

Farrow, N., D. Miller, P. Cmielewski, M. Donnelley, R. Bright, and D. W. Parsons. 2013. "Airway gene transfer in a non-human primate: Lentiviral gene expression in marmoset lungs." *Sci Rep* 3:1287. doi:10.1038/srep01287.

Felgner, P. L., T. R. Gadek, M. Holm, R. Roman, H. W. Chan, M. Wenz, J. P. Northrop, G. M. Ringold, and M. Danielsen. 1987. "Lipofection: A highly efficient, lipid-mediated DNA-transfection procedure." *Proc Natl Acad Sci U S A* 84 (21):7413–7417.

Ferrari, S., U. Griesenbach, A. Iida, R. Farley, A. M. Wright, J. Zhu, F. M. Munkonge et al. 2007. "Sendai virus-mediated CFTR gene transfer to the airway epithelium." *Gene Ther* 14 (19):1371–1379. doi:10.1038/sj.gt.3302991.

Ferrari, S., U. Griesenbach, T. Shiraki-Iida, T. Shu, T. Hironaka, X. Hou, J. Williams et al. 2004. "A defective nontransmissible recombinant Sendai virus mediates efficient gene transfer to airway epithelium in vivo." *Gene Ther* 11 (22):1659–1664. doi:10.1038/sj.gt.3302334.

Ferreira, V., H. Petry, and F. Salmon. 2014. "Immune responses to AAV-vectors, the Glybera example from bench to bedside." *Front Immunol* 5:82. doi:10.3389/fimmu.2014.00082.

Fischer, A. C., C. I. Smith, L. Cebotaru, X. Zhang, F. B. Askin, J. Wright, S. E. Guggino, R. J. Adams, T. Flotte, and W. B. Guggino. 2007. "Expression of a truncated cystic fibrosis transmembrane conductance regulator with an AAV5-pseudotyped vector in primates." *Mol Ther* 15 (4):756–763. doi:10.1038/sj.mt.6300059.

Flotte, T. R., A. C. Fischer, J. Goetzmann, C. Mueller, L. Cebotaru, Z. Yan, L. Wang, J. M. Wilson, W. B. Guggino, and J. F. Engelhardt. 2010. "Dual reporter comparative indexing of rAAV pseudotyped vectors in chimpanzee airway." *Mol Ther* 18 (3):594–600. doi:10.1038/mt.2009.230.

Flotte, T. R., P. L. Zeitlin, T. C. Reynolds, A. E. Heald, P. Pedersen, S. Beck, C. K. Conrad et al. 2003. "Phase I trial of intranasal and endobronchial administration of a recombinant adeno-associated virus serotype 2 (rAAV2)-CFTR vector in adult cystic fibrosis patients: A two-part clinical study." *Hum Gene Ther* 14 (11):1079–1088. doi:10.1089/104303403322124792.

Foged, C. 2012. "siRNA delivery with lipid-based systems: promises and pitfalls." *Curr Top Med Chem* 12 (2):97–107.

Gao, G., L. H. Vandenberghe, M. R. Alvira, Y. Lu, R. Calcedo, X. Zhou, and J. M. Wilson. 2004. "Clades of Adeno-associated viruses are widely disseminated in human tissues." *J Virol* 78 (12):6381–6388. doi:10.1128/jvi.78.12.6381-6388.2004.

Geller, D. E., and S. Madge. 2011. "Technological and behavioral strategies to reduce treatment burden and improve adherence to inhaled antibiotics in cystic fibrosis." *Respir Med* 105 (Suppl 2):S24–S31. doi:10.1016/s0954-6111(11)70024-5.

Giljohann, D. A., D. S. Seferos, A. E. Prigodich, P. C. Patel, and C. A. Mirkin. 2009. "Gene regulation with polyvalent siRNA-nanoparticle conjugates." *J Am Chem Soc* 131 (6):2072–2073. doi:10.1021/ja808719p.

Gottlieb, J., M. R. Zamora, T. Hodges, A. W. Musk, U. Sommerwerk, D. Dilling, S. Arcasoy et al. 2016. "ALN-RSV01 for prevention of bronchiolitis obliterans syndrome after respiratory syncytial virus infection in lung transplant recipients." *J Heart Lung Transplant* 35 (2):213–221. doi:10.1016/j.healun.2015.08.012.

Griesenbach, U., and E. W. Alton. 2009. "Gene transfer to the lung: Lessons learned from more than 2 decades of CF gene therapy." *Adv Drug Deliv Rev* 61 (2):128–139. doi:10.1016/j.addr.2008.09.010.

Griesenbach, U., and E. W. Alton. 2013. "Expert opinion in biological therapy: Update on developments in lung gene transfer." *Expert Opin Biol Ther* 13 (3):345–360. doi:10.1517/14712598.2013.735656.

Griesenbach, U., S. Ferrari, D. M. Geddes, and E. W. Alton. 2002. "Gene therapy progress and prospects: Cystic fibrosis." *Gene Ther* 9 (20):1344–1350. doi:10.1038/sj.gt.3301791.

Griesenbach, U., D. M. Geddes, and E. W. Alton. 2006. "Gene therapy progress and prospects: Cystic fibrosis." *Gene Ther* 13 (14):1061–1067. doi:10.1038/sj.gt.3302809.

Griesenbach, U., M. Inoue, C. Meng, R. Farley, M. Chan, N. K. Newman, A. Brum et al. 2012. "Assessment of F/HN-pseudotyped lentivirus as a clinically relevant vector for lung gene therapy." *Am J Respir Crit Care Med* 186 (9):846–856. doi:10.1164/rccm.201206-1056OC.

Guo, S., Y. Huang, Q. Jiang, Y. Sun, L. Deng, Z. Liang, Q. Du et al. 2010. "Enhanced gene delivery and siRNA silencing by gold nanoparticles coated with charge-reversal polyelectrolyte." *ACS Nano* 4 (9):5505–5511. doi:10.1021/nn101638u.

Halbert, C. L., J. M. Allen, and A. D. Miller. 2001. "Adeno-associated virus type 6 (AAV6) vectors mediate efficient transduction of airway epithelial cells in mouse lungs compared to that of AAV2 vectors." *J Virol* 75 (14):6615–6624. doi:10.1128/jvi.75.14.6615-6624.2001.

Halbert, C. L., J. M. Allen, and A. D. Miller. 2002. "Efficient mouse airway transduction following recombination between AAV vectors carrying parts of a larger gene." *Nat Biotechnol* 20 (7):697–701. doi:10.1038/nbt0702-697.

Ibraheem, D., A. Elaissari, and H. Fessi. 2014. "Gene therapy and DNA delivery systems." *Int J Pharm* 459 (1–2):70–83. doi:10.1016/j.ijpharm.2013.11.041.

Ihara, D., N. Hattori, Y. Horimasu, T. Masuda, T. Nakashima, T. Senoo, H. Iwamoto, K. Fujitaka, H. Okamoto, and N. Kohno. 2015. "Histological quantification of gene silencing by intratracheal administration of dry powdered small-interfering RNA/chitosan complexes in the Murine Lung." *Pharm Res* 32 (12):3877–3885. doi:10.1007/s11095-015-1747-6.

Inoue, M., Y. Tokusumi, H. Ban, T. Kanaya, T. Tokusumi, Y. Nagai, A. Iida, and M. Hasegawa. 2003. "Nontransmissible virus-like particle formation by F-deficient sendai virus is temperature sensitive and reduced by mutations in M and HN proteins." *J Virol* 77 (5):3238–3246.

Jaafar-Maalej, C., A. Elaissari, and H. Fessi. 2012. "Lipid-based carriers: Manufacturing and applications for pulmonary route." *Expert Opin Drug Deliv* 9 (9):1111–1127. doi:10.1517/17425247.2012.702751.

Jensen, D. K., L. B. Jensen, S. Koocheki, L. Bengtson, D. Cun, H. M. Nielsen, and C. Foged. 2012. "Design of an inhalable dry powder formulation of DOTAP-modified PLGA nanoparticles loaded with siRNA." *J Control Release* 157 (1):141–148. doi:10.1016/j.jconrel.2011.08.011.

Kapoor, M., and D. J. Burgess. 2012. "Physicochemical characterization of anionic lipid-based ternary siRNA complexes." *Biochim Biophys Acta* 1818 (7):1603–1612. doi:10.1016/j.bbamem.2012.03.013.

Kasper, J. C., C. Troiber, S. Kuchler, E. Wagner, and W. Friess. 2013. "Formulation development of lyophilized, long-term stable siRNA/oligoaminoamide polyplexes." *Eur J Pharm Biopharm* 85 (2):294–305. doi:10.1016/j.ejpb.2013.05.010.

Khalil, H., T. Chen, R. Riffon, R. Wang, and Z. Wang. 2008. "Synergy between polyethylenimine and different families of antibiotics against a resistant clinical isolate of Pseudomonas aeruginosa." *Antimicrob Agents Chemother* 52 (5):1635–1641. doi:10.1128/aac.01071-07.

Kircheis, R., L. Wightman, and E. Wagner. 2001. "Design and gene delivery activity of modified polyethylenimines." *Adv Drug Deliv Rev* 53 (3):341–358.

Koehler, D. R., H. Frndova, K. Leung, E. Louca, D. Palmer, P. Ng, C. McKerlie, P. Cox, A. L. Coates, and J. Hu. 2005. "Aerosol delivery of an enhanced helper-dependent adenovirus formulation to rabbit lung using an intratracheal catheter." *J Gene Med* 7 (11):1409–1420. doi:10.1002/jgm.797.

Koping-Hoggard, M., K. M. Varum, M. Issa, S. Danielsen, B. E. Christensen, B. T. Stokke, and P. Artursson. 2004. "Improved chitosan-mediated gene delivery based on easily dissociated chitosan polyplexes of highly defined chitosan oligomers." *Gene Ther* 11 (19):1441–1452. doi:10.1038/sj.gt.3302312.

Lam, J. K., W. Liang, and H. K. Chan. 2012. "Pulmonary delivery of therapeutic siRNA." *Adv Drug Deliv Rev* 64 (1):1–15. doi:10.1016/j.addr.2011.02.006.

Lee, R. J., and L. Huang. 1996. "Folate-targeted, anionic liposome-entrapped polylysine-condensed DNA for tumor cell-specific gene transfer." *J Biol Chem* 271 (14):8481–8487.

Li, J., Y. C. Chen, Y. C. Tseng, S. Mozumdar, and L. Huang. 2010. "Biodegradable calcium phosphate nanoparticle with lipid coating for systemic siRNA delivery." *J Control Release* 142 (3):416–421. doi:10.1016/j.jconrel.2009.11.008.

Li, S., and L. Huang. 2000. "Nonviral gene therapy: Promises and challenges." *Gene Ther* 7 (1):31–34. doi:10.1038/sj.gt.3301110.

Li, Y., B. Li, C. J. Li, and L. J. Li. 2015. "Key points of basic theories and clinical practice in rAd-p53 (Gendicine) gene therapy for solid malignant tumors." *Expert Opin Biol Ther* 15 (3):437–454. doi:10.1517/14712598.2015.990882.

Liang, M. 2012. "Clinical development of oncolytic viruses in China." *Curr Pharm Biotechnol* 13 (9):1852–1857.

Limberis, M. P., and J. M. Wilson. 2006. "Adeno-associated virus serotype 9 vectors transduce murine alveolar and nasal epithelia and can be readministered." *Proc Natl Acad Sci U S A* 103 (35):12993–12998. doi:10.1073/pnas.0601433103.

Liu, X., M. Luo, C. Trygg, Z. Yan, D. C. Lei-Butters, C. I. Smith, A. C. Fischer et al. 2007. "Biological differences in rAAV transduction of airway epithelia in humans and in old world non-human primates." *Mol Ther* 15 (12):2114–2123. doi:10.1038/sj.mt.6300277.

Lu, C., D. J. Stewart, J. J. Lee, L. Ji, R. Ramesh, G. Jayachandran, M. I. Nunez et al. 2012. "Phase I clinical trial of systemically administered TUSC2(FUS1)-nanoparticles mediating functional gene transfer in humans." *PLoS One* 7 (4):e34833. doi:10.1371/journal.pone.0034833.

Luo, Y., X. Zhai, C. Ma, P. Sun, Z. Fu, W. Liu, and J. Xu. 2012. "An inhalable beta(2)-adrenoceptor ligand-directed guanidinylated chitosan carrier for targeted delivery of siRNA to lung." *J Control Release* 162 (1):28–36. doi:10.1016/j.jconrel.2012.06.005.

Lv, H., S. Zhang, B. Wang, S. Cui, and J. Yan. 2006. "Toxicity of cationic lipids and cationic polymers in gene delivery." *J Control Release* 114 (1):100–109. doi:10.1016/j.jconrel.2006.04.014.

Mao, S., W. Sun, and T. Kissel. 2010. "Chitosan-based formulations for delivery of DNA and siRNA." *Adv Drug Deliv Rev* 62 (1):12–27. doi:10.1016/j.addr.2009.08.004.

Markman, J. L., A. Rekechenetskiy, E. Holler, and J. Y. Ljubimova. 2013. "Nanomedicine therapeutic approaches to overcome cancer drug resistance." *Adv Drug Deliv Rev* 65 (13–14):1866–1879. doi:10.1016/j.addr.2013.09.019.

Meng, H., M. Liong, T. Xia, Z. Li, Z. Ji, J. I. Zink, and A. E. Nel. 2010. "Engineered design of mesoporous silica nanoparticles to deliver doxorubicin and P-glycoprotein siRNA to overcome drug resistance in a cancer cell line." *ACS Nano* 4 (8):4539–4550. doi:10.1021/nn100690m.

Misra, A., K. Jinturkar, D. Patel, J. Lalani, and M. Chougule. 2009. "Recent advances in liposomal dry powder formulations: Preparation and evaluation." *Expert Opin Drug Deliv* 6 (1):71–89. doi:10.1517/17425240802652309.

Mitomo, K., U. Griesenbach, M. Inoue, L. Somerton, C. Meng, E. Akiba, T. Tabata et al. 2010. "Toward gene therapy for cystic fibrosis using a lentivirus pseudotyped with Sendai virus envelopes." *Mol Ther* 18 (6):1173–1182. doi:10.1038/mt.2010.13.

Morales, J. O., K. R. Fathe, A. Brunaugh, S. Ferrati, S. Li, M. Montenegro-Nicolini, Z. Mousavikhamene, J. T. McConville, M. R. Prausnitz, and H. D. C. Smyth. 2017. "Challenges and future prospects for the delivery of biologics: Oral mucosal, pulmonary, and transdermal routes." *AAPS J* 19 (3):652–668. doi:10.1208/s12248-017-0054-z.

Moroz, E., S. Matoori, and J. C. Leroux. 2016. "Oral delivery of macromolecular drugs: Where we are after almost 100years of attempts." *Adv Drug Deliv Rev* 101:108–121. doi:10.1016/j.addr.2016.01.010.

Moss, R. B., C. Milla, J. Colombo, F. Accurso, P. L. Zeitlin, J. P. Clancy, L. T. Spencer et al. 2007. "Repeated aerosolized AAV-CFTR for treatment of cystic fibrosis: A randomized placebo-controlled phase 2B trial." *Hum Gene Ther* 18 (8):726–732. doi:10.1089/hum.2007.022.

Mueller, C., and T. R. Flotte. 2013. "Gene-based therapy for alpha-1 antitrypsin deficiency." *Copd* 10(Suppl 1):44–49. doi:10.3109/15412555.2013.764978.

Mullard, A. 2016. "EMA greenlights second gene therapy." *Nat Rev Drug Discov* 15 (5):299. doi:10.1038/nrd.2016.93.

Munier, S., I. Messai, T. Delair, B. Verrier, and Y. Ataman-Onal. 2005. "Cationic PLA nanoparticles for DNA delivery: Comparison of three surface polycations for DNA binding, protection and transfection properties." *Colloids Surf B Biointerfaces* 43 (3–4):163–173. doi:10.1016/j.colsurfb.2005.05.001.

Mura, S., H. Hillaireau, J. Nicolas, S. Kerdine-Romer, B. Le Droumaguet, C. Delomenie, V. Nicolas, M. Pallardy, N. Tsapis, and E. Fattal. 2011. "Biodegradable nanoparticles meet the bronchial airway barrier: How surface properties affect their interaction with mucus and epithelial cells." *Biomacromolecules* 12 (11):4136–4143. doi:10.1021/bm201226x.

Newman, S. P. 2005. "Principles of metered-dose inhaler design." *Respir Care* 50 (9):1177–1190.

Nunes, C., A. M. Pereira, and M. Morais-Almeida. 2017. "Asthma costs and social impact." *Asthma Res Pract* 3:1. doi:10.1186/s40733-016-0029-3.

Okuda, T., D. Kito, A. Oiwa, M. Fukushima, D. Hira, and H. Okamoto. 2013. "Gene silencing in a mouse lung metastasis model by an inhalable dry small interfering RNA powder prepared using the supercritical carbon dioxide technique." *Biol Pharm Bull* 36 (7):1183–1191.

Oliveira, C., A. J. Ribeiro, F. Veiga, and I. Silveira. 2016. "Recent advances in nucleic acid-based delivery: From bench to clinical trials in genetic diseases." *J Biomed Nanotechnol* 12 (5):841–862.

Ostedgaard, L. S., T. Rokhlina, P. H. Karp, P. Lashmit, S. Afione, M. Schmidt, J. Zabner, M. F. Stinski, J. A. Chiorini, and M. J. Welsh. 2005. "A shortened adeno-associated virus expression cassette for CFTR gene transfer to cystic fibrosis airway epithelia." *Proc Natl Acad Sci U S A* 102 (8):2952–2957. doi:10.1073/pnas.0409845102.

Park, S. C., J. P. Nam, Y. M. Kim, J. H. Kim, J. W. Nah, and M. K. Jang. 2013. "Branched polyethylenimine-grafted-carboxymethyl chitosan copolymer enhances the delivery of pDNA or siRNA in vitro and in vivo." *Int J Nanomedicine* 8:3663–3677. doi:10.2147/ijn.s50911.

Patel, B., N. Gupta, and F. Ahsan. 2015. "Particle engineering to enhance or lessen particle uptake by alveolar macrophages and to influence the therapeutic outcome." *Eur J Pharm Biopharm* 89:163–174. doi:10.1016/j.ejpb.2014.12.001.

Patil, S. D., D. G. Rhodes, and D. J. Burgess. 2004. "Anionic liposomal delivery system for DNA transfection." *AAPS J* 6 (4):e29. doi:10.1208/aapsj060429.

Patil, Y. B., S. K. Swaminathan, T. Sadhukha, L. Ma, and J. Panyam. 2010. "The use of nanoparticle-mediated targeted gene silencing and drug delivery to overcome tumor drug resistance." *Biomaterials* 31 (2):358–365. doi:10.1016/j.biomaterials.2009.09.048.

Patton, J. S., C. S. Fishburn, and J. G. Weers. 2004. "The lungs as a portal of entry for systemic drug delivery." *Proc Am Thorac Soc* 1 (4):338–344. doi:10.1513/pats.200409-049TA.

Perricone, M. A., J. E. Morris, K. Pavelka, M. S. Plog, B. P. O'Sullivan, P. M. Joseph, H. Dorkin et al. 2001. "Aerosol and lobar administration of a recombinant adenovirus to individuals with cystic fibrosis. II. Transfection efficiency in airway epithelium." *Hum Gene Ther* 12 (11):1383–1394. doi:10.1089/104303401750298544.

Pilcer, G., and K. Amighi. 2010. "Formulation strategy and use of excipients in pulmonary drug delivery." *Int J Pharm* 392 (1–2):1–19. doi:10.1016/j.ijpharm.2010.03.017.

Pol, J., G. Kroemer, and L. Galluzzi. 2016. "First oncolytic virus approved for melanoma immunotherapy." *Oncoimmunology* 5 (1):e1115641. doi:10.1080/2162402x.2015.1115641.

Putnam, D. 2006. "Polymers for gene delivery across length scales." *Nat Mater* 5 (6):439–451. doi:10.1038/nmat1645.

Qiu, Y., J. K. Lam, S. W. Leung, and W. Liang. 2016. "Delivery of RNAi therapeutics to the airways-from bench to bedside." *Molecules* 21 (9). doi:10.3390/molecules21091249.

Raemdonck, K., K. Braeckmans, J. Demeester, and S. C. De Smedt. 2014. "Merging the best of both worlds: Hybrid lipid-enveloped matrix nanocomposites in drug delivery." *Chem Soc Rev* 43 (1):444–472. doi:10.1039/c3cs60299k.

Rawlins, E. L., and B. L. Hogan. 2008. "Ciliated epithelial cell lifespan in the mouse trachea and lung." *Am J Physiol Lung Cell Mol Physiol* 295 (1):L231–L234. doi:10.1152/ajplung.90209.2008.

Riordan, J. R., J. M. Rommens, B. Kerem, N. Alon, R. Rozmahel, Z. Grzelczak, J. Zielenski et al. 1989. "Identification of the cystic fibrosis gene: Cloning and characterization of complementary DNA." *Science* 245 (4922):1066–1073.

Rubin, B. K., and J. B. Fink. 2005. "Optimizing aerosol delivery by pressurized metered-dose inhalers." *Respir Care* 50 (9):1191–1200.

Sakuma, T., M. A. Barry, and Y. Ikeda. 2012. "Lentiviral vectors: Basic to translational." *Biochem J* 443 (3):603–618. doi:10.1042/bj20120146.

Schuster, B. S., A. J. Kim, J. C. Kays, M. M. Kanzawa, W. B. Guggino, M. P. Boyle, S. M. Rowe, N. Muzyczka, J. S. Suk, and J. Hanes. 2014. "Overcoming the cystic fibrosis sputum barrier to leading adeno-associated virus gene therapy vectors." *Mol Ther* 22 (8):1484–1493. doi:10.1038/mt.2014.89.

Schuster, B. S., J. S. Suk, G. F. Woodworth, and J. Hanes. 2013. "Nanoparticle diffusion in respiratory mucus from humans without lung disease." *Biomaterials* 34 (13):3439–3446. doi:10.1016/j.biomaterials.2013.01.064.

Seguin, R. M., and N. Ferrari. 2009. "Emerging oligonucleotide therapies for asthma and chronic obstructive pulmonary disease." *Expert Opin Investig Drugs* 18 (10):1505–1517. doi:10.1517/13543780903179294.

Siegel, R., D. Naishadham, and A. Jemal. 2013. "Cancer statistics, 2013." *CA Cancer J Clin* 63 (1):11–30. doi:10.3322/caac.21166.

Sinn, P. L., A. C. Arias, K. A. Brogden, and P. B. McCray, Jr. 2008. "Lentivirus vector can be readministered to nasal epithelia without blocking immune responses." *J Virol* 82 (21):10684–10692. doi:10.1128/jvi.00227-08.

Sirninger, J., C. Muller, S. Braag, Q. Tang, H. Yue, C. Detrisac, T. Ferkol, W. B. Guggino, and T. R. Flotte. 2004. "Functional characterization of a recombinant adeno-associated virus 5-pseudotyped cystic fibrosis transmembrane conductance regulator vector." *Hum Gene Ther* 15 (9):832–841. doi:10.1089/hum.2004.15.832.

Son, S., R. Namgung, J. Kim, K. Singha, and W. J. Kim. 2012. "Bioreducible polymers for gene silencing and delivery." *Acc Chem Res* 45 (7):1100–1112. doi:10.1021/ar200248u.

Stein, S. W., and C. G. Thiel. 2017. "The history of therapeutic aerosols: A chronological review." *J Aerosol Med Pulm Drug Deliv* 30 (1):20–41. doi:10.1089/jamp.2016.1297.

Su, W. P., F. Y. Cheng, D. B. Shieh, C. S. Yeh, and W. C. Su. 2012. "PLGA nanoparticles codeliver paclitaxel and Stat3 siRNA to overcome cellular resistance in lung cancer cells." *Int J Nanomedicine* 7:4269–4283. doi:10.2147/ijn.s33666.

Summerford, C., and R. J. Samulski. 1998. "Membrane-associated heparan sulfate proteoglycan is a receptor for adeno-associated virus type 2 virions." *J Virol* 72 (2):1438–1445.

Tang, B. C., M. Dawson, S. K. Lai, Y. Y. Wang, J. S. Suk, M. Yang, P. Zeitlin, M. P. Boyle, J. Fu, and J. Hanes. 2009. "Biodegradable polymer nanoparticles that rapidly penetrate the human mucus barrier." *Proc Natl Acad Sci U S A* 106 (46):19268–19273. doi:10.1073/pnas.0905998106.

Toietta, G., D. R. Koehler, M. J. Finegold, B. Lee, J. Hu, and A. L. Beaudet. 2003. "Reduced inflammation and improved airway expression using helper-dependent adenoviral vectors with a K18 promoter." *Mol Ther* 7 (5 Pt 1):649–658.

Tosi, M. F., A. van Heeckeren, T. W. Ferkol, D. Askew, C. V. Harding, and J. M. Kaplan. 2004. "Effect of Pseudomonas-induced chronic lung inflammation on specific cytotoxic T-cell responses to adenoviral vectors in mice." *Gene Ther* 11 (19):1427–1433. doi:10.1038/sj.gt.3302290.

Trewyn, B. G., S. Giri, I. I. Slowing, and V. S. Lin. 2007. "Mesoporous silica nanoparticle based controlled release, drug delivery, and biosensor systems." *Chem Commun (Camb)* (31):3236–3245. doi:10.1039/b701744h.

Ungaro, F., I. d'Angelo, A. Miro, M. I. La Rotonda, and F. Quaglia. 2012a. "Engineered PLGA nano- and micro-carriers for pulmonary delivery: challenges and promises." *J Pharm Pharmacol* 64 (9):1217–1235. doi:10.1111/j.2042-7158.2012.01486.x.

Ungaro, F., D. De Stefano, C. Giovino, A. Masuccio, A. Miro, R. Sorrentino, R. Carnuccio, and F. Quaglia. 2012b. "PEI-engineered respirable particles delivering a decoy oligonucleotide to NF-kappaB: Inhibiting MUC2 expression in LPS-stimulated airway epithelial cells." *PLoS One* 7 (10):e46457. doi:10.1371/journal.pone.0046457.

van Rijt, S. H., D. A. Bolukbas, C. Argyo, S. Datz, M. Lindner, O. Eickelberg, M. Konigshoff, T. Bein, and S. Meiners. 2015. "Protease-mediated release of chemotherapeutics from mesoporous silica nanoparticles to ex vivo human and mouse lung tumors." *ACS Nano* 9 (3):2377–2389. doi:10.1021/nn5070343.

Villaflor, V. M., and R. Salgia. 2013. "Targeted agents in non-small cell lung cancer therapy: What is there on the horizon?" *J Carcinog* 12:7. doi:10.4103/1477-3163.109253.

Virella-Lowell, I., B. Zusman, K. Foust, S. Loiler, T. Conlon, S. Song, K. A. Chesnut, T. Ferkol, and T. R. Flotte. 2005. "Enhancing rAAV vector expression in the lung." *J Gene Med* 7 (7):842–850. doi:10.1002/jgm.759.

Wagner, J. A., I. B. Nepomuceno, A. H. Messner, M. L. Moran, E. P. Batson, S. Dimiceli, B. W. Brown et al. 2002. "A phase II, double-blind, randomized, placebo-controlled clinical trial of tgAAVCF using maxillary sinus delivery in patients with cystic fibrosis with antrostomies." *Hum Gene Ther* 13 (11):1349–1359. doi:10.1089/104303402760128577.

Walters, R. W., T. Grunst, J. M. Bergelson, R. W. Finberg, M. J. Welsh, and J. Zabner. 1999. "Basolateral localization of fiber receptors limits adenovirus infection from the apical surface of airway epithelia." *J Biol Chem* 274 (15):10219–10226.

Wang, T., J. R. Upponi, and V. P. Torchilin. 2012. "Design of multifunctional non-viral gene vectors to overcome physiological barriers: dilemmas and strategies." *Int J Pharm* 427 (1):3–20. doi:10.1016/j.ijpharm.2011.07.013.

Watanabe, N., K. Yano, K. Tsuyuki, T. Okano, and M. Yamato. 2015. "Re-examination of regulatory opinions in Europe: Possible contribution for the approval of the first gene therapy product Glybera." *Mol Ther Methods Clin Dev* 2:14066. doi:10.1038/mtm.2014.66.

Watts, J. K., and D. R. Corey. 2010. "Clinical status of duplex RNA." *Bioorg Med Chem Lett* 20 (11):3203–3207. doi:10.1016/j.bmcl.2010.03.109.

Weber, S., A. Zimmer, and J. Pardeike. 2014. "Solid lipid nanoparticles (SLN) and nanostructured lipid carriers (NLC) for pulmonary application: A review of the state of the art." *Eur J Pharm Biopharm* 86 (1):7–22. doi:10.1016/j.ejpb.2013.08.013.

Willis, L., D. Hayes, Jr., and H. M. Mansour. 2012. "Therapeutic liposomal dry powder inhalation aerosols for targeted lung delivery." *Lung* 190 (3):251–262. doi:10.1007/s00408-011-9360-x.

Wu, Z., E. Miller, M. Agbandje-McKenna, and R. J. Samulski. 2006. "Alpha2,3 and alpha2,6 N-linked sialic acids facilitate efficient binding and transduction by adeno-associated virus types 1 and 6." *J Virol* 80 (18):9093–9103. doi:10.1128/jvi.00895-06.

Yeh, G. Y., and R. Horwitz. 2017. "Integrative medicine for respiratory conditions: Asthma and chronic obstructive pulmonary disease." *Med Clin North Am* 101 (5):925–941. doi:10.1016/j.mcna.2017.04.008.

Yin, H., R. L. Kanasty, A. A. Eltoukhy, A. J. Vegas, J. R. Dorkin, and D. G. Anderson. 2014. "Non-viral vectors for gene-based therapy." *Nat Rev Genet* 15 (8):541–555. doi:10.1038/nrg3763.

Yla-Herttuala, S. 2012. "Endgame: Glybera finally recommended for approval as the first gene therapy drug in the European union." *Mol Ther* 20 (10):1831–1832. doi:10.1038/mt.2012.194.

Zabner, J., M. Seiler, R. Walters, R. M. Kotin, W. Fulgeras, B. L. Davidson, and J. A. Chiorini. 2000. "Adeno-associated virus type 5 (AAV5) but not AAV2 binds to the apical surfaces of airway epithelia and facilitates gene transfer." *J Virol* 74 (8):3852–3858.

Zamora, M. R., M. Budev, M. Rolfe, J. Gottlieb, A. Humar, J. Devincenzo, A. Vaishnaw et al. 2011. "RNA interference therapy in lung transplant patients infected with respiratory syncytial virus." *Am J Respir Crit Care Med* 183 (4):531–538. doi:10.1164/rccm.201003-0422OC.

Zhang, L., A. Bukreyev, C. I. Thompson, B. Watson, M. E. Peeples, P. L. Collins, and R. J. Pickles. 2005. "Infection of ciliated cells by human parainfluenza virus type 3 in an in vitro model of human airway epithelium." *J Virol* 79 (2):1113–1124. doi:10.1128/jvi.79.2.1113-1124.2005.

Zhang, L., F. X. Gu, J. M. Chan, A. Z. Wang, R. S. Langer, and O. C. Farokhzad. 2008. "Nanoparticles in medicine: Therapeutic applications and developments." *Clin Pharmacol Ther* 83 (5):761–769. doi:10.1038/sj.clpt.6100400.

Zhang, Y., L. Peng, R. J. Mumper, and L. Huang. 2013a. "Combinational delivery of c-myc siRNA and nucleoside analogs in a single, synthetic nanocarrier for targeted cancer therapy." *Biomaterials* 34 (33):8459–8468. doi:10.1016/j.biomaterials.2013.07.050.

Zhang, Y., N. M. Schwerbrock, A. B. Rogers, W. Y. Kim, and L. Huang. 2013b. "Codelivery of VEGF siRNA and gemcitabine monophosphate in a single nanoparticle formulation for effective treatment of NSCLC." *Mol Ther* 21 (8):1559–1569. doi:10.1038/mt.2013.120.

16

Genome Editing for Genetic Lung Diseases

Ying Zhang and Hao Yin

CONTENTS

16.1 Introduction of Genome Editing

16.1.1 Principles of Genome Editing

Genome editing is a type of DNA engineering which allows precise modifications in the genomic DNA. Genome editing is mediated through programmable nucleases which recognize and bind specific sequences in the genome.[1,2] Once binding, the nucleases can be engineered to cut targeted genomic DNA, resulting in double-strand breaks (DSBs), which are efficiently repaired by non-homologous end joining (NHEJ) or homology-directed repair (HDR) in the presence of a donor DNA template.[1–5] NHEJ is error-prone, often introducing small or large insertions or deletions (indels) at the DNA cut site.[6] Depending on the types and positions, indels that shift the open reading frame (ORF) can lead to the mRNA degradation or production of abnormal and non-functional proteins.[7] Genome editing nucleases-mediated NHEJ is able to introduce long-term disruption of disease-prone genes.[8] It is also feasible to engineer nucleases-mediated NHEJ to restore ORF of a malfunctioning gene.[9–13] For example, mutations in dystrophin gene can lead to ORF shifting and severe disruption or deletion of dystrophin protein, to cause Duchenne muscular dystrophy. Disruption of the ORF-shifted exons to restore the ORF can rescue the function of dystrophin for treating Duchenne muscular dystrophy.[9–13] In contrast to error-prone NHEJ pathway, HDR-mediated genome editing enables precise modifications by incorporation of the donor DNA with homologous sequences.[14] Genome editing via HDR pathway could be used to precisely repair mutations or knock-in sequences at the desired loci.[15–17] Besides introducing DSBs, genome editing nucleases (e.g. Cas9) can be engineered to enable many different modifications, including epigenetic modification of targeted sequences, induction or suppression of gene expression, base editing, imaging of genomic locus, and many others.[8,18–25]

16.1.2 Introduction of ZFN, TALEN, and CRISPR

Zinc-finger nucleases (ZFNs) were discovered as one of the first useful tools for genome editing.[3,26] A zinc-finger protein (ZFP) is composed of at least three zinc-finger domains, which provide sequence specificity by recognizing 3-bp DNA sequence through each domain.[3,26] To create ZFN, ZFP is fused with the non-specific cleavage domain of the FokI endonuclease.[3,26] A pair of ZFNs generate DSBs of DNA with the dimerization of the cleavage domain.[3,26] In past decades, the editing efficiency of ZFNs has been significantly enhanced, and the engineering process has been considerably improved.[3] However, sophisticated protein engineering is still required to target new genomic sequences.[3] Later on, another powerful genome editing platform named transcription activator-like effector nucleases (TALENs) were developed.[27] Each monomer of the DNA binding domain recognizes one specific nucleotide of the target sequence.[27] The simplicity of one monomer-one nucleotide rule allows a faster design and assembly process of TALENs than ZFNs.[27,28]

Clustered regularly interspaced short palindromic repeats/associated endonuclease (CRISPR/Cas) systems are essentially RNA-guided nucleases.[4,5,29,30] Class 2 CRISPR/Cas systems use a single Cas endonuclease that cleaves DNA upon target recognition by CRISPR RNA (crRNA).[4,5,29,30] A target specific crRNA and a trans-activating CRISPR RNA (tracrRNA) of Cas9 could be fused to form a single guide RNA (sgRNA).[4,5,29,30] The Cas endonucleases bind a protospacer adjacent motif (PAM) sequence, and use a RNA guide sequence located in the crRNA to recognize the complementary DNA sequence.[4,5,29,30] By changing the guide sequences, it is very simple to target most genomic sequences, making CRISPR/Cas system a powerful genome editing tool. Cas9 system, in particular Streptococcus pyrogenes Cas9 (SpCas9), has a simple PAM requirement (NGG, indicating GG or CC are required) and high potency and, thus, is now broadly used in biomedical research and drug development.[4,5,29,30]

16.2 Biomolecular Delivery to the Lung

16.2.1 The Targets of Genome Editing

Genetic lung diseases are devastating disorders, usually resulting in high morbidity and mortality.[31–34] Some of the well-known congenital diseases, such as cystic fibrosis, alpha-1 antitrypsin (AAT) deficiency, and surfactant protein (SP) deficiency disorders, are caused by monogenic mutations.[31–33] Current studies mainly focus on developing small molecules or supporting therapies to alleviate disease manifestation. Direct exposure of the lung to the air allows for selective targeting of pulmonary cell lineages via "local" delivery method, which is attractive due to convenient inhalation method and patient compliance.[35] To reach long-term therapeutic outcome, it is ideal to target pulmonary stem/progenitor cells, including alveolar type II cells for SP deficiency disorders and basal cells for cystic fibrosis.[36–38] However, the levels of editing efficiency required to observe a positive outcome in clinical setting is still unknown.[36–38] Based on the results from gene transfer in animal studies, it was speculated that at least 20%–25% of surface ciliated cells need to be corrected to support the normal lung function of cystic fibrosis patients.[39]

16.2.2 Lessons from Gene Therapy

Gene therapy or gene replacement therapy for genetic diseases has been an on-going research for over 30 years.[35,40] Despite such long history, there is no FDA approved gene replacement therapy for lung diseases yet. Theoretically, genetic materials via viral or non-viral vectors can be administrated to the epithelial surface of the lung via airway. However, the complexity of human lung anatomy is the physical barrier for successful "local" gene delivery. The airways of human start with the trachea and divide to the bronchi and bronchioles, which continuously divide about 23 generations.[41] The details of the lung anatomy are described elsewhere in the book. Due to its extensive surface and airway architecture, it is difficult to evenly distribute genetic materials to the entire human lung.

Most preclinical gene replacement therapy studies use animal models. Genetically modified mice are widely used for preclinical studies of lung gene therapy. Due to the striking differences of the lung biology among various species, studies in animal models, in particular mice, may not always translate to the results in patients.[42–44] For gene replacement therapy for the lung, repetitive administration or targeting the progenitor population may provide sustained therapeutic effect. However, anti-vector immunity is a major challenge for repeat dosing.[45,46] Recombinant adeno-associated virus (rAAV) is widely used for *in vivo* gene therapy due to its low immunogenicity and high transduction efficiency for a number of tissues.[47] rAAV is considered safe given the fact that it rarely integrates into genome and persists as episomal DNA in the nucleus. rAAV can transduce both dividing and non-dividing cells, and its expression gets diluted out in dividing cells since it doesn't replicate. Repeat dosing of rAAV activates adaptive immunity in human, making the second dose ineffective.[47] Thus, using rAAV for transgene expression might not be suitable for lung diseases which require persistent protein expression in progenitor cells or fast-turnover epithelial cells under chronic injury.[47–49] On the other hand, rAAV could be an efficient vehicle to carry genome editing proteins to transduce progenitor cells, as transient expression of those nucleases is sufficient enough to correct genetic mutations.[50–52]

Recombinant adenoviruses have a natural tropism for respiratory tract and have a large enough size to carry Cas9 and gRNA gene in one vector.[53] They are able to transfer gene *in vivo* in several animal models.[54,55] A key challenge is that adenovirus vectors are immunogenic, limiting gene expression to a few weeks.[47,55–57] Despite this limitation, adenoviruses have been tested in a number of clinical trials for lung diseases, including CF trials, and they were found to be well tolerated in most studies.[58,59] However, additional research is still required to enable safe and efficacious use of adenoviruses to deliver genome editing nucleases.

Retroviral and lentiviral vectors have been widely used for *ex vivo* cell therapy.[47,60,61] Up to 8 kb transgene can be inserted, making them attractive for gene transfer.[47,50,60,61] The RNA genomes of those viruses are reverse transcribed to DNA that integrate into the host genome.[47,50,60,61] Both viruses can effectively transduce dividing cells, but only lentiviral vectors are able to successfully transduce non-dividing cells.[47,50,53] Single dose of lentivirus is able to induce persistent gene expression and repeated dosing is less likely to introduce an inhibitory immune response.[62,63] Despite these advantages, the transduction efficiency of lentivirus in lung tissue is still low. The cell receptors required for viral entry are expressed more abundantly on the basolateral surface, rather than apical surface of lung epithelial cells.[64,65] The protection of tight junctions makes those receptors less accessible to the viral vectors.[64,65] Pseudotyped virus with modified viral envelopes or mutated viral proteins by directed evolution hold the potential to overcome this challenge.[64,65]

In addition to the viral vectors described above, a number of other viruses, including polyomaviruses, vaccinia virus, and baculovirus, have been tested for gene transfer into lung in preclinical models.[66–68] It will be interesting to evaluate the potential ability of those viruses to deliver the genome editing nucleases to various types of cells from the lung.

Gene therapy using plasmid DNA via lipid- or polymer-based non-viral vectors have been evaluated in preclinical models and multiple clinical trials.[40] Non-viral vectors can also be used to deliver mRNA and microRNA for gene therapy in lung tissue.[40,69,70] Compared to DNA, mRNA delivery is superior in terms of safety and transfection efficiency, but it requires more frequent administrations than DNA.[69–71] By endocytosis or membrane fusion, non-viral vectors significantly boost translocation of nucleic acids into the cytosol.[40] Non-viral vectors likely overcome several limitations of the viral vectors, such as immunogenicity, size limitation of the cargo, and mutagenesis.[40] However, the transfection efficiency of non-viral vectors is low *in vivo*, restricting its successful clinical development.[40,72]

16.2.3 Delivery Route: Local versus Systemic

Most lung gene therapies used delivery route via the airways, including nebulization, intratracheal administration, and bronchoscopy.[54,73–75] Theoretically, the local delivery strategy is ideal for lung epithelial disorders, such as cystic fibrosis (Table 16.1). A number of preclinical studies for the lung gene therapy have been carried out in wild-type and disease animal models.[54,73–76] Intratracheal administration

TABLE 16.1

Comparison of Local versus Systemic Delivery Targeting the Lung

Route	Pros	Cons	References
Local Delivery	• Site-specific delivery: maximized presence at the site of action • Minimal systemic exposure to reduce side effects such as immunogenicity • Large absorptive surface area	• Needs to overcome enzymatic and physical barrier (e.g. thick layer of mucus in cystic fibrosis patients) • Physical instability of drug formulation during inhalation delivery due to attrition and temperature increase • Potentially heterogeneous delivery	83–88
Systemic Delivery	• Possible access to all organs • Suitable for all types of modalities • Reproducible pharmacokinetics • Commonly used and clinically proven delivery route for gene and cell therapies • Not limited by volume	• Difficult to deliver into lung epithelial and basal cells • High manifestation of off-target toxicity • Dose dilution effect upon administration • May requires frequent hospital visits	89,90

of lentivirus, adeno-associated virus, or adenovirus carrying the human cystic fibrosis transmembrane conductance regulator (CFTR) gene to mice and pigs led to a clear detection of CFTR mRNA expression in part of nasal and lung epithelium.[47,57,63,64,77,78] Engineered viral vectors improved the efficiency of transfection for bronchioles epithelial cells.[64,65,79] Besides viral delivery, a proof-of-concept study used liposomes to deliver a plasmid encoding CFTR, resulting in its expression in the lung for up to 4 weeks.[80] Subsequently, a number of studies tested a collection of non-viral vectors to transfer the CFTR gene into the lung of small and large animal models.[81,82]

Based on the successful results that adenoviral vectors were able to transfect human bronchial epithelial cells *in vitro*, a clinical trial to transfer CFTR gene to the lung started in early 90s.[91] To date, more than 25 gene therapy trials for cystic fibrosis have been completed.[42,91] CFTR gene delivery was generally tolerated, but limited efficiency was observed.[42,91] Numerous challenges remain for delivery of genetic materials to the lung. Although CFTR gene can be transferred into lung cells, the percentage of transduced cells and the expression level need to be further improved.[47,57,64,65,77,78] Moreover, studies to characterize the transduced cells and to understand the fate of those cells could provide the key information for improving intracellular delivery. Results from linage tracing studies indicate that airway epithelial cells of mice have a half-life of 17 months.[92] However, those animals were under clean air environment, and the turnover rate of these cells in human is not exactly known.[92] To maintain the persistent expression in the right cell type, either repeated injection or targeting the lung progenitor cells are preferred.[70,93] However, immune responses are likely induced by repeated administration, and it is not clear that "local" delivery via the airway could efficiently transduce the lung progenitor cells.[40,94]

Although lung problems are the main causes for the most cases of morbidity and mortality of cystic fibrosis patients, CFTR mutations also affect intestine, liver, and several other organs.[32,53,59] Thus, systemic delivery via intravenous administration is attractive. Transfection of pulmonary endothelial cells *in vivo* was demonstrated by intravenous injection of polymer-based nanoparticles.[95,96] However, it remains to be determined whether the lung basal cells and the intestinal cells can be accessed by those vectors. In AAT deficiency or Pompe disease, the desired therapeutics are secreted and systemically circulated.[97,98] Therefore, the idea of delivery of transgenes or genome editing proteins to the liver or muscle to work as a "protein factory" in generating the right form of proteins for the lung is very attractive.[97,98]

16.2.4 Challenges of *Ex Vivo* Therapy and *In Vivo* Therapy

To bypass the *in vivo* delivery challenge, *ex vivo* therapy transplanting the genetically modified (via gene transfer or gene editing) stem cells or progenitor cells has been considered.[37] One of the key challenges for *ex vivo* therapy is the successful engraftment of gene-corrected cells to the lung.[37] The standards of

TABLE 16.2

Key Benefits and Challenges for *In Vivo* and *Ex Vivo* Genome Editing for Lung Diseases

	Challenges	Benefits	References
Ex vivo	• High cost, quality control, and complicated process of manufacture for autologous cell therapy (stem cells or lung progenitor cells) • Transplantation barriers • Limited understanding of biological consequences	• Avoidance of delivery barriers • Low immunogenicity	102–105
In vivo	• Complicated delivery barriers • Potential off-target effects in the tissue • Potential toxicity from delivery vectors • Immunogenicity and genome instability	• Known process of manufacture • Available viral and non-viral delivery vectors	

genetically engineered stem cells for autologous cell transplant need to be further established, and the safety of transplantation must be comprehensively evaluated. Despite these difficulties, the combinations of CRISPR-mediated gene editing, induced pluripotent stem cells (iPSCs), lung organoids, and biomaterials for scaffold provide great opportunities to advance the cell-based therapies for treating various types of lung diseases.[99,100]

As a barrier organ to communicate with external environment, the lung can be targeted via intratracheal or intranasal routes.[42,56,59] However, *in vivo* delivery of genetic materials to the "right" cell populations is still a challenge (Table 16.2). For example, it is extremely challenging to deliver into the basal cells, which are the target progenitor cells for treating cystic fibrosis. Mucus and even lung epithelial cells greatly restrict the access of delivery vectors to basal cells.[36,64,92,101] Moreover, the polarity of the lung epithelial cells and the basal cells further prevent the entry of vectors.[64,65] Under pathological circumstances, the adherent-solidified mucus plaques on airway surfaces further represent an additional barrier for *in vivo* delivery via the airway.[101] Alternatively, using systemic delivery via IV injection, it is also critical to overcome endothelium barriers to approach the progenitor cells embedded beneath the pulmonary vasculature.

16.3 Current Research, Preclinical, and Clinical Efforts of Genome Editing for the Lung

16.3.1 Applications in Biomedical Research

Lung cancer involves a large collection of genetic alterations in tumor suppressor genes and oncogenes.[106–109] Mouse lung cancer models provide great platforms to study the underlying mechanisms of tumor and to screen for new and effective chemotherapies. Traditionally, it takes in average 1 year–2 year to generate new a lung cancer model relying on homologous recombination in mouse Embryonic Stem (ES) Cells, germline transmission, and multiple generations of genetic cross to get the target genotype. *In vivo* delivery of CRISPR/Cas9 with the lentivirus or AAV targeting the tumor suppressors generated loss-of-function mutations in *Lkbl* and *p53* genes, which are frequently mutated in lung adenocarcinoma.[107,110] Besides gene knock out, HDR-mediated *Kras* (G12D) mutations could also be generated in Cas9-expressing transgenic mice via AAV delivery of sgRNA and a donor template.[110] The initial HDR-mediated Kras mutation was as low as 0.1%, but it was sufficient to promote tumor initiation and progression.[110] A fusion between DNA sequences of anaplastic lymphoma kinase (ALK) and echinoderm microtubule-associated protein like 4 (EML4) was detected in a portion of human non-small cell lung cancers (NSCLC).[111] *In vivo* viral delivery of CRISPR/Cas9 targeting these two genes induced the specific chromosomal rearrangements and generated the Eml4-Alk-driven lung cancer in mice.[111] CRISPR-mediated *in vivo* gene manipulation allow systematically dissecting the complex network of mutations identified in lung cancer.[107,110] A combination of CRISPR-mediated genome editing and a barcode sequencing is a powerful tool in understanding the functional consequence of genomic alternation in lung cancer.[112,113]

16.3.2 Preclinical and Clinical Studies of Therapeutic Genome Editing for Lung Diseases

Alpha-1 antitrypsin (AAT) deficiency causes progressive lung diseases due to the loss of AAT function and results in significant liver injury due to toxic gain-of-function mutations of AAT.[114,115] Injection of two AAVs, one for Cas9 and the other for AAT guide RNA plus HDR template, partially restored the right form of AAT protein expression in hepatocytes, suggesting an effective approach for the clinical applications.[114,115] The CRISPR/Cas9 approach was used to correct the mutated CFTR gene via HDR in the cultured intestinal stem cells from CF patients.[116] The corrected allele expressed the fully functional CFTR protein in clonally expanded organoids and provided the proof-of-concept support for HDR-mediated gene correction in adult stem cells from patients with hereditary defects.[116] In another study, induced pluripotent stem cells (iPSCs) were generated from CF patients with the deltaF508 mutation genotype in the CFTR gene.[117] Using CRISPR, mutated CFTR is corrected in iPSCs, and the edited iPSCs are able to differentiate into airway epithelial cells with restored function of CFTR protein.[117]

A combinational approach of non-viral and viral vectors was used to treat SP-B deficiency in mice.[70] Specifically, they used a non-viral vector to deliver the chemically modified mRNA encoding ZFN which was complexed with the chitosan-coated poly (lactic-co-glycolic) acid to form biodegradable nanoparticles.[70] rAAV6, a viral vector which has high tropism towards lung, was used to carry a repair template.[70] Transgenic surfactant protein B (SP-B) mice intratracheally treated with the combination of AAV6 and nanoparticles yielded the site-specific genome editing *in vivo,* resulting in prolonged life of experimental animals.[70] However, due to natural turnover of lung epithelial cells, the rescue effect was only transient.[70]

16.4 Perspective and Challenges for Therapeutic Genome Editing for the Lung

16.4.1 Delivery Barriers

In vivo intracellular delivery of genome editing proteins exhibits numerous challenges.[50,53] First, similar to gene transfer, the size of genome editing proteins needs to fit into the delivery vector.[50] The size of ZFNs is relatively small (~1 kb each, two molecules).[3] TALENs are a pair of molecules ~3 kb each, and CRISPR is about 3.2 kb–4.5 kb.[27] Viral vectors hold a maximal size limit of genetic sequences that they can pack.[47] For example, AAV has a package limit of ~4.7 kb. It is difficult to pack Cas9, sgRNA, and a donor template into one AAV vector.[118] Dual AAV vectors and smaller forms of Cas9 (e.g. Staphylococcus aureus Cas9, saCas9) are often used for *in vivo* delivery.[9,11,12,118] In contrast to viral delivery, the payload size is less pertinent for non-viral-mediated delivery.[50] For example, several polymer nanoparticles were demonstrated to be flexible with their payload from a small interfering RNA to a large 10 kb mRNA.[119,120]

Second, the cellular and endosomal membranes are the physical barriers to entry.[40] Large and charged molecules such as mRNA, DNA, and proteins cannot efficiently pass through hydrophobic cellular membranes.[40] If injecting systemically, they are subject to immediate degradation by nucleases circulating in the blood and likely to activate the immune system.[40] Besides degradation, the therapeutic biomolecules have to pass through the lung endothelial cells and the extracellular matrix between the lung endothelial and epithelial cells. If the therapeutic biomolecules are administrated via the airway, they have to be broadly distributed to cover bigger surface area for maximum therapeutic effects. The viscous mucus layer, in particular under pathological condition of lung, is another crucial barrier to overcome for successful airway delivery.[101,121,122] The uneven distribution of surface receptors for viral vectors entry to the cells require additional engineering of the viral surface protein.[64,65] For both, gene transfer and genome editing, efficient targeting of the "right" cell type is the key to provide a long-term therapeutic effect.[36,38,123] Nevertheless, as it stands right now, delivery is the rate-limiting step for successful therapeutic genome editing and gene transfer for the lung and many other organs and tissues.

Immune response is another worrisome concern for biomolecule delivery. A large number of delivery vectors after airway administration may be taken by residential macrophages in the lung, that get activated in promoting inflammatory responses.[42,59,124] Repeat injection of viral and non-viral vectors might induce adaptive immune reactions and inflammation.[40,47] Moreover, restoration of a protein, which has never been exposed to the immune system, is another factor that may provoke autoimmune reactions.[47,125] Another important point is that neutralization antibodies against saCas9 and spCas9 have been detected in more than 50% of human population tested, raising the concerns of long-term expression of CRISPR in patients and delivery of CRISPR in protein format.[126,127]

16.4.2 Short- and Long-Term Efficiency

The potential to provide long-term effect is a great advantage of therapeutic genome editing over small molecule drugs.[8,17] However, the duration of therapeutic outcome depends on the type and turnover of gene edited cells.[8,17] The ciliated cells in cystic fibrosis patients have a high turnover rate of several weeks.[92] The half-life of human lung epithelial cells in healthy population remains to be determined.[92] Thus, the gene editing of lung progenitor cells rather than the differentiated ciliated cells is likely to provide a long-term benefit. On the other hand, repeated dosing of non-viral vectors carrying genome editing nucleases to target the fast turnover lung epithelial cells might provide a sustained benefit.

16.4.3 Off-Target Effects and Safety

Off-target gene modification is one of the key concerns for genome editing therapy. Many studies investigated on how to precisely measure the frequencies and locations of off-target sites, and how to minimize the off-target effects.[128–136] Extensive screening for guide RNA sequences, ZFN and TALEN, and optimized delivery methods can dramatically reduce off-target effect of genome editing nucleases.[51,137–139] Moreover, engineering the guide RNA and the structure of Cas9 can further reduce the off-target effects.[128–136] Results from genome-wide, cell-based off-target analysis suggested that very few or no off-target sites were detected under optimized conditions with improved sgRNA and Cas proteins.[128–136] It is worth noting that oncogenic mutations in some somatic cells might trigger cancer. Nevertheless, the off-target effects in patient tissues from the incoming clinical trials remain to be determined.

Besides off-target, the genome editing nucleases may induce other unexpected side effects. For example, two recent studies on cell line or human pluripotent cells suggested that the CRISPR/Cas9 delivery induced an activation of p53-mediated DNA damage response and thus lead to cell death.[140,141] Primary cells such as lung progenitors could be more sensitive to DSBs created through nucleases. It is crucial to monitor the long-term effects of engineered progenitor cells and their ability of self-renewal and differentiation after *ex vivo* and *in vivo* gene editing.[70]

The repair of DSBs by NHEJ is semi-random, resulting in various indel sizes, inversions, or chromosomal translocation.[142–145] One strategy to minimize unexpected repair outcome is based on deactivated or nickase version of Cas9.[146–152] Rather than generating DSBs, deactivated or nickase Cas9 only binds to target sequence or results a single strand break, respectively.[146–152] Fusion of deactivated Cas9 with the transcriptional activation domain VP64 was demonstrated to enhance expression of targeted gene.[146,147] Using deactivated Cas9 alone or its fusion with a transcriptional repressor resulted in suppression of gene expression.[146] A fusion of Cas proteins with a cytidine deaminase converts cytidine to uridine. Engineered Cas9 base editors can make changes of cytosine (C) to thymine (T) or guanine (G) to adenine (A) substitution within a 5-nt window of the gRNA sequence.[21,153,154] Adenine base editors (ABEs) were then created to convert A•T base pairs to G•C in mammalian cells.[22] These expanded Cas9 tools provide a programmable introduction of genomic modifications without introducing DSBs. Thus, these therapeutic applications may hold a great potential to reduce the side effects associated with DSBs.

16.4.4 Competition with Other Therapeutic Platforms

Although it is attractive to transform the precise genome editing therapy into clinics, the therapeutic genome editing for lung diseases faces strong competitions from small molecule drugs, protein replacement therapy, and RNA inference therapy. It is likely that the next generation of CFTR protein correctors, presented as small molecules, would benefit more than 90% of cystic fibrosis patients carrying one or both copies of delta508 mutations, leaving 6%–8% patients without effective treatment.[155] Infusion of AAT protein, gene transfer of AAT, or a potential AAT protein corrector might treat all AAT disorders.[31,97,156,157] Although small interfering RNAs did not obtain statistically significant outcome in a phase II trial for treating respiratory syncytial virus (RSV) infection, a more potent and stable form of siRNA has been developed.[158,159] Nevertheless, a successful genome editing program may make use of undruggable targets and/or provide a better therapeutic outcome.

16.4.5 Cost, Benefit, and Target Populations

Genome editing targets rare or ultra-rare lung genetic diseases. A genome editing treatment can be as expensive as a cell therapy or a gene therapy treatment due to the small patient population, the complicated drug development process, and the high cost of manufacture. A key consideration during clinical translation is how to make drug development profitable and how to bring such types of drug to the market with affordable price. A universal gene editing strategy to treat as many patients as possible would significantly reduce the cost. For example, a targeted insertion of the entire or a large fragment of CFTR gene would benefit most of patients without a copy of delta508 mutation.[59] A combination of gene deletion and gene correction of AAT might be suitable for a large number of AAT patients.[114,115] Considering the potential of one-time treatment for a life-time benefit and life-saving outcome, the social cost of the therapeutic genome editing treatment could be potentially lower than the current treatments of alleviating/halting the disease manifestation and symptom such as continuous hospitalization and chronic treatment with small molecule drugs.

REFERENCES

1. Doudna, J.A. & Charpentier, E. Genome editing. The new frontier of genome engineering with CRISPR-Cas9. *Science (New York, N.Y.)* **346**, 1258096 (2014).
2. Kim, H. & Kim, J.-S. A guide to genome engineering with programmable nucleases. *Nature Reviews Genetics* **15**, 321–334 (2014).
3. Urnov, F.D., Rebar, E.J., Holmes, M.C., Zhang, H.S. & Gregory, P.D. Genome editing with engineered zinc finger nucleases. *Nature Reviews Genetics* **11**, 636–646 (2010).
4. Cong, L. et al. Multiplex genome engineering using CRISPR/Cas systems. *Science (New York, N.Y.)* **339**, 819–823 (2013).
5. Mali, P. et al. RNA-guided human genome engineering via Cas9. *Science (New York, N.Y.)* **339**, 823–826 (2013).
6. Lieber, M.R., Ma, Y., Pannicke, U. & Schwarz, K. Mechanism and regulation of human non-homologous DNA end-joining. *Nature Reviews Molecular Cell Biology* **4**, 712–720 (2003).
7. Isken, O. & Maquat, L.E. Quality control of eukaryotic mRNA: Safeguarding cells from abnormal mRNA function. *Genes & Development* **21**, 1833–1856 (2007).
8. Cox, D.B., Platt, R.J. & Zhang, F. Therapeutic genome editing: Prospects and challenges. *Nature Medicine* **21**, 121–131 (2015).
9. Tabebordbar, M. et al. In vivo gene editing in dystrophic mouse muscle and muscle stem cells. *Science (New York, N.Y.)* **351**, 407–411 (2016).
10. Xu, L. et al. CRISPR-mediated genome editing restores dystrophin expression and function in mdx mice. *Molecular Therapy* **24**, 564–569 (2016).
11. Nelson, C.E. et al. In vivo genome editing improves muscle function in a mouse model of Duchenne muscular dystrophy. *Science (New York, N.Y.)* **351**, 403–407 (2016).
12. Long, C. et al. Postnatal genome editing partially restores dystrophin expression in a mouse model of muscular dystrophy. *Science (New York, N.Y.)* **351**, 400–403 (2016).

13. Long, C. et al. Prevention of muscular dystrophy in mice by CRISPR/Cas9-mediated editing of germline DNA. *Science (New York, N.Y.)* **345**, 1184–1188 (2014).
14. Rouet, P., Smih, F. & Jasin, M. Introduction of double-strand breaks into the genome of mouse cells by expression of a rare-cutting endonuclease. *Molecular and Cellular Biology* **14**, 8096–8106 (1994).
15. Sadelain, M., Papapetrou, E.P. & Bushman, F.D. Safe harbours for the integration of new DNA in the human genome. *Nature Reviews Cancer* **12**, 51–58 (2012).
16. Li, H. et al. In vivo genome editing restores haemostasis in a mouse model of haemophilia. *Nature* **475**, 217–221 (2011).
17. Yin, H. et al. Genome editing with Cas9 in adult mice corrects a disease mutation and phenotype. *Nature Biotechnology* **32**, 551–553 (2014).
18. Baeumler, T.A., Ahmed, A.A. & Fulga, T.A. Engineering synthetic signaling pathways with programmable dCas9-based chimeric receptors. *Cell Reports* **20**, 2639–2653 (2017).
19. Billon, P. et al. CRISPR-mediated base editing enables efficient disruption of eukaryotic genes through induction of STOP codons. *Molecular Cell* **67**, 1068–1079.e4 (2017).
20. Chen, B. et al. Dynamic imaging of genomic loci in living human cells by an optimized CRISPR/Cas system. *Cell* **155**, 1479–1491 (2013).
21. Komor, A.C., Kim, Y.B., Packer, M.S., Zuris, J.A. & Liu, D.R. Programmable editing of a target base in genomic DNA without double-stranded DNA cleavage. *Nature* **533**, 420 (2016).
22. Gaudelli, N.M. et al. Programmable base editing of A•T to G•C in genomic DNA without DNA cleavage. *Nature* **551**, 464 (2017).
23. Nishida, K. et al. Targeted nucleotide editing using hybrid prokaryotic and vertebrate adaptive immune systems. *Science (New York, N.Y.)* **353** (2016).
24. Fellmann, C., Gowen, B.G., Lin, P.C., Doudna, J.A. & Corn, J.E. Cornerstones of CRISPR-Cas in drug discovery and therapy. *Nature Reviews Drug Discovery* **16**, 89–100 (2017).
25. Gootenberg, J.S. et al. Nucleic acid detection with CRISPR-Cas13a/C2c2. *Science (New York, N.Y.)* **356**, 438–442 (2017).
26. Porteus, M.H. & Carroll, D. Gene targeting using zinc finger nucleases. *Nature Biotechnology* **23**, 967–973 (2005).
27. Joung, J.K. & Sander, J.D. TALENs: A widely applicable technology for targeted genome editing. *Nature Reviews Molecular Cell Biology* **14**, 49–55 (2013).
28. Gaj, T., Gersbach, C.A. & Barbas, C.F., 3rd ZFN, TALEN, and CRISPR/Cas-based methods for genome engineering. *Trends in Biotechnology* **31**, 397–405 (2013).
29. Jinek, M. et al. A programmable dual-RNA-guided DNA endonuclease in adaptive bacterial immunity. *Science (New York, N.Y.)* **337**, 816–821 (2012).
30. Jinek, M. et al. RNA-programmed genome editing in human cells. *eLife* **2**, e00471 (2013).
31. Green, C.E. et al. PiSZ alpha-1 antitrypsin deficiency (AATD): pulmonary phenotype and prognosis relative to PiZZ AATD and PiMM COPD. *Thorax* **70**, 939–945 (2015).
32. Spoonhower, K.A. & Davis, P.B. Epidemiology of cystic fibrosis. *Clinics in Chest Medicine* **37**, 1–8 (2016).
33. Hamvas, A. Inherited surfactant protein-B deficiency and surfactant protein-C associated disease: clinical features and evaluation. *Seminars in Perinatology* **30**, 316–326 (2006).
34. Nogee, L.M. Genetic basis of children's interstitial lung disease. *Pediatric Allergy, Immunology, and Pulmonology* **23**, 15–24 (2010).
35. Rosenfeld, M.A. et al. In vivo transfer of the human cystic fibrosis transmembrane conductance regulator gene to the airway epithelium. *Cell* **68**, 143–155 (1992).
36. Crystal, R.G., Randell, S.H., Engelhardt, J.F., Voynow, J. & Sunday, M.E. Airway epithelial cells: Current concepts and challenges. *Proceedings of the American Thoracic Society* **5**, 772–777 (2008).
37. Harrison, P.T., Hoppe, N. & Martin, U. Gene editing & stem cells. *Journal of Cystic Fibrosis* **17**, 10–16 (2018).
38. Nadkarni, R.R., Abed, S. & Draper, J.S. Stem cells in pulmonary disease and regeneration. *Chest* **153**, 994–1003 (2018).
39. Griesenbach, U., Pytel, K.M. & Alton, E.W. Cystic fibrosis gene therapy in the UK and elsewhere. *Human Gene Therapy* **26**, 266–275 (2015).
40. Yin, H. et al. Non-viral vectors for gene-based therapy. *Nature Reviews Genetics* **15**, 541–555 (2014).

41. Kim, N., Duncan, G.A., Hanes, J. & Suk, J.S. Barriers to inhaled gene therapy of obstructive lung diseases: A review. *Journal of Controlled Release* **240**, 465–488 (2016).
42. Conese, M. et al. Gene and cell therapy for cystic fibrosis: From bench to bedside. *Journal of Cystic Fibrosis* **10 Suppl 2**, S114–S128 (2011).
43. Liu, X. et al. Comparative biology of rAAV transduction in ferret, pig and human airway epithelia. *Gene Therapy* **14**, 1543–1548 (2007).
44. Liu, X., Yan, Z., Luo, M. & Engelhardt, J.F. Species-specific differences in mouse and human airway epithelial biology of recombinant adeno-associated virus transduction. *American Journal of Respiratory Cell and Molecular Biology* **34**, 56–64 (2006).
45. Oakland, M., Sinn, P.L. & McCray, P.B., Jr. Advances in cell and gene-based therapies for cystic fibrosis lung disease. *Molecular Therapy* **20**, 1108–1115 (2012).
46. Chirmule, N. et al. Immune responses to adenovirus and adeno-associated virus in humans. *Gene Therapy* **6**, 1574–1583 (1999).
47. Kay, M.A. State-of-the-art gene-based therapies: The road ahead. *Nature Reviews Genetics* **12**, 316–328 (2011).
48. Ayuso, E. Manufacturing of recombinant adeno-associated viral vectors: New technologies are welcome. *Molecular Therapy – Methods & Clinical Development* **3**, 15049 (2016).
49. Sumner-Jones, S.G., Gill, D.R. & Hyde, S.C. Lack of repeat transduction by recombinant adeno-associated virus type 5/5 vectors in the mouse airway. *Journal of Virology* **81**, 12360–12367 (2007).
50. Yin, H., Kauffman, K.J. & Anderson, D.G. Delivery technologies for genome editing. *Nature Reviews Drug Discovery* **16**, 387–399 (2017).
51. Yin, H. et al. Therapeutic genome editing by combined viral and non-viral delivery of CRISPR system components in vivo. *Nature Biotechnology* **34**, 328–333 (2016).
52. Bak, R.O., Dever, D.P. & Porteus, M.H. CRISPR/Cas9 genome editing in human hematopoietic stem cells. *Nature Protocols* **13**, 358–376 (2018).
53. Driskell, R.A. & Engelhardt, J.F. Current status of gene therapy for inherited lung diseases. *Annual Review of Physiology* **65**, 585–612 (2003).
54. Cannizzo, S.J. et al. Augmentation of blood platelet levels by intratracheal administration of an adenovirus vector encoding human thrombopoietin cDNA. *Nature Biotechnology* **15**, 570–573 (1997).
55. Rosenfeld, M.A. et al. Adenovirus-mediated transfer of a recombinant alpha 1-antitrypsin gene to the lung epithelium in vivo. *Science (New York, N.Y.)* **252**, 431–434 (1991).
56. Koehler, D.R. et al. Aerosol delivery of an enhanced helper-dependent adenovirus formulation to rabbit lung using an intratracheal catheter. *The Journal of Gene Medicine* **7**, 1409–1420 (2005).
57. Koehler, D.R. et al. Protection of Cftr knockout mice from acute lung infection by a helper-dependent adenoviral vector expressing Cftr in airway epithelia. *Proceedings of the National Academy of Sciences of the United States of America* **100**, 15364–15369 (2003).
58. Bellon, G. et al. Aerosol administration of a recombinant adenovirus expressing CFTR to cystic fibrosis patients: A phase I clinical trial. *Human Gene Therapy* **8**, 15–25 (1997).
59. Hart, S.L. & Harrison, P.T. Genetic therapies for cystic fibrosis lung disease. *Current Opinion in Pharmacology* **34**, 119–124 (2017).
60. Cartier, N. et al. Hematopoietic stem cell gene therapy with a lentiviral vector in X-linked adrenoleukodystrophy. *Science (New York, N.Y.)* **326**, 818–823 (2009).
61. Sessa, M. et al. Lentiviral haemopoietic stem-cell gene therapy in early-onset metachromatic leukodystrophy: An ad-hoc analysis of a non-randomised, open-label, phase ½ trial. *Lancet (London, England)* **388**, 476–487 (2016).
62. Sinn, P.L., Arias, A.C., Brogden, K.A. & McCray, P.B., Jr. Lentivirus vector can be readministered to nasal epithelia without blocking immune responses. *Journal of Virology* **82**, 10684–10692 (2008).
63. Sakuma, T., Barry, M.A. & Ikeda, Y. Lentiviral vectors: Basic to translational. *The Biochemical Journal* **443**, 603–618 (2012).
64. Cooney, A.L. et al. Lentiviral-mediated phenotypic correction of cystic fibrosis pigs. *JCI Insight* **1**, e88730 (2016).
65. Steines, B. et al. CFTR gene transfer with AAV improves early cystic fibrosis pig phenotypes. *JCI Insight* **1**, e88728 (2016).
66. Hu, Y.C. Baculovirus vectors for gene therapy. *Advances in Virus Research* **68**, 287–320 (2006).
67. Vera, M. & Fortes, P. Simian virus-40 as a gene therapy vector. *DNA and Cell Biology* **23**, 271–282 (2004).

68. Guo, Z.S. & Bartlett, D.L. Vaccinia as a vector for gene delivery. *Expert Opinion on Biological Therapy* **4**, 901–917 (2004).
69. Robinson, E. et al. Lipid nanoparticle-delivered chemically modified mRNA restores chloride secretion in cystic fibrosis. *Molecular Therapy* **26**, 2034–2046 (2018).
70. Mahiny, A.J. et al. In vivo genome editing using nuclease-encoding mRNA corrects SP-B deficiency. *Nature Biotechnology* **33**, 584–586 (2015).
71. Yin, H. et al. Structure-guided chemical modification of guide RNA enables potent non-viral in vivo genome editing. *Nature Biotechnology* **35**, 1179–1187 (2017).
72. Rezaee, M., Oskuee, R.K., Nassirli, H. & Malaekeh-Nikouei, B. Progress in the development of lipopolyplexes as efficient non-viral gene delivery systems. *Journal of Controlled Release* **236**, 1–14 (2016).
73. Alton, E.W. et al. Non-invasive liposome-mediated gene delivery can correct the ion transport defect in cystic fibrosis mutant mice. *Nature Genetics* **5**, 135–142 (1993).
74. Hyde, S.C. et al. Correction of the ion transport defect in cystic fibrosis transgenic mice by gene therapy. *Nature* **362**, 250–255 (1993).
75. Tian, D. et al. Therapeutic effect of intratracheal administration of murine IL-4 receptor antagonist on asthmatic airway inflammation. *The Journal of Asthma* **45**, 715–721 (2008).
76. Aguero, J. et al. Intratracheal gene delivery of SERCA2a ameliorates chronic post-capillary pulmonary hypertension: A large animal model. *Journal of the American College of Cardiology* **67**, 2032–2046 (2016).
77. Ostedgaard, L.S. et al. The DeltaF508 mutation causes CFTR misprocessing and cystic fibrosis-like disease in pigs. *Science Translational Medicine* **3**, 74ra24 (2011).
78. Rogers, C.S. et al. Production of CFTR-null and CFTR-DeltaF508 heterozygous pigs by adeno-associated virus-mediated gene targeting and somatic cell nuclear transfer. *The Journal of Clinical Investigation* **118**, 1571–1577 (2008).
79. Walters, R.W. et al. Basolateral localization of fiber receptors limits adenovirus infection from the apical surface of airway epithelia. *The Journal of Biological Chemistry* **274**, 10219–10226 (1999).
80. Yoshimura, K. et al. Expression of the human cystic fibrosis transmembrane conductance regulator gene in the mouse lung after in vivo intratracheal plasmid-mediated gene transfer. *Nucleic Acids Research* **20**, 3233–3240 (1992).
81. Konstan, M.W. et al. Compacted DNA nanoparticles administered to the nasal mucosa of cystic fibrosis subjects are safe and demonstrate partial to complete cystic fibrosis transmembrane regulator reconstitution. *Human Gene Therapy* **15**, 1255–1269 (2004).
82. McLachlan, G. et al. Pre-clinical evaluation of three non-viral gene transfer agents for cystic fibrosis after aerosol delivery to the ovine lung. *Gene Therapy* **18**, 996–1005 (2011).
83. Kuzmov, A. & Minko, T. Nanotechnology approaches for inhalation treatment of lung diseases. *Journal of Controlled Release* **219**, 500–518 (2015).
84. Sanjar, S. & Matthews, J. Treating systemic diseases via the lung. *Journal of Aerosol Medicine* **14 Suppl 1**, S51–S58 (2001).
85. Agu, R.U., Ugwoke, M.I., Armand, M., Kinget, R. & Verbeke, N. The lung as a route for systemic delivery of therapeutic proteins and peptides. *Respiratory Research* **2**, 198–209 (2001).
86. Labiris, N.R. & Dolovich, M.B. Pulmonary drug delivery. Part I: Physiological factors affecting therapeutic effectiveness of aerosolized medications. *British Journal of Clinical Pharmacology* **56**, 588–599 (2003).
87. Depreter, F., Pilcer, G. & Amighi, K. Inhaled proteins: Challenges and perspectives. *International Journal of Pharmaceutics* **447**, 251–280 (2013).
88. Orson, F.M. et al. Gene delivery to the lung using protein/polyethylenimine/plasmid complexes. *Gene Therapy* **9**, 463–471 (2002).
89. Trang, P. et al. Systemic delivery of tumor suppressor microRNA mimics using a neutral lipid emulsion inhibits lung tumors in mice. *Molecular Therapy* **19**, 1116–1122 (2011).
90. Xue, W. et al. Small RNA combination therapy for lung cancer. *Proceedings of the National Academy of Sciences* (2014). doi:10.1073/pnas.1412686111.
91. Burney, T.J. & Davies, J.C. Gene therapy for the treatment of cystic fibrosis. *The Application of Clinical Genetics* **5**, 29–36 (2012).
92. Rawlins, E.L. & Hogan, B.L. Ciliated epithelial cell lifespan in the mouse trachea and lung. *American Journal of Physiology – Lung Cellular and Molecular Physiology* **295**, L231–L234 (2008).

93. Alton, E. et al. Repeated nebulisation of non-viral CFTR gene therapy in patients with cystic fibrosis: A randomised, double-blind, placebo-controlled, phase 2b trial. *The Lancet Respiratory Medicine* **3**, 684–691 (2015).
94. Nakanishi, M. & Otsu, M. Development of Sendai virus vectors and their potential applications in gene therapy and regenerative medicine. *Current Gene Therapy* **12**, 410–416 (2012).
95. Khan, O.F. et al. Endothelial siRNA delivery in nonhuman primates using ionizable low-molecular weight polymeric nanoparticles. *Science Advances* **4**, eaar8409 (2018).
96. Dahlman, J.E. et al. In vivo endothelial siRNA delivery using polymeric nanoparticles with low molecular weight. *Nature Nanotechnology* **9**, 648–655 (2014).
97. Brantly, M.L. et al. Phase I trial of intramuscular injection of a recombinant adeno-associated virus serotype 2 alphal-antitrypsin (AAT) vector in AAT-deficient adults. *Human Gene Therapy* **17**, 1177–1186 (2006).
98. Brantly, M.L. et al. Sustained transgene expression despite T lymphocyte responses in a clinical trial of rAAV1-AAT gene therapy. *Proceedings of the National Academy of Sciences of the United States of America* **106**, 16363–16368 (2009).
99. Barkauskas, C.E. et al. Lung organoids: Current uses and future promise. *Development (Cambridge, England)* **144**, 986–997 (2017).
100. Wang, H.X. et al. CRISPR/Cas9-based genome editing for disease modeling and therapy: Challenges and opportunities for nonviral delivery. *Chemical Reviews* **117**, 9874–9906 (2017).
101. Mastorakos, P. et al. Highly compacted biodegradable DNA nanoparticles capable of overcoming the mucus barrier for inhaled lung gene therapy. *Proceedings of the National Academy of Sciences of the United States of America* **112**, 8720–8725 (2015).
102. Kotton, D.N. & Morrisey, E.E. Lung regeneration: Mechanisms, applications and emerging stem cell populations. *Nature Medicine* **20**, 822–832 (2014).
103. Donne, M.L., Lechner, A.J. & Rock, J.R. Evidence for lung epithelial stem cell niches. *BMC Developmental Biology* **15**, 32 (2015).
104. Lau, A.N., Goodwin, M., Kim, C.F. & Weiss, D.J. Stem cells and regenerative medicine in lung biology and diseases. *Molecular Therapy* **20**, 1116–1130 (2012).
105. Kanasty, R., Dorkin, J.R., Vegas, A. & Anderson, D. Delivery materials for siRNA therapeutics. *Nature Materials* **12**, 967–977 (2013).
106. Xue, W. et al. CRISPR-mediated direct mutation of cancer genes in the mouse liver. *Nature* **514**, 380–385 (2014).
107. Sanchez-Rivera, F.J. et al. Rapid modelling of cooperating genetic events in cancer through somatic genome editing. *Nature* **516**, 428–431 (2014).
108. Snyder, E.L. et al. Nkx2-1 represses a latent gastric differentiation program in lung adenocarcinoma. *Molecular Cell* **50**, 185–199 (2013).
109. Herbst, R.S., Heymach, J.V. & Lippman, S.M. Lung cancer. *The New England Journal of Medicine* **359**, 1367–1380 (2008).
110. Platt, R.J. et al. CRISPR-Cas9 knockin mice for genome editing and cancer modeling. *Cell* **159**, 440–455 (2014).
111. Maddalo, D. et al. In vivo engineering of oncogenic chromosomal rearrangements with the CRISPR/Cas9 system. *Nature* **516**, 423–427 (2014).
112. Rogers, Z.N. et al. Mapping the in vivo fitness landscape of lung adenocarcinoma tumor suppression in mice. *Nature Genetics* **50**, 483–486 (2018).
113. Shalem, O., Sanjana, N.E. & Zhang, F. High-throughput functional genomics using CRISPR-Cas9. *Nature Reviews Genetics* **16**, 299–311 (2015).
114. Shen, S. et al. Amelioration of alpha-1 antitrypsin deficiency diseases with genome editing in transgenic mice. *Human Gene Therapy* **29**, 861–873 (2018).
115. Song, C.Q. et al. In vivo genome editing partially restores alphal-antitrypsin in a murine model of AAT deficiency. *Human Gene Therapy* **29**, 853–860 (2018).
116. Schwank, G. et al. Functional repair of CFTR by CRISPR/Cas9 in intestinal stem cell organoids of cystic fibrosis patients. *Cell Stem Cell* **13**, 653–658 (2013).
117. Firth, A.L. et al. Functional gene correction for cystic fibrosis in lung epithelial cells generated from patient iPSCs. *Cell Reports* **12**, 1385–1390 (2015).
118. Ran, F.A. et al. In vivo genome editing using Staphylococcus aureus Cas9. *Nature* **520**, 186–191 (2015).

119. Chahal, J.S. et al. An RNA nanoparticle vaccine against Zika virus elicits antibody and CD8+ T cell responses in a mouse model. *Scientific Reports* **7**, 252 (2017).
120. Chahal, J.S. et al. Dendrimer-RNA nanoparticles generate protective immunity against lethal Ebola, H1N1 influenza, and Toxoplasma gondii challenges with a single dose. *Proceedings of the National Academy of Sciences of the United States of America* **113**, E4133–E4142 (2016).
121. Kim, A.J. et al. Use of single-site-functionalized PEG dendrons to prepare gene vectors that penetrate human mucus barriers. *Angewandte Chemie (International ed. in English)* **52**, 3985–3988 (2013).
122. Lai, S.K. et al. Rapid transport of large polymeric nanoparticles in fresh undiluted human mucus. *Proceedings of the National Academy of Sciences of the United States of America* **104**, 1482–1487 (2007).
123. Desai, T.J., Brownfield, D.G. & Krasnow, M.A. Alveolar progenitor and stem cells in lung development, renewal and cancer. *Nature* **507**, 190–194 (2014).
124. Zhang, D., Wu, M., Nelson, D.E., Pasula, R. & Martin Ii, W.J. Alpha-1-antitrypsin expression in the lung is increased by airway delivery of gene-transfected macrophages. *Gene Therapy* **10**, 2148 (2003).
125. Nathwani, A.C. et al. Long-term safety and efficacy of factor IX gene therapy in hemophilia B. *The New England Journal of Medicine* **371**, 1994–2004 (2014).
126. Charlesworth, C.T. et al. Identification of pre-existing adaptive immunity to Cas9 proteins in humans. *bioRxiv* (2018).
127. Wang, D. et al. Adenovirus-mediated somatic genome editing of pten by CRISPR/Cas9 in mouse liver in spite of Cas9-specific immune responses. *Human Gene Therapy* **26**, 432–442 (2015).
128. Ran, F.A. et al. Double nicking by RNA-guided CRISPR Cas9 for enhanced genome editing specificity. *Cell* **154**, 1380–1389 (2013).
129. Tsai, S.Q. et al. Dimeric CRISPR RNA-guided FokI nucleases for highly specific genome editing. *Nature Biotechnology* **32**, 569–576 (2014).
130. Guilinger, J.P., Thompson, D.B. & Liu, D.R. Fusion of catalytically inactive Cas9 to FokI nuclease improves the specificity of genome modification. *Nature Biotechnology* **32**, 577–582 (2014).
131. Slaymaker, I.M. et al. Rationally engineered Cas9 nucleases with improved specificity. *Science (New York, N.Y.)* **351**, 84–88 (2016).
132. Kleinstiver, B.P. et al. High-fidelity CRISPR-Cas9 nucleases with no detectable genome-wide off-target effects. *Nature* **529**, 490–495 (2016).
133. Bolukbasi, M.F. et al. DNA-binding domain fusions enhance the targeting range and precision of Cas9. *Nature Methods* **12**, 1150–1156 (2015).
134. Fu, Y., Sander, J.D., Reyon, D., Cascio, V.M. & Joung, J.K. Improving CRISPR-Cas nuclease specificity using truncated guide RNAs. *Nature Biotechnology* **32**, 279–284 (2013).
135. Chen, J.S. et al. Enhanced proofreading governs CRISPR–Cas9 targeting accuracy. *Nature* **550**, 407 (2017).
136. Yin, H. et al. Partial DNA-guided Cas9 enables genome editing with reduced off-target activity. *Nature Chemical Biology* **14**, 311 (2018).
137. Kim, S., Kim, D., Cho, S.W., Kim, J. & Kim, J.S. Highly efficient RNA-guided genome editing in human cells via delivery of purified Cas9 ribonucleoproteins. *Genome Research* **24**, 1012–1019 (2014).
138. Veres, A. et al. Low incidence of off-target mutations in individual CRISPR-Cas9 and TALEN targeted human stem cell clones detected by whole-genome sequencing. *Cell Stem Cell* **15**, 27–30 (2014).
139. Lee, C.M., Cradick, T.J., Fine, E.J. & Bao, G. Nuclease target site selection for maximizing on-target activity and minimizing off-target effects in genome editing. *Molecular Therapy* **24**, 475–487 (2016).
140. Haapaniemi, E., Botla, S., Persson, J., Schmierer, B. & Taipale, J. CRISPR-Cas9 genome editing induces a p53-mediated DNA damage response. *Nature Medicine* **24**, 927–930 (2018).
141. Ihry, R.J. et al. p53 inhibits CRISPR-Cas9 engineering in human pluripotent stem cells. *Nature Medicine* **24**, 939–946 (2018).
142. Ghezraoui, H. et al. Chromosomal translocations in human cells are generated by canonical nonhomologous end-joining. *Molecular Cell* **55**, 829–842 (2014).
143. Vanoli, F. et al. CRISPR-Cas9-guided oncogenic chromosomal translocations with conditional fusion protein expression in human mesenchymal cells. *Proceedings of the National Academy of Sciences of the United States of America* **114**, 3696–3701 (2017).
144. Choi, P.S. & Meyerson, M. Targeted genomic rearrangements using CRISPR/Cas technology. *Nature Communications* **5**, 3728 (2014).

145. Bauer, D.E., Canver, M.C. & Orkin, S.H. Generation of genomic deletions in mammalian cell lines via CRISPR/Cas9. *Journal of Visualized Experiments* **95**, e52118 (2014).
146. Gilbert, L.A. et al. Genome-scale CRISPR-mediated control of gene repression and activation. *Cell* **159**, 647–661 (2014).
147. Gilbert, L.A. et al. CRISPR-mediated modular RNA-guided regulation of transcription in eukaryotes. *Cell* **154**, 442–451 (2013).
148. Qi, L.S. et al. Repurposing CRISPR as an RNA-guided platform for sequence-specific control of gene expression. *Cell* **152**, 1173–1183 (2013).
149. Larson, M.H. et al. CRISPR interference (CRISPRi) for sequence-specific control of gene expression. *Nature Protocols* **8**, 2180–2196 (2013).
150. Cheng, A.W. et al. Multiplexed activation of endogenous genes by CRISPR-on, an RNA-guided transcriptional activator system. *Cell Research* **23**, 1163–1171 (2013).
151. Zalatan, J.G. et al. Engineering complex synthetic transcriptional programs with CRISPR RNA scaffolds. *Cell* **9**, 1–12 (2015).
152. Konermann, S. et al. Genome-scale transcriptional activation by an engineered CRISPR-Cas9 complex. *Nature* **517**, 583–588 (2015).
153. Zafra, M.P. et al. Optimized base editors enable efficient editing in cells, organoids and mice. *Nature Biotechnology* **36**, 888–893 (2018).
154. Li, X. et al. Base editing with a Cpf1-cytidine deaminase fusion. *Nature Biotechnology* **36**, 324–327 (2018).
155. Taylor-Cousar, J.L. et al. Tezacaftor-ivacaftor in patients with cystic fibrosis homozygous for Phe508del. *The New England Journal of Medicine* **377**, 2013–2023 (2017).
156. Mueller, C. et al. Sustained miRNA-mediated knockdown of mutant AAT with simultaneous augmentation of wild-type AAT has minimal effect on global liver miRNA profiles. *Molecular Therapy* **20**, 590–600 (2012).
157. Chiuchiolo, M.J. & Crystal, R.G. Gene therapy for alpha-1 antitrypsin deficiency lung disease. *Annals of the American Thoracic Society* **13 Suppl 4**, S352–S369 (2016).
158. Adams, D. et al. Patisiran, an RNAi therapeutic, for hereditary transthyretin amyloidosis. *The New England Journal of Medicine* **379**, 11–21 (2018).
159. Foster, D.J. et al. Advanced siRNA designs further improve in vivo performance of GalNAc-siRNA conjugates. *Molecular Therapy* **26**, 708–717 (2018).

17

Inhalation Drug Products Containing Nanomaterials

Sandro R.P. da Rocha, Rodrigo S. Heyder, Elizabeth R. Bielski, Ailin Guo, Martina Steinmaurer, and Joshua J. Reineke

CONTENTS

17.1 An Overview

In drug products, nanomaterials can be either the active pharmaceutical ingredients (APIs) themselves, carriers for the APIs, or alternatively, they may function as excipients. Since 1970[1] there have been a total of 359 applications for drug products containing nanomaterials (DPCNs) submitted to the Center for Drug Evaluation and Research (CDER) at the US Food and Drug Administration (FDA) (D'Mello et al. 2017). Approximately 19% of all 234 investigational new drugs (INDs, which are submissions to determine if a drug product is reasonably safe before initiating clinical trials) related to DPCNs resulted in new drug applications (NDAs, which are submissions of a new drug product to gain approval for marketing in the United States). Of these 44 NDAs, 34 have been approved, thus representing a similar rate of approval as all other drug products (D'Mello et al. 2017). These numbers strongly support the view that DPCNs represent attractive, translatable strategies for the development of enhanced drug products.

The majority of DPCNs to date have been indicated for i.v. administration (59%), while 21% were intended for oral administration. Applications related to inhalation DPCNs (IDPCNs) correspond to only

[1] Statistics collected until 2015 (D'Mello et al. 2017).

approximately 4% of all those submissions (D'Mello et al. 2017). Interestingly, this is slightly higher than the net worth share of the global pulmonary drug market (3%) compared to the global drug delivery market as a whole (MAM 2017).

In a search for clinical trials related to IDPCNs, 37 studies were found.[2] All but two of those studies involved the use of liposomes as the nanomaterial in the drug product; and, in all those trials, liposomes worked as drug carriers to improve the characteristics of the formulations. Liposomes are also the most prevalent nanomaterials when surveying all DPCNs' submissions (33%) taken all routes of administration together (D'Mello et al. 2017). The dominance of liposomes in DPCNs can be attributed to their early success, safety, and versatility, as well as the expiration of patent protections (D'Mello et al. 2017). It is of interest to note here that abbreviated new drug applications (ANDAs, submissions for a generic version of an existing approved drug) can include nanomaterials even if the reference listed drug (RLD) does not. This may happen when the size of the active or inactive ingredients is not specified in the RLD (D'Mello et al. 2017).

The majority (65%) of clinical trials of IDPCNs has focused on treatment of infections, while 16% were related to cancer. That differs significantly to the overall focus of DPCNs' submissions where the most common application (35%) has been cancer related (D'Mello et al. 2017). Clinical trials of IDPCNs indicate not only that liposomal formulations are safe, but also that toxicities typically associated with APIs (e.g. antibacterial, antifungal, chemotherapy) when administered through conventional routes can be significantly reduced when APIs are delivered in liposomal formulations.

When you combine those findings with the fact that lung cancer is the leading cause of cancer death among both men and women in the United States and worldwide (Siegel et al. 2018), we conclude that there are still significant opportunities to explore liposomal formulations for the efficient local delivery of chemotherapeutics to the lungs—at the minimum as adjuvant therapies to enhance conventional (i.v./oral) chemotherapies. Initial success with liposomal fentanyl also points to the potential of IDPCNs for the systemic delivery of therapeutics through the lungs. Limitations in this particular instance stem from the fact that the nanocarrier itself is likely not capable of translocating intact across the pulmonary epithelium (Abdelbary 2017). Therefore, the favorable characteristics of nanocarriers cannot be carried over to impact the drug behavior when in systemic circulation, such as long circulating times or targeting, as one could potentially achieve if the same liposome system were to be delivered i.v. (Allen and Cullis 2013, Caracciolo 2018).

That brings us to another limitation of clinical studies related to IDPCNs performed to date, which is the fact that few advancements/studies have been seen/performed for other types of nanomaterials. It is clear and important to note that liposomes (or any other single nanomaterial for that matter) should not be seen as the silver bullet to improve therapeutic efficacy and/or decrease toxicity for all classes of drugs and/or disease applications. It is also important to consider that indiscriminate use of liposomes, as we have seen in all but two of the clinical trials related to IDPCNs to date, may lead to overall disappointment in IDPCNs in general as trials fail to lead to commercial products—and create a significant set-back to the field.

In summary, the current landscape of studies related to IDPCNs suggest that liposomal formulations have a robust, favorable safety profile for the delivery of a variety of therapeutics directly to the pulmonary tract. The information discussed below also suggest that the field is mature enough for the consideration of more complex, second generation nanomaterials as their toxicity profiles are addressed.

17.2 Nanomaterials in Drug Products

17.2.1 Definition of Nanomaterials as It Relates to Drug Products

According to the FDA, a drug product involves the application of nanotechnology when: (i) "a material or end product is engineered to have at least one external dimension, or an internal or surface structure, in the nanoscale range (approximately 1 nm to 100 nm)" OR (ii) "a material or end product is engineered to exhibit properties or phenomena, including physical or chemical properties or biological effects, that are attributable to its dimension(s), even if these dimensions fall outside the nanoscale range, up to one micrometer (1,000 nm)." The European Medicine Agency (EMA) operates on a similar definition of a

[2] Search terms: "inhalation" or "pulmonary" and "micelle" or "dendrimer" or "polymeric" or "nanoparticle(s)" or "liposome" or "solid lipid" or "microemulsion" latest search carried out January 2018.

nanomaterial except that it must satisfy BOTH of the criteria listed above AND also meet the definition of a medicinal product, which is a "substance or combination of substances that is intended to treat, prevent or diagnose a disease, or to restore, correct or modify physiological functions by exerting a pharmacological, immunological or metabolic action" (EMA 2018). These DPCNs can find use in prophylaxis, as therapeutic agents, or in diagnostics.

17.2.2 Classification of Nanomaterials Used in Drug Products

There is a wide range of nanomaterials used in drug products (Doane and Burda 2012, Hubbell and Langer 2013, Kharisov et al. 2015, Peltonen and Hirvonen 2018, Quader and Kataoka 2017). One way to classify nanomaterials is regarding to their function in the drug product. According to a recent publication (D'Mello et al. 2017), the FDA's Office of Pharmaceutical Quality at CDER classifies nanomaterials as: (i) APIs (e.g. nanocrystals, drug nanoparticles); (ii) drug carriers (e.g. drug encapsulated liposomes); (iii) excipients (e.g. drug-metal complexes), or (iv) complex/conjugates (e.g. drug-protein).

Those nanomaterials *include:* (i) lipid-based systems (including liposomes, solid-lipid nanoparticles, and drug-lipid complexes), (ii) API nanocrystals and nanoparticles, (iii) polymer-based systems formed by complexation, encapsulation, or conjugation of the API (including proteins, other natural polymers, or synthetic materials), (iv) self-assembled systems with amphiphilic materials (such as nanoemulsions, micelles); (v) inorganic nanomaterials (including silica, iron-polymer, and other metal complexes, nanotubes); (vi) viral nanoparticles; (vii) natural membrane nanoparticles (as for example exosomes); and (viii) hybrid systems.

While recent trends suggest that more complex systems are making their way into submissions of drug containing nanomaterials, liposomal formulations (carriers) continue to be the most common nanomaterial in drug products (33%). These formulations are followed by nanocrystals (API, 23%). Other common submissions include emulsions, iron-polymer complexes, and micelles (14%, 9%, and 6%, respectively), while all other nanomaterials make up the other 14% of submissions (D'Mello et al. 2017).

17.2.3 Important Attributes of Nanomaterials Used in Drug Products

The physicochemical and biological attributes of nanomaterials and how they may relate to their quality, safety, and performance should be an important consideration in the selection of nanomaterials for use in drug products. In order to *describe* the nanomaterials, information including size, charge, morphology, and composition are essential, as well as their functionality (e.g. as carrier or targeting). It is also important to identify the nanomaterial's critical quality attributes (CQAs) and how they may impact performance. The quality may be unique to each material and will usually include attributes such as size distribution and physical stability and may also be non-material specific, such as impurities.

According to the FDA (FDA 2017), the following attributes should be described and measured for any nanomaterial in a drug product: (i) chemical composition; (ii) average particle size; (iii) particle size distribution (PSD); (iv) shape and morphology; (v) physical stability; and (vi) chemical stability. The following additional attributes may also be needed to describe nanomaterials, including: (vii) assay and distribution of the API (bound/conjugated to the carrier versus free); (viii) structural attributes that relate to function (e.g. core-shell); (ix) surface properties (surface area, surface charge, ligand); (x) coating properties, including how coatings are bound to nanomaterials; (xi) porosity; (xii) particle concentration; (xiii) *in vitro* release; (xiv) crystal form; (xv) impurities; and (xvi) sterility and endotoxin levels. These measured attributes are in addition to characterizations required for all medical products of similar intended application (e.g. efficacy, toxicity).

A wide range of techniques are available to evaluate each of the above characteristics including nuclear magnetic resonance spectroscopy (NMR), light scattering, scanning and transmission electron microscopy, spectroscopy, surface plasmon resonance (SPR), and others, but the appropriateness of each specific technique may be dependent on the material being characterized and/or the nanomaterial application. Neither the FDA nor EMA have mandated standardized testing protocols, although both agencies recognize the importance of standardized characterization and have solicited input from the research community. To provide guidance for companies developing nanomaterial-based medicines, the National Institutes of Health (NIH) established the Nanomedicine Characterization Lab (NIH-NCL) in 2004 with the aim of increasing successful translation of nanomedicines. The European Union later followed suit and in 2015 established the EU-NCL. Both NCLs have developed assay cascades that include *in vitro* characterization of physicochemical properties and *in vivo* procedures to evaluate the biological interactions (EUNCL 2018, NIH 2018b). Beyond the pre-clinical characterization, there is also the importance of batch quality control assessment for approved products on the market. This is an area where further development and guidance is needed (Coty and Vauthier 2018).

17.3 Considerations for Inhalation Drug Products Containing Nanomaterials (IDPCNs)

17.3.1 Deposition of Nanoparticles from IDPCNs in the Lungs

One important aspect in the development of IDPCNs is the ability to formulate those products in a way that they can be efficiently delivered to the lungs. Because optimal aerosol diameter for deep lung deposition falls outside the nano range (ca. 0.5 μm–5 μm) (Patton 2007), it is important to consider the selection of nanomaterials and how they will be formulated early in the development stage.

So far, most clinical studies of IDPCNs have been performed with liposomes as the nanomaterial and with nebulizers as the inhalation devices (NIH 2018a). Liposomes containing the APIs are typically dispersed in an aqueous medium and, with the help of either a jet or ultrasound, droplets of the aqueous medium containing liposomes are aerosolized and subsequently inhaled (Carvalho and McConville 2016). Formulations in nebulizers are relatively simple, as their use as (in their simplest form) nebulizers require only use of tidal breathing for inhalation of the drug product. However, they typically require extended periods of time for the administration of desired doses and have relatively low lung deposition profiles and high losses (Martin and Finlay 2015), which may represent a challenge for high potency drugs or costly drug products such as biologics and potentially IDPCNs. While some lipid-based nanomaterials may be formulated in traditional portable inhalers such as dry powder inhalers (DPIs) and pressurized metered-dose inhalers (pMDIs), liposomes cannot be directly formulated in such portable inhalers as they require an aqueous environment to be formed. Portable soft-mist inhalers, which are propellentless, metered dose devices (Dalby et al. 2011), offer new opportunities in this area.

Outside the clinical trials described above, there is an abundant literature on pre-clinical studies discussing the formulation of alternative nanomaterials (that are not liposomes) in portable inhalers. Formulation strategies of IDPCNs in DPIs typically revolve around particle engineering strategies where the nanomaterial, such as polymeric nanoparticles, are encapsulated within a shell that is expected to break down when in contact with the fluid lining the lung epithelium, thus releasing the nanocarrier system (Carter and Puig-Sellart 2016, Chen et al. 2017, Kamal et al. 2017). Alternatively, loose aggregation of the nanomaterial may also be utilized to achieve an appropriate (micron range) aerodynamic diameter for deep lung deposition (Eleftheriadis et al. 2018, Parikh and Dalwadi 2014).

DPIs are very important inhalation devices as they are portable and very flexible in terms of the drug product that can be formulated in such devices. However, DPI formulations that rely on drug-carrier interactions (typically lactose as carrier) are more complex, difficult to study, typically show poor lung deposition, and may also experience significant batch to batch variability (Healy et al. 2014). Carrier-free systems that employ engineered particles or *in situ* (as they travel in the airways) nanoparticle growth strategies (de Boer et al. 2017) may help overcome such limitations.

pMDIs represent another class of portable inhalers for the formulation of IDPCNs. Similar to DPIs, there are also advantages and challenges in the development of IDPCNs in pMDIs (Myrdal et al. 2014). They are attractive as they do not rely on patient inspiration to deposit the aerosol particle to the lungs (may work even when lung function is compromised), but typical pMDIs have shown relatively low drug deposition in the lungs, and patients may have difficulty in coordinating device actuation and inhalation (Aggarwal and Gogtay 2014, Nicolas and Richard 2016).

Several studies have reported the formulation of IDPCNs in pMDIs, including polymeric nanoparticles and dendrimers that can be used as carriers for small molecules and biologics and with lung depositions reported upwards of 90% of the emitted dose (Conti et al. 2014, Heyder et al. 2017). However, a major limitation of pMDIs is the relatively low dose that can be delivered per actuation (Bell and Newman 2007).

Formulation strategies include engineering of nanocarriers in microparticles in order to enhance deep lung deposition and physical stabilization in the propellant (Bharatwaj et al. 2010) and also polymer solubilization in the propellant with subsequent phase separation *in situ* in the aerosol droplet, leading to appropriate aerodynamic diameters for deep lung deposition in spite of their small size (Zhong and da Rocha 2016).

There are significant opportunities in the development of IDPCNs in portable inhalers due to their ease of use and versatility. A strength of DPIs is the potential to deliver high drug doses while pMDIs may be reliably employed to deliver high potency drugs (at lower doses) even in patients with compromised air flow. There are also significant opportunities for the development of formulation of IDPCNs in the portable soft-mist inhalers (Brand et al. 2008), an area that has seen relativity little activity so far.

17.3.2 Clearance of Nanoparticles from IDPCNs from the Lungs

The clearance mechanisms of nanoparticles from the lungs will be dependent on both the deposition and the material properties of the IDPCNs. Mechanisms have been thoroughly reviewed elsewhere (Geiser and Kreyling 2010, Geiser 2010, Weber et al. 2014) and are discussed briefly here for context. Generally, clearance mechanisms can be divided into absorptive (macrophage uptake, systemic uptake) and non-absorptive clearance (macrophage uptake, mucociliary elimination, enzymatic degradation).

The lung epithelial cells of the upper conducting airways are ciliated and covered by a periciliary fluid layer and mucus layer. The cilia gradually move the mucus layer, and any particulate matter entrapped by the mucus, towards the larynx, and they are eliminated in the gastrointestinal tract. This mucociliary escalator pathway is the major non-absorptive clearance mechanism of inhaled particulates; particularly those with upper airway deposition. Playing a lesser role is enzymatic degradation of degradable particles. The lung route has a much lower enzymatic activity relative to the oral route, which is an advantage of IDPCNs. Degradation happens by proteases and peptidases, expressed on the extracellular membrane, in addition to intracellular degradation mechanisms within lysosomes (Zarogoulidis et al. 2012).

In the respiratory airways of the lungs, alveolar macrophages are the major contributor to nanoparticle clearance. Particles deposited in the alveolar region that are engulfed by alveolar macrophages will either be degraded by enzymes in lysosomes or transported to lymph nodes via lymphatics. A small proportion of particle-carrying alveolar macrophages will migrate from alveolar regions to the start of the ciliated airways where they are cleared by mucociliary clearance. Activation of alveolar macrophages may cause the release of immunological mediators (e.g. IL-1b, IL-8, TNF-a) that can cause subsequent pulmonary inflammation (Manke et al. 2013). The choice of nanoparticles in IDPCNs should be selected to minimize such inflammatory interactions. Macrophage uptake may be limited for nanoparticles <100 nm as epithelial uptake is more efficient (Zhang et al. 2011) for this size range. Additionally, surface modification approaches (such as PEGylation) may reduce/delay macrophage uptake (Kolte et al. 2017).

Absorptive elimination through systemic absorption is attributed to the large lung surface area, high vascularity, and good epithelial permeability. A rapid elimination by systemic absorption results in suboptimal local effect and may cause adverse side effects. On the other hand, the systemic effect is achieved when inhaled drugs cross the epithelia into interstitium and then into the blood stream. The air to blood translocation of inhaled particles highly depends on their nature, such as size, molecular weight, lipophilicity/hydrophobicity, and surface properties. In general, small lipophilic particles are rapidly absorbed from lung to systemic circulation via passive diffusion (El-Sherbiny et al. 2015, Ryan et al. 2013, Zhong et al. 2016).

17.4 Clinical Studies of IDPCNs

17.4.1 Liposomes: The Most Common Nanomaterials in IDPs

As mentioned earlier, several IDPCNs have successfully reached clinical trials. A list of all trials of IDPCNs found at https://clinicaltrials.gov[3] are listed in Table 17.1. Out of the 37 trails, not surprisingly, the vast majority (35) refer to the use of liposomes as drug carrier systems. Liposomes represent the

[3] Search terms: "inhalation" or "pulmonary" and "micelle" or "dendrimer" or "polymeric" or "nanoparticle(s)" or "liposome" or "solid lipid" or "microemulsion" latest search carried out January. 2018. Does not include viral vectors.

TABLE 17.1
Clinical Trials of Inhalation Formulations Involving Nanomaterials

Nanocarrier	API	Clinical Stage	Status	Condition(s)	Dosage Form	Ref
Nanosilver	Silver	Observational	Withdrawn	Inflammatory Disease	nebulizer	NCT02408874
@HPMC	Oxymetazoline	Phase 2	Withdrawn	Inflammatory disease	nebulizer	NCT02408874
Liposome	Amikacin[1]	Phase 1/2	Completed	Cystic fibrosis	nebulizer	NCT00558844
Liposome	Amikacin[1]	Phase 1/2	Completed	Bronchiectasis	nebulizer	NCT00775138
Liposome	Amikacin[1]	Phase 1/2	Completed	Cystic fibrosis	nebulizer	NCT00777296
Liposome	Amikacin	Phase 2	Recruiting	Mycobacterium infections, NTM, Atypical	nebulizer#	NCT03038178
Liposome	Amikacin	Phase 2	Completed	Mycobacterium infections, NTM	eFLOW® nebulizer	NCT01315236
Liposome	Amikacin[2]	Phase 3	Completed	*P. aeruginosa* infections	eFLOW® nebulizer	NCT01315678
Liposome	Amikacin	Phase 3	Active, not recruiting	Mycobacterium infections, NTM	nebulizer#	NCT02344004
Liposome	Amikacin	Phase 3	Completed	Cystic fibrosis	eFLOW® nebulizer	NCT01316276
Liposome	Amikacin[2]	Phase 3	Withdrawn	Cystic fibrosis	eFLOW® nebulizer	NCT01315691
Liposome	Amikacin	Phase 3	Enrolling by Invitation	NTM, lung infections due to MAC	nebulizer#	NCT02628600
Liposome	Fentanyl[3]	Phase 1	Completed	Healthy	AeroEclipse BAN nebulizer	NCT00708318
Liposome	Fentanyl[3]	Phase 1	Completed	Healthy	AeroEclipse BAN nebulizer	NCT00709254
Liposome	Fentanyl[3]	Phase 1	Completed	Healthy	nebulizers (various)	NCT00794209
Liposome	Fentanyl[3]	Phase 2	Completed	Pain, post-operative pain	nebulizer	NCT00791804
Liposome	Fentanyl[3]	Phase 2	Completed	Pain	nebulizer	NCT00286065
Liposome	Ciprofloxacin[4]	Phase 2	Completed	Non-cystic fibrosis bronchiectasis	nebulizer	NCT00889967
Liposome	Ciprofloxacin	Phase 1/2	Withdrawn	Cystic fibrosis (w/*P. aeruginosa*)	nebulizer	NCT01090908
Liposome	Ciprofloxacin (dual release)[5]	Phase 3	Completed	Non-cystic fibrosis bronchiectasis	nebulizer#	NCT01515007
Liposome	Ciprofloxacin[5]	Phase 3	Completed	Non-cystic fibrosis bronchiectasis	nebulizer	NCT02104245
Liposome	Amphotericin B[6]	Phase 2/3	Completed	Aspergillosis	nebulizer	NCT00263315
Liposome	Amphotericin B[6]	Phase 2	Suspended	Lung Transplant	nebulizer#	NCT01254708
Liposome	Amphotericin B[6]	Phase 3	Completed	Lung transplant, fungal infections	nebulizer	NCT00177710
Liposome	Amphotericin B[6]	Phase 4	Unknown	Invasive pulmonary aspergillosis	nebulizer	NCT00986713
Liposome	Amphotericin B[7]	Phase 2	Completed	Invasive pulmonary aspergillosis, lymphoblastic and myeloblastic leukemia,	nebulizer	NCT01615809
Liposome	Amphotericin B[7]	Phase 3	Completed	lung transplant, fungal infections	nebulizer	NCT00177684

(*Continued*)

TABLE 17.1 (*Continued*)

Clinical Trials of Inhalation Formulations Involving Nanomaterials

Nanocarrier	API	Clinical Stage	Status	Condition(s)	Dosage Form	Ref
Liposome	Amphotericin B[7]	Phase 3	Terminated	Lung transplant, lung diseases	nebulizer	NCT00235651
Liposome	Cyclosporine	Phase 3	Terminated	Bronchiolitis obliterans		NCT01439958
Liposome	Cyclosporine	Phase 2/3	Terminated	Bronchiolitis obliterans	nebulizer	NCT01334892
Liposome	Cyclosporine	Phase 1/2	Completed	Disorder related to lung transplant, bronchiolitis obliterans, decreased immunologic activity, chronic rejection of lung transplant	nebulizer	NCT01650545
Liposome	9-Nitro-20 (S)-Camptothecin	Observational	Completed	Corpus uteri, lung cancer	nebulizer[#]	NCT00277082
Liposome	9-Nitro-20 (S)-Camptothecin	Phase 2	Completed	Corpus uteri, endometrial cancer	nebulizer[#]	NCT00249990
Liposome	9-Nitro-20 (S)-Camptothecin	Phase 2	Completed	Lung diseases, cancer	nebulizer[#]	NCT00250068
Liposome	9-Nitro-20 (S)-Camptothecin	Phase 2 (withdrawn)	Completed	Lung diseases, cancer	nebulizer[#]	NCT00250120
Liposome	LipoAerosol©	Interventional	Completed	Tracheostomy complication	nebulizer	NCT02157129
Liposome	Cisplatin	Phase 1/2	Completed	Osteosarcoma metastatic	nebulizer	NCT00102531

[@] HPMC = hydroxyl-propyl-methyl cellulose powder; [1] Arikace®; [2] Arikayce®; [3] AeroLEF®; [4] ARD-3100®; [5] ARD-3150, Pulmaquin®; [6] AmBisome®; [7] Abelcet®; NTM = non-tuberculous mycobacterium; MAC = mycobacterium avium complex; Data compiled January 2018.

nanomaterials of choice for IDPs at a much larger extent than compared to other more mature routes of administration where several other nanomaterials have made it into clinical trials and have received approval (Cipolla et al. 2013, D'Mello et al. 2017).

Due to established safety profiles, liposomes have been the obvious first choice to bring IDPCNs to clinical trials (D'Mello et al. 2017, Loira-Pastoriza et al. 2014). Only one trial is related to nasal route, which is in phase 2, and involves the use of hydroxyl-propyl-methyl cellulose (HPMC) powder for the sustained release of oxymetazoline (topical decongestant) for the treatment of allergic rhinitis (Valerieva et al. 2015). The other clinical trial not involving liposomes relates to the use of nanosilver as the active ingredient. Nanosilver has been used in antimicrobial cleaning supplies and fabrics and claims have been made it can boost the immune system (Chen and Schluesener 2008, Małaczewska 2011, Pishbin et al. 2013). The goal of the clinical study discussed here related to silver as nanomaterial was to assess the impact that inhaled nanosilver may have on the lung's immune system. However, this clinical trial was withdrawn. The status of those 37 trials includes 25 completed, two recruiting/enrolling by invitation, two active, three withdrawn, one suspended, three terminated, and one unknown trial. Of the 37 trials, one was in phase 4, 11 were in phase 3, 19 were in phase 1/2, 2, or 2/3, and the others were in phase 1, observational or interventional.

17.4.2 Nebulizers: The Most Common Devices Used to Deliver IDPCNs in Clinical Trials

It is worth noting that nebulizers are the most commonly used devices for delivering IDPCNs. Only one clinical trial (nasal formulation with HPMC) does not reference the use of nebulizers. All other drug products, including nanosilver, were tested in the clinic with nebulizers. Nebulizers are the device of choice for liposomal formulations due to the ease of formulation in preparation of large volumes without the need of complicated techniques (Elhissi et al. 2014).

17.4.3 Liposomal Formulations in IDPCNs in Clinical Trials

Liposomes can by prepared with lipids that are endogenous to the lung or are very similar to mammalian pulmonary surfactants (Elhissi et al. 2014, Loira-Pastoriza et al. 2014). The biocompatibility profiles of liposomes in the lungs have been extensively reported, and they have been, therefore, the nanomaterials of choice for the preparation of IDPCNs (Elhissi et al. 2014, Loira-Pastoriza et al. 2014). Lipids used in the formulation of liposomes contain a polar hydrophilic head group and a hydrophobic tail that lead to the formation of lipid bilayers (Loira-Pastoriza et al. 2014). The lipid bilayers can be composed of different phospholipids and cholesterol (CHOL) to modulate the stability of the liposome and rate of drug release (Loira-Pastoriza et al. 2014). Some common lipids used in formulations include 1,2-dipalmitoyl-sn-glycero-3-phosphocholine (DPPC), hydrogenated soy phosphatidylcholine (HSPC), distearoylphosphatidyl glycerol (DSPG), dimyristoyl phosphatidylcholine (DMPC), dimyristoyl phosphatidylglycerol (DMPG), and dilauroylphosphatidylcholine (DLPC). Liposomes have the ability to encapsulate a wide range of APIs, including hydrophilic, hydrophobic, small molecules, and biologics (Elhissi 2017, Sercombe et al. 2015). Liposomal inhalation drug products are used to localize the API to the targeted lung tissue, thus prolonging therapeutic effect in the lungs while decreasing systemic side effects to other organs (Elhissi et al. 2014, Loira-Pastoriza et al. 2014). The possibility of using inhalation drug products containing liposomes for the treatment of lung diseases including infections, transplantations, and cancers have been explored in the trials discussed above. There is only one clinical trial in which inhalation drug products containing liposomes were investigated for the systemic delivery of therapeutics through the lungs—pain relief from knee surgery. The associated drugs that were encapsulated in these studies include antibiotics, antifungal medications, immunosuppressant's, opioids, lipids, and chemotherapeutics.

Trends in IDPs containing nanomaterials can be compared to those seen for the aggregate (all routes of delivery) submissions where 94% are related to treatment of medical conditions—only 6% for imaging (D'Mello et al. 2017). The majority the IDP submissions containing nanomaterials was related to products that focus on infections (24 of 37% = 65%), likely driven by the significant need to address pulmonary infections. In comparison, when looking in aggregate (all routes), only 12% of drug products have been reported to be related to infections (D'Mello et al. 2017). On the other hand, only six out of 37 IDP submissions are related to cancer (16%), while in aggregate (all routes) the numbers are much greater (35%) (D'Mello et al. 2017).

17.4.4 Drug Classes in IDPs Containing Liposomes in Clinical Trials

17.4.4.1 Antibiotics

17.4.4.1.1 Liposomal Amikacin for Inhalation (LAI, Arikace™, Arikayce)

Of these pulmonary liposomal drug formulations in clinical trials, liposomal amikacin for inhalation (LAI, Arikace™, Arikayce) delivered by nebulization remains the most studied, comprising of ten of the 37 (27%) clinical trials (Table 17.1). Of these, five (50%) reached phase 3.

Amikacin is an aminoglycoside antibiotic used for the treatment of multidrug resistant gram-negative bacteria (*Pseudomonas aeruginosa* associated with cystic fibrosis) and resistant strains of Mycobacterium tuberculosis (Caster et al. 2017, Elhissi 2017). It irreversibly binds to 30S subunit of bacterial ribosomes blocking protein synthesis (Ehsan and Clancy 2015). It is generally reserved for severe infections, can induce severe renal and neurologic toxicity, requiring frequent blood monitoring, and has a relatively short half-life (Caster et al. 2017, Elhissi 2017). The LAI (Arikace™, Arikayce) was designed with the hope to address these limitations.

LAI is made by encapsulating amikacin in vesicles made from DPPC and CHOL, and the resulting liposomes have sizes of ca. 300 nm (Elhissi 2017, Meers et al. 2008). The phospholipid DPPC is the main component of mammalian lung surfactant while cholesterol is a main constituent of cellular membranes making this formulation highly biocompatible with and of low toxicity to the lung tissue (Elhissi 2017). When delivered to the lungs, the LAI can localize the action of amikacin in the lung with enhanced retention time and antibacterial effect, reduced systemic side effects, and enhanced penetration into the bacterial biofilm (Ehsan and Clancy 2015, Elhissi 2017). Also, the use of liposomes themselves can help within the nebulization process as lung deposition is promoted by increasing the fine particle fraction (FPF) as compared with the drug alone (Elhissi 2017).

Within clinical trials, LAI has been delivered through an optimized Pari eFlow vibrating-mesh nebulizer for the treatment of *pseudomonas* infections in cystic fibrosis patients, patients with bronchiectasis, and, more recently, the treatment of non-tuberculosis mycobacterium lung infections (Ehsan and Clancy 2015, Elhissi 2017). The treatment strategy usually consisted of doses ranging from 70 mg–560 mg once daily for 28 days (Ehsan and Clancy 2015). The phase 1–3 clinical trials for treatment of *pseudomonas* infection in cystic fibrosis patients have shown no visible toxicity between drug treatment groups and placebo groups (Caster et al. 2017, Ehsan and Clancy 2015). The formulation allowed for sustained release, localized drug release in the lungs, enhanced penetration of the drug into the biofilm, and release of the drug at the localized bacterial site (Ehsan and Clancy 2015, Elhissi 2017). The prolonged deposition allowed for a maintained effect on lung function when not in treatment. Improvement in respiratory symptoms and forced expiratory volumes (FEV) and decreased *Pseudomonas aeruginosa* burden were reported (Ehsan and Clancy 2015, Bilton et al. 2014). LAI was also compared to tobramycin inhalation solution (TIS) and shown to be safe, well-tolerated, and similar effects on FEVs and baseline *P. aeruginosa* sputum density, achieving a primary endpoint of a non-inferiority margin of 5% which allowed the FDA to fast-tract designation status and has been granted orphan drug status in United States and Europe for cystic fibrosis patients with *pseudomonas* infections (Ehsan and Clancy 2015, Konstan et al.).

Due to its success in treatment of *P. aeruginosa* in cystic fibrosis patients, the clinical trials have now extended for treatment of non-tuberculosis mycobacterium lung infections. A phase 2 study investigated the efficacy and safety of LAI in treatment by adding treatment of 590 mg once daily for 84 days to patients already on a multidrug regimen and could receive open-label LAI for an additional 84 days (Olivier et al. 2017). The results of the study revealed negative sputum cultures were achieved early in treatment and were sustained over time. Improvements in patients' functional capacity with limited systemic toxicity and best treatment effect was seen in patients without cystic fibrosis and with *mycobacterium avium* complex (MAC) and sustained effect for 1 year after LAI treatment (Olivier et al. 2017). It was concluded that the addition of LAI could be an effective option for treatment of non-tuberculosis mycobacterium lung infections (Olivier et al. 2017).

The success of LAI and the fundamental difference between LAI and other inhaled antibiotic formulations has been attributed to the incorporation of nanotechnology to the drug product in the form of liposomes (Ehsan and Clancy 2015). Multiple factors have been linked to the liposomal formulation success including the shielding penetration of the amikacin into the bacterial biofilm and cystic fibrosis sputum allowing the antibiotic to reach the desired site of action (Ehsan and Clancy 2015). Additionally, the size and the use of endogenous phospholipid components (DPPC and CHOL) of the liposomes provide a stable formulation during the nebulization process (Elhissi 2017). The vibrating mesh nebulizer provides a platform for the delivery of LAI as a suitable aerosol formulation consisting of a relatively gentle shearing mechanism resulting in higher retention of drug in the lungs compared to air-jet nebulizers (Elhissi 2017). Therefore, the utilization of inhalation drug products containing liposomes delivered using nebulizers hold great promise in the treatment of these and other pulmonary disorders.

17.4.4.1.2 Ciprofloxacin for Inhalation (Lipoquin, Pulmaquin)

The testing of liposomal formulation of ciprofloxacin (Lipoquin™) and a mixture of unencapsulated ciprofloxacin with the liposomal form (Pulmaquin™) is another example liposomal antibiotic formulation tested in clinical trials. Ciprofloxacin is a broad-spectrum antibiotic which inhibits bacterial DNA gyrase and topoisomerase IV involved in separation of DNA required for bacterial DNA replication, transcription, repair, and recombination, thus inhibiting cell division (Cartlidge and Hill 2017). The clinical trials were used for the treatment of non-cystic fibrosis bronchiectasis and severe *P. aeruginosa* infections.

An initial phase 2 clinical trial was attempted with Lipoquin with 36 patients to test two different doses (3 mL–150 mg, 6 mL–300 mg). The phase 2 trial of Lipoquin over 4 weeks delivered once daily with patients with bronchiectasis infected with *P. aeruginosa* demonstrated a lowering of *P. aeruginosa* colony forming units/g during and 1 week after treatment (Cartlidge and Hill 2017). However, the higher dose led to one possible drug-related adverse reaction, while no difference between respiratory treatment emergent adverse events between treatment and placebo groups were reported (Cartlidge and Hill 2017). This pushed for a subsequent series of trials known as ORBIT: Once Daily Respiratory Bronchiectasis Inhalation Treatment. ORBIT-1 was a phase 2b clinical trial (double-blind, placebo-controlled) where Lipoquin at 100 mg at 2 mL and 150 mg at 3 mL was tested against patients with chronic *P. aeruginosa* infections. A significant mean change decrease in *P. aeruginosa* colony forming units/g (CFU/g) with no significant difference between the two doses was reported. The 3 mL dose was considered the optimal dose (Cartlidge and Hill 2017). The ORBIT-2 phase 2b clinical trial (Australian/New Zealand) expanded time to 168 days with 42 adult patients experiencing bronchiectasis with chronic *P. aeruginosa* infection using a dose of 210 mg/6 mL (150 mg/3 mL—Liposomal ciprofloxacin, 60 mg/3 mL—free ciprofloxacin) of the Pulmaquin formulation delivered once daily for 28 days on/28 days off (Cartlidge and Hill 2017, Serisier et al. 2013). A reduction in CFU/g of *P. aeruginosa* was found at day 28 and delayed time to first pulmonary exacerbation and demonstrated potent antipseudomonal microbial efficacy. The treatment was also found to be well tolerated with fewer pulmonary adverse events (Serisier et al. 2013). Overall, these phase 2 clinical trials demonstrate appropriate safety and efficacy.

Based on the success of these phase 2 clinical trials, phase 3 clinical trials (ORBIT-3 and ORBIT-4) were conducted for Pulmaquin for the treatment of non-cystic fibrosis bronchiectasis infected with *pseudomonas aeruginosa* in 582 patients (ORBIT-3, NCT01515007, $n = 278$; ORBIT-4, NCT02104245, $n = 304$) (Haworth et al. 2017). A 6-cycle, 28 days on/28 days off treatment with open-label extension was given to patients receiving Pulmaquin. The results of the phase 3 clinical trials demonstrated that Pulmaquin was deemed safe and well tolerated in patients with no significant change in lung function or irritation (Pecota 2016). There was significant reduction in pulmonary exacerbations and annual exacerbation frequency in patients and a decrease in *P. aeruginosa* density with a maintenance of antibiotic activity throughout each treatment cycle (Pecota 2016, Haworth et al. 2017). These results are promising as there is currently no drug approved for the treatment of non-cystic fibrosis bronchiectasis (Pecota 2016).

Pulmaquin has been given orphan drug status in United States for treatment of non-cystic fibrosis bronchiectasis and deemed a qualified infectious disease product (QIDP) by the FDA, allowing it to obtain fast track designation (Pecota 2016). It has also been considered a product candidate for the treatment of cystic fibrosis and non-tuberculous mycobacteria and bioterrorism infections (inhaled tularemia, pneumonic plague, melioidosis, Q fever, and inhaled anthrax) (Pecota 2016). Currently, longer-term studies to determine the viability of the drug remain to be completed as well as cost-effectiveness (Cartlidge and Hill 2017).

17.4.4.2 Antifungal Therapeutics

There have been two different liposomal formulations of Amphotericin B: AmBisome® and Abelcet® that have gone through clinical trials to treat pulmonary fungal infections (*Aspergillosis*), for lung transplantations, and for leukemia. The main ingredient in Amphotericin B is a fungicidal against many human yeast and mold pathogens including *Aspergillus*, *Candida*, *Mucor*, *Rhizopus*, *Cryptococcus*, and against dimorphic fungi (Adler-Moore et al. 2017). The main mechanism of action is the binding of amphotericin B to ergosterol in fungal cell membranes forming pores that increase permeability to small molecules irreversibly damaging the fungal cell (Aversa et al. 2017). Its main limitation of use is due to its nephrotoxicity. Therefore, liposomal formulations were produced to limit the toxicity and improve solubility, resulting in improved clinical efficacy (Aversa et al. 2017). The two liposomal formulations that have been translated for pulmonary delivery and tested in clinical trials are AmBisome® and Abelcet®.

17.4.4.2.1 Liposomal Amphotericin B

AmBisome® (L-AmB) is one of the liposomal formulations of Amphotericin B which has been on the market for over 25 years as a treatment for a variety of fungal infections and Leishmaniasis parasite infection, administered via i.v. injection (Adler-Moore et al. 2017). The formulation is composed of hydrogenated soy HSPC, CHOL, and DSPG in a 2:1:0.8 ratio, respectively, encapsulating amphotericin B to form ~80 nm liposomes (Adler-Moore et al. 2017, Jensen 2017, Aversa et al. 2017). DSPG was added to the formulation since it has a fatty acid side chain similar to that of HSPC. It also contains a similar length to the hydrophobic region of Amphotericin B and can form an ion pair with it as well. The Amphotericin B binds to the CHOL present in the liposome to form stable nanoparticles. The success of this formulation led for its commercialization in the early 1990s (Jensen 2017).

Clinical development of L-AmB by the Gilead Sciences (United States) continued including the aerosolized form delivered by nebulization to prevent fungal infections, including four clinical trials: two completed, one suspended, and one unknown outcome. The L-AmB formulation was aerosolized via a nebulizer in these clinical trials. The first clinical trial tests were a randomized, placebo-controlled phase 2/3 trial conducted in the treatment of invasive pulmonary *aspergillosis* (IPA) in patients with chemotherapy-induced prolonged neutropenia (Rijnders et al. 2008). A total of 271 eligible adult patients with hematologic disease were included in the trial. Inhaled L-AmB was induced to be a preventative measure to protect from development of IPA in these patients. The inhalation L-AmB included a 5 mg/mL solution with a total volume of 2.5 mL. This solution was nebulized for 30 minutes per day on 2 consecutive days per week. This weekly regimen continued until neutrophil recovery was confirmed (>300 cells/mm^3), with a maximum of 12 inhalations given per neutropenic episode (Rijnders et al. 2008). The nebulizer utilized was an advanced adaptive aerosol delivery system (HaloLite AAD or Prodose AAD; Romedic/Medic-Aid) adapting to the breathing patterns of the individual ensuring adequate deposition. Additionally, aerosolized particles were of an average diameter 1.9 µm; optimally sized for deep lung deposition (Rijnders et al. 2008). Of the 271 patients studied, the intent-to-treatment analysis displayed that 18 of 132 patients developed IPA in the placebo group compared to 6 of 139 patients developed IPA in the treatment group, while 13 of 97 in placebo and 2 of 91 in treatment group developed IPA when using on-treatment analysis. Therefore, it was concluded that inhalation of L-AmB significantly reduced the incidence of IPA in high-risk patients from 14% to 4% ($P = 0.005$) (Rijnders et al. 2008). No major adverse effects or systemic toxicity from the inhalation therapy was seen, thus avoiding the renal toxicity seen with i.v. administration of Amphotericin B. However, there were some adverse effects of coughing during inhalation treatment, suggesting some inhalation effort in some patients was an obstacle and did lead to their discontinuation of treatment. Despite this finding, it was concluded that, with further study, nebulized L-AmB could provide an alternative treatment for preventative treatment of IPA for patients with prolonged neutropenia (Rijnders et al. 2008).

Further studies of the pharmacokinetics and safety of L-AmB was conducted to prevent *Aspergillus* infection for those receiving lung transplantations. Of the conducted studies, one did not report any results (NCT00177710), and another was suspended due to shortage of funding (NCT01254708). However, results of similar work were presented elsewhere (Monforte et al. 2009, Monforte et al. 2010). Pharmacokinetics and safety of L-AmB was assessed after pulmonary inhalation given to patients who received lung transplants. The dose consisted of 25 mg of L-AmB in 6 mL of sterile water and nebulized by a jet nebulizer (Ventstream or Sidestream, Respironics) with a CR60 compressor (air pressure: 27.2 psi; flow: 7.3 liters/min) for 10 minutes–15 minutes up to three times a week up to 60 days post-transplantation, once per week between days 60 post-transplantation–180 post-transplantation, and once every 2 weeks after 180 days post-transplantation. Bronchoscopies were conducted to evaluate drug concentration in lungs, that remained relatively high up to 14 days, adequate enough for prophylaxis of *Aspergillus* infection with no significant systemic absorption being detected (Monforte et al. 2009). The FEV remained the same before and after treatment of nebulized L-AmB indicating no adverse effect on respiratory function (Monforte et al. 2009). This provides an incentive for further studies with aerosolized L-AmB for the potential treatment/prevention of *Aspergillus* infection, as well as provides a less expensive alternative to conventional treatments.

Further study on this liposomal formulation was conducted by the same group where nebulized L-AmB was used for the prevention of *Aspergillus* lung infection after lung transplantation and compared to nebulized free drug (Amphotericin B deoxycholate—n-ABD) (Monforte et al. 2010). The dose, nebulizers, and treatment plan remained the same as the previous study and frequency of *Aspergillus* infection was measured (Monforte et al. 2010). The incidence of *Aspergillus spp.* was 7.7% with 1.9% of invasive disease when prophylaxis treatment with nebulized L-AmB was given, a significantly lower rate of invasive disease incidence of 15% when no prophylaxis treatment is given (Monforte et al. 2010). Similar rates of *Aspergillus* incidence (10.2%) and invasive infection (4.1%) were seen with n-ABD treatment. The treatment of nebulized L-AmB was also seen as well-tolerated with only 2.9% of patients requiring treatment-withdrawal due to adverse effects (bronchospasm or nausea) (Monforte et al. 2010). This allows for the formulation to have the potential for long-term treatment, if required, since systemic side effects and issues with nephrotoxicity are avoided due to direct lung delivery and liposomal formulation. Nebulized L-AmB also holds an advantage to n-ABD due to providing a more convenient administration regimen, which can result in better adherence to treatment. Despite the cost for treatment with nebulized L-AmB potentially being more than n-AMD, it will be lower than other alternative conventional drugs. Therefore, nebulizer L-AmB was found to be effective, safe, and convenient for the preventative treatment of *Aspergillus* infection with the advantage of the potential for prolonged administration if required (Monforte et al. 2010). However, the most suitable treatment for prophylaxis in lung transplantation remains to be seen as a comparison of other drugs in clinical trials could elucidate the best treatment strategy.

17.4.4.2.2 Lipid Complex Amphotericin B

A competing formulation of Amphotericin B is a lipid complex of Amphotericin B known as Abelcet®. Abelcet® comprises of ribbon-like structures with sizes ranging from 1.6 µm–11 µm with a 1:1 molar ratio between Amphotericin B and lipids, the lipids comprising of 70:30 of dimyristoyl phosphatidylcholine and dimyristoyl phosphatidylglycerol, respectively (Aversa et al. 2017, Adler-Moore et al. 2017). Abelcet®, as with L-AmB, has been a long-standing conventional antifungal therapy for the management of invasive fungal infections via i.v. route. Studies in the early 2000s allowed for more serious expansion and study of Abelcet® to be delivered via pulmonary route (Mesco 2003, Palmer et al. 2001). These studies demonstrated the safety and tolerability of Abelcet® in lung/heart and lung transplants of 51 patients with measurement of incidence of fungal infections (Palmer et al. 2001). The regimen included 100 mg/20 mL solution for ventilated patients and 50 mg/10 mL solution for patients delivered using a face mask jet nebulizer (Hudson RCI Up-Draft model 1724) at an oxygen flow rate of 7 L/min–8 L/min inhaled over a 15 minute–30 minute period given once every day for 4 consecutive days, then once per week for a minimum of 2 months (Palmer et al. 2001). It was found that aerosolized Abelcet® was well tolerated in 98% of the patients treated with no significant adverse events. The pulmonary function declined by 20% or more in less than 5% of the treatments administered, which was considered well-tolerated. The incidence of pulmonary fungal infection was 4%, while extrapulmonary fungal infection occurred at 8% (Palmer et al. 2001). Questions concerning dose and efficacy pushed further studies, including a comparison of aerosolized Amphotericin B deoxycholate (AmBd) and Abelcet® in lung transplant recipients for prevention of invasive fungal infections (Drew et al. 2004). The dose and regimen remained the same for Abelcet® as in the previous study by this group, with AmBd at half the dose. The drug intolerance was lower in treatment group that received Abelcet® compared to AmBd at 5.9%–12.2%, respectively (Drew et al. 2004). Those receiving AmBd were also more likely to receive an adverse event compared to patients receiving Abelcet®, and a lower incidence of fungal infection was seen (14.3% for AmBd versus 11.8% for Abelcet®) (Drew et al. 2004). Therefore, the lower incidence of adverse events compared to conventional AmBd demonstrated potential benefit of safety and tolerance and further clinical benefit of Abelcet® (Mesco 2003).

Due to the success in safety, tolerance, and efficacy of Abelcet®, a continuance of clinical testing occurred, including combination treatment with fluconazole (Alexander et al. 2006, Borro et al. 2008). The addition of fluconazole to nebulized Abelcet® was tested in patients at high risk of invasive fungal infections including patients receiving hematopoietic stem cell transplants (HSCTs) (Alexander et al. 2006) and those receiving lung transplants (Borro et al. 2008). The treatment for 40 patients receiving an allogeneic HSCT were tested with nebulized Abelcet® (50 mg/10 mL in Hudson RCI Up-Draft, Model No 1724 Nebulizer) starting 2 days after transplantation, once a day for 4 days, followed by once a week for 13 weeks with the addition of 400 mg of fluconazole given orally/intravenously once daily for 100 days (Alexander et al. 2006). Pulmonary function decrease (≥20%) was seen in 5.2% of Abelcet® administrations, however, none required discontinuation from study or use of bronchodilators. Only four mild adverse events were considered as possibly related to treatment, and no severe adverse events were seen. Only 1 of 40 patients developed an invasive fungal infection during treatment, demonstrating combination of aerosolized Abelcet® with fluconazole a promising regimen for antifungal prophylaxis in these HSCT patients (Alexander et al. 2006). Those patients receiving a lung transplant received a dose of 50 mg/10 mL nebulized for 10 minutes–15 minutes administered on alternating days, once a day, for the first 2 weeks after transplantation followed by once a week for up to 13 weeks (Borro et al. 2008). Fuconazole (200 mg) was also administered intravenously for first dose followed by oral administration every 12 hours for the first 3 weeks after transplantation (Borro et al. 2008). The prophylaxis efficiency and safety of treatment was assessed after 6 months from first drug dose administration. It was demonstrated that prophylaxis was 98.3% efficient with only one patient developing invasive fungal infection and four patients having adverse effects (nausea/vomiting) (Borro et al. 2008). It was considered a success in prevention of invasive fungal infection as well during early stages post-transplantation. Therefore, the combination therapy of Abelcet® with fluconazole seemed a promising route for prevention of invasive fungal infection for these patients.

Further study into the lung deposition (Corcoran et al. 2006) and pharmacokinetics (Husain et al. 2010) was conducted. To study lung deposition, a radiolabeled Abelcet® (35 mg/7 mL, with ~4 mCi–6 mCi) was administered once with a AeroEclipse nebulizer (Monaghan Medical) with 8650D Compressor (Sunrise Medical) set to 40 psig. Images with a gamma camera captured the distribution of drug after administration and monitored for 20 minutes to determine lung clearance (Corcoran et al. 2006). The study was able to demonstrate that the drug is well distributed within the lungs of patients with single or double lung transplant. However, drug delivered to the native lung was suboptimal, especially in patients with idiopathic pulmonary fibrosis (Corcoran et al. 2006). This demonstrated the importance in understanding different pulmonary disease states so that the aerosol drug delivery techniques can be optimized for each population group and disease state (Corcoran et al. 2006). The pharmacokinetics of lung deposition was also monitored (measuring dose in epithelial lining fluid and plasma) in lung transplant patients where a dose of 1 mg/kg nebulized via breath actuated AeroEclipse nebulizer (Monaghan Medical Corporation) with a 8650D air compressor (Sunrise Medical) set to 40 psig 1 every 24 hours for a total of 4 days (Husain et al. 2010). It was concluded that the concentration of Amphotericin B could be maintained above the minimum inhibitory concentration of *Aspergillus* and was achieved at 168 hours after the last dose was administered as well as being well tolerated (Husain et al. 2010). Therefore, it is possible to use this treatment and regimen to serve for the prophylaxis against invasive fungal infections in lung transplant patients (Husain et al. 2010). However, the long-term efficacy and safety still needs to be established. Also, the comparison of other drugs or drug formulations or combinations still need to be assessed to optimize the best long-term strategy for treatment of patients who are susceptible to invasive fungal infections in the lung.

17.4.4.3 Analgesic

17.4.4.3.1 Liposome Encapsulated Fentanyl, AeroLEF

Fentanyl was introduced in the 1950s and is a synthetic opioid analgesic used as an anesthetic adjunct during surgery and for acute and chronic pain management. It has an enhanced analgesic effect with fewer side effects compared to morphine or meperidine (Oprea). A liposome-encapsulated formulation of fentanyl was developed to provide a controlled, sustained release of the fast-acting fentanyl (Oprea). AeroLEF is a mixture of free and liposomal fentanyl for aerosolization via nebulizers for pain management. Phase I and II clinical trials were conducted both on healthy patients and for treatment of post-operative pain following anterior cruciate ligament (ACL) knee surgery or orthopedic surgery. AeroLEF represents the first aerosolized drug containing nanomedicine tested clinically whose main focus was for the drug to reach systemic circulation.

The first few clinical trials were phase I clinical trials to test the bioavailability, safety, pharmacokinetics, and pharmacodynamics of AeroLEF when given as a single or multiple dose and compared to intravenous dose of fentanyl. A single dose of AeroLEF at 1500 µg (3 mL of 500 µg/mL) was nebulized using a breath-actuated AeroEclipse BAN device over a 7 minute–15 minute period and compared to i.v. dose of fentanyl at 200 µg (Hung et al. 2004, Hung and Pliura 2008). Maximum plasma concentrations of fentanyl were seen to be similar for both i.v. dose and AeroLEF and was seen shortly after the completion of AeroLEF administration demonstrating rapid absorption of the drug from the lung (Hung and Pliura 2008). Plasma levels of the drug remained in the effective range for several hours when AeroLEF was delivered, which was not seen in the i.v. delivery of fentanyl (Hung and Pliura 2008). No severe adverse events were seen in both treatment groups and no significant changes in lung function (Hung et al. 2004, Hung and Pliura 2008). Therefore, it was determined that AeroLEF was safe and well tolerated at the dose given as well as it was able to prolong effective fentanyl amounts allowing for sustained release (Hung et al. 2004, Hung and Pliura 2008).

Based on these promising results, phase 2 clinical trials were initiated for the treatment of post-surgical pain following ACL surgery (Clark et al. 2008) or orthopedic surgery (Brull and Chan 2008). A total of 19 patients were treated after ACL surgery whom had moderate to severe pain and were instructed to self-administer AeroLEF via breath actuated nebulizer until they achieved relief, dose-limiting side effects, or completed a maximum of two doses (3 mL with 500 μg/mL of fentanyl per dose) (Clark et al. 2008). The median time of effective analgesia was 17 minutes after dose administered with a mean duration of analgesia of 3.7 hours. Patients' requests for additional doses were associated with a decrease in mean plasma levels to 0.887 ng/mL, which were comparable to reported minimal effective dose in post-surgical patients. However, mean plasma levels of fentanyl varied among patients 6.5-fold with a 9-fold dosing range selected by patients in order to obtain analgesia, demonstrating the patient variability in opioid use (Clark, et al. 2008). Also, adverse events were mild compared to those generally associated with opioid use. Another larger study involving 99 patients undergoing orthopedic surgery were randomized to receive 1,500 μg of AeroLEF or placebo during each treatment session where a second nebulizer was permitted per session (Brull and Chan 2008). Up to three treatment sessions were allowed over an 8 hour–12-hour time-span. No significant respiratory problems were found between AeroLEF and placebo group. More patients who received the AeroLEF treatment reported mild or no pain after administration and moderate-to-complete pain relief (with statistical significance, 60% versus 32% of patients, $P < 0.02$) (Brull and Chan 2008). This suggests that AeroLEF administration can provide effective and safe pain relief after surgery.

Despite the promising outcomes from these clinical trials, the pursuit of AeroLEF formulation was discontinued. Another study was suspended in phase I for cancer pain in 2010. The successes of the trials suggest the potential of the proposed strategy. The use of second generation nanomaterials that can help manipulate biodistribution and pharmacokinetics in systemic circulation upon pulmonary administration can be potentially used to enhance circulation times and tissue targeting in a way not possible with liposomes.

17.4.4.4 Immunosuppressant

17.4.4.4.1 Liposomal Cyclosporine

The peptide Cyclosporine A (CsA) is a potent immunosuppressive drug that works by inhibition of T-lymphocytes, including pulmonary T-lymphocytes (Waldrep et al. 1998). Therefore, the direct delivery of CsA to the lungs could potentially improve treatment of immunologically mediated lung diseases including allergy, chronic severe asthma, obliterative bronchiolitis, and pulmonary sarcoidosis (Waldrep et al. 1998, Behr et al. 2009). Among pulmonary complications, obliterative bronchiolitis is the most common non-infectious respiratory complication for patients after a hematopoietic stem cell transplantation, and it is thought to be the major contributing factor in the activation of T-lymphocytes by major histocompatibility alloantigens (Behr et al. 2009). Direct delivery of CsA to the lungs may allow for high local concentration of the drug to sufficiently suppress lung T-lymphocytes (Behr et al. 2009).

Various inhalation formulations of CsA have been tested. Previous clinical trials for a propyleneglycol-based solution of CsA aerosolized were hindered by bad tolerability (Behr et al. 2009). In the late 1990s, a liposomal formulation of CsA made of DLPC was tested clinically in ten healthy patients administered in AeroTech II nebulizer (CIS-US, Inc) (Gilbert et al. 1997). This study demonstrated the safety and tolerability of nebulized liposomal-CsA formulations. More recently, a new liposomal formulation of CsA (L-CsA) was prepared and tested for prevention of bronchiolitis obliterans syndrome (BOS) following lung transplantation (Behr et al. 2009). The L-CsA formulation included a non-ionic surfactant and phospholipids to form liposomes ~50 nm in diameter (Behr et al. 2009). Doses of 10 mg/2 mL or 20 mg/4 mL was delivered using an eFlow® nebulizer to 12 patients who received lung transplants, and the deposition of drug within the lungs was evaluated (Behr et al. 2009). The lung deposition was found to be 40 ± 6% for the 10 mg dose and 33 ± 7% for the 20 mg dose with no statistical difference in patients who received a single- or double-lung transplant. The inhalation treatment was also seen to be well-tolerated with no drug side effects observed and with only minor, however, statistically significant changes in lung function. A dose of 10 mg once or twice a day was recommended to obtain sufficient peripheral lung deposition above 15 mg per week as their target dose (Behr et al. 2009).

A longer-term study starting in 2012 was conducted to assess the safety and efficacy of L-CsA for BOS and ended in August of 2015 (Iacono et al. 2016). A total of 22 lung transplant recipients (either single- or double-lung transplants) with stage 1 or 2 BOS were randomized to receive the standard of care (SOC) alone (triple drug immunosuppressants—Tacrolimus, mycophenolate mofetil, prednisone) or L-CsA + SOC for 24 weeks with a 12-month follow-up. The L-CsA was given twice daily via PARI Pharma's eFlow® nebulizer system at a dose of 5 mg/1.25 mL for single-lung transplant recipients or 10 mg/2.5 mL for double-lung transplant recipients (Iacono et al. 2016). The study concluded that the addition of L-CsA was well-tolerated and in combination with SOC for treatment of BOS and had an overall better outcome for patients when compared to SOC alone (Iacono et al. 2016). However, more assessment and analysis of the trial is needed.

17.4.4.5 Chemotherapeutics

17.4.4.5.1 Liposomal 9-Nitro-20 (S)-Camptothecin (L9NC)

Aerosolized liposomal 9-nitro-20 (S)-camptothecin (L9NC) has been studied in clinical trials. The chemotherapeutic 9-nitro-20 (S)-camptothecin (9NC) is a water-insoluble camptothecin analogue topoisomerase-I inhibitor which has shown to have potent antitumor effects in mice and modest anti-tumor effects when administered orally (Verschraegen et al. 2004, Verschraegen 2006). The idea to improve upon formulation with liposomes and use an alternative route of delivery could potentially improve the therapeutic index of 9NC (Verschraegen 2006). The formulation included 9NC mixed with DLPC to form a liposomal-complex formulation (L9NC) with an aerosol droplet size of 1 μm–3 μm.

Phase I and phase II clinical trials were conducted on patients with primary or metastatic lung cancer (Verschraegen et al. 2000, Verschraegen et al. 2004, Verschraegen 2006). The treatment strategy included nebulized L9NC from AeroMist nebulizer (CIS-US) at a flow rate of 10 L/min for 30 minutes and delivered twice daily for 5 consecutive days/week for 1 week, 2 weeks, 4 weeks, or 6 weeks followed by 2 weeks of rest at a dose of 6.7 μg/kg/day. Stepwise dose escalation was also used with doses ranging from 6.7 μg/kg/day to 26.6 μg/kg/day delivered Monday through Friday for 8 weeks followed by 2 weeks of rest (Verschraegen et al. 2004). It was concluded that aerosolized L9NC was safe to use with minimal side effects. Plasma levels of drug were seen to be comparable to those when drug is given orally, but with less side effects. An optimal dose was found to be 13.3 μg/kg/day (0.5 mg/m^2/day) with two consecutive 30 minute nebulizations/day with a concentration of 4 mg/mL of 9NC given from Monday–Friday for 8 weeks with 2 weeks rest (total 10 weeks) (Verschraegen et al. 2004). Responses were observed in patients who had endometrial cancer within the lungs seeing partial remission as well as partial remissions in liver metastasis demonstrating potential of lung treatment as well as systemically (Verschraegen et al. 2004, Verschraegen 2006). There was a lack of hematologic toxicity as seen previously with oral administration (Verschraegen 2006). Phase II studies for non-small lung cancer and endometrial cancer were initiated, however, due to a small amount of patients, data were inconclusive to determine efficacy of treatment (Verschraegen 2006). In conclusion, L9NC demonstrated potential of liposomal inhaled therapeutics for treatment of lung cancers, metastatic cancers to the lung, and in some cases, cancer treatment to other sites as well. However, more robust and larger clinical trials need to be run to further address the efficacy of such treatment plans for patients.

17.4.4.5.2 Sustained Release Lipid Inhalation Targeting (SLIT) Cisplatin/Inhaled Lipid Cisplatin (ILC)

The other chemotherapeutic that was tried as an aerosolized lipid formulation was cisplatin. Cisplatin is a very common and widely used chemotherapeutic and is the first-line chemotherapeutic for advanced non-small cell lung cancer (Wittgen et al. 2007). SLIT cisplatin initially was investigated as a formulation for inhalation of cisplatin that could reduce unwanted side effects of drug including nephrotoxicity and increase clinical benefit (Wittgen et al. 2007). SLIT cisplatin comprises of cisplatin encapsulated in lipid vesicles dispersed in a 0.9% NaCl solution. The liposome composition comprises of DPPC and CHOL (Wittgen et al. 2007). The nebulization process provides immediate release of 40%–50% of cisplatin while the rest remains encapsulated allowing for prolonged release (Wittgen et al. 2007).

Initial phase I clinical trials were assessed to determine dose, toxicity, safety, and pharmacokinetics of SLIT cisplatin on 18 patients with primary or metastatic carcinoma in the lung (Wittgen et al. 2007). The dose given per week ranged from 1 mg to 80 mg per week and was administered 1–4 consecutive days in 3-week treatment cycles. The PARI LC Star nebulizer was used and set to nebulize 0.2 mL/min–0.3 mL/min with time of nebulization over 20 minutes with a maximum of two sessions per day with a minimum of 2-hour rest per session. Cycles were repeated every 3 weeks with number of cycles ranging from two to eight. Doses were increased by 20% until dose limiting toxicity was observed (Wittgen et al. 2007). The results from this study revealed no DLT was reached at maximum tolerated dose. No adverse events as seen with systemic delivery of cisplatin (hematologic toxicity, nephrotoxicity, ototoxicity, or neurotoxicity) were seen. However, some adverse events were reported, including changes in pulmonary function in a few patients (Wittgen et al. 2007). There were very low plasma platinum levels revealed by the pharmacokinetic data, and plasma platinum was only seen in patients with the longest and repeated inhalation regimen. An optimal dose was not considered to have been reached due to not reaching the dose limiting toxicity of this SLIT cisplatin. Overall, 12 patients were seen to have stabilized the disease, while in four patients the disease progressed (Wittgen et al. 2007). Therefore, the overall conclusion was nebulized SLIT cisplatin is a feasible treatment strategy and safe.

Since the initial clinical trials initiated by Transave, Inc., it was absorbed by Insmed, Inc. in 2010. Following this merger, Eleison Pharmaceuticals LLC was given exclusive rights to patent applications covering SLIT cisplatin in 2012 (Rudokas et al. 2016). Since then, Eleison Pharmaceuticals developed a liposomal formulation of cisplatin termed inhaled lipid cisplatin (ILC), in which a phase 2 clinical trial to characterize the safety and efficacy of ILC was initiated for 19 patients with relapsed or progressive osteosarcoma metastatic to the lung (Chou et al. 2013). The treatment scheme was reported as similar to the previous investigation done by Transave, Inc. (Wittgen et al. 2007), with ILC being administered on an every 2 week cycle (Chou et al. 2013). If possible, metastasectomy was performed in patients after two cycles. Few adverse events were seen with one patient having nausea/vomiting, and one patient experiencing a respiratory problem (not associated with drug). However, no toxicity common with i.v. delivery of cisplatin was seen. In terms of patient response, three patients (16%) had a complete response to the therapy, one (5%) had partial response, seven (37%) had stable disease, and eight (42%) had progressive disease (Chou et al. 2013). The patients who showed sustained benefit were those whose pulmonary lesions were smaller than 2 cm and those who underwent complete surgical resection, demonstrating efficacy for those patients. Therefore, nebulized ILC was found to be safe and potentially effective for treatment of osteosarcoma metastatic to the lung at low tumor burden or utilized as an adjuvant therapy (Chou et al. 2013). The study of this formulation still remains in the early clinical stages. Whether this will reach marketable stages remains to be seen.

17.5 Concluding Remarks, Challenges, and Opportunities

A significant number of IDPCNs have made it to clinical trials, with some of those technologies having received fast track designation from the FDA. Most of these pioneering studies have focused on the use of liposomes as the drug carrier and nebulizers as the inhalation device. The safety profiles of liposomal IDPs have now been firmly established, with a significant number of trials having progressed to phase 2 and 3. Also important to note is that plasma concentration levels of therapeutics delivered to the lungs using IDPCNs can be maintained at comparable levels (or better) to i.v. administered therapeutics, and that IDPCNs can thus be used to treat diseases whose targets are not the lungs (e.g. case of fentanyl and 9-nitro-20(S)-camptothecin). These results should come as a strong incentive for sponsors to continue submitting IND applications for IDPs containing liposomes as they apply for the treatment of different diseases and different classes of drugs, for both local delivery to the lungs and systemic delivery through the lungs.

At the same time, as the potential of liposomes in IDPs has now been established, one should note that there is no single nanomaterial that will be able to address all the needs in this area. The selection and design (optimization) of nanomaterials for use in IDP needs to be based on the drug target site (down to the organelle and/or molecular target) and physiological barriers of the lungs (either diseased tissue for locally targeted drugs or healthy lungs if the target is systemic circulation). For example, liposomes are not expected to translocate into systemic circulation upon pulmonary administration. Alternative nanomaterials need to be considered, in that case, to explore their beneficial properties such as improved circulation times or targeting. There are, therefore, tremendous opportunities to study second generation nanomaterials for the development of IDPCNs to treat relevant diseases of the lungs and systemic disorders as well. These advancements are expected to materialize as ongoing clinical studies through more traditional routes (i.v./oral) help determine the safety profiles of these various nanomaterials. Finally, the clinical study of IDPNCs in portable devices may also open up new opportunities in terms of treatment of chronic disorders of the lungs and also for systemic delivery.

REFERENCES

Elhissi, A. 2017. "Liposomes for pulmonary drug delivery: The role of formulation and inhalation device design." *Current Pharmaceutical Design* 23 (3):362–372. doi:10.2174/1381612823666161116114732.

Adler-Moore, JP., RT. Proffitt, JA. Olson, and GM. Jensen. 2017. "Tissue pharmacokinetics and pharmacodynamics of AmBisome® (L-AmBis) in uninfected and infected animals and their effects on dosing regimens." *Journal of Liposome Research* 27 (3):195–209. (just-accepted):1–53.

Aggarwal, B. and J. Gogtay. 2014. "Use of pressurized metered dose inhalers in patients with chronic obstructive pulmonary disease: review of evidence." *Expert Review of Respiratory Medicine* 8 (3):349–356. doi: 10.1586/17476348.2014.905916.

Alexander, BD., ES. Dodds Ashley, RM. Addison, JA. Alspaugh, NJ. Chao, and JR. Perfect. 2006. "Non-comparative evaluation of the safety of aerosolized amphotericin B lipid complex in patients undergoing allogeneic hematopoietic stem cell transplantation." *Transplant Infectious Disease* 8 (1):13–20.

Allen, TM., and PR. Cullis. 2013. "Liposomal drug delivery systems: From concept to clinical applications." *Advanced Drug Delivery Reviews* 65 (1):36–48. doi:10.1016/j.addr.2012.09.037.

Aversa, F., A. Busca, A. Candoni, S. Cesaro, C. Girmenia, M. Luppi, A. M. Nosari, L. Pagano, L. Romani, and G. Rossi. 2017. "Liposomal amphotericin B (AmBisome®) at beginning of its third decade of clinical use." *Journal of Chemotherapy* 29 (3):131–143.

Behr, J., G. Zimmermann, R. Baumgartner, H. Leuchte, C. Neurohr, P. Brand, C. Herpich, K. Sommerer, J. Seitz, and G. Menges. 2009. "Lung deposition of a liposomal cyclosporine A inhalation solution in patients after lung transplantation." *Journal of Aerosol Medicine and Pulmonary Drug Delivery* 22 (2):121–130.

Bell, J. and S Newman. 2007. "The rejuvenated pressurised metered dose inhaler." *Expert Opinion on Drug Delivery* 4 (3):215–234. doi:10.1517/17425247.4.3.215.

Bharatwaj, B., L. Wu, JA. Whittum-Hudson, and SRP. da Rocha. 2010. "The potential for the noninvasive delivery of polymeric nanocarriers using propellant-based inhalers in the treatment of Chlamydial respiratory infections." *Biomaterials* 31 (28):7376–7385. doi:10.1016/j.biomaterials.2010.06.005.

Bilton, D., T. Pressler, I. Fajac, JP. Clancy, Predrag Minic, Marco Cipolli, Ivanka Galeva, Amparo Solé, L. Dupont, N. Mayer-Hamblett Torchio, S.; McGinnis, JP; Eagle, G. and Konstan, M., Journal of Cystic Fibrosis. 2014. "Analysis of long-term liposomal amikacin for inhalation in patients with cystic fibrosis and chronic infection from pseudomonas aeruginosa." *Pediatric Pulmonology* 49:317–318. Supplement: 38 Meeting Abstract 284.

Borro, JM., A. Sole, M. De la Torre, A. Pastor, R. Fernandez, A. Saura, M. Delgado, E. Monte, and D. Gonzalez. 2008. "Efficiency and safety of inhaled amphotericin B lipid complex (Abelcet) in the prophylaxis of invasive fungal infections following lung transplantation." *Transplantation Proceedings* 40 (9):3090–3093.

Brand, P., B. Hederer, G. Austen, H. Dewberry, and T. Meyer. 2008. "Higher lung deposition with Respimat® Soft Mist™ Inhaler than HFA-MDI in COPD patients with poor technique." *International Journal of Chronic Obstructive Pulmonary Disease* 3 (4):763–770.

Brull, R., and V. Chan. 2008. "(265) A randomized controlled trial demonstrates the efficacy, safety and tolerability of aerosolized free and liposome-encapsulated fentanyl (AeroLEF) via pulmonary administration." *The Journal of Pain* 9 (4):42.

Caracciolo, G. 2018. "Clinically approved liposomal nanomedicines: Lessons learned from the biomolecular corona." *Nanoscale* 10 (9):4167–4172. doi:10.1039/C7NR07450F.

Carter, KC., and M. Puig-Sellart. 2016. "Nanocarriers made from non-ionic surfactants or natural polymers for pulmonary drug delivery." *Current Pharmaceutical Design* 22 (22):3324–3331. doi:10.2174/1381612822666160418121700.

Cartlidge, MK., and AT. Hill. 2017. "Inhaled or nebulised ciprofloxacin for the maintenance treatment of bronchiectasis." *Expert Opinion on Investigational Drugs* 26 (9):1091–1097.

Carvalho, TC., and JT. McConville. 2016. "The function and performance of aqueous aerosol devices for inhalation therapy." *Journal of Pharmacy and Pharmacology* 68 (5):556–578. doi:10.1111/jphp.12541.

Caster, JM., AN. Patel, T. Zhang, and A. Wang. 2017. "Investigational nanomedicines in 2016: A review of nanotherapeutics currently undergoing clinical trials." *Wiley Interdisciplinary Reviews: Nanomedicine and Nanobiotechnology* 9 (1):e1416.

Chen, R., L. Xu, Q. Fan, M. Li, J. Wang, L. Wu, W. Li, J. Duan, and Z. Chen. 2017. "Hierarchical pulmonary target nanoparticles via inhaled administration for anticancer drug delivery." *Drug Delivery* 24 (1):1191–1203. doi:10.1080/10717544.2017.1365395.

Chen, X., and HJ. Schluesener. 2008. "Nanosilver: A nanoproduct in medical application." *Toxicology Letters* 176 (1):1–12. doi:10.1016/j.toxlet.2007.10.004.

Chou, AJ., R. Gupta, MD. Bell, KOD. Riewe, PA. Meyers, and R. Gorlick. 2013. "Inhaled lipid cisplatin (ILC) in the treatment of patients with relapsed/progressive osteosarcoma metastatic to the lung." *Pediatric Blood & Cancer* 60 (4):580–586.

Cipolla, D., I. Gonda, and HK. Chan. 2013. "Liposomal formulations for inhalation." *Therapeutic Delivery* 4 (8):1047–1072. doi:10.4155/tde.13.71.

Clark, A., M. Rossiter-Rooney, and F. Valle-Leutri. 2008. "(264) Aerosolized liposome-encapsulated fentanyl (AeroLEF) via pulmonary administration allows patients with moderate to severe post-surgical acute pain to self-titrate to effective analgesia." *The Journal of Pain* 9 (4):42.

Conti, DS., D. Brewer, J. Grashik, S. Avasarala, and SRP da Rocha. 2014. "Poly(amidoamine) dendrimer nanocarriers and their aerosol formulations for siRNA delivery to the lung epithelium." *Molecular Pharmaceutics* 11 (6):1808–1822. doi:10.1021/mp4006358.

Corcoran, TE., R. Venkataramanan, KM. Mihelc, AL. Marcinkowski, J. Ou, BM. McCook, L. Weber, ME. Carey, DL. Paterson, and JM. Pilewski. 2006. "Aerosol deposition of lipid complex amphotericin-B (Abelcet) in lung transplant recipients." *American Journal of Transplantation* 6 (11):2765–2773.

Coty, J. and C. Vauthier. 2018. "Characterization of nanomedicines: A reflection on a field under construction needed for clinical translation success." *Journal of Controlled Release* 275:254–268. doi:10.1016/j.jconrel.2018.02.013.

D'Mello, SR., CN. Cruz, ML. Chen, M. Kapoor, SL. Lee, and KM. Tyner. 2017. "The evolving landscape of drug products containing nanomaterials in the United States." *Nature Nanotechnology* 12 (6):523–529.

Dalby, RN., J. Eicher, and B. Zierenberg. 2011. "Development of Respimat® Soft Mist™ Inhaler and its clinical utility in respiratory disorders." *Medical Devices (Auckland, N.Z.)* 4:145–155. doi:10.2147/MDER.S7409.

de Boer, A. H., P. Hagedoorn, M. Hoppentocht, F. Buttini, F. Grasmeijer, and HW. Frijlink. 2017. "Dry powder inhalation: past, present and future." *Expert Opinion on Drug Delivery* 14 (4):499–512. doi:10.1080/17425247.2016.1224846.

Doane, TL., and C. Burda. 2012. "The unique role of nanoparticles in nanomedicine: Imaging, drug delivery and therapy." *Chemical Society Reviews* 41 (7):2885–2911. doi:10.1039/C2CS15260F.

Drew, RH., ED. Ashley, DK. Benjamin Jr, RD. Davis, SM. Palmer, and JR. Perfect. 2004. "Comparative safety of amphotericin B lipid complex and amphotericin B deoxycholate as aerosolized antifungal prophylaxis in lung-transplant recipients." *Transplantation* 77 (2):232–237.

Ehsan, Z. and JP. Clancy. 2015. "Management of pseudomonas aeruginosa infection in cystic fibrosis patients using inhaled antibiotics with a focus on nebulized liposomal amikacin." *Future Microbiology* 10 (12):1901–1912.

El-Sherbiny, IM., NM. El-Baz, and MH. Yacoub. 2015. "Inhaled nano- and microparticles for drug delivery." *Global Cardiology Science and Practice* 2015:2. doi:10.5339/gcsp.2015.2.

Eleftheriadis, GK., M. Akrivou, N. Bouropoulos, J. Tsibouklis, IS. Vizirianakis, and DG. Fatouros. 2018. "Polymer–Lipid microparticles for pulmonary delivery." *Langmuir* 34 (11):3438–3448. doi:10.1021/acs.langmuir.7b03645.

Elhissi, A., SR. Dennison, W. Ahmed, KMG. Taylor, and DA. Phoenix. 2014. "New delivery systems–Liposomes for pulmonary delivery of antibacterial drugs." *Novel Antimicrobial Agents and Strategies*:387–406.

EMA. 2018. European Medicines Agency, accessed 06/2018. http://www.ema.europa.eu/ema/index.jsp?curl=pages/regulation/general/general_content_000334.jsp&mid=WC0b01ac05800ba1d9.

EUNCL, European Nanomedicine Characterization Laboratory. 2018. "Assay Cascade." accessed 06/2018. http://www.euncl.eu/about-us/assay-cascade/.

FDA, U.S. Food and Drug Administration. 2017. *Drug Products, Including Biological Products, That Contain Nanomaterials—Guidance for Industry.* Silver Spring, MD: U.S. Department of Health and Human Services.

Geiser, M. 2010. "Update on macrophage clearance of inhaled micro- and nanoparticles." *Journal of Aerosol Medicine and Pulmonary Drug Delivery* 23 (4):207–217. doi:10.1089/jamp.2009.0797.

Geiser, M., and W. G. Kreyling. 2010. "Deposition and biokinetics of inhaled nanoparticles." *Particle and Fibre Toxicology* 7:2. doi:10.1186/1743-8977-7-2.

Gilbert, BE., C. Knight, FG. Alvarez, JC. Waldrep, JR. Rodarte, V. Knight, and WL. Eschenbacher. 1997. "Tolerance of volunteers to cyclosporine A-dilauroylphosphatidylcholine liposome aerosol." *American Journal of Respiratory and Critical Care Medicine* 156 (6):1789–1793.

Haworth, C., A. Wanner, J. Froehlich, T. O'Neal, A. Davis, I. Gonda, and A. O'Donnell. 2017. "Inhaled liposomal ciprofloxacin in patients with bronchiectasis and chronic pseudomonas aeruginosa infection: Results from two parallel phase III trials (ORBIT-3 And-4)." In *b14. Clinical trials across pulmonary disease, Am Thoracic Soc.* A7604–A7604.

Healy, AM., MI. Amaro, KJ. Paluch, and L. Tajber. 2014. "Dry powders for oral inhalation free of lactose carrier particles." *Advanced Drug Delivery Reviews* 75:32–52. doi:10.1016/j.addr.2014.04.005.

Heyder, RS., Q. Zhong, RC. Bazito, and SRP. da Rocha. 2017. "Cellular internalization and transport of biodegradable polyester dendrimers on a model of the pulmonary epithelium and their formulation in pressurized metered-dose inhalers." *International Journal of Pharmaceutics* 520 (1):181–194. doi:https://doi.org/10.1016/j.ijpharm.2017.01.057.

Hubbell, JA., and R. Langer. 2013. "Translating materials design to the clinic." *Nature Materials* 12:963. doi:10.1038/nmat3788.

Hung, O., and D. Pliura. 2008. "(243) Comparative phase I PK study of aerosolized free and liposome-encapsulated fentanyl (AeroLEF) demonstrates rapid and extended plasma fentanyl concentrations following inhalation." *The Journal of Pain* 9 (4):36.

Hung, OR., EM. Sellers, HL. Kaplan, and MK. Romach. 2004. "Phase Ib clinical trial of aerosolized liposome encapsulated fentanyl (AeroLEF™)." *Clinical Pharmacology & Therapeutics* 75 (2):P4–P4.

Husain, S., B. Capitano, T. Corcoran, SM. Studer, M. Crespo, B. Johnson, JM. Pilewski, K. Shutt, DL. Pakstis, and S. Zhang. 2010. "Intrapulmonary disposition of amphotericin B after aerosolized delivery of amphotericin B lipid complex (Abelcet; ABLC) in lung transplant recipients." *Transplantation* 90 (11):1215–1219.

Iacono, A., M. Terrin, K. Rajakopal, J. McGrain, E. Barr, J. Rinaldi, A. Patel, I. Timofte, J. Kim, and Z. Kon. 2016. "A single center, randomized, open-label, controlled pilot study to demonstrate efficacy and safety of the addition of inhaled liposomal cyclosporine (L-CSA) therapy versus standard therapy alone in the treatment of bronchiolitis obliterans syndrome (BOS) following lung transplantation." *The Journal of Heart and Lung Transplantation* 35 (4):S44–S45.

Jensen, GM. 2017. "The care and feeding of a commercial liposomal product: Liposomal amphotericin B (AmBisome®)." *Journal of Liposome Research* 27 (3):173–179. doi:10.1080/08982104.2017.1380664.

Kamal, D., B. Mary, A. Rajendra, KT. Rakesh, T. Muktika, G. Gaurav, P. Terezinha De Jesus Andreoli, and M. Hansbro Philip. 2017. "Application of chitosan and its derivatives in nanocarrier based pulmonary drug delivery systems." *Pharmaceutical Nanotechnology* 5 (4):243–249. doi:10.2174/2211738505666170808095258.

Kharisov, B., O. Kharissova, and U. Ortiz-Mendez. 2015. *CRC Concise Encyclopedia of Nanotechnology.* Boca Raton, FL: CRC Press.

Kolte, A., S. Patil, P. Lesimple, JW. Hanrahan, and A. Misra. 2017. "PEGylated composite nanoparticles of PLGA and polyethylenimine for safe and efficient delivery of pDNA to lungs." *International Journal of Pharmaceutics* 524 (1–2):382–396. doi:10.1016/j.ijpharm.2017.03.094.

Konstan, M., I. Fajac, T. Pressler, JP. Clancy, D. Sands, P. Minic, M. Cipolli, I. Galeva, A. Solé, and R. Monroe. "Long-term study of liposomal amikacin for inhalation in patients with cystic fibrosis and chronic pseudomonas aeruginosa infection."

Loira-Pastoriza, C., J. Todoroff, and R. Vanbever. 2014. "Delivery strategies for sustained drug release in the lungs." *Advanced Drug Delivery Reviews* 75:81–91.

Małaczewska, J. 2011. "Effect of silver nanoparticles on splenocyte activity and selected cytokine levels in the mouse serum." *Bulletin of the Veterinary Institute in Puławy* 55:317–322.

MAM, Markets and Markets. 2017. Drug Delivery Technology Market worth 1,669.40 Billion USD by 2021.

Manke, A., L. Wang, and Y. Rojanasakul. 2013. "Mechanisms of nanoparticle-induced oxidative stress and toxicity." *BioMed Research International* 2013:942916. doi:10.1155/2013/942916.

Martin, AR., and WH. Finlay. 2015. "Nebulizers for drug delivery to the lungs." *Expert Opinion on Drug Delivery* 12 (6):889–900. doi:10.1517/17425247.2015.995087.

Meers, P., M. Neville, V. Malinin, AW. Scotto, G. Sardaryan, R. Kurumunda, C. Mackinson, G. James, S. Fisher, and WR. Perkins. 2008. "Biofilm penetration, triggered release and in vivo activity of inhaled liposomal amikacin in chronic Pseudomonas aeruginosa lung infections." *Journal of Antimicrobial Chemotherapy* 61 (4):859–868.

Mesco, S., D. Walsey. 2003. *Important Role of ABELCET® in Antifungal Management Highlighted at Infectious Disease Conference.* Fujisawa, Japan: Evaluate Ltd., Enzon Pharmaceuticals, Gilead Sciences, Duke University.

Monforte, V., P. Ussetti, J. Gavaldà, C. Bravo, R. Laporta, O. Len, C. López García-Gallo, L. Tenorio, J. Solé, and A. Román. 2010. "Feasibility, tolerability, and outcomes of nebulized liposomal amphotericin B for Aspergillus infection prevention in lung transplantation." *The Journal of Heart and Lung Transplantation* 29 (5):523–530.

Monforte, V., P. Ussetti, R. López, J. Gavaldà, C. Bravo, A. de Pablo, L. Pou, A. Pahissa, F. Morell, and A. Román. 2009. "Nebulized liposomal amphotericin B prophylaxis for Aspergillus infection in lung transplantation: Pharmacokinetics and safety." *The Journal of Heart and Lung Transplantation* 28 (2):170–175.

Myrdal, PB., P. Sheth, and SW. Stein. 2014. "Advances in metered dose inhaler technology: Formulation development." *AAPS PharmSciTech* 15 (2):434–455. doi:10.1208/s12249-013-0063-x.

Nicolas, R., and DPN. Richard. 2016. "The evolution of pressurized metered-dose inhalers from early to modern devices." *Journal of Aerosol Medicine and Pulmonary Drug Delivery* 29 (4):311–327. doi:10.1089/jamp.2015.1232.

NIH, National Institute of Health—National Library of Medicine. 2018a. "Clinical trials." accessed 06/2018. https://clinicaltrials.gov/.

NIH, National Institute of Health—NCL Protocols. 2018b. "Assay cascade protocols." accessed 06/2018. https://ncl.cancer.gov/resources/assay-cascade-protocols.

Olivier, KN., DE. Griffith, G. Eagle, JP. McGinnis, L. Micioni, K. Liu, CL. Daley, KL. Winthrop, S. Ruoss, and DJ. Addrizzo-Harris. 2017. "Randomized trial of liposomal amikacin for inhalation in nontuberculous mycobacterial lung disease." *American Journal of Respiratory and Critical Care Medicine* 195 (6):814–823.

Oprea, D. 2010. "Inhaled fentanyl." In R. Sinatra, J. Jahr, and J. Watkins-Pitchford (Eds.), *The Essence of Analgesia and Analgesics* (pp. 444–447). Cambridge, UK: Cambridge University Press. doi:10.1017/CBO9780511841378.111.

Palmer, SM., RH. Drew, JD. Whitehouse, VF. Tapson, RD. Davis, RR. McConnell, SS. Kanj, and JR. Perfect. 2001. "Safety of aerosolized amphotericin B lipid complex In lung transplant recipients12." *Transplantation* 72 (3):545–548.

Parikh, R., and S. Dalwadi. 2014. "Preparation and characterization of controlled release poly-ε-caprolactone microparticles of isoniazid for drug delivery through pulmonary route." *Powder Technology* 264:158–165. doi:10.1016/j.powtec.2014.04.077.

Patton, JS. 2007. "Inhaling medicines: Delivering drugs to the body through the lungs." *Nature Reviews Drug Discovery* 6 (1):67–74.

Pecota, N., Aradigm Corporation. 2016. Aradigm announces top-line results from two phase 3 studies evaluating Pulmaquin for the chronic treatment of non-cystic fibrosis bronchiectasis patients with lung infections with Pseudomonas aeruginosa. *BusinessWire*: Acquire Media. https://www.businesswire.com/news/home/20161201005450/en/Aradigm-Announces-Top-Line-Results-Phase-3-Studies.

Peltonen, L. and J. Hirvonen. 2018. "Drug nanocrystals—Versatile option for formulation of poorly soluble materials." *International Journal of Pharmaceutics* 537 (1):73–83. doi:10.1016/j.ijpharm.2017.12.005.

Pishbin, F., V. Mouriño, JB. Gilchrist, DW. McComb, S. Kreppel, V. Salih, MP. Ryan, and AR. Boccaccini. 2013. "Single-step electrochemical deposition of antimicrobial orthopaedic coatings based on a bioactive glass/chitosan/nano-silver composite system." *Acta Biomaterialia* 9 (7):7469–7479. doi:10.1016/j.actbio.2013.03.006.

Quader, S. and K. Kataoka. 2017. "Nanomaterial-enabled cancer therapy." *Molecular Therapy* 25 (7):1501–1513. doi:10.1016/j.ymthe.2017.04.026.

Rijnders, BJ., JJ. Cornelissen, L. Slobbe, MJ. Becker, JK. Doorduijn, WC. Hop, EJ. Ruijgrok et al. 2008. "Aerosolized liposomal amphotericin B for the prevention of invasive pulmonary aspergillosis during prolonged neutropenia: A randomized, placebo-controlled trial." *Clinical Infectious Diseases* 46 (9):1401–1408.

Rudokas, M., M. Najlah, MA. Alhnan, and A. Elhissi. 2016. "Liposome delivery systems for inhalation: A critical review highlighting formulation issues and anticancer applications." *Medical Principles and Practice* 25 (Suppl 2):60–72. doi:10.1159/000445116.

Ryan, GM., LM. Kaminskas, BD. Kelly, DJ. Owen, MP. McIntosh-, and CJ. Porter. 2013. "Pulmonary administration of PEGylated polylysine dendrimers: Absorption from the lung versus retention within the lung is highly size-dependent." *Molecular Pharmaceutics* 10 (8):2986–2995. doi:10.1021/mp400091n.

Sercombe, L., T. Veerati, F. Moheimani, SY. Wu, AK. Sood, and S. Hua. 2015. "Advances and challenges of liposome assisted drug delivery." *Frontiers in Pharmacology* 6 (286). doi:10.3389/fphar.2015.00286.

Serisier, DJ., D. Bilton, A De Soyza, PJ. Thompson, J. Kolbe, HW. Greville, D. Cipolla, P. Bruinenberg, I. Gonda, and ORBIT-2 investigators. 2013. "Inhaled, dual release liposomal ciprofloxacin in non-cystic fibrosis bronchiectasis (ORBIT-2): A randomised, double-blind, placebo-controlled trial." *Thorax* 68 (9):812–817.

Siegel, RL., KD. Miller, and A. Jemal. 2018. "Cancer statistics, 2018." *CA: A Cancer Journal for Clinicians* 68 (1):7–30.

Valerieva, A., TA. Popov, M. Staevska, T. Kralimarkova, E. Petkova, E. Valerieva, T. Mustakov, T. Lazarova, V. Dimitrov, and MK. Church. 2015. "Effect of micronized cellulose powder on the efficacy of topical oxymetazoline in allergic rhinitis." *Allergy and Asthma Proceedings* 36 (6):e134–e139.

Verschraegen, CF. 2006. "Aerosolized liposomal 9-Nitro-20 (S)-Camptothecin in patients with advanced malignancies in the lungs." *Pneumologie* 60 (07):A2.

Verschraegen, CF, BE. Gilbert, AJ. Huaringa, R. Newman, N. Harris, FJ. Leyva, L. Keus, K. Campbell, T. Nelson-Taylor, and V. Knight. 2000. "Feasibility, phase I, and pharmacological study of aerosolized liposomal 9-Nitro-20 (S)-Camptothecin in patients with advanced malignancies in the lungs." *Annals of the New York Academy of Sciences* 922 (1):352–354.

Verschraegen, CF., BE. Gilbert, E. Loyer, A. Huaringa, G. Walsh, RA. Newman, and V. Knight. 2004. "Clinical evaluation of the delivery and safety of aerosolized liposomal 9-nitro-20 (s)-camptothecin in patients with advanced pulmonary malignancies." *Clinical Cancer Research* 10 (7):2319–2326.

Waldrep, JC., J. Arppe, KA. Jansa, and M. Vidgren. 1998. "Experimental pulmonary delivery of cyclosporin A by liposome aerosol." *International Journal of Pharmaceutics* 160 (2):239–249.

Weber, S., A. Zimmer, and J. Pardeike. 2014. "Solid lipid nanoparticles (SLN) and nanostructured lipid carriers (NLC) for pulmonary application: A review of the state of the art." *European Journal of Pharmaceutics and Biopharmaceutics* 86 (1):7–22. doi:10.1016/j.ejpb.2013.08.013.

Wittgen, BPH., PWA. Kunst, KVD. Born, AW. Van Wijk, W. Perkins, FG. Pilkiewicz, R. Perez-Soler, S. Nicholson, GJ. Peters, and PE. Postmus. 2007. "Phase I study of aerosolized SLIT cisplatin in the treatment of patients with carcinoma of the lung." *Clinical Cancer Research* 13 (8):2414–2421.

Zarogoulidis, P., E. Chatzaki, K. Porpodis, K. Domvri, W. Hohenforst-Schmidt, EP. Goldberg, N. Karamanos, and K. Zarogoulidis. 2012. "Inhaled chemotherapy in lung cancer: Future concept of nanomedicine." *International Journal of Nanomedicine* 7:1551–1572. doi:10.2147/IJN.S29997.

Zhang, J., L. Wu, HK. Chan, and W. Watanabe. 2011. "Formation, characterization, and fate of inhaled drug nanoparticles." *Advanced Drug Delivery Reviews* 63 (6):441–455. doi:10.1016/j.addr.2010.11.002.

Zhong, Q., OM. Merkel, JJ. Reineke, and SR. da Rocha. 2016. "Effect of the route of administration and PEGylation of poly(amidoamine) dendrimers on their systemic and lung cellular biodistribution." *Molecular Pharmaceutics* 13 (6):1866–1878. doi:10.1021/acs.molpharmaceut.6b00036.

Zhong, Q., and Sandro RP. da Rocha. 2016. "Poly(amidoamine) dendrimer–doxorubicin conjugates: In vitro characteristics and pseudosolution formulation in pressurized metered-dose inhalers." *Molecular Pharmaceutics* 13 (3):1058–1072. doi:10.1021/acs.molpharmaceut.5b00876.

Section VI

Devices

18

Pressurized Metered-Dose Inhalers

Sandro R.P. da Rocha, Balaji Bharatwaj, Rodrigo S. Heyder, and Lin Yang

CONTENTS

18.1 Pressurized Metered-Dose Inhalers (pMDIs): The Basics

pMDIs are complex *drug-device* combination products that are widely used to treat lung diseases. pMDIs may also be advantageously employed to deliver active pharmaceutical ingredients (APIs) to the systemic circulation *through* the lungs (Hickey 2013). The *device* component of a typical pMDI is comprised of a canister, a metering valve, and an actuator—Figure 18.1 (Stein et al. 2014), while the *drug* component consists of the formulation (Myrdal et al. 2014), which is contained within the canister by the valve. A pMDI formulation is composed of the API and excipients, including a liquid propellant and (typically) co-solvents and/or surfactants. pMDIs may be in the form of solution (API dissolved in liquid propellant) or suspension (API particles dispersed in liquid propellant) formulations.

18.2 Aerosol Generation in pMDIs

Propellant droplets containing the API (and any other excipients) are formed at the actuator nozzle as the patient presses the valve, thus opening the channel between the metering chamber within the valve (which is held at saturation pressure of the propellant-excipient mixture) and the atmosphere—Figure 18.1 (Zhu et al. 2015). Large aerosol droplets with high initial velocities are initially formed. As the aerosol cloud travels towards the patient's mouth, the liquid propellant evaporates and cools, and the droplets decrease in size and reduce their velocity. Particles that possess appropriate aerosol characteristics are subsequently deposited in the pulmonary tract. Both device design and formulation have a dramatic impact on the quality of the aerosol and, therefore, on the deposition of the API in the lungs. Hardware design and formulation will be discussed in detail in this chapter.

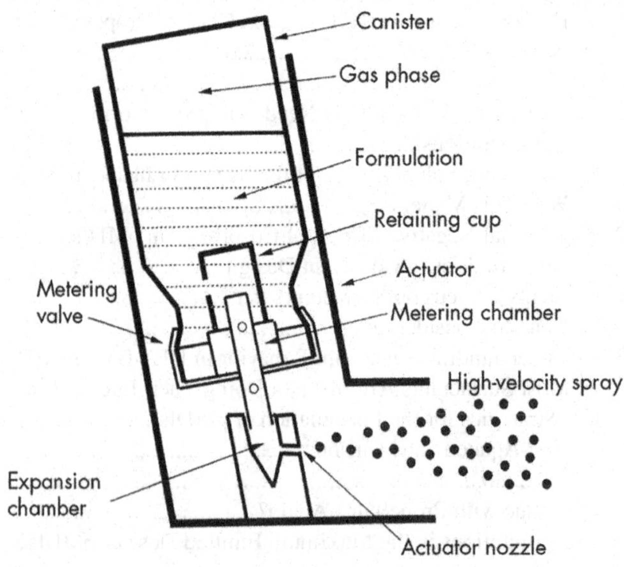

FIGURE 18.1 Schematic diagram of the basic components of a pMDI and aerosol generated upon device actuation. (Adapted from Fromer, L. et al., 2010. *Postgraduate Medicine*, 122, 83–93, 2010. With permission.)

TABLE 18.1
A Complete List of the HFA-Based pMDI Drug Products Approved by the FDA Currently in the Market

Year	Product Name	Drug	Manufacturer
1996	Proventil HFA	Albuterol sulfate	3M
2000	QVAR	Beclomethasone diproprionate	3M
2001	Ventolin HFA	Albuterol sulfate	GlaxoSmithKline
2004	ProA ir HFA	Albuterol sulfate	Ivax
2004	Atrovent HFA	Ipratropium bromide	Boehringer Ingelheim
2005	Xopenex HFA	Levalbuterol tartrate	Sepracor
2006	Aerospan	Flunisolide	Forest
2006	Advair HFA	Fluticasone propionate/salmeterol	GlaxoSmithKline
2006	Flovent HFA	Fluticasone propionate	GlaxoSmithKline
2006	Symbicort	Budesonide/formoterol	AstraZeneca
2008	Alvesco	Ciclesonide	AstraZeneca
2010	Dulera	Mometasone/formoterol fumarate	Merck
2014	Asmanex HFA	Mometasone fuorate	Merck
2016	Bevespi Aerosphere	Glycopyrrolate/formoterol fumarate	Astra Zeneca

18.3 A Brief History of pMDIs

pMDIs were invented in 1950s at the Reiker Laboratories, Inc. (now 3M) as a response to a need to efficiently deliver drugs to the lungs. The first pMDI drug products were solution formulations of epinephrine and isoproterenol in chlorofluorocarbon (CFC) propellants and co-solvent ethanol, and were approved by the FDA a year after the invention of pMDIs (Anderson 2005). This new invention that allowed targeting of drugs to the lungs was followed by the approval of more than 20 CFC-based pMDIs within the next four decades. For a detailed historical perspective of therapeutic aerosols, including pMDIs, the readers are directed to (Stein and Thiel 2017). A new phase for pMDIs started with the signing of the Montreal Protocol in 1987, which represented the beginning of the phase out of the ozone depleting CFCs. Hydrofluoroalkane (HFA) propellants were then introduced in the market, leading to innovations in device and materials for pMDIs, and new materials and particle engineering concepts for their (re)formulation. A number of HFA-based pMDIs have been introduced in the US market since then—a complete list[1] of the HFA-based pMDIs in the US is shown in Table 18.1.

Since their invention, pMDIs have become the most widely used device for pulmonary drug delivery (Stein and Thiel 2017). pMDIs occupy ca. 70% of the respiratory inhaler devices market share, which is composed mostly of pMDIs, dry powder inhalers (DPIs), and nebulizers, and are expected to continue their dominance in the foreseeable future (FMI 2017).

18.4 Challenges That Have Pushed Technological Advances in the Field of pMDIs

Technological advances that built upon the initial concept of pMDIs first came about from the realization that such devices were relatively inefficient in delivering drugs to the lungs. High inertial impaction of large aerosol particles that had high velocities resulted in significant oropharyngeal losses. Such challenges led to the development and use of spacers (*add-on devices*). Difficulty in

[1] https://www.accessdata.fda.gov/scripts/cder/ob/index.cfm—search: "aerosol, metered"

synchronization between patient inhalation and dose actuation was also identified early on as a significant challenge in the field of pMDIs. The answer to this problem came with the development of *breath-actuated pMDIs*, which were commercially introduced in 1970 (Thiel 1996). Another significant challenge that continues to stimulate technological advancements in the area of pMDIs are ongoing issues with the propellants used in these drug-device combinations. The phase out of CFCs led to the use of HFA propellants in pMDIs. While HFAs are non-ozone depleting, they have significantly different physicochemical properties compared to CFCs. HFAs have a dual character, in that they are somewhat lipophobic and hydrophobic at the same time (Peguin and da Rocha 2008). As a consequence of this ambivalence, most drugs have very low solubility in the HFA propellants used in FDA approved formulations. In order to formulate solution formations in pMDIs, cosolvents are thus usually necessary. Cosolvents may also be necessary to enhance the solubility of surfactants for the development of dispersion formulations. Such need arises as the surfactants used in FDA approved formulations were originally optimized to be used with CFC propellants that are significantly less polar than HFAs. Stimulated by these challenges, significant new knowledge was developed in terms of *excipient design* (cosolvent and surfactants) (Conti et al. 2012, Myrdal et al. 2014) and *particle engineering strategies* for the formulation of suspension-based formulations (Wu et al. 2008, Dexter and Hak-Kim 2015, Liang et al. 2015). Because propellants are in direct and prolonged contact with the pMDI canister and valve, their interaction with those materials is also a consideration and has led to innovation in the *hardware design* as well (Stein et al. 2014).

18.5 Device (Hardware) Design

18.5.1 Metering Valves

The metering valve is at the heart of pMDIs. A detail representation of the components of a retention-type metering valve used in pMDIs is shown in Figure 18.2. In its most common form, metering valves can meter, hold and discharge pressurized formulation, and can do so consistently for over 200 doses. Advances in regulatory, technology and market awareness demand that metering valves in use in pMDIs meet a long list of requirements including good stability performance, low leachables/extractables, good barrier capability with low moisture ingress and leak rate, and low drug absorption, accurately and uniformly metering of the formulation, reasonable actuation force, and they also need to be economical. Such requirements demand a certain degree of complexity and clever engineering in the metering valve

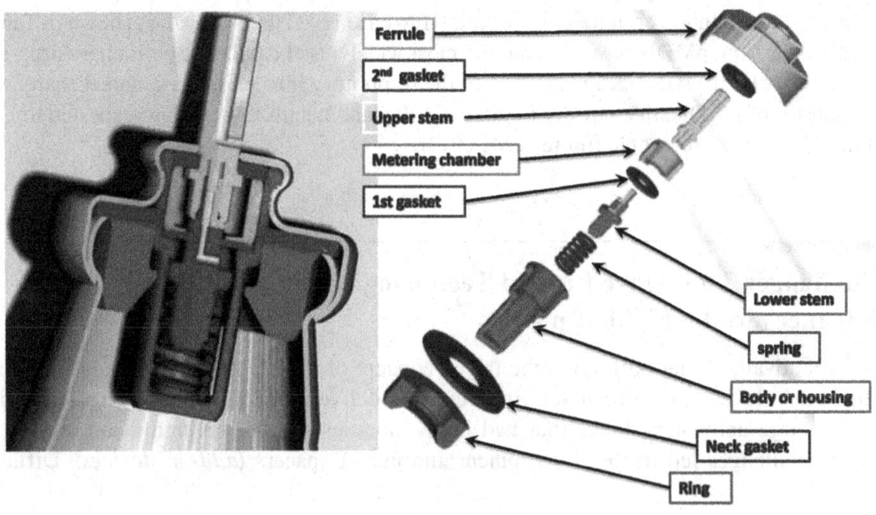

FIGURE 18.2 Typical components of retention type metering valve. (Courtesy of Aptar Group Inc.)

design. It is thus of interest to review some of the most recent advances in metering valve technology, and revisit some of the challenges together with opportunities related to metering valves for use in pMDIs.

18.5.1.1 Basic Mechanism of Operation

The vast majority of the pMDI metering valves on the market have been retention valves. When depressed, the valve stem's side opening goes in the metering chamber, thus connecting the formulation inside the metering chamber to the atmosphere. The formulation will then be self-propelled and a dose discharged. The valve stem returns to its rest position after an actuation, with the metering chamber then being closed to the atmosphere and connected to the formulation bulk through a refill pathway. As the metering chamber is close to atmospheric pressure, the pressure differential between the formulation bulk and the metering chamber will drive the formulation into the metering chamber. The formulation will fill in the metering chamber as it evaporates in the metering chamber trying to reach saturation pressure and a vapor bubble will exist in the end of the refill process. Defined by a few factors including formulation pressure and viscosity, refill pathway geometry, metering chamber volume and shape, the size of the vapor bubble should be reproducible for each refill within a certain temperature range. The refill pathway between the metering chamber and the formulation bulk is typically small and tortuous—giving rise to capillary forces that are enough to stop the formulation in the metering chamber to flow back into the bulk even when the canister is reversed (in the valve up position), most of the time.

In spite of its dominant presence in the pMDI industry, retention valves have certain shortcomings:

Loss of prime (LOP) is characterized by a first dose with low drug content, which is usually followed by a second dose with high drug content. Although the exact cause of LOP is still unclear, and in reality may differ from case to case, there are a few likely causes: (1) thermal fluctuations: it is hypothesized that when temperature fluctuates, the metering chamber's extra thermal barrier cause it to have a temperature and thus pressure differential over the bulk, which drives some of the formulation out of the metering chamber, in spite of the capillary effect; (2) leakage from metering chamber top gasket may also contribute to the loss of prime; (3) over the storage period, drug may get localized in the metering chamber and thus cannot be aerosolized during actuation; (4) it may simply be that the dose just gets "shook out" by the patient. The LOP contributes to some of the marketed product whose "one dose" is composed of two actuations—to even out the lower first dose and higher second dose. Most pMDIs on the market, suspension or solution, need to be primed and re-primed after prolonged periods of non-use. It is worth mentioning that some valves have a "retention cap," which is supposed to help in preventing LOP when the valve is reversed.

Rise/fall of dose through canister life is another commonly observed effect seen during the development of pMDIs that use retention valves. The effect of the headspace compensation concentrating effect is known to cause rise of dose through canister life. On top of that, and unique to the retention valve, is non-uniformly metered dose for the suspension formulation; the refill of the retention valve's metering chamber happens after an actuation, the time gap between shaking to releasing the valve stem and refilling (typically 2–10 seconds) might be enough for the development of inhomogeneity for some formulations. The result is either increase or decrease of the dose toward end of canister life, depending on the suspension characteristics (sedimenting or creaming suspension).

Given these shortcomings of retention valves, there have been significant efforts from valve manufacturers to develop primeless valves. Valois's ACT valve, Bespak's easifill and 3M's Face Seal valves are examples of primeless valves. At rest, the metering chamber is wide open to the formulation bulk, the "metering" happens just when an actuation is made right after shaking—when the valve stem is being pressed, the metering chamber forms and discharges the dose simultaneously. By design, there is no need for priming/re-priming. These valves can thus be favorably used in breath actuated inhaler designs. Moreover, because there is no delay in shaking and metering, the potential for non-uniformly metered dose is much lower. A comparison between a retention and primeless valve geometry is shown in Figure 18.3.

18.5.1.2 Materials Used in Metering Valves

Gasket materials: gaskets materials are usually identified as the most critical components in metering valves. There are typically three gaskets in the metering valve that are: (i) neck gasket; (ii) metering

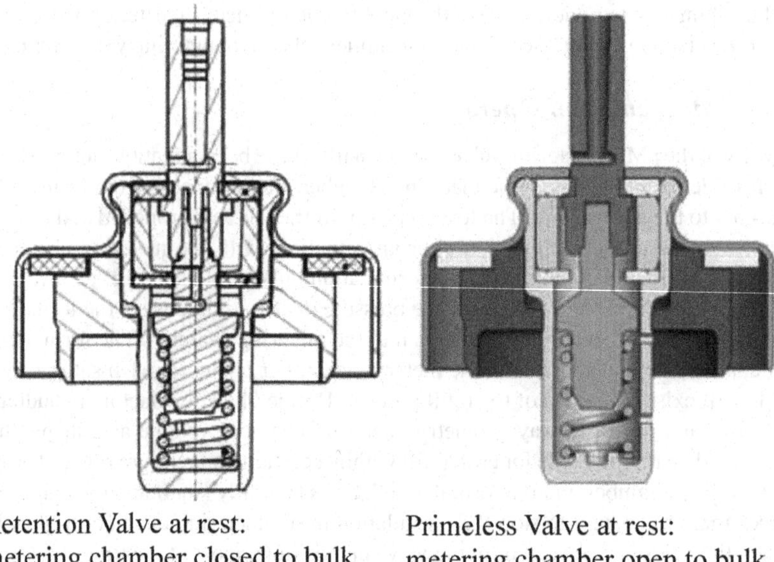

FIGURE 18.3 Schematic diagram of a retention and a primeless valve. (Courtesy of Aptar Group Inc.)

chamber top gasket; (iii) and metering chamber bottom gasket. The metering chamber gaskets are dynamic parts in that they have to retain their radial and axial sealing properties while enabling the valve stem to travel hundreds of times. The metering chamber bottom gasket also needs to have the right amount of rigidness so that when the right amount of pressure is applied from inside the metering chamber, it could deform slightly to create a filling pathway to enable pressure filling—the mainstay of the industry nowadays, and seal again when the pressure is removed. Besides the mechanical requirements, dynamic gaskets also have to have good compatibility, low extractable/leachables, good barrier properties, and good stability behavior. Given such demanding tasks, the pool of elastomers that one can rely on narrows down to only a few. Currently, the majority of valves are made from elastomers selected from Nitrile (Nitrile Butadiene Rubber), Ethylene Propylene Diene Monomer (EPDM), butyl/halobutyl and polychloroprene rubber.

The neck gasket is a static part which is less demanding on the mechanical properties. As a result, the neck gasket can be selected from another pool of materials with different merit. A good example is Aptar's use of COCe gasket in the DF-30 plus valves, which is predicted to have less extractable/leachables, and much better barrier property—less moisture ingress and less leakage.

Currently, the industry is also exploring the use of gaskets made of polymer blends. The idea is to combine the advantages of different rubber materials to more accurately target the desired properties. Different blends of hydrogenated nitrile, polyolefine elastomer and bromobutyl have been discussed.

Plastic materials: Similar to the gasket materials used in metering valves, other polymeric materials used in the functional parts of the metering valves also have to meet a long list of requirements including a pharmaceutically acceptable extractable/leachable profile, propellant compatible, and mechanically robust. As a result, the materials that can be used for the metering chamber or the valve stem are limited to only acetal resins and polyesters. It is worth noting that because of lower surface energy displayed by stainless steel in comparison to acetal and polyester resins, it may be advantageous for some suspension formulations to use stainless steel metering chamber/valve stem, to reduce drug adhesion to the surface.

Plasma processes can also be used to create low friction surfaces by adding layers of highly cross-linked fluorocarbons to the relevant surfaces or by direct fluorination of polymers or rubbers. The result is the elimination of the need for silicones that are traditionally used to lubricate the valves' dynamic parts. Such coatings on the metering valves can also, to some degree, reduce the adhesion of drugs onto the valve component.

18.5.1.3 Looking Ahead

Since pMDIs are projected to maintain their dominance in the inhalation market in the foreseeable future, suppliers and pharmaceutical companies are expected to continue to make improvements on the valve technologies used in pMDIs. Most advances are likely to be incremental, as for example materials with less extractables/leachables, better dosing performance, and better barrier performance. Some innovations may be also seen where novel drugs/formulations are developed. However, little is expected to be changed in the valves' basic form as the industry supply chain and market both have significant inertia.

Just as the transition from CFCs to HFAs has resulted in the redesign of pMDI valves, the next generation propellants are also expected to lead to a redesign of pMDI valves. There are currently also more and more biomolecules being considered for dosing through the inhalation route. Although not considered as the device of choice for the delivery of macromolecules to the lungs (as DPIs/nebulizers), pMDIs do have certain advantages. pMDIs are less demanding in terms of the patient inhalation effort, and have considerably better container closure for superior stability of the drug. It is conceivable that pMDI valves with larger metering chambers, yet slower discharging rates, when combined with coordinated efforts on formulation and actuator development could potentially represent an answer to the delivery of biomacromolecules to the lungs.

18.5.2 Canisters

Canisters used in pMDIs are made from either aluminum or stainless steel. The focus in technological advancements in canisters is mostly on minimizing formulation—canister interactions. A class of fluorocarbon coatings is widely used to minimize formulation—canister interactions. The result is less loss of drug to the canister walls for the suspension formulation, better stability profile for solution formulation that are susceptible to degradation in the presence of aluminum, and better anti-corrosion properties for the canister where acid is used in the formulation (Young et al. 2003, Traini et al. 2006, Brouet et al. 2006). Monomers with high fluorine content are preferred for coatings like perfluoroalkoxyalkylene (PFA) and polytetrafluoroethylene (PTFE). Other coating types include expoxy—phenol resins or even glass thin films.

There is an array of canister coating techniques including pre-coating, spray coating, dipping, and electrostatic dry powder coating (Brouet et al. 2006, Turner 2010). Special stainless steel compositions are also developed to be compatible with some of the more corrosive formulations. The gas plasma processing is a more recent technique that involves constant or pulsed excitation of gas by either radio frequency or microwave field to produce energetic plasma. With the right control of the plasma coating process, including a combination of gas/monomer configuration and electric field that is customized to the can geometry, a thin layer of coating can be developed that is uniform, of submicron thickness, of high crosslink density, and devoid of any solvents, being practically extractable free (Turner 2010, Stevenson 2016). The plasma coating has been evaluated for different drugs in both solution and suspension formulations, and has shown to be able to reduce drug deposition to the wall as well as reduce drug degradation (Baron et al. 2014).

With a variety of new drugs being considered for delivery via the inhalation route, there are cases where smaller than usual canister sizes may be desirable. It may be related to the need for small doses, or controlled substances, or ultra-long acting LAMA/LABA. The industry has developed smaller canisters with a base which makes it possible to use smaller content with regular pMDI valves and actuators, yet not to suffer from head space effect.

It is worth mentioning that there are ongoing efforts to integrate dose indicating solutions into the canister design. Presspart Quantum Dose Indicator® is one of such example where dose indication is achieved via biased weight distribution of the canister, such that with different amounts of formulation inside, the canister will reach balance in a different rotational orientation.

18.5.3 Actuators

Actuators have been an integral part of the pMDI ensemble since its inception in 1956 (Anderson et al. 2017). They are, in simple terms, the conduit that facilitates the exit of the aerosol from the canister via the metering chamber. Actuators are available in different sizes to accommodate canisters of

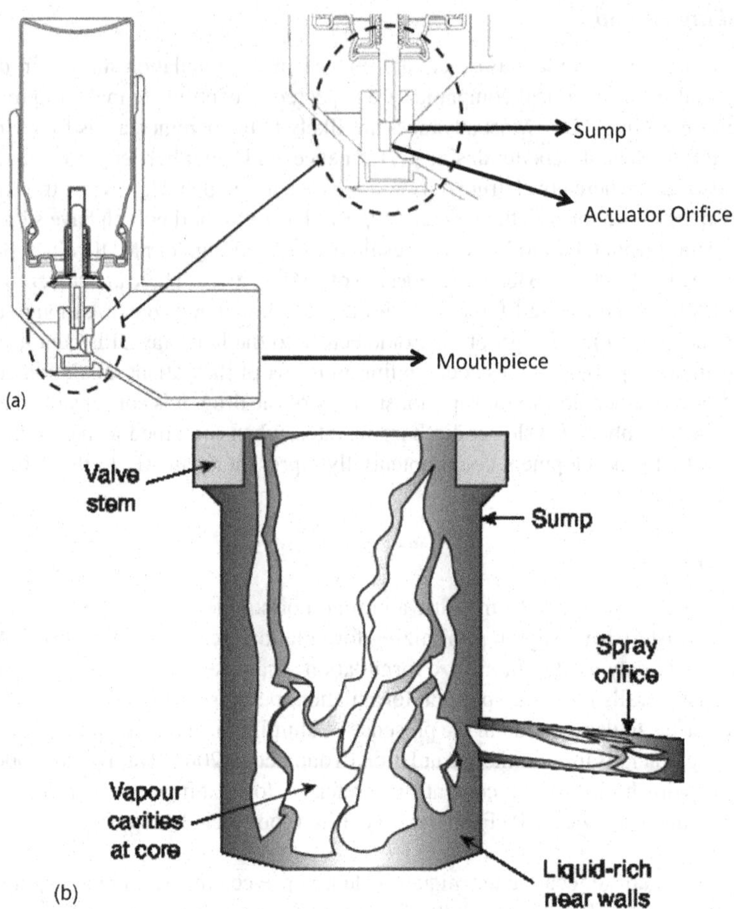

FIGURE 18.4 (a) Illustration of a press and breathe MDI actuator cross section. (Adapted from Stein, S.W. et al., *AAPS PharmSciTech*, 15, 326–338, 2015.); (b) A pictographic depiction of the atomization process occurring within the core components of the actuator. (Courtesy of David Lewis, 2007.)

different volumes. The actuator is comprised of the spray nozzle or actuator orifice, the sump, and the actuator mouthpiece (Lewis 2007). Additionally, actuators come with a dust cap to maintain mouthpiece cleanliness. Some of the major commercial manufacturers of actuators include Bespak, H&T Presspart, 3M and Coster. A detailed schematic of a press and breath actuator is given in Figure 18.4a (Stein et al. 2015).

The pMDI canister is mated with an actuator to enable the patient to inhale the formulation emanating from the canister (Stein et al. 2015). Atomization of the pMDI formulation within the actuator is fundamental to creating a respirable dose. In a typical actuation process, the formulation exits the metering valve, through the valve stem, actuator sump and over the length of the actuator orifice causing expansion of the liquid formulation followed by flashing of the volatile propellant as the dose is emitted from the actuator's mouthpiece into the patient's mouth (Chen et al. 2015, Stein et al. 2015). An analogous representation is shown in Figure 18.4b (Lewis 2007).

Actuators exercise significant influence over the delivery of the formulation from the canister. Actuator parameters like nozzle diameter and path length, expansion chamber's shape and size and shape and length of the mouthpiece in conjunction with actuator attachments like spacers all have an important role to play in the administration of medications from pMDI formulations (Lewis 2007, Stein et al. 2015). Even though current actuators remain quite similar in their overall design compared to their predecessors, several improvements have been made and introduced.

18.5.3.1 Actuator Design and Geometry

As detailed earlier, the actuator of a metered dose inhaler comprises of mouthpiece, sump and an orifice. The design and dimensions of the actuator can have a profound impact on the aerodynamic characteristics of the emitted aerosol and the subsequent lung deposition (Lewis 2007, Chen et al. 2015, Ivey et al. 2015). The sections below provide some insight into the impact of the actuator geometry on the aerosol performance of pMDIs.

Actuator orifice diameter and shape. The actuator orifice or nozzle is the orifice through which the formulation exits the metering chamber into the mouthpiece and it exerts significant influence on the dynamics of the atomizing aerosol (Ivey et al. 2015, Stein et al. 2015). Aerosol particle size varies directly with the nozzle diameter and can have an impact on the lung deposition of the formulation. Typical orifice diameters vary between 0.14 and 0.6 mm (Stein et al. 2015). It has also been reported that the fine particle fraction (FPF) of solution pMDI formulations varies inversely with nozzle diameters (ND) as shown for the HFA134a formulation in Figure 18.5.

Equation 18.1 provides an empirical correlation between FPF and ND.

$$\mathrm{FPF} = 2.1\times 10^{-5}\ a^{-1.5} v^{-0.25} C^{3} \tag{18.1}$$

where a is the orifice diameter (in mm), v is the metered dose volume (in µL) and C is the propellant content (Lewis 2007). The most efficient delivery (high FPFs) of solution pMDI formulations of HFA134a was obtained when nozzles with smaller diameter and small valve sizes (metering valve volume) were used (Stein et al. 2015). Interestingly, a similar relationship was observed when the nozzle diameter was reduced in the case of suspension pMDI aerosols of HFA227. This could be attributed to a combination of the smaller initial droplet size (to some extent) and the decreased momentum imparted to the exiting aerosol, that results in reduced deposition in the oropharyngeal region (Stein et al. 2015). Although a reduction in actuator size can improve overall product performance, there are other practical limitations viz. patient inhalation profiles, nozzle clogging etc., that need to be considered. Most commercial actuators have a nozzle diameter greater than 0.3 mm (Lewis et al. 2006, Stein et al. 2015).

In addition to the nozzle diameter, other orifice parameters that have been explored include nozzle shape configurations and exit geometries (Lewis et al. 2006, Stein et al. 2015). Despite evaluating multiple nozzle configurations *in vitro*, no significant improvement in the aerosol characteristics have been ascertained

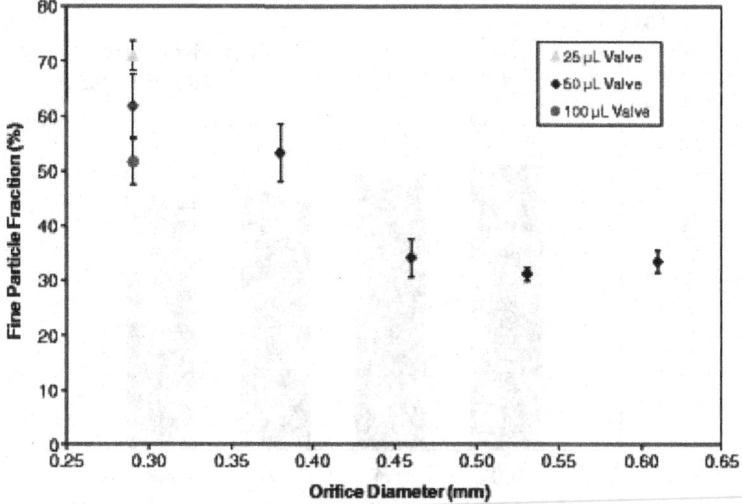

FIGURE 18.5 The effect of nozzle/orifice diameter on the fine particle fraction of a solution MDI formulation of Beclomethasone dipropionate in HFA134a. The API concentration was 0.167% (w/w) and ethanol concentration was 8%. (Reproduced from Stein, S.W. et al., *AAPS PharmSciTech*, 15, 326–338, 2015. With permission.)

relative to the conventional round nozzle geometry. However, exit geometries have been shown to have an impact on the aerodynamic properties of the formulation due to the impact they have on the electrostatic charge of the atomized particles. Typically, most of the exit geometries of the nozzle are conical. However, additional configurations like flat, spout and double cones have also been studied (Newman 2005, Lewis 2007, Stein et al. 2015). The effect of orifice length (ranges between 0.6 and 0.7 mm) on the pMDI performance was also examined and found to be formulation dependent (Lewis 2007).

Actuator Sump. Another important component in the actuator ensemble is the actuator sump, which can potentially influence the ratio of liquid and vapor phases during atomization. However, studies have shown that the sump volume has minimal effect on aerosol delivery characteristics when the volume is varied two fold or six fold. This is likely due to the relatively large dead volume inside of a valve stem, which will mask the seemingly drastic sump volume change. Interestingly, the actuator sump geometry in conjunction with the orifice geometry has been shown to alleviate blockage of the actuator (Lewis 2007). Specific formulations tend to be influenced by the geometry of the actuator sump, in that they minimize accumulation of the drug around the nozzle, thereby ensuring consistency in drug delivery. Ideally, the actuator sumps are designed to have smooth and round interiors to promote continuous flow of the formulation out of the metering valve into the orifice. Additional properties that actuator sumps have shown to influence include the spray pattern and plume geometry (Lewis 2007, Stein et al. 2015).

Mouthpiece configuration. The mouthpiece of the original actuator when the pMDI was introduced was 3 to 4 times longer than the ones that are commonly in use today. While a longer mouthpiece tends to improve lung deposition and minimize oropharyngeal deposition, it makes the actuator bulky, causing portability and packaging constraints. Add on devices like spacers and valve holding chambers have been incorporated to overcome some of the aforementioned impediments and improve aerosol deposition in the lungs (Newman 2005, Lewis 2007). Altering the mouthpiece configuration of the actuator can influence the particle disposition. For instance, increasing the length would increase deposition in the mouthpiece which would potentially surmount several disadvantages plaguing the device including high oropharyngeal deposition, high plume velocity and poor breath coordination among patients (Lewis et al. 2006, Stein et al. 2015). Indeed, it was shown that a modest increase in the mouthpiece length of a Bespak actuator reduced the non-respirable dose significantly while largely maintaining the respirable dose for a solution pMDI formulation as depicted in Figure 18.6 (Lewis et al. 2006, Lewis 2007).

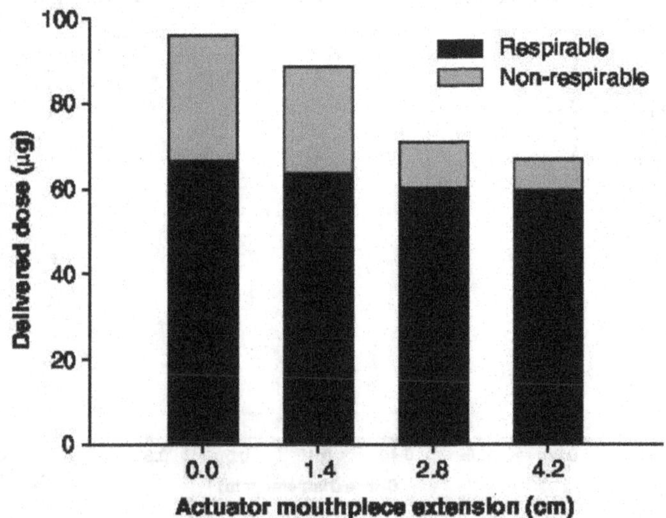

FIGURE 18.6 The effect of altering mouthpiece length on delivered dose of beclometasone dipropionate formulated as a solution MDI in HFA134a. (Courtesy of David Lewis, 2007).

18.5.3.2 Recent Innovations in Actuators

Innovation in the realm of actuators has been centered on improving patient breath coordination and reducing oropharyngeal deposition. Tempo inhaler developed at MAP pharma/Allergan incorporates a porous mouthpiece that facilitates entry of air perpendicular to the mouthpiece to minimize deposition (Shrewsbury et al. 2007). Other systems that have been developed to minimize mouth throat deposition are devices from Bespak and 3M where incoming air has been utilized to slow down the aerosol plume resulting in retardation of the spray, which reduces oropharyngeal deposition in patients. Despite the multitude of benefits offered, these designs that tend to decrease mouthpiece deposition also lend to additional complexity and cost of the actuator, which hamper their widespread use (Lewis et al. 2006, Stein et al. 2015).

Some of the drawbacks of press and breath inhalers have been addressed through the development of breath-actuated inhalers. Breath-actuated devices sense the inhalation of the patient through the actuator and triggers the dose release from the canister (Bell and Newman 2007, Stein et al. 2015). If used correctly, patients have been shown to have better management of asthma when using breath actuated devices instead of the conventional pMDIs (Newman 2005, Stein et al. 2015). The introduction of such devices were reported in 1960s and since then several iterative design changes have been made to such devices with a majority of innovation focusing on modifications to the actuator housing. Some of the breath actuated devices that have been launched include 3M's Autohaler®, IVAX's Easi-breathe™, and MD Turbo by Respirics (Lewis 2007).

18.5.4 Add On Devices

18.5.4.1 Spacers

Spacers are add on devices connected to the mouthpieces of pMDIs, and help minimize oropharyngeal deposition by retaining larger particles within them, potentially increasing lung deposition and improving breathing coordination by reducing requirement for the synchrony between inhalation and actuation—this might be particularly useful for pediatric and geriatric patient population (Anderson et al. 2017). As a consequence, various national and international obstructive lung disease guidelines stipulate the use of spacers in patient subgroups prone to pMDI handling errors (Newman 2004). They are connected to a pMDI at one end and contain a mouthpiece or a facemask at the other. Numerous studies have shown that utilizing spacers as add on devices greatly minimize oropharyngeal deposition and reduce unwanted systemic side effects. Parameters that impact drug delivery via spacers include spacer dimensions and geometry and the charge (Newman 2004). For instance, electrostatic charge on the surface of the spacer can reduce drug delivery efficiency (Dissanayake and Suggett 2018) (Figure 18.7).

The types of spacers include simple tubular systems affixed to the actuator mouthpiece, holding chambers that have a one way valve to prevent the user from blowing the dose away and reverse flow systems where the aerosol is actuated away from the patient (Newman 2004, Stein et al. 2015). Typical volumes of commercially available spacers vary between 20 and 750 mL (Anderson et al. 2017). Some of the commonly marketed spacers include Aerochamber and Aerochamber Plus (Trudell), Optichamber (Phillips), Babyhaler (GSK), Volumatic (GSK) and Nebuhaler (AZ). In terms of flexibility, it must be mentioned that while some spacer devices have universal adapters that make them amenable to any pMDI, there are others that are rigid and can only be utilized with certain inhalers (Stein et al. 2015).

18.5.4.2 Dose Counters

Among multiple factors, one thing that stands out as a culprit to poor asthma control is patient adherence (Conner and Buck 2013). While this could be attributed to poor technique and in some cases patients forgetting to take the medication, there are several instances where nonadherence can be inadvertent

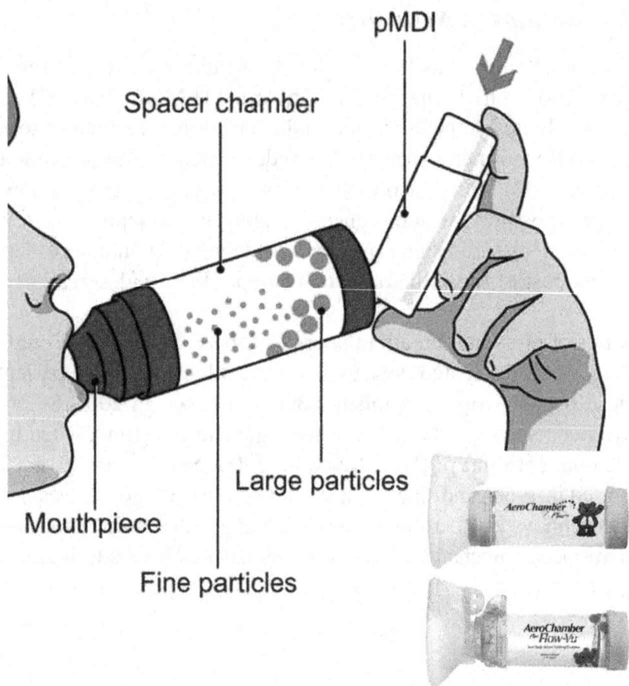

FIGURE 18.7 An illustration showing the incorporation of a pMDI into a spacer device. (Adapted from Anderson, G. et al., *Expert Opin. Drug Deliv.*, 15, 419–430, 2017. With permission.) (inset) Aerochamber plus® spacer with a face-mask. (Adapted from Dissanayake, S., and Suggett, J., *Ther. Adv. Respir. Dis.*, 12, 1–14, 2018. With permission.)

(Conner and Buck 2013, Kaur et al. 2015). Within the context of pMDIs this can happen frequently, especially since the formulation is encased within an opaque canister and a situation could arise wherein the patients actuate and inhale a near empty or a completely empty device (Bell and Newman 2007, Kaur et al. 2015). In a survey conducted prior to the introduction of dose counters, 52% of the respondents reported that they were not sure if there is medication remaining in their inhaler. To circumvent this issue, it was mandated to incorporate dose counters within the pMDI ensemble. Dose counters are the most reliable and robust way for the patients to assess the amount of medicine remaining in the pMDIs. FDA issued guidance documents in 2003 around the integration of dose counters in inhalers in the form of numeric characters or other indicator mechanisms (color coding for example). Important rules governing the requirements of dose counter are appropriately summarized in the following reference (Stein et al. 2015). With the introduction of dose counters, 97.4% of the patients were certain when to replace their inhaler underscoring their importance for patients dependent on pMDIs for their medicine (Stein et al. 2015).

The issuance of the new guidance has led to several innovations in this space. While correlating remaining dose after accurately measuring the mass of the inhaler after administering the medication would be ideal for a dose counter, the approach is prohibitively expensive (Kaur et al. 2015). Indirect methods of measuring dose remaining in an inhaler are either by force driven or displacement driven means (Kaur et al. 2015, Stein et al. 2015). In both cases, dose counters need to be designed such that they overcount/increment a dose as soon as the canister is depressed. This would mean ensuring that the force and displacement to fire a valve is a critical quality attribute that needs to be within specification (lot-to-lot variability to be minimum) for the dose counter functionality to be accurate (Kaur et al. 2015). Some of the commercially available dose counters are listed in Table 18.2.

Ultimately, the role of the dose counter is to ensure patient safety. A comprehensive review of dose counters can be found in the following publications (Kaur et al. 2015, Stein et al. 2015).

TABLE 18.2

Table Listing Popular Dose Counters Used in Commercial pMDI Products

Brand/Name	Company	Type	Characteristics	Integrated
Aerocount	Trudell	Force driven	Counts down/color coding	No
Landmark	Aptar	Displacement driven	Counts down/color coding	Yes
3M Integrated dose counter/Indicator	3M	Displacement driven	Counts down/color coding	Yes
Evohaler	GSK	Displacement driven	Counts down	Yes
On Can design and in-actuator dose counter	Presspart	Displacement driven	Electronic	No

Source: Stein, S.W. et al., *AAPS PharmSciTech*, 15, 326–338, 2015; Kaur, I. et al., *Expert Opin. Drug Deliv.*, 12, 1301–1310, 2015.

18.6 Drug Component (Formulation) Design for pMDIs

As discussed earlier, the drug component of pMDIs (the formulation) is contained within a canister that is isolated form the atmosphere by a valve. The major component of the formulation is the *propellant*, which is at its saturation pressure after being loaded into the canister (Figure 18.1). The *API(s)* in commercial formulations are either solubilized or suspended (particle form) in the liquid phase of the propellant. Other common components of the formulation are *co-solvents* (typically ethanol) that are commonly employed to enhance the solubility of the API in solution formulations, or of other excipients, as for example *surfactants*, which may be employed in both solution formulations (e.g. for valve lubrication) and also in dispersion formulations (e.g. as surface-active species for preventing aggregation of the API particles).

18.6.1 The Propellant

The propellant has two main functions in a pMDI: (i) provide the necessary energy to generate the aerosol containing the API when the valve is opened to the atmosphere; (ii) serves as a medium where the API can be either solubilized or dispersed before actuation. In the canister, the propellant is at its saturation pressure (there is a vapor-liquid interface) and the drug is solubilized or dispersed in the liquid phase. The propellant is not present as a compressed liquid or else its solvent quality (characteristics of the liquid phase) would change throughout the life of the product thus affecting formulation stability and aerosol characteristics.

18.6.1.1 Hydrofluoroalkanes (HFAs)

With the signing of the Montreal Protocol in 1987, HFAs have been selected as replacements to CFCs, which were the first propellants to be used in pMDIs. Two HFAs are currently widely used as propellants in the pMDIs approved by the FDA: in 1,1,1,2-tetrafluoroethane (HFA-134a) and 1,1,1,2,3,3,3-heptafluo ropropane (HFA-227). Some key physicochemical and environmental properties of CFCs and HFAs are listed in Table 18.3.

The fact that HFAs have zero ozone depleting potential (ODP) meant that they were good candidates to replace CFCs. However, they still have high global warming potential (GWP).

Besides significant differences in environmental impact of HFAs compared to CFCs, the physicochemical properties of HFAs are also significantly different, and that has led to new developments in the area. pMDIs with the new HFA propellants had to be redesigned as the aerosol characteristics of the drug product were impacted, the interaction between propellant and the device materials were altered, and last by not least, the ability to formulate the APIs in the new propellant were also affected.

TABLE 18.3

Physical Properties of Semi-Fluorinated Alkanes (HFAs) and Olefins (HFOs), and of Chlorofluorocarbons (CFCs)

	P^{sat}*(bar)	ρ_1*(g•ml^{-1})	μ(D)	ε	ODP	GWP
CFC 11 (CCl_3F)[a]	0.87	1.49	0.46	2.3	HIGH	HIGH
CFC 12 (CF_2Cl_2)[b]	5.60	1.33	0.51	2.1	HIGH	8100
CFC 114 (CF_2Cl_2)[c]	1.81	1.47	0.50	2.3	HIGH	HIGH
HFA 134a (CF_3CH_2F)[d]	5.72	1.23	2.06	9.5	None	1430
HFA 227 (CF_3CFHCF_3)[e]	3.90	1.42	0.93	4.1	None	3200
HFO-1234ze (CH(F)=$CHCF_3$)[f]	4.81[@]	1.12	1.44	/	None	6
HFO-1234yf (CH_2=$CFCF_3$)[g]	5.96[&]	1.09	2.54	/	None	4
HFA-152a (CH_3CF_2(H))[h]	4.16	0.911*	2.30	/	None	138

[&] ρ = density; μ = dipole moment; ε = dielectric constant; ODP = ozone depleting potential; GWP = global warming potential, relative to that of CO_2. * at 20°C; [@] at 25°C; [&] at 21.1°C

[a] Csonka et al. (2012), Morris-Cohen et al. (2012), Nagy et al. (2012), Esposito et al. (2012), Quinones et al. (2012), Ikpi et al. (2012).

[b] Esposito et al. (2012), Morris-Cohen et al. (2012), Quinones et al. (2012), Ikpi et al. (2012), Csonka et al. (2012), Nagy et al. (2012).

[c] Esposito et al. (2012), Morris-Cohen et al. (2012), Quinones et al. (2012), Ikpi et al. (2012), Csonka et al. (2012), Nagy et al. (2012)

[d] Wang et al. (2012).

[e] Hughes et al. (2012).

[f] Mendoza and Ujevic (2012), Foell et al. (2012).

[g] Ling et al. (2012), Foell et al. (2012).

[h] Chemours (2017), Myrdal et al. (2014).

In terms of impact of the new propellant in the formulation of pMDIs, perhaps the most notable difference compared to CFCs is the fact that HFAs have a dual character, being somewhat lipophobic and hydrophobic at the same time. The implication of this unique character is that most molecules either polar or non-polar have poor solubility in HFAs. Most macromolecules, including biologics, also have low solubility in HFAs. As a consequence, the majority of APIs of interest cannot be formulated as solutions in HFAs, unless co-solvents are added to the formulation. However, cosolvents may negatively impact the chemical and physical stability of the formulation and the aerosol characteristics as discussed later in this chapter. Dispersion formulations (micron-sized drug/drug-containing particles), the alternative to solution pMDIs, were also impacted with the transition from CFCs to HFAs, as most surfactants used in the CFC-based pMDIs are also poorly soluble in HFAs.

While we are still trying to understand the unique properties of HFA propellants, and how they impact our ability to formulate in HFA-based pMDIs, recent regulations and the signing of the Kigali amendment to the Montreal Protocol (UN 2016), which proposes the phase out of HFAs staring in 2019, has lead the industry to look at the next generation of propellants/refrigerants alternatives to HFAs.

18.6.1.2 Hydrofluoroolefins (HFOs): Next Class of Propellants for Medicinal Aerosols?

Given their zero ODP and unique low GWP (Table 18.3), HFOs have emerged as potential alternatives to HFA propellants. While the refrigerant and auto industry have made significant progress in transitioning from HFAs to HFOs (Mota-Babiloni et al. 2015, Daviran et al. 2017), largely driven by tighter environmental regulations, particularly in Europe, studies highlighting the potential of HFOs as medicinal aerosols are lagging behind.

Two HFO propellants are currently being produced in large scale: 1,3,3,3-tetrafluoropropene (HFO-1234ze) and 2,3,3,3-tetrafluoropropene (HFO-1234yf). In a comparison between HFO-1234ze and HFA-134a both showed similar toxicity profiles (Schuster et al. 2009, Rusch et al. 2013), thus paving the way for the consideration of HFOs as medicinal aerosols (Zyhowski and Brown 2011). While new studies regarding the solvent quality of HFOs compared to HFAs are just emerging, it seems that the solvation forces for HFO-1234ze are comparable to that for HFA-134a (Yang and da Rocha 2014). This happens in spite of the lower dipole moment of HFO-1234ze (1.14D) compared to HFA-134a (2.12D), behavior attributed to the greater number of heavy atoms (dispersion forces) in HFO-1234ze. Similar solvating behavior of HFO-1234ze and HFA134a propellants can be seen as a good indicator of its potential to replace HFA in pMDIs. Results suggest that dispersions in HFO-1234ze may be just as capable of yielding viable formulations as those based on HFA-134a (Yang and da Rocha 2014). Detailed toxicological studies will be needed, however, to fully understand their potential in medicinal aerosols. As we move forward with HFOs as the next generation propellants in various industries, it is also important to carefully consider the potential environmental impact of the breakdown products of HFOs such as trifluoroacetate.

It is clear that the development of HFA-alternatives for medicinal aerosols is an area of tremendous potential. While it is clear that extensions to the Kigali amendment may be provided to HFAs for use in medicinal aerosols, in case necessary, in a similar fashion to what happened to CFCs, eventually, HFAs are expected to be phased out. Later in this chapter we discuss potential strategies on how this problem could be potentially mitigated in the shorter term with the selection of HFAs that have a lower carbon foot print compared to HFA-134a and HFA-227.

18.6.2 The Cosolvent

18.6.2.1 Why May Cosolvents Be Needed in pMDI Formulations and General Considerations

Given the propellant characteristics described above, cosolvents are typically added to HFA-based pMDIs to enhance the solubility of APIs (for solution formulations) or other excipients (both solution and dispersion formulations). They may also help mediate particle-particle interactions by changing the solvent environment, and can also be used to enhance valve function (Stein et al. 2014). The most common co-solvent used in pMDIs is ethanol (Myrdal et al. 2014). The only other excipient listed as cosolvent for HFA-based pMDIs is water (Atrovent HFA®). However, other components in HFA-based pMDIs such as polyethylene glycol 1000 Da (PEG 1000) (Symbicort®) and propylene glycol (that have found use as suspension aids), may also be potentially considered as a solubilization enhancer.

Several studies have addressed experimentally the solubility enhancement of APIs and excipients in propellant HFA in the presence of cosolvent ethanol (Hoye and Myrdal 2008). While the solubility of such compounds can be enhanced hundreds of fold with the aid of cosolvents (and this behavior is shown and expected for most compounds), there is no correlation that has been developed to date to predict the extent of solubility enhancement in propellant HFA upon the addition of cosolvent based solely on the chemistry of the solute. Solubility enhancement thus needs to be determined experimentally for each compound/API.

18.6.2.2 Enhancing Solubility is Not the Same as Enhancing Solvation ... and Why This Matters

One key aspect that has been largely overlooked is that enhancement in solubilization upon addition of a cosolvent does not necessarily imply an equal level of enhancement in *solvation* of the solute. This is particularly important when cosolvents are being used to promote the solubility of surfactants whose function is to stabilize drug particle suspension in pMDIs. Chemical force microscopy (CFM) results have shown that while the addition of ethanol helps decrease cohesive forces between surfaces representative of surfactant-tail groups found in approved pMDIs (alkyl-based), those forces are not fully screened even when a high volume percent of ethanol cosolvent is added to HFA (in this case liquid HFA—HPFP to allow for experimentation using an AFM) (Conti et al. 2012). The implication of such results is that while the solubility of surfactants with alky-based tails commonly employed in pMDIs such as lecithin, oleic acid, sorbitan trioleate and Tween 80, can be enhanced in HFAs upon addition of ethanol, their ability to stabilize particles in this propellant-cosolvent mixture will never be at its fullest compared to an alkane solvent that ideally solvates such tails. Similar CFM studies indicate that cohesive forces can, however, be completely screened (within accuracy of measurement) for designer chemistries that have improved interactions with HFAs (Conti et al. 2012). Those studies suggest that CFM may be a powerful strategy for the design of both new cosolvents and also new chemistries that may serve as the base for surfactants for pMDIs.

18.6.2.3 Potential Negative Effects of Cosolvents in pMDIs

The presence of cosolvents (and other species less volatile then the propellant) also brings about negative effects. These excipients are less volatile than the HFA propellants and impact key properties of this propellant-cosolvent mixture including density, saturation pressure, surface tension and others that in turn negatively impact the quality of the aerosol being generated (Stein and Myrdal 2006).

The effect of ethanol on the quality of aerosols from HFA-based pMDIs shows that the initial droplets mass median aerodynamic diameter (MMAD) increases with an increase in percent of ethanol. The larger particles and slower rates of droplet evaporation in the presence of ethanol leads to a decrease in fine particle fraction (FPF)—the respirable fraction of the dose (Gupta et al. 2003, Myrdal et al. 2004, Stein and Myrdal 2006, Mason-Smith et al. 2017). This suggests that careful consideration is needed when deciding whether or not to add cosolvents and how much to add. Addition of ethanol leads to increase in solubility but decrease in lung deposition (FPF), with the two effects negating each other.

A potential way out is to use other solubilization aids (alone or in combination with ethanol) that promote solubility of the compound of interest while decreasing the overall amount of cosolvent, and thus reducing the impact of the less volatile components on the aerosol quality. Examples include functionalized PEG and oligomers of esters that have a synergistic effect with ethanol in enhancing solubility of certain solutes (Stefely et al. 2000, 2002, Scherrer et al. 2003, Stein et al. 2004, Myrdal et al. 2014).

18.6.2.4 Opportunities in Cosolvent Design

This is an area that seems to have significant opportunities for further development/studies, particularly as new propellants alternatives to HFA-134a and HFA-227 are phased in for use in pMDIs. Screening of new cosolvents that are also generally recognized as safe (GRAS) substances could offer a good start. Important here is the ability to develop techniques to support the understanding of the effects of cosolvents that go beyond simply measuring the enhancement in solubility of APIs and other excipients of interest, but that will help understand their impact on solvation forces as for example the use of CFM as discussed earlier.

18.6.3 Other Excipients—Focus on Surfactants

18.6.3.1 General Considerations

While cosolvents are typically needed when formulators believe the best way forward is with a solution-based pMDI product, surfactants are the go to excipients for dispersion-based pMDIs. Because of the cohesive nature of particles of APIs when dispersed in HFA propellants, surfactants are used to screen particle-particle interactions so as to minimize flocculation/aggregation, which is deleterious to the physical stability of the formulations, and impact the quality of the aerosol (Williams et al. 2007). Surfactants can also be used in both solution and dispersion formulations for valve lubrication and to reduce adhesion between drug particles and canister walls.

A simple but important requirement for surfactants to be used in pMDI formulations is that they need to have appreciable solubility in the HFA propellants. There is a relatively small list of surfactants that are part of FDA-approved pMDI formulations. Those include lecithin, oleic acid, sorbitan trioleate and Tween 80—all designed for CFC-based inhalers, and thus have relatively poor solubility in HFA propellants due to mostly their highly hydrophobic tail groups. Other excipients like Poly(vinylpyrrolidone) (PVP) and PEG are also listed in pMDI formulations. While PVP's solubility is still fairly limited, the solubility of PEG in HFAs (and HFA in PEG) is very high. For an extensive compilation of surfactant solubility in HFAs the readers are referred to (Myrdal et al. 2014). For surfactants that have poor solubility in HFAs, one potential strategy is to use cosolvents such as ethanol to enhance their solubility, or design API particle processing strategies with the surfactant of interest before loading into the canisters.

18.6.3.2 Understanding Surfactant Behavior in HFA-Based pMDIs—and Why Most Surfactants Are Just Not Doing Their Intended Job Very Well!

There are several experimental strategies that can be utilized to qualitatively and quantitatively understand the behavior of surfactants in suspension formulations as they relate to the stabilization of the drug particles. For example, surfactant effects on particle stability can be assessed by loading desired amounts of surfactant and drug particles to a pressure-proof glass container, and subsequently adding a known mass of propellant so to achieve a desired final drug and surfactant concentration. Particle sedimentation/creaming after mechanical energy input provides for an opportunity to understand the ability of the excipient to screen cohesive forces between particles—Figure 18.8a. The density of the sedimented/creamed front also provides qualitative information regarding the ability of the surfactant to screen attractive forces between particles/loose aggregates

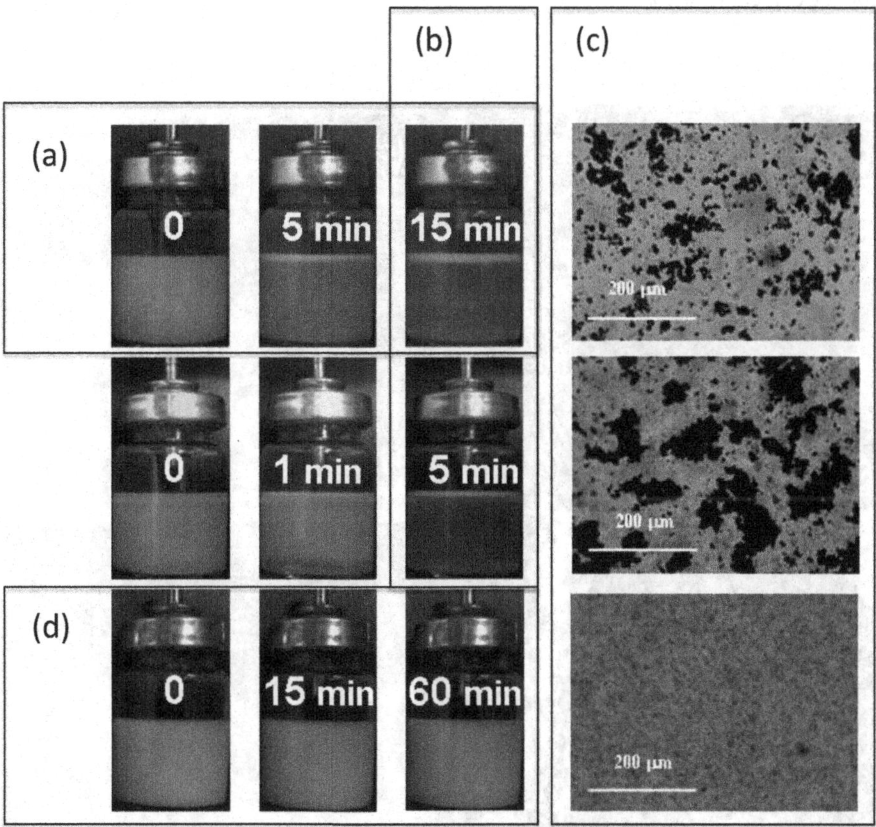

FIGURE 18.8 Visual assessment of the ability of excipients to enhance physical stability of particle suspensions in pMDIs. (a) creaming of flocculated particles as a function of time after mechanical agitation of the system; (b) compactness of the creaming front; (c) optical micrographs in a high-pressure optical cells; (d) example of enhanced stability of drug suspension. Formulation at 2mg/mL API and (a) no and (b) high concentration of stabilization agent. Dark spots on micrographs represents groups of flocculated particles of APIs. (Adapted from Wu, L. and da Rocha, S.R.P., *Langmuir*, 27, 10501–10506, 2011.)

that have phase separated from the propellant due to gravitational forces—Figure 18.8b. High pressure optical microscopy can also be utilized to assess the bulk system but at the particle level—Figure 18.8c.

While the solubility of surfactants can be enhanced in HFAs upon the addition of cosolvents, the solvation of the surfactant tail group, which is expected to be responsible for screening particle cohesive forces (F_{co}) may not be fully addressed simply by adding the cosolvent. To clarify this point, we present some colloidal force microscopy (CFM) results next. CFM is an AFM-based technique (Wu and da Rocha 2008). An AFM cantilever is modified with the particle of the API of interest, and the F_{co} between this cantilever and a single crystal of the same API is measured in a mimic liquid HFA (HPFP) in the presence and absence of excipients as illustrated in Figure 18.9.

In this experiment, the F_{co} between salbutamol particle and single crystal was measured first in liquid HFA in the absence of any excipient, resulting in an attractive force with a magnitude of 12.1nN—Table 18.4. The addition of ethanol cosolvent alone somewhat screens the attractive forces between particles lowering the F_{co} down to 6.3nN. The addition of oleic acid and ethanol, while further reducing F_{co} to 1.5nN, does not completely screen attractive forces, and the corresponding formulation shows the formation of aggregates. Surfactants designed especially for HFAs (designer surfactant) can, however, completely screen particle forces resulting in a formulation with long term stability—resists creaming. Similar strategy (CPM or CFM) can be used to design a range of excipients for HFA-based pMDIs, both in terms of suspension stabilizers or cosolvents (Traini et al. 2005, Peguin et al. 2007, Peguin and da Rocha 2008, Conti et al. 2012).

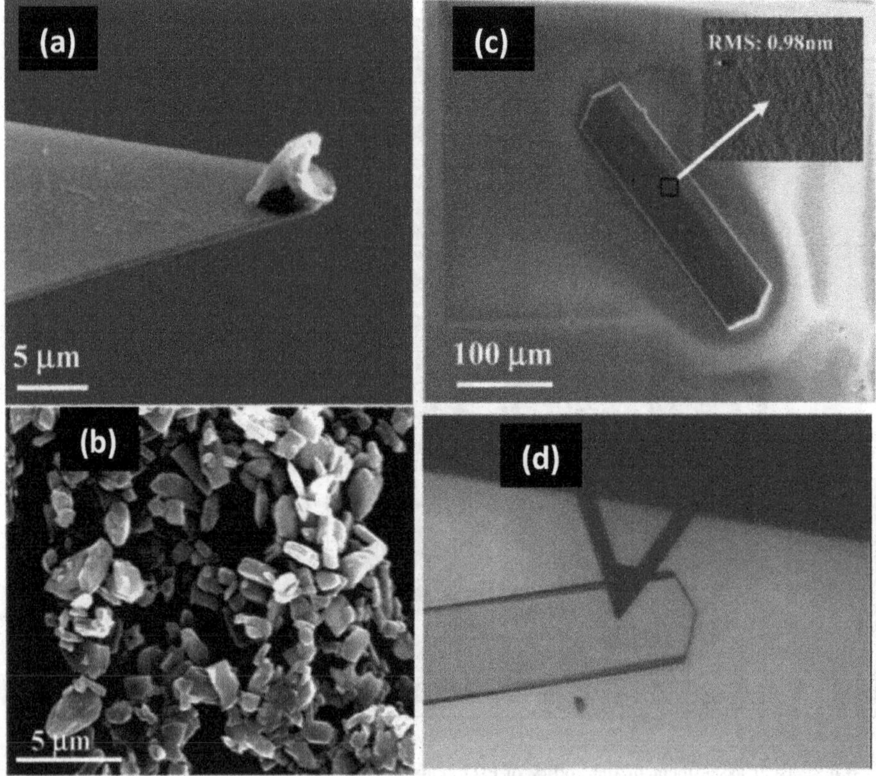

FIGURE 18.9 (a) SEM image of a single salbutamol particle-modified AFM cantilever; (b) SEM image of the micronized salbutamol; (c) SEM image of a single salbutamol recrystallized from ethanol; (d) optical image of the cantilever in (a) interacting with the single crystal in (c)—colloidal probe measurement in liquid HFA (HPFP). (Adapted from Wu, L. and da Rocha, S.R.P., *Langmuir*, 23, 12104–12110, 2007.)

TABLE 18.4

Average Force of Cohesion (F_{co}) Between the Salbutamol-Modified Atomic Force Microscope (AFM) Cantilever and a Smooth Salbutamol Substrate Single Crystal, as Determined by Colloidal Probe Microscopy (CPM) in Presence of Excipients. F_{co} Measured in Liquid HFA (model propellant HPFP) in the Absence (first column) and Presence of Various Excipients with a Single Cantilever (same drug particle-substrate).

Surfactant	Ethanol	F_{co} (nN)
none	None	12.1
none	7% (v/v)	6.3
Oleic acid (1mM)	7% (v/v)	1.5
Designer surfactant (1mM)	None	0

Source: Wu, L. and da Rocha, S.R.P., *Langmuir*, 23, 12104–12110, 2007.

18.6.4 Alternative Strategies for the Formulation of pMDIs

As described above, traditional dispersion-based formulations in HFAs are inherently unstable due to the cohesive forces between particles and also due to the gravitational fields. Surfactants are generally required in traditional pMDIs in order to overcome particle–particle interactions. However, most amphiphiles in pMDIs approved by the FDA have extremely low solubility in HFAs due to a mismatch between the hydrogenated nonpolar surfactant tails and the hydrophobic and lipophobic nature of the HFA propellants (Ridder et al. 2005, O'Donnell and Williams 2013). Cosolvents are, therefore, generally required in order to enhance surfactant solubility but may negatively impact the formulations.

In order to address these limitations, several studies have focused on the design of amphiphiles for conventional HFA-based pMDIs (Butz et al. 2002, Looker et al. 2003a, 2003b, Rogueda 2004, Stein et al. 2004). More recently, alternatives to traditional dispersion formulations have also been proposed. Those can be generally classified as (i) non-aqueous and (ii) aqueous systems—for a review the reader is directed to the previous edition of this book (Hickey 2003) and other more recent publications (Huang et al. 2017, Ngan and Asmawi 2018). Here we provide a general overview of those strategies and a brief description the colloidal science behind them.

18.6.4.1 Non-Aqueous Suspensions

Non-aqueous suspensions can be further broken down as (i) *density matching*, (ii) *particle surface modification;* (iii) *non-adsorbing excipients*; and (iv) *nanocarrier-based systems.*

- *Density Matching*: The stability of insoluble drugs in HFAs can be significantly improved by incorporating the drug into a carrier with a resulting particle density closely matching that of the propellant medium. Crosslinking of chitosan, a potential carrier for small molecules and biologics, may lead to density matching with the propellants and improve suspension stability (Williams III et al. 1998). Another approach is the preparation of highly porous microspheres (Dellamary et al. 2000). The propellant is capable of penetrating the open pores of the spheres thus modifying their apparent density, leading to a density matching between the particle and the propellant medium. Such strategies may require changes in the morphology of the API for their formulation.

- *Particle Surface Modification*: Direct modification of particles with stabilizing agents may provide for a simple way to screen van der Waals cohesive forces between particles in the propellant, thus stabilizing the suspension. Surface modification strategies include coating APIs with lipids and alkylpolyglycoside using spray drying (Columbano et al. 2003, Tarara et al. 2004), or physically trapping HFA-philic moieties onto particle surfaces, during their preparation by techniques such as emulsification diffusion (Wu et al. 2008a). Formation of core-shell

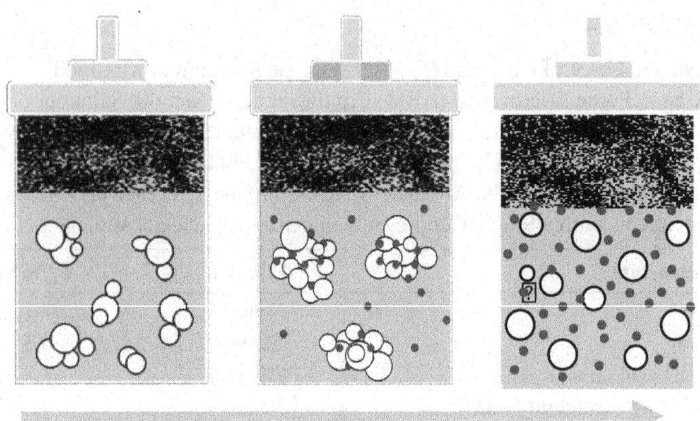

FIGURE 18.10 Schematic diagram of the mechanism of stabilization of suspension formation in pMDIs using highly dispersible, non-adsorbing nanoparticles. LHS panel: left to their own device, micrometer-sized drug particles suspended in pure propellant HFAs will tend to flocculate due to the strong cohesive forces. Center panel: Because of entropic depletion forces, the addition of extremely small amounts (low volume fraction) of nanoparticles will tend to induce further instability in the particle dispersion. RHS panel: Depletion attraction in a system composed of spheres of different sizes comes from an entropic gain achieved by excluding the smaller spheres from the region between two large spheres that approach each other within a distance equivalent to the diameter of the smaller spheres; this is the so-called "excluded volume" to the smaller spheres. However, as the nanoparticle concentration increases, flocculation can be suppressed.

particles with a shell that acts as a steric stabilizer for the drug particles may provide opportunities to encapsulate small molecular weight hydrophilic and hydrophobic compounds, drug crystals and biologics as well (Wu et al. 2008b). Some of these strategies are limited by the type of drugs that can be formulated or require changes in the API crystal structure or both, so they would have to be considered on a case-by-case basis.

- *Non-adsorbing excipients* represent an exciting strategy as they can be used without need to alter the physical state of the API (will work for crystalline or amorphous APIs as prepared during synthesis or purification), and may be applied to both small molecules and biologics. Moreover, because they are not designed to interact with the particle surface, they serve as a general platform for the stabilization of any API; i.e., they do not need to be optimized for each formulation (Cantor et al. 2008, Wu and da Rocha 2011). One such example is the use of non-adsorbing nanoparticles (NPs) of a biodegradable polymer (Wu and da Rocha 2011). When chitosan oligomers are grafted with oligolactic acid, particles of such co-oligomers can be formed and are highly dispersed in the propellant HFAs. Such biodegradable and water-soluble NPs of 80–100 nm in diameter have been shown to act as physical barrier preventing API microparticles from interacting to each other and aggregating. A schematic diagram of how this mechanism is thought to work is shown in Figure 18.10.

18.7 Future Perspectives

There seem to be a few existential questions regarding the future of pMDIs. The short answer, however, from our perspective is that pMDIs are here to stay and every new challenge will continue to present itself as an opportunity to spur technological advances in this area. Some opportunities for furthering pMDIs (formulation and device) have been discussed earlier in this chapter. Other important considerations relative to the future of pMDIs will be addressed next.

18.7.1 What Is the Issue with Propellants Again?

Propellant is the major constituent of pMDIs. Propellants used in pMDIs need not only be safe for human use, but they also need to have appropriate physicochemical properties to serve their function as the liquid medium to solubilize/disperse the drug product and also as energy source for the generation of the aerosol upon valve actuation.

Another requirement for propellants is that they need to be environmentally acceptable. While volumes of propellants used in the manufacture of medicinal aerosols are very small (ca. 2%) compared to other industries (CMR 2017), it is clear that HFAs will be eventually phased out due to environmental issues. Another strong motivator for phase out of HFAs is the fact that alternative propellants for other industries have already been identified and are in use (Harby 2017). There is, therefore, a decreasing motivation for the industry to continue producing HFAs for medicinal aerosols as it becomes less cost effective due to smaller production volumes. Clearly, phasing out HFAs does not mean interrupting the supply of HFA-based pMDIs. Similarly to CFCs, we can expect extensions on their use for medicinal purposes if necessary. The question is then how soon will they be phased out. The answer is that it really depends on how much effort and resources the industry and federal governments are willing to invest in the study of alternative propellants for medicinal aerosols. It is worth noticing that the reformulation of all pMDI products in other forms of portable inhalers, even if possible, may also take significant time, cost and effort, not to mention challenges in acceptability and patient compliance.

One interesting and promising alternative HFA chemistry not currently in use in commercial pMDIs is HFA-152a (1,1-difluorethane) (Myrdal et al. 2014). Initial safety considerations suggest the potential use of HFA-152a in humans at doses of exposure typically found in pMDIs, but more extensive investigations are necessary for a direct comparison with HFA-134a/HFA-227 as it relates to toxicity (Ernstgård et al. 2012, Vance et al. 2012). Similarly, it is likely that new development in materials for pMDIs will be necessary, even though preliminary studies also showed good compatibility. While flammability in the context of production seems to be of concern, the physicochemical properties of HFA-152a seem to be amenable for use in the formulation of pMDIs (Corr and Noakes 2012). Bench-filled salbutamol sulfate pMDIs were shown to have similar (or better) emitted dose and aerosol performance compared to HFA-134a (Corr and Noakes 2013). It is important to note that HFA-152a has zero ODP and a GWP of 138. That is a relatively large number, but compares very favorably to the GWP of 1300 and 3350 for HFA-134a and HFA-227 (see Table 18.3), respectively.

In the big scheme of things—when truly and honestly considering our environment, a more appropriate discussion in terms of viability of HFAs and particularly HFA-152a for use in medicinal aerosols needs to take into account the overall carbon footprint to produce such drug-device combinations. Carbon footprint analysis indicates a reduction in the footprint for the whole device from ca. 19 $kgCO_2$ (per 100 dose) for a canister of HFA-134a to ca. 2 $kgCO_2$ (per 100 dose) for a canister with HFA-152a. Interestingly, this number is smaller than the carbon footprint for a 200 dose DPI device (Noakes and Corr 2016). The carbon foot print for either pMDI can be also put in the context to the current carbon footprint for the average daily commute to work in the US of 13.2 $kgCO_2$! (16 miles each way, (ABC-NEWS 2005) with a 411gCO_2 emission per mile in a 21.6 miles/gallon automobile (EPA 2018b)). The carbon footprints for the DPI mentioned above or the HFA-152a pMDI are also smaller than the carbon footprint of the cheeseburger one may get on the drive back from work—ca. 3 $kgCO_2$ (EPA 2018a). It seems plausible, therefore, that temporary solutions and environmentally sound alternatives to existing HFA-134a and HFA-227 pMDIs may emerge from within the HFA family itself as we work on developing the next class of medicinal propellants that will have no ODP, ultra-low GWP and also low overall environmental impact (water/soil as well).

18.7.2 Addressing Limitations in the Maximum Emitted Dose of pMDIs

One of the universal limitations for pMDI products is the maximum emitted dose. Bounded by valve performance, patient usability and aerosol performance considerations, pMDIs traditionally have a dose delivery range from several micrograms to sub-milligram. This dosing range has worked well for locally acting drugs for asthma and COPD.

However, as biological molecules are considered for the inhalation route of delivery, with some locally acting and some with potential of systemic targeting, it would be of interest to open up the dosing range of traditional pMDIs to the milligrams, or even higher. This can only be achieved by coordinated effort in formulation, valve, and actuator design, to either increase the formulation concentration, or the volume of formulation delivered by the valve and actuator.

If the concentration of drug in either suspension of solution formulation is increased by 10 fold, co-solvents and excipients systems need to be developed to maintain the physical and chemical stability of the formulation at such concentration. With higher concentrations in the formulation, the aerosol generation process will predictably perform very differently. The valve and actuator combined, would need to be optimized to prevent clogging, and to have desirable aerosol performance.

Alternatively, larger dosing capability can be achieved by increasing the volume of formulation delivered by the valve and actuator. With larger volumes being delivered, the duration will be longer, coupled with more pronounced cooling effect caused by larger volumes of propellant being expanded. The challenge here is that patients have a certain inspiration volume and duration. There are a few directions proposed here: (i) the use of spacers/valve holding chambers can help delivery efficiency and minimize the effect of chilling; (ii) use multiple actuations to deliver a dose; (iii) the use of breath coordinated device, to better utilize the patient inspiration window; (iv) or simply reconsidering the traditional metering system of pMDIs.

18.7.3 Making the Case for Diversifying pMDIs

The global pulmonary drug delivery market is projected to grow from ca. U$ 36.1 billion in 2016 to U$ 52.4 billion by 2021 (MAM 2017b). pMDIs occupy ca. 70% of the respiratory inhaler devices market share (in volume), and are expected to continue their dominance in the foreseeable future (Myrdal et al. 2014). While this suggests a comfortable position for pMDIs, one should note the following: while the overall pulmonary drug delivery market growth represents a healthy 6.5% compound annual growth rate (CAGR), it is projected to grow at a slower pace than the global drug delivery market, which is expected to have a CAGR of 7.2%, increasing to U$ 17 trillion by 2021 (MAM 2017a). In fact, therefore, the pulmonary market is expected to occupy a smaller footprint relative to the global market.

The point here is that new technologies for pMDIs that can disrupt the market and innovative ideas that can alleviate inertial forces preventing the implementation of such technologies are badly needed so that we can expand the market share of orally inhaled product. Examples of such technologies include: (i) *formulation development*: such as diversification of therapeutics being delivered with pMDIs that need to go beyond the (very limited) classes of compounds shown in Table 18.1. Examples include other classes of drugs/drug containing materials such as biologics, high potency drugs, local vs. systemic delivery to the lungs, nanomaterials; and (ii) *device innovation* such as developing technologies to overcome dose limitation of pMDIs to make the delivery of other classes of drug more viable.

18.7.4 pMDIs and the Digital World

While inhalation devices like pMDIs, DPIs and nebulizers are the most important tools available to treat pulmonary ailments, they are plagued by adherence and compliance issues that lead to them being improperly used or underutilized—both of which cause immense burden to the healthcare system as a whole (Newman 2014). Addressing the lack of adherence through digital means is beginning to take shape and respiratory devices are some of the earliest adopters of the transition to the digital/electronic era. Incorporation of electronic sensors, chips and Bluetooth into pMDIs have transformed those products from a simple marriage of a canister, metering valve and an actuator to a more advanced digital platform. 3M's Intelligent Inhaler, Presspart's eMDI and the Hailie™ Solution by Adherium are some of the innovations that have occurred in the recent past to bring pMDIs into the electronic realm. In fact, Adherium's platform received clearance for use with Astrazeneca's Symbicort® pMDI in September 2017 and 3M Intelligent Inhaler has begun with several digital devices in clinical trials. For more information, readers are directed to these two excellent articles that detail some of the developments that have occurred in this space over the past few years (Kikidis et al. 2016, Anderson 2017).

DEDICATION

This chapter is in honor of Professor Paul B. Myrdal and his outstanding accomplishments in the field of pMDIs.

REFERENCES

ABC-NEWS. 2005. "A look under the hood of a nation on wheels." https://abcnews.go.com/images/Politics/973a2Traffic.pdf.

Anderson, G., N. Johnson, A. Mulgirigama, and B. Aggarwal. 2017. "Use of spacers for patients treated with pressurized metered dose inhalers: Focus on the VENTOLIN™ mini spacer." *Expert Opinion on Drug Delivery* 15 (4):419–430.

Anderson, W. C. III. 2017. Incorporating technology to advance asthma controller adherence. *Current Opinion in Allergy and Clinical Immunology* 17 (2):153–159.

Anderson, P. J. 2005. "History of aerosol therapy: Liquid nebulization to MDIs to DPIs." *Respiratory Care* 50 (9):1139–1150.

Baron, C., B. Grosjean, D. Heyworth, E. Robins, A. Sule, R. Turner, and G. Williams. 2014. "Evaluation of powder adhesion and stability of pMDIs with different canister types including plasma treated canisters." *Respiratory Drug Delivery* 2:349–354.

Bell, J., and S. Newman. 2007. "The rejuvenated pressurised metered dose inhaler." *Expert Opinion on Drug Delivery* 4 (3):215–234.

Brouet, G., E. Robins, S. Hall, G. Butterworth, J. Hemy, and R. Turner. 2006. "Developing new container closure options: A suppliers perspective." *Respiratory Drug Delivery-X. River Grove IL: Davis Horwood* 111–120.

Butz, N., C. Porté, H. Courrier, M. P. Krafft, and Th F. Vandamme. 2002. "Reverse water-in-fluorocarbon emulsions for use in pressurized metered-dose inhalers containing hydrofluoroalkane propellants." *International Journal of Pharmaceutics* 238 (1):257–269. doi:10.1016/S0378-5173(02)00086-8.

Cantor, A. S., J. S. Stefely, P.A. Jinks, J. R. Baran, J. M. Ganser, and Mueting. M. W. 2008. "Modifying interparticulate interactions using surface-modified excipient nanoparticles." *Respiratory Drug Delivery* 1:309–318.

Chemours. 2017. HP 152a–Aerosol Propellant–Technical Information.

Chen, Y., P. M. Young, D. M. Fletcher, H. K. Chan, E. Long, D. A. Lewis, T. Church, and D. Traini. 2015. "The effect of actuator nozzle designs on the electrostatic charge generated in pressurised metered dose inhaler aerosols." *Pharmaceutical Research* 32:1237–1248.

CMR. 2017. Aerosol propellants market by product and application. Crystal Market Research.

Columbano, A., G. Buckton, and P. Wikeley. 2003. "Characterisation of surface modified salbutamol sulphate-alkylpolyglycoside microparticles prepared by spray drying." *International Journal of Pharmaceutics* 253 (1):61–70. doi:10.1016/S0378-5173(02)00634-8.

Conner, J. B., and P. O. Buck. 2013. "Improving asthma management: The case for mandatory inclusion of dose counters on all rescue bronchodilators." *Journal of Asthma* 50 (6):658–663.

Conti, D. S., J. Grashik, L. Yang, L. Wu, and S. R. da Rocha. 2012. "Solvation in hydrofluoroalkanes: How can ethanol help?" *Journal of Pharmacy and Pharmacology* 64 (9):1236–1244. doi:10.1111/j.2042-7158.2011.01398.x.

Corr, S., and T. J. Noakes. 2012. Pharmaceutical Compositions. edited by World Intellectual Property Organization: Mexichem Amanco Holding S.A. de C.V.

Corr, S., and T. J. Noakes. 2013. Compositions Comprising Salbutamol. edited by World Intellectual Property Orgarnization: Mexichem Amanco Holding S.A. de C. V.

Csonka, S., I. Weymann, and G. Zarand. 2012. "An electrically controlled quantum dot based spin current injector." *Nanoscale* 4 (12):3635–3639. doi:10.1039/c2nr30399j.

Daviran, S., A. Kasaeian, S. Golzari, O. Mahian, S. Nasirivatan, and S. Wongwises. 2017. "A comparative study on the performance of HFO-1234yf and HFC-134a as an alternative in automotive air conditioning systems." *Applied Thermal Engineering* 110:1091–1100. doi:10.1016/j.applthermaleng.2016.09.034.

Dellamary, L. A., T. E. Tarara, D. J. Smith, C. H. Woelk, A. Adractas, M. L. Costello, H. Gill, and J. G. Weers. 2000. "Hollow porous particles in metered dose inhalers." *Pharmaceutical Research* 17 (2):168–174. doi:10.1023/a:1007513213292.

Dexter, D., and C. Hak-Kim. 2015. "A review of methods for evaluating particle stability in suspension based pressurized metered dose inhalers." *Current Pharmaceutical Design* 21 (27):3955–3965. doi:10.2174/1381612821666150820110153.

Dissanayake, S., and J. Suggett. 2018. "A review of the *in vitro* and *in vivo* valved holding chamber (VHC) literature with a focus on the AeroChamber Plus Flow-Vu Anti-static VHC." *Therapeutic Advances in Respiratory Disease* 12:1–14.

EPA. 2018a. "Carbon footprint calculator." USA Environmental Protection Agency, Accessed June 2018. https://www3.epa.gov/carbon-footprint-calculator/.

EPA. 2018b. "Green vehicle guide." USA Environmental Protection Agency, Accessed June 2018. https://www.epa.gov/greenvehicles/greenhouse-gas-emissions-typical-passenger-vehicle.

Ernstgård, L., B. Sjögren, W. Dekant, T. Schmidt, and G. Johanson. 2012. "Uptake and disposition of 1,1-difluoroethane (HFC-152a) in humans." *Toxicology Letters* 209 (1):21–29. doi:10.1016/j.toxlet.2011.11.028.

Esposito, M., N. Kumar, K. Lindenberg, and C. Van den Broeck. 2012. "Stochastically driven single-level quantum dot: A nanoscale finite-time thermodynamic machine and its various operational modes." *Phys Review E Statistical Nonlinear, and Soft Matter Physics* 85 (3 Pt 1):031117.

FMI, Future Market Insights. 2017. Respiratory inhaler devices market. Future Marketing Insights.

Foell, C. A., E. Schelew, H. Qiao, K. A. Abel, S. Hughes, F. C. van Veggel, and J. F. Young. 2012. "Saturation behaviour of colloidal PbSe quantum dot exciton emission coupled into silicon photonic circuits." *Optics Express* 20 (10):10453–10469. doi:10.1364/OE.20.010453.

Fromer, L., E. Goodwin, and J. Walsh. 2010. "Customizing inhaled therapy to meet the needs of COPD patients." *Postgraduate Medicine* 122 (2):83–93. doi:10.3810/pgm.2010.03.2125.

Gupta, A., S. W. Stein, and P. B. Myrdal. 2003. "Balancing ethanol cosolvent concentration with product performance in 134a-based pressurized metered dose inhalers." *Journal of Aerosol Medicine* 16 (2):167–174. doi:10.1089/089426803321919924.

Harby, K. 2017. "Hydrocarbons and their mixtures as alternatives to environmental unfriendly halogenated refrigerants: An updated overview." *Renewable and Sustainable Energy Reviews* 73:1247–1264. doi:10.1016/j.rser.2017.02.039.

Hickey, A. J. 2003. *Pharmaceutical Inhalation Aerosol Technology.* Edited by Anthony J. Hickey. Boca Raton, FL: CRC Press.

Hickey, A. J. 2013. "Back to the future: Inhaled drug products." *Journal of Pharmaceutical Sciences* 102 (4):1165–1172. doi:10.1002/jps.23465.

Hoye, J. A., and P. B. Myrdal. 2008. "Measurement and correlation of solute solubility in HFA-134a/ethanol systems." *International Journal of Pharmaceutics* 362 (1):184–188. doi:10.1016/j.ijpharm.2008.06.020.

Huang, Z., H. Wu, B. Yang, L. Chen, Y. Huang, G. Quan, C. Zhu, X. Li, X. Pan, and C. Wu. 2017. "Anhydrous reverse micelle nanoparticles: New strategy to overcome sedimentation instability of peptide-containing pressurized metered-dose inhalers." *Drug Delivery* 24 (1):527–538. doi:10.1080/10717544.2016.1269850.

Hughes, B. K., D. A. Ruddy, J. L. Blackburn, D. K. Smith, M. R. Bergren, A. J. Nozik, J. C. Johnson, and M. C. Beard. 2012. "Control of PbSe quantum dot surface chemistry and photophysics using an alkylselenide ligand." *ACS Nano* 6 (6):5498–506. doi:10.1021/nn301405j.

Ikpi, M. E., P. Atkinson, S. P. Bremner, and D. A. Ritchie. 2012. "Fabrication of a self-aligned cross-wire quantum-dot chain light emitting diode by molecular beam epitaxial regrowth." *Nanotechnology* 23 (22):225304. doi:10.1088/0957-4484/23/22/225304.

Ivey, J. A., R. Vehring, and W. H. Finlay. 2015. "Understanding pressurized metered dose inhaler performance." *Expert Opinion on Drug Delivery* 12 (6):901–916.

Kaur, I., B. Aggarwal, and J. Gogtay. 2015. "Integration of dose counters in pressurized metered-dose inhalers for patients with asthma and chronic obstructive pulmonary disease: Review of evidence." *Expert Opinion on Drug Delivery* 12 (8):1301–1310.

Kikidis, D., Konstantinos, V., Tzovaras, D., Usmani, O.S. 2016. "The digital asthma patient: The history and future of inhaler based health monitoring devices." *Journal of Aerosol Medicine and Pulmonary Drug Delivery* 29 (3):219–232.

Lewis, D. A., B. J. Meakin, and G. Brambilla. 2006. "New actuators versus old: Reasons and results for actuator modifications for HFA solution MDIs." *Respiratory Drug Delivery* 1:101–110.

Lewis, D. 2007. "Metered-dose inhalers: Actuators old and new." *Expert Opinion on Drug Delivery* 4 (3):235–245.

Liang, Z., R. Ni, J. Zhou, and S. Mao. 2015. "Recent advances in controlled pulmonary drug delivery." *Drug Discovery Today* 20 (3):380–389. doi:10.1016/j.drudis.2014.09.020.

Ling, H. S., S. Y. Wang, W. C. Hsu, and C. P. Lee. 2012. "Voltage-tunable dual-band quantum dot infrared photodetectors for temperature sensing." *Opt Express* 20 (10):10484–10489. doi:10.1364/OE.20.010484.

Looker, B. E., C. J. Lunnins, and A. J. Redgrave. 2003a. Carboxylic acid compounds for use as surfactants. edited by World Intellectual Property Organization: Glaxo Group Limited, London, UK.

Looker, B. E., C.J. Lunnins, and A. J. Redgrave. 2003b. Compounds for use as surfactants. edited by World Intellectual Property Organization: Glaxo Group Limited, London, UK.

MAM, Markets and Markets. 2017a. Drug Delivery Technology Market worth 1,669.40 Billion USD by 2021.

MAM, Markets and Markets. 2017b. "Pulmonary/Respiratory Drug Delivery Market by Formulation, Device Type, Canister, End User, Applications–Forecasts to 2021."

Mason-Smith, N., D. J. Duke, A. L. Kastengren, D. Traini, P. M. Young, Y. Chen, D. A. Lewis, D. Edgington-Mitchell, and D. Honnery. 2017. "Revealing pMDI spray initial conditions: Flashing, atomisation and the effect of ethanol." *Pharmaceutical Research* 34 (4):718–729. doi:10.1007/s11095-017-2098-2.

Mendoza, M., and S. Ujevic. 2012. "Magneto-conductance fingerprints of purely quantum states in the open quantum dot limit." *Journal of Physics: Condensed Matter* 24 (23):235302. doi:10.1088/0953-8984/24/23/235302.

Morris-Cohen, A. J., K. O. Aruda, A. M. Rasmussen, G. Canzi, T. Seideman, C. P. Kubiak, and E. A. Weiss. 2012. "Controlling the rate of electron transfer between a quantum dot and a tri-ruthenium molecular cluster by tuning the chemistry of the interface." *Physical Chemistry Chemical Physics* 14 (40):13794–13801. doi:10.1039/c2cp40827a.

Mota-Babiloni, A., J. Navarro-Esbrí, Á. Barragán-Cervera, F. Molés, B. Peris, and G. Verdú. 2015. "Commercial refrigeration–An overview of current status." *International Journal of Refrigeration* 57:186–196. doi:10.1016/j.ijrefrig.2015.04.013.

Myrdal, P. B., K. L. Karlage, S. W. Stein, B. A. Brown, and A. Haynes. 2004. "Optimized dose delivery of the peptide cyclosporine using hydrofluoroalkane-based metered dose inhalers." *Journal of Pharmaceutical Sciences* 93 (4):1054–1061. doi:10.1002/jps.20025.

Myrdal, P. B., P. Sheth, and S. W. Stein. 2014. "Advances in metered dose inhaler technology: Formulation development." *AAPS PharmSciTech* 15 (2):434–455. doi:10.1208/s12249-013-0063-x.

Nagy, A., A. Steinbruck, J. Gao, N. Doggett, J. A. Hollingsworth, and R. Iyer. 2012. "Comprehensive analysis of the effects of CdSe quantum dot size, surface charge, and functionalization on primary human lung cells." *ACS Nano* 6 (6):4748–4762. doi:10.1021/nn204886b.

Newman, S. 2014. "Improving inhaler technique, adherence to therapy and the precision of dosing: Major challenges for pulmonary drug delivery." *Expert Opinion on Drug Delivery* 11 (3):365–378. doi:10.1517/17425247.2014.873402.

Newman, S. P. 2004. "Spacer devices for metered dose inhalers." *Clinical Pharmacokinetics* 43 (6):349–360.

Newman, S. P. 2005. "Principles of inhaled metered dose design." *Respiratory Care* 50 (9):1177–1190.

Ngan, C. L., and A. A. Asmawi. 2018. "Lipid-based pulmonary delivery system: A review and future considerations of formulation strategies and limitations." *Drug Delivery and Translational Research* 8 (5):1527–1544. doi:10.1007/s13346-018-0550-4.

Noakes, T., and S. Corr. 2016. Metered Dose Inhaler Propellants. Mexichem–Propellants. Press Release. 2016 Noakes, T., and S. Corr. Metered Dose Inhaler Propellants. Company: Mexichem–Propellants

O'Donnell, K. P., and R. O. Williams. 2013. "Pulmonary dispersion formulations: The impact of dispersed powder properties on pressurized metered dose inhaler stability." *Drug Development and Industrial Pharmacy* 39 (3):413–424. doi:10.3109/03639045.2012.664145.

Peguin, R. P. S., and S. R. P. da Rocha. 2008. "Solvent–solute interactions in hydrofluoroalkane propellants." *The Journal of Physical Chemistry B* 112 (27):8084–8094. doi:10.1021/jp710717s.

Peguin, R. P. S., L. Wu, and S. R. P. da Rocha. 2007. "The ester group: How hydrofluoroalkane-philic is it?" *Langmuir* 23 (16):8291–8294. doi:10.1021/la700996x.

Quinones, G. A., S. C. Miller, S. Bhattacharyya, D. Sobek, and J. P. Stephan. 2012. "Ultrasensitive detection of cellular protein interactions using bioluminescence resonance energy transfer quantum dot-based nanoprobes." *Journal of Cellular Biochemistry* 113 (7):2397–2405. doi:10.1002/jcb.24111.

Ridder, K. B., C. J. Davies-Cutting, and I. W. Kellaway. 2005. "Surfactant solubility and aggregate orientation in hydrofluoroalkanes." *International Journal of Pharmaceutics* 295 (1):57–65. doi:10.1016/j.ijpharm.2005.01.027.

Rogueda, P. G. 2004. "Pushing the bounderies: Searching for novel HFA suspension formulations." *Respiratory Drug Delivery* 1:117–124.

Rusch, G. M., A. Tveit, H. Muijser, M.-M. Tegelenbosch-Schouten, and G. M. Hoffman. 2013. "The acute, genetic, developmental and inhalation toxicology of trans-1,3,3,3-tetrafluoropropene (HFO-1234ze)." *Drug and Chemical Toxicology* 36 (2):170–180. doi:10.3109/01480545.2012.661738.

Scherrer, R. A., J. S. Stefely, and Stephen W. Stein. 2003. Medicinal Aerosol Formulations Comprising Ion Pair Complexes. World Intellectual Property Organization: 3M Innovative Properties Company. WO 2003/059316.

Schuster, P., R. Bertermann, G. M. Rusch, and W. Dekant. 2009. "Biotransformation of trans-1,1,1,3-tetrafluoropropene (HFO-1234ze)." *Toxicology and Applied Pharmacology* 239 (3):215–223. doi:10.1016/j.taap.2009.06.018.

Shrewsbury, S. B., R. O. Cook, G. Taylor, C. Edwards, and N. B. Ramadan. 2007. "Safety and pharmacokinetics of dihydroergotamine mesylate administered via a novel tempo inhaler." *Headache* 48 (3):355–367.

Stefely, J. S., B. Brown, D. M. Hammerbeck, and Stephen W. Stein. 2002. "Equipping the MDI for the 21st century by expanding its formultion options." *Respiratory Drug Delivery* 1:207–214.

Stefely, J. S., D. C. Duan, Paul B. Myrdal, D. L. Ross, D. W. Schultz, and C. L. Leach. 2000. "Design and utility of a novel class of biocompatible excipients for HFA based MDIs." *Respiratory Drug Delivery* 7:83–90.

Stein, S. W., P. A. Sheth, D. A. Hodson, and P. B. Myrdal. 2015. "Advances in metered dose inhaler technology: Hardware development." *AAPS PharmSciTech* 15 (2):326–338.

Stein, S. W., B. R. Forsyth, J. S. Stefely, J. D. Christensen, T. D. Alband, and P.A. Jinks. 2004. "Expanding the dosing range of metered dose inhalers through formulation and hardware optimization." *Respiratory Drug Delivery* 1:125–134.

Stein, S. W., and P. B. Myrdal. 2006. "The relative influence of atomization and evaporation on metered dose inhaler drug delivery efficiency." *Aerosol Science and Technology* 40 (5):335–347. doi:10.1080/02786820600612268.

Stein, S. W., P. Sheth, P. D. Hodson, and P. B. Myrdal. 2014. "Advances in metered dose inhaler technology: Hardware development." *AAPS PharmSciTech* 15 (2):326–338. doi:10.1208/s12249-013-0062-y.

Stein, S. W., and C. G. Thiel. 2017. "The history of therapeutic aerosols: A chronological review." *Journal of Aerosol Medicine and Pulmonary Drug Delivery* 30 (1):20–41. doi:10.1089/jamp.2016.1297.

Stevenson, P. 2016. "Controlling surface performance characteristics of medical devices: A critical review of the latest industrial techniques." *Respiratory Drug Delivery* 1:147–156.

Tarara, T. E., M. S. Hartman, H. Gill, A. A. Kennedy, and J. G. Weers. 2004. "Characterization of suspension-based metered dose inhaler formulations composed of spray-dried budesonide microcrystals dispersed in HFA-134a." *Pharmaceutical Research* 21 (9):1607–1614. doi:10.1023/B:PHAM.0000041455.13980.f1.

Thiel, C. G. 1996. "From Susie's question to CFC-free: An inventor's perspective on forty years of MDI development and regulation." *Respiratory Drug Delivery* 115–123.

Traini, D., P. Rogueda, P. Young, and R. Price. 2005. "Surface energy and interparticle force correlation in model pMDI formulations." *Pharmaceutical Research* 22 (5):816–825. doi:10.1007/s11095-005-2599-2.

Traini, D., P. M. Young, P. Rogueda, and R. Price. 2006. "The use of AFM and surface energy measurements to investigate drug-canister material interactions in a model pressurized metered dose inhaler formulation." *Aerosol science and technology* 40 (4):227–236.

Turner, R. 2010. "Modifying MDI canister surfaces to improve drug stability & drug delivery." *PressPart.*http://www.ondrugdelivery.com/.

UN, Environment. 2016. "The Kigali amendment to the montreal protocol: Another Commitment to stop climate change." Accessed June 2018. https://www.unenvironment.org/news-and-stories/news/kigali-amendment-montreal-protocol-another-global-commitment-stop-climate.

Vance, C., C. Swalwell, and I. M. McIntyre. 2012. "Deaths involving 1,1-difluoroethane at the San Diego county medical examiner's office." *Journal of Analytical Toxicology* 36 (9):626–633. doi:10.1093/jat/bks074.

Wang, J., H. Han, X. Jiang, L. Huang, L. Chen, and N. Li. 2012. "Quantum dot-based near-infrared electrochemiluminescent immunosensor with gold nanoparticle-graphene nanosheet hybrids and silica nanospheres double-assisted signal amplification." *Analytical Chemistry* 84 (11):4893–4899. doi:10.1021/ac300498v.

Williams III, R. O., M. K. Barron, M. J. Alonso, and C. Remuñán-López. 1998. "Investigation of a pMDI system containing chitosan microspheres and P134a." *International Journal of Pharmaceutics* 174 (1):209–222. doi:10.1016/S0378-5173(98)00266-X.

Williams, R. O., D. R. Taft, and J. T. McConville. 2007. *Advanced Drug Formulation Design to Optimize Therapeutic Outcomes*. Boca Raton, FL: CRC Press.

Wu, L., M. Al-Haydari, and S. R. P. da Rocha. 2008a. "Novel propellant-driven inhalation formulations: Engineering polar drug particles with surface-trapped hydrofluoroalkane-philes." *European Journal of Pharmaceutical Sciences* 33 (2):146–158. doi:10.1016/j.ejps.2007.10.007.

Wu, L., B. Bharatwaj, J. Panyam, and S. R. P. da Rocha. 2008b. "Core–shell particles for the dispersion of small polar drugs and biomolecules in hydrofluoroalkane propellants." *Pharmaceutical Research* 25 (2):289–301. doi:10.1007/s11095-007-9466-2.

Wu, L., and S. R. P. da Rocha. 2007. "Biocompatible and biodegradable copolymer stabilizers for hydrofluoroalkane dispersions: A colloidal probe microscopy investigation." *Langmuir* 23 (24):12104–12110. doi:10.1021/la702108x.

Wu, L., and S. R. P. da Rocha. 2008. "Applications of the atomic force microscope in the development of propellant-based inhalation formulations." *KONA Powder and Particle Journal* 26:106–128. doi:10.14356/kona.2008011.

Wu, L., and S. R. P. da Rocha. 2011. "Nanoparticle-stabilized colloids in compressible hydrofluoroalkanes." *Langmuir* 27 (17):10501–10506. doi:10.1021/la201906f.

Yang, L., and S. R. P. da Rocha. 2014. "Understanding solvation in the low global warming hydrofluoroolefin HFO-1234ze propellant." *The Journal of Physical Chemistry B* 118 (36):10675–10687. doi:10.1021/jp5059319.

Young, P. M., R. Price, D. Lewis, S. Edge, and D. Traini. 2003. "Under pressure: Predicting pressurized metered dose inhaler interactions using the atomic force microscope." *Journal of Colloid and Interface Science* 262 (1):298–302.

Zhu, B., D. Traini, and P. Young. 2015. "Aerosol particle generation from solution-based pressurized metered dose inhalers: a technical overview of parameters that influence respiratory deposition." *Pharmaceutical Development and Technology* 20 (8):897–910. doi:10.3109/10837450.2014.959176.

Zyhowski, G., and A. Brown. 2011. Low global warming fluids for replacement of HFC-245fa and HFC-134a in ORC applications. *1st International Seminar on ORC Power Systems*, Delft, the Netherlands.

19

Dry Powder Inhalation

Anne H. de Boer and Floris Grasmeijer

CONTENTS

19.1 Introduction

Intuitively the solid state may not seem to be the most obvious form in which a therapeutic aerosol can be taken. Vapors and mists are ostensibly more appropriate for inhalation as they can be created easily by evaporation and atomization of the drug or drug solution, respectively. Besides, the inhalation of "fine particles" has a bad reputation ever since air pollution due to the large-scale burning of coal during the Industrial Revolution became a health problem. For the creation of wet aerosols (or spays), a variety of different nebulization principles are available. Some of them were already developed in the eighteenth and nineteenth century for inhaling thermal waters and are still in use. Physicians and patients became aware of the importance of wet nebulization after Philip Stern acknowledged in 1764 that "the only possible way of applying medicines directly to the lung is through the windpipe" (Sanders 2007). Developments for therapeutic use benefitted particularly from inventions made for spraying fungicides against grapevine diseases. Since Stern made his statement, it took more than 100 years before Alfred Newton patented the first dry powder inhaler (DPI) for the delivery of pulverized potassium chloride to the lung. His device was never manufactured on an industrial scale, however, and the Aerohalor™ (launched by Abbott in 1948) for the delivery of penicillin and norethisterone is considered the first commercially available DPI instead (Sanders 2007). Despite this slow development, dry powder inhalation has several advantages over nebulization. Only recently, it has been recognized that the aerodynamic particle size distribution (APSD) of the aerosol is of utmost importance for adequate lung deposition (Lippmann et al. 1980). Dry powders are interesting in this respect because their APSD can be well controlled with a variety of different preparation techniques. Dry powders have much better chemical stability than drug solutions and are, therefore, more appropriate for use in warm climates. They can also effectively be dispersed with the energy derived from the inhaled air stream. This enables to keep DPIs simple and cheap without the use of auxiliary power units, which is a great advantage considering the continuing pressure on health budgets. Being cheap makes DPIs potentially disposable for various one-off applications like vaccination and rescue medication. Compared to nebulization, the inhalation of high powder doses takes considerably less time. Irrespective of all these and other advantages of the solid state, the greatest boost to the development of dry powder inhalers was first given in the late 1900s when the use of chlorofluorocarbon (CFC) propellants for pressurized metered dose inhalers (pMDIs) was banned. Hence, alternatives had to be found for this popular type of inhalation device. As a result of all this, dry powder inhalation is relatively new and the technology used for delivering dry powder aerosols to the respiratory tract is still in its infancy. Nowadays dry powder inhalation seems to be first choice for many applications, and it is well recognized that the inhalation of a therapeutic "dust" may not lead to more complaints than inhaling wet aerosols although much depends on the chemical nature of the drug and its APSD in this respect.

19.2 Particle Interaction Mechanisms

In dry powder inhalation technology, powder formulation, dose measuring, and powder dispersion are key operations. Numerous publications in the past decades witnessed the tremendous effort put in understanding and controlling the properties of the powder formulation with the drug. The focus is directed mainly to properties that determine the powder density, flowability, and dispersibility, which are all relevant to pulmonary drug delivery. They control the accuracy and reproducibility of dose measuring as well as the quantity and properties of the delivered aerosol, and they depend on the physical interactions between the particles in the powder. Forces of different nature can be responsible for these interactions, including van der Waals, Coulombic and capillary forces, but also the force of gravity plays an important role. It is the force of gravity (F_G) that makes powders flow. Being proportional to the third power of the particle diameter, F_G increases much more rapidly with increasing particle diameter than any of the attraction forces. Particles become free flowing at diameters larger than 30 μm to 100 μm depending on several other particle properties, however. The narrower the size distribution, the smaller the median diameter is at which F_G generally exceeds the attraction forces. The nature of the van der Waals, and other attraction forces, has been described before (Hinds 1982; Visser 1989) and in powders for inhalation Coulombic and capillary forces are preferably excluded as they are too strong for effective dispersion of the powder during inhalation. van der Waals forces are proportional to the first power of the particle diameter, but the magnitude of the force of cohesion (or adhesion) between two particles depends on the chemical nature of the components too. It furthermore depends strongly on physical particle properties like the particles' shape and surface texture (Hickey et al. 1994; Kawashima et al. 1998). They influence the surface area per contact point and the distance between adjacent particles. The strength of a powder in which multiple contact points between particles exist varies furthermore with the number of contact points (coordination number) per particle which is related to the packing density of the powder and affected by the size and shape distributions of the particles, too. The mixing process finally can change the particle surface properties and the size of individual contact points between particles. Mixing may also be responsible for various other effects like the formation or break-down of drug particle agglomerates. The great effect of the particle properties on the powder cohesiveness is the rationale for manipulating shape and surface texture of particles for inhalation. The techniques used to obtain the desired surface and bulk properties have been described and reviewed extensively before and are not the subject of this chapter (e.g. Shoyele and Cawthorne 2006; Vehring 2008; Weers and Miller 2015).

The size distribution of particles for inhalation offers less possibilities for variation than their shape and surface texture as the particles need to be smaller than 3 μm to 5 μm aerodynamically in order to be able to pass the oropharynx. They also are preferably larger than 1 μm for effective deposition by sedimentation in the lower respiratory tract. An exception is for low dose drugs in the microgram range that are mixed with much coarser particles to increase the dose volume and improve the flow properties of the powder. In such mixtures, the micronized drug particles adhere to the surface of the coarser "carrier" particles which are mostly lactose crystals in a size range varying between 10 μm and 300 μm. During inhalation, the carrier and drug particles have to be separated from each other to render the drug particles in the desired aerodynamic size distribution. In many studies the basic interaction forces between pure drug-drug and drug-lactose combinations has been studied (e.g. Begat et al. 2004). However, the value of such studies may be questioned considering the effect of the mixing process on the adhesive force and the presence of surface impurities on the lactose crystals, including water of adsorption. Also, the unknown surface area per contact point and coordination numbers in the mixture make prediction of the interparticulate forces uncertain. A deliberate use of an impurity on the contact area between particles in inhalation formulations is made with so-called force control agents (FCAs) like l-leucine and magnesium stearate (Begat et al. 2009). Such film-forming excipients form a molecular barrier between the contacting particles and reduce the force of attraction. The same forces that are responsible for particle-particle interaction also determine the adhesion of particles onto inhaler walls.

19.3 Powder Dispersion

A variety of different aerodynamic dispersers for cohesive powders exists, and the principles used depend on the application and desired fineness of the powder. Principles designed for the dispersion of such powders mostly make use of shear flow and rapid acceleration and/or deceleration of powder agglomerates in air streams. Also inertial forces from vibration, particle-particle collisions, or particle impaction against bodies placed in the air stream are used (Kousaka et al. 1979). Examples of such dispersers are eductors, Venturi's, nozzles, capillary tubes, and orifice impactors (Calvert et al. 2009) (Figure 19.1).

Such principles are often operated at high pressures resulting in high air velocities through the devices. Complete dispersion of cohesive powders in the gas phase is generally difficult for particles

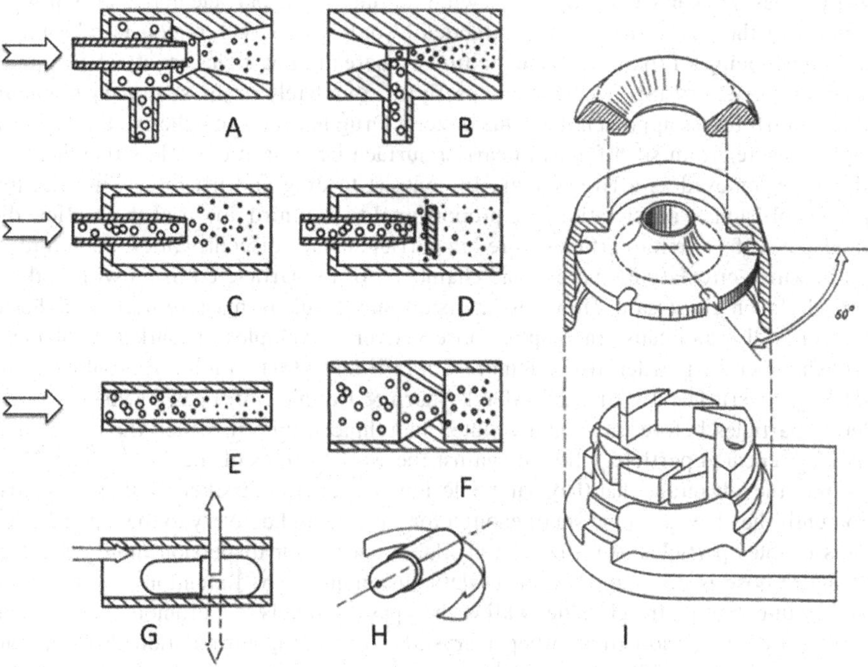

FIGURE 19.1 Different powder dispersion principles (schematically), A. eductor type, B. Ventüri type, C. nozzle type, D. nozzle with impaction plate, E. capillary tube, F. orifice plate. The examples G and H are applied in capsule inhalers. G shows the principle of the Boehringer HandiHaler having the capsule with the drug formulation in a narrow air channel. When the inhaled air stream passes through the channel, and partly through the two-sided pierced capsule, the capsule moves quickly to the side along which the air flows due to the Bernoulli effect. This displaces the air stream to the opposite capsule side where the same effect occurs, and as a result of that repeating action the capsule starts to oscillate in the narrow channel at high frequency to fluidize the powder inside. Example H shows a (pierced) spinning capsule from which the drug formulation is removed during inhalation by the action of the centrifugal force. Example I is a circulation chamber in which powder particles circulate at high velocity while colliding with other particles and with the cylindrical wall sections of the chamber (example Meda Novolizer®).

smaller than 10 µm to 20 µm, however, because of the high interparticulate attraction forces compared to the separation forces (Hinds 1982; Young et al. 2007). For dry powder inhalation, the most optimal APSD is in the narrow size range between 1 µm and 3 µm. Moreover, the flow rate through dry powder inhalers delivering the energy for dispersion should preferably be limited to ≤60 L/min in order to minimize the drug losses in the oropharynx by inertial deposition (Usmani et al. 2005). Mostly, the inhaled air flow is accelerated locally within the DPI through narrow passageways to increase its kinetic energy in the dispersion zone. Also, the velocity that can be achieved is limited as the DPI resistance to air flow should not make it impossible for the patient to generate a sufficiently high flow rate through the device. Mostly 30 L/min or more is needed to entrain the powder from the dose (measuring) compartment and to deliver the entire dose to the lung. Too narrow air passageways increase the resistance to unacceptable values. This also makes it impossible for the patient to inhale long enough for total drug dose transport into the deep lung. Narrow channels, furthermore, bear the risk of clogging by particle agglomerates. Therefore, making an appropriate choice for the type of dispersion force to be used for dispersion of inhalation powders is of utmost importance. This choice depends on the type of formulation used which can either be a carrier-based (adhesive) mixture (see Paragraph 19.5), a soft pellet formulation, or unformulated powder. Dispersion efficacy of all types of formulations in all types of dispersers mentioned may be influenced by the relative air humidity: at low humidity, electrostatic forces may become of influence, whereas at high humidity, capillary forces may take over (Young et al. 2007).

The different types of forces that can be used for dispersion differ in the order of magnitude and their efficacy for different formulation types. Drag forces acting on particles are proportional to the first power (Stokes' law) or second power (Newton regime) of the particle diameter. For micronized drug particles in the size range ≤5 µm, practically only the Stokes region is relevant (particle Reynolds number being <1.0). In adhesive mixtures, where drug particles are attached to the surface of much larger carrier crystals, particles are partly or completely in the stationary boundary layer where drag and lift forces approach the value of zero. Drug particles in adhesive mixtures may also find complete shelter from such forces in carrier surface irregularities, unless they are agglomerated and can be removed as a large chunk. In contrast to drag and lift forces, inertial forces, as from particle collision or acceleration, are proportional to the third power of the particle diameter. They can also be effective for particles stored in carrier surface discontinuities. Such forces can be generated in whirl, circulation, and cyclone chambers, or by particle collision with bodies placed in the particle laden air stream. However, collision may result in massive particle adhesion onto the impaction bodies and cause incomplete dose delivery. Examples of marketed inhalers with a circulation chamber for powder dispersion are Conix™ DPI (3M) with a reverse-flow cyclone and NEXThaler® (Chiesi). The Twisthaler® (Merck Sharp & Dohme Corp) has a swirl nozzle chamber to accelerate particles before they enter a fluted mouthpiece tube in which the actual dispersion takes place by repeated particle collision against the wall sections of the mouthpiece. Circulation chambers have the advantage that they can be designed as an air classifier which keeps particles in circulation until they have become small enough for passage and delivery to the lung (de Boer et al. 2003). This enables particles to utilize the available energy for dispersion more effectively than when the entire dose is discharged from the DPI instantaneously. Retention in classifiers can be minimized by interrupting the classifier wall with bypass channels that promote the air and particle circulation, or by adding so-called sweeper crystals to the drug formulation that wipe adhering drug particles off the classifier walls. Such sweeper crystals are not released from the classifier and, thus, not inhaled by the patient when they are larger than the classifier's cut-off value (de Boer et al. 2006). Air classifier technology has been applied in the Genuair® (AstraZeneca) and Twincer® (PureIMS) dry powder inhalers. A dispersion principle based on impaction and internal shear of soft agglomerates is found in the Turbuhaler® (AstraZeneca). In this inhaler, the drug agglomerates are dragged by the inhaled air stream through a narrow spiral-shaped channel (Wetterlin 1979). During passage they make contact with the inner wall of that channel by the action of the centrifugal force. This causes friction and internal shear of the pellets. A distinct group of inhalers are the capsule-based DPIs (see also Paragraph 19.4). They carry a single dose in a hard gelatin or hydroxypropyl methycellulose (HPMC) capsule which is discharged after piercing the capsule wall to create

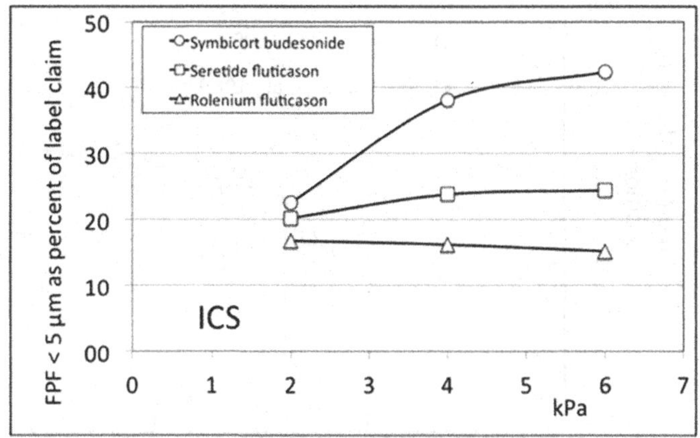

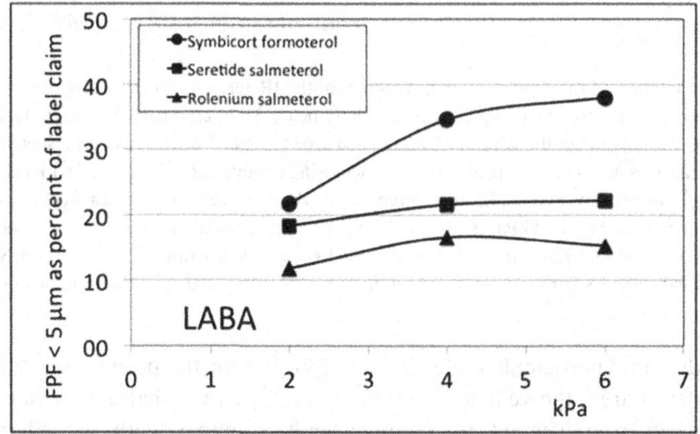

FIGURE 19.2 Different output modes for the fine particle fraction (FPF < 5 µm) from three dry powder inhalers. The examples shown are for drug combinations of an inhaled cortico steroid (ICS; top figure) and a long acting beta2 agonist (LABA; bottom figure). The AstraZeneca Symbicort® Turbuhaler delivers a higher fine particle dose when the flow rate through the inhaler is increased to compensate (at least partly) for the shift in deposition towards larger airways in the respiratory tract. For the GSK Seretide® Diskus and Rolenium® Elpenhaler® the fine particle fraction is fairly independent of the inhaled flow rate.

openings for the powder to escape. For this type of inhaler, the inhaled air stream is primarily used to bring the capsule into spinning (e.g. Cyclohaler®), shaking and twisting (e.g. Turbospin®), or oscillation (e.g. HandiHaler®). Dispersion of the powder in capsule devices is either by acceleration, shear flow and impaction, or by a combination of these forces.

Dry powder inhalers can roughly be divided into two different groups depending on the type of dispersion principle used: those delivering more or less the same fine particle dose at all flow rates, and those producing more fine particles when the flow rate is increased (Figure 19.2).

Being independent of the flow rate has intuitively long been considered an advantage because it suggests a patient independent therapy. In reality, the opposite is more likely (Demoly et al. 2014). Increasing the flow rate through the DPI is increasing the velocity (U) at which the particle enters the respiratory tract. This increases particle momentum ($m.\ U$, where the particle mass m equals $\pi/6.D^3$ for spherical particles), and a higher momentum will result in more inertial deposition in the upper airways, including the oropharynx, where most inhaled drug particles are not needed. To keep the momentum the same, the particle mass has to be halved when its velocity is doubled, but because particle mass is proportional to the third power of the particle diameter, theoretically, only a 21% smaller particle diameter (D) is needed. This is very well achievable with effective dispersion principles, such as air classifiers, as it corresponds, for example, to a relatively small decrease in diameter from 3 µm to 2.38 µm. Practically, the impaction parameter (IP) is frequently used to predict particle deposition. IP is the product of the

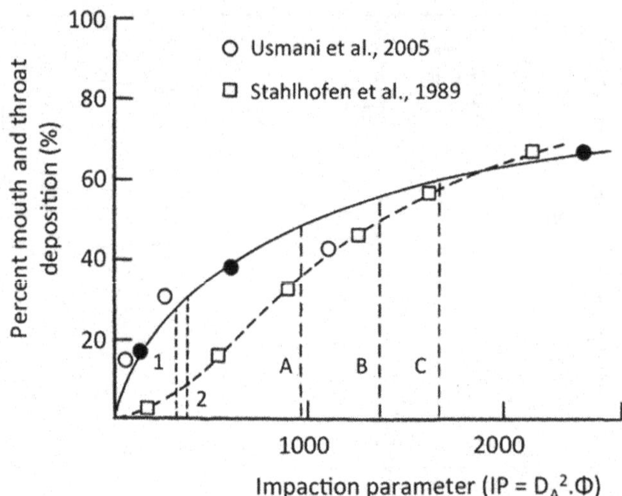

FIGURE 19.3 Percent mouth and throat deposition as function of the IP derived from two different studies. For the study of Usmani et al. the open symbols are for monodisperse 1.5 micron particles, 3.0 micron particles, and 6.0 micron particles inhaled at 30.8 L/min; the closed symbols are for the same particles inhaled at 67.1 L/min. Vertical lines represent the IP-values of aerosols from the (medium resistance) AstraZeneca Eklira® Genuair when being operated at 2 kPa (1) and 6 kPa (2). This inhaler delivers a finer aerosol at higher flow rates. The lines A, B, and C represent the IP-values of the (low resistance) Cyclohaler capsule DPI for the same Eklira formulation at 2 kPa (A), 4 kPa (B), and 6 kPa (C). Computations of the IP-values for the aerosols from the inhalers were based on the mass median aerodynamic diameters of the fine particle fractions < 6 μm. (From Stahlhofen, W. et al., *J. Aerosol. Med.*, 2, 285–308, 1989; Usmani, O.S. et al., *Am. J. Respir. Crit. Care Med.*, 172, 1497–1504, 2005.)

square of the aerodynamic particle diameter (D_A^2) and U, but for the particle deposition from inhalers in the mouth and throat area, the velocity is often replaced by the inhaled flow rate (Φ). This has the consequence that results from different studies are difficult to compare with each other because the same flow rate may result in different velocities (and flow patterns) depending on the shape and geometry of the inhaler's mouthpiece (Figure 19.3). Figure 19.3 shows that IP-values higher than 500 to 1000, as for aerosols consisting of relatively large particles delivered at high velocity, are unwanted because of the high drug losses in the oropharynx. High IP-values also cause a shift in deposition in upper and central airways where inertial deposition is dominant. The figure furthermore shows the IP-values and (to be expected) corresponding oropharyngeal losses for the aerosols from two different dry powder inhalers, the Genuair and the Cyclohaler (ISF) inhaler both tested with the Eklira® formulation from the Genuair at 2 kPa, 4 kPa, and 6 kPa. For the low resistance, Cyclohaler high IP-values (A, B, and C) are computed at the high flow rates through this device of 75 L/min (at 2 kPa), 105 L/min, and 129 L/min (at 6 kPa), respectively, and there is little compensation from the median diameter of the fine particle aerosol which is almost the same (approx. 3.6 μm) at all flow rates. For the Genuair, with much lower flow rates of 48 L/min, 67 L/min, and 82 L/min and a decreasing median aerosol diameter from 2.63 (at 48 L/min) to 2.16 (at 82 L/min), the IP-values (1 and 2) for the most extreme flow rates are almost the same.

One aspect that needs to be considered for all types of dispersion principles is that they may become overloaded by high powder feed rates to the principle. This could affect the type of principle to be used for high drug doses.

19.4 Classic DPI Design and Its Shortcomings

For adequate delivery of powder aerosols to the respiratory tract a complex set of variables has to be fine-tuned. To this purpose, the design of the drug formulation and the inhaler device as well as the performance of the patient all play a crucial role. During drug delivery, the inhaler device has to generate powder dispersion forces that surmount the particle interaction forces in the drug formulation for obtaining a suitable aerosol for inhalation. This requires a proper balancing of the particle interaction and separation forces. Additionally, as explained in the previous paragraph, good balancing between the particle separation and lung deposition forces is needed. Increasing the flow rate through the inhaler device makes more energy available for dispersion, but also increases the velocity with which the aerosol is delivered. For the example of the Genuair in Figure 19.3, not only the median diameter of the fine particle aerosol decreases at a higher flow rate; also the mass percent of fine particles increases from 33% (at 2 kPa) to 39% of the label claim (at 6 kPa). To meet the prerequisites for good performance, a DPI needs to consist of four well-matched primary functional parts: the powder formulation with the drug, a dose (measuring) system, a powder dispersion principle, and the housing encasing previously mentioned parts. To achieve this balanced DPI performance, integrated formulation-device development is to be recommended. However, when the first classic DPIs were developed, the state of the art technology of the 1960s was used for their design, and this resulted in an arbitrary combination of functional inhaler parts. The existence of what were named "ordered mixtures" after their discovery was reported shortly after scanning electron microscopy became available (e.g. Travers and White 1971). It was Hersey (1975) who recognized the high degree of homogeneity and physical stability of such mixtures in which micronized particles adhere strongly to the surface of coarser particles in an ordered arrangement. This high degree of homogeneity of ordered mixtures seemed to make them particularly suitable for reproducible measuring of small drug doses in dry powder inhalers, but the high degree of stability appeared to impede good dispersion. First, after mixing was presented as a dynamic process in which adhesive (cohesive) and non-adhesive mixing exist together (Staniforth 1981 and 1987), it was realized that the outcome of the mixing process can be driven in a desired direction in which adhesive and non-adhesive are the extremes. Taking this recognition and other aspects into consideration, it was, therefore, recommended to replace the name ordered mixtures by adhesive mixtures (Staniforth 1987). By changing the mixing conditions and the properties of the particles in the mixture, the outcome can be shifted towards either non-adhesive, having the lowest degree of homogeneity, or adhesive, having the highest degree of homogeneity, but also the highest physical stability. This ambivalence between high homogeneity and high stability (including poor dispersibility) of the powder makes adhesive mixtures less suitable for inhalation, unless an inhaler with a powerful dispersion principle is used.

Hard gelatin capsules were selected as unit-dose compartment because adequate filling apparatus was already available for this type of powder container. Early formulation studies focused more on content uniformity, delivered dose consistency, and good capsule emptying than on dispersion efficacy and delivering a high fraction of the metered dose as suitable aerosol for inhalation (e.g. Bell et al. 1971). As explained in Paragraph 19.3 capsule DPIs do not have a distinct dispersion principle; emptying of the capsule and aerosolization of the powder occurs simultaneously in the same maneuver. As a result, fine particle doses from adhesive mixtures are limited to the range between 20% and 40% of the label claim. Capsule inhalers have low resistances that yield flow rates of 100 L/min or more at a moderate pressure drop of 4 kPa. Such high flow rates are often needed for complete emptying of the capsule in a reasonable inhalation time, and this has the disadvantage that substantial drug deposition occurs in the oropharynx. In addition to that, hard gelatin, but also HPMC, capsules frequently fragment during circulation at flow rates higher than 60 L/min. Patients can inhale fragments of damaged capsules and fragmentation can hinder complete emptying. Capsules also require a secondary packaging to protect the drug formulation against a high relative air humidity capsule. Finally, it has occasionally been reported that patients inhale oral capsules that fit in their DPI. In spite of all these disadvantages of the classic DPI design, many capsule-based inhalers are still on the market and even more concepts of the same basic principle are newly introduced. To improve their performance drug (and carrier), particle engineering and blending of the drug or drug-carrier mixture with so-called force control agents are applied (Paragraphs 19.5 and 6).

19.5 Low Dose Drug Formulation: State of the Art

Low dose drug formulations for dry powder inhalation are generally formulations containing several micrograms to a few hundred micrograms of a potent drug for the treatment of asthma or chronic obstructive pulmonary disease. As explained in previous paragraphs, reproducible dosing of such small drug amounts requires the use of excipients which dilute the drug and improve the flowability of the powder bulk. With the exception of only one marketed product, so far this is always achieved by adhesion of the drug particles to coarse carrier particles consisting of alpha lactose monohydrate in adhesive mixtures. The simplicity of spontaneous adhesion of micron-sized drug particles to coarse lactose carrier particles during mixing conceals a tremendous complexity associated to adhesive mixtures for inhalation. Despite over 20 years of active research into the influence of variables concerning the drug and excipient starting materials, the mixing process, and the process of dispersion, it is generally acknowledged that a fundamental understanding of adhesive mixtures has yet to be obtained (Marriott and Frijlink 2012). As a result, low-dose drug formulation for dry powder inhalation appears to be more of an art than a science. Fortunately, appearances may be deceiving and some steps towards the fundamental understanding of adhesive mixtures for inhalation have been made indeed. However, one should not expect that such an understanding results in straightforward answers regarding the influence of certain formulation or dispersion variables. On the contrary, it leads one to understand that straightforward answers are very rare, as most effects are highly situation dependent. It is a basic and well established notion that the dispersion performance of adhesive mixtures depends on the balance between adhesion and dispersion forces, and that these forces are governed by factors concerning the particles' surface, their size distribution and bulk properties, the mixing process, as well as the dispersion principle and the inhalation flow rate applied. Logically, this has resulted in numerous studies concerning the influence on dispersion performance of, for example, carrier surface roughness (Kawashima et al. 1998; Young et al. 2002; Flament et al. 2004), added fine excipient (Lucas et al. 1998; Jones and Price 2006; Grasmeijer et al. 2014a), carrier, drug or fine excipient material (Tee et al. 2000; Hooton at al. 2006), drug content (Kulvanich and Stewart 1987a; Grasmeijer et al. 2013a; Young et al. 2005), or mixing time (Kulvanich and Stewart 1987b; Dickhoff et al. 2003; Grasmeijer et al. 2013b). However, for all of these variables, the influence on mixture dispersion performance is inconsistent throughout the literature (Grasmeijer et al. 2015). Even for a factor such as surface free energy, which according to basic theory should be proportional to the force of adhesion and, therefore, inversely related to dispersion performance, inconsistent results are obtained (Hickey et al. 2007a). With reference to this basic theory, many have undoubtedly proclaimed "it should, all other things being equal, still be of influence on dispersion performance as expected" Except, in practice not all other things are equal. This may be because of linkage between variables, i.e. when one variable inevitably causes the change of another variable, as explained by de Boer et al. (2012). This may also be simply because of a different choice of study conditions. These differences in "things" or variables within and between studies cause interactions, and it is these interactions which are more and more held accountable for the observed inconsistencies throughout literature (Jones et al. 2010; de Boer et al. 2012; Grasmeijer et al. 2015). Understanding these interactions therefore appears to be paramount to obtaining a fundamental understanding of adhesive mixtures.

Due to interactions, individual studies that have investigated single variables under a specific set of conditions may appear to be valuable only when in practice those specific conditions are met. However, when considered together, the whole body of scientific literature on adhesive mixtures for inhalation may reveal the interactions occurring and, more importantly, their underlying mechanisms. Recently, a theoretical framework that explains the interplay between variables was proposed based on a literature review for the most widely studied formulation variables (Grasmeijer et al. 2015). It was suggested that four principle factors of the powder exist, i.e. the size distribution of the drug particles (including drug/drug and drug/fine excipient particles) as they are detached from the carrier surface; the degree of compression of the drug particles onto the carrier surface; the distribution in "activity" of carrier sites that are occupied by drug particles; and the tensile strength or fluidization behavior of the mixture. Every interaction between variables is supposedly the result of a change in the relevance of alterations in these factors (type 1 interactions) or of a change in how these factors are altered (type 2 interactions). It is noteworthy that the "energy ratio distributions" used by Grasmeijer et al. to explain type 1 interactions in adhesive mixtures, i.e. an interaction with flow rate (Grasmeijer and de Boer 2014b; Grasmeijer et al. 2015), bear close resemblance to the powder strength distribution used to understand a similar interaction in the dispersion of fine lactose powders by Das et al. (2012). Such a resemblance between rather distinct powder formulations suggests a more universal applicability of this approach.

Modeling approaches such as computational fluid dynamics (CFD, especially large eddy simulations, LES) and discrete element models (DEM) are used more and more to better understand the dispersion process of adhesive mixtures in dry powder inhalers (Cui et al. 2014; van Wachem et al. 2017). They provide insights into the relevance of detachment mechanisms such as aerodynamic lift or inertial detachment due to particle-particle or particle-inhaler wall collisions. Furthermore, the drug-carrier interaction models, although never capturing the full complexity of reality, can provide valuable insights into the relevance of particle properties such as their hardness or adhesive and cohesive behavior. Theoretical frameworks and models require validation in order to determine their value. Many of the particle and powder properties that are supposedly relevant to the performance of adhesive mixtures in the framework and models mentioned are difficult to measure (Grasmeijer and de Boer 2014b; Grasmeijer et al. 2015; Hickey et al. 2007b). New or improved characterization techniques will, therefore, likely be necessary to further advance the fundamental understanding of adhesive mixtures.

19.6 High-Dose Drug Formulation

The most fundamental difference between high (mg-range) and low (µg-range) dose drug formulations is the necessity to incorporate excipients in the latter to achieve the desired dose reproducibility. Without excipient, the volume is too small for accurate measuring. For high dose formulations, the use of filler excipient is to be rejected, particularly when the drug dose is already 50 mg or more. Single capsules for inhalation can carry doses up to approx. 50 mg to 60 mg of powder depending on its density, and adding excipient(s) to the drug formulation increases the powder volume. This mostly leads to a larger number of capsules to be inhaled for a single dose. Obviously, this increases the burden of the therapy for the patient, particularly because most capsules need to be inhaled at least twice for complete emptying. Two new inhaler types, Twincer and Orbital® multi-breath dry powder inhaler, are also capable of delivering high drug doses up to 50 mg–100 mg and 100 mg–400 mg, respectively (de Boer et al. 2006; Young et al. 2014). For the Twincer, delivery is in one single inhalation maneuver, whereas the Orbital requires a number of subsequent inhalations for complete emptying of the dose compartment. The maximal amount of powder to be delivered in one single breath is also limited by what the patient can bear. Little is still known about patient acceptance regarding the maximal dose weight, but it has been reported that this may depend on the chemical nature of the drug (Westerman et al. 2004) as well as on the particle size distribution of the aerosol. By comparing the patient acceptance of the Turbospin (Colobreathe®, Teva) and Twincer for pure colistimethate sodium with each other, it was found that offering a finer aerosol without capsule fragments at a lower flow rate to the patient, as from the Twincer, can minimize cough reactions considerably (Hagedoorn et al. 2016). This is likely the result of a lower deposition in the throat where the cough reflex is initiated.

There exists a similarity between low and high dose formulations for inhalation in the pursuance of increasing the dispersibility of the powder. Some of the approaches to understand and control the drug-to-carrier interaction forces in low dose adhesive mixtures have been summarized in Paragraph 19.5. Approaches used for high dose formulations are basically the same, but the engineering techniques to achieve the desired particle properties may partly be different. For reasons of stability and processing (mixing), spray drying is less favorable for drugs in drug-carrier mixtures. On the contrary, spray drying is a well-established technique for high dose drugs to control particle shape, density, and surface properties (Vehring 2008). A large variety of favorable properties relevant to dispersion may be obtained (Figure 19.4) by varying the process conditions and excipients, which are frequently only needed in small quantities (<2% by mass) for this purpose.

Examples of particle engineering for increased dispersibility of high dose drugs have been reviewed extensively in literature (Shoyele and Cawthorne 2006; Pilcer and Amighi 2010; Weers and Miller 2015) and can be found elsewhere in this book. Particle engineering techniques may also be needed to achieve better dissolution (or controlled release) of the drug, target (or escape the uptake by), macrophages, muco-adhesion, delay (or promote), water uptake, etc. They are not the scope of this chapter and may require complex multi-step processes and the use of a range of different excipients. For any of these applications, the question should be asked whether the end justifies the means. For several excipients mentioned in

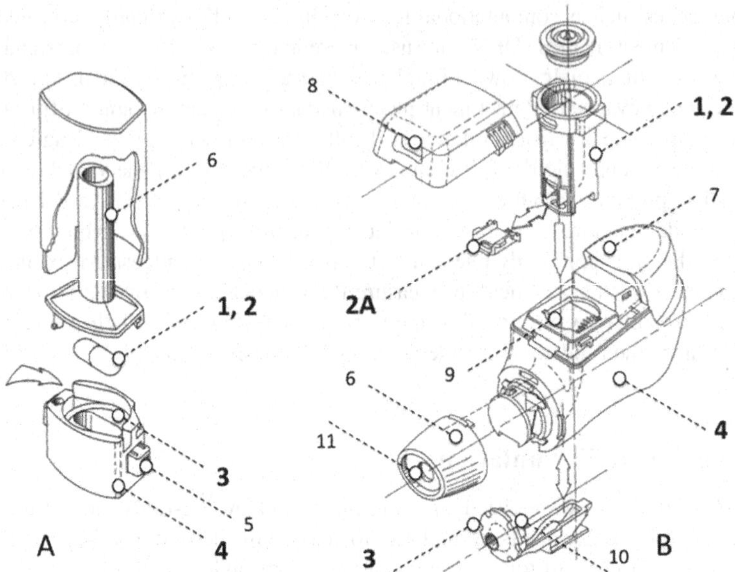

FIGURE 19.4 Examples of particle properties being relevant to inhalation. Example A shows the effect of particle shape on the contact area and number of contact points between two particles. Examples B1 and B2 present the effect of surface texture (rugosity) on the difference in separation distance (δ) to a flat surface for particles with a completely smooth (B1) and irregular surface (B2). Example B3 shows how drug particles in adhesive mixtures can find shelter from separation forces in the irregular surface of the carrier particles. Example D shows different types of particles with a low density having the same aerodynamic diameter as solid particles (with the same weight: C1), but much larger geometric diameters (C2–C4). Such large porous particles can be hollow (C3, with or without aperture in the shell), have voids internally (C2), or externally in wrinkled shells (C4).

various studies, the long term safety has not (yet) been demonstrated. Being endogenous is not an undisputable justification for their use. So are sodium chloride and cholesterol, but an ongoing high intake may on the long term cause serious health problems. Moreover, it took several decades to recognize this. Excipients may not only increase the dose weight, but also the volume of the powder when highly porous particles are produced. As already mentioned, this may have a negative effect on patient's compliance with the instructions and adherence to the therapy. Particle engineering for improved dispersion may not be needed as this goal can also be achieved from designing better inhalers.

19.7 Multi-Dose, Reservoir DPIs: Functional Parts and Considerations

Multi-dose DPIs can be divided into multiple-unit dose inhalers (mostly making use of blisters) and multi-dose reservoir devices. Both types need an operating system for transport of the blister strip (or disk) and the slide (or cylinder) that has the cavity for measuring single doses from the powder mass in the reservoir, respectively. This makes the design of multi-dose DPIs more complex than that of single dose devices (Figure 19.5).

Multi-dose inhalers have the advantage that the patient does not have to carry single capsules or blisters around. Unless the inhaler is empty, a dose is always available. It also eliminates the risk of physical damage of the (loose) dose compartments, which can hinder complete emptying during inhalation and accidental administration of (oral) capsules that are not meant for inhalation with the device. Furthermore, it prevents incorrect assembling of the inhaler parts after a capsule or blister has been inserted. Multiple-unit dose inhalers carry accurately and reproducibly premetered powder quantities as single doses in aluminum blister pockets sealed with a lidding foil. Such blisters mostly provide good protection against moisture uptake by the drug formulation. The apparatus to be used for their filling, and

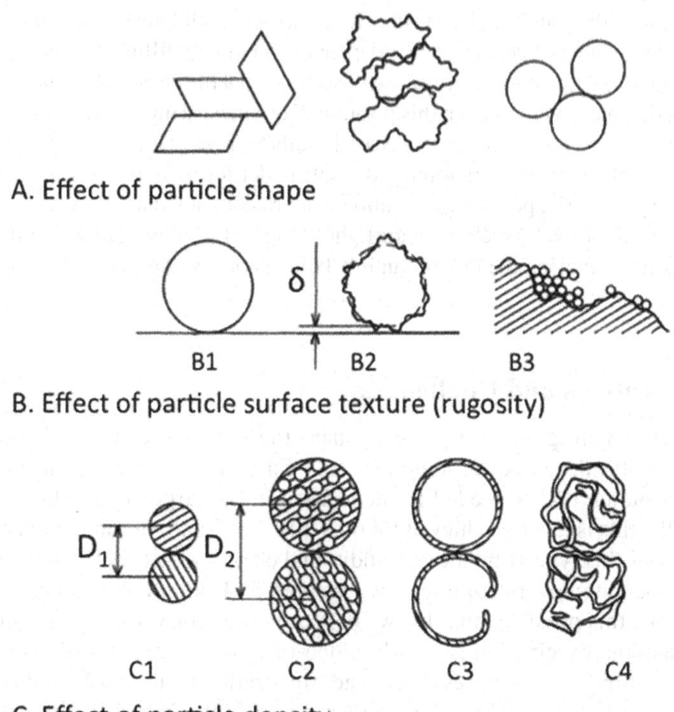

FIGURE 19.5 Comparison of the designs of a single dose capsule inhaler (A: Cyclohaler) and a multi-dose reservoir dry powder inhaler (B: Novolizer). The bold figures represent the primary functional inhaler parts (see the text). For the Cyclohaler, part 3 is the circulation chamber in which the (pierced) capsule spins during inhalation to deliver and disperse the powder formulation, 5 is the knob to pierce the capsule, and 6 is the mouthpiece channel. For the Novolizer, part 2A is the measuring slide for the drug formulation, 7 is the knob bringing the measured dose in the powder channel towards the classifier when being pressed, 8 is a window that changes color upon correct inhalation, 9 is a valve mechanism operated by the inhaled air stream to reset the dose measuring slide, 10 are bypass slots to control the inhaler resistance to air flow, and 11 is an opening providing a sheath of clean air around the aerosol cloud.

that of other types of dose compartments, may impose special properties on the drug formulation, however, which can influence dispersion and the consistency of delivered (fine particle) dose. Reproducible administration also depends on accurate emptying of the blisters during inhalation. Mostly, this requires that the lidding foil is completely removed before inhalation. Local rupture, as from piercing, may bring fragments of lidding foil into the way out for the drug formulation and leave powder residues in the blister compartment. The number of blisters for adhesive mixtures is quite limited (e.g. GSK Diskhaler®). The number of blisters on a strip can be much higher, but the transport mechanism for such devices is considerably more complex (e.g. GSK Diskus®).

Multi-dose reservoir inhalers can hold the largest number of doses in supply. Their relatively large powder reservoirs make them eminently suitable for high doses, but so far no high dose multi-dose reservoir DPI has reached the market. Reservoir DPIs mostly have a rather complex design, but this includes various secondary inhaler features, such as signaling to the patient about correct inhalation (e.g. Genuair, NEXThaler). In contrast with nearly all capsule and multiple-unit dose inhalers, multi-dose reservoir inhalers also have a distinct and mostly highly effective dispersion principle for the powder formulation. This renders generally a much higher fine particle dose from the same type of formulation, but its design imposes several additional demands on the powder formulation too. In addition to good dispersion, good flowability is needed to guarantee reproducible filling of the dose cavity in the measuring slide or cylinder. Good physical and mechanical stability are also needed in order to withstand violent inhaler movements. Dropping, shaking, or vibration of the inhaler may not influence the dose measuring accuracy. Segregation of drug and carrier in adhesive mixtures should not occur and neither may soft pellets clump into one large lump of powder. Being dependent on gravity filling, the inhaler must in principle be held in the correct upright position during dose measuring, but the design of the dose measuring system has to allow a considerable deviation from this position. Dose measuring accuracy may be supported by a puff of air through the dose compartment (e.g. Easi-Breathe®, Teva). Only the Turbuhaler has a different dose measuring principle with scrapers forcing the soft pellet formulation into small conical holes in a disk. Moisture protection of the powder formulation is more complex than in multiple-unit dose inhalers and may require special measures such as an air tight cap (e.g. Turbuhaler) in which the inhaler is stored when not used. Finally, preparing the DPI for an inhalation should be simple.

19.8 New Applications and Challenges

All types of pulmonary drug delivery systems share the same challenge in improvement of their efficacy. Only part of the drug or drug solution is transformed into particles within the narrow aerodynamic size distribution that is needed for deposition in the target area, which is quite often the deep lung. For DPIs, this is mostly achieved for only 10%–40% and, in some rare cases, up to 60% of the weighed dose. For this type of inhaler, an additional challenge is to achieve the desired improvement at a low to moderate flow rate, preferably less than 50 L/min to 60 L/min. New technological inventions may make this possible, and this will open the way for various new applications such as pulmonary vaccination. Vaccination is mostly a one-off administration and also taking a booster dose is not a daily routine. This requires that the administration is successful and reliable or the vaccinee will not be protected. Also, for antibiotic therapies, a high efficacy is mandatory. Underdosing may result in bacterial resistance development, and considering the extreme drug gradient over the entire lung to be expected from pulmonary administration, good drug targeting is needed or underdosing will occur in the most distal airways. Currently, most antibiotics against diseases like tuberculosis cannot be inhaled as a dry powder because of the huge quantities involved. Although for some drugs the pulmonary dose can be decreased by a factor of 10 compared to oral administration, this still challenges DPI engineers to the extreme for antibiotics given orally in amounts of ≥1 g. For treatment with currently marketed DPIs, this requires multiple inhalations and only increasing the efficacy of delivery may further decrease the inhaled dose. Improvement of patient adherence to the therapy and compliance with the instructions for use are two other major challenges to face for antibiotic therapy with DPIs. Although drug administration with DPIs is much faster, easier, and more convenient for the patient than with nebulizers, many errors are made. Incorrect inhaler use by patients can lead to poor adherence to the therapy and treatment failure (Newman and Busse 2002). Minimizing the number of steps to complete an inhalation and simplifying the inhaler use by making self-intuitive device designs need to be primary objectives for future developments. Good feedback to the patient about his or her inhalation performance may also help to improve the compliance and inform the physician about the patient's attitude towards the therapy if the inhalation data can be stored. Many feedback systems, some as add-on device, are being developed, but some standardization is required for convenience of the health care professionals. Uniform operation procedures and instructions may also reduce the errors made by patients using different types of DPIs with different drugs for their therapy. Administration of systemically acting drugs via the pulmonary route is also a major challenge for inhalation therapy with DPIs. Many of these drugs are biopharmaceuticals that cannot withstand the high shear forces during atomization with nebulizers or MDIs, whereas they can be very instable in solution. Drugs like levodopa or loxapine are in development or already approved by the FDA as inhalation powder, and there is an interest in developing a large variety of other drugs for inhalation too. But perhaps the greatest challenge of all is in keeping the inhalers cheap. Considering the increasing pressure on health budgets and the ageing populations in the industrialized countries, the need for cheap, but effective medication will rapidly grow. There is also a growing need for inhaled medicines in developing countries and both needs can be met only with simple, but highly cost-effective DPIs.

19.9 Innovations in Dry Powder Inhaler Technology

There is a difference between innovations in dry powder inhaler technology and innovations in the techniques and methods used to design and develop this technology (see Paragraph 19.10). Some innovations in inhaler technology of the past have already been mentioned in previous paragraphs like the use of carrier free formulations for low dose drugs in the Turbuhaler. Also various particle engineering techniques and the use of force control agents to minimize the interparticulate interaction forces have been referred to in previous paragraphs. Remarkably, most of the innovations in dry powder inhalation technology are in the drug formulation and only few are in device design. Some device innovations of the past were not very successful, like the application of electro-mechanical energy for aerosol generation (e.g. Spiros® DPI, Dura Pharmaceuticals). Battery driven impellers, and also pressurized air (e.g. Exubera®, Pfizer), offer a constant amount of energy for powder dispersion (Han et al. 2002; Harper et al. 2007). This results in largely the same aerosol properties at all flow rates. In spite of what has frequently been claimed, this does not guarantee a patient independent deposition however, as the deposition shifts towards higher airways at a higher flow rate (Paragraph 19.3). The Spiros and Exubera inhaler were also quite complex and expensive devices and particularly the Exubera device required a large number of preparation steps before a dose could be inhaled. Whether this is the reason why these devices have failed to find a reasonable market share has not become very clear. For the Exubera inhaler, a lack of discretion has been mentioned as an important reason for not wanting to use the device (Heinemann 2008). Patients do not wish to draw attention when they take their insulin dose, and the Exubera was not only cumbersome to use, but also large and, thus, difficult to operate unnoticed. Also the high price of the device, safety concerns for long term use, limited dose flexibility, and the use of unconventional dosage units (in milligrams instead of international units) contributed to a poor acceptance of the device by both patients and physicians. The Exubera example shows that being small, simple, cheap, effective, and safe are key features for a DPI to become successful. A device innovation of the present is the development of feedback systems providing information to the patient about correct use of the DPI. They have been mentioned in paragraph 19.8 and are often presented as an add-on device (e.g. Pilcher et al. 2015).

Some recent DPI developments include the 3M™ Taper DPI (Sitz 2010) and the Jethaler® or Ultrahaler® (Newman and Busse 2002). The Taper DPI has a micro-structured carrier tape to store up to 120 metered 1 mg doses of an active pharmaceutical ingredient. This proprietary 3M technology for low dose drugs makes carrier lactose redundant, but the system has limited flexibility in respect of dose weight. The Jethaler (Mundipharma GmbH) is a scraper DPI, having the drug in a ring-shaped tablet compressed from an adhesive mixture with coarse lactose crystals and the micronized drug (de Boer et al. 2004). During inhalation, part of the tablet is aerosolized into the inhaled air stream by a spring-driven ceramic disk with sharp projections scraping over the surface of the tablet upon pressing a release button. A breath-actuated version (Auto-Jethaler alias MAGhaler®) of this principle has also been developed (Steiss et al. 2007). Another recent development to be considered as a DPI innovation is the Staccato® technology (Alexza Pharmaceuticals). With this technology, a thin film of pure drug in the solid state on a metallic substrate is rapidly evaporated (within 0.2 seconds to approx. 400°C) and subsequently condensated to particles in the appropriate size distribution for inhalation (Noymer et al. 2010). Staccato has been tested for a number of different drugs and will be launched first for loxapine. Currently, DPI development is focused furthermore on pulmonary delivery of high doses, but so far only two new devices have been tested successfully for that. Most powder formulations for high dose drugs were developed for existing capsule inhalers and in most cases this required the use of particle engineering with a considerable amount of excipients increasing either the powder mass, the powder volume, or both. Only the Twincer platform (de Boer et al. 2006) and Orbital Multi-Breath DPI (Young et al. 2014) were developed specifically to administer high doses to the lungs, of which, the Twincer was designed to be used primarily for excipient-free formulations primarily.

Innovations in drug formulation refer particularly to various particle engineering techniques for inhalation powders. Particle engineering is most frequently applied to control of the particle's density, surface properties, and shape. One of the first studies regarding engineered powders for inhalation was from Edwards et al. (1997), who presented the advantages of so-called "large porous particles." Such particles prepared with emulsion solvent evaporation technique have improved dispersion behavior thanks to a low mass density (<0.4 g/cm^3) and a large geometric diameter (>5 µm). By preparing them with poly(lactic acid-co-glycolic acid), they can escape the lungs' natural clearance mechanisms (macrophage uptake) and deliver their drug content before they are biodegraded. Supercritical fluid (SCF) drying has been proposed as an alternative for micronization (Rehman et al. 2004). Supercritical fluid drying particles have reduced surface energy parameters compared to mechanically comminuted particles and, for instance, for terbutalin sulphate particles, an improved fine particle fraction could be obtained with this technique. The spray drying process enables to produce a large variety of different particle morphologies and shapes (Vehring 2008), and one of the most innovative formulations prepared by spray drying are the PulmoSphere® powders (Dellamary et al. 2000; Duddu et al. 2002). In the field of the powder formulation, a noteworthy innovation is also "excipient enhanced growth" (EEG) of inhaled drug particles (Tian et al. 2013). This technique enables to inhale small particles in order to avoid substantial oropharyngeal deposition. Such particles are in a formulation with a hygroscopic excipient that absorbs water in the moist environment of the airways during transportation towards the deep lung. This results in particle growth and, thus, in mass increase which improves the efficiency of sedimentation deposition in the most distal airways. Promising innovations in drug formulation are also the Technosphere® (MannKind) and iSPERSE™ (Pulmatrix) technologies. Technosphere formulations make use of self-assembling (fumaryl diketopiperazine, FDKP) carrier particles with a large surface area for absorbing large active molecules. The carrier particles are small enough to be inhaled with the drug. Therefore, separation of the active component and the excipient in the inhaled air stream is not needed (Richardson and Boss 2007). They are administered with a new inhaler (DreamBoat) and have been developed for Technosphere Insulin (AFREZZA®). iSPERSE powders consist of highly dispersible, dense salt-containing particles in the appropriate size range for inhalation (Lipp and Sung 2015). They do not need blending with lactose, and iSPERSE powders contain typically less than 20% excipient in the formulation with the drug or drug combination. Finally, new therapeutic strategies affect the powder formulation. Already in 2006, the results from clinical studies showed that superior control and reduced severe exacerbations of asthma and COPD can be obtained from the synergistic effect of two drugs used in combination (Miller-Larson and Selroos 2006). Generally, drug combinations include an inhaled corticosteroid (ICS) and a long acting beta2-agonist (LABA). More recently also the advantages of triple therapy have been reported. By adding a long acting muscarinic receptor antagonist (LAMA) to the fixed ICS/LABA combination, an improved efficacy of the pharmacological treatment of patients with particularly severe to very severe chronic obstructive pulmonary disease (COPD) has been obtained (Montuschi et al. 2016). These changes in therapeutic strategy make new demands on the formulations to be used in DPIs and so does the therapy with extrafine drug particles (Corradi et al. 2014). Such extrafine particles, of which a significant mass fraction is in the submicron range, cannot be dispersed effectively without adding previously mentioned force control agents like magnesium stearate to the formulation (see Paragraph 19.2).

19.10 Innovations in Techniques for DPI Design and Development

Innovations in various techniques used for design, development, and testing of DPIs are highly relevant to the improvement and understanding of the device performance, but they are not really the scope of this chapter. Therefore, some of the most noteworthy innovations are only briefly mentioned in this paragraph. For the dispersion of adhesive mixtures, the division of the total drug mass in single particles and small agglomerates and their spatial distribution over the carrier surface are of utmost importance. Recently, it has been shown that coherent anti-stokes Raman spectroscopy (CARS) (Fussell et al. 2014), X-ray photoelectron spectroscopy (XPS), and time of flight secondary ion mass spectroscopy (TOF-SIMS) (Wang et al. 2016) can become useful techniques for studying these aspects. However, increasing the resolution and refining the data processing and interpretation are necessary. For device design and development, computer aided design (CAD) and manufacturing (CAM) have become the standard. Three-dimensional (3D) overnight modeling techniques are frequently applied to produce models for device handling experiments. The manufacturing of DPIs can meet the required high standards thanks to precision molding with high quality tooling. With new computer software being developed, the desire grows to study the entire inhalation process in silico. Computational fluid dynamics (CFD) and discrete element method (DEM) models have been used to study the effect of inhaler design modifications on their performance (e.g. Coates et al. 2004, 2006; Leung et al. 2016). As already mentioned in Paragraph 19.5 CFD and large eddy simulation (LES) are also used to simulate dispersion of adhesive mixtures during inhalation (Cui et al. 2014; van Wachem et al. 2017), particle deposition in the lungs (e.g. Horemans et al. 2012), and the effect of drug deposition on airway geometry and resistance (e.g. de Backer et al. 2011). These studies benefit from the developments in airway imaging techniques like (high-resolution) computed tomography, (HR)CT, and combining CT-scans with images from single photon emission computed tomography (SPECT/CT). Computer simulation of processes may give good insight in the importance and role of certain process variables. However, many mechanisms (physical and physiological effects and events) involved in the array of process steps between aerosol generation and the therapeutic effect have still to be further unraveled and understood. Without this understanding, incorrect starting points for the simulations may be chosen and rather meaningless outcomes may be obtained. Therefore, further experimental exploration is inevitable. Testing of inhaler performance during the development phase has received a strong impulse from laser diffraction technique. Although this technique does not yield aerodynamic particle diameters, in contrast with cascade impactors, it enables fast and highly accurate comparative evaluation between the primary PSD of the formulation and the PSD of the aerosol from the inhaler, particularly when no excipients are involved.

19.11 Future Perspectives

Future perspectives for the long term can hardly be given. Yet unforeseen breakthroughs in aerosolization technique may enable applications that are currently even beyond imagination. Much depends also on the affordability, stability, and safety of future inhalation devices. For instance large-scale programs for mass vaccination via the pulmonary route in developing countries, where the need is highest, depend on the availability of cheap devices with stable drug formulations. In most cases this requires dry powder formulations which, in contrast with liquid drug formulations, do not need cold chain solutions for transport, storage, and local distribution. For the short term, the expectations in addition to vaccination seem highest for pulmonary administration of systemically acting drugs and antibiotics against infectious diseases in or via the lungs. Like vaccines, many of the new drugs in development for systemic action are biopharmaceuticals. Also similar to vaccines, they are mostly instable in solution and for that reason preferably administered as inhalation powders. This requires that they are stabilized in sugar glasses which technique increases the inhaled powder mass and volume considerably (Saluja et al. 2010). Also the antibiotics that seem interesting for pulmonary administration against infectious diseases such as tuberculosis are high to extremely high dose. As for vaccines (e.g. against measles, influenza, Q-fever, pertussis, and also tuberculosis), there exists a global need for antibiotics treatment of tuberculosis, including the multi-drug- and extensively drug-resistant phenotypes, and other infectious lung diseases. Particularly against drug-resistant strains, inhalation may offer new possibilities as bacterial resistance depends on whether the minimum inhibitory concentration (MIC-value) for the antibiotic can be achieved or not. Via the pulmonary route much higher local drug concentrations can be achieved without increasing the adverse systemic side effects compared to oral and parenteral administration. For many applications the inhalers are preferably disposable, particularly when the drug formulation is hygroscopic or the administration is one-off, as for vaccination. Safety, efficacy, and reliability are served best with simple devices with a highly patient-independent delivery. To this purpose, various conditions must be met. The steps to prepare and operate the inhaler must be simple too and small in number for maximal compliance with the instructions and adherence to the therapy. Compliance and adherence are both efficacy and safety aspects, particularly when antibiotics and vaccines are involved. This includes that the inhalation requires acceptable inspiratory effort to the patient and that the number of inhalations per single dose is minimized. Correct inhaler use must also be intuitive, particularly when well skilled health care personnel are absent for instructions. The aerosol properties must compensate for the flow rate; a finer aerosol or a larger fine particle dose needs to be delivered at a higher flow rate. And, finally, to keep DPIs affordable for a wide population of patients, their design and production costs must be low.

REFERENCES

Begat P, Morton DAV, J Shur et al. 2009. The role of force control agents in high-dose dry powder inhaler formulations. *J Pharm Sci* 98: 2770–2783.

Begat P, Morton DAV, JN Staniforth et al. 2004. The cohesion-adhesion balance in dry powder inhaler formulations I: Direct quantification by atomic force microscopy. *Pharm Res* 21: 1591–1597.

Bell JH, Hartley PS, and JSG Cox. 1971. Dry powder aerosols I: A new powder inhalation device. *J Pharm Sci* 60: 1559–1564.

Calvert G, Ghadir M, and R Tweedie. 2009. Aerodynamic dispersion of cohesive powders: A review of understanding and technology. *Adv Powd Technol* 20: 4–16.

Coates MS, Fletcher DF, H-K Chan et al. 2004. Effect of design on the performance of a dry powder inhaler using computational fluid dynamics. Part 1: Grid structure and mouthpiece length. *J Pharm Sci* 93: 2863–2876.

Coates MS, and HK Chan. 2006. Effect of design on the performance of a dry powder inhaler using computational fluid dynamics. Part 2: Air inlet size. *J Pharm Sci* 95: 1382–1392.

Corradi M, Chrystyn H, BG Cosio et al. 2014. NEXThaler, an innovative dry powder inhaler delivering an extrafine fixed combination of beclomethasone and formoterol to treat large and small airways in asthma. *Exp Opin Drug Deliv* 11:1497–1506.

Cui Y, Schmalfuss S, S Zellnitz et al. 2014. Towards the optimisation and adaption of dry powder inhalers. *Int J Pharm* 470: 120–132.

Das SC, Behara SRB, JB Bullita et al. 2012. Powder strength distributions for understanding de-agglomeration of lactose powders. *Pharm Res* 29: 2926–2935.

De Backer LA, Vos WG, R Salgado et al. 2011. Functional imaging using computer methods to compare the effect of salbutamol and ipratropium bromide in patient-specific airway models of COPD. *Int J COPD* 6: 637–646.

de Boer AH, Chan HK, and R Price. 2012. A critical view on lactose-based drug formulation and device studies for dry powder inhalation: Which are relevant and what interactions to expect? *Adv Drug Deliv Rev* 64: 257–274.

de Boer AH, Gjaltema D, P Hagedoorn et al. 2004. Comparative in vitro performance evaluation of the Novopulmon® 200 Novolizer® and Budesonid-ratiopharm® Jethaler: Two novel budesonide dry powder inhalers. *Pharmazie* 59: 692–699.

de Boer AH, Hagedoorn P, D Gjaltema et al. 2003. Air classifier technology (ACT) in dry powder inhalation Part 1: Introduction of a novel force distribution concept (FDC) explaining the performance of a basic air classifier on adhesive mixtures. *Int J Pharm* 260: 187–200.

de Boer AH, Hagedoorn P, PPH Le Brun et al. 2006. Design and in vitro performance testing of multiple air classifier technology in a new disposable inhaler concept (Twincer) for high powder doses. *Eur J Pharm Sci* 28: 171–178.

Dellamary LA, Tarara TE, BJ Smith et al. 2000. Hollow porous particles in metered dose inhalers. *Pharm Res* 17: 168–174.

Demoly P, Hagedoorn P, AH de Boer et al. 2014. The clinical relevance of dry powder inhaler performance for drug delivery. *Resp Med* 108: 1195–1203.

Dickhoff BHJ, de Boer AH, D Lambregts et al. 2003. The effect of carrier surface and bulk properties on drug particle detachment from crystalline lactose carrier particles during inhalation, as function of carrier payload and mixing time. *Eur J Pharm Biopharm* 56: 291–302.

Duddu SP, Sisk SA, YH Walter et al. 2002. Improved lung delivery from a passive dry powder inhaler using an engineered PulmoSphere powder. *Pharm Res* 19: 689–695.

Edwards DA, Hanes J, G Caponetti et al. 1997. Large porous particles for pulmonary drug delivery. *Science (AAAS)* 276: 1868–1871.

Flament M-P, Leterne P, and A Gayot. 2004. The influence of carrier roughness on adhesion, content uniformity and the in vitro deposition of terbutaline sulphate from dry powder inhalers. *Int J Pharm* 275: 201–209.

Fussell AL, Grasmeijer F, HW Frijlink et al. 2014. CARS microscopy as a tool for studying the distribution of micronized drugs in adhesive mixtures for inhalation. *J Raman Spectrosc* 45: 495–500.

Grasmeijer F, and AH de Boer. 2014b. The dispersion behaviour of dry powder inhalation formulations cannot be assessed at a single flow rate. *Int J Pharm* 465: 165–168.

Grasmeijer F, Grasmeijer N, P Hagedoorn et al. 2015. Recent advances in the fundamental understanding of adhesive mixtures for inhalation. *Curr Pharm Des* 21: 5900–5914.

Grasmeijer F, Hagedoorn P, HW Frijlink et al. 2013a. Drug content effects on the dispersion performance of adhesive mixtures for inhalation. *PLoS One* 8: e71339.

Grasmeijer F, Hagedoorn P, HW Frijlink et al. 2013b. Mixing time effects on the dispersion performance of adhesive mixtures for inhalation. *PLoS One* 8: e69263.

Grasmeijer F, Lexmond AJ, M van den Noort et al. 2014a. New mechanisms to explain the effects of added lactose fines on the dispersion performance of adhesive mixtures for inhalation. *PLoS One* 9: e87825.

Hagedoorn P, Grasmeijer F, M Hoppentocht et al. 2016. In vitro evaluation of the Twincer colistin dry powder inhaler as a non-cough inducing alternative to Colobreathe. *Eur Respir J* 48(Suppl 60): PA2561.

Han R, Papadopoulos G, and BJ Greenspan. 2002. Investigation of powder dispersion inside a Spiros® dry powder inhaler using particle image velocimetry. *Powd Technol* 125: 266–278.

Harper NJ, Gray S, J De Groot et al. 2007. The design and performance of the Exubera pulmonary insulin delivery system. *Diabetes Technol Ther* 9(Suppl 1): S16–S27.

Heinemann L. 2008. The failure of Exubera: Are we beating a dead horse? *J Diabetes Sci Technol* 2: 517–529.

Hersey JA. 1975. Ordered mixing: A new concept in powder mixing practice. *Powd Technol* 11: 41–44.

Hickey AJ, Concessio NM, MM Van Oort et al. 1994. Factors influencing the dispersion of dry powders as aerosols. *Pharm Technol* 18: 58–82.

Hickey AJ, Mansour HM, MJ Telko et al. 2007a. Physical characterization of component particles included in dry powder inhalers. I. Strategy review and static characteristics. *J Pharm Sci* 96: 1282–1301.

Hickey AJ, Mansour HM, MJ Telko et al. 2007b. Physical characterization of component particles included in dry powder inhalers. II. Dynamic characteristics. *J Pharm Sci* 96: 1302–1319.

Hinds WC. 1982. *Aerosol Technology. Properties, Behavior, and Measurement of Airborne Particles.* New York: John Wiley & Sons, pp. 127–132.

Hooton JC, Jones MD, and R Price. 2006. Predicting the behaviour of novel sugar carriers for dry powder inhaler formulations via the use of a cohesive-adhesive balance approach. *J Pharm Sci* 95: 1288–1297.

Horemans B, Van Holsbeke C, W Vos et al. 2012. Particle deposition in airways of chronic respiratory patients exposed to an urban aerosol. *Environ Sci Technol* 46: 12162–12169.

Jones MD, and R Price. 2006. The influence of fine particle excipients on the performance of carrier-based dry powder inhalation formulations. *Pharm Res* 23: 1665–1674.

Jones MD, Santo JGF, B Yakub et al. 2010. The relationship between drug concentration, mixing time, blending order and ternary dry powder inhalation performance. *Int J Pharm* 391: 137–147.

Kawashima Y, Serigano T, Y Hino et al. 1998. Effect of surface morphology of carrier lactose on dry powder inhalation property of pranlukast hydrate. *Int J Pharm* 172: 179–188.

Kousaka Y, Okuyama K, A Shimizu et al. 1979. Dispersion mechanism of aggregate particles in air. *J Chem Eng Japan* 12: 152–159.

Kulvanich P, and PJ Stewart. 1987a. The effect of particle size and concentration on the adhesive characteristics of a model drug-carrier interactive system. *J Pharm Pharmacol* 39: 673–678.

Kulvanich P, and PJ Stewart. 1987b. The effect of blending time on particle adhesion in a model interactive system. *J Pharm Pharmacol* 39: 732–733.

Leung CM, Tong Z, QT Zhou et al. 2016. Understanding the different effects of inhaler design on the aerosol performance of drug-only and carrier-based DPI formulations. Part 1: Grid structure. *AAPS J* 18: 1159–1167.

Lipp MM, and JC Sung. 2015. Monovalent metal cation dry powders for inhalation. US patent 0231066A1.

Lippmann M, Yeates DB, and RE Albert. 1980. Deposition, retention and clearance of inhaled particles. *British J Inhaled Med* 37: 337–361.

Lucas P, Anderson K, and J Staniforth. 1998. Protein deposition from dry powder inhalers: Fine particle multiplets as performance modifiers. *Pharm Res* 15: 562–569.

Marriott C, and HW Frijlink. 2012. Lactose as a carrier for inhalation products: Breathing new life into an old carrier. *Adv Drug Deliv Rev* 64: 217–219.

Miller-Larsson A, and O Selroos. 2006. Advances in asthma and COPD treatment: Combination therapy with inhaled corticosteroids and long acting beta2-agonists. *Curr Pharm Des* 12: 3261–3279.

Montuschi P, Malerba M, G Macis et al. 2016. Triple inhaled therapy for chronic obstructive pulmonary disease. *Drug Discov Today* 21: 1820–1827.

Newman SP, and WW Busse. 2002. Evolution of dry powder inhaler design, formulation and performance. *Resp Med* 96: 293–304.

Noymer P, Meyers D, M Glazer et al. 2010. The staccato system: Inhaler design characteristics for rapid treatment of CNS disorders. *Resp Drug Deliv* 1: 11–20.

Pilcer G, and K Amighi. 2010. Formulation strategy and use of excipients in pulmonary drug delivery. *Int J Pharm* 392: 1–19.

Pilcher J, Shirtcliffe P, M Patel et al. 2015. Three-month validation of a Turbuhaler electronic monitoring device: Implications for asthma clinical trial use. *BMJ Open Resp Res* doi:10.1136/bmjresp-2015-000097.

Rehman M, Shekunov BY, P York et al. 2004. Optimisation of powders for pulmonary delivery using supercritical fluid technology. *Eur J Pharm Sci* 22: 1–17.

Richardson PC, and AH Boss. 2007. Technosphere insulin technology. *Diabetes Technol Ther* 9: S65–S72.

Saluja V, Amorij J-P, JC Kapteyn et al. 2010. A comparison between spray drying and freeze drying to produce an influenza subunit vaccine for inhalation. *J Control Release* 144: 127–133.

Sanders M. 2007. Inhalation therapy: A historical review. *Prim Care Respir J* 16: 71–81.

Shoyele SA, and S Cawthorne. 2006. Particle engineering techniques for inhaled biopharmaceuticals. *Adv Drug Deliv Rev* 58: 1009–1029.

Sitz R. 2010. Current innovations in dry powder inhalers. *Ondrugdelivery* 10–12. Available from www.ondrugdelivery.com.

Stahlhofen W, Rudolf G, and AJ James. 1989. Intercomparison of experimental regional aerosol deposition data. *J Aerosol Med* 2: 285–308.

Staniforth JN. 1981. Total mixing. *Int J Pharm Tech & Prod Mfr* 2: 7–12.

Staniforth JN. 1987. Order out of chaos. *J Pharm Pharmacol* 39: 329–334.

Steiss JO, Heckmann M, B Jödicke et al. 2007. A new breath actuated dry powder inhaler (Auto-jethaler). *Klin Pädiatrie* 219: 66–69.

Tee SK, Marriott C, XM Zeng et al. 2000. The use of different sugars as fine and coarse carriers for aerosolized salbutamol sulphate. *Int J Pharm* 208: 111–123.

Tian G, Longest PW, X Li et al. 2013. Targeting aerosol deposition to and within the lung airways using excipient enhanced growth. *J Aerosol Med Pulm Drug Deliv* 26: 248–265.

Travers DN, and White RC. 1971. The mixing of micronized sodium bicarbonate with sucrose crystals. *J Pharm Pharmacol* 23: 260S–261S.

Usmani OS, Biddiscombe MF, and PJ Barnes. 2005. Regional lung deposition and bronchodilator response as a function of β_2-agonist particle size. *Am J Respir Crit Care Med* 172: 1497–1504.

van Wachem B, Thalberg K, J Remmelgas et al. 2017. Simulation of dry powder inhalers: Combining micro-scale, meso-scale and macro-scale modeling. *AIChE J* 63: 501–506.

Vehring R. 2008. Pharmaceutical particle engineering via spray drying. *Pharm Res* 25: 999–1022.

Visser J. 1989. Van der Waals and other cohesive forces affecting powder fluidization. *Powd Technol* 58: 1–10.

Wang W, Zhou QT, and SP Sun. 2016. Effects of surface composition on the aerosolisation and dissolution of inhaled antibiotic combination powders consisting of colistin and rifampicin. *AAPS J* 18: 371–384.

Weers JG, and DP Miller. 2015. Formulation design of dry powders for inhalation. *J Pharm Sci* 104: 3259–3288.

Westerman EM, Le Brun PPH, DJ Touw et al. 2004. Effect of nebulized colistin sulphate and colistin sulphomethate on lung function in patients with cystic fibrosis: A pilot study. *J Cyst Fibros* 3: 23–28.

Wetterlin K. 1979. Aerosol inhalation device. US-patent 4,137,914.

Young PM, Cocconi D, P Colombo et al. 2002. Characterization of a surface modified dry powder inhalation carrier prepared by "particle smoothing." *J Pharm Pharmacol* 54: 1339–1344.

Young PM, Crapper J, G Philips et al. 2014. Overcoming dose limitations using the Orbital multi-breath dry powder inhaler. *J Aerosol Med Pulm Drug Del* 27: 138–147.

Young PM, Edge S, D Traini et al. 2005. The influence of dose on the performance of dry powder inhalation systems. *Int J Pharm* 296: 26–33.

Young PM, Sung A, D Traini et al. 2007. Influence of humidity on the electrostatic charge and aerosol performance of dry powder inhaler carrier based system. *Pharm Res* 24: 963–970.

20

Nebulizers

John N. Pritchard, Dirk von Hollen, and Ross H.M. Hatley

CONTENTS

20.1 A Brief History of Nebulizers

The nebulizer has a long history of use for the administration of aerosols to the lungs, following the production of devices such as the Sales-Girons nebulizer in the late 1850s (Anderson 2005, Dessanges 2001). Early devices were often made of glass and powered by a rubber hand-bulb compressor (Grossman 1994). However, these devices produced aerosol droplets/particles that were often too large to reach the lower airways and delivered varying amounts of solution with each squeeze of the hand-bulb (Nikander and Saunders 2010). The production of alternating current (AC) powered electric compressors in the 1930s (Sanders 2007), which could produce a greater, more consistent flow of compressed air, and the introduction of durable plastic nebulizers, turned the jet nebulizer into a reliable piece of medical equipment capable of consistent generation of aerosol droplets/particles of a size suitable for delivery to the lungs (Rau 2005). Compressor-powered jet nebulizers subsequently became the delivery system of choice for inhaled medications until the mid 20th century when they were overtaken by the introduction of portable inhalers. Dry powder inhalers (DPIs) were introduced in the late 1940s (Pritchard 2015a, Inhalatorium) and pressurized metered dose inhalers (pMDIs) in 1956 (Dolovich et al. 2005). The obvious advantages of pocket-sized portable inhalers that could deliver doses of aerosol within seconds might have led to the eradication of the nebulizer as an aerosol delivery option. However, aerosol delivery via nebulizer still confers some significant advantages over portable inhalers such as pMDIs and DPIs. Nebulizers can be used by a wider range of patients as delivery is usually accomplished using tidal breathing, so fine motor skills and coordination of complicated breathing maneuvers are not required for correct use (Taffet et al. 2014). This led to the nebulizer remaining the preferred aerosol drug delivery modality for the very young and the very old. Nebulizers have also become the device of choice in specialized treatment areas such as cystic fibrosis and pulmonary hypertension where the patient numbers are smaller and delivered doses are higher. From a pharmaceutical development viewpoint, nebulizers are capable of delivering a larger range of doses, formulations are easier to develop for early stage clinical trials in drug development and are more likely to be used when commercializing drugs for niche patient groups (Pritchard 2015a). Recently, market trends in the Far East have led to increasing use of nebulized therapy for aerosol delivery to the lungs (Pritchard 2017).

20.2 Current Types of Nebulizer

The process of spraying a liquid in aerosol form into a gas for inhalation can be achieved by a number of different mechanisms (Ari 2015). The key requirement is that the size of the droplets produced by the aerosolization process be such that they will penetrate the upper airways and deposit in the smaller airways and periphery of the lungs (Chapter 2 Aerosol Critical Attributes). The three main types of nebulizer technology currently available to patients all use different mechanisms of aerosol generation, these mechanisms of aerosol generation are described in the sections below. Table 20.1 shows the key characteristics of each type of nebulizer (Figure 20.1). In recent years another class of liquid aerosol delivery device has been developed, namely, the soft mist inhaler. Soft mist inhalers differ from nebulizers in that the aerosol dose is delivered in between 1 breath and 3 breaths, and they contain an integral multi-dose drug cartridge, which may be replaceable. Soft mist inhalers are dealt with in Chapter 21.

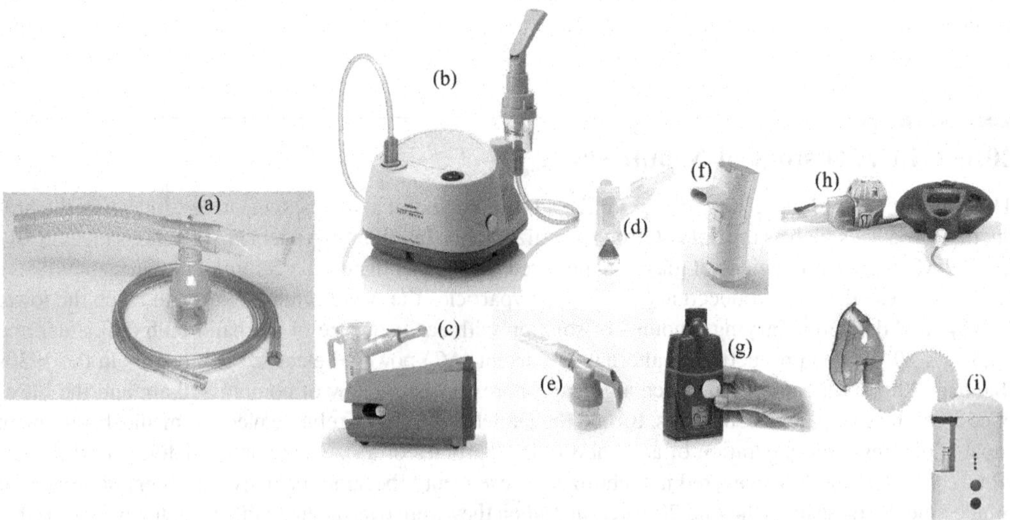

FIGURE 20.1 Montage of different types of nebulizer, photos shown to approximately similar scale. (a) Salter 8900 conventional nebulizer with T piece and tubing, (b) Philips SideStream open vent nebulizer shown with InnoSpire Elegance compressor, (c) Pari LC Plus breath-enhanced nebulizer shown with compact compressor, (d) Salter NebuTech breath-enhanced nebulizer, (e) Philips SideStream Plus breath-enhanced nebulizer, (f) Philips InnoSpire Go mesh nebulizer, (g) Philips I-neb AAD System breath activated mesh nebulizer, (h) Pari eFlow rapid mesh nebulizer, and (i) Mabis Mist II ultrasonic nebulizer with tubing and mask. (Salter images courtesy of Salter Labs, Philips images courtesy of Respironics Respiratory Drug Delivery (UK) Ltd, Pari images courtesy of Pari GmbH, and Mabis Mist II image by Irina Rogova, shutterstock.com.)

TABLE 20.1

Key Features of Jet, Ultrasonic, and Mesh Nebulizers

Type	Features	Advantages	Disadvantages
Jet	Most common and the cheapest form of nebulizer in any market Almost all models are general purpose nebulizers designed for delivery of general purpose drugs such as short-acting beta$_2$ agonists and corticosteroids. Piston compressor supplies air for nebulization, a jet of compressed air entrains the liquid drug and produces a polydisperse aerosol, only about 5% of the aerosol is respirable, the remainder is removed by impaction and returned to the reservoir. This multiple cycle generation process is inherently inefficient. Medication cooled during nebulization Requires baffles to aid droplet breakup. Large minimum fill volume (~2 mL) Power requirement ~50 W–250 W Cleaning is typically rinse after each use and boil wash weekly Nebulizer replacement typically after 30 days (disposable) or 6 months (durable)	Relatively insensitive to changes in viscosity/surface tension Insensitive to changes in osmolality Classed as general purpose nebulizers that can be used interchangeably with drugs approved for nebulization	Limited portability (alternating current or large battery pack required) Heavy and bulky (compressor/tubes/nebulizer) Loud noise when operating Typically long treatment times (10 minutes–15 minutes) Concentration of medication can increase over time due to evaporation Large residual volume (1 mL–1.5 mL) Performance depends on compressor/nebulizer pairing Large variability in dose delivery between different makes/models Many parts to clean/maintain (compressor including air filter/tubes/nebulizer)
Ultrasonic	Electricity powers piezo element for nebulization via fountain Requires baffles to exclude large droplets from aerosol output Medication heated during nebulization Large residual volume (1 mL–1.5 mL) Drug released to environment during exhalation Particle sizes approximately 4 µm–7 µm (salbutamol) Ultrasonic waves in KHz transmitted into the liquid drug formulation Power requirement ~50 W	Portable (AC or battery) Faster than jet nebulizers, shorter treatment times Quieter than jet nebulizers	Not suitable for suspension formulations Unsuitable for thermolabile medications due to medication heating Few treatments from one charge/set of batteries Need to replace coupling liquid on a (daily/weekly) basis
Mesh	Model determines whether used with general purpose only or also with model specific drugs (drug–device combination) Piezo element vibrates the mesh, this vibration pumps liquid drug through the mesh, the liquid is emitted from the mesh in droplets generating the aerosol, and nominally 100% of the aerosol produced by the mesh is respirable No baffles—Aerosol generation on 1st pass Low minimum fill volume (0.3 mL–2 mL) Power requirement ~1.5 W Cleaning regimes vary widely depending on model, but typically comprise rinse after use, wash daily, and boil weekly, often using distilled water Mesh replacement typically after 6 or 12 months	Portable (AC or battery) Energy efficient—Many treatments from 1 charge/set of batteries Fast (high output rate), short treatment times (3 minutes–10 minutes) Possibility of low residual volume (0.1 mL–1.25 mL) Quiet Electronic platform allows inclusion of advanced drug delivery features (breath activated/feedback/adherence) Few parts to clean/maintain Continuity of care using the same aerosol generator Drug subjected to low shear and single pass through mesh thereby retaining biological activity of macromolecules Selection of Mass Median Aerodynamic Diameter (MMAD) of aerosol output possible	Some models only available for specific drugs (drug-device combinations) Potential for loss of performance with inadequate cleaning regime (liquids that crystalize when dried) Performance can be formulation dependent

20.2.1 Jet Nebulizers

Jet nebulizers rely upon compressed gas, supplied either via a piston compressor or typically in hospitals via gas piped from compressed gas cylinders (Ari 2012). The gas at high pressure is fed into the nebulizer, and passes through a narrow orifice, where the gas velocity increases, and it is emitted from the orifice as a fast moving jet of air, which causes a reduction in atmospheric air pressure near the orifice due to mixing of the stationary air in the immediate vicinity of the orifice with the fast moving jet. Jet nebulizers capitalize on this reduction in air pressure by positioning a liquid feed tube, which extends down to the liquid reservoir; the liquid is thus pushed up the tube and entrained into the fast moving jet of air, the fast moving air breaks up the liquid into droplets as a result of turbulence. These droplets are polydisperse in size, typically with a mass median diameter in the range 16 µm–400 µm (Nerbrink et al. 1994), and the majority of the mass of the liquid aerosolized in this way is far too large to avoid inertial impaction both on the walls of the nebulizer and baffles placed some distance from the jet to ensure that these large droplets do not exit the nebulizer. The large droplets hit the baffles, coalesce, and are returned to the fluid reservoir as a constant stream of liquid, to be sucked back up the liquid uptake tube and repeat the process of aerosol generation. In this process, only about 5% of the liquid is in smaller droplets (<10 µm) which are carried by the airflow past the baffles and can exit the nebulizer. In a conventional jet nebulizer, the only flow for carrying the aerosol droplets out of the nebulizer is the flow supplied to the jet of the nebulizer, which is typically between 6 L/min–8 L/min. This relatively low flow means the small aerosol droplets have time to coalesce with other droplets, reducing the output efficiency of small droplets. The constant recirculation of liquid droplets back to the reservoir gives rise to a number of undesirable consequences. The first of these is that the exposure of such a large surface area of the liquid to the air passing through the nebulizer cup leads to evaporation of the liquid and, hence, concentration of the drug formulation dissolved or suspended in the liquid over the course of nebulization (Mercer et al. 1968). The second, which is dependent upon the design of the nebulizer, relates to the fate of the droplets that are not carried out of the nebulizer by the airflow. As described earlier, these droplets will impact the baffles and walls of the nebulizer, but may be trapped on the walls of the nebulizer and will form part of the residual volume of drug left in the nebulizer cup at the end of nebulization. The amount thus trapped will depend upon the internal surface area of the nebulizer and the surface tension of the drug formulation (Smye et al. 1991) and typically lies between 1 mL–1.5 mL (Elphick et al. 2015). The open vent jet nebulizer is a development of the conventional jet nebulizer that uses the low pressure in the vicinity of the jet to dual effect; in addition to entraining liquid from the feed tube, the same low pressure is used to draw ambient air into the nebulizer via a specially incorporated flow-path, typically increasing the total output flow from 6 L/min to 16 L/min (Shah et al. 1997). This reduces the residence time of small droplets in the nebulizer and thus reduces the chance of coalescence. A further increase in airflow through the nebulizer can be achieved with breath-enhanced nebulizers, these use a pair of one way valves to allow the patient to inhale through the nebulizer; but direct exhaled flow away from the nebulizer (O'Callaghan and Barry 1997). As patient inhalation flows are typically in the region of 0 L/min–90 L/min (Nikander and Denyer 2000), this increases the aerosol output still further, and this type of design has been adopted by a number of jet mesh nebulizer manufacturers (Gardenhire et al. 2013). Although this design boosts aerosol output during inhalation, in common with conventional and open vent nebulizers, aerosol output continues during exhalation (Figure 20.2), which leads to a large amount of wasted drug. The solution to drug waste during exhalation was provided by the breath-activated jet nebulizer (Leung et al. 2004). Breath-activated nebulizers only generate aerosol during the inspiratory portion of patient breathing. The most common type of breath-activated jet nebulizer uses the pressure difference created by inspiratory flow through the nebulizer to actuate a diaphragm that moves a pin down to above the jet orifice. Air is then deflected past the liquid feed tube and aerosol generation occurs in a similar way to the jet nebulizers described earlier. As actuation is dependent upon the patient's inhalation flow, this type of breath-activated nebulizer is unsuitable for patients with low inhalation flows (Rubin 2011).

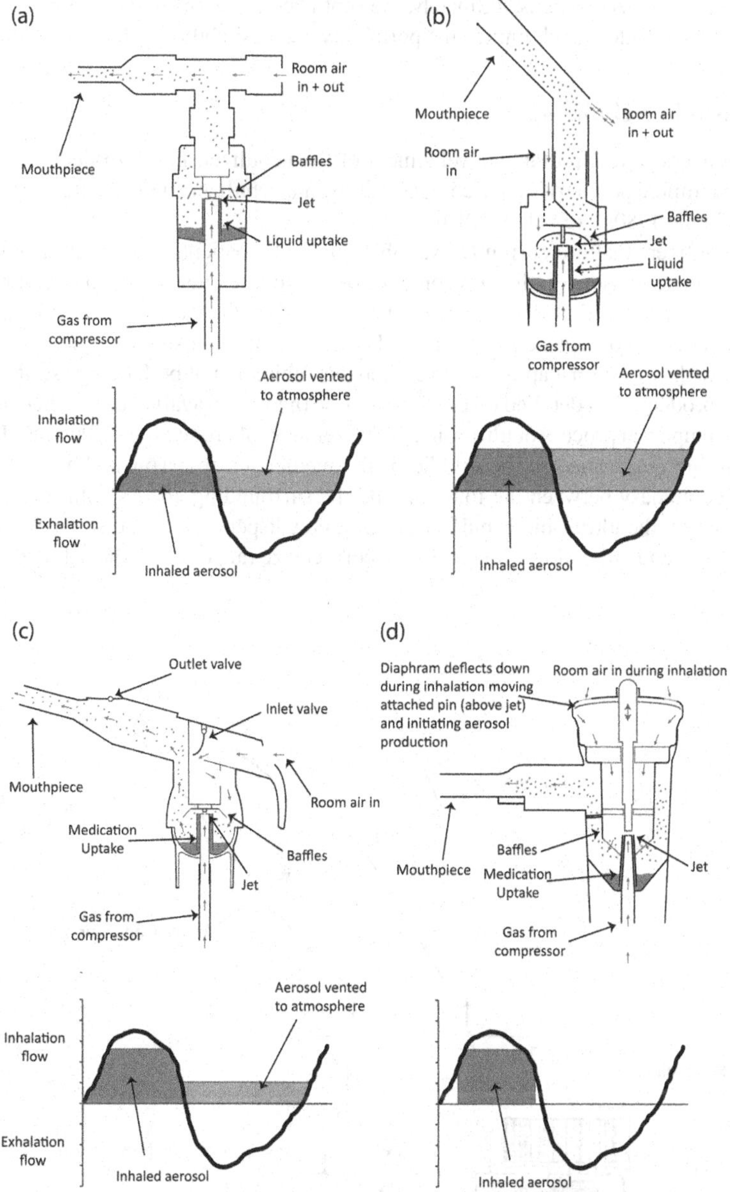

FIGURE 20.2 Main sub-types of jet nebulizer (a) conventional, (b) open vent, (c) breath–enhanced, and (d) breath–activated.

Jet nebulizers are prone to wear of the jet orifice (Nerbrink and Dahlbäck 1994) and require regular cleaning to prevent blockage of the jet. Although such cleaning should ensure reproducible performance over the recommended life of the nebulizer (Standaert et al. 1998), patients often fail to comply with cleaning, replacement, and maintenance recommendations of both nebulizer and the compressor used to supply the compressed air (Boyter and Carter 2005). Despite the improvements from conventional through to breath-activated jet nebulizer designs, ultimately, the continued requirement for a bulky compressor driven by either AC or a large battery pack limited the portability and desirability of the jet nebulizer.

20.2.2 Ultrasonic Nebulizers

Ultrasonic nebulizers were a portable development of the nebulizer, first introduced in 1949, however, they only gained limited popularity once compact ultrasonic nebulizers with a battery life of several days were produced in the 1980s (Yeo et al. 2010).

Ultrasonic nebulizers that are currently available for use by patients rely on ultrasonic waves generated by a piezoelectric transducer; the ultrasonic waves are focused inside a reservoir of medication, and aerosol droplets are produced at the surface of the medication. Generally, the piezo element is a fixed part of the design that is not replaced by the user. The precise mechanism of droplet formation is subject to some debate, with cavitation, capillary waves, and a combination of both being ascribed to be responsible for aerosol production; a detailed discussion of these theories is available elsewhere (Rau 2002, Yeo et al. 2010). The empirical process of ultrasonic nebulizer aerosol production is illustrated in Figure 20.3, which shows a fountain formed in the middle of the medication reservoir and aerosol droplets being produced at the boundary between the fountain and the surrounding air. As with the jet nebulizer, the droplets produced by the ultrasonic nebulizer are of a polydisperse size, and so baffles are required to classify the droplets and only allow droplets in the correct size range to exit the nebulizer. Unlike the jet

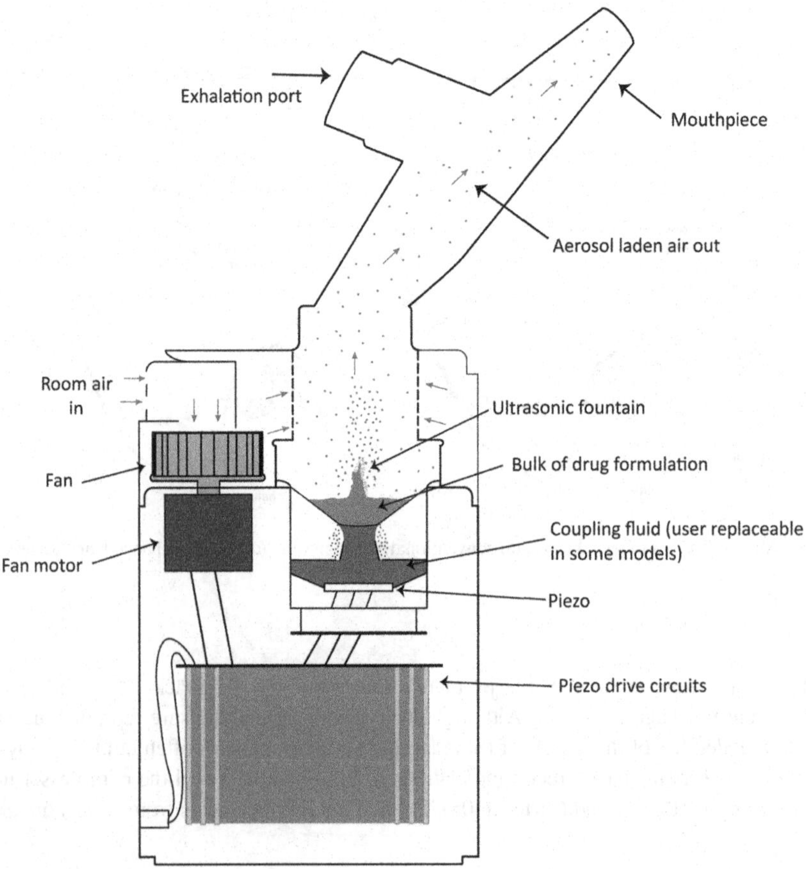

FIGURE 20.3 Ultrasonic nebulizer.

nebulizer, there is no driving flow of gas, so the aerosol droplets produced in the vicinity of the fountain are generally transported to the exit of the nebulizer by a current of air generated by an internal fan (Hess 2000). The ultimate popularity of ultrasonic nebulizers was hampered by the inefficiency of the nebulization of suspensions (Nikander et al. 1999) and the heating of the fluid within the nebulizer cup during nebulization that could damage thermolabile drugs (Rau 2002).

20.2.3 Mesh Nebulizers

It was not until the mesh nebulizer was introduced to the market in the mid 1990s that nebulizer technology was revolutionized by providing a portable, quiet, and efficient means of nebulizing aqueous drug formulations. Mesh nebulizers also rely on a piezoelectric transducer for creation of the aerosol droplets, but instead of using the power of the ultrasonic waves to break the surface of the liquid apart, the vibrations from the piezo are used in combination with a fine mesh constructed of a thin substrate punctured with many holes. At the time of publication, the two main methods for mesh production were electroplating and laser cutting techniques; both are used to produce a tapered hole. A tapered hole is required to optimize mesh performance it amplifies flow at the nozzle and reduces viscous losses. The electroplating method relies on the use of a lithographic plate, and the eventual size of the mesh holes is determined by the duration of the electroplating process; the holes get smaller as the metal is deposited on the edge of the hole over time. Laser cutting involves the use of a laser beam to cut the mesh holes in a thin sheet of metal or polymer material; laser cutting metal can result in molten material being deposited around the hole, which is then removed by electropolishing. Most mesh nebulizer meshes are constructed from either metal alloy or ceramic materials, to give the rigidity, mass, durability, and inert chemical properties required for the aerosolization of different drug formulations, though some manufacturers have opted for laser drilled polymer meshes.

Mesh nebulizers can be divided into two sub-types, passive and active, and two different geometries of mesh are generally used. Passive mesh nebulizers use a horn connected to the piezoelectric transducer, the other end of the horn is located in close proximity to the mesh, with a thin fluid layer between them; vibrations are conducted through the horn and fluid layer to the mesh. The vibrations are associated with an alternating cycle of pressure in the liquid behind the mesh which first causes a column of liquid to be extruded from the front of the mesh and, as the pressure cycle reverses, the end of the column separates as a liquid droplet. This process results in much more efficient conversion of input energy into the creation of the surface energy of the droplets, meaning that mesh nebulizers can be powered by small batteries. The size of the droplet is approximately twice the size of the mesh hole, as predicted in Rayleigh's theory (Rayleigh 1878). Most passive mesh nebulizers use a flat mesh geometry (Figure 20.4a); only the mesh is replaced during use, the piezo lasts the life of the nebulizer. Active mesh nebulizers generally involve the piezo element being bonded directly to the mesh substrate, which is in contact with a reservoir of fluid; the piezo vibrates the mesh directly and an alternating pressure cycle is induced which pushes the fluid through the holes in the mesh (Figure 20.4b). Both the piezo element and mesh that it is bonded to are replaced after a period of use. Many active mesh nebulizers use a domed mesh geometry because the rigidity of the mesh structure is important to prevent oscillations of varying amplitude across the surface of the mesh, which could result in inconsistent aerosolization performance (Figure 20.4c).

Because size of the aerosol droplets generated at the surface of the mesh is dictated primarily by the size of the holes in the mesh, the aerosol droplets created have a much smaller range in size compared with the primary droplets created by jet and ultrasonic nebulizers. The aerosol is created in a "1st pass" through the mesh, and baffles are not required to remove large droplets, and there is no recirculation of liquid past the point of aerosol generation as is seen with jet and ultrasonic nebulizers. The low energy consumption required to vibrate the piezo element, combined with the efficient 1st pass aerosol generation, means that mesh nebulizers can be designed as small handheld units that are virtually silent in operation. The lack of baffles and other impaction surfaces combined with the fact that drug solution lies adjacent to, or on top of the mesh, and that the mesh holes are micron-sized, means that mesh nebulizers can aerosolize virtually all of the solution placed into the drug chamber, resulting in smaller residual volumes than jet or ultrasonic nebulizers (Elphick et al. 2015).

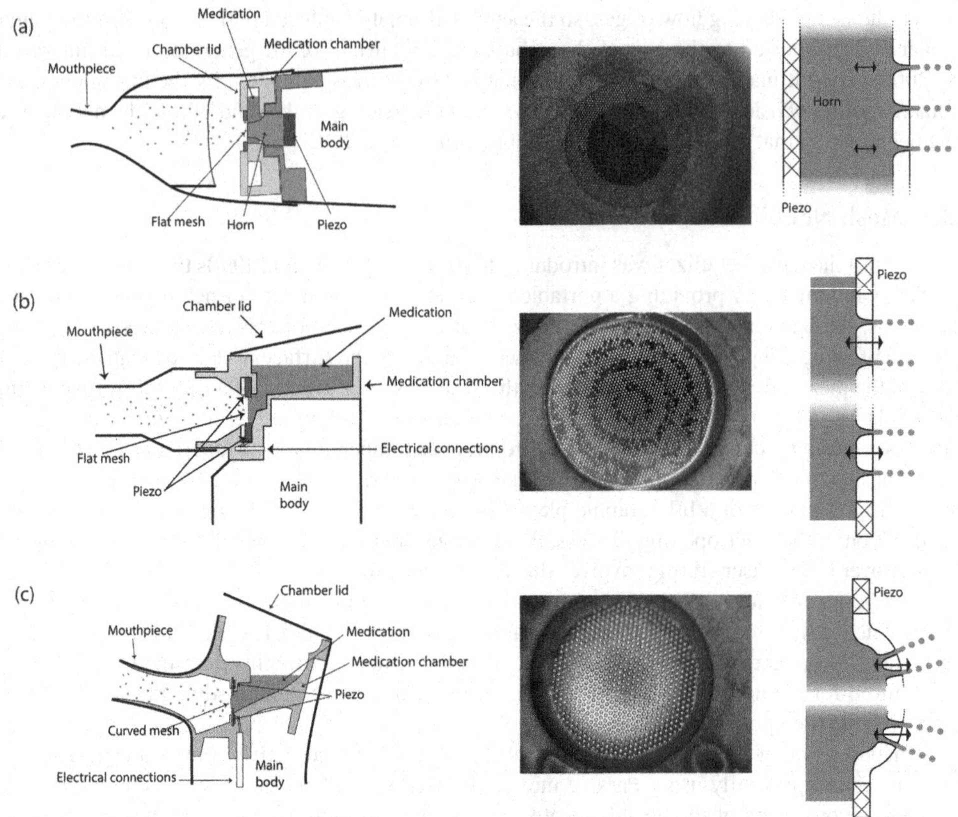

FIGURE 20.4 Three designs of mesh nebulizer (a) passive flat mesh, (b) active flat mesh, and (c) active curved mesh. All have removable medication chambers for mesh replacement, but as the piezo is included in the main body of the passive design (a), only the mesh is replaced for this type of design. For active mesh nebulizers (b and c), when the mesh is replaced so is the piezo, so an electrical connection is required between the medication chamber and the main body. There are two sizes of mesh holes for the passive mesh design (A middle) with no holes in the centre of the mesh, whereas the active mesh designs use a single hole size across the surface of the mesh.

The mesh nebulizer is not without its limitations compared with other types of nebulizer. The range in surface tension and viscosity of the liquid drug formulations that can be nebulized efficiently is smaller than for jet nebulizers (Pritchard 2017), and the size of the mesh holes precludes nebulization of suspensions in which the size of the smallest axis of the suspended particles are larger than the size of the hole. As with other types of nebulizer, compliance with the recommended cleaning regime is important, as blockage of a number of the mesh holes, through lack of cleaning, can impair performance (Rottier et al. 2009). Concerns over cleaning and nebulization of suspensions have not prevented the popularity of the mesh nebulizer increasing rapidly in recent years (Pritchard et al. 2018).

20.2.4 Advanced Nebulizers

The advantage of the nebulizer in being able to deliver aerosol to all patients via tidal breathing was historically partially offset by the up to tenfold differences in jet nebulizer system performance (Boe et al. 2001), and the wastage of drug due to the large residual which resulted in a larger cost per dose than an inhaler. In combination, these factors inhibited preference for nebulized aerosol delivery for new pharmaceutical developments. Before the advent of mesh nebulizers, this dosing issue was addressed by advanced forms of jet nebulizer such as: (a) the HaloLite and Prodose Adaptive Aerosol

Delivery systems (Denyer and Dyche 2010), that monitored the patient's breathing and only delivered aerosol into inhalation, and (b) the AKITA Jet nebulizer system that delivered aerosol according to a smart card preprogrammed with the patient's optimal inhalation profile (Bennett 2005). Systems such as these allowed repeatable doses of aerosol to be delivered, but involved additional cost of electronics and electro-mechanical control systems to be added to the compressor systems powering the jet nebulizers, and so retained the disadvantages of bulkiness and requirement for an AC power supply, with increased cost of manufacture and sale.

The introduction of mesh technology with its first pass aerosol generation allowed a reduction in the volume of drug required and is built upon a base of micro-electronic control circuitry that is required to generate the frequencies required to operate the piezo element. The inherent micro-processor controlled nature of mesh nebulizer designs offers significant benefits in terms of the cost effective inclusion of advanced features such as, breath activation, automatic detection of end-of-treatment, monitoring inhalation flow, feedback during/after treatment, and the inclusion of recording and feedback of adherence to regimen and compliance with correct use of the device. Some of these features will be examined in further detail below.

20.2.4.1 Features of Advanced Nebulizers

The primary strength of the nebulizer in being able to deliver aerosol into the tidal breathing of all patient groups also led to a significant drawback for constant output jet nebulizer designs, i.e. the potential for a large proportion of the aerosolized dose to be wasted to the local atmosphere during patient exhalation (O'Callaghan and Barry 1997). This had significant implications for the magnitude of the dose received by the patient, as well as for caregivers and others in the vicinity of someone receiving nebulized treatment (Gardenhire et al. 2013). The repercussions of aerosol emitted into the local atmosphere are relatively minor for pharmaceutical entities such as beta-agonists, but become more of an issue for drugs such as antibiotics and antivirals (Tsai et al. 2015). Waste of large amounts of drug could also be an issue for expensive pharmaceuticals where the cost of manufacture makes the minimization of fill dose a desirable property. Breath activation ensures that aerosol is only produced during the inspiratory phase of breathing, so eliminating the waste associated with constant output nebulizers. Breath-activated nebulizers are available in both jet and mesh technologies, but the jet variety confers less advantage in delivery efficiency due to the high residual volume of jet nebulizers, and are not suitable for those with insufficient inhalation flow to trigger the mechanism (Rubin 2011). Mesh varieties with low residual volumes and the rapid onset of aerosol generation can utilize the micro-processor control system to incorporate algorithms that optimize delivery of aerosol into the maximum amount of the time spent inhaling, while also stopping aerosol production before the end of the breath to reduce the amount of aerosol exhaled (Denyer and Dyche 2010).

Feedback mechanisms can also be incorporated to provide audible, visual, or even tactile signals to the patient during and after treatment. One example of how feedback can be used to improve both drug delivery during the treatment and the patient experience of the overall treatment is provided by the target inhalation mode (TIM) feature of the I-neb AAD system (Denyer et al. 2010). The feedback mechanisms used in TIM guide the patient via vibrations pulsed down the nebulizer mouthpiece to encourage a long slow inhalation, thereby extending their inhalation cycle up to their individually determined physiologically comfortable level. This has been shown to result in reduced treatment times (McCormack et al. 2011) and aid penetration of the aerosol deep into the lungs (Nikander et al. 2010). Restricting the flowrate at which aerosol is inhaled reduces the momentum of aerosol droplets/particles and, hence, reduces impaction of these droplets/particles within the upper levels of the labyrinthine morphology of the lungs, evolved specifically to filter out particulate pollution. As the volume of a sphere is related to the radius cubed, penetration of larger droplets of drug containing liquid can increase drug delivery significantly. Recent nebulizer developments, such as the Micro (Respironics Respiratory Drug Delivery (United Kingdom) Ltd.) and FOX (Vectura Group plc, Chippenham, United Kingdom) nebulizers, are equipped to monitor the inhalation flow and provide visual feedback to the patient to inform them whether they are inhaling too rapidly or too slowly, to optimize the delivery of aerosol into the lungs.

Indication of end-of-treatment by automatic cessation of aerosol production and audible and visual feedback, which in some models of mesh nebulizer is synonymous with indication that the required dose has been delivered, is also a useful feedback feature. It can result in treatment times that are much shorter than when having to make a highly subjective determination of end of treatment when using jet nebulizers.

The aforementioned advances in the convenience, speed, and efficiency of treatment all help to ensure that the required dose of aerosolized drug reaches the intended target sites in a patient's lungs, but if the patient does not use the device then disease control will obviously suffer (Mäkelä et al. 2013). Adherence with all forms of medication regime has been shown to be low (Sabate 2003), due to a variety of factors (Restrepo et al. 2008), and patients have been shown to struggle at all stages, from collection of the prescription to maintaining a regular dosing schedule (Bårnes and Ulrik 2015). Modern electronic nebulizers also include the facility to record the date and time that treatments are started and whether the treatment was taken to completion (Pritchard and Nicholls 2015). This information can be transmitted to secure servers for access by the patients, clinicians, and support personnel, such as relatives to help identify patterns in missed treatments and find solutions to aid the patient to maintain their treatment regime (Pritchard and Nicholls 2015).

20.3 Current Nebulized Therapies

The advantage of nebulization as a form of aerosol drug delivery is the ease with which aerosol can be inhaled into both tidal breathing and also during an exacerbation. Nebulized therapies are typically used for the domiciliary treatment of patients who may struggle with the defined inhalation maneuvers required for use of pMDIs and DPIs, such as young children and the elderly. An additional benefit for the elderly, who may have degraded fine motor skills, coordination, dexterity, and hand muscle strength issues, is that nebulizers are easier for them to use than inhalers (Taffet et al. 2014). Nebulized therapy is also the favored form of aerosol delivery in the treatment of lung diseases with smaller patient populations such as cystic fibrosis and pulmonary hypertension where the doses required are larger than can be delivered by pMDI or DPI inhalers. Nebulizers are also widely used in emergency departments for the treatment of patients with asthma and Chronic Obstructive Pulmonary Disease (COPD) admitted following an exacerbation; as a result of this, they can become associated in these patients minds with being the most effective type of device, as they are the device used to aid their recovery when feeling at their worst. This may provide an incentive for patients to persist with this treatment upon discharge to the home environment, and nebulized therapy may be prescribed preferentially to patients with COPD upon discharge due to the reduced likelihood of errors in use. Recent research has shown that upon discharge from hospital, patients with COPD and peak inspiratory flow below 60 L/min prescribed a nebulizer, were found to have lower readmission rates than those prescribed a DPI (Loh et al. 2017).

However, most of the nebulized therapies available today for the treatment of asthma and COPD were developed in the last century for administration via low efficiency jet nebulizer and comprise short-acting antimuscarinics and short-acting beta$_2$-agonists as well as corticosteroids and antibiotics (Table 20.2).

The exception to this are the long-acting beta$_2$-agonists formoterol and arformoterol available in the United States, in contrast to this, at the time of writing there were around 27 long-acting drugs or drug combinations in late stage development or recently launched in inhaler form for the treatment of asthma and COPD. Long-acting formulations decrease the burden of disease upon the patient, adherence is improved with once daily medication compared with 2 times, 3 times, or 4 times a day (Falagas et al. 2015) and the likelihood of readmission is reduced (Bollu et al. 2013). Therefore, the lack of nebulized options for the treatment of the sickest asthma and COPD patients who may struggle with correct use of inhalers is unlikely to persist in the competitive market of inhaled therapy. There are signs that the development of handheld mesh nebulizers, with most of the convenience of inhalers and additional benefits of

TABLE 20.2

Nebulized Therapies Available in the United Kingdom and United States for Use with General Purpose Nebulizers

Class	Drug	Concentration (mg)/mL	Nebule Volume (mL)
Antimuscarinic	Ipratropium bromide	0.25[1], 0.5[2]	1[1], 2[1], 2.5[2]
Antimuscarinic and SABA	Ipratropium with salbutamol	0.5/2.5[3]	2.5[1], 3[2]
Short-acting beta$_2$–agonist	Salbutamol	(1, 2, 5)[1], (0.63, 1.25, 2.5)[2]	2.5[1], 3[2]
Short-acting beta$_2$–agonist	Terbutaline sulfate	2.5[1]	2[1]
Long-acting beta$_2$–agonist	Formoterol fumarate	0.2[2]	2[2]
Long-acting beta$_2$–agonist	Arformoterol tartrate	0.15[2]	2[2]
Corticosteroid	Budesonide	0.25[3], 0.5[3], 1[2]	2[3]
Corticosteroid	Fluticasone propionate	0.25[1], 1[1]	2[1]
Mucolytic	Dornase alfa	1[3]	2.5[3]
Aminoglycoside antibiotic	Tobramycin	60[2], 75[3]	4[3], 5[2]
Polymixin antibacterial	Colistimethate sodium	1 MIU[1]	–

1 = UK, 2 = USA, 3 = UK & USA

adherence monitoring, is resulting in the development of many new drug formulations in nebulized form (Santus et al. 2017, Quinn et al. 2018). For example, Sunovion recently received approval in the United States for their nebulized long-acting muscarinic.

20.4 Opportunities for Nebulizers in the Drug Development Process

The background to the lack of development of new nebulized drug formulations may lie in the dominance of jet nebulizers that were considered to be an unattractive means of bringing a new drug product to market. The obvious disadvantages of jet nebulizers already discussed (Table 20.1) outweighed their universal applicability, so before the advent of portable, fast mesh nebulizers, nebulization was not perceived to be an attractive route for commercialization of new drug entities. Also, because of the need to establish the correct dose, late nebulizer development represents a significant investment in a new clinical development programme, which might have limited returns if started too late, when drug patent life is limited. The arrival of mesh nebulizers that have the convenience of inhalers, with the possibility of added e-health capability, can be expected to upset the drug delivery development paradigm that has been predominant over the past couple of decades.

Perhaps surprisingly, as illustrated in Figure 20.5a, this development paradigm has often included the use of nebulized formulations for early stage development, which were dropped after proof-of-principle in favor of the pMDI or DPI formulations intended for commercialization. The reasons for this substitution lie in the relative simplicity of early stage (phase I–IIa) development of water soluble drug compounds for nebulization, compared with development of pMDI or DPI formulations on a small scale in these early stages, along with the high levels of attrition seen in inhaled product development (around 48% fail in phase I), which meant minimizing early costs was important to the economics of the overall development pipeline. However, once the early stages of development had been passed successfully and the proof-of-principle for the new drug had been proved using the nebulized formulation, the development would then be reset onto a pMDI/DPI development path, with a consequent need to repeat a portion of the development work. Although this development paradigm gets faster market access for the more commonly prescribed pMDI/DPI inhalers, recent work has shown that a better return on investment may be obtained by continuing the nebulized development through to market (Pritchard 2015b, 2016). The development of a new drug in a nebulized format also has the advantage that, currently, nebulizer users tend to be patients with more severe disease.

This means the clinical trials can be run with a greater chance of showing clinically and statistically significant changes and so provide the best chance of success, as well as establishing the drug as a valuable addition to the physician's armamentarium.

In Figure 20.5b, the net present value (NPV) represents the value in today's terms of cash flows expected in the future. In order to calculate the net present value of a project, the value of expected profits must first be discounted to the present value. The expected NPV (eNPV) is used if the project only has a probability of success, the NPV is scaled down by the likelihood of success. In the event that different revenue streams are possible, the probability of each is multiplied by the NPV of that outcome and summed to give the total expected NPV.

This new development paradigm has been made attractive due to the advances in nebulizer technology mentioned earlier, so that the all-important first arrival of the new drug into the marketplace is made via a convenient, user-friendly delivery device that is designed to ensure correct delivery and can be supplemented with advanced features such as feedback and integrated electronic monitoring.

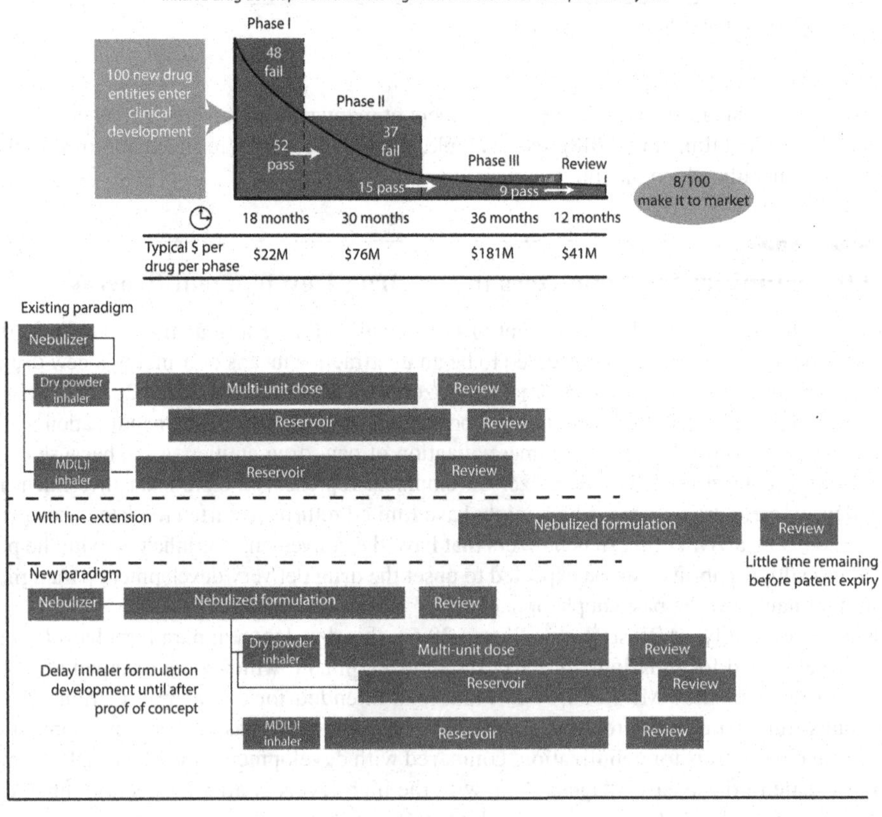

FIGURE 20.5 Drug commercialization paradigms. (a) Inhaled drug development involves high risk and cost over time periods of years. *(Continued)*

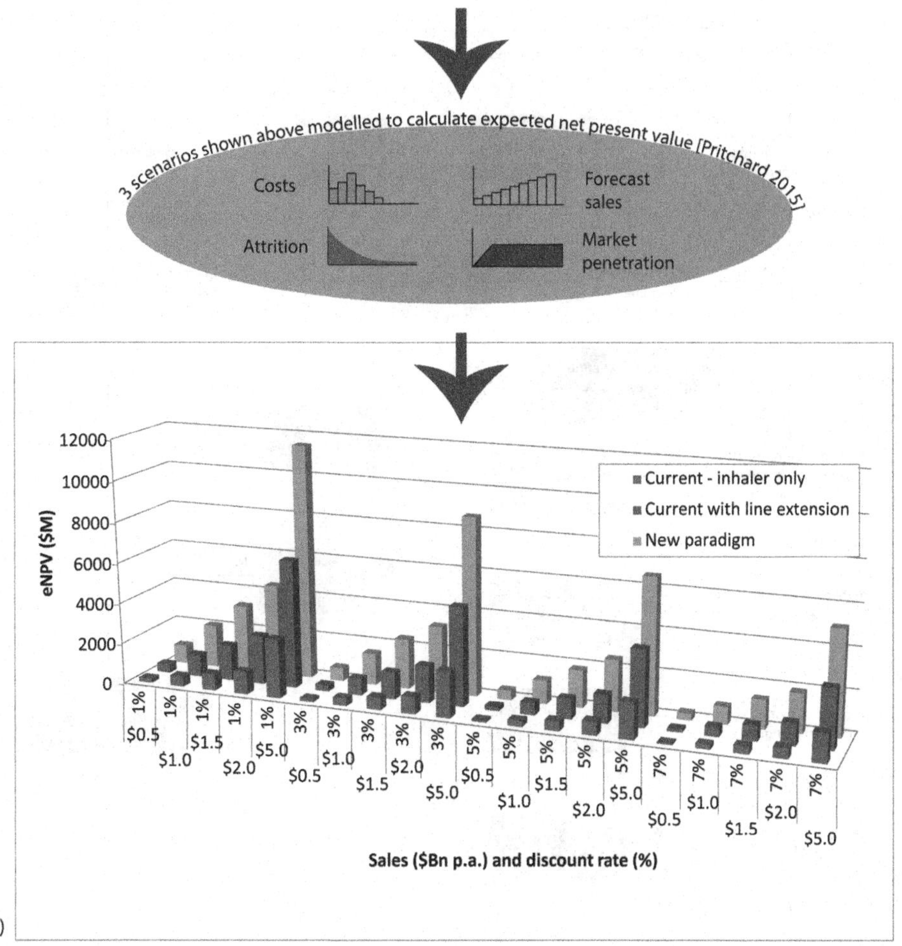

(b)

FIGURE 20.5 (Continued) Drug commercialization paradigms. (b) Three scenarios shown in part (a) modeled to calculate expected net present value. (With kind permission from Taylor & Francis: *Int J Pharm.*, Rethinking the paradigm for the development of inhaled drugs, 496(2), 2015b, 1069 –1072, Pritchard, J.N.)

Indeed, features such as integrated electronic monitoring are also useful during the development process, as good clinical practice requires patient usage of drug to be monitored and adherence to be reported (The European Medicines Evaluation Agency 1997). A recent examination of clinical trial databases has shown that since the development of mesh nebulizer technology, mesh nebulizers have rapidly overtaken jet and ultrasonic nebulizers as the technology of choice for use in clinical trials sponsored by pharmaceutical companies (Pritchard et al. 2018).

The options available to pharmaceutical companies developing new drug compounds now cover a full range of commercial considerations, from low value, simple solution formulated drugs aimed at a mass market to more complex formulations with specific physiochemical and dosing requirements (Figure 20.6).

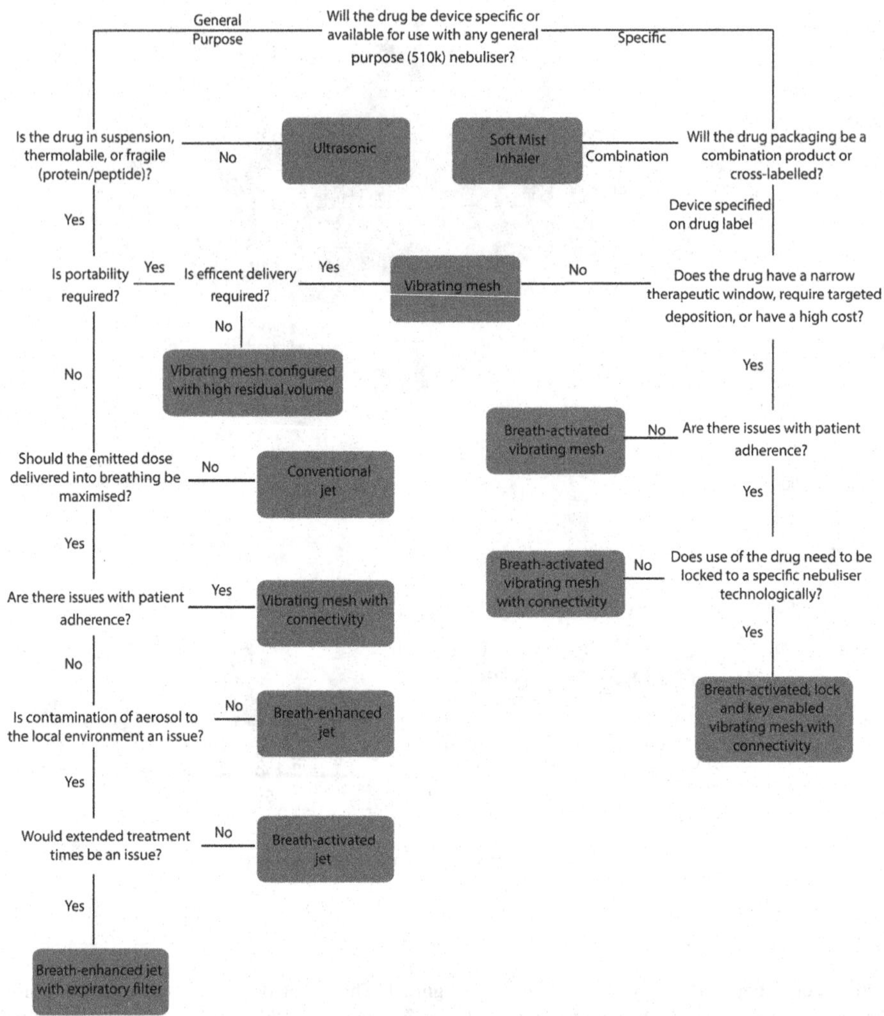

FIGURE 20.6 Nebulizer selection options for pharmaceutical drug developments.

20.5 Demonstrating Performance

The flexibility of the nebulizer in delivering aerosol into all types of breathing pattern complicates the demonstration of performance, as the range of conditions under which the nebulizer must reliably deliver aerosol is much wider than for inhalers that must be used with specific inhalation maneuvers. Despite the long history of nebulized therapy, a dedicated nebulizer test standard was not established until publication of the British Standard BS 7711-3 in 1994, which used sodium fluoride tracer to determine output to a filter and residual left in the nebulizer chamber, along with laser diffraction to measure droplet size (Dennis 2009). Up to the introduction of this standard, weight loss was commonly used to define aerosol output from a nebulizer, but this gravimetric method did not take into account the significant amount of evaporation that can occur within a jet nebulizer during nebulization, leading to concentration of the remaining drug within the nebulizer fluid remaining in the nebulizer cup. Once standardized testing was established, the international standards evolved to provide ever-more relevant testing, with introduction of the European Standard EN 13544-1 in 2001 followed by the European Pharmacopoeia chapter 2.9.44 and ISO 27427:2013, each time improving the simplified test model approximations of the fate of aerosol in the clinical situation. Today these standards involve the measurement of actual drug delivered onto a filter during simulated breathing, with aerosol droplet/particle size characterization by cascade impaction, which provides a closer approximation of the real-life fate of aerosol droplets/particles entering the lungs compared with the mathematical basis of laser diffraction used in earlier standards. However, despite the improvements in these standard test methods, the relevance of these simplified models, developed with a background of the need to characterize constant output jet nebulizers, is likely to recede without significant update to account for recent developments in nebulizer design and operation. Features such as breath activation and guidance of the user to perform optimized breathing cycles have the potential to improve day to day drug delivery, but it is important that the test standards keep pace with the way in which these advanced devices are used so that the advantages built into these advanced devices are not overlooked when using in vitro tests. A recent study investigated the variability in delivered and respirable delivered doses from nine different models of nebulizer when the simulated breathing patterns defined in the test standards were tested along with modifications of the patterns to reflect the inhalation/exhalation ratios that are representative of patients with a range of airflow obstruction/restriction (Hatley and Byrne 2017). The results showed a difference of up to 2.5 times the delivered dose and a four-fold difference in respirable delivered dose between the nebulizers when using the test breathing pattern defined in the standards. However, the results also showed a reduction of up to 60% in respirable delivered dose from the non-breath-activated nebulizers, compared with a respirable delivered dose that was independent of I:E ratio for the breath-activated mesh nebulizer.

The wide range in delivered dose seen with nebulizers has been acceptable in the past due to the predominant use of these nebulizers to deliver drugs with wide therapeutic indexes (Table 20.2). These devices colloquially known as general purpose nebulizers are increasingly being supplanted by a new generation of advanced nebulizers that will be referenced on the drug label. Although technically classified as a drug-device combination product, since the nebulizer is required to deliver the drug, unless it is chosen to develop the nebulizer for one drug only and label the entire device only for use with that drug, it would not fall under the cross-labeled drug-device combination classification. A cross-labeled product requires a two way drug-device and device-drug unique link (Food and Drug Administration 2017a). Not being a cross-labeled product enables the device and drug to be developed under the separate drug and device good manufacturing practices and quality systems. Thus, the nebulizer would remain as a class 2a product, and not a class 3 medical device, as required for drug-device combinations. In the future, as new drugs are developed with more specific dosing requirements, the choice of nebulizer used for delivery will initially be restricted to the device used during the drug development programme. The initial restriction may over the lifecycle of the licensed drug be expanded to allow other devices to be used. This could include alternative devices developed to deliver the drug even in the absence of a partnership between the drug and device companies, if the device company could demonstrate a range of safety and handling aspects of the device with the drug (Food and Drug Administration 2017b). Devices should therefore have a wide combination of features if the drug company is to be able to minimize the loss of control of the effectiveness of the drug, as initially tested, when delivered by alternative devices. As nebulizers become more sophisticated in dose delivery while maintaining the important attribute of universal usability, then demonstration of performance and development of standards will need to evolve to match the variation in patient groups the nebulizers are used to treat.

20.6 The Future of Nebulization

Technological advances typically go through an adoption period between first release to market and widespread adoption. In the case of medical devices, the adoption period can be lengthened by both the demands of existing regulations and standards as well as the differing infrastructure of healthcare models used around the world.

20.6.1 Mesh Nebulizer Development

The launch of the 1st mesh nebulizer in 1993 was followed by a tortuous negotiation of technical, regulatory, mass manufacturing, and existing healthcare infrastructure, supply and reimbursement considerations that had to be overcome before the mesh nebulizer became the preferred choice for new aerosolized pharmaceutical developments (Pritchard 2017), many of which are still to come to market. The widespread adoption of mesh technology means that the mesh nebulizer now has an established place in the nebulizer market. In addition to new drug-device combinations being released, driven by the expansion into different therapy areas previously dominated by pMDI and DPI inhalers (Pritchard 2015b, Santus et al. 2017, Quinn et al. 2018), there will also be opportunities in improving the design for both mass manufacture and user convenience. Although mesh technology has become successfully established as a new route for nebulized therapy, it is currently in a phase of technological improvement. One such development of the mesh nebulizer is the photo-defined aperture plate (PDAP), which uses a novel mesh wafer architecture to reduce the droplet size, increase the output rate of aerosol, and broaden the range of liquid viscosity that mesh nebulizers could be used to nebulize (Fink et al. 2016). Instead of a single layer mesh with continuously tapering orifices, the photo-defined aperture plate utilizes a two layer mesh; the upper layer consists of large diameter apertures sunk into a thick substrate, and the lower much thinner layer has up to 20 small apertures within the diameter of the upper layer aperture. Early tests have demonstrated aerosol production with droplet sizes in the region of 1 μm while achieving an output rate of around 0.3 mL/min, equivalent to high performance mesh nebulizers with much larger droplet sizes. Flat plate technology may also be a potential future development. In this design of mesh nebulizer, the piezo transducer is separated from the mesh with a resonant cavity approximately 1 mm–3 mm deep. This design would allow just the mesh component to be easily replaced which could simplify device cleaning and reduce service costs (Hijlkema and Leppard 2015). Another area of intense research concerns fabrication of the meshes fitted to mesh nebulizers, which are currently mainly made from metal alloys and are expensive to fabricate. In the future, the development of alternative materials such as plastic may reduce the cost of manufacture, and provide an option for disposable meshes that could be changed on a weekly or even daily basis, reducing the burden of cleaning and providing the user with convenience akin to replacing the sensor strip on their glucose monitor before each use.

20.6.2 Other Aerosol Generation Technologies

In addition to improvements in established nebulizer technologies, there is also potential for the development of nebulizers based on improved aerosol generators that could offer improvements in ease of cleaning, output rate (faster and tailored to the medication/user), droplet size (smaller and tailored to the medication/user), and droplet size geometric standard deviation (monodisperse).

There are a range of novel aerosolization technologies in early stage development, many of which blur the boundary between nebulizer, inhaler, and soft mist inhaler. Devices such as Omega Life Science's Alphazer nebulizer and MEway Pharma's UltraFlow Nebulizer are named as nebulizers, but share some characteristics with inhalers and soft mist inhalers. Many novel devices in early stage development will fail during the decade that it typically takes to get a new technology ready for starting clinical trials. The Battelle Mystic drug delivery platform uses an electro hydrodynamic mechanism to generate an aerosol and has been under consideration for delivery of a number of compounds since 1999, but a commercially available product has yet to see the light of day.

Completely new aerosol generator technologies such as surface acoustic wave and capillary aerosol generators seem to hold promise for successful development. The phenomena of surface acoustic waves, used for signal processing and bandpass filtering for decades, also has promise for use in micro-fluidics for applications such as mixing, propagation, jetting, and atomization (Yeo and Friend 2009, Luong and Nguyen 2010). The application of surface acoustic waves for atomization offers the same level of power efficiency as mesh nebulizers, but without the requirement for the thousands of tolerance-critical mesh holes contained within a mesh that must be bonded to the piezo element consistently and that have the potential to clog with inadequate cleaning. Surface acoustic wave atomization relies on the leakage of a MHz frequency wave into a liquid sat on a piezoelectric substrate. The wave leakage causes acoustic streaming within the liquid and at powers similar to mesh nebulizers (~1 W), capillary waves are generated at the surface of the liquid which leads to atomization once the capillary stress has been overcome (Yeo and Friend 2009).

Thermal energy has also been used to generate aerosol. The capillary aerosol generator uses a heated micro-capillary to vaporize nebulizer liquid pumped through the capillary, the vapor is emitted into surrounding cool air, whereupon it supersaturates, and a nuclei is formed. Condensation occurs onto the nuclei, which results in aerosol droplets. Control of the surrounding air allows control of coagulation, evaporation, and hygroscopic growth, which influences the eventual droplet size of the aerosol (Hong et al. 2002). A drawback with this method of aerosol production is the temperature of the vapor, which can reach between 150 degrees centigrade to 200 degrees centigrade (Carvalho and McConville 2016), and, hence, limits the drug formulations to those that are both volatile and thermally stable. The first part of the process (vaporization in a micro-capillary) is similar to the method used in some models of electronic cigarette; however, in an electronic cigarette the liquid is drawn from the bulk container via a wick, with little control over the amount of liquid (dose) emitted apart from the user determined heater activation time. The universal adoption of condensation aerosols for the delivery of nicotine, in electronic cigarettes, where most of these developments have been outside of the normal pharmaceutical approval process, has resulted in new regulations being imposed on these products as they become wildly available to the public. They are also being considered for other applications such as the delivery of cannabis-based products, and this may lead to a crossover of the technology into the pharmaceutical industry. Though the technology has some potential limitations for traditional pharmaceuticals, the huge investment in this technology for the delivery of nicotine and the increased regulation may result in low cost delivery technologies that are suitable for a wider range of pharmaceuticals.

20.6.3 Future Features of Nebulizers

The monitoring and feedback features built into the more advanced nebulizer systems today compare favorably with features available for other types of inhaler, which tend to focus only on monitoring adherence and not technique (Kikidis et al. 2016). The wider range of feedback and monitoring signals and parameters provided by nebulizer systems are most likely a consequence of the ease with which these features can be added to these electrically powered devices. However, monitoring and feedback are still in the early stages of adoption, and it can be expected that as the challenges of engineering-improved aerosol generators are conquered, manufacturers will also expand on the sensor capabilities and analytical capability built into devices to provide more features. Research into the use of physiological parameter monitoring to predict exacerbations in patients with COPD is underway (Al Rajeh and Hurst 2016), and it is feasible to imagine variables such as respiratory rate, peak expiratory flow rate, and forced expiratory volume in 1 second being monitored and tested by sensors built-in into the nebulizer. When combined with other parameters measured by the patient's smartphone, exchanged via wireless connectivity, advanced nebulizer features could give a wide scope to provide useful patient self-management tools to both patients and healthcare professionals.

20.7 Conclusion

Nebulizers represent the original medical means of delivering liquid aerosolized medication to the lungs, but were supplanted by pMDI and DPI inhalers in the mid to late twentieth century. There has been a recent resurgence in nebulized therapy due to the arrival of mesh nebulizers that offer patient convenience akin to that of inhalers along with the ability to deliver larger doses of drug, and the ability of patients to use nebulizers successfully without the need to perform the specific breathing maneuvers that are required for the correct use of inhalers. These advantages coupled with both the popularity of the nebulizer in the Far East and the opportunities for incorporation of advanced nebulizer features such as adherence and physiological parameter monitoring as well as improvements in the speed of nebulization imply an increasing role for nebulized therapy in inhaled medication delivery in the future.

REFERENCES

Al Rajeh, A.M., and Hurst, J.R. 2016. Monitoring of physiological parameters to predict exacerbations of chronic obstructive pulmonary disease (COPD): A systematic review. *J Clin Med.* 5(12). pii: E108.

Anderson, P.J. 2005. History of aerosol therapy: Liquid nebulization to MDIs to DPIs. *Respir Care.* 50(9):1139–1150.

Ari, A. 2012. Aerosol delivery device selection for spontaneously breathing patients: 2012. *Respir Care.* 57(4):613–626.

Ari, A. 2015. Aerosol therapy in pulmonary critical care. *Respir Care.* 60(6):858–879.

Bårnes, C.B., and Ulrik, C.S. 2015. Asthma and adherence to inhaled corticosteroids: Current status and future perspectives. *Respir Care.* 60(3):455–468.

Bennett, W.D. 2005. Controlled inhalation of aerosolised therapeutics. *Expert Opin Drug Deliv.* 2(4):763–767.

Boe, J., Dennis, J.H., and O'Driscoll, B.R., et al. 2001. European respiratory society guidelines on the use of nebulizers. *Eur Respir J.* 18:228–242.

Bollu, V., Ernst, F.R., and Karafilidis, J., et al. 2013. Hospital readmissions following initiation of nebulized arformoterol tartrate or nebulized short-acting beta-agonists among inpatients treated for COPD. *Int J Chron Obstruct Pulmon Dis.* 8:631–639. doi:10.2147/COPD.S52557

Boyter, A.C. and Carter, R. 2005. How do patients use their nebulizer in the community? *Respir Med.* 99:1413–1417.

Carvalho, T.C., and McConville, J.T. 2016. The function and performance of aqueous aerosol devices for inhalation therapy. *J Pharm Pharmacol.* 68:556–578.

Dennis, J. 2009. Evolution of evaporative understanding within nebulizer standards. *J Aerosol Med Pulm Drug Deliv.* 22(1):5–8.

Denyer, J., and Dyche, T. 2010. The adaptive aerosol delivery (AAD) technology: Past, present, and future. *J Aerosol Med Pulm Drug Deliv.* 23(Suppl 1):S1–S10.

Denyer, J., Black, A., and Nikander, K., et al. 2010. Domiciliary experience of the target inhalation mode (TIM) breathing maneuver in patients with cystic fibrosis. *J Aerosol Med Pulm Drug Deliv.* 23(Suppl 1):S45–S54.

Dessanges, J.F. 2001. A history of nebulization. *J Aerosol Med.* 14(1):65–71.

Dolovich, M.B., Ahrens, R.C., and Hess, D.R., et al. 2005. Device selection and outcomes of aerosol therapy: Evidence-based guidelines. *Chest.* 127(1):335–371.

Elphick, M., von Hollen, D., and Pritchard, J.N., et al. 2015. Factors to consider when selecting a nebulizer for a new inhaled drug product development program. *Expert Opin Drug Deliv.* 12(8):1375–1387.

Falagas, M.E., Karagiannis, A.K., and Nakouti, T., et al. 2015. Compliance with once-daily versus twice or thrice-daily administration of antibiotic regimens: A meta-analysis of randomized controlled trials. *PLoS One.* 10(1):e0116207. doi:10.1371/journal.pone.0116207

Fink, J.B., MacLoughlan, R., and Telfer, C., et al. 2016. Developing inhaled drugs for critically ill patients: A platform for all ages. In *Respiratory Drug Delivery 2016* (Volume 2). Dalby, R.N., Byron, P.R., Peart, J., et al. (Eds.), Richmond, VA: Virginia Commonwealth University, 249–252.

Food and Drug Administration. 2017a. Code of federal regulations Title 21. https://www.accessdata.fda.gov/scripts/cdrh/cfdocs/cfcfr/CFRSearch.cfm?fr=3.2.

Food and Drug Administration. 2017b. Devices Referencing Drugs; Public Hearing; Request for Comments. Webcast recording. https://www.fda.gov/NewsEvents/MeetingsConferencesWorkshops/ucm572528.htm.

Gardenhire, D.S., Ari, A., and Hess, D., et al. 2013 A guide to aerosol delivery devices for respiratory therapists, 3rd edition. American Association for Respiratory Care, 2013. Available at: [http://www.aarc.org/resources/clinical-resources/aerosol-resources/#rt] accessed 13th December 2017.

Grossman, J. 1994. The evolution of inhaler technology. *J Asthma.* 31(1):55–64.

Hatley, R.H., and Byrne, S.M. 2017. Variability in delivered dose and respirable delivered dose from nebulizers: Are current regulatory testing guidelines sufficient to produce meaningful information? *Med Devices (Auckl).* 10:17–28.

Hess, D.R. 2000. Nebulizers: Principles and performance. *Respir Care.* 45(6):609–622.

Hijlkema, M., and Leppard, M.J.R., inventors. 2015. Nebulizer and a method of manufacturing a nebulizer. United States Patent US2015/0144128 A1.

Hong, J.N., Hindle, M., and Byron, P.R. 2002. Control of particle size by coagulation of novel condensation aerosols in reservoir chambers. *J Aerosol Med.* 15(4):359–368.

Inhalatorium. Abbott's Aerohaler DPI. http://www.inhalatorium.com/wpcproduct/abbotts–aerohalor–dry–powder–inhaler/

Kikidis, D., Konstantinos, V., and Tzovaras, D. 2016. The digital asthma patient: The history and future of inhaler based health monitoring devices. *J Aerosol Med Pulm Drug Deliv.* 29(3): 219–232.

Leung, K., Louca, E., and Coates, A.L. 2004. Comparison of breath-enhanced to breath-actuated nebulizers for rate, consistency, and efficiency. *Chest.* 126:1619–1627.

Loh, C.H., Peters, S.P., and Lovings, T.M., et al. 2017. Suboptimal inspiratory flow rates are associated with chronic obstructive pulmonary disease and all-cause readmissions. *Ann Am Thorac Soc.* 14(8):1305–1311.

Luong, T.D., and Nguyen, N.T. 2010. Surface acoustic wave driven microfluidics—A review. *Micro and Nanosystems.* 2. 217–225. https://www.researchgate.net/publication/230852272_Surface_Acoustic_Wave_Driven_Microfluidics_-_A_Review. (Accessed December 14, 2017)

Mäkelä, M.J., Backer, V., and Hedegaard, M., et al. 2013. Adherence to inhaled therapies, health outcomes and costs in patients with asthma and COPD. *Respir Med.* 107:1482–1490.

McCormack, P., McNamara, P.S., and Southern, K.W. 2011. A randomised controlled trial of breathing modes for adaptive aerosol delivery in children with cystic fibrosis. *J Cyst Fibros.* 10(5):343–349.

Mercer, T.T, Tillery, M.I, and Chow, H.Y. 1968. Operating characteristics of some compressed air nebulizers. *Am Ind Hyg Assoc J.* 29(1):66–67.

Nerbrink, O., and Dahlbäck, M. 1994. Basic nebulizer function. *J Aerosol Med.* 7(Suppl 1):S7–S11.

Nerbrink, O., Dahlbäck, M., and Hansson, H.C. 1994. Why do medical nebulizers differ in their output and particle size characteristics? *J Aerosol Med.* 7(3):259–276.

Nikander, K., and Denyer, J. 2000. Breathing patterns. *Eur Respir Rev.* 10(76):576–579.

Nikander, K., Prince, I., and Coughlin, S. 2010. Mode of breathing-tidal or slow and deep-through the I-neb Adaptive Aerosol Delivery (AAD) system affects lung deposition of (99m)Tc-DTPA. *J Aerosol Med Pulm Drug Deliv.* 23(Suppl 1):S37–S43.

Nikander, K., and Saunders, M. 2010. The early evolution of nebulizers. *Medicamundi.* 54(3):47–53.

Nikander, K., Turpeinen, M., and Wollmer, P. 1999. The conventional ultrasonic nebulizer proved inefficient in nebulizing a suspension. *J Aerosol Med.* 12(2):47–53.

O'Callaghan, C., and Barry, P.W. 1997. The science of nebulized drug delivery. *Thorax.* 52(Suppl 2): S31–S44.

Pritchard, J.N. 2015a. Industry guidance for the selection of a delivery system for the development of novel respiratory products. *Expert Opin Drug Del.* 12(11):1755–1765.

Pritchard, J.N. 2015b. Rethinking the paradigm for the development of inhaled drugs. *Int J Pharm.* 496(2):1069–1072.

Pritchard, J.N. 2016. Maximizing the effectiveness of the inhaled drug development process. In *Respiratory Drug Delivery 2016* (Volume 3). Dalby, R.N., Byron, P.R., Peart, J., et al. (Eds.), Richmond, VA: Virginia Commonwealth University. 497–502.

Pritchard, J.N. 2017. Nebulized drug delivery in respiratory medicine: What does the future hold? *Ther Del.* 8(6):391–399. doi:10.4155/tde-2017-0015.

Pritchard, J.N., Hatley, R.H.M., and Denyer, J., et al. 2018. Mesh nebulizers have become the first choice for new nebulized pharmaceutical drug developments. *Ther Deliv.* 9(2):121–136.

Pritchard, J.N., and Nicholls, C. 2015. Emerging technologies for electronic monitoring of adherence, inhaler competence, and true adherence. *J Aerosol Med Pulm Drug Deliv.* 28(2):69–81.

Quinn, D., Barnes, C.N., and Yates, W., et al. 2018. Pharmacodynamics, pharmacokinetics and safety of revefenacin (TD-4208), a long-acting muscarinic antagonist, in patients with chronic obstructive pulmonary disease (COPD): Results of two randomized, double-blind, phase 2 studies. *Pulm Pharmacol Ther.* 48:71–79.

Rau, J.L. 2002. Design principles of liquid nebulization devices currently in use. *Respir Care.* 47(11):1257–1278.

Rau, J.L. 2005. The inhalation of drugs: Advantages and problems. *Respir Care.* 50(3):367–382.

Rayleigh, J.W. 1878. On the instability of jets. *Proc London Math Soc.* 10(1):4–13.

Restrepo, R.D, Alvarez, M.T., and Wittnebel, L.D., et al. 2008. Medication adherence issues in patients treated for COPD. *Int J Chron Obstruct Pulmon Dis.* 3(3):371–384.

Rottier, B.L., Van Erp, C.J.P., Sluyter, T.S., et al. 2009. Changes in performance of the Pari eFlow® Rapid and Pari LC Plus™ during 6 months use by CF patients. *J Aerosol Med Pulm Drug Deliv.* 22(2):1–7.

Rubin, B.K. 2011. Pediatric aerosol therapy: New devices and new drugs. *Respir Care.* 56(9):1411–1421.

Sabate, E. 2003. *Adherence to Long-Term Therapies: Evidence for Action*. Geneva, Switzerland: World Health Organization. Available at http://www.who.int/chp/knowledge/publications/adherence_report/en/. Accessed December 13, 2017.

Sanders, M. 2007. Inhalation therapy: An historical review. *Prim Care Respir J.* 16:71–81.

Santus, P., Radovanovic, D., and Cristiano, A., et al. 2017. Role of nebulized glycopyrrolate in the treatment of chronic obstructive pulmonary disease. *Drug Des Devel Ther.* 11:3257–3271.

Shah, P.L., Scott, S.F., and Geddes, D.M., et al. 1997. An evaluation of two aerosol delivery systems for rhDNase. *Eur Respir J.* 10:1261–1266.

Smye, S.W., Jollie, M.I., and Littlewood, J.M., 1991. A mathematical model of some aspects of jet nebulizer performance. *Clin Phys Physiol Meas.* 12(3):289–300.

Standaert, T.A., Morlin, G.L., Williams-Warren, J., et al. 1998. Effects of repetitive use and cleaning techniques of disposable jet nebulizers on aerosol generation. *Chest.* 114(2):577–586.

Taffet, G.E., Donohue, J.F., and Altman, P.R. 2014. Considerations for managing chronic obstructive pulmonary disease in the elderly. *Clin Interv Aging.* 9:23–30.

The European Medicines Evaluation Agency. 1997. *International Conference on Harmonisation ICH topic E8: General Considerations for Clinical Trials.* http://www.emea.europa.eu (accessed December 14, 2017).

Tsai, R.J., Boiano, J.M., and Steege, A.L., et al. 2015. Precautionary practices of respiratory therapists and other health-care practitioners who administer aerosolized medications. *Respir Care.* 60(10):1409–1417.

Yeo, L.Y., and Friend, J.R. 2009. Ultrafast microfluidics using surface acoustic waves. *Biomicrofluidics.* 3(1):12002. doi:10.1063/1.3056040 (accessed December 14, 2017).

Yeo, L.Y., Friend, J.R., and McIntosh, M.P., et al. 2010. Ultrasonic nebulization platforms for pulmonary drug delivery. *Expert Opin Drug Deliv.* 7(6):663–679.

21

Soft Mist Inhalers

Stefan Leiner, David Cipolla, Joachim Eicher, Wilbur de Kruijf, and Herbert Wachtel

CONTENTS

21.1 Introduction

As inhalation medicine often needs to be taken daily and for the long term, an ideal inhaler should provide efficient, reliable, and well-tolerated drug delivery, while also offering convenience to the patient. For the efficient delivery to the lungs, a drug needs to be administered either as a liquid or solid aerosol. Limitations of traditional inhaler devices, such as metered-dose inhalers (MDIs) and dry powder inhalers (DPIs) (outlined below), and a need for a convenient propellant-free inhaler allowing for effective delivery of aerosols from solutions prompted the development of a new technology that generates a single-breath, inhalable aerosol from a drug solution (Dalby et al. 2011).

Soft mist inhalers (SMIs)–so-called to describe both the mechanism of aerosol generation and the qualities of the aerosol cloud–are non-pressurized MDIs using microfluidic technology, characterized by a metering function that allows delivery of distinct doses (Cipolla and Gonda 2011; Wachtel 2016). To the authors' knowledge, as of mid-2017, one type of soft mist inhaler is commercially available (Respimat® Soft Mist™ Inhaler; Boehringer Ingelheim, Ingelheim, Germany) and two have reached a late development stage (AERx Essence®; Aradigm, Hayward, CA; Aqueous Droplet Inhaler [ADI®]; Pharmaero, Copenhagen, Denmark, a subsidiary of SHL Group and Xellia Pharmaceuticals; nozzle for the ADI produced by Medspray, Enschede, the Netherlands). A fourth device, the Ecomyst (Aero Pump, Hochheim, Germany), which also uses the Medspray nozzle, is in early clinical development. This chapter therefore focuses on these four inhaler systems. A comparison of the key features and specifications of these inhalers is shown in Table 21.1.

In the United States Pharmacopeia 41—National Formulary 36 (United States Pharmacopeial Convention 2017), the regulatory term for soft mist inhaler products is "inhalation spray." In contrast, the regulatory term in the European Union (described in the European Pharmacopoeia 9th Edition)

TABLE 21.1

Comparison of Key Features and Specifications of Soft Mist Inhalers Currently Either on the Market or in Clinical Development

Specification	Respimat	AERx Essence	Medspray Nozzle (Ecomyst and Aqueous Droplet Inhaler)
Generation of aerosol	Uniblock (two nozzle outlets fed by multiple fine filter channels)	Single-use nozzle; integral array of submicrometer-sized nozzle holes	Nozzle composed of round orifices in very thin membranes
Manufacturing method	Etched into a silicon wafer and bonded to glass. Uniblock chips are produced on wafer scale, then singulated (diced), controlled, picked, and placed by a robot into the uniblock holder	Manufactured with solid-state lasers, producing nozzle arrays with submicrometer-sized exit holes	Nozzle chips are produced on wafer scale, more than 10,000 units per wafer, then singulated (diced), picked, and placed by a robot with a heated bond head into the medical-grade plastic nozzle holder
Output droplet size and distribution	Predominantly in fine particle range (between 65%–80% < 5.8 μm)	90% < 4.95 μm	Mean mass aerodynamic diameter of approximately 5 μm–6 μm
Exit velocity of aerosol cloud	0.8 m/s	Entrained into inhalation flow at 30 L/min	Individual jets: 40 m/s, entrained into inhalation flow at 15 L/min.
Delivery rate	~10 μL in 1 second	~40 μL in 1 second	~15 μL in 1 second

is "non-pressurized metered dose inhalers" (European Directorate for the Quality of Medicines and Healthcare 2017). This term—"non-pressurized metered dose inhalers"—nicely combines two of their characteristics: the non-reliance on propellants and the ability to deliver distinct doses. Their ability to meter and deliver distinct doses by the integrated inhaler differentiates SMI products from preparations for nebulization (inhalation solutions or inhalation suspensions), e.g. in unit dose vials.

21.2 Advantages and Disadvantages of SMIs over Pressurized MDIs and DPIs

Before the development of SMIs, the most common inhalers were pressurized MDIs (pMDIs) and DPIs. Effective use of hydrofluoroalkane pMDIs requires slow and controlled inhalation for optimal drug deposition because of its high aerosol velocity of 2 m/s–8 m/s (Hochrainer et al. 2005), as well as adequate coordination for synchronized actuation and inhalation by the patient (Dalby et al. 2011). In DPIs, the fine particle dose generated is largely dependent on inspiratory airflow and absolute lung capacity, which can be highly variable between patients (Cipolla et al. 2010). In contrast, SMIs have inherent advantages relating to lung deposition and ease of use. SMIs are active systems not requiring any propellants, meaning that the energy for the generation of the aerosol originates from the inhaler and is therefore independent of patient inspiratory effort (Wachtel et al. 2017). By delivering a defined volume of a drug dissolved in solution from a reservoir or a single-use dosage form, dose-to-dose reproducibility of SMIs is more consistent compared with delivery of a small quantity of suspension released by a pMDI or with powder from a DPI. For a soft mist inhaler, the drug is dissolved in solution and therefore less vulnerable to moisture ingress compared with dry powders, making SMIs suitable for use in places with humid ambient conditions. The relatively low velocity and long spray duration of SMIs makes the aerosol easier to inhale reproducibly. However, for SMIs, it is generally a requirement that the drug is soluble and stable in solution unless specific formulation technologies are applied.

21.3 Available Technologies to Generate Soft Mist Out of Liquid

To generate an inhalable aerosol from a drug solution, the solution needs to be converted into droplets of appropriate size. Several technical methods are available to develop a pocket-sized device that can aerosolize a drug solution into a transient mist containing a full dose; these include piezoelectric vibration, extrusion through micron- or submicron-sized holes with Rayleigh break-up (Medspray system, AERx system), electrohydrodynamics (Zierenberg and Eicher 2003; Dalby et al. 2011), capillary forces, and thermoelectrics. The required energy is provided either as electrical energy from a battery or by the transformation of mechanical energy into droplet-generating energy.

Typically, SMIs harness mechanical power from a spring, which causes a piston to squeeze the drug solution through a small nozzle or an array of nozzle holes to create an aerosol.

Optimal deposition of the drug in the peripheral airways by SMIs is determined by physical parameters such as particle (droplet) size, aerosol speed at the point of droplet generation and subsequent entrainment into the inspiration airstream, and duration of cloud extrusion (Dalby et al. 2011).

21.4 Considerations for Formulations

In all known SMIs, the generation of the primary droplets takes place in the close vicinity of the nozzle system. Depending on the mechanism of droplet creation, the formulations that can be used may face constraints with respect to viscosity, surface tension, density, and vapor pressure (the most relevant physico-chemical properties). As the devices include a metering function, it is mandatory that the formulation stays homogeneous on a macroscopic scale, which is required for metering and for avoiding clogging in the microfluidic channels. For the AERx technology, the nozzles are an integral part of each single-use dosage form, which ensures that they are pristine prior to each administration event. Local or temporal changes in drug concentration may generate severe challenges if they affect dosing; therefore, in most cases, solutions are selected as formulations of choice.

Due to the size of the nozzles and internal filter systems, SMIs are often limited to drugs that are soluble or create stable suspensions. The Respimat and AERx system have been successfully used to atomize nanosuspensions (Boehringer Ingelheim, data on file; Chattopadhyay et al. 2007); however, the aerosolization of nanosuspensions with SMIs has yet to be reported in clinical practice.

Suitable solvents include water or water/ethanol formulations (Pritchard 2015). To allow drug delivery within a single breath, the metered volume per actuation is limited to a volume of 10 µL–100 µL based on liquid flow rate through the nozzle system, aerosol concentration, and possible droplet coalescence.

Besides the active ingredient and the solvent, formulations may contain pH adjusters, other stabilizers, and isotonicity agents. Similar to other dosage forms, the drug solution has to be compatible with the components of the inhaler. Surfactants, present in many pMDI formulations, are not required.

In Section 21 CFR 200.51, the United States Food and Drug Administration requires all aqueous-based drug products for oral inhalation to be manufactured as sterile products (Food and Drug Administration 2000). Therefore, SMI formulations and their container closure systems must also be designed to afford manufacturing processes that guarantee sterility, e.g. terminal sterilization or aseptic manufacture. When the dosage form is a multi-dose form, care must also be given to guarantee an appropriate microbiological quality during patient use, e.g. by adding preservatives to ensure microbial stability.

Regulatory aspects for the development of SMIs are summarized in Table 21.2.

TABLE 21.2

Regulatory Considerations for the Development of Soft Mist Inhalers

Quality Guidelines	
US	US-FDA: Guidance for Industry—Nasal Spray and Inhalation Solution, Suspension, and Spray Drug Products—Chemistry, Manufacturing, and Controls Documentation (June 2002)
	Combination product regulations
EU	European Medicines Agency: Guideline for the Pharmaceutical Documentation of Inhalation and Nasal Products (June 2006); EMEA/CHMP/QWP/49313/2005 Corr
	Medical Device Regulation 2017/745
Specific Aspects	
Homogeneity within a spray	Because of the long spray duration, a consistent droplet distribution over the spray duration must be demonstrated
Metering and dosing system	Because the metering and dosing system of SMIs is more complex than that of pMDIs, robustness of the metering and dosing system against dropping, vibration, transport, and during patient use must be assured
Leachables and extractables	Liquid formulations, even if aqueous, are more susceptible towards leachables than solid formulations. Stringent purity controls of the container closure system components for extractables are mandatory
Sterility of formulation	Aqueous-based formulations for inhalation (including those for SMIs) are regulated under section 21 CFR 200.51 of the US-FDA and required to be manufactured as sterile products
Microbial quality of formulation over use	Products where the formulation is presented as bulk solution need to pay attention to maintaining an appropriate microbiological quality over the duration of use

21.5 The Respimat System

The Respimat is the only commercially available propellant-free soft mist inhaler. The device was designed with the aim of improving the patient experience of taking inhaled medication, and patients have indicated in clinical trials and in studies using self-report instruments that they found the Respimat easy to operate and preferable over pMDIs or DPIs (Wachtel et al. 2017).

The key elements of the Respimat are shown in Figure 21.1. Medication to be delivered by the Respimat is stored in a cartridge, i.e. an aluminum cylinder with a double-walled, collapsible plastic bag on the inside that contracts once the solution has been withdrawn (Anderson 2006). This ensures that the Respimat capillary is always immersed in the solution until the last actuation, and there is no tailing-off effect as the cartridge is depleted. The Respimat has a locking mechanism and a built-in dose indicator, which reminds patients when a new prescription is required. Currently, in the US, the device and the inserted cartridge need to be replaced after 120 actuations; however, in the EU, three products have been approved recently with a reusable Respimat device. The addition of a preservative to the drug solution prevents microbial contamination once the cartridge has been inserted by the patient prior to first use (Dalby et al. 2004).

The accuracy of the delivered dose is set by the precision of the Respimat parts that determine the metering properties and by the reproducibility of the aerosolization process of the metered volume *ex uniblock* (approximately 15 μL for the approved products) to give the delivered volume *ex mouthpiece.* Dose reproducibility using data from ten devices from three different batches has been demonstrated, confirming spray volume uniformity of the doses delivered by the Respimat over 120 actuations without tail-off (Dalby et al. 2004, 2011).

Twisting the clear base of the Respimat by 180° compresses the spring, moves the cartridge with the inserted capillary downwards, and transfers a predefined metered volume of drug solution from the

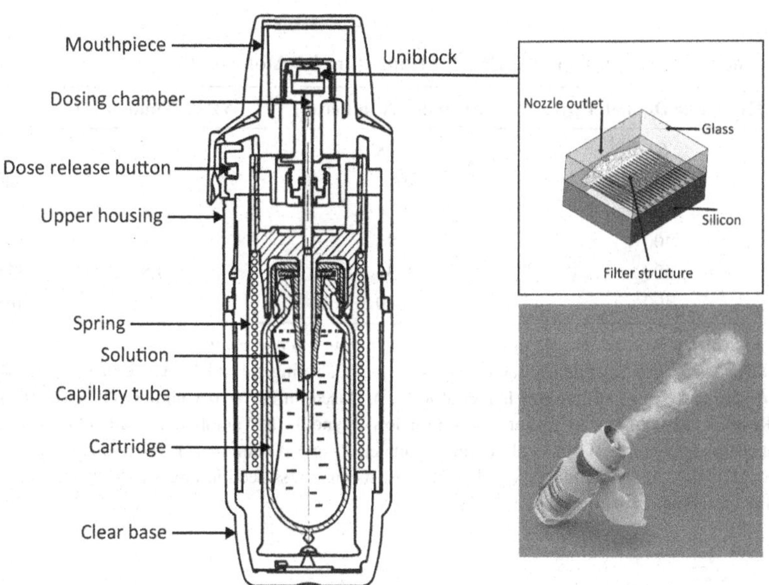

FIGURE 21.1 The Respimat® Soft Mist™ inhaler with the key components of the device and details of the uniblock.

cartridge via the capillary tube into the dosing chamber. By pressing the release button, the metered volume of drug solution is forced by the released energy of the spring through the uniblock.

The uniblock, shown in Figure 21.1, is a key component of the Respimat. It consists of two nozzle outlets (5.6 µm × 8 µm) that are fed by multiple extremely fine filter channels. The drug solution is forced through the two-channel nozzle, resulting in the solution being split into two jets that converge at a carefully controlled angle. The impact causes the drug solution to disintegrate into a slow-moving aerosol (soft mist) composed of inhalable droplets (Zierenberg et al. 1996; Zierenberg and Eicher 2003).

The channel structure is etched into a silicon wafer based on microchip production technology, which allows for high precision and large-scale production of the units (Dalby et al. 2004).

The liquid flow through the uniblock and the subsequent atomization is characterized by two non-dimensional parameters: (Equation 21.1) the Weber number and (Equation 21.2) the Reynolds number (Wachtel 2016):

$$We = \rho u_j^2 D / \sigma \tag{21.1}$$

$$Re = \rho u_j D / \mu \tag{21.2}$$

whereby ρ stands for liquid density, D for jet diameter, u_j for mean jet velocity, σ for surface tension, and μ for the viscosity of the liquid.

The operating data for the Respimat in the field of impinging jet atomizers are shown in Table 21.3, with a graphical illustration of the different flow regimes shown in Figure 21.2. At very low flow rates, large surface drops grow in front of the nozzle exits and prevent the generation of jets and droplets. When the flow rate is increased, a liquid chain structure is formed (a). If the jet velocity is increased even further, a liquid sheet is generated, which is enclosed by a thicker closed rim (b). Further increases in velocity and a reduction in the surface tension of the liquid lead to the rim opening up and an increase of the Weber number (c). This unstable rim (d) is suitable for the generation of droplets; however, the impact wave regime shown in (e) is preferred for optimum droplet formation (Wachtel 2016).

The uniblock of the Respimat has been designed using Quality by Design aspects. The fine particle fraction can be set by the impaction angle and the hydraulic diameter (defined as 4 * area/circumference) of the uniblock outlets (Pañao and Delgado 2013). Increasing the impaction angle increases the

TABLE 21.3

Operating Regime of the Respimat in the Field of Impinging Jet Atomizers

Case	Hydraulic Diameter (μm)	Reynolds Number (–)	Weber Number (–)	Assessment
Respimat	6.6	738	1840	Impact wave (*We*)
(a)	400	1000	27.5	Liquid chain
(b)	400	40.4	58.8	Closed rim
(c)	400	294	152	Open rim
(d)	400	3536	343.5	Unstable rim
(e)	400	5000	687	Impact wave

Source: Reproduced from Wachtel, H., Respiratory drug delivery, in *Microsystems for Pharmatechnology: Manipulation of Fluids, Particles, Droplets, and Cells*, ed. A. Dietzel, p. 257, Springer, Heidelberg, Germany, 2016. With permission.

Assessment of cases (a) to (e) according to Chen et al. (2013). Based on the Weber number (*We*), the Respimat generates impact waves. Respimat's micro-jets are responsible for the low Reynolds (*Re*) number, indicating highly laminar flow. (The *Re* and *We* numbers are quoted from Chen et al. [diameter-related *Re* and *We* numbers]). The hydraulic diameter of the outlet channels is defined as 4 * area/circumference, whereby area means cross-section area of the channel and circumference means the length of the boundary around the area.

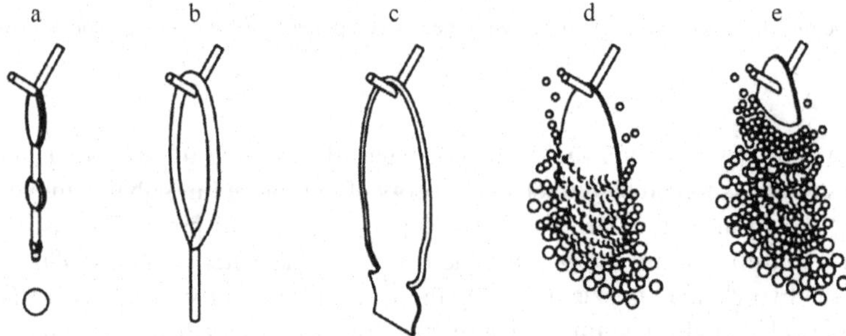

FIGURE 21.2 Graphical illustration of the different flow regimes encountered when increasing the Weber number of impinging jet atomizers. (a) liquid sheet, (b) closed rim, (c) open rim, (d) unstable rim, and (e) impact wave. (Reproduced from Wachtel, H., Respiratory drug delivery, in *Microsystems for Pharmatechnology: Manipulation of Fluids, Particles, Droplets, and Cells*, ed. A. Dietzel, p. 257, Springer, Heidelberg, Germany, 2016. With permission.)

impaction energy, which results in a higher fine particle fraction. The increase of the hydraulic diameter reduces the resistance in the uniblock outlets and leads to a higher fine particle fraction, overcompensating the geometrical size effect of the diameter. The configuration of the outlet channels in the uniblock configuration of the approved products leads to a high proportion of the particles generated falling into the fine particle fraction (<5.8 μm; between 65%–80%) (Dalby et al. 2004), depending on whether aqueous or ethanolic solutions are used. A typical example of the particle distribution generated by Respimat using an aqueous drug solution, as determined by Andersen Cascade Impactor, is shown in Figure 21.3. The fine particle fraction is almost double the value reported for aerosols generated by pMDIs and DPIs.

In addition to the high fine particle fraction described earlier, the soft mist that emerges from the uniblock has a velocity of 0.8 m/s, which is 3 times–10 times slower than that observed with pMDIs (Hochrainer et al. 2005). The Respimat, therefore, has a relatively long spray duration compared with pMDIs (1.2 seconds versus 0.15 seconds–0.36 seconds, respectively), allowing for a better coordination of the actuation/inhalation maneuver by the patient (Wachtel et al. 2017). Overall, the

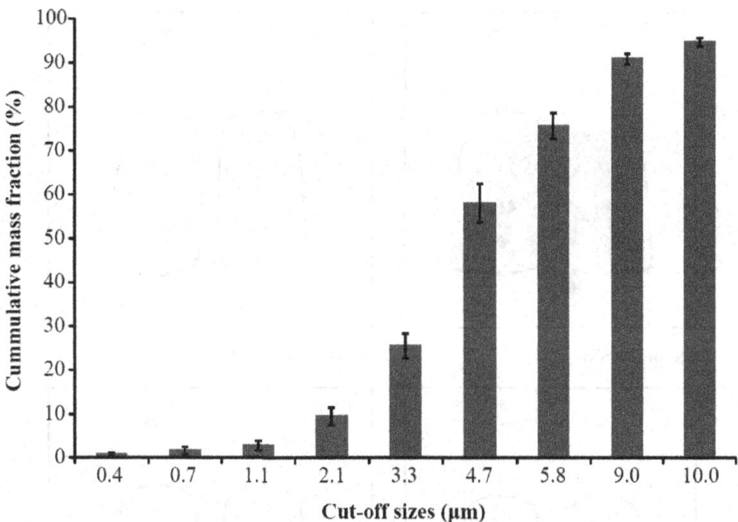

FIGURE 21.3 Typical distribution of aerodynamic particles of an aqueous solution released by the Respimat into an Anderson Cascade Impactor at 90% ambient relative humidity (cumulative mass fraction, % ± standard deviation). (Reproduced from Spallek, M. et al., *Respir. Drug Deliv. VIII*, 2, 375–378, 2002. With permission. Virginia Commonwealth University and RDD Online.)

combination of lower velocity, smaller particle size, and longer duration of the aerosol cloud suggests improved coordination of inhalation and actuation, higher drug deposition in the lung, and less loss in the oropharyngeal tract (Anderson 2006); this was clinically proven by scintigraphic studies in humans (see below).

21.5.1 Clinical Performance of the Respimat

Early studies using radiolabeled drug particles and gamma scintigraphy have found improved lung deposition of drug aerosols administered by the Respimat (Newman et al. 1998; Pitcairn et al. 2005). In a comparison of the Respimat and a conventional pMDI with or without a valved holding chamber in healthy non-smoking volunteers, significantly more fenoterol was delivered to the lungs by the Respimat (39.2% versus 11% and 9.9% for Respimat, pMDI without and with valved holding chamber, respectively; $p < 0.01$) and significantly less drug was deposited in the oropharynx (Newman et al. 1998). Equally, the Respimat achieved significantly higher deposition of flunisolide in the lungs compared with the MDI plus valved holding chamber (44.6% versus 26.4%, respectively; $p < 0.01$), with similar oropharyngeal deposition. A comparison of patients with mild-to-moderate asthma using either the Respimat (containing budesonide solution), Turbuhaler® (AstraZeneca; containing budesonide dry powder), or a pMDI (containing beclomethasone dipropionate) found significantly greater mean whole-lung deposition from the Respimat compared with the Turbuhaler (at both fast or slow inhaled flow rates) or the pMDI (Figure 21.4). Drug administration by the Respimat resulted in a more peripheral deposition pattern compared with the Turbuhaler (Pitcairn et al. 2005).

The Respimat is currently approved as a component of products that deliver tiotropium (Spiriva®) and fixed-dose combinations of ipratropium/fenoterol (Berodual®; the Netherlands and Germany) in patients with asthma or chronic obstructive pulmonary disease (COPD), olodaterol (Striverdi®), and fixed-dose combinations of olodaterol/tiotropium (Spiolto® [Stiolto® in the United States]) and ipratropium/albuterol (Combivent®) for the treatment of COPD.

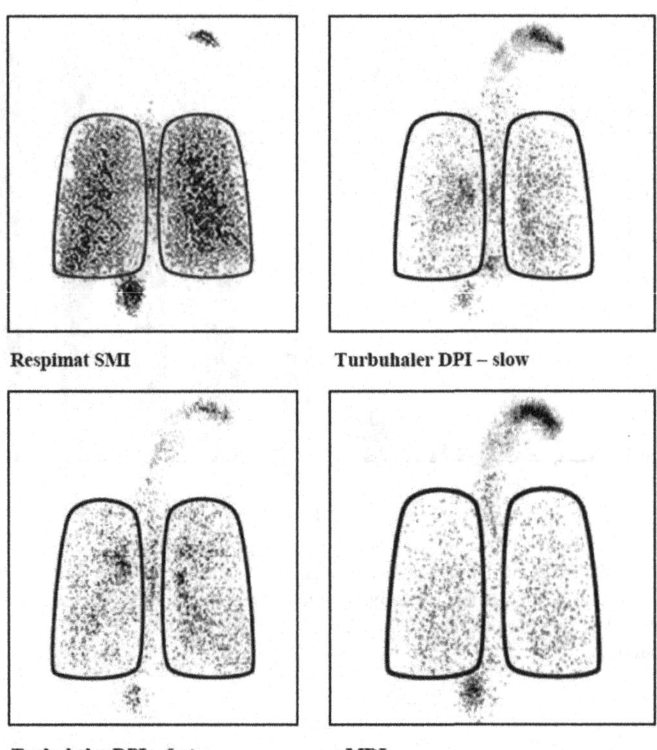

FIGURE 21.4 Example of scintigraphic images for Respimat, Turbuhaler DPI (slow and fast inhaled flow rates), and a pMDI containing chlorofluorocarbon, comparing the deposition of corticosteroid aerosol in the human lung. (From Pitcairn, G. et al., *J. Aerosol Med.*, 18, 264–272, 2005; Reprinted from Mary Ann Liebert, Inc., New Rochelle, New York. With permission.)

A number of randomized dose-finding studies have compared the efficacy and safety of tiotropium soft mist administered with the Respimat with tiotropium as dry powder administered by the HandiHaler® device (Boehringer Ingelheim). These studies found that tiotropium Respimat 5 μg has a comparable pharmacokinetic (PK), efficacy, and safety profile compared with tiotropium 18 μg administered in dry powder form using the HandiHaler (Caillaud et al. 2007; van Noord et al. 2009; Ichinose et al. 2010; Hohlfeld et al. 2014).

In the TIOSPIR trial, a large-scale phase III study in patients with COPD treated with tiotropium Respimat (5 μg or 2.5 μg) or tiotropium HandiHaler (18 μg), a similar efficacy and safety profile was found for the Respimat and HandiHaler despite the lower doses of tiotropium administered by Respimat (Wise et al. 2013), thus confirming the efficacy of the device. *Post hoc* and pooled analyses from the TIOSPIR trial across a range of patient subtypes provided further evidence that both tiotropium inhalers were comparable with regards to overall lung function, exacerbation risk, quality of life, and safety (Dahl and Kaplan 2016).

An extensive study of the PK properties of tiotropium found a lower systemic exposure (determined by mean plasma concentration at steady state) in patients with COPD treated with once-daily tiotropium Respimat 5 μg compared with patients treated with once-daily tiotropium HandiHaler 18 μg (Hohlfeld et al. 2014). The five-way crossover study consisted of five 4-week periods and also included tiotropium Respimat doses of 1.25 μg and 2.5 μg. A 4-week treatment period was considered sufficient to reach PK and pharmacodynamic steady states. The mean plasma concentrations of tiotropium from 2 minutes to 6 hours post-dosing for tiotropium Respimat 1.25 μg, 2.5 μg, and 5 μg and tiotropium HandiHaler 18 μg are shown in Figure 21.5.

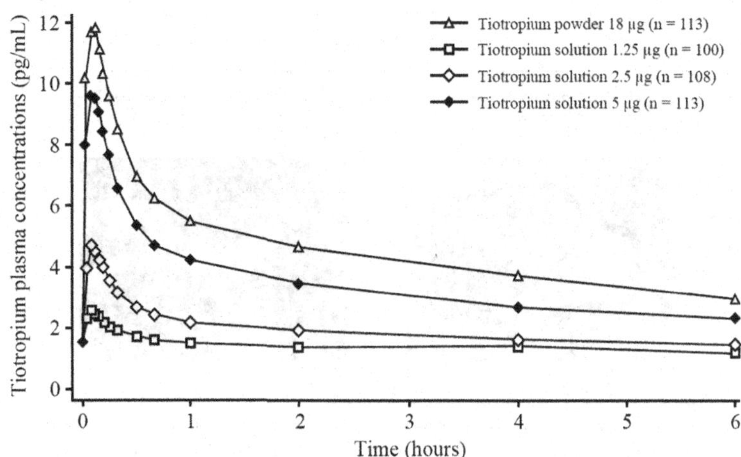

FIGURE 21.5 Geometric mean tiotropium plasma concentration–time profile following multiple inhalations of tiotropium Respimat or tiotropium HandiHaler. (Reproduced from Hohlfeld, J. M. et al., *J. Clin. Pharmacol.*, 54, 405–414, 2014. With permission.)

21.6 The AERx System

The AERx platform of small handheld devices includes both an electromechanical device, which was developed first, and the battery-free, all-mechanical AERx Essence, with both reusable devices utilizing the same dosage form (strip) technology (Figure 21.6).

The single-use, disposable dosage form contains an integral array of submicrometer-sized nozzle holes separated from a sealed compartment containing the sterile drug formulation. Upon actuation by the user, the device extrudes the drug formulation through the precisely drilled nozzle array to create the aerosol spray, thus ensuring uniformity of the aerosol particle size distribution and the amount of drug in the aerosol droplets. Furthermore, the single-use nozzle array cannot be compromised by prior use, and there is no requirement for preservatives in the formulation.

The electromechanical device was developed primarily to address the treatment burden of patients who have to inject themselves frequently with their medications, e.g. patients with diabetes who require multiple insulin injections daily (Thipphawong et al. 2002) or patients with breakthrough pain episodes connected to intravenous opiates. These devices provided complete disease management capabilities, including compliance management and electronic key/lockout mechanisms to prevent abuse and overdosing of opiates. Using an inhaled technology to address systemic indications with narrow therapeutic windows like those described above necessitated devices with high precision of delivery to the peripheral lung, which was not possible at the time using other inhalation technologies. Thus, a new inhaled technology had to be developed.

The AERx electromechanical device enables automatic user coordination of inhalation with actuation and reduces the impact of anatomical variability on lung deposition. The electromechanical device prompts and trains the user to inhale at the optimal flow rate and only delivers the aerosol early in the inspiration event, ensuring that over 90% of the emitted aerosol avoids the oropharynx and deposits in the lung (Sangwan et al. 2001; for topical treatment with a protein). For morphine, a small molecule, over 90% of the emitted dose deposits in the lung and rapidly enters the systemic circulation (Cipolla and Johansson 2008).

The electromechanical device also has the capability to titrate fractional doses from the insulin strip by controlling the depth of the stroke of the piston, allowing patients with diabetes to modulate each dose, resulting in glucose control comparable or superior to injection (Thipphawong et al. 2002). Clinical evaluation of the electromechanical AERx device included small molecule drugs, peptides, proteins, and gene therapeutic agents (Cipolla and Johansson 2008).

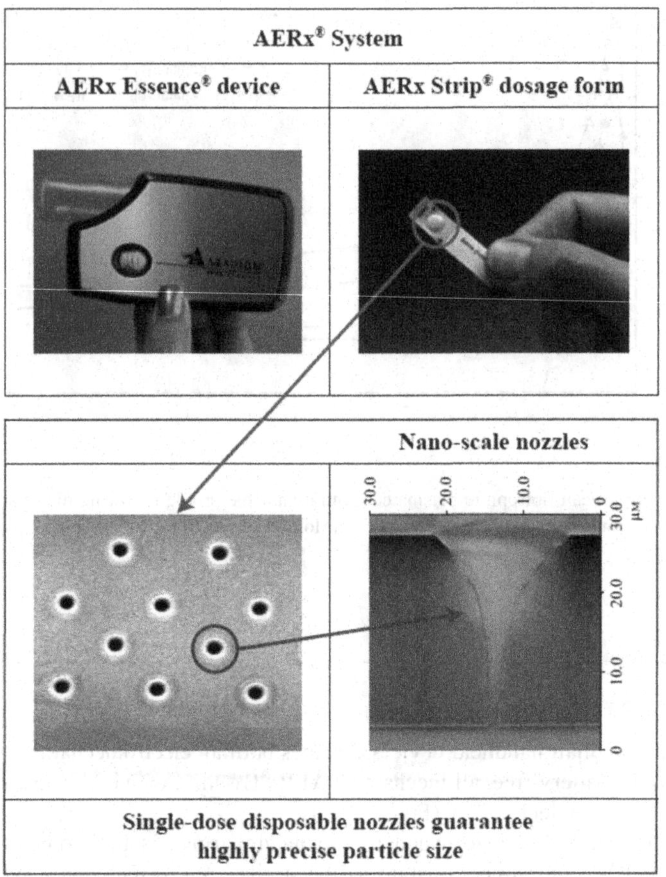

FIGURE 21.6 The AERx Essence® device, dosage form, and nozzle array.

The AERx Essence device utilized many of the same guiding principles as the electromechanical device so as to minimize aerosol deposition in the oropharynx and maximize delivery to the lung, but accomplished this by using simple, mechanical elements (Cipolla and Johansson 2008). The AERx Essence was developed to address topical lung disease that required greater precision or higher doses than could be delivered by MDIs, as well as for select systemic applications. This device generates very fine aerosols using nozzles that are manufactured with solid state lasers, producing nozzle arrays with submicrometer-sized exit holes. In contrast, the electromechanical device requires a heater to facilitate reduction in droplet size for efficient and precise delivery to the lung.

21.6.1 Clinical Performance of the AERx Essence

The AERx Essence system has been evaluated in the clinic for delivery of treprostinil for patients with pulmonary hypertension (Cipolla et al. 2011) and nicotine for smoking cessation (Cipolla and Gonda 2015). In those trials, the aerosol-emitted dose was approximately 50% of the loaded dose in the strip, compared with 70% for the electromechanical device. However, the device control features still enabled 91.6% ± 7.9% (mean ± SD; n = 14) of the treprostinil emitted dose to deposit in the lung with greater uniformity and a lower central:peripheral ratio (1.39) than for the nebulizer (3.96) (Cipolla et al. 2011). To improve smoking cessation effectiveness, AERx Essence provides more rapid peak plasma nicotine levels than nicotine replacement therapies (e.g. gums, patches, and nasal spray) and even e-cigarettes

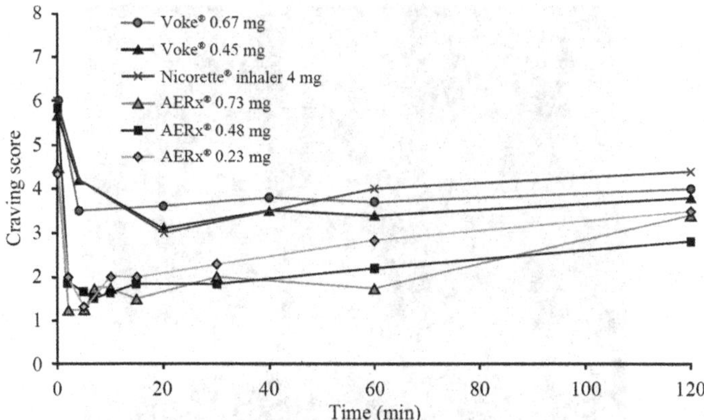

FIGURE 21.7 Reduction in craving from the AERx Essence® system compared with the Voke® inhaler and Nicorette® inhalator. The sample sizes are $n = 5$, 6, and 5 for AERx Essence 0.73, 0.48, and 0.23 mg nicotine, respectively, and $n = 24$ for both Voke groups and the Nicorette Inhalator. (Reprinted from Cipolla, D., and Gonda, I., *Asian J. Pharm. Sci.*, 10, 472–480, 2015. With permission.)

(Cipolla and Gonda 2015). Thus, it has the potential to provide the same physiological response that smokers receive from cigarettes and so may successfully address the craving episodes and other symptoms of nicotine withdrawal (Figure 21.7).

21.7 Devices Based on Medspray Nozzles

Two devices based on spray nozzle technology from Medspray are currently in clinical trials and planned to enter the market in 2019. The Ecomyst device (Figure 21.8A), developed in collaboration with Aero Pump, looks similar to a pMDI and is based on a preservative-free pump system, designed to compete with current pMDI systems with propellants (De Kruijf 2017; De Kruijf and Garbin 2017). The ADI (Figure 21.8B)

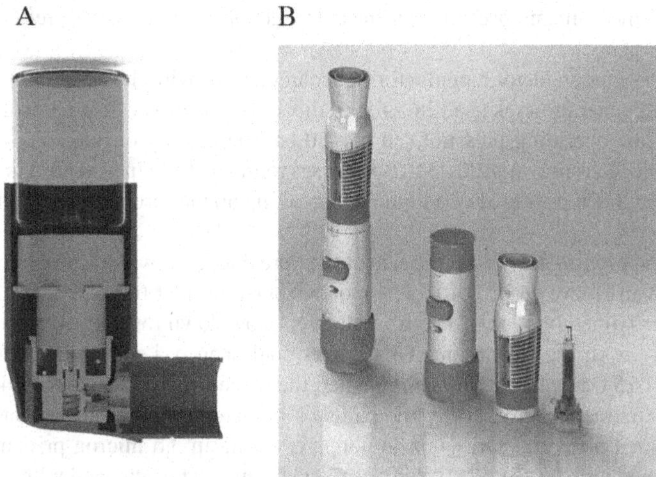

FIGURE 21.8 Devices incorporating the Medspray nozzle. (A) The Ecomyst® device (Aero Pump): the device is based on a 25 microliter, preservative-free, airless, or vented pump system (vented system shown here, airless system has a shrinking inner bag in the container). (Courtesy of Aero Pump.) (B) The Aqueous Droplet Inhaler® device (Pharmaero). The mouthpiece is a daily disposable and contains a 1 mL glass syringe with the drug formulation. The mechanical base part with the spring-driven dosing mechanism can be reused during 1 month. (Courtesy of Pharmaero.)

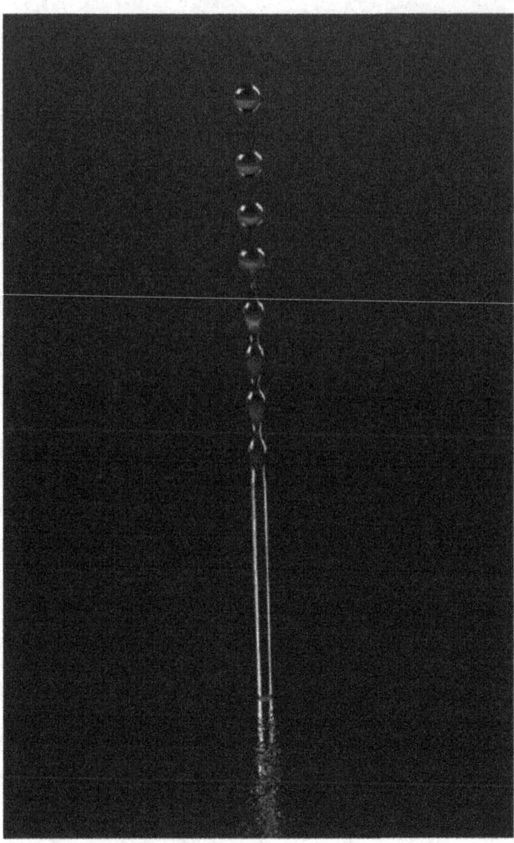

FIGURE 21.9 Rayleigh or capillary wave break-up. The droplet size is approximately 2 times the size of the spray pore. No formation of satellite droplets. (Courtesy of Medspray.)

is based on dosing mechanisms used in pen injector technology and uses a prefilled glass syringe as primary package.

Using silicon and semiconductor manufacturing techniques (as with the Respimat), but using Rayleigh break-up for droplet generation (as used in AERx), this device is a soft mist aerosol generator that can work at relatively low operating pressure (20 bar–50 bar, depending on viscosity of the formulation; 1 mPa·s–5 mPa·s). For the spray nozzles, Medspray uses round orifices in very thin membranes, approximately 1 micron thin. Each pore creates a liquid jet, breaking up into droplets by capillary wave break-up (Figure 21.9).

The droplets are approximately twice the size of the pore diameter, with minimal formation of smaller satellite droplets (Van Hoeve et al. 2010). The monodisperse droplet trains exit the 2 μm nozzle pores at a velocity of approximately 40 m/s. The front droplets slow down instantly as they are "in the wind," while the pursuers are in the slipstream. This causes coalescence, i.e. droplets merging together (the double-drop has a 1.25 times larger droplet diameter, the triple-drop diameter is 1.44 times larger, etc.). Adding turbulent airstreams, invoked by the patient's inhalation maneuver, can prevent such coalescence. Starting from 1.8 micron spray nozzle pores, resulting in 3.6 micron primary droplet trains, a median mass aerodynamic diameter between 5 μm and 6 μm can be achieved with such an aerosol mix chamber (as described in Medspray patent WO 2014/137215 A1) (De Kruijf et al. 2014).

Medspray's nozzle units are designed for mass fabrication. The nozzle chips are produced on a wafer scale (more than 10,000 units per wafer) before being singulated, picked, and placed by a robot with a heated bond head into the medical-grade plastic nozzle holder. This means that no glue is used, which is crucial as the nozzle is part of the primary package of the drug. Both the ADI and the Ecomyst devices

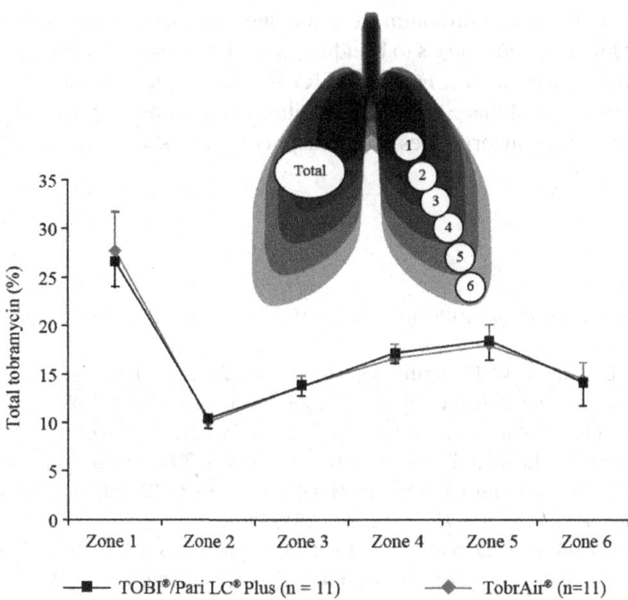

FIGURE 21.10 Distribution of tobramycin throughout the different lung zones. Scintigraphic measurements with TobrAir® (grey diamonds) and Pari LC® Plus (black squares); mean ± SD. (Reprinted from Beckert, M. et al., A phase I pharmacoscintigraphic study in healthy volunteers comparing the delivery of tobramycin using the TobrAir compared to the delivery of tobramycin nebulizer solution (Tobi) by Pari LC Plus, *Poster presented at the North American Cystic Fibrosis Conference*, Phoenix, AZ. With permission.)

feature a high airflow resistance (190 √Pa L/min), nudging the patients to a target inhalation airflow of approximately 15 L/m (De Kruijf 2017; De Kruijf and Garbin 2017). This way, an aerosol with a median mass aerodynamic diameter of 5.5 μm and a geometric standard deviation of 1.5 μm results in a lung dose of >50% of the metered dose and an alveolar dose of >30% of the metered dose (Aerosol Research Laboratory of Alberta calculator) (ICRP Publication 66 1994; Finlay and Martin 2008). Large medicine doses can be achieved by longer actuation times, e.g. 3 seconds–4 seconds inhalation, resulting in a drug flow rate of approximately 12 μL/s–15 μL/s.

Clinical phase I trials with TobrAir®, a product based on the ADI and filled with a viscous 150 mg/mL tobramycin formulation, have shown a scintigraphically determined lung dose of more than 50% of the metered volume of 50 μL and a lung distribution very similar to the Pari LC® Plus Nebulizer, with corresponding PKs (Beckert et al. 2015) (Figure 21.10).

Investigator-driven trials with an early version of the Ecomyst device show a pharmacodynamic effect of salbutamol at emitted doses 5 times lower than current pMDI systems, with a 6 μm median mass aerodynamic diameter soft mist aerosol (Munnik et al. 2009).

21.8 Conclusion

SMIs provide an innovative approach to inhalation therapy, using mechanisms to generate a slow-moving aerosol cloud from a dosed volume of drug solution by means of mechanical energy, without the need for propellants or electric power sources and independent of interpersonal variations. Compared with traditional inhalers, the soft mist device delivers an aerosol spray with improved particle characteristics, leading to an increased percentage of dose deposition in the lungs and less loss in the oropharyngeal area. SMIs are not sensitive to environmental humidity, and perform in a consistent and repeatable manner, regardless of ambient temperatures or pressure. To be suitable for use in an SMI, a drug needs to be soluble in either water or ethanol, and available at a concentration that achieves the target dose once aerosolized. Clinical studies with tiotropium Respimat have provided evidence that the improved lung deposition allows for lower absolute doses to be administered, with similar efficacy and safety outcomes compared with tiotropium with a DPI. For the AERx Essence device, human PK and lung deposition imaging data have demonstrated that >90% of the emitted aerosol dose deposits in the lung. Early clinical reports of the ADI, which incorporates the Medspray nozzle, show comparable lung deposition of tobramycin with a nebulizer.

REFERENCES

Anderson, P. 2006. Use of Respimat soft mist inhaler in COPD patients. *International Journal of Chronic Obstructive Pulmonary Disease* 1, no. 3:251–259.

Beckert, M., P. Evans, L. Patrick, W. De Kruijf, and T. Norling. 2015. A phase I pharmacoscintigraphic study in healthy volunteers comparing the delivery of tobramycin using the TobrAir compared to the delivery of tobramycin nebuliser solution (Tobi) by Pari LC Plus. Poster 36, *Journal of Cystic Fibrosis* 15:S60

Caillaud, D., C. Le Merre, Y. Martinat, B. Aguilaniu, and D. Pavia. 2007. A dose-ranging study of tiotropium delivered via Respimat soft mist inhaler or HandiHaler in COPD patients. *International Journal of Chronic Obstructive Pulmonary Disease* 2, no. 4:559–565.

Chattopadhyay, P., B. Y. Shekunov, D. Yim, D. Cipolla, B. Boyd, and S. Farr. 2007. Production of solid lipid nanoparticle suspensions using supercritical fluid extraction of emulsions (SFEE) for pulmonary delivery using the AERx system. *Advanced Drug Delivery Reviews* 59, no. 6:444–453.

Chen, X., D. Ma, V. Yang, and S. Popinet. 2013. High-fidelity simulations of impinging jet atomization. *Atomization Sprays* 23, no. 1079:1101.

Cipolla, D., P. Bruinenberg, I. Gonda et al. 2011. Deeper lung pulmonary delivery of treprostinil is associated with delayed systemic absorption. *Journal of Aerosol Medicine and Pulmonary Drug Delivery* 24:16.

Cipolla, D., H. K. Chan, J. Schuster, and D. Farina. 2010. Personalizing aerosol medicine: Development of delivery systems tailored to the individual. *Therapeutic Delivery* 1, no. 5:667–682.

Cipolla, D., and I. Gonda. 2011. Formulation technology to repurpose drugs for inhalation delivery. *Drug Discovery Today: Therapeutic Strategies* 8:123–130.

Cipolla, D., and I. Gonda. 2015. Inhaled nicotine replacement therapy. *Asian Journal of Pharmaceutical Sciences* 10:472–480.

Cipolla, D., and E. Johansson. 2008. AERx pulmonary drug delivery systems. In *Modified Release Drug Delivery Technology*, ed. M. J. Rathbone, J. Hadgraft, M. S. Roberts and M. Lane, pp. 563–572. New York: Informa Healthcare.

Dahl, R., and A. Kaplan. 2016. A systematic review of comparative studies of tiotropium Respimat® and tiotropium HandiHaler® in patients with chronic obstructive pulmonary disease: Does inhaler choice matter? *BMC Pulmonary Medicine* 16, no. 1:135.

Dalby, R., J. Eicher, and B. Zierenberg. 2011. Development of Respimat(®) soft mist inhaler and its clinical utility in respiratory disorders. *Medical Devices (Auckland, N.Z.)* 4:145–155.

Dalby, R., M. Spallek, and T. Voshaar. 2004. A review of the development of Respimat soft mist inhaler. *International Journal of Pharmaceutics* 283, no. 1–2:1–9.

De Kruijf, W. 2017. Development of a propellant-free metered dose inhaler. Poster P100, *Journal of Aerosol Medicine and Pulmonary Drug Delivery* 30, no. 3:A-23.

De Kruijf, W., and N. Garbin. 2017. Usability test results with high resistance inhalers. Poster P16, *Journal of Aerosol Medicine and Pulmonary Drug Delivery* 30, no. 3:A-20.

De Kruijf, W., W. Nijdam, J. M. Wissing, and T. V. Huijgen. 2014. Aerosol generator for generating an inhalation aerosol. Patent PCT/NL2014/050136.

European Directorate for the Quality of Medicines and Healthcare. 2017. European Pharmacopoeia (Ph. Eur.) 9th edition. https://www.edqm.eu/en/european-pharmacopoeia-9th-edition.

Finlay, W. H., and A. R. Martin. 2008. Recent advances in predictive understanding respiratory tract deposition. *Journal of Aerosol Medicine and Pulmonary Drug Delivery* 21:189–205.

Food and Drug Administration. 2000. Sec. 200.51 aqueous-based drug products for oral inhalation. https://www.ecfr.gov/cgi-bin/text-idx?SID=35844250aa537621dbdf71035f5428f5&mc=true&node=se21.4.200_151&rgn=div8.

Hochrainer, D., H. Hölz, C. Kreher, L. Scaffidi, M. Spallek, and H. Wachtel. 2005. Comparison of the aerosol velocity and spray duration of Respimat soft mist inhaler and pressurized metered dose inhalers. *Journal of Aerosol Medicine: The Official Journal of the International Society for Aerosols in Medicine* 18, no. 3:273–282.

Hohlfeld, J. M., A. Sharma, J. A. van Noord et al. 2014. Pharmacokinetics and pharmacodynamics of tiotropium solution and tiotropium powder in chronic obstructive pulmonary disease. *Journal of Clinical Pharmacology* 54, no. 4:405–414.

Ichinose, M., T. Fujimoto, and Y. Fukuchi. 2010. Tiotropium 5microg via Respimat and 18microg via HandiHaler; efficacy and safety in Japanese COPD patients. *Respiratory Medicine* 104, no. 2:228–236.

ICRP Publication 66. 1994. Human respiratory tract model for radiological protection. *Annals of the ICRP* 24:1–3.

Munnik, P., A. H. de Boer, J. Wissink et al. 2009. In vivo performance testing of the novel Medspray wet aerosol inhaler. *Journal of Aerosol Medicine and Pulmonary Drug Delivery* 22, no. 4:317–321.

Newman, S. P., J. Brown, K. P. Steed, S. J. Reader, and H. Kladders. 1998. Lung deposition of fenoterol and flunisolide delivered using a novel device for inhaled medicines: Comparison of Respimat with conventional metered-dose inhalers with and without spacer devices. *Chest* 113, no. 4:957–963.

Pañao, M. R. O., and J. M. D. Delgado. 2013. Characteristics of multijet impingement sprays for water applications." *ILASS-Americas 25th Annual Conference on Liquid Atomization and Spray Systems*, Pittsburgh, PA:1–10.

Pitcairn, G., S. Reader, D. Pavia, and S. Newman. 2005. Deposition of corticosteroid aerosol in the human lung by Respimat soft mist inhaler compared to deposition by metered dose inhaler or by turbuhaler dry powder inhaler. *Journal of Aerosol Medicine: The Official Journal of the International Society for Aerosols in Medicine* 18, no. 3:264–272.

Pritchard, J. N. 2015. Industry guidance for the selection of a delivery system for the development of novel respiratory products. *Expert Opinion on Drug Delivery* 12, no. 11:1755–1765.

Sangwan, S., J. M. Agosti, L. A. Bauer et al. 2001. Aerosolized protein delivery in asthma: Gamma camera analysis of regional deposition and perfusion. *Journal of Aerosol Medicine: The Official Journal of the International Society for Aerosols in Medicine* 14, no. 2:185–195.

Spallek, M., D. Hochrainer, and H. Wachtel. 2002. Optimizing nozzles for SMIs. *Respiratory Drug Delivery* VIII 2:375–378.

Thipphawong, J., B. Otulana, P. Clauson, J. Okikawa, and S. J. Farr. 2002. Pulmonary insulin administration using the AERx insulin diabetes system. *Diabetes Technology & Therapeutics* 4, no. 4:499–504.

United States Pharmacopeial Convention. 2017. *United States Pharmacopeia 41 - National Formulary 36.* Rockville, MD: United States Pharmacopeial Convention.

van Hoeve, W., S. Geckle, J. Snoeijer, M. Versluis, M. Brenner, and D. Lohse. 2010. Breakup of diminutive Rayleigh jets. *Physics of Fluids* 22:1222003.

van Noord, J. A., P. J. Cornelissen, J. L. Aumann, J. Platz, A. Mueller, and C. Fogarty. 2009. The efficacy of tiotropium administered via Respimat soft mist inhaler or HandiHaler in COPD patients. *Respiratory Medicine* 103, no. 1:22–29.

Wachtel, H. 2016. Respiratory drug delivery. In *Microsystems for Pharmatechnology: Manipulation of Fluids, Particles, Droplets, and Cells*, ed. A. Dietzel, p. 257. Heidelberg, Germany: Springer.

Wachtel, H., S. Kattenbeck, and S. Dunne. 2017. The Respimat® development story: Patient-centered innovation. *Pulmonary Therapy* 3:19.

Wise, R. A., A. Anzueto, D. Cotton et al. 2013. Tiotropium Respimat inhaler and the risk of death in COPD. *New England Journal of Medicine* 369, no. 16:1491–1501.

Zierenberg, B., and J. Eicher. 2003. The Respimat, a new soft mist inhaler for delivering drugs to the lungs. In *Modified-Release Drug Delivery Technology*, ed. M. J. Rathbone, J. Hadgraft and M. S. Roberts, pp. 925–932. Boca Raton, FL: Marcel Dekker.

Zierenberg, B., J. Eicher, S. Dunne, and B. Freund. 1996. Boehringer Ingelheim nebulizer Bineb®: A new approach to inhalation therapy. *Respiratory Drug Delivery* 1:187–194.

Section VII

Drug Product Testing

22

Quality by Design Considerations

William Craig Stagner and Anthony J. Hickey

CONTENTS

22.1 Introduction

Quality by design has long been a component of pharmaceutical process engineering and has been a focus of the United States Food and Drug Administration since the turn of the Millennium (FDA 2006a; Lionberger et al. 2008; Yu et al. 2014). Pharmaceutical inhalation aerosol products are complex dosage forms that require risk management to ensure their quality and performance. In this context, statistical experimental design principles can be applied to manufacturing and process analytical technology to monitoring critical quality attributes known to correlate with desired outcomes linked to the quality of the product (FDA 2004; Hickey and Ganderton 2010; Hickey 2018).

Quality is built into the final product and is critically dependent on the integration of the formulation, manufacturing process, and container closure system design (inhalation drug delivery system) (FDA 2009a). In the case of pharmaceutical inhalation aerosol dosage forms, the formulation components and manufacture, metering system (components and indexing mechanism), and device (flow path, baffles, and aerosol dispersion mechanism) all require consideration.

Adequate control of components and processes can only be achieved through appropriate validated analytical techniques. Depending on the nature of the process, particularly whether they are batch or continuous manufacturing, assembly, or packaging processes, these techniques can be used off-line, on-line, or in-line. As the names suggest the techniques can be applied with greater or lesser proximity to the process which has implications for the speed at which corrections can be made to deviations. The tools employed to evaluate the component or process may scrutinize the chemistry of the drug or additive or the mechanics of the device assembly and performance.

The product development considerations are broken into the composition of the formulation. The qualitative (components) and quantitative (concentrations) elements must be defined. Manufacturing controls must be established on unit operations such as milling, mixing or blending, and filling. The quality environment current good manufacturing practice (CGMP) in which drug manufacturing files, protocols, and standard operating procedures ensure accuracy, and reproducibility links directly to subsequent preclinical toxicology pharmacokinetic and pharmacodynamic studies that are also conducted with quality standards current good laboratory practice and current good clinical practice (CGLP and CGCP).

The target product profile (TPP) is defined in terms of the key components that define performance to meet the clinical need (FDA 2007). The evolution of the TPP depends on knowledge gained in development and is therefore subject to modification within parameters that assure the final performance. In response to the TPP, critical quality attributes emerge that must be monitored and controlled to assure the quality and performance of the product and ultimately its safety and efficacy.

Risk management is usually achieved through a comprehensive understanding of the product and processes which can be achieved using the principles of statistical experimental design to establish design and process space within which the product or process are invariant with respect to input variables (FDA 2006b). The broader the operating space with respect to manufacturing variables, the lower the risk of failure. The product can also be challenged through failure mode and effects analysis. Monitoring of product and processes allows for out of specification analysis with contingencies for correction as a step before discarding product.

Adopting a quality by design approach through the application of process analytical technology allows critical quality attributes to be managed to address the target product profile mitigating risks of product and process failure. The knowledge gained through these activities facilitate lifecycle management and continual improvement to ensure the safety and efficacy of product brought to the clinic and to market (FDA 2009b).

22.2 QbD Product Design Quality Elements

22.2.1 Quality Target Product Profile

The ultimate beneficiary of the quality target product profile (QTPP) is the patient. The QTPP is a strategic prospective compilation of product characteristics aimed to ensure desired safety, efficacy, and commercial success. A target product profile is typically developed by a multidisciplinary team. The TPP is a "living" document that is reviewed and revised throughout the various development phases. Each team member is responsible for being a patient advocate. The team composition varies depending if the drug is a small molecule or a biotechnology-derived product. Disciplines often represented are molecular biology, chemistry research and development, bioengineering, pharmacology, toxicology/drug safety, metabolism, pharmacokinetics, formulation design and manufacturing, clinical development, commercial manufacturing, and marketing.

A detailed TPP is often 12 pages–15 pages. The time and effort to prepare a TPP should be balanced with the risk of the product failing critical milestones. The FDA has issued a guidance document providing an example TPP listing the 17 key product labeling sections provided in a product monograph (FDA, 2007). Formulation scientists would be most involved with discussions involving indications and usage; dosage and administration; dosage forms and strengths; use in specific populations; description; clinical pharmacology; clinical studies; how supplied; and patient counseling information TPP sections.

The indication will dictate whether treatment is expected to provide systemic or local drug effect which in turn may impact the desired drug particle size. The drug strength, dose, expected dose range, dose duration, dosing interval, and age related dosing all affect the type of delivery system chosen. Use in special populations such as pediatrics (neonates, infants, children, and adolescents) and geriatrics impact the selection of the inhalation device. The clinical pharmacology drug properties like permeability, absorption, pharmacokinetics, and pharmacodynamics impact formulation design. For example, a short half-life may require a higher drug dose that is given at a higher dosing frequency. This could affect the amount of drug substance required for development. A higher dose may make a dry powder inhaler the preferred delivery system. Clinical studies significantly impact the product design effort. The study population and dose criteria need to be defined (age, number of subjects, national or international trials, escalating drug strength, dose, dosing interval, timing, and more). This information will help the product design team decide to keep development inside the company or look for external partners for some or all the development and clinical requirements The "how supplied" section of the TPP will be a function of the inhalation drug delivery device, the selected strength or strengths supported by the clinical studies, and the product stability which is often a function of the device (metered dose, dry power, nebulizer, soft mist, and so on). Patient counseling information is very important for orally inhaled products. Most orally inhaled drug delivery systems require very specific patient use instructions. Intuitively, the simpler the inhalation device, the simpler the patient use instructions, the patient is more compliant, and the medical outcomes are better.

22.2.2 Critical Quality Attributes

Orally inhaled drug product design is complex and multifactorial. Formulation design, process design, container closure, and drug delivery design are inextricably linked. The final product is referred to as *inhalation drug delivery system.* A product design specific TPP is based on the critical quality attributes of the drug substance, excipients, container closure system (CCS)/device delivery system, and drug product. The product design specific TPP can document the drug's physicochemical properties (appearance, odor, taste, morphology, particle size, density, surface area, melting point, moisture content, polymorphism, amorphous content, hygroscopicity, impurities, residual solvents, bacterial endotoxins, pKa, solid and solution state stability, lot-to-lot variability, and others) and their product design and TTP implications. The lungs of the patient population using orally inhaled drug products are often sensitive to inhaling foreign materials. This requires a thorough characterization and rigorous effort to set tight excipient quality control specifications. Much like the physicochemical characterization for drugs, a similar in-depth characterization is required for orally inhaled excipients. The CCS/delivery system critical quality attributes include the device components and their material composition. The size, shape, and geometry of the components such as valves, metering chamber, actuators, mouth piece, and orifice. The trigger flow rate is an important critical quality attribute for breath-actuated devices. The extensive FDA Drug Product specifications and characterization requirements for orally inhaled pMDI, DPI, and liquid sprays are summarized in Tables 22.1 and 22.2.

22.2.3 Quality Risk Management

Risk management involves risk assessment and risk control. Risk assessment identifies potential variables that could affect product quality. Risk assessment also evaluates the likelihood of a critical quality failure and consequences of such a failure. Risk control explicitly states how variables are going to be controlled and to what level.

22.2.3.1 Risk Assessment

The ultimate stakeholder in risk assessment is the patient. The company also has an invested interest in eliminating product recalls and preventing product performance failures. Risk assessment involves asking three fundamental questions: "What can go wrong?" This leads to risk identification: "What is the probability of going wrong?" These risks are often expressed as a probably of occurring or by rank ordering the risks by likelihood of occurring; and: "What are the consequences?" This is the evaluation phase of risk assessment. An Ishikawa diagram can be used to identify variables that have a potential to

TABLE 22.1

Summary of FDA Critical Quality Attribute Tests for Orally Inhaled Aerosols: Specifications for Drug Products

Drug Product Specifications			
Attribute Test	**pMDIs**	**DPIs**	**Liquid Sprays**[a]
Description	+[b],[c]	+	+
• Appearance of the container closure system			
• Color United States Pharmacopeia (USP) <631> and clarity <641> (for solutions)			
Identification	+	+	+
• Two independent methods to identify the drug			
Assay	+	+	+
• Stability indicating method for drug content			
Impurities and degradation products	+	+	+
• Validated analytical methods			
• Individual and total impurities and degradation products			
Preservatives and other stabilizing excipients[d]	+[d]	+[d]	+[d]
• Chemical content using specific assay			
• Antimicrobial preservative effectiveness testing USP<51>,[e] Antimicrobial Agents—contents USP <341>, microbial enumeration test <61>[f]			
Sterility USP <71>	−	−	+
Valve delivery/pump delivery amount and reproducibility	+	−	+
Spray content uniformity (SCU)[g]	+	−	+
Spray pattern and plum geometry (size and shape)	+	−	+
• Evaluated on a routine basis			
Droplet size distribution for solutions USP <429> and <786>	+	−	+
Particle size distribution of emitted dose USP <429> and <786>	+	+	+
Particulate matter USP <788> for solutions	+	−	+
Microbial limits[h] UPS <61>	+	+	+
Weight loss on stability (upright and inverted or horizontal)	+	−	+
Net content USP minimum fill <751>	+	−	+
Number of doses	+	+	−
Leachables (stability)[i]	+	−	+
pH USP <791>	−	−	+
Osmolality USP <785>	−	−	+
Viscosity if suspending or viscosity agent is used USP <911–914>	−	−	+
Mass median aerodynamic diameter and geometric standard deviation[j]	+	+	+
Water or moisture USP <921> and Karl Fischer USP <610>	+	+	−

(Continued)

TABLE 22.1 (*Continued*)

Summary of FDA Critical Quality Attribute Tests for Orally Inhaled Aerosols: Specifications for Drug Products

Drug Product Specifications			
Attribute Test	**pMDIs**	**DPIs**	**Liquid Sprays**[a]
Dose content uniformity (see Guidance)	+	+	–
Dose content uniformity through container life (see Guidance)	+[k]	+[k]	+[k]
Microscopic examination	+	+	–
Pressure testing[l]	+	–	–
Value delivery (shot weight)	+	–	–
Leak rate	+	–	–

Source: Al-Achi, A. et al., Aerosol product design, in *Integrated Pharmaceutics: Applied Preformulation, Product Design, and Regulatory Science*, 1st ed., John Wiley & Sons, Hoboken, NJ, pp. 451–454, 2013; Aerosol product design, in *Integrated Pharmaceutics: Applied Preformulation, Product Design, and Regulatory Science*, 1st ed., John Wiley & Sons, Hoboken, NJ, pp. 447–450, 2013; FDA, Guidance for industry, Metered dose inhaler (MDI) and dry powder inhaler (DPI) drug products, https://www.fda.gove/downloads/drugs/guidances/ucm070573.pdf, 1998; Guidance for industry, Nasal spray and inhalation solution, suspension, and spray drug products—chemistry, manufacturing, and controls documentation, https://www.fda.gov/downloads/drugs/guidancecomplianceregulatoryinformation/guidances/ucm070575.pdf, 2002.

[a] Inhalation solutions, suspensions, sprays, and soft mists (usually aqueous based)
[b] + indicates the attribute test is required
[c] – indicates the attribute test is not required
[d] Use only the minimum level of excipients
[e] For liquid sprays
[f] For pMDIs, DPIs, and liquid sprays
[g] Spray discharged through the actuator for drug content from beginning, middle, and end (for an individual container, among containers, and across batches)
[h] Show that product does not support growth of microorganism
[i] USP elastomer closures for injections <381>; Containers—plastics <661>; Biological reactivity tests *in vitro* <87>; Biological reactivity tests *in vivo* <88>
[j] Suspensions or solids USP <601>
[k] For device-metered DPI and liquids
[l] When using a cosolvent or more than one propellant

TABLE 22.2

Summary of FDA Attribute Tests for Orally Inhaled Aerosols: Characterization of Drug Product

Attribute Tests	pMDI	DPI	Liquid Sprays[a]
Priming and repriming (multiple use products) • Instructions should be developed for priming and repriming after different periods of non-use in the upright and horizontal configurations	+	–	+
Effect of resting time (multiple use products) • Determine the effect of increase resting time of the first spray of unprimed units (6 hours, 12 hours, 24 hours, 48 hours)	+	–	+
Temperature cycling	+[b]	–	+[c]
Effect of moisture • Determine effect of low and high humidity on spray content uniformity (SCU) and particle size distribution	–	+	–
In vitro dose proportionality (for multiple strengths)	+	+	+
Drug deposition on mouth piece • Determine amount of drug deposited on the mouth piece, adapters, and other accessories	+	+	–
Cleaning instructions • In-use studies need to determine the frequency of cleaning • Cleaning instruction should be provided	+	+	+
Device (as part of the container closure system) robustness • Performance should be studied for in-use (shaking, high temperature, low temperature, low humidity, high humidity), inadvertent use (dropping), and transportation (vibration and environmental conditions)	–	+	+
Effect of dosing orientation	+	+	+
Profiling of sprays near container exhaustion (trail off characteristics)	+	+	+
Effect of varying inspiratory flow rates • Determine the effect flow rates by children, adults, patients with severe lung disease and when spacers and other accessories are used. Breath-actuated triggering flow-rates	+	+	+
Effect of storage on particle size • Primary concern is for suspensions	+	+	+
Plume geometry • Complementary to the spray pattern test • Determines the shape of the entire plume • Plume geometry can be evaluated by high speed flash photography to allow the monitoring of the plume development over time. Not required as a routine test	+	–	+
Preservative effectiveness and sterility maintenance • Preservation must be maintained at a lower limit preservative level	–	–	+
Liquid sprays must maintain their sterility throughout the life of the product	–	–	+
Microbial challenge • Confirm product will not support the growth microbes	+	–[d]	+
Photostability • Performed for products whose primary package allows light exposure	+	+	+
Stability of primary (unprotected) package • Applies to products that have a protective secondary package (foil for low density polyethylene [LDPE] nebulizer solutions, or foil for dry powder inhalers) • Data should confirm use time for unprotected product in the primary container	–	+	–

Source: Al-Achi, A. et al., Aerosol product design, in *Integrated Pharmaceutics: Applied Preformulation, Product Design, and Regulatory Science*, 1st ed., John Wiley & Sons, Hoboken, NJ, pp. 451–454, 2013; FDA, Guidance for industry, Metered dose inhaler (MDI) and dry powder inhaler (DPI) drug products, https://www.fda.gove/downloads/drugs/guidances/ucm070573.pdf, 1998; Guidance for industry, Nasal spray and inhalation solution, suspension, and spray drug products—chemistry, manufacturing, and controls documentation, https://www.fda.gov/downloads/drugs/guidancecomplianceregulatoryinformation/guidances/ucm070575.pdf, 2002.

[a] Inhalation solutions, suspensions, sprays, and soft mists (usually aqueous based).

[b] Three or four 6-hour cycles per between subfreezing temperatures and 40°C for up to 6 weeks.

[c] 12-hour cycles, freezer (–10°C–20°C) and for at least 4 weeks.

[d] Not mentioned in Guidance for characterization, but is mentioned in Specification section.

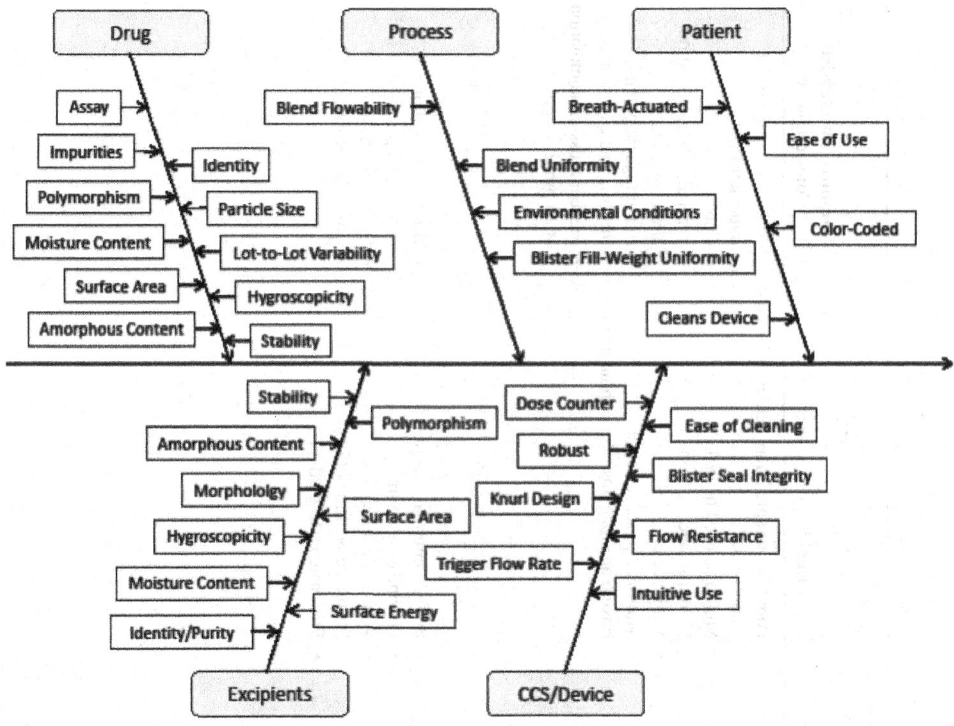

FIGURE 22.1 Ishikawa diagram illustrating the identification of variables that can affect a correct DPI dose.

impact a particular quality attribute. Figure 22.1 is an Ishikawa diagram for a DPI. In this example, it is used to identify potential variables that can affect a correct dose.

22.2.3.2 Risk Control and Control Strategy

The purpose of risk control is to manage the risk of product failure to an acceptable level. This is a difficult challenge requiring a balance among risk consequences, resources, and mitigating or avoiding the risk. Risk control undergoes a continual review cycle. Risk control identifies variables that can impact product quality and places appropriate controls to ensure product performance. Table 22.3 provides a risk control strategy for orally inhaled drug products. It identifies the risk factors (formulation, product process, CCS/device, CCS/formulation interactions, and patient considerations) and the key performance targets (dose reproducibility, prevent product adulteration, enable proper use, and minimize unintended effects).

22.2.4 Design Space

The design space (DS) defines the interrelationships between material attributes and process parameters (input variables) and acceptable critical product attributes (CPAs). These interrelationships are multidimensional and involve the combination and interaction of the input variables. Critical product quality attributes are expected to be met when the material attributes and process parameters are kept inside the DS. Likewise, product attribute failure is expected to occur when the input variables fall outside the DS. Making changes to the input variables within the DS is not considered a change from a regulatory perspective.

TABLE 22.3
Risk Control Strategy for Orally Inhaled Drug Products

	Performance Targets			
Risk Factors	**Assure Reproducible Dose**[a]	**Prevent Product Adulteration**	**Enable Proper Use**	**Minimize Unintended Consequences**
Formulation	• Control drug purity • Control drug properties • Maximize drug stability • Control excipient properties • Control excipient performance • Maintain suspension uniformity • Optimize blend flow	• Control drug purity • Control excipient purity • Maintain drug stability • Use stable excipients • Minimize leaching • Unit dose for sterility • Use effective preservatives	• Poor taste or smell may decrease compliance • Minimize need to shake • Minimize need to prime • Minimize resting effect • Minimize position effect • Ensure accurate dose throughout use	• Address lung potential hypersensitivity • Consider tonicity, particulate load, irritation, allergenic, and immunogenic potential of the drug and excipients
Product Process	• Control environmental moisture levels • Maintain uniform suspension • Control blend uniformity • Control fill weight • Eliminate leaks	• Maintain sterile area • Stop microbial ingress • GMP facility cleaning • GMP equipment cleaning • GMP cleaning of parts • Prevent dust generation		• Prevent cross-contamination at all process steps
CCS[b]**/Device**	• Precise and robust valves • Prevent moisture ingress • Aerosolization energy independent of patient disease state • Reliable robust power • Rugged design • Environmentally robust • Minimize resting • Minimize position effect	• Prevent "suck back" • Minimize leachables • Minimize foreign non-viable particles • Prevent microbe ingress • Easily cleaned	• Provide intuitive design • Provide dose counter • Warn patient near end of dosing • Eliminate position effect • Eliminate resting effect	• Breath-actuated or self-actuated systems • Should not misfire • Eliminate priming
CCS/Form-ulation Interactions	• Dose proportionality • Consistent spray • Consistent plume geometry • Robust over temperature ranges • Minimize static charge • Minimize crystal deposition • Prevent valve sticking	• Minimize leachables • Minimize preservative loss to CCS		

(Continued)

TABLE 22.3 (*Continued*)
Risk Control Strategy for Orally Inhaled Drug Products

	Performance Targets			
Risk Factors	**Assure Reproducible Dose[a]**	**Prevent Product Adulteration**	**Enable Proper Use**	**Minimize Unintended Consequences**
Patient Factors	• Coordinate inspiration • Use education- • Use instructions • Robust product design • Harsh weather worthy	• Device cleaning education • Cleaning instructions	• Remove dose build-up • Eliminate a required use orientation • Coordinate inspiration • Use education • Use instructions • Robust product design • Harsh weather worthy	• Eliminate excess drug doses when dose counter is at "0" • Consider how to avoid patient taking two or more drugs with different dosing regimens, leading to mix-ups

Source: Al-Achi, A. et al., Aerosol product design, in *Integrated Pharmaceutics: Applied Preformulation, Product Design, and Regulatory Science*, 1st ed., John Wiley & Sons, Hoboken, NJ, pp. 447–450, 2013; Horhota, S.T. and Leiner, S., Developing performance specifications for pulmonary drug delivery, in *Controlled Pulmonary Drug Delivery*, eds. H.D.C. Smyth and A.J. Hickey, Springer, New York, pp. 529–541, 2011.

[a] As measured by aerodynamic particle size distribution and content uniformity.

[b] CCS (container closure system).

A number of statistical and chemometric tools can be used to describe the DS. One of the most popular approaches uses a combination of choosing statistical experimental design (design of experiments), performing randomized experiments, analyzing the data to determine significant factors, and finally defining the DS using response contour/surface plots and regression models. Chemometric tools such as principle component analysis, partial least squares analysis, and partial least squares regression are useful in qualitatively and quantitatively assessing the effect of material attributes and process parameters on CPAs. Both the response surface regression models and partial least squares regression models can evaluate the main factor effects, interaction effects, and curvilinear effects on the product traits.

A funnel can be used as an analogy for defining the DS. At the top of the funnel are the many possible factors that could impact the CPAs. As steps are taken to become more informed about which factors/parameters/variables are most likely to impact the product, the process of defining the DS moves towards the narrow opening. By the time the process reaches the bottom of the funnel, the DS is defined. The acceptability of the DS is confirmed by verification experiments.

A chemometrics approach to defining the DS would generally begin with identifying factors that could potentially impact the CPAs. This preliminary parameter identification draws upon prior experience, knowledge, risk assessments, and CPAs. Experimentation and principle component analysis could be used to provide qualitative factor screening to identify the most impactful factors. Principle component analysis provides a visual way to interpret the data, which is often helpful with complex data sets. With a reduced set of factors, partial least squares analysis and partial least squares regression can be used to model data and determine acceptable parameter ranges. These model equations are used to define the DS.

The design space can be defined in multiple ways such as linear parameter ranges, mathematical relationships, time dependent functions, and mathematical models from multivariate methods. The contour/surface plots provide a means to visualize the design space and is an easy way to identify desirable target values for the input variables.

A case study is presented to illustrate the use of statistical tools and multicriteria optimization to specify the DS (Vinjamuri et al., 2016). The purpose of the study was to design orally inhalable ipratropium bromide microparticles using a spray drying process. A 2^{7-3} fractional factorial screening design, requiring 16 experimental runs, was used evaluate seven factors (% lactose, % leucine, % ethanol, spray gas pressure, aspiration %, feed flow rate, and inlet temperature) on four CPAs [yield %, volume median diameter (VMD), span, and outlet temperature (OT)]. Sensitivity analysis showed that lactose (L), spray gas pressure, feed flow rate, and inlet temperature had the greatest impact on the CPAs. A three level response surface custom design was used to identify the critical individual, interaction, and curvilinear effects. Twenty experiments were required for this design. Aspiration was held constant at 100% with a drying air flow rate of 35 m^3/h. Least squares of effects model equations and multicriteria optimization were used to determine the DS. Statistically significant predictive models were developed for yield % ($p = 0.0020$, adjusted $R^2 = 0.9320$), VMD ($p = 0.0001$, adjusted $R^2 = 0.9938$), span ($p = 0.0278$, adjusted $R^2 = 0.7912$), and OT ($p = 0.0082$, adjusted $R^2 = 0.8768$). Figure 22.2 shows the multicriteria optimization contour plot for yield, VMD, span, and OT. The lower and upper spray gas pressures studied were 20 mm–64 mm. The lower and upper range of % lactose was 2% to 15% w/w. The response surface plots in the upper right hand corner clearly show the non-linear response of the four CPAs. In this particular case, the DS (white space) occupies a very small region of the study design. An independent verification batch confirmed the model's predictive capability. The predicted and actual values were in good agreement. VMD was 3.32 ± 0.09 μm (4.7% higher than predicted). Span was determined to be 1.71 ± 0.18, which was 5.3% higher than the predicted value. The process yield was found to be 50.3%, compared to the predicted value of 65.3%. The OT was 100°C versus the predicted value of 105°C.

22.2.5 Lifecycle Management and Continual Improvement

The product lifecycle stages include product design, technology transfer, commercial manufacturing, and product discontinuation. Product design is a complicated, multivariate process that integrates patient drug therapy with formulation, manufacturing (process), and container closure system design. The product design goal is to gain timely regulatory approval for a drug product that consistently meets the needs of patients, health care providers, and payers.

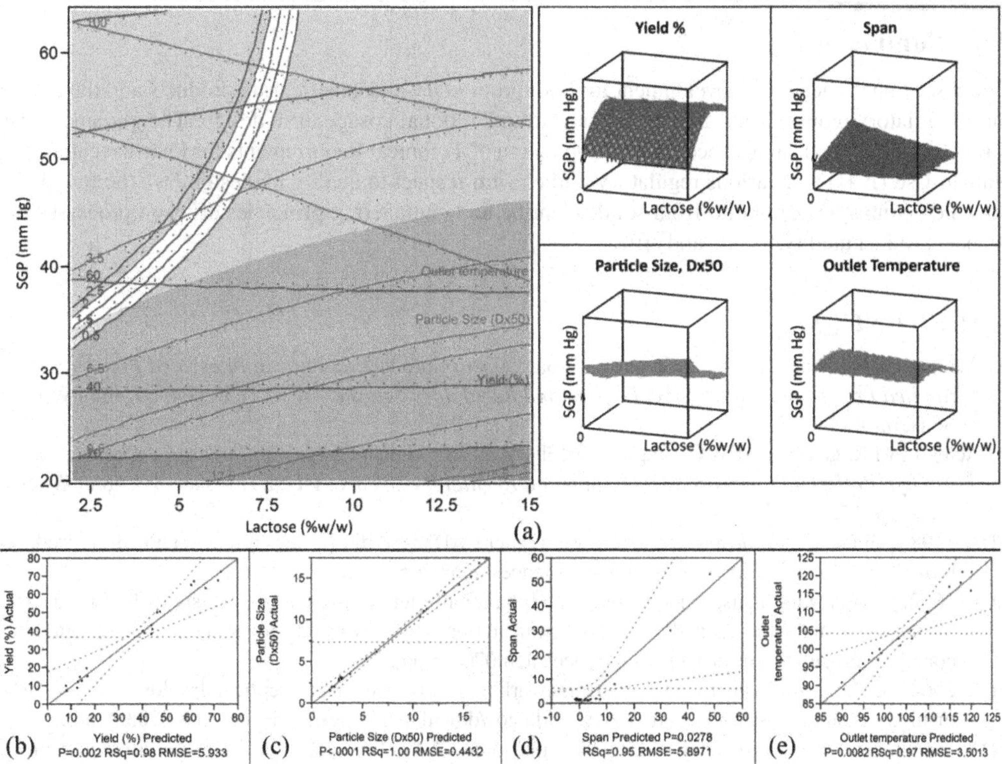

FIGURE 22.2 Response surface custom design and multicriteria optimization (a) contour plot and response surface plots of predicted yield %, particle size [μm], span, outlet temperature [°C] as a function of spray gas pressure [mm Hg] and lactose concentration [% w/w]; and prediction plots for (b) yield %, (c) particle size [μm], (d) span, and (e) outlet temperature [°C]. The unshaded white region in Fig. 22.2a, 2-dimensional SGP-Lactose plot, contour plot represents the multicriteria optimized design space for desired process and product criterion.

A second product lifecycle stage is product technology transfer. Technology transfer often involves scaling the formulation and process form 1 kg–5 kg small scale to 10 kg–50 kg pilot scale. Dimensionless numbers such as the Reynolds number, Newton number, or Froude number are used to scale up and scale down processes. Other empirical methods such as statistical design of experiments accompanied by model regression analysis is also employed. In some cases like spray drying, models based on the first principles of mass and heat transfer can be used to successfully scale up or down. A second technology transfer phase takes place from pilot scale to commercial manufacturing scale. A third technology transfer phase may occur between manufacturing sites. The technology transfer goal is to transmit all formulation, process, container closure system knowledge explicitly to the receiving site in the form of official reports and transfer records. The product history and knowledge is also transferred by members of the transfer team during the actual scale-up and product manufacture. Once several batches are manufactured successfully, an official sign-off by the transfer team and receiving unit is made.

At the commercial manufacturing stage, product should be routinely produced that consistently meets or exceeds product specifications. Opportunities to improve the acceptable ranges of CPAs are sought and rewarded as part of quality improvement culture.

The goal of product discontinuation is to thoughtfully and professionally terminate the manufacture and distribution a drug product. Stakeholder communication is critical to a smooth discontinuation. Retention of all critical documents and samples is paramount.

22.3 Summary

The cost of pharmaceutical development for both proprietary and generic drug products and the need to meet regulatory requirements creates urgency around rational dosage form design. The guidance given through International Conference for Harmonization of Technical Requirements for Pharmaceuticals for Human Use (ICH) and various regulatory bodies with respect to quality by design lays the foundation on which companies can build from solid scientific and engineering principles efficient processes that support product quality, safety, and efficacy.

REFERENCES

Al-Achi A., M.R. Gupta, and W.C. Stagner. 2013a. "Aerosol product design," in *Integrated Pharmaceutics: Applied Preformulation, Product Design, and Regulatory Science*, 1st ed. Hoboken, NJ: John Wiley & Sons, pp. 451–454.

Al-Achi A., M.R. Gupta, and W.C. Stagner. 2013b. "Aerosol product design," in *Integrated Pharmaceutics: Applied Preformulation, Product Design, and Regulatory Science*, 1st ed. Hoboken, NJ: John Wiley & Sons, pp. 447–450.

FDA. 1998. Guidance for industry, metered dose inhaler (MDI) and dry powder inhaler (DPI) drug products. https://www.fda.gove/downloads/drugs/guidances/ucm070573.pdf.

FDA. 2002. Guidance for industry, nasal spray and inhalation solution, suspension, and spray drug products—chemistry, manufacturing, and controls documentation. https://www.fda.gov/downloads/drugs/guidance complianceregulatoryinformation/guidances/ucm070575.pdf.

FDA. 2004. Guidance for industry, PAT—A framework for innovative pharmaceutical development, manufacturing, and quality assurance. https://www.fda.gov/downloads/drugs/guidances/ucm070305.pdf.

FDA. 2006a. Guidance for industry, quality systems approach to pharmaceutical CGMP regulations. https://www.fda.gov/downloads/Drugs/Guidances/UCM070337.pdf.

FDA. 2006b. Guidance for industry, Q9 quality risk management. https://www.fda.gov/downloads/Drugs/Guidances/ucm073511.pdf.

FDA. 2007. Guidance for industry, target product profile—a strategic development process tool. https://www.fda.gov/downloads/drugs/guidancecomplianceregulatoryinformation/guidances/ucm080593.pdf.

FDA. 2009a. Guidance for industry, Q8(R2) pharmaceutical development. https://www.fda.gov/downloads/drugs/guidances/ucm073507.pdf.

FDA. 2009b. Guidance for industry, Q10 pharmaceutical quality system. https://www.fda.gov/downloads/drugs/guidances/ucm073517.pdf.

Hickey A.J. 2018. "Regulatory strategy," in *Inhaled Pharmaceutical Product Development Perspectives*. New York: Elsevier, pp. 73–84.

Hickey A.J., and D. Ganderton. 2010. "Process analytical technology," in *Pharmaceutical Process Engineering*. New York: Informa Healthcare, pp. 202–206.

Horhota S.T., and S. Leiner. 2011. "Developing performance specifications for pulmonary drug delivery," in *Controlled Pulmonary Drug Delivery*, eds. H.D.C. Smyth and A.J. Hickey. New York: Springer, pp. 529–541.

Lionberger R.A., S.L. Lee, L.M. Lee, A. Raw, and L.X. Yu. 2008. "Quality by design: Concepts for ANDAs." *AAPS J*, 10: 268–276.

Vinjamuri P.B., R.V. Haware, and W.C. Stagner. 2016. "Inhalable ipratropium bromide particle engineering with multicriteria optimization." *AAPS PharmSciTech*. doi:10.1208/s12249-016-0668-y.

Yu L.X., G. Amidon, M.A. Khan, S.W. Hoag, J. Polli, G.K. Raju, and J. Woodcock. 2014. "Understanding pharmaceutical quality by design." *AAPS J*, 16: 771–783.

23

Solid State Testing of Inhaled Formulations

Philip Chi Lip Kwok and Hak-Kim Chan

CONTENTS

23.1 Introduction

Drugs and excipients are incorporated as solids in dry powder inhalers (DPIs). A thorough understanding of their physicochemical characteristics is crucial in ensuring the stability and performance of the products. The relevant solid state properties for inhalable powders include particle shape, surface morphology, particle density, porosity, specific surface area, powder density, powder flow, interparticulate cohesion/adhesion, surface energy, thermodynamic behavior, crystallinity, water content, uniformity of delivered dose, and particle size distribution. A wide variety of techniques are used to examine these properties throughout all stages of research and development. However, some tests are utilized more often in the preformulation or early formulation phase while others are conducted routinely for the quality control of the developed product. These are discussed in turn in this chapter.

23.2 Preformulation and Early Formulation Tests

A number of tests are performed in the early stages of the research and development of inhalable dry powder formulations. They focus on the solid state characterization of the drug and excipient powders before they are incorporated into, and tested with, the inhaler.

23.2.1 Particle Shape

Particle shape can affect powder flow, aerosolization, and particle deposition (Hassan and Lau 2009, Chan 2008). The most direct method of visualizing particle shape is microscopy. The British, European, and United States Pharmacopeial monographs on optical microscopy state that "information on particle shape" must be included with particle size data for irregularly shaped (i.e. non-spherical) particles (*British Pharmacopoeia* 2017, *European Pharmacopoeia* 2017, *United States Pharmacopeia 40-National Formulary 35* 2017). The information on particle shape referred to in the pharmacopoeias is qualitative, using descriptive terms such as acicular, columnar, flake, etc. Various quantitative geometric shape factors have been adopted to express certain characteristics of the shape of particles, such as aspect ratio, sphericity, and circularity (Shekunov et al. 2007, Lau and Chuah 2013). However, these shape factors are derived from geometric measurements by microscopy and image analysis so they are number-based rather than mass-based. Generally, mass-based parameters and statistics are preferred for drug particles because they can be related directly to doses. Furthermore, the static nature of these geometric shape factors conveys no information on the influence of particle shape on the aerodynamics of particles.

The most relevant shape factor used for pharmaceutical aerosols is the dynamic shape factor (χ), which is the ratio of the drag force exerted on the particle of interest to that exerted on a sphere with the same volume when both particles move at the same velocity in the same fluid (Fuchs 1964, Lau and Chuah 2013). Therefore, the more sphere-like the particle, the closer the dynamic shape factor is to 1.0. Except for some streamline-shaped particles, the dynamic shape factor for most particles is larger than 1.0 (Hinds 1999). Since the drag force is affected by the orientation of an irregularly shaped particle with respect to the direction of movement, so is the dynamic shape factor. Usually the dynamic shape factor is averaged over all orientations, as is the case for most particles travelling in laminar flow (Hinds 1999). The dynamic shape factor relates the physical diameter of a particle to its aerodynamic diameter:

$$d_a = d_v \sqrt{\frac{\rho}{\rho_0 \chi}} \tag{23.1}$$

where d_a is the aerodynamic diameter, d_v the volumetric (physical) diameter, ρ the particle density (more specifically, the granular density; see Section 23.2.3), and ρ_0 unit density (1 g/cm^3). Geometric shape factors cannot be used in place of χ because they do not account for aerodynamic effects, as mentioned above. The dynamic shape factor can be calculated by first measuring ρ (by mercury porosimetry), d_v, and d_a (by laser diffraction, and cascade impaction, respectively), then substituting them into Equation 23.1 and solve for χ (Hickey and Edwards 2018). The experimental techniques for measuring these parameters are discussed in Sections 23.2.3 and 23.3.2.

23.2.2 Surface Morphology

Aerosol performance of dry powders can be controlled by varying the surface morphology of the particles (Chan 2008). In general, dispersibility increases with surface roughness (Kwok et al. 2011, Adi et al. 2008, Young et al. 2009, Chew et al. 2005, Adi et al. 2008, Chan 2008). The surface morphology of micron-sized particles for pulmonary delivery can be qualitatively evaluated by scanning electron microscopy (SEM), the spatial resolution of which is in the nanometer range. High-resolution SEM can even resolve structures in the angstrom range. Images of the particle surface architecture is generated by scanning of the specimen with a focused beam of accelerated electrons. Besides high-resolution imaging, another advantage of SEM is that only a small amount of powder (< 1 mg) is required as a specimen, which is desirable if the powder is expensive or limited in quantity. Most inhalable drugs and excipients are organic compounds with low electrical conductivity. Therefore, the specimens must be sputter coated with an electrically conducting material (e.g. gold, platinum, gold/palladium) to avoid the charging, and subsequent deformation, of the particles due to the accumulation of high energy electrons from the scanning. This metallic coating should be thin, typically 2 nm–20 nm thick, because overly thick coatings will mask and smoothen particle surface features.

While particle surface morphology can be qualitatively examined from SEM images, surface roughness can be quantitatively measured using atomic force microscopy (AFM) or white-light interferometry. In AFM, the particle surface is raster scanned with a cantilever, the position of which is detected and used to generate a three-dimensional topographical image of the surface (De Oliveira et al. 2012, Raposo et al. 2007). The spatial resolution depends on the geometry and dimensions of the cantilever tip, but it is in the nanometer to angstrom range. The sharper the cantilever tip, the higher the resolution. The height data of the scan can be statistically analyzed to calculate the surface roughness. The two most commonly used roughness parameters are average roughness (R_a) and root mean square roughness (R_q or R_{RMS}). The former is the arithmetic average of the absolute vertical heights from the mean plane of the surface, whereas the latter is the root mean square of those heights. The equations for both roughness parameters are shown below (De Oliveira et al. 2012, Raposo et al. 2007).

$$R_a = \frac{1}{n}\sum_{i=1}^{n}\left|z_i - \bar{z}\right| \tag{23.2}$$

$$R_q = \sqrt{\frac{1}{n}\sum_{i=1}^{n}\left(z_i - \bar{z}\right)^2} \tag{23.3}$$

where $z_i - \bar{z}$ is the vertical height between point i on the scanned surface to the mean plane in a scan with n points (Figure 23.1). The R_q is better than R_a for indicating undulations on the particle surface because it is more sensitive to peaks and valleys (i.e. deviations from the mean plane) due to the squaring of the heights in the calculation. The R_q has been shown to correlate positively with aerosol performance of dry powder formulations (Adi et al. 2008, Kwok et al. 2011).

White-light interferometry is a non-contact, optical profilometry technique that can quantify roughness by measuring the interference pattern of split light beams scanning a surface (Adi et al. 2008). A white light beam is split into two beams, one travels to the sample and the other to a reference mirror inside the interferometer. The two beams are then relayed to the image sensor to form a pixelated interference pattern because the pathlengths travelled by the two beams are unequal. The constructive interference fringes (degree of coherence) at each pixel indicate the height at that point (Adi et al. 2008). The advantage of this technique is that it is fast and does not damage/change the sample surface. Its height and lateral resolutions are 0.1 nm and 150 nm, respectively. The working distance can be up to 10 mm so large areas with many particles can be covered in one scan. The three-dimensional images and R_q values of micron-sized particles and carrier particles measured by white-light interferometry and AFM have been shown to be comparable (Adi et al. 2008).

23.2.3 Particle Density, Porosity, and Specific Surface Area

Particle density, porosity, and surface area provide information on the structure of the particles. They are relevant in the engineering of the particles for optimizing aerosol performance or dissolution. As shown in Equation 23.1, aerodynamic diameter can be reduced by decreasing particle density or increasing porosity. In turn, porous particles have large specific surface areas (surface area-to-mass ratios) that can facilitate dissolution, which is beneficial for drugs with low aqueous solubility. The methods for measuring these three particle parameters involve adsorption of a gas or liquid onto the particles.

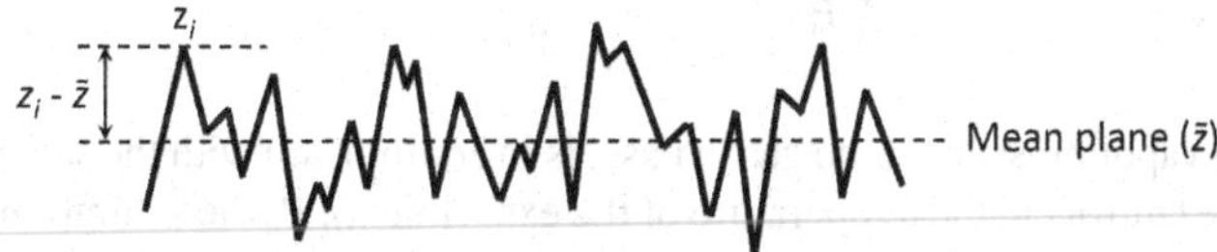

FIGURE 23.1 Profile of a solid surface scanned by atomic force microscopy. The vertical height of point *i* from the mean plane is shown.

Density equals mass divided by volume. However, there are several types of densities with regards to solids, depending on what volume is included in the measurement. *True density* of a compound is the mass divided by the volume of the atomic or molecular unit cell in a crystal, without voids. It can be derived from X-ray diffraction data on the composition and volume of a unit cell (*British Pharmacopoeia* 2017, *European Pharmacopoeia* 2017). *Pycnometric density* is obtained by measuring the volume occupied by a powder in a gas displacement pycnometer (*British Pharmacopoeia* 2017, *European Pharmacopoeia* 2017, *United States Pharmacopeia 40-National Formulary 35* 2017). There are two chambers in the gas pycnometer, namely, a calibrated test chamber with volume V_c and an expansion chamber with volume V_r. They are connected by a valve in between. A known mass of powder is first put into the test chamber. After closing the pycnometer and with the valve open between the two chambers, the reference pressure (P_r) is recorded. That valve is then closed and the test chamber is filled with a gas to an initial pressure P_i. Helium is usually used because it can fill small pores due to its high diffusivity. Then the valve between the two chambers is opened and the final pressure within the two connected chambers becomes P_f. The volume occupied by the sample (V_{sample}) can be calculated as below (*British Pharmacopoeia* 2017, *European Pharmacopoeia* 2017, *United States Pharmacopeia 40-National Formulary 35* 2017):

$$V_{\text{sample}} = V_c - \frac{V_r}{\left(\dfrac{P_i - P_r}{P_f - P_r}\right) - 1} \tag{23.4}$$

V_{sample} excludes the volume occupied by open pores, but includes that occupied by closed pores (i.e. pores isolated from the external environment) or very fine open pores that the gas cannot fill. If the particles have minimal closed voids, then the pycnometric density should be very similar to the true density. *Granular density* is obtained by mercury porosimetry, in which the pressure of mercury against the particle surface is measured. Since mercury has high surface tension, the applied pressure can be controlled to coat the particle surface, but not fill the open pores (Rouquerol et al. 2012, Lowell and Shields 1991). The volume of the particles determined thus includes the volume occupied by closed pores and open pores not filled by mercury. Those unfilled open pores have an upper size limit that depends on the applied pressure on the mercury. Therefore, different granular densities with particular pore size limits can be measured on the same sample at various applied pressures. By the same way, particle porosity can be examined using mercury porosimetry. The pressures needed to fill the pores of different size limits can be measured to obtain a pore size distribution on the particles (Rouquerol et al. 2012).

A common method for measuring specific surface area is by adsorbing an inert gas (nitrogen or krypton) onto the surface of the sample (Lowell and Shields 1991). The experiment is conducted in a liquid nitrogen bath (77.4 K) because the amount of adsorbed gas at a given pressure increases with decreasing temperature (*British Pharmacopoeia* 2017, *European Pharmacopoeia* 2017, *United States Pharmacopeia 40-National Formulary 35* 2017). The gas molecules form layers on the particle surfaces by van der Waals forces. The volume of the adsorbed gas is then used to calculate the surface area with the Brunauer, Emmett, and Teller equation:

$$\frac{1}{V_a\left(\dfrac{P}{P_0} - 1\right)} = \frac{C-1}{V_m C} \times \frac{P}{P_0} + \frac{1}{V_m C} \tag{23.5}$$

where P is the partial vapor pressure of the gas in pascals in equilibrium with the sample surface at 77.4 K (boiling point of liquid nitrogen, the temperature of the experiment), P_0 the saturation pressure of the gas in pascals at the same temperature, V_a the volume of gas in milliliters adsorbed at standard temperature and pressure (273.15 K and 1.013×10^5 Pa), V_m the volume of gas in milliliters adsorbed at standard temperature and pressure to form a monomolecular layer on the surface, and C dimensionless constant that is related to the enthalpy of adsorption (*British Pharmacopoeia* 2017, *European Pharmacopoeia* 2017, *United States Pharmacopeia 40-National Formulary 35* 2017). V_a is measured at a series of P/P_0 values. The left hand side of Equation 23.5 is plotted against P/P_0. This plot should be linear between 0.05-0.3 for P/P_0. The slope and y-intercept will then be $(C-1)/V_mC$ and $1/V_mC$, respectively. After V_m is solved, it is used to calculate the specific surface area by using:

$$S = \frac{V_m Na}{22400m} \tag{23.6}$$

where S is the specific surface area in m^2/g, N the Avogadro constant (6.022×10^{23} mol^{-1}), a the effective cross-sectional area of one gas molecule in m^2 (1.62×10^{-10} m^2 for nitrogen and 1.95×10^{-10} m^2 for krypton), and m the mass of the powder (*British Pharmacopoeia* 2017, *European Pharmacopoeia* 2017, *United States Pharmacopeia 40-National Formulary 35* 2017). The Brunauer, Emmett, and Teller method is suitable for determining the specific surface area of micronized drug and large carrier particles. However, it should be noted that not all the surface area measured on the carrier particles can interact with drug particles (Zeng et al. 2000). For example, surfaces inside pores or channels on the carrier particles that are physically narrower than the drug particles will not be able to contact the drug.

23.2.4 Powder Density

Bulk and tapped densities are the two densities relevant for powders. They are calculated by dividing the mass of a powder by the volume that the powder occupies before and after tapping, respectively. Both these densities include the void volume between particles so they are necessarily lower than the true density of the particles. Tapped density has a lower interparticulate void volume than bulk density because tapping increases particle packing. Bulk and tapped density can be used to predict powder flowability (see Section 23.2.5), which can affect dosing of DPIs during manufacturing and aerosolization.

The measurement procedure is simple and is specified in the pharmacopoeias (*British Pharmacopoeia* 2017, *European Pharmacopoeia* 2017, *United States Pharmacopeia 40-National Formulary 35* 2017). Essentially, a powder is poured freely into a 250 mL graduated measuring cylinder so that the untapped filling volume is 150 mL–250 mL. The mass of, and volume occupied by, the powder in the cylinder are then used to calculate the bulk density. The cylinder is then tapped for 10 taps, 500 taps, and 1250 taps by a tapping apparatus (*British Pharmacopoeia* 2017, *European Pharmacopoeia* 2017, *United States Pharmacopeia 40-National Formulary 35* 2017). The volumes occupied by the powder after each tapping episode are recorded. If the difference in the volumes after 500 taps and after 1250 is ≤2 mL, then the volume after 1250 taps is the tapped volume. Otherwise, repeat the tapping in increments of 1250 taps until the difference between two consecutive tapping episodes is ≤2 mL. The tapped volume is then used to calculate the tapped density.

A special method for measuring bulk density is to form and weigh a powder puck. This is done because it is the way powders are filled on drum fillers in the pharmaceutical industry (Ung et al. 2016). The density obtained is called *puck density*. Powder is sampled by vacuum into a dosing wand with a cylindrical cavity of known volume and consolidated into a compact disc (puck). The puck is then ejected by positive air pressure and weighed (Ung et al. 2016). The puck density equals the puck mass divided by the dosing wand cavity volume. This density is more relevant for the performance of DPI products whose formulation is in the form of pucks packaged in blister strips/disks because it is the puck, rather than a loose powder, that is dispersed into an aerosol.

23.2.5 Powder Flow

As mentioned before, powder flow can affect dosing, filling into capsules/blisters for DPIs, and aerosolization so it should be evaluated during formulation development. It can be measured directly or assessed indirectly using some relevant flow indicators.

Powder flow can be determined directly by measuring the flow rate of a powder through an orifice by gravity or by measuring shear parameters in a shear cell or powder rheometer. The first method is simply the measurement of the mass of powder flowing out from a container, which may be a hopper, funnel, or cylinder (*British Pharmacopoeia* 2017, *European Pharmacopoeia* 2017, *United States Pharmacopeia 40-National Formulary 35* 2017). The mass flow over time can be monitored using an electronic balance coupled to recording equipment. The disadvantage of this method is that the flow rate measured is experiment-specific. Besides particle-related factors (e.g. particle size, shape, surface morphology, density, etc.), the powder flow rate is also affected by the experimental setup and procedure (geometry/dimensions of container, size and shape of the orifice, amount of powder tested, etc.) (*British Pharmacopoeia* 2017, *European Pharmacopoeia* 2017, *United States Pharmacopeia 40-National Formulary 35* 2017). Therefore, flow rate data obtained using different setups cannot be directly compared. Furthermore, there is limited control in the manner the powder flows besides letting it flow freely by gravity.

The second powder flow measurement method measures the forces exerted on a powder as it is moved inside a shear cell or powder rheometer. Although shear cells have well-defined geometries, they are available commercially with different designs and modes of operation. Therefore, it is important to include details of the instrument and procedure with shear cell data because the setup can affect the measurement, as mentioned above. Nevertheless, shear cells offer more experimental control so the testing conditions can be well-defined. In one example, the force needed to shear the powder bed by a shear shell ring inside the cell is measured (*British Pharmacopoeia* 2017, *European Pharmacopoeia* 2017, *United States Pharmacopeia 40-National Formulary 35* 2017). Other flow parameters and indices can also be measured using this method. The FT4 Powder Rheometer from Freeman Technology is a novel equipment that determines powder flow by forcing a twisted blade through a powder bed along a programmed helical path (Freeman 2007, Leturia et al. 2014, Hare et al. 2015, Lu et al. 2017). The forces and energy exerted by the blade in traversing through the powder are measured. Different flow patterns can be investigated by varying the speed and direction of the moving blade so the powder rheometer offers more flexibility and control in examining powder flow dynamics (Freeman 2007, Leturia et al. 2014, Hare et al. 2015).

Some indicators that can be used to predict powder flow include the compressibility index, Hausner ratio, and angle of repose. While these do not describe powder flow rate per se, they have been shown to correlate with flowability. The compressibility index and Hausner ratio are calculated as:

$$\text{Compressibility index} = 100 \times \frac{\rho_{\text{tapped}} - \rho_{\text{bulk}}}{\rho_{\text{tapped}}} \tag{23.7}$$

$$\text{Hausner ratio} = \frac{\rho_{\text{tapped}}}{\rho_{\text{bulk}}} \tag{23.8}$$

where ρ_{tapped} and ρ_{bulk} are the tapped and bulk densities, respectively (*British Pharmacopoeia* 2017, *European Pharmacopoeia* 2017, *United States Pharmacopeia 40-National Formulary 35* 2017). The angle of repose experiment is conducted by letting a powder flow freely from a container onto a flat, vibration-free platform to form a symmetrical powder cone. The height (h) and base (b) of the cone are then measured and used to calculate the angle of repose (α) using the following equation:

$$\alpha = \tan^{-1}\left(\frac{h}{0.5b}\right) \tag{23.9}$$

The correlation between compressibility index, Hausner ratio, angle of repose, and powder flow is shown in Table 23.1. It should be noted that the value of these three flow indicators depend on the experimental method. However, they can be used to compare between different powders measured with the same setup and procedure.

TABLE 23.1

Correlation Between Compressibility Index, Hausner Ratio, Angle of Repose and Powder Flowability

Type of Flow	Compressibility Index (%)	Hausner Ratio	Angle of Repose (°)
Excellent	1–10	1.00–1.11	25–30
Good	11–15	1.12–1.18	31–35
Fair	16–20	1.19–1.25	36–40
Passable	21–25	1.26–1.34	41–45
Poor	26–31	1.35–1.45	46–55
Very poor	32–37	1.46–1.59	56–65
Very, very poor	>38	>1.60	>66

Source: *United States Pharmacopeia 40-National Formulary 35*, 2017.

23.2.6 Interparticulate Cohesion/Adhesion and Surface Energy

Interparticulate cohesion and adhesion affects the dispersibility of dry powder formulations (Zeng et al. 2000). AFM can be applied to directly measure these interactive forces. In such applications, the technique is also known as colloidal probe microscopy (Weiss et al. 2015). A drug particle of interest can be mounted onto a tipless AFM cantilever with an adhesive by a micromanipulation technique (D'Sa et al. 2014, Islam et al. 2014, Weiss et al. 2015, Young et al. 2003). The mounted particle thus acts as a probe for measuring interactive forces. It is crucial that only one particle is mounted because multiple mounted particles will introduce artifacts in the measurements due to the interference from multiple "probes" (D'Sa et al. 2014). The substrate is the material that the probe is supposed to test against and is loaded onto the AFM sample stage. It can be the same type of particle as the probe (to investigate cohesion) or another type of particle/solid surface such as carrier particles or inhaler material (to investigate adhesion). During a raster scan conducted in the same manner as an AFM topographical scan (see Section 23.2.2), the probe contacts the substrate surface and is then pulled off. The force-distance curve of this maneuver is recorded and provides the cohesion/adhesion force and separation energy at each contact point. These parameters can also be mapped in the scanned region or statistically analyzed. The measurement can be conducted at controlled relative humidity (RH) to investigate the effect of moisture on interparticulate forces (Young et al. 2003, Young et al. 2006).

Although interparticulate forces can be directly characterized by colloidal probe microscopy, the measurements are sensitive to the nature of the contact points so data reproducibility is difficult. Moreover, due to constraints in the area size that can be scanned, the data may not be representative for the whole powder, especially if its surface properties are heterogeneous (Tong et al. 2006). Inverse gas chromatography is an indirect, but sensitive, method that examines the energetics of the whole powder surface. The interaction between a powder sample and various adsorbate molecules (also known as probes) is measured by this technique to derive surface energetic parameters that can be used to quantify cohesion and adhesion. The probes are volatile organic solvents that are polar (e.g. chloroform, acetone, ethyl acetate) or non-polar (alkanes). The powder is packed in a hollow column with an inert internal surface. Adsorbate vapors are then injected individually at different vapor pressures into the column. The probe molecules are carried through the powder (the stationary phase) via an inert carrier gas, usually nitrogen (the mobile phase). The retention time of the peaks of the eluted probes in the chromatogram is the main parameter measured in inverse gas chromatography (Mohammadi-Jam and Waters 2014, Ho and Heng 2013). It indicates the molecular interactive forces between the probe and the powder surface. Together with other experimental information (e.g. the elution dead time, the mass of the powder, the specific surface area of the powder, carrier gas flow rate, temperature, etc.), various surface energetic parameters can be calculated, including Gibbs free energy of adsorption (ΔG_A), enthalpy of adsorption (ΔH_A), dispersive component of free energy of the solid (γ_s^D), interaction parameter (φ), and cohesive/adhesive interactions. The calculations and theory for these parameters are covered in detail elsewhere (Mohammadi-Jam and Waters 2014, Ho and Heng 2013). Inverse gas chromatography has been applied to characterize the surface energy of inhalable powders and its relation to aerosol performance (Das et al. 2009, Tong et al. 2006, Cline and Dalby 2002, Davies et al. 2005, Wagner et al. 2005). Aerosol performance of the drug was found to be better when drug-carrier adhesion was stronger than drug-drug cohesion (Tong et al. 2006, Cline and Dalby 2002) or when the total surface energy of the powder was reduced (Das et al. 2009).

23.2.7 Thermodynamic Behavior

Thermodynamic behaviours, specifically the mass and energy changes that occur in a solid upon heating, can indicate solid state changes, chemical changes, and the presence of impurities. The two major thermal analysis techniques are thermogravimetric analysis (TGA) and differential scanning calorimetry (DSC).

TGA monitors the mass of a sample upon heating from room temperature at a constant heating rate (typically 5°C/min–10°C/min) (*British Pharmacopoeia* 2017, *European Pharmacopoeia* 2017). Adsorbed/solvated water, residual organic solvents, or sublimable compounds in the sample will be released as vapors upon heating and the sample mass thereby decreasing. The data are presented as a mass versus temperature or time plot. The mass loss indicates the presence and total amount of evaporative compounds in the sample. However, TGA cannot identify or differentiate between those compounds. Karl Fischer coulometric titration (see Section 23.2.9) and gas chromatography are selective methods to assay for adsorbed water and residual organic solvents, respectively (*British Pharmacopoeia* 2017, *European Pharmacopoeia* 2017, *United States Pharmacopeia 40-National Formulary 35* 2017).

DSC monitors the difference in the energy input between a sample and a reference as both are heated or cooled to the same temperature (Höhne et al. 2003). Usually the sample is kept inside a crimped crucible so an empty crucible serves as the reference. Heat to the sample will be increased or reduced if an endothermic or exothermic phase transition event occurs, respectively. These events appear as peaks or deviations from the baseline in the thermogram as a heat flow versus temperature plot. The area under the curve is proportional to the enthalpy of the event (*British Pharmacopoeia* 2017, *European Pharmacopoeia* 2017, *United States Pharmacopeia 40-National Formulary 35* 2017). Its onset and peak temperature can also be obtained from the thermogram. A list of common phase transition events is shown in Table 23.2. The type of phase transition observed provides information on the solid state (e.g. crystalline or amorphous) the sample was originally in. For example, an endothermic peak at a temperature corresponding to the melting point of the compound implies that the sample is crystalline. On the other hand, amorphous solids show a glass transition step instead of a melting peak. Thus, DSC data can be complemented with other data to confirm the crystallinity of the solid (see Section 23.2.8). The temperature range and heating rate can be explored in preliminary runs to scan for phase transitions of interest before deciding on an optimized scheme. Multiple heating-cooling cycles can also be employed to examine more intricate thermal events.

TABLE 23.2
Phase Transition Events Observed in Differential Scanning Calorimetry

Solid to solid	Desolvation	Endothermic
	Polymorphic change	Endothermic or exothermic
	Glass transition	Second order event
	Crystallization from amorphous state	Exothermic
Solid to liquid	Melting	Endothermic
Solid to gas	Sublimation	Endothermic
Liquid to solid	Crystallization	Exothermic
	Freezing	Exothermic
Liquid to gas	Vaporization	Endothermic

Source: United States Pharmacopeia 40-National Formulary 35, 2017.

Although DSC is adequate for the investigation of common thermal behaviors, it cannot show the individual processes in a thermal event that consists of weak, complex, and/or concurrent phase transitions because the heating rate is constant. A newer technique called modulated DSC overcomes this problem by superimposing a temperature modulation scheme (i.e. temperature oscillations) over a constant heating rate and measuring the response to multiple heating rates simultaneously (Knopp et al. 2016). Sensitivity and resolution are improved by this method. Weak and overlapping phase transitions can also be detected and distinguished.

23.2.8 Crystallinity

Crystallinity is the degree of order in the molecular arrangement in the solid. All molecules are in the correct lattice position in a perfect crystal, while all long-range order is lost in an amorphous solid. No real solids belong to these two extremes. Even the most ordered crystals and the most disordered amorphous solids possess low levels of disordered and ordered domains, respectively. The crystallinity and polymorphic form of a drug can affect its particle shape, dissolution rate, stability, and aerosol performance (Zeng et al. 2000), so their characterization is needed in product development (*Guidance for Industry: Metered Dose Inhaler (MDI) and Dry Powder Inhaler (DPI) Drug Products* 1998, *Guideline on the Pharmaceutical Quality of Inhalation and Nasal Products* 2006). Many pharmacopoeial methods can be used to determine crystallinity, namely, X-ray powder diffraction, DSC, microcalorimetry, solution calorimetry, near-infrared spectroscopy, infrared absorption spectrophotometry, Raman spectrometry, solid-state nuclear magnetic resonance, and optical microscopy (*British Pharmacopoeia* 2017, *European Pharmacopoeia* 2017, *United States Pharmacopeia 40-National Formulary 35* 2017). Optical microscopy is a simple, qualitative method in which the particles are viewed using a polarizing microscope. Crystalline particles show birefringence interference colors when the polariser or sample is turned. The most common methods for crystallinity determination are X-ray powder diffraction, DSC, microcalorimetry, and dynamic gravimetric water sorption.

X-ray powder diffraction involves the detection of the X-ray diffraction pattern of a randomly oriented powder. The diffraction patterns of highly crystalline solids show sharp peaks, while those of amorphous solids show broad halo patterns (Figure 23.2). The angular positions of the peaks are characteristic to the compound, and polymorphic form thus can serve as a "fingerprint" for identification. Peak intensity is affected by the preferred orientation and crystallinity of the particles. Preferred orientation is a particularly a problem for acicular and plate-like particles. One way of increasing the orientation randomness in the powder bed is particle size reduction (*British Pharmacopoeia* 2017, *European Pharmacopoeia* 2017, *United States Pharmacopeia 40-National Formulary 35* 2017). However, too much milling may reduce the crystallinity, change the polymorphic form, or cause other solid state reactions so it should be avoided.

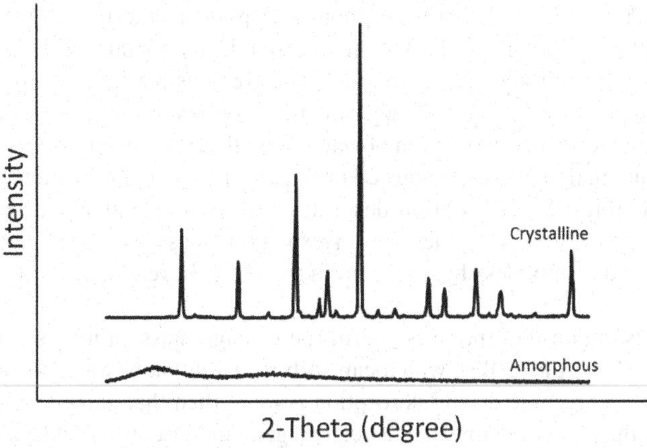

FIGURE 23.2 Typical X-ray diffraction patterns of crystalline and amorphous solids.

Particles in the inhalable size range (1 μm–5 μm) should have less issues with preferred orientation because they can pack better than large particles.

The crystallinity of a sample can be quantified by comparing the peak intensity of its diffraction pattern to that from a reference powder of known crystallinity. This is possible if the sample and reference are of the same polymorphic form and there is no preferred orientation. Another method involves the calculation of three areas in the diffraction pattern:

A is the total area of the crystalline peaks

B is the total area under the diffraction pattern excluding the crystalline peaks

C is the background area from the equipment, air scattering, etc.

The percentage of crystallinity can then be estimated as 100A/(A + B − C) (*British Pharmacopoeia* 2017, *European Pharmacopoeia* 2017, *United States Pharmacopeia 40-National Formulary 35* 2017). This value is not the absolute crystallinity, but it is helpful for comparing between samples.

DSC can be used to indicate crystallinity because crystalline solids show an endothermic melting peak upon heating, followed by decomposition and evaporation if heating continues. On the other hand, amorphous solids show glass transition instead of melting.

Microcalorimetry is very sensitive in measuring the amorphicity of solids. Depending on the compound and testing conditions, amorphicity of less than 1% can be detected (*British Pharmacopoeia* 2017, *European Pharmacopoeia* 2017, *United States Pharmacopeia 40-National Formulary 35* 2017). This technique measures the heat of recrystallization upon exposing the sample to high relative humidity or organic vapor inside a sealed ampule. The mass of the sample and the type of vapour are chosen so that a sharp recrystallization peak can be measured by the microcalorimeter. The amorphous content can be calculated by comparing the area of this peak to that obtained from an amorphous standard (*British Pharmacopoeia* 2017, *European Pharmacopoeia* 2017, *United States Pharmacopeia 40-National Formulary 35* 2017). The recrystallization dynamics are affected by the nature of the solid and its immediate environment. For example, physical mixtures of fully crystalline and amorphous solids will recrystallizing differently to a partially amorphous solid (*British Pharmacopoeia* 2017, *European Pharmacopoeia* 2017, *United States Pharmacopeia 40-National Formulary 35* 2017). This should be noted when choosing standards and comparing data between samples.

Inhalable drug particles have large specific surface areas due to their small size (1 μm–5 μm). This is even more so for rough and porous particles. Such large surface areas promote potential interactions with water vapor in the environment, especially if the drug is hygroscopic. Adsorbed or absorbed water can cause physical changes in the solid, such as changes in the particle size distribution and polymorphic form, aggregation due to interparticulate capillary force, or recrystallization of amorphous regions.

Dynamic vapor sorption can be performed to examine solid-water interactions by monitoring the mass change of the sample as a function of RH. The RH is programmed to step up and down sequentially at a constant temperature to obtain sorption-desorption isotherms (Ward and Schultz 1995, Buckton and Darcy 1995). The sample mass increases and decreases during the sorption and desorption phases, respectively. Water absorbed into amorphous regions may act as a plasticizer and lowers the glass transition temperature. This may trigger the recrystallization of these regions and results in a sudden mass loss due to the partial desorption of water upon the formation of crystalline regions, which have lower water affinity than their amorphous counterparts. The recrystallization event can be verified by running the sample through two sorption-desorption cycles. If the recrystallization of amorphous regions was completed in the first cycle, then the corresponding mass loss should not recur in the second cycle. The sample should also be less hygroscopic in the second cycle because it is crystalline (Ward and Schultz 1995).

Hysteresis in the adsorption-desorption isotherm (percentage mass gain versus RH plot) can imply an amorphous sample (Lau et al. 2017), which can sorb relatively more water. Hysteresis occurs when the amount of water in the sample during desorption is more than that gained during sorption or vice versa. This is because the pores and amorphous regions gain and lose water under different equilibrium conditions. It may also be caused by a change in the extent of solid-vapor interaction due to a change in the solid state of the sample (e.g. polymorphic change, crystallization, etc.).

Dynamic vapor sorption using an organic solvent (*n*-octane) instead of water to generate the vapor has been used to quantify the amorphous content of powders (Young et al. 2007). This technique is advantageous if the drug of interest can form a hydrate with water vapor, but cannot form a solvate with the vapor of a particular organic solvent. If that is the case, organic adsorption is preferred because the mass change as a function of partial vapor pressure is not confounded by other phase transition events. The amorphous content of salbutamol sulfate and lactose was shown to correlate positively with the percentage mass gain at 90% partial vapor pressure of *n*-octane (Young et al. 2007).

23.2.9 Water Content

The amount of adsorbed moisture in inhalable powders should be controlled to prevent solid state changes in the powder (*Guidance for Industry: Metered Dose Inhaler (MDI) and Dry Powder Inhaler (DPI) Drug Products* 1998). Therefore, the water content needs to be determined. If water is deemed to be the only evaporative species in the powder, then a loss on drying experiment (e.g. TGA) can be performed because the percentage loss in mass may be interpreted as the water content of the sample. However, this method is not selective for water so it will be unsuitable if other residual solvents or compounds with low vapor pressure are present in the sample.

The most common selective and sensitive method for water content determination is Karl Fischer coulometric titration (MacLeod 1991). The principle of operation involves a reaction of water with iodine and sulfur dioxide in the presence of an alcohol (e.g. methanol) and an organic base (e.g. imidazole). Automated instruments and reagents containing all the necessary chemicals offer convenience and simplify the operation of the titration. The reagent is kept in a tightly sealed reaction cell with a large anode and a small cathode that conducts an electrical current through the cell. Iodine is generated by electrolysis by the anode and reacts with the water in the reagent. The reaction consumes water stoichiometrically until no more water is present (MacLeod 1991, *British Pharmacopoeia* 2017, *European Pharmacopoeia* 2017, *United States Pharmacopeia 40-National Formulary 35* 2017). There will then be an excess of iodine, which is detected by a change in the electrical conductivity in the cell, signifying the titration end point. The electrical current needed to generate the iodine during the titration is used to calculate the amount of water present (MacLeod 1991, *British Pharmacopoeia* 2017, *European Pharmacopoeia* 2017, *United States Pharmacopeia 40-National Formulary 35* 2017).

To measure the water content of a powder, it may be dissolved in anhydrous methanol or other suitable solvents before introducing into the reaction cell (*United States Pharmacopeia 40-National Formulary 35* 2017). Otherwise, the sample should be heated in an external oven that is connected to the reaction cell. The desorbed water vapor is carried into the cell as a continuous stream by an inert and dry gas (e.g. nitrogen). Heating of the sample should be controlled to avoid the generation of water from decomposition (*United States Pharmacopeia 40-National Formulary 35* 2017). Thus, data from TGA and DSC (see Section 23.2.7) will be helpful to choose an appropriate heating profile.

23.3 Product Quality Control Tests

Pharmaceutical regulatory authorities, such as the Food and Drug Administration and European Medicines Agency (EMA), have issued detailed guidelines for the industry on the quality control requirements for inhaler products (*Guidance for Industry: Metered Dose Inhaler (MDI) and Dry Powder Inhaler (DPI) Drug Products* 1998, *Guideline on the Pharmaceutical Quality of Inhalation and Nasal Products* 2006). The aim of the quality control tests is to examine the aerosol performance of marketed products and those used in clinical trials. Some quality control tests stipulated in the guidelines have been covered in Section 23.2 (e.g. crystallinity, water content), so this section will focus on the tests that pertain to aerosolized dose and particle size measurement.

23.3.1 Uniformity of Delivered Dose

The delivered dose generated from a DPI product should be consistent. In other words, the inter-dose variation should be small. This is tested with a dose collection apparatus described in the pharmacopoeias (*British Pharmacopoeia* 2017, *European Pharmacopoeia* 2017, *United States Pharmacopeia 40-National Formulary 35* 2017). Essentially it is a cylinder with a filter at one end that is connected to a vacuum pump (Figure 23.3). The air flow should be adjusted to establish a 4 kPa pressure drop across the inhaler. The duration of sampling is the time taken to draw 2.0 L or 4.0 L of air at this flow rate according to the United States Pharmacopeia and British/European Pharmacopoeias, respectively (*British Pharmacopoeia* 2017, *European Pharmacopoeia* 2017, *United States Pharmacopeia 40-National Formulary 35* 2017). If the flow rate at 4 kPa pressure drop exceeds 100 L/min, then 100 L/min is used. The specified pressure drop and sampled volume requirements are supposed to standardize the experimental conditions and are deemed to be representative. However, there are many DPIs with different airflow resistances and aerosolization efficiencies. Furthermore, patients can achieve a wide range of flow rates on these inhalers clinically that may be different to the pharmacopoeial standard (Buttini et al. 2016). Therefore, testing all of them at one pressure drop may not be realistic. It is becoming obvious that there is no unique, optimal pressure drop/flow rate that is generalizable to all DPIs (Demoly et al. 2014). Therefore, although all pharmacopoeias recommend measuring the delivered dose uniformity and fine particle dose (see Section 23.3.2) of DPIs at a pressure drop of 4 kPa, the Food and Drug Administration and EMA recommend evaluating these at different flow rates (*Guidance for Industry: Metered Dose Inhaler (MDI) and Dry Powder Inhaler (DPI) Drug Products* 1998, *Guideline on the Pharmaceutical Quality of Inhalation and Nasal Products* 2006). This will provide useful information on the flow dependence of the product. The range of flow rates employed should be realistic and justified by those observed clinically and experimentally for the inhaler concerned (*Guideline on the Pharmaceutical Quality of Inhalation and Nasal Products* 2006).

The number of doses that constitutes the minimum recommended dose is sampled for each run (*British Pharmacopoeia* 2017, *European Pharmacopoeia* 2017, *United States Pharmacopeia 40-National Formulary 35* 2017). The dose collection apparatus is then disassembled, and the drug deposits on the filter and internal surfaces of the collector are dissolved in a solvent and assayed using an appropriate analytical method (e.g. ultraviolet-visible spectrophotometry or liquid chromatography). Ten runs should be conducted for products with pre-metered doses. On the other hand, three, four, and three doses need to be sampled individually at the beginning, in the middle, and at the end of the life of reservoir-based products. The product complies with the test if nine out of ten results are within ± 25% of the mean dose and all within ± 35%.

Environmental RH may affect the performance of DPI formulations (Zeng et al. 2000). In particular, poor emission, de-aggregation, and/or hygroscopic growth may occur at high RH, especially if the particles are hygroscopic. Therefore, the temperature and RH of the air for testing the uniformity of delivered

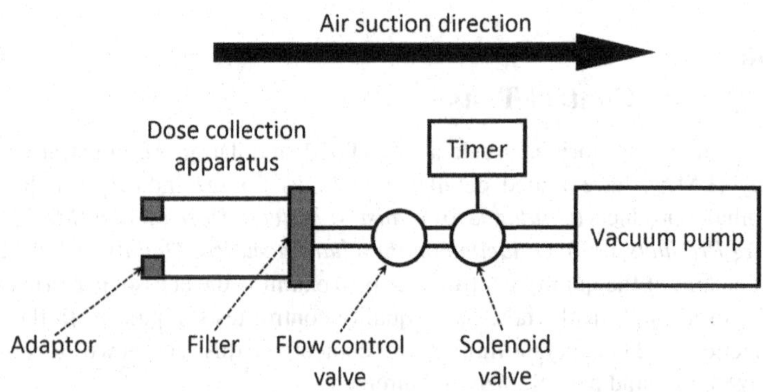

FIGURE 23.3 Schematic of the setup for the uniformity of delivered dose test.

dose and aerodynamic size (see Section 23.3.2) should be controlled to minimize variability from these factors (*Guideline on the Pharmaceutical Quality of Inhalation and Nasal Products* 2006). This can be achieved by conducting the experiments inside an environment control box or room.

23.3.2 Particle Size Distribution

Particle size distribution is a very important attribute of inhalation products because it directly affects the site of deposition and consequently the delivery efficiency. The volumetric and aerodynamic diameters are of particular interest because the former is the size of the primary particles and the latter the size of the agglomerates/particles after dispersion from an inhaler. The standard techniques for measuring these are laser diffraction and cascade impaction, respectively. Both are pharmacopoeial methods.

The laser diffraction method is based on the International Organization for Standardization Standard 13320:2009 (*British Pharmacopoeia* 2017, *European Pharmacopoeia* 2017, *United States Pharmacopeia 40-National Formulary 35* 2017, *ISO 13320:2009 Particle Size Analysis—Laser Diffraction Methods* 2009). It is an indirect sizing technique because the particle size distribution is derived from the diffraction pattern obtained when particles pass through a laser beam. The Fraunhofer or Mie diffraction models are commonly employed for the data conversion. The Fraunhofer model is simpler and does not require knowledge of refractive indices, but it is less accurate for sizing small particles (<10 μm). On the other hand, the Mie model is preferred if the particles are relatively small, using a measured or estimated refractive index of the particle material. An imaginary refractive index (usually 0.01–0.1) is also included to account for light absorbance by the particles (*British Pharmacopoeia* 2017). The technique is suitable for measuring volumetric particle diameters from 0.1 μm to 3 mm, but this range can be extended above and below these sizes with special conditions and instrumentation (*ISO 13320:2009 Particle Size Analysis—Laser Diffraction Methods* 2009). The principle assumption of laser diffraction is that all the particles measured are un-agglomerated and spherical (*British Pharmacopoeia* 2017, *European Pharmacopoeia* 2017). Since laser diffraction cannot distinguish between single particles and agglomerates, the powder samples need to be fully dispersed in air or in a non-solvent liquid for the measurement. A small amount of surfactant (e.g. Tween 80, Span 80) may be added to the suspension to facilitate dispersion (Jaffari et al. 2013). The typical size indicators are the 10th (D_{10}), 50th (D_{50}), and 90th (D_{90}) percentiles of the cumulative volume diameter distribution. Another name for D_{50} is the median volume diameter. The broadness of the distribution is expressed as the span, which is $(D_{90} - D_{10})/D_{50}$. Other size indicators such as the percentage of particles under 5 μm (the fine particle fraction) or 10 μm can also be obtained. Since distributions by volume are the same as those by mass, the data can also be considered as mass-based. The size data of non-spherical and/or agglomerated particles should be interpreted with caution because it is the equivalent spherical diameter that is being measured (Shekunov et al. 2007). Those irregular particles may also have preferred orientations to the laser beam and in the dispersion medium (air or liquid), which can influence the measurement. Regardless of particle shape, the size data should be checked against SEM images because the size of the primary particles evident from the images help to check whether agglomerates were present during laser diffraction measurement. This might be the case if the particle sizes measured by laser diffraction were significantly larger than those seen in SEM images.

Aerodynamic particle size testing is covered in detail in Chapter 24. Thus, only the major points will be discussed here. Multi-stage cascade impactors or impingers collect and fractionate particles generated from an inhaler into a series of aerodynamic size fractions. The design and usage procedure of various aerodynamic sizing apparatus are described in the pharmacopoeias (Table 23.3) (*British Pharmacopoeia* 2017, *European Pharmacopoeia* 2017, *United States Pharmacopeia 40-National Formulary 35* 2017). A right-angled induction port is used with the apparatus to mimic the throat. Not all apparatus are listed in all pharmacopoeias. The twin-stage glass impinger is listed in the British and European Pharmacopoeias, but not in the United States Pharmacopeia and vice versa for the Marple Miller Impactor. Impingers require a solvent to be dispensed into the stages to dissolve the drug deposits, whereas the impactors are used dry. However, since there is a risk of bounce from impactor stages and subsequent re-entrainment for particles from DPIs, impactor stages should be coated with a sticky material (e.g. silicone grease or glycerol in a volatile solvent) as a preventive measure (Nasr et al. 1997,

TABLE 23.3

Pharmacopoeial Aerodynamic Particle Sizing Apparatus

	BP 2017, Ph Eur 9.1	USP 40-NF 35
Glass Impinger	Apparatus A	Not included
Multi-stage Liquid Impinger	Apparatus C	Apparatus 4
Andersen Cascade Impactor	Apparatus D	Apparatus 1 (without pre-separator) Apparatus 3 (with pre-separator)
Next Generation Impactor	Apparatus E	Apparatus 5 (with pre-separator) Apparatus 6 (without pre-separator)
Marple Miller Impactor	Not included	Apparatus 2

Source: *British Pharmacopoeia*, 2017; *European Pharmacopoeia*, 2017; *United States Pharmacopeia 40-National Formulary 35*, 2017.

BP: British Pharmacopoeia, Ph Eur: European Pharmacopoeia, USP: United States Pharmacopeia, NF: National Formulary.

Kamiya et al. 2004, Kamiya et al. 2009, Mitchell 2013). As for uniformity of delivered dose tests, the dispersion flow rate should be set to generate a pressure drop of 4 kPa across the inhaler or 100 L/min maximum (see Section 23.3.1). The duration of sampling is the time taken to draw 4.0 L of air at this flow rate (*British Pharmacopoeia* 2017, *European Pharmacopoeia* 2017, *United States Pharmacopeia 40-National Formulary 35* 2017). The drug deposits on each part of the experimental setup are dissolved in a solvent and chemically assayed.

The primary data from cascade impaction are the drug mass deposited on the various parts, from the dose loading site (e.g. capsule), inhaler, adaptor, and throat, to all the stages in the impactor or impinger. Depending on the inhaler design, the drugs in the dose loading site and inhaler may or may not be assayed. Some inhalers contain multiple doses in a blister strip (e.g. Diskus from GlaxoSmithKline) or reservoir (e.g. Turbuhaler from AstraZeneca) inside the device body (Dunbar et al. 1998), which preclude the dismantling and assaying of those parts. The EMA requires the drug mass on each stage and the cumulative undersize data to be provided instead of the emitted fraction only (percentage of drug emitted from the inhaler) because they can show variations within the various size fractions (*Guideline on the Pharmaceutical Quality of Inhalation and Nasal Products* 2006). The fine particle dose under 5 µm can be interpolated from the cumulative undersize distribution (*British Pharmacopoeia* 2017, *European Pharmacopoeia* 2017). The fine particle fraction can then be calculated by dividing the fine particle dose by the loaded or emitted dose. If the aerodynamic particle size distribution is monomodal and log-normal, then the mass median aerodynamic diameter and geometric standard deviation can also be derived (*British Pharmacopoeia* 2017, *European Pharmacopoeia* 2017).

The minimum number of doses sampled in an impactor run depends on the sensitivity of the assay method (*British Pharmacopoeia* 2017, *European Pharmacopoeia* 2017, *United States Pharmacopeia 40-National Formulary 35* 2017, *Guidance for Industry: Metered Dose Inhaler (MDI) and Dry Powder Inhaler (DPI) Drug Products* 1998). The amount of drug deposits on each part must be enough for reliable quantification, but the number of doses sampled should be minimized to avoid masking inter-dose variations. The EMA specifically requires the testing of the single dose fine particle dose, determined by using the minimum recommended dose for the product (*Guideline on the Pharmaceutical Quality of Inhalation and Nasal Products* 2006). Justification is required if a higher number of doses is required for testing and that the resultant data are equivalent to those obtained using the minimum recommended dose (*Guideline on the Pharmaceutical Quality of Inhalation and Nasal Products* 2006). Furthermore, if the product has different strengths, proportionality of the fine particle dose and the dose in other size fractions should also be compared between the strengths (*Guideline on the Pharmaceutical Quality of Inhalation and Nasal Products* 2006). Mass balance should be calculated for each impactor run by totaling the drug masses assayed on all parts of the experimental setup and divided by the number of sampled doses in the run to verify the validity of the experiment. The British and European Pharmacopoeias state that the total recovered drug mass should be ±25% of the average delivered dose determined from the dose uniformity test (*British Pharmacopoeia* 2017, *European Pharmacopoeia* 2017). On the other hand, the United States Pharmacopeia and Food and Drug Administration require that the recovered drug mass should be ±15% of the labeled dose (*United States Pharmacopeia 40-National Formulary 35* 2017, *Guidance for Industry: Metered Dose Inhaler (MDI) and Dry Powder Inhaler (DPI) Drug Products* 1998).

23.4 Quality by Design and Process Analytical Technology

Quality by design is a modern concept of pharmaceutical manufacturing and product quality that is covered in Chapter 22. The main principle is that quality cannot be guaranteed by testing a finished product. Rather, it should be built into the product by integrating monitor and feedback mechanisms into the manufacturing process. These built-in mechanisms can be automated and provide real-time data that can prompt adjustments in the manufacturing if the quality of the product or its components is suboptimal. This will improve the efficiency of production and decrease wastage of resources and labour.

The characterization techniques discussed above are traditionally conducted discretely. However, with the move towards quality by design, some of them have been, or are being, developed to be used as process analytical technology (PAT) to measure real-time critical quality parameters and performance attributes during product development and manufacturing. For example, an in-line laser diffraction setup has been shown to be an alternative to impactor runs for particle sizing to show the dynamic behavior of particles during and after dispersion from a DPI (Shekunov et al. 2007). This in-line sizing method provided dynamic data, which are more informative than the static data conventionally obtained from an impactor. The dynamic data can be used to send feedback to the production process to adjust the quality of the formulation accordingly through changing the relevant production parameters. Although some PATs have not yet been demonstrated on DPI formulations, they are potentially applicable. Real-time Raman spectrophotometry has been used to detect the end point of crystallization and quantitate the polymorphic fraction in a solid product (Helmbach et al. 2013). Real-time near-infrared spectroscopy has been employed to assess the homogeneity of powder blends (Jamrógiewicz et al. 2013). These may be integrated into DPI product manufacturing to monitor the crystallinity of a drug and the mixing of a drug-carrier blend. Thus, more PATs are expected to be developed for inhaler products in the near future.

23.5 Conclusion

A wide range of product testing techniques have been reviewed in this chapter. They examine different aspects of the DPI product, from solid state properties of the particles to the dispersibility of the powder from the inhaler. Data obtained from these tests complement each other and provide a more complete picture on the characteristics and quality of the product. With the advancement of the industry towards quality by design, more of these tests would be applied as PATs in DPI product development and manufacturing.

REFERENCES

Adi, H, D Traini, H-K Chan, and P M Young. 2008. "The influence of drug morphology on the aerosolisation efficiency of dry powder inhaler formulations." *Journal of Pharmaceutical Sciences* 97:2780–2788.

Adi, S, H Adi, H-K Chan, P M Young, D Traini, R Yang, and A Yu. 2008. "Scanning white-light interferometry as a novel technique to quantify the surface roughness of micron-sized particles for inhalation." *Langmuir* 24:11307–11312.

Adi, S, H Adi, P Tang, D Traini, H-K Chan, and P M Young. 2008. "Micro-particle corrugation, adhesion and inhalation aerosol efficiency." *European Journal of Pharmaceutical Sciences* 35:12–18.

British Pharmacopoeia. 2017. London, UK: Stationery Office.

Buckton, G, and P Darcy. 1995. "The use of gravimetric studies to assess the degree of crystallinity of predominantly crystalline powders." *International Journal of Pharmaceutics* 123:265–271.

Buttini, F, G Brambilla, D Copelli, V Sisti, A G Balducci, R Bettini, and I Pasquali. 2016. "Effect of flow rate on *in vitro* aerodynamic performance of NEXThaler® in comparison with Diskus® and Turbohaler® dry powder inhalers." *Journal of Aerosol Medicine and Pulmonary Drug Delivery* 29:167–178.

Chan, H-K. 2008. "What is the role of particle morphology in pharmaceutical powder aerosols?" *Expert Opinion on Drug Delivery* 5:909–914.

Chew, N Y K, P Tang, H-K Chan, and J A Raper. 2005. "How much particle surface corrugation is sufficient to improve aerosol performance of powders?" *Pharmaceutical Research* 22:148–152.

Cline, D, and R Dalby. 2002. "Predicting the quality of powders for inhalation from surface energy and area." *Pharmaceutical Research* 19:1274–1277.

Das, S, I Larson, P Young, and P Stewart. 2009. "Surface energy changes and their relationship with the dispersibility of salmeterol xinafoate powders for inhalation after storage at high RH." *European Journal of Pharmaceutical Sciences* 38:347–354.

Davies, M, A Brindley, X Chen, M Marlow, S W Doughty, I Shrubb, and C J Roberts. 2005. "Characterization of drug particle surface energetics and Young's modulus by atomic force microscopy and inverse gas chromatography." *Pharmaceutical Research* 22:1158–1166.

Demoly, P, P Hagedoorn, A H de Boer, and H W Frijlink. 2014. "The clinical relevance of dry powder inhaler performance for drug delivery." *Respiratory Medicine* 108:1195–1203.

De Oliveira, R R L, D A C Albuquerque, T G S Cruz, F M Yamaji, and F L Leite. 2012. "Measurement of the nanoscale roughness by atomic force microscopy: Basic principles and applications." In *Atomic Force Microscopy: Imaging, Measuring and Manipulating Surfaces at the Atomic Scale*, edited by V Bellito. Rijeka, Croatia: InTech, pp. 147–174.

D'Sa, D J, H-K Chan, and W Chrzanowski. 2014. "Attachment of micro- and nano-particles on tipless cantilevers for colloidal probe microscopy." *Journal of Colloid and Interface Science* 426:190–198.

Dunbar, C A, A J Hickey, and P Holzner. 1998. "Dispersion and characterization of pharmaceutical dry powder aerosols." *Kona*:7–45.

European Pharmacopoeia. 2017. Sainte-Ruffine, France: Maisonneuve.

Freeman, R. 2007. "Measuring the flow properties of consolidated, conditioned and aerated powders—A comparative study using a powder rheometer and a rotational shear cell." *Powder Technology* 174:25–33.

Fuchs, N A. 1964. *The Mechanics of Aerosols*. New York, NY: Pergamon Press.

Guidance for Industry: Metered Dose Inhaler (MDI) and Dry Powder Inhaler (DPI) Drug Products. 1998. Rockville, MD: Center for Drug Evaluation and Research, Food and Drug Administration.

Guideline on the Pharmaceutical Quality of Inhalation and Nasal Products. 2006. London, UK: European Medicines Agency.

Hare, C, U Zafar, M Ghadiri, T Freeman, J Clayton, and M J Murtagh. 2015. "Analysis of the dynamics of the FT4 powder rheometer." *Powder Technology* 285:123–127.

Hassan, M S, and R W M Lau. 2009. "Effect of particle shape on dry particle inhalation: Study on flowability, aerosolization, and deposition properties." *AAPS PharmSciTech* 10:1252–1262.

Helmbach, L, M P Feth, and J Ulrich. 2013. "Integration of process analytical technology tools in pilot-plant setups for the real-time monitoring of crystallizations and phase transitions." *Organic Process Research & Development* 17:585–598.

Hickey, A J, and D A Edwards. 2018. "Density and shape factor terms in Stokes' equation for aerodynamic behavior of aerosols." *Journal of Pharmaceutical Sciences* 107:794–796.

Hinds, W C. 1999. *Aerosol Technology*. New York, NY: John Wiley & Sons.

Ho, R, and J Y Y Heng. 2013. "A review of inverse gas chromatography and its development as a tool to characterize anisotropic surface properties of pharmaceutical solids." *Kona* 30:164–180.

Höhne, G, W F Hemminger, and H-J Flammersheim. 2003. *Differential Scanning Calorimetry*. New York: Springer-Verlag.

Islam, N, R A Tuli, G A George, and T R Dargaville. 2014. "Colloidal drug probe: Method development and validation for adhesion force measurement using atomic force microscopy." *Advanced Powder Techonology* 25:1240–1248.

ISO 13320:2009 Particle Size Analysis – Laser Diffraction Methods. 2009. Geneva, Switzerland: International Organization for Standardization.

Jaffari, S, B Forbes, E Collins, Barlow D J, G P Martin, and D Murnane. 2013. "Rapid characterisation of the inherent dispersibility of respirable powders using dry dispersion laser diffraction." *International Journal of Pharmaceutics* 447:124–131.

Jamrógiewicz, M, K Cal, M Gruszecka, and A Ciesielski. 2013. "Determination of API content in a pilot-scale blending by near-infrared spectroscopy as a first step method to process line implementation." *Acta Poloniae Pharmaceutica – Drug Research* 70:419–429.

Kamiya, A, M Sakagami, M Hindle, and P R Byron. 2004. "Aerodynamic sizing of metered dose inhalers: An evaluation of the Andersen and next generation pharmaceutical impactors and their USP methods." *Journal of Pharmaceutical Sciences* 93:1828–1837.

Kamiya, A, M Sakagami, and P R Byron. 2009. "Cascade impactor practice for a high dose dry powder inhaler at 90 L/min: NGI versus modified 6-stage and 8-stage ACI." *Journal of Pharmaceutical Sciences* 98:1028–1039.

Knopp, M M, K Löbmann, D P Elder, T Rades, and R Holm. 2016. "Recent advances and potential applications of modulated differential scanning calorimetry (mDSC) in drug development." *European Journal of Pharmaceutical Sciences* 87:164–173.

Kwok, P C L, A Tunsirikongkon, W Glover, and H-K Chan. 2011. "Formation of protein nano-matrix particles with controlled surface architecture for respiratory drug delivery." *Pharmaceutical Research* 28:788–796.

Lau, M, P M Young, and D Traini. 2017. "Co-milled API-lactose systems for inhalation therapy: Impact of magnesium stearate on physico-chemical stability and aerosolization performance." *Drug Development and Industrial Pharmacy* 43:980–988.

Lau, R, and H K L Chuah. 2013. "Dynamic shape factor for particles of various shapes in the intermediate settling regime." *Advanced Powder Techonology* 24:306–310.

Leturia, M, M Benali, S Lagarde, I Ronga, and K Saleh. 2014. "Characterization of flow properties of cohesive powders: A comparative study of traditional and new testing methods." *Powder Technology* 253:406–423.

Lowell, S, and J E Shields. 1991. *Powder Surface Area and Porosity*. New York: John Wiley & Sons.

Lu, X-Y, L Chen, C-Y Wu, H-K Chan, and T Freeman. 2017. "The effects of relative humidity on the flowability and dispersion performance of lactose mixtures." *Materials* 10:592.

MacLeod, S K. 1991. "Moisture determination using Karl Fischer titrations." *Analytical Chemistry* 63:557A–566A.

Mitchell, J P. 2013. "Good cascade impactor practices." In *Good Cascade Impactor Practices, AIM and EDA for Orally Inhaled Products*, edited by T P Tougas, J P Mitchell, and S A Lyapustina. New York: Springer.

Mohammadi-Jam, S, and K E Waters. 2014. "Inverse gas chromatography applications: A review." *Advances in Colloid and Interface Science* 212:21–44.

Nasr, M M, D L Ross, and N C Miller. 1997. "Effect of drug load and plate coating on the particle size distribution of a commercial albuterol metered dose inhaler (MDI) determined using the Andersen and Marple-Miller cascade impactors." *Pharmaceutical Research* 14:1437–1443.

Raposo, M, Q Ferreira, and P A Ribeiro. 2007. "A guide for atomic force microscopy analysis of soft-condensed matter." In *Modern Research and Educational Topics in Microscopy*, edited by A Méndez-Vilas and J Diaz. Badajoz, Spain: Formatex.

Rouquerol, J, G Baron, R Denoyel, H Giesche, J Groen, P Klobes, P Levitz, A V Neimark, S Rigby, R Skudas, K Sing, M Thommes, and K Unger. 2012. "Liquid intrusion and alternative methods for the characterization of macroporous materials (IUPAC Technical Report)." *Pure and Applied Chemistry* 84:107–136.

Shekunov, B Y, P Chattopadhyay, H H Y Tong, and Albert H L Chow. 2007. "Particle size analysis in pharmaceutics: Principles, methods and applications." *Pharmaceutical Research* 24:203–227.

Tong, H H Y, B Y Shekunov, P York, and Albert H L Chow. 2006. "Predicting the aerosol performance of dry powder inhalation formulations by interparticulate interaction analysis using inverse gas chromatography." *Journal of Pharmaceutical Sciences* 95:228–233.

Ung, K T, N Rao, J G Weers, D Huang, and H-K Chan. 2016. "Design of spray dried insulin microparticles to bypass deposition in the extrathoracic region and maximize total lung dose." *International Journal of Pharmaceutics* 511:1070–1079.

United States Pharmacopeia 40-National Formulary 35. 2017. Rockville, MD: United States Pharmacopeial Convention.

Wagner, K G, U Dowe, and J Zadnik. 2005. "Highly loaded interactive mixtures for dry powder inhalers: Prediction of the adhesion capacity using surface energy and solubility parameters." *Pharmazie* 60:339–344.

Ward, G H, and R K Schultz. 1995. "Process-induced crystallinity changes in albuterol sulfate and its effect on powder physical stability." *Pharmaceutical Research* 12:773–779.

Weiss, C, P McLoughlin, and H Cathcart. 2015. "Characterisation of dry powder inhaler formulations using atomic force microscopy." *International Journal of Pharmaceutics* 494:393–407.

Young, P M, H Chiou, T Tee, D Traini, H-K Chan, F Thielmann, and D Burnett. 2007. "The use of organic vapor sorption to determine low levels of amorphous content in processed pharmaceutical powders." *Drug Development and Industrial Pharmacy* 33:91–97.

Young, P M, M J Tobyn, R Price, M Buttrum, and F Dey. 2006. "The use of colloid probe microscopy to predict aerosolization performance in dry powder inhalers: AFM and *in vitro* correlation." *Journal of Pharmaceutical Sciences* 95:1800–1809.

Young, P M, P Kwok, H Adi, H-K Chan, and D Traini. 2009. "Lactose composite carriers for respiratory delivery." *Pharmaceutical Research* 26:802–810.

Young, P M, R Price, M J Tobyn, M Buttrum, and F Dey. 2003. "Investigation into the effect of humidity on drug-drug interactions using the atomic force microscope." *Journal of Pharmaceutical Sciences* 92:815–822.

Zeng, X M, G P Martin, and C Marriott. 2000. *Particulate Interactions in Dry Powder Formulations for Inhalation*. Boca Raton, FL: CRC Press.

24

Aerodynamic Particle Size Testing

Jolyon Mitchell

CONTENTS

24.1 Introduction

The aerodynamic particle size distribution (APSD) of an orally inhaled product is understood to be a critical quality attribute by the regulatory agencies (Health Canada 2006, European Medicines Agency 2006, United States Food and Drug Administration 2018) because airborne particle aerodynamic diameter is correlated with the likely deposition location in the human respiratory tract (Hinds 1999, Rudolph et al. 1990, Heyder and Svartengren 2002). Particle inertia dominates the motion of aerosols in the size range from about 0.4 µm–10 µm aerodynamic diameter typically produced by inhaled aerosols (Heyder et al. 1986), and the detection of differences in inertia is therefore the most widely used approach that is utilized to size-separate particles to measure their APSD (Marple and Liu 1974).

After outlining the underlying theory of inertial particle size separation, the development of methodologies for the determination of APSD in product quality control is explored, focusing primarily on those procedures involving the pharmacopeial multi-stage cascade impactors (US Pharmacopeial Convention 2018a, US Pharmacopeial Convention 2018b, European Directorate for Quality in Medicines (EDQM) 2018a, European Directorate for Quality in Medicines (EDQM) 2018b). Key aspects affecting the use of these apparatuses are reviewed. The Abbreviated Impactor Measurement and Effective Data Analysis concepts are intended to simplify the existing approaches to measurement and assessment of APSDs, respectively, from orally inhaled products (Tougas et al. 2011). Both concepts are therefore presented, examining the evidence for both their suitability as well as their limitations as product quality control tools. The almost universal application of cascade impactor-based methodologies has in the past 20 years created a need for guidance on both the maintenance and system suitability verification of these apparatuses. This process has resulted in the development of the Good Cascade Impactor Practices (GCIP) concept, which is therefore next examined in some detail.

Tension currently exists between the relatively simple-in-concept apparatuses for APSD determination associated with product quality control and the more elaborate approaches that have been developed in order to make these measurements more relevant in support of the clinical program during the product lifecycle (Tougas et al. 2011). The applicability of these developments at different points in the product lifecycle is therefore assessed, illustrating how clinically relevant APSD measurements can augment their equivalents made for quality control purposes. Examples of more clinically relevant measurements in association with APSD determinations are:

1. The development of age-appropriate idealized oropharyngeal inlets (Stapleton et al. 2000, Golshahi and Finlay 2012, Carrigy et al. 2014);
2. The creation of a range of small, medium, and large adult anatomically accurate oropharyngeal models (McRobbie et al. 2003); and
3. The use of a novel laminar flow-based mixing inlet that enables the inhaler to be operated connected to a breathing simulator while the cascade impactor samples at its required fixed flow rate for effective operation (Miller 2002).

The likelihood is greatly improved for achieving meaningful *in vitro-in vivo* correlations (IVIVCs) for orally inhaled products if all three measures are put in place (Olsson et al. 2013).

Although complicated and time-consuming to use (Bonam et al. 2008), the multi-stage cascade impactor has been adopted as the apparatus of choice for APSD determinations because, as well as determining particle aerodynamic size directly, the active pharmaceutical ingredient(s) in the formulation being aerosolized can be recovered and assayed quantitatively (Mitchell and Nagel 2003). Nevertheless, there is continued interest in determining aerodynamic size-relevant measures more rapidly and with greater size resolution. This chapter therefore concludes with an examination of two alternative techniques that more closely meet these criteria. The first is based on particle time-of-flight (TOF) in an accelerating flow field (Mitchell and Nagel 1999, Mitchell et al. 2011a). This aerodynamic particle size measurement methodology, though providing far higher size-resolution than available using a cascade impactor, is not generally favored by the regulatory agencies, since until recently there has been no capability to recover and assay the active pharmaceutical ingredient(s) present (Mitchell et al. 2011a). The development of single particle aerodynamic mass spectrometry (SPAMS) offers the prospect of Active Pharmaceutical Ingredient (API)-specific identification combined with individual particle aerodynamic size measurement (Morrical et al. 2015, Jetzer et al. 2017). This additional capability may alter the situation, particularly in early stage product development, if the cost of the equipment can be made comparable with cascade impactor-based methods. Likewise, laser diffractometry (LD) (Mitchell et al. 2011a), which is the second alternative approach to aerosol sizing, also offers significant advantages in terms of user interface simplicity, size resolution, and measurement rapidity. LD, although a light scattering- and not an inertial-based method, has applicability in particular to the assessment of nebulizing systems, since the API-containing aqueous droplets that nebulizers typically disperse have aerodynamic diameters that are equivalent to physical (geometric) diameters obtainable by techniques such as microscopy-image analysis.

24.2 Theory of Inertial Particle Size Fractionation

Cascade impactors provide measures of the size distribution of the sampled aerosol in terms of particle aerodynamic diameter, rather than the size scale based on physical dimensions (D_p) that is often acquired by microscopy-image analysis. D_p is most conveniently expressed in terms of volume equivalent diameter (D_v) to take into account the usual situation for inhaled aerosol particles, in which the 3-dimensional particle shape is non-spherical (Merkus 2009). It follows that $D_p = D_v$ for perfectly spherical particles.

Aerodynamic diameter (D_{ae}) represents the size scale that takes into account the effect of both particle density and shape on mobility when in motion in an associated flow field. D_{ae} is related to D_p through the expression:

$$D_{ae} = \left[\frac{\rho_p}{\rho_0 \chi}\right]^{1/2} D_p C_c \tag{24.1}$$

in which ρ_p and ρ_0 are the particle density and reference density (i.e. that for water = 1.00 g cm^{-3}), respectively, χ is the dynamic shape factor that takes into account deviations in shape from spherical (χ = 1.00), and C_c is the Cunningham slip correction factor (Hinds 1999), given by:

$$C_c = 1 + 0.5Kn_p\left[2.34 + 1.05\exp\left(-0.195Kn_p\right)\right] \tag{24.2}$$

Kn_p is the dimensionless particle Knudsen number, relating D_p to the mean free path length of a molecule of the surrounding air (λ), where:

$$Kn_p = {}^{2\lambda}\!/_{D_p} \tag{24.3}$$

For particle sizes larger than a few micrometers, Kn_p decreases towards zero, describing motion in the continuum regime, in which the value of C_c approaches unity. Equation 24.1 can then be simplified to:

$$D_{ae} = \left[\frac{\rho_p}{\rho_0 \chi}\right]^{1/2} D_p \tag{24.4}$$

which, for practical purposes, provides the relationship between the aerodynamic and physical size scales, when measuring the APSD of aerosols emitted from all classes of orally inhaled product.

All types of impactors share the common feature that they are intended to operate at a constant flow rate. The flow rate is set such that the incoming aerosol enters the stages within a flow of air having a fixed velocity profile that is ideally laminar (flow Reynolds number, Re_f <2000). As will be shown later, the fixed flow rate criterion is intentionally not met when testing dry powder inhalers (DPIs) (US Pharmacopeial Convention 2018a, European Directorate for Quality in Medicines (EDQM) 2018a), because it is necessary to mimic an inhalation maneuver in order to disperse the powder from its source (either a bulk powder reservoir, capsule, or blister) in order to convey the medication to the user via the mouthpiece of the inhaler.

Before going on to discuss the operation of a multi-stage cascade impactor, it is worthwhile to examine the underlying operating principle of a single stage impactor, and Figure 24.1 illustrates its essential features. The stage comprises a nozzle plate of diameter, *W*, that is located a fixed distance (*S*) from a collection surface. A vacuum is applied to the exit of the assembly, such that the aerosol particle stream enters the nozzle at a fixed flow rate, *Q*. The trajectories of three different sized particles are considered. The largest particle has too much inertia to avoid its trajectory separating substantially from the flow streamline as the flow direction changes abruptly at the nozzle exit, such that the particle arrives at the impaction surface where it remains collected. The trajectory of the medium sized particle is also perturbed, but by an amount that is insufficient to prevent it from remaining in the airflow that moves adjacent to, and passing over, the impaction surface. Likewise, the perturbation of the trajectory of the smallest particle is too small for it to be collected there. The dimensionless Stokes number (*St*), which is the ratio of the stopping distance of a particle to a characteristic dimension, in this case the nozzle diameter, *W* (or average diameter, for a multi-orifice stage) describes the process analytically. *St* is related to *W* through the expression:

$$St = \frac{\rho_p C_c D_p^2 U}{9\eta W} \tag{24.5}$$

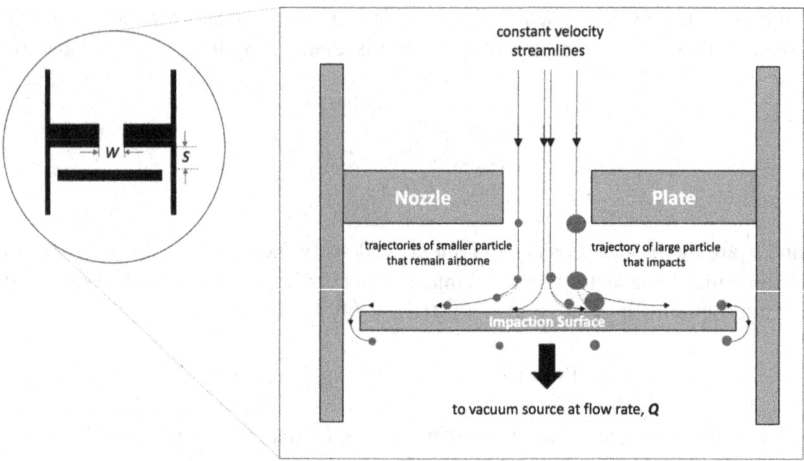

FIGURE 24.1 Idealized single stage inertial impactor showing three sizes of particles passing through, the largest has too much inertia to avoid collection on the impaction surface, the smaller particles have insufficient inertia to deviate enough from the flow streamlines, and therefore pass beyond the impaction surface.

where η is the gas (air) viscosity and defines St in terms of the ratio of the stopping distance of the particle, which is related to its inertia, to the nozzle radius, $W/2$ (Marple and Willeke 1976). On this basis, St is related to D_{ae} by combining Equations 24.1 and 24.5 as follows:

$$St = \frac{\rho_p C_{ae} D_{ae}^2 U}{9\eta W \chi} \tag{24.6}$$

The value of $\sqrt{St}$ at which particles impact rather than remain in the flow is about 0.49 for circular nozzles (Marple and Liu 1974).

In well-designed multi-stage apparatuses, such as the Next Generation Impactor (NGI) (Marple et al. 2003a), the first stage comprises a single nozzle aligned on-axis to the incoming flow, much as illustrated in Figure 24.1. This design feature avoids the potential for maldistribution of the incoming flow affecting the uniformity of particle deposition associated with this stage. Such flow maldistribution has recently been observed upstream of the widely used 8-stage Andersen non-viable cascade impactor (ACI) (Roberts and Mitchell 2017). In this configuration, the nozzle plate of the first stage contains 96 circular nozzles arranged in four concentric circles located at increasing lateral distances perpendicular to the incoming flow axis. Beyond the first stage, most impactor designs contain multiple nozzles associated with each stage, so that the incoming aerosol can be distributed more evenly to each collection surface. Roberts (2009) has shown that the aerodynamic properties of such a stage can be described in terms of the effective diameter (W_{eff}), defined in terms of the area mean (W_{mean}), and area median (W_{median}) diameter of the nozzle array:

$$W_{eff} = \left[\left(W_{mean}\right)^{2/3} \cdot \left(W_{median}\right)^{1/3} \right] \tag{24.7}$$

This finding has implications concerning how the diameters of multi-nozzle stages are periodically checked by image analysis combined with microscopy (stage mensuration), in order to verify that the manufacturer's intended performance has been maintained within specification. This process is discussed in more detail later in this chapter.

If a given single stage impactor is regarded as a particle size fractionator, its most important property, regardless of the number of nozzles, is the function that describes the change in collection efficiency (E) with particle aerodynamic size. E is conveniently expressed as a percentage that varies smoothly from 0%, where all small particles pass through the stage without impacting there, to 100%, where all incoming particles within a larger size range impact at that stage. The collection efficiency curve for an ideal size fractionator increases in a step-wise manner between limits of zero to 100% at a single, fixed size (curve A of Figure 24.2). In practice, however, the relationship between E and either D_{ae} or D_p is a monotonic sigmoidal function that increases steeply from E ≈ 0% to > 95%, reaching its maximum steepness when E is 50% (curve B of Figure 24.2). The size corresponding to $E_{50\%}$ is often termed the cut-point size (D_{50}), also known as the effective cut-off diameter. D_{50} is related to $\sqrt{St_{50}}$ through the expression:

$$D_{50}\sqrt{C_{c,50}} = \left[\frac{9\pi\mu n W_{\text{eff}}^3}{4\rho_0 Q}\right]^{1/2} \sqrt{St_{50}} \tag{24.8}$$

for a multi-orifice stage comprising n circular nozzles. An important outcome of this equation is that impactors are designed to operate at a fixed volumetric flow rate, Q (Marple and Liu 1974). This requirement is in conflict with an inhalation maneuver needed to operate passive DPIs, and the continuously varying flow rate-time profiles associated with respiration (Mitchell and Nagel 2003). In practice, it is assumed that the time for the flow rate through the impactor to stabilize after applying vacuum at the start of sampling is a sufficiently small portion of the total time to collect the 4 L sample defined by the pharmacopeial methodologies for DPI testing, that the non-ideal flow rate ramp-up to stability can be ignored (US Pharmacopeial Convention 2018a, European Directorate for Quality in Medicines [EDQM] 2018a).

The two shaded areas in Figure 24.2 depict the mass of larger particles that should have impacted on the stage, but instead passed through (area 1) and the mass of smaller particles that should have passed through the stage, but instead were collected (area 2). These areas are approximately equal with well-designed stages (Marple and Willeke 1976), so that the impactor can be treated as if its size-fractionating performance is ideal with D_{50} for each stage defined by the size at which it collects particles with 50% collection efficiency, as assumed by Equation 24.8.

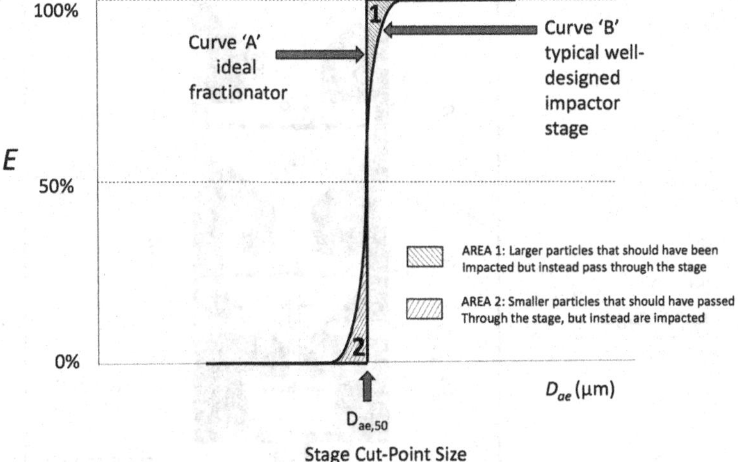

FIGURE 24.2 Collection efficiency curves for a single stage impactor; curve (A) illustrates ideal behavior in which the collection efficiency is a step function of particle size (perfect size selectivity); curve (B) depicts a more realistic situation in which the collection efficiency gradually increases from zero to 100%, with the greatest rate of change at the stage cut-point size, corresponding to 50% collection efficiency.

The size selectivity of the stage can be defined in terms analogous to the geometric standard deviation (GSD) of the cumulative form of the APSD (Mitchell and Nagel 2003), namely:

$$GSD_{stage} = \sqrt{\frac{D_{84.1}}{D_{15.9}}} \tag{24.9}$$

in which $D_{84.1}$ and $D_{15.9}$ represent the sizes at which the stage collection efficiency for the incoming aerosol particles are 84.1% and 15.9%, respectively. Roberts and Mitchell (2013) have shown theoretically that the error introduced by the step change assumption is larger for certain stages of the ACI than for the NGI. However, the error is sufficiently small to be inconsequential, unless the APSD is nearly monodisperse (GSD $\leq$ 1.2), a condition that is unlikely to occur with aerosols emitted by almost all orally inhaled products.

Multi-stage cascade impactors are created by combining several stages in series, as illustrated by Figure 24.3 (Marple and Liu 1974). A back-up filter is normally located behind the final size-fractionating stage to collect any fines that may have penetrated beyond that stage. The design of each successive impaction stage progressively increases the flow velocity, resulting in particles of increasingly finer size being collected. This process is achieved by decreasing W_{eff} from one stage to the next, so that the incoming flow velocity to the stage is correspondingly increased. In this way, the critical value of $\sqrt{St}$ of 0.49 is achieved with successively finer particles as the aerosol passes through the apparatus. The mass of particulate collected on each stage, as well as the mass deposited on so-called "non-sizing" components of the sampling train, such as the inlet (induction port) and pre-separator (if used), represent the entire sub-divided aerosol emitted from the inhaler (Dunbar and Mitchell 2005). This is the deposition profile and represents the raw data that are obtained from the measurement apparatus. The sum of each deposited mass throughout all locations in the sampling train is the mass balance associated with the determination. This mass balance had, until recently, been regarded by the United States Food and Drug Administration (USFDA) as a measure or product quality for pressurized metered dose inhaler (pMDI) and DPI products, having indicated limits between 85% and 115% label claim mass/actuation

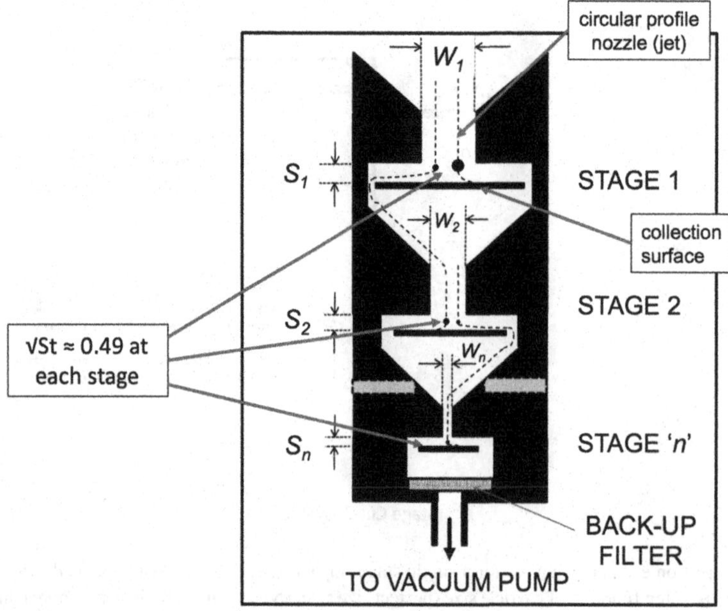

FIGURE 24.3 Multi-stage cascade impactor concept: The aerosol flow velocity is progressively increased from stage-to-stage throughout the sequence by decreasing W_{eff}, and $\sqrt{St}$ is about 0.49 at each successive stage for circular profile nozzles; the outcome is a deposition profile comprising progressively finer particles from which the APSD can be constructed.

(United States Food and Drug Administration 1998). However, the wider consensus is that the mass balance outcome should be used primarily to assert system suitability for each determination, given the complexity of the cascade impaction methodology (Wyka et al. 2007, Bagger-Jörgensen et al. 2005). In the most recent update to their draft reviewer guidance on pMDI and DPI drug products chemistry, manufacturing, and controls documentation, there has been a shift in USFDA thinking towards considering system suitability in the event that a mass balance value outside these limits is obtained (United States Food and Drug Administration 2018). An out-of-specification mass balance result provides the opportunity to follow an ordered process to ascertain its cause(s) (Wyka et al. 2007).

Until the early 1990s, cascade impactors were individually calibrated with monodisperse, spherical aerosol particles of known aerodynamic diameter at the flow rate(s) of use (Mitchell et al. 1987, Vaughan 1989, Asking and Olsson 1997). However, the process is both time-consuming and exacting to complete. Nowadays, stage mensuration is the preferred approach to verify that the aerodynamic performance of each impactor stage is within the manufacturer's specifications. In 2003, a single so-called "archival" NGI whose individual stage nozzles were manufactured as close as possible to their nominal sizes, was calibrated at 30 L/min, 60 L/min, and 100 L/min (Marple et al. 2003b) for use with pMDI and DPI products to provide reference data against which other NGI apparatus could be validated by mensuration. The same impactor was later calibrated by the same process at 15 L/min for use primarily with nebulizing systems (Marple et al. 2004). In both instances, monodisperse particles were generated as calibrant aerosols, whose sizes were traceable to national standards in order to provide a reference point for comparison of other impactors of this type. The archival impactor has not been used since it was calibrated, so that it is potentially available should it be necessary at some date in the future to re-validate this apparatus. All other cascade impactor designs rely on manufacturer-specified D_{50} values that are related to nominal nozzle diameters for each stage.

Tables 24.1 through 24.4 contain the nominal stage D_{50} values for the pharmacopeial impactors at the recommended flow rates for use. However, a given impactor may need to operate at a flow rate intermediate between values for which calibration data are available, in particular for DPI testing, since the final flow rate attained in the sampling process following the procedures in the pharmacopeial compendia is dependent upon the flow resistance of the inhaler (Van Oort 1995). Equation 24.10 can therefore be used to estimate the D_{50} values at the intermediate flow rate (Marple and Willeke 1976):

$$D_{50,\mathrm{int}} = D_{50,\mathrm{cal}}\sqrt{\frac{Q_{\mathrm{cal}}}{Q_{\mathrm{int}}}} \quad (24.10)$$

TABLE 24.1

Values of D_{50} (μm) for the Size Fractionating Stages of the ACI at (a) Q = 28.3 L/min, (b) 60 L/min*, and (c) 90 L/min*

	Nominal Flow Rate (L/min)		
Stage	**28.3**	**60.0**	**90.0**
–2	Not applicable	Not applicable	8.0
–1	Not applicable	8.6	6.5
0	9.0	6.5	5.2
1	5.8	4.4	3.5
2	4.7	3.2	2.6
3	3.3	1.9	1.7
4	2.1	1.2	1.0
5	1.1	0.5	0.22
6	0.7	0.26	Not applicable
7	0.4	Not applicable	Not applicable

Source: United States Pharmacopeial Convention.

* Special stage –0 which has a modified outer upper section, so that an additional stage instead of the inlet cone can be inserted above it, is inserted when testing at either 60.0 L/min or 90.0 L/min.

TABLE 24.2

Values of D_{50} (μm) for the Size Fractionating Stages of the NGI at (a) $Q = 15$ L/min, (b) 30 L/min, (c) 60 L/min, and (d) 90 L/min

	Nominal Flow Rate (L/min)			
Stage	**15**	**30**	**60**	**100.0**
1*	14.1	11.7	8.06	6.12
2	8.61	6.40	4.46	3.42
3	5.39	3.99	2.82	2.18
4	3.30	2.30	1.66	1.31
5	2.08	1.36	1.17	0.72
6	1.36	0.83	0.55	0.40
7	0.98	0.54	0.34	0.24

Source: United States Pharmacopeial Convention.

* Values for stage 1 assume this stage is preceded by USP/Ph. Eur. induction port—these ECDs are slightly different if a pre-separator is also used (Marple et al. 2003b).

TABLE 24.3

Values of D_{50} (μm) for the Size Fractionating Stages of the Various Versions of the MMI for Use at Different Values of Q

Stage	**Model and Flow Rate for Which Calibration Data Are Available**				
	150P*	**150P***	**150**	**160**	**160**
Q (L/min) =	4.9	12	30	60	90
1	10.0	10.0	10.0	10.0	8.1
2	7.2	4.7	5.0	5.0	4.0
3	4.7	3.1	2.5	2.5	2.0
4	3.1	2.0	1.25	1.25	1.00
5	0.77	0.44	0.63	0.63	0.50

Source: United States Pharmacopeial Convention.

* Model 150P developed for pediatric applications.

TABLE 24.4

Values of D_{50} (μm) for the Size Fractionating Stages of the MSLI at $Q = 60$ L/min

Stage	D_{50}
1	13.0
2	6.8
3	3.1
4	1.7

Source: United States Pharmacopeial Convention.

in which $D_{50,cal}$ and $D_{50,int}$ are the cut-point sizes at the calibration (Q_{cal}) and intermediate (Q_{int}) flow rates, respectively. Here, the effect of the Cunningham slip correction factor (C_c) can be ignored, as it is close to unity at the size range of interest when measuring aerosols from orally inhaled products. A more generalized form of this equation, taking the form:

$$D_{50,int} = A\left[\frac{60}{Q_{int}}\right]^B \tag{24.11}$$

TABLE 24.5

Values of Constants "A" and "B" in Equation 24.11 to Calculate NGI Stage D_{50} Values at Intermediate Values of Q Between 30 L/min and 100 L/min

Stage	A	B
1	8.06	0.54
2	4.46	0.52
3	2.82	0.50
4	1.66	0.47
5	0.94	0.53
6	0.55	0.60
7	0.34	0.67

Source: Marple, V.A. et al., *J. Aerosol Med.*, 16, 301–324, 2003b; Mary Ann Liebert, Inc., publishers, New Rochelle, New York.

has been used to enable values of D_{50} to be calculated at intermediate flow rates ($D_{50,\text{int}}$) from the archival calibration data for the NGI obtained at 60 L/min, where values of the constants A and B for each stage are listed in Table 24.5. The equation used to calculate $D_{50,\text{int}}$ for the pre-separator, which was also archivally calibrated is:

$$D_{50,\text{int}} = 12.8 - 0.07\left(Q_{\text{int}} - 60\right) \tag{24.12}$$

The micro-orifice collector (MOC) does not have a complete collection efficiency curve, as its purpose is to capture any fines penetrating the last impaction stage, offering an alternative and more rapid to use option to the normal back-up filter. Its size at which 80% of the incoming particle mass is collected (D_{80}) was defined by the expression, analogous to Equation 24.11:

$$D_{80,\text{int}} = 0.14\left[\frac{60}{Q_{\text{int}}}\right]^{1.36} \tag{24.13}$$

There may be concern that the back-up capability of the MOC alone may be inadequate, when sizing products that produce aerosols with a substantial portion of the APSD contained in particles finer than about 1 μm aerodynamic diameter (Marple et al. 2003a). Under these circumstances, a separate back-up filter can either be used following the MOC, or the MOC may be replaced by an internal filter.

24.3 The Pharmacopeial Cascade Impactor Apparatuses

24.3.1 Measuring APSDs of pMDIs and Soft Mist Inhalers

Currently, there are two different apparatuses (Figure 24.4) described in Chapter <601> of the United States Pharmacopeia for the assessment of pMDI-derived aerosols (US Pharmacopeial Convention 2018a). These are:

1. The 8-stage ACI without pre-separator operated at 28.3 L/min and
2. The 7-stage NGI without pre-separator operated at 30 L/min.

The same apparatuses are listed in Monograph 2.91.8 of the European Pharmacopeia (European Directorate for Quality in Medicines (EDQM) 2018a).

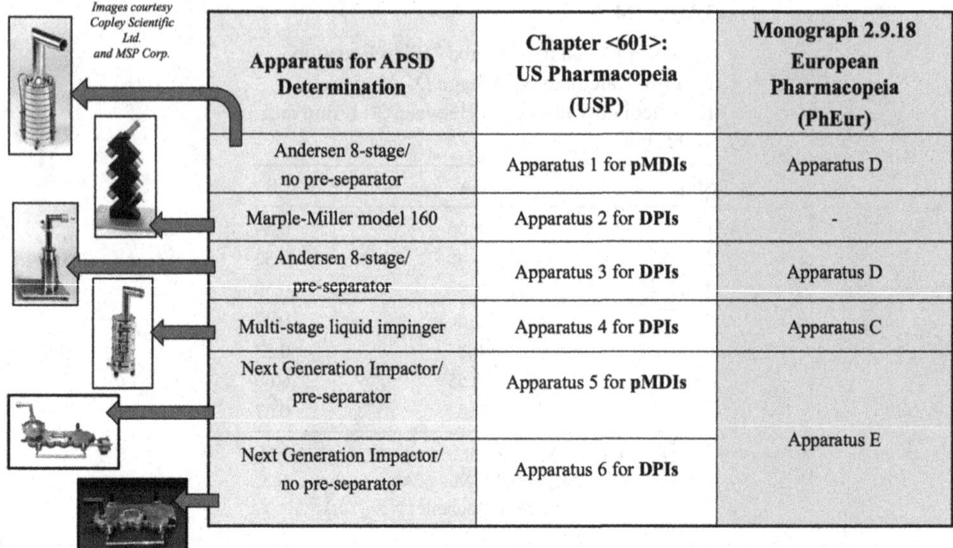

Apparatus for APSD Determination	Chapter <601>: US Pharmacopeia (USP)	Monograph 2.9.18 European Pharmacopeia (PhEur)
Andersen 8-stage/ no pre-separator	Apparatus 1 for **pMDIs**	Apparatus D
Marple-Miller model 160	Apparatus 2 for **DPIs**	-
Andersen 8-stage/ pre-separator	Apparatus 3 for **DPIs**	Apparatus D
Multi-stage liquid impinger	Apparatus 4 for **DPIs**	Apparatus C
Next Generation Impactor/ pre-separator	Apparatus 5 for **pMDIs**	Apparatus E
Next Generation Impactor/ no pre-separator	Apparatus 6 for **DPIs**	

FIGURE 24.4 Measurement apparatuses defined for the measurement of pMDI- and DPI-emitted aerosol APSD in Chapter <601> of the United States Pharmacopeia and Monograph 2.9.18 of the European Pharmacopeia.

Although not specifically mentioned in the pharmacopeias, the recently introduced soft mist inhaler class of orally inhaled product, of which the Respimat® (Dalby et al. 2004) (Boehringer Ingelheim AG & Ko. KG) is currently the most widely encountered member, is included with the pMDI class for the purpose of defining test apparatuses. This is because the soft mist inhaler generates the aerosol internally, rather than requiring the patient to inhale to make it function, as is the case with passive DPIs. In consequence, it is used much like a pMDI, in terms of the requirement to actuate the device before the aerosol is emitted (Dalby et al. 2004).

The collection surfaces of the ACI are circular plates whose periphery is slightly raised (Figure 24.5A). These plates are available in either aluminum or stainless steel, but the latter are preferred because of the avoidance of corrosion during handling and cleaning between uses. The plates can be used with the raised edge facing upwards where a significant amount of particulate is anticipated to be collected, but are normally used with the edges facing downwards to avoid turbulence in the flow passing to the next stage that might increase internal losses to the exterior walls of the flow pathway. The plates used with the first two stages are annular (Figure 24.5B), based on a development that took place by McFarland et al. (1977) in an attempt to reduce internal losses with this impactor design. An 81-mm diameter filter is used in the final stage of the ACI.

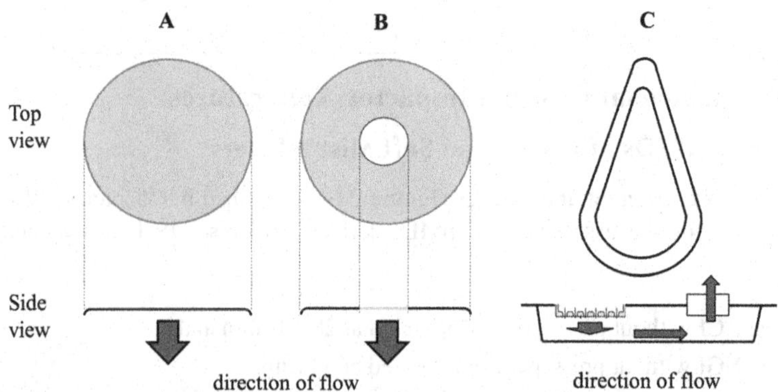

FIGURE 24.5 Top and side views of collection plates for (A) lowermost six stages of the ACI; (B) uppermost two stages of the ACI; and (C) one of the six standard collection cups for the NGI.

Coating of cascade impactor stage surfaces with an agent to improve particle adhesion is well understood to be necessary to avoid particle bounce and subsequent re-entrainment in the flow passing from a particular stage to the remainder of the apparatus (Rao and Whitby 1978a, 1978b). In the past, when testing pMDI-based products, the collection surfaces of the impaction stages of the ACI were often used without coating, as many inhalers of this type were formulated containing surfactant as an excipient, thereby mitigating potential of bias arising from particle bounce and re-entrainment. Since the replacement of chlorofluorocarbon with hydrofluoroalkane propellants, however, many pMDI-delivered formulations do not contain surfactant, so that coating with a material capable of providing a tacky surface to incoming particles has become normal practice (Mitchell and Nagel 2003).

In contrast with the ACI, the collection surfaces of each stage of the NGI are shallow stainless steel, pear-shaped cups (Figure 24.5C), having a surface roughness between 0.5 µm and 2 µm. The diameter of the cup for the first stage is larger than for the other size-fractionating stages to minimize impaction of the largest particles entering the impactor, near the vertical wall of the cup (Marple et al. 2003a). The MOC comprises 4032 nozzles nominally of 70 µm mean diameter, and is located above its own cup, having the same larger size as the cup located below the first stage. Nowadays, surface coating of these collection cups is normal practice, for the reasons already given in connection with the use of the ACI.

Figure 24.6 illustrates schematically the basic configuration needed to evaluate aerosols from this class of orally inhaled product using either the ACI or the NGI. In the case of the ACI, used at 28.3 L/min the induction port is attached to the entry of a short entrance cone that sits on top of the vertical stack of impaction stages labeled "0" through "7," with the back-up filter stage located beneath stage "7" (Figure 24.7). When using the NGI (Figure 24.8), the inlet is inserted directly into the inlet port for stage 1 without the need for an expansion cone. This cascade impactor has its stages oriented in the horizontal plane to improve its capability for automated use (Marple et al. 2003a). The collection cups are conveniently loaded onto a tray that is inserted on the bottom frame, and the lid containing the seal body is affixed to the tray via a purpose-designed mechanism operated by a handle that is pulled down in order to seal the flow passageway from ingress of ambient air via leak pathways when sampling an inhaler-generated aerosol.

In operation, either design of impactor is first assembled in accordance with manufacturer instructions, before connecting its outlet to a vacuum source via a flow control needle valve using a short length of suitable-sized tubing. After attaching the induction port, the needle valve is used to adjust the volumetric flow rate to the appropriate value, by means of a suitable flow meter located at the entry to the inlet. The flow meter is then detached from the apparatus. The pMDI is prepared for actuation following the manufacturer's instructions concerning priming, if appropriate, then the mouthpiece is inserted on axis into the entry to the induction port, using a suitable adapter. The pMDI is then actuated once, allowing at least 30 seconds to elapse before the next actuation. The rubric in the FDA draft guidance for

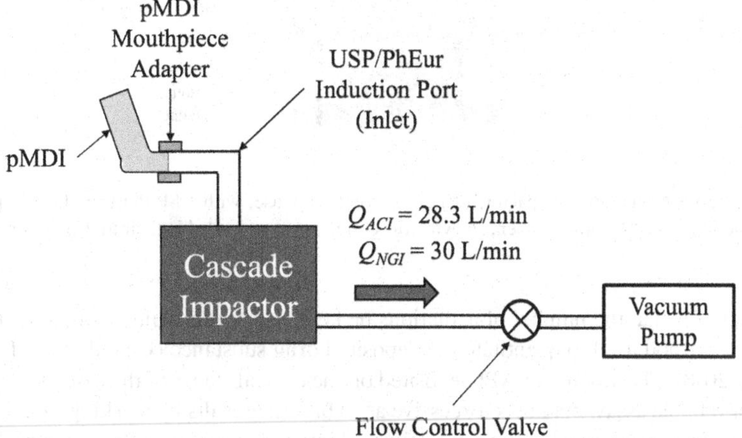

FIGURE 24.6 Apparatus configuration for the evaluation of APSD of pMDI-generated aerosols in accordance with the methodology in Chapter <601> of the United Stated Pharmacopeia or Monograph 2.9.18 of the European Pharmacopeia.

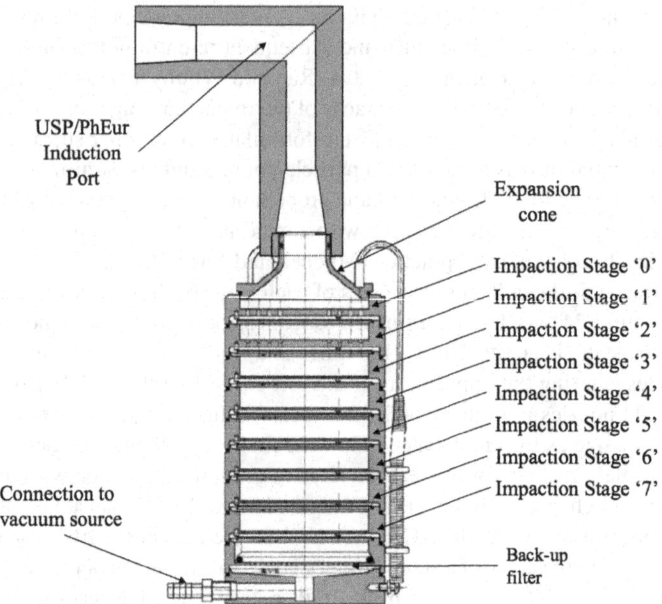

FIGURE 24.7 The Andersen 8-stage cascade impactor in the configuration used at 28.3 L/min; the induction port is connected directly to a short expansion cone that sits on top of the vertical stack containing the impaction stages, with the stage containing a back-up filter underneath the bottom impaction stage.

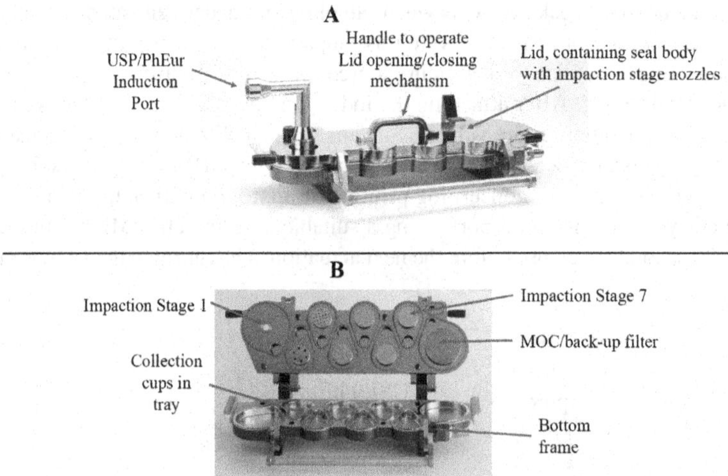

FIGURE 24.8 The next generation impactor: (A) closed ready for use, with USP/PhEur induction port attached to entry port to impaction stage "1" and (B) open, showing the collection cups loaded in their tray. (Courtesy of MSP Corp., Minneapolis, MN.)

pMDI testing advises that the number of actuations be kept to the minimum, justified by the sensitivity of the analytical method used to quantitate the deposited drug substance (United States Food and Drug Administration 2018). The amount of API deposited on the critical stages of the cascade impactor should be sufficient for reliable assay, but not so excessive as to bias the results by masking individual actuation variation. In practice, up to five actuations are delivered into the apparatus before switching power off to the vacuum source to terminate the measurement. However, where the API is highly potent, as many as ten actuations may be needed to collect sufficient mass on the lighter-loaded collection surfaces.

24.3.2 Measuring APSDs of DPI-Based Products

Currently, there are four apparatuses (Figure 24.4) described in Chapter <601> of the United States Pharmacopeia for the assessment of pMDI- and DPI-derived aerosols. These are:

1. The 5-stage Marple-Miller impactor (MMI) operated at 60 L/min;
2. The 8-stage ACI with pre-separator operated at 60 L/min;
3. The 4-stage Multi-Stage Liquid Impinger (MSLI) operated at 60 L/min; and
4. The NGI with pre-separator operated at higher flow rates (60 L/min and 100 L/min).

Currently, neither the MMI (Figure 24.9) nor the MLSI (Figure 24.10) are in widespread use because they do not offer sufficient size-resolution to meet requirements for a minimum of five size-fractionating

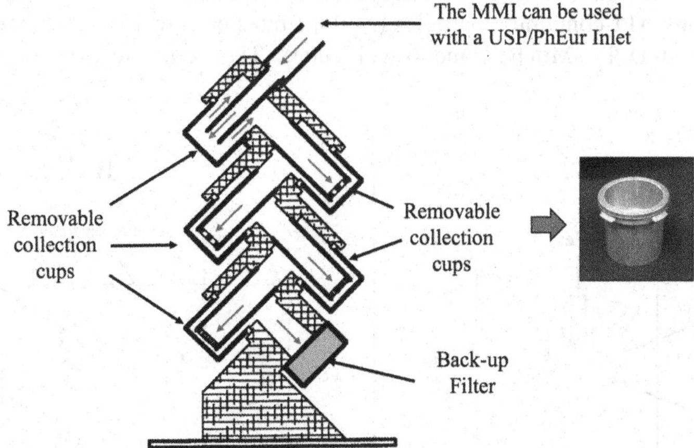

FIGURE 24.9 MMI, the size-fractionated aerosol particles are collected in deep cups located beneath the five impaction stages. (Courtesy of MSP Corp., Minneapolis, MN.)

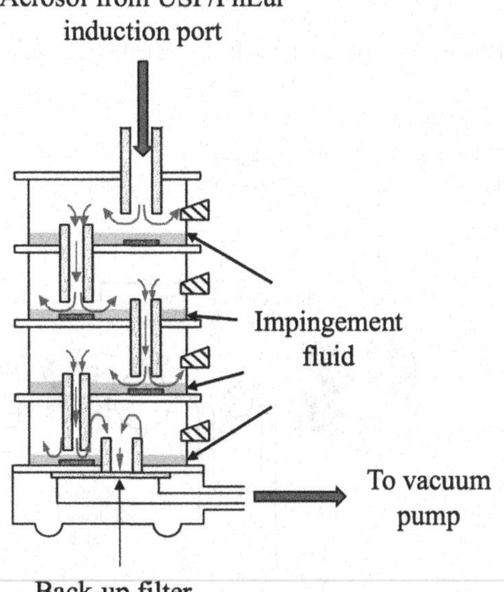

FIGURE 24.10 MSLI, the size fractionated aerosol particles impinger into a shallow liquid layer located beneath each impaction stage.

stages with cut-points between 0.5 µm and 5.0 µm aerodynamic diameter (Marple et al. 2003a). However, in the past, the MSLI was popular in Europe because it has the distinct advantage that by collecting the impinged particles in a liquid medium, the potential for APSD bias to finer sizes, associated with particle bounce on the hard surfaces associated with the other impactor designs, is avoided altogether (Asking and Olsson 1997). Furthermore, the collection medium can be chosen to be suitable for API recovery and quantitative assay without the need for any intermediate steps.

In contrast with pMDI testing, which is undertaken at a constant flow rate throughout the aerosol sampling period, the aerosol generation process and release of the aerosol bolus from the DPI in either bulk powder (reservoir) or single-dose format is accomplished by simulating a highly standardized inhalation maneuver. When working with either the ACI or NGI, a pre-separator (Figure 24.11) is normally used to remove carrier particles, such as lactose, when present, as their aerodynamic size is an order of magnitude greater than the API-containing particles that become separated as part of the powder dispersion processes (Nichols et al. 2013, Dunbar and Hickey 2000). The pre-separator also serves to capture any API-containing particles (agglomerates etc.) that may be released particularly from reservoir-based DPIs (Mitchell and Nagel 2003). The complete system (Figure 24.12) is

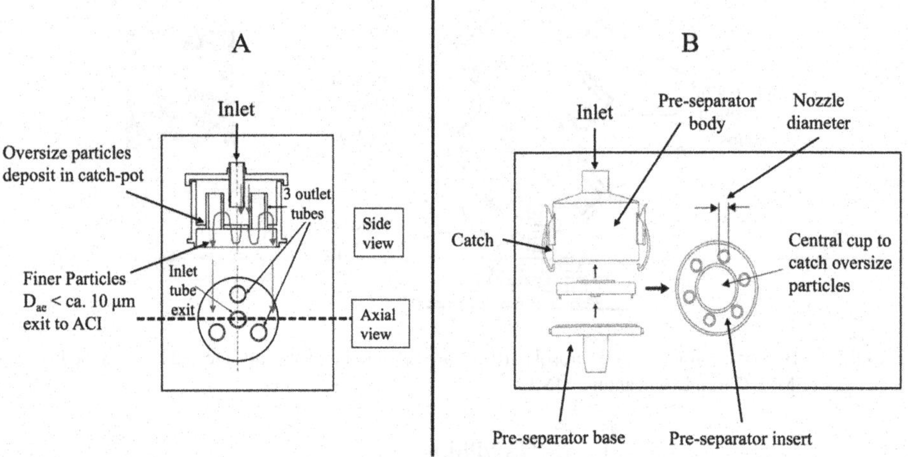

FIGURE 24.11 Pre-separators for use with (A) the ACI and (B) the NGI. ([B] Courtesy of MSP Corp., Minneapolis, MN.)

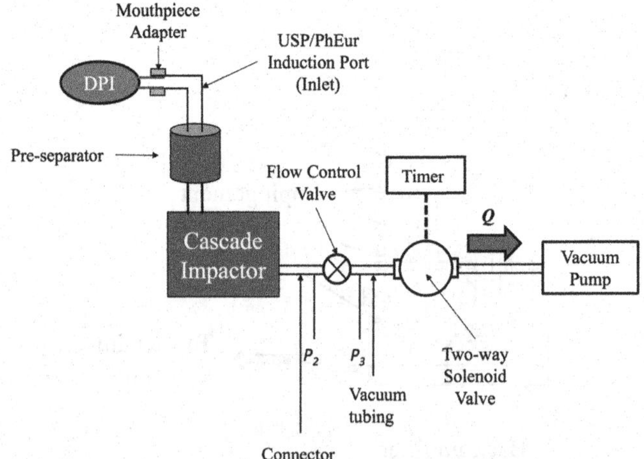

FIGURE 24.12 Apparatus configuration for the evaluation of APSD for DPI-generated aerosols in accordance with the methodology in Chapter <601> of the United Stated Pharmacopeia or Monograph 2.9.18 of the European Pharmacopeia.

connected to a vacuum pump via a flow controller containing a critical orifice that eliminates the impact of fluctuations caused by variations in pump performance. The capacity of the vacuum pump is chosen such that the ratio of pressures downstream (P_3) and upstream (P_2) of the flow control valve can be maintained at ≤0.5 to ensure critical (sonic velocity) flow after the initial rise from zero to a stable flow rate. This control valve is also used to adjust the flow rate to provide a 4 kPa pressure drop at the device. Once the apparatus has been prepared in accordance with the manufacturer's instructions, the mouthpiece of the DPI is coupled to the entrance of the induction port. Actuation of the DPI takes place by initiating the flow by means of a timer-operated solenoid valve. The vacuum propagates backwards from the vacuum pump, through the impactor, pre-separator, and induction port, and finally through the DPI. In the pharmacopeial methodologies, the timer is set such that a 4 L sample is taken before the vacuum is shut off from the impactor, terminating the sample collection process (US Pharmacopeial Convention 2018a, European Directorate for Quality in Medicines (EDQM) 2018a). This volume is necessary to ensure that the entire aerosol dispersed from the DPI has had sufficient time to traverse the entire apparatus (Mohammed et al. 2012), which is especially important with the NGI, whose dead space, including the pre-separator, is 2.025 L (Copley et al. 2005).

It is not necessary to change the physical configuration of the NGI to sample DPI products at flow rates different from those at which calibration data are available. The MMI for DPI testing does not have a pre-separator and is calibrated for use at either 60 L/min or 90 L/min (Marple et al. 1995). Likewise, the MSLI does not have its own pre-separator and is calibrated for use only at 60 L/min (Asking and Olsson 1997). In order to extend the operating range of the ACI for DPI testing, Nichols et al. (1998) developed and calibrated an alternative configuration of the ACI for use at a higher flow rate (60 L/min) than the design flow rate of 28.3 L/min for the original apparatus (Table 24.6). In the higher flow rate configuration, stage "0" is replaced by a version containing the same nozzle plate configuration, but with the external surface modified to accept a stage "–1" above instead of the expansion cone. Stage "7" is discarded to maintain the same number of impaction stages. The same process was applied to a further extension of the concept, intended for use at 90 L/min, where stage "–2" is now inserted above stage "–1" of the 60 L/min apparatus, and stage "6" is simultaneously removed.

It is most important to apply a coating of a tacky substrate to the collection surfaces of the cascade impactor, when sampling DPI-generated aerosols (see Section 24.3.1). This procedure should also

TABLE 24.6
Cut-Point Sizes (D_{50}, µm) for the Various Configurations of the Andersen 8-Stage Cascade Impactor

	Nominal Flow Rate (L/min)		
Stage	**28.3**	**60**	**90**
–2	N/A	N/A	8.0
–1	N/A	7.2	6.5
0	9.0	6.4	5.2
1	5.8	3.9	3.5
2	4.7	2.9	2.6
3	3.3	1.9	1.7
4	2.1	1.2	1.0
5	1.1	0.55	0.22
6	0.7	0.22	N/A
7	0.4	N/A	N/A

Source: United States Pharmacopeial Convention.
N/A = not applicable in this configuration.

include the pre-separator for the most accurate work. It should be noted that the collection surface of the insert for the NGI pre-separator contains a cup-like space aligned on axis with the incoming flow, to contain a small amount (typically 15 mL) of a suitable liquid to act as an impingement medium as an alternative to a tacky coating (Marple et al. 2003a).

24.3.3 Nebulizers and Add-On Devices for Use with pMDIs

The NGI without pre-separator is the recommended apparatus for the evaluation of aqueous products or preparations for nebulization Figure 24.13, described in Chapter <1601> of the United States Pharmacopeia (US Pharmacopeial Convention 2018b). The content of this chapter is largely harmonized with Monograph 2.9.44 of the European Pharmacopeia (European Directorate for Quality in Medicines (EDQM) 2018b). The entire flow from the nebulizer-on-test is sampled into the USP/PhEur induction port (Figure 24.14). However, this flow rate should ideally not exceed 15 L/min to avoid increased potential for measurement bias from evaporative effects associated with increased mixing of unsaturated ambient air with the droplet stream from the nebulizer (Dennis et al. 2000). Furthermore, impactors, such as the NGI that have significant thermal mass should be cooled to about +5°C in order to mitigate heat transfer-related evaporation (Stapleton and Finlay 1999, Dennis et al. 2008).

An alternative sampling arrangement in which a low-flow impactor, such as the Marple 298/6X Personal Sampler that operates at 2 L/min is used to extract a portion of the droplet stream sampled at 15 L/min from the nebulizer (Figure 24.14A) was initially developed as part of a European Standard (European Committee for Standardization (CEN) 2009) and later adopted into an international standard for the assessment of nebulizing systems and components as an optional method for APSD measurement (International Standards Organization [ISO] 2013). However, it is important to appreciate that removing the sample without taking the precaution to sample isokinetically (Nerbrink et al. 2003) may result in size-related bias (Wilcox 1956). An example of an isokinetic sampling arrangement is illustrated in Figure 24.14B.

Nebulizing systems differ from the other orally inhaled products because they provide the API(s) in a continuous stream of aqueous droplets for the duration of the treatment period, instead of delivering a bolus of medication following actuation or when the user inhales (Hess 2000). Typical treatment times for nebulizer-based therapies are often many minutes in duration. Nebulizer-generated aqueous droplets generally do not require coated collection surfaces when sampled by cascade impactor, as they adhere strongly to the collection surface once impacted there. The determination of the sampling time for an APSD determination is therefore limited by the droplet delivery rate of the nebulizer, the fill of liquid containing medication in its reservoir and, most importantly, the need to avoid overloading the collection surfaces of the impactor stages with collected droplets. It is self-evident that cascade impactors that make use of collection plates are more vulnerable to stage overload rather than those apparatuses that use cups to collect the impacted droplets. A pilot study to establish a suitable sampling time per determination

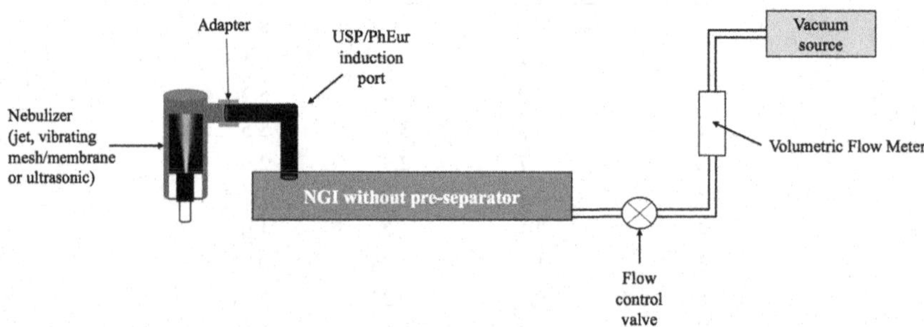

FIGURE 24.13 APSD measurement of products/preparations for nebulization in accordance with the United States and European Pharmacopeial harmonized method; all the droplet stream from the nebulizer is sampled by the NGI at 15 L/min.

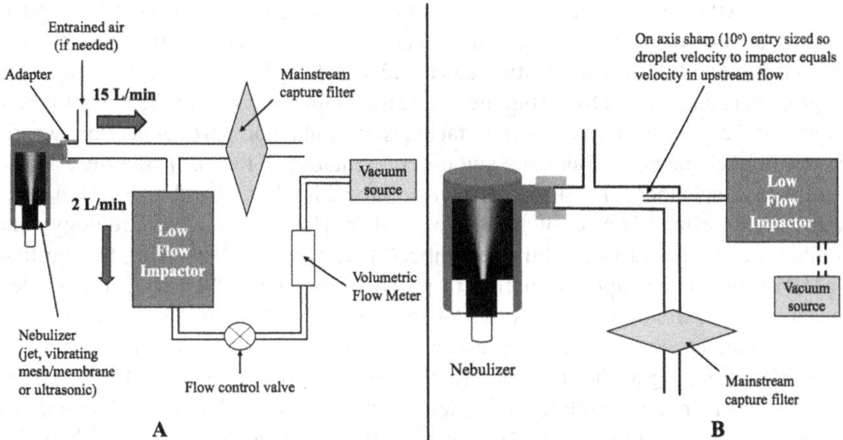

FIGURE 24.14 APSD measurement of nebulizer-generated droplets (A) in accordance with the methodology in EN13544:2009/ISO 27427:2013 and (B) adaptation to establish isokinetic sampling to the low flow impactor.

is therefore a prudent precaution in method development involving nebulizer testing, especially when an impactor with collection plates is chosen.

Care is also needed to avoid introducing bias by unwanted evaporation, particularly when additional air is introduced to make up the 15 L/min flow rate (Nerbrink et al. 2003). Evaporative effects are likely to be most apparent either with continuous, non-entrainment jet nebulizers, or vibrating mesh/membrane devices in which sub-saturated ambient air carries the droplet stream via the patient interface (mouthpiece of facemask) to the cascade impactor. Jet nebulizers that incorporate air entrainment to increase their output are less vulnerable to evaporation-related bias because the entrained air acquires moisture from the droplet stream in milliseconds, providing a saturated or near-to-saturated shroud around the droplets as they enter the sampling system (Dennis 2007).

24.3.4 Spacers and Valved Holding Chambers for Use with pMDIs

Spacers and valved holding chambers substantially modify the APSD of the emitted aerosol from all types of pMDIs by removing the bulk of the coarse particulate that would otherwise deposit in the oropharynx of the patient (Dolovich et al. 2000, 2005), with certain API classes (i.e. some corticosteroids) to cause adverse topical effects such as dysphonia (62) and oral candidiasis (Galván and Guarderas 2012). Until recently, the pharmacopeial compendia were silent about the laboratory testing of these add-ons, considering them to be devices rather than drug products. Recognizing the absence of guidance concerning an important group of adjunct devices for this class of orally inhaled products, the Canadian Standards Association developed a local standard in 2002, revising it in 2008, and reaffirming it without further change in 2016 (Canadian Standards Association [CSA] 2016). Its content, including the *in vitro* test methodology for aerosol APSD, was reviewed by Dolovich and Mitchell (2004) at the time of its development. More recently, increasing USFDA interest in how these add-on devices are evaluated led to the development of Chapter <1602> of the USP, that became official text in 2017 (US Pharmacopeial Convention 2018c). Either apparatus 1 or 5, as defined in Chapter <601> of the USP, is recommended for the evaluation of add-on devices intended for adult use. In the case of add-on devices for infant or small child use, the low-flow version of the MMI that operates at either 4.9 L/min or 12.0 L/min (Olson et al. 1998) may be used. This chapter currently has no equivalent monograph in the European Pharmacopeia, although interest has been expressed from the British Pharmacopoeia in developing a monograph to cover the evaluation of spacers and valved holding chambers (Mitchell and Suggett 2014).

Measurement of APSD with valved holding chambers equipped with a facemask is undertaken by removing the facemask so that the device can be readily interfaced either directly to the inlet of the USP/PhEur induction port or to an apparatus used to create a delay between inhaler actuation and sampling. This process is undertaken by fitting the facemask adapter directly to the entry to the sampling apparatus without the complication of a direct facemask-to-induction port connection, where internal dead space would likely be both ill-defined and unrepresentative of the "in-patient-use" condition.

The sampling arrangement for testing a spacer or valved holding chamber is based on the methodologies already described in Section 24.3.1 for pMDIs. However, the methodology contains the important addition that for valved holding chambers, that as well as sampling the emitted aerosol from the pMDI immediately upon actuation to provide baseline APSD data, a short delay takes place between inhaler actuation and the onset of sampling. Delay testing is recommended because valved holding chambers are frequently prescribed for patients who have difficulty coordinating the need to initiate inhaling at the time of actuating their inhaler (Crompton 1982). The European Medicines Agency has indicated the need for delay testing for valved holding chambers, recognizing the importance of evaluating the performance of these products as they are likely to be used, both in terms of assurance of product quality (European Medicines Agency 2006) and in support of clinical programs (European Medicines Agency 2009). It is impractical to evaluate aerosol delivery from pMDI-open-tube spacer combinations, because much, if not all of the aerosol emitted from the inhaler will have dispersed to the ambient environment during the waiting interval (US Pharmacopeial Convention 2018c).

Figure 24.15 illustrates an apparatus that has been employed successfully to simulate delayed inhalation when evaluating valved holding chambers (Mitchell and Suggett 2014). In use, the patient interface (mouthpiece or facemask adapter) of the valved holding chamber is attached to the upstream side of the delay apparatus. The vertical shutter gate is initially in the upward position blocking the exit pathway from the valved holding chamber, so that flow to the impactor takes the pathway of least resistance, bypassing the chamber altogether. After a prescribed delay interval that is typically in the range from 1 second to 10 seconds, a timer/controller operates a solenoid that withdraws the pin supporting the shutter so that the latter drops rapidly to the downward position. The aerosol contained in the chamber can then be sampled by the cascade impactor via the now open port in the shutter gate that has aligned on-axis with the chamber exit. This apparatus has the advantage that flow to the cascade impactor can already be at steady-state before the shutter drops, meeting the requirement to operate the cascade impactor at constant flow rate for the duration of the measurement process (Mitchell and Suggett 2014). In an alternative approach that involves more manual dexterity in execution, the

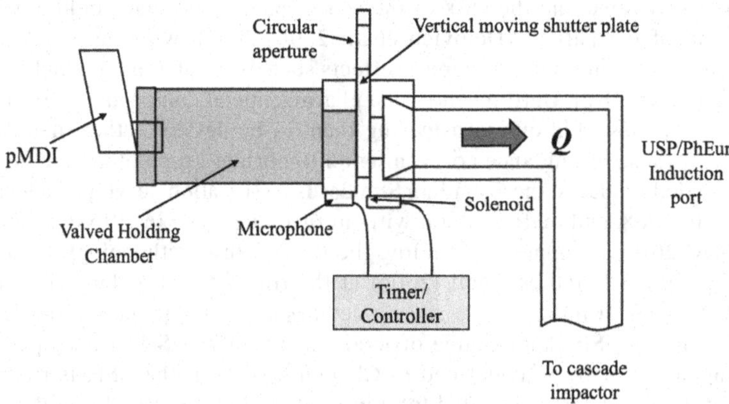

FIGURE 24.15 Apparatus for introducing delayed sampling when evaluating the APSD from a pMDI with valved holding chamber; the vertical shutter plate is initially in the upward position so that flow to the impactor bypasses the chamber. After the prescribed delay interval, the timer/controller operates a solenoid that withdraws the pin supporting the shutter so that it drops to the downward position, in which the aerosol contained in the chamber can be sampled by the cascade impactor.

pMDI-valved holding chamber combination is uncoupled from the cascade impactor at the time of pMDI actuation, so that the aerosol from the inhaler is retained within the chamber, by means of its shut inhalation valve. After the pre-determined time has elapsed, the chamber exit is manually coupled to the induction port entry. This procedure opens the valve of the chamber, thereby allowing the aerosol contained within to be sampled.

The effect of a short delay on key metrics derivable from the aerosol APSD is illustrated in general terms by Figure 24.16; actual changes in the individual metrics presented are valved holding chamber, pMDI product, and delay duration dependent. The derivation of these metrics will be discussed later in this chapter. For now, total emitted mass (TEM) from the pMDI alone is often regarded as representing the label claim mass per actuation ex mouthpiece, if internal losses of particles to the walls of the measurement apparatus are ignored. Impactor-sized mass (ISM) is that portion of TEM which penetrates to the first impaction stage whose upper bound size is known. The sub-fractions, fine particle mass (FPM) and extra-fine particle mass (EPM) are often defined in terms of particles finer than about 5 μm and 1 μm aerodynamic diameter, respectively. The presence of a holding chamber greatly reduces the coarse particle mass (CPM), where:

$$\text{CPM} = \text{ISM} - \text{FPM} \tag{24.14}$$

thereby resulting in a noticeable decrease in ISM, whereas the magnitudes of both FPM and EPM are barely affected when pMDI actuation is coincident with the onset of sampling. Removal of CPM occurs in the valved holding chamber primarily as the result of inertial impaction and turbulent deposition of the spray droplets on the distal valve and interior walls, combined with further evaporation of any liquid propellant that may be present initially (Mitchell and Dolovich 2012). FPM ex valved holding chamber may slightly increase, primarily as the result of evaporation of residual co-solvent, typically ethanol that is present with some formulations (Stein 2008). When a delay is present, gravitational sedimentation operates to remove preferentially the largest remaining airborne particles in the chamber (Mitchell and Dolovich 2012). Both ISM and FPM decrease, but EPM remains largely unaffected, since this deposition mechanism is largely ineffective for the removal of sub-micrometer-sized particles. Typical data for a wide range of currently available pMDI-delivered products using a particular valved holding chamber family have been provided by Mitchell et al. (2009a, 2016).

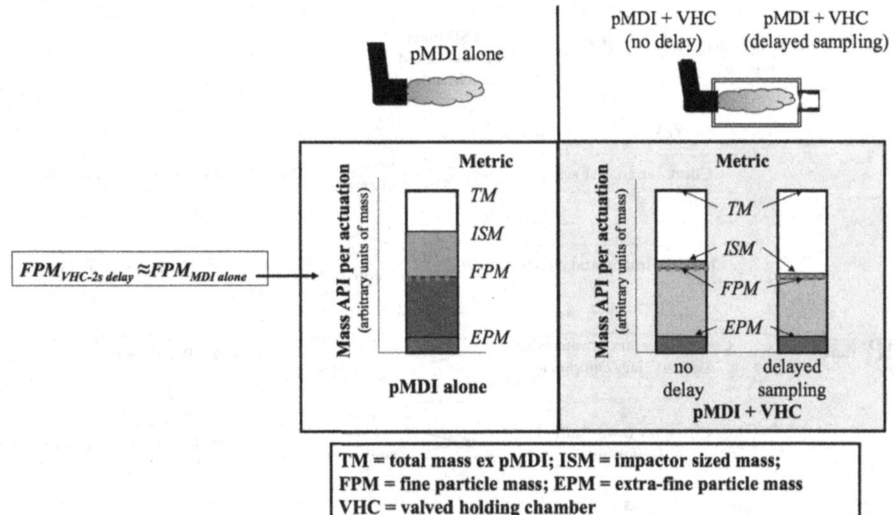

FIGURE 24.16 The effect of a short delay on the APSD various metrics related to the aerosol sampled by cascade impactor from a pMDI-valved holding chamber combination. The left-most figure illustrates the behavior of the pMDI alone, and the rightmost two images represent the pMDI with valved holding chamber with no delay and with delayed sampling. (Courtesy of American Association of Pharmaceutical Scientists, Arlington, VA.)

24.4 The Good Cascade Impactor Practices Concept

The idea of developing a structured approach to the day-to-day management of cascade impactors arose from a Product Quality Research Institute initiative that took place in the early 2000s, in connection with assertion of the mass balance that has already been mentioned as being obtained as part of the APSD determination in accordance with pharmacopeial methodologies. The Product Quality Research Institute initiative addressed the "what if" situation, in the case that a mass balance determination was found to be out of specification as proposed by the USFDA in their original draft guidance for industry MDI and DPI drug products chemistry, manufacturing, and controls documentation (United States Food and Drug Administration 1998). The outcome was a fault diagnosis tree (Figure 24.17), in which a logical approach can be applied when attempting to isolate the cause (Christopher et al. 2003). In the original publication, GCIP applied specifically to the checking for errors associated with the cascade impactor and its auxiliary equipment.

There are currently two main considerations in the current development of GCIP:

1. Removal of sources of bias in measurements (in-use) and
2. Maintenance of the measurement apparatus components.

In use aspects are as follows:

1. Assertion of correct assembly;
2. Precautions to mitigate particle bounce and re-entrainment;
3. Precautions to mitigate bias arising from electrostatic charge;
4. Precautions to mitigate leakage of the apparatus;
5. Flow rate setting before *each* determination;
6. Cleaning and storage between uses; and
7. Wall/interior loss management.

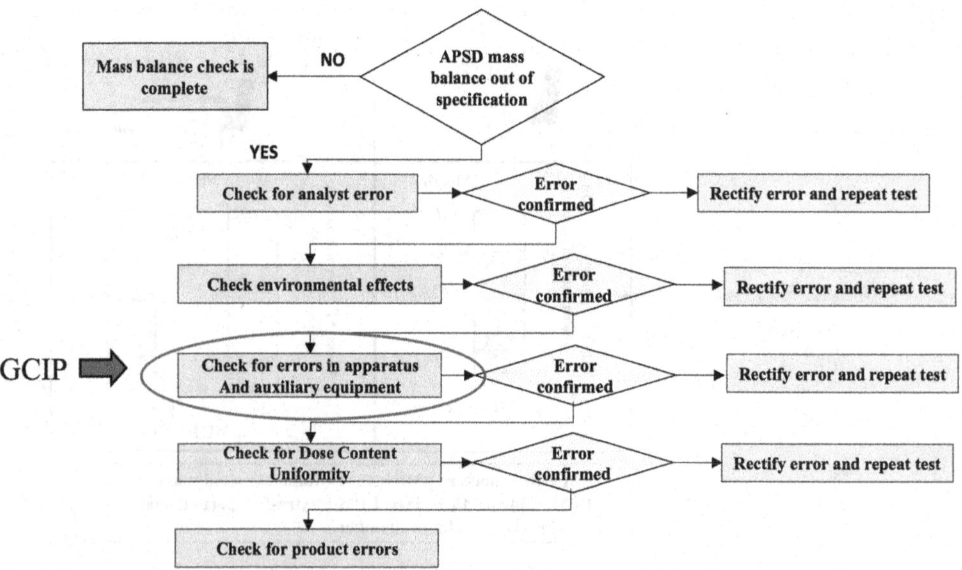

FIGURE 24.17 Failure investigation tree for a mass balance determination associated with the APSD measurement of orally inhaled product generated aerosols by cascade impactor. (Adapted from Christopher, D. et al., *J. Aerosol. Med.*, 16, 235–247, 2003.)

There is anecdotal evidence that incorrect assembly of certain types of cascade impactor is quite common, especially in laboratories in which many impactors of the same type are in use at the same time. Assertion that the impactor has been assembled correctly is most important for apparatuses in which stages can be separated from the body of the impactor, as is the case with the ACI. Unless each stage is uniquely identified by some form of marking to belong to a particular impactor stack, an ACI can easily be assembled from components coming from more than one original impactor apparatus. It is also easy to assemble the stages in the incorrect order. It is therefore highly recommended that each impactor assembly be assigned its own identity, by engraving the impactor apparatus identification and stage number on each stage, including the back-up filter, as part of the installation qualification process.

Particle bounce and re-entrainment are encountered sources of measurement bias with all types of cascade impactor (Esmen and Lee 1980, Mitchell and Nagel 2003). The most obvious sign of this phenomenon is if more than the expected mass fraction of the sampled aerosol is recovered from the back-up filter/MOC. The application of a coating to the collection surfaces to mitigate particle bounce has already been mentioned in Sections 24.3.1 and 24.3.2, in connection with size-classifying pMDI- and DPI-delivered aerosols. Collection surface coating methodologies form a key component of in-use GCIP because of the widespread prevalence of this potential source of bias, unless precautions are taken.

When dealing with the potential for bias associated with electrostatic charge, it is important to be aware that many pMDI- and DPI-generated aerosols are highly charged (Kwok and Chan 2005). Some formulations contain charges of just one sign (positive or negative), whereas others may have bi-polar charge distributions (Kwok and Chan 2005, 2008). Such charge retention can be highly dependent upon the local relative humidity of the environment in which the inhaler is being used (Kwok and Chan 2008). Furthermore, spacers and valved holding chambers often acquire substantial charge in manufacture and/or by subsequent handling, unless manufactured from electrically conducting or charge dissipative (antistatic) polymeric materials (Mitchell et al. 2007). In consequence, the advice associated with GCIP is to ground (maintain at earth potential) the complete cascade impactor apparatus. Likewise, operators should be grounded and wearing charge dissipative laboratory coats and gloves to avoid the possibility of charge transfer when handling the inhaler and any add-on device, if present.

Assertion that the cascade impactor assembly is free from ingress(es) of ambient air other than by the intended inlet pathway is also an important part of in-use qualification. Leak testing needs to be done before each measurement of APSD is undertaken, especially with impactor configurations that involve the correct assembly of a stack of impaction stages on top of the back-up filter stage, such as the ACI. Cracked or perished seals are common sources of leaks, so that seal rings should be regularly inspected and replaced if visible defects are apparent. Leakages are generally unpredictable and are potentially the most serious in stages more distal within the impactor, where the pressure drop below atmospheric pressure is largest. Ambient air ingress reduces the sampling flow rate at the entry to the apparatus (Q), resulting in systematic increases to the D_{50} values for each stage upstream of the leak and consequential bias towards finer sizes in the measured deposition profile and APSD.

Figure 24.18 summarizes a strategy that Nichols et al. (2013) proposed could be used for implementing such a practice. In the design of the NGI, a leak rate smaller than 1.6 kPa/min was defined as constituting a "good seal" for the assembled impactor (Marple et al. 2003a). Nichols et al. (2013) therefore suggested maximum acceptable leakage rates would therefore be of the order of 10 kPa/min for systems using the NGI and slightly higher at close to 15 kPa/min for ACI-based systems, and leakage rates <1 kPa/min are likely to be of no consequence. The detection of leak rates of this order is readily possible with a digital pressure gauge and stop-clock. A GCIP-compatible strategy would be: (a) check the pressure drop (ΔP) across the entire apparatus before each measurement, (b) set the inlet flow rate (Q) after the leakage check, and (c) regularly check the pressure drop across each stage as part of an inspection of seals, with replacement if found to be defective.

The operating flow rate of the cascade impactor is as important a determinant of the stage cut-point sizes as are the values of W_{eff} for the stages (see Equations 24.7 and 24.8), so that ensuring that the flow rate through the apparatus is set correctly is an essential component of in-use GCIP. Guidance concerning the selection of appropriate flow rates for testing the different classes of orally inhaled product has been provided in Section 24.3 of this chapter. However, the focus of GCIP is on how and when the flow

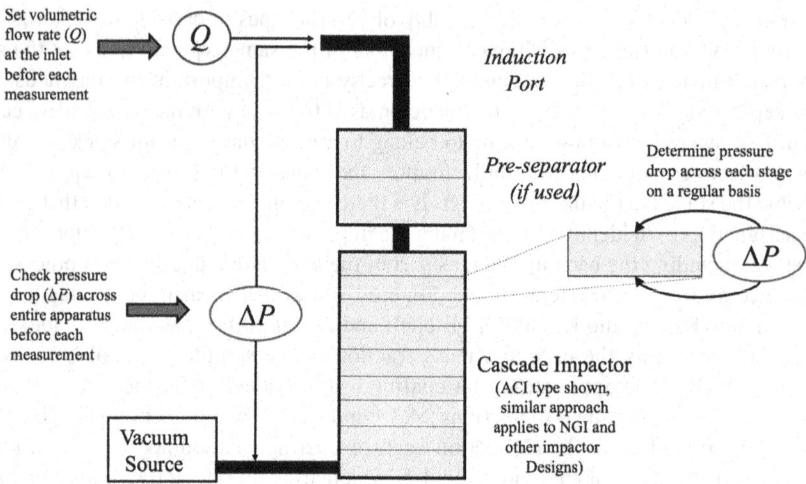

FIGURE 24.18 Strategy for leakage testing of a generic apparatus train for determining APSD of aerosols from orally inhaled products. (Adapted from Nichols, S.C., *AAPS PharmSciTechnol.*, 14, 375–390, 2013. With permission from American Association of Pharmaceutical Scientists.)

rate should be measured. Olsson and Asking (2003) have reviewed the methods for setting the flow rate, pointing out that there are the following essential requirements:

1. The flowmeter is calibrated for the *volumetric* flow exiting the meter;
2. The flow rate is set with the flowmeter attached to the entry to the apparatus (normally the induction port); and
3. Critical (sonic) flow is maintained in the regulating flow control valve (Figure 24.12), when testing DPIs following the compendial method.

In connection with requirement (3), Olsson and Asking (2003) observed that direct measurements have demonstrated that when critical flow exists in the regulating valve, the volumetric flow rate downstream from a resistor at the inlet of an impactor is rendered insensitive (±1%) to changes in flow resistance over a broad range of elicited pressure drops (up to at least 12 kPa). This outcome validates the pharmacopeial method of temporarily replacing the DPI with a flow meter as part of the flow rate setting process before making an APSD measurement.

The interval between cleaning each impactor should logically be the choice of the user, given the wide range of operating conditions. This interval is likely to be dependent upon the frequency of APSD determinations, as well as the physicochemical properties of the aerosol particles (e.g. surface tackiness) that affect the accumulation of internal wall deposits. Cleaning would not be a concern in cases where the API recovered from adjacent walls is added to the mass recovered from each impaction stage. However, this process adds further complexity to the overall APSD measurement process. Furthermore, there are indications from a calibration study involving monodisperse particles in the micrometer size range, that the deposition locations of particles deposited to the walls of the ACI may be much more widespread spatially within the impactor than that of similar sized particles that are impacted almost entirely on specific stages (Mitchell et al. 1987). The practice is therefore likely unwise. In overall terms, internal losses associated with either pMDI or DPI testing should not exceed 5% of the label claim mass/actuation (US Pharmacopeial Convention 2018a, European Directorate for Quality in Medicines (EDQM) 2018a). The pharmacopeias are silent concerning the limits applicable for the evaluation of products/preparations for nebulization. However, given that the magnitude of internal losses is largely the result of the internal geometry of the cascade impactor, it would be reasonable to apply the same limit for the evaluation of nebulizing systems as well as add-on devices for pMDIs. A key component of GCIP is therefore to advise on a strategy to evaluate internal losses and establish an appropriate cleaning regimen.

GCIP associated with maintenance of the hardware relates to the following aspects:

1. Stage mensuration, measurement traceability, and mensuration interval;
2. Replacement of damaged/deformed collection plate or cups; and
3. Replacement of damaged stages or the seal body in the case of the NGI.

Impactor stage nozzle sizes change from their "as supplied" condition, either by mechanical plugging or through chemical corrosion. Although stage mensuration is described in the relevant pharmacopeial chapters (US Pharmacopeial Convention 2018a, European Directorate for Quality in Medicines (EDQM) 2018a), the only guidance provided is that the process be carried out on a regular basis (i.e. undefined time interval). It is difficult to be specific about choice of time interval between successive mensuration procedures, because the amount of wear or corrosion associated with the nozzles of a specific impactor stage is, to a large extent, dependent upon the material within which the nozzle set is formed, as well as the exposure received by the nozzles to particles and cleaning/API recovery solvents in use. However, the consensus from a survey of members of the European Pharmaceutical Aerosol Group (EPAG) undertaken a few years ago was that an annual inspection is the norm (Mitchell 2005). In a more recent article attempting to define the scope for GCIP, Nichols et al. (2013) suggested the following strategy could apply for stage mensuration:

1. Confirmation on receipt of a new complete cascade impactor as part of installation qualification, demonstrating conformance with the manufacturer specifications comprising the nominal values of nozzle diameter with associated tolerance or a given impactor stage and
2. Periodic establishment of stage nozzle measurements associated with time-in-service, as part of operation qualification.

These processes should also be supported by visual inspection of each stage for gross defects, for instance, nozzle plugging, as part of the daily preparation for use.

Stage mensuration is important in verification of cascade impactor performance because the effective diameter of the nozzles for a given impaction stage (W_{eff}) from Equation 24.7 has been shown by Roberts (2009) to be related to the stage D_{50} value, from Equation 24.8, by the expression:

$$W_{eff} = \left(\frac{Q}{n}\right)^{1/3} \left(\frac{4C_{50}\rho_p}{9\pi\eta St_{50}}\right)^{1/3} \left(D_{50}\right)^{2/3} \tag{24.15}$$

W_{eff} is easily calculated from measures of nozzle diameter using automated image analysis combined with precision microscopy (Copley 2008). This is a service that is provided by most cascade impactor manufacturers and which can ultimately be made traceable to international length standard through the use of calibration reticles for the microscope/image analyzer system (Chambers et al. 2010). Values of D_{50}, together with their associated tolerances, are available in the pharmacopeial compendia (US Pharmacopeial Convention 2018a, European Directorate for Quality in Medicines (EDQM) 2018a), as well as in the article by Nichols et al. (2013), making it a practical proposition to define in-use limits for W_{eff} as part of impactor qualification.

Current designs of cascade impactor are tolerant of small scratches to the collection surfaces (Marple and Willeke 1976, Mitchell and Nagel 2003). However, larger deformation/distortion will affect the nozzle-to-collection surface distance (S). If the ratio $S/W_{eff} < 1.0$, the D_{50} value of the stage will become sensitive to changes in this ratio, potentially affecting the overall accuracy of APSD determinations. Regular, inspection followed by replacement of damaged/deformed collection plate or cups should therefore form part of a GCIP regimen. Likewise, in the unlikely event that impaction stages, or the seal body in the case of the NGI, become damaged, replacement/refurbishment by the manufacturer would be the consequence. Such a situation is more likely to arise through chemical attack rather than mechanical deformation due to mishandling, because these components are mechanically robust.

24.5 Data Analysis in Connection with the APSD Determination

The raw data from the cascade impactor and associated non-sizing components is the mass deposition profile. At its simplest, the deposition profile relates mass of a single API recovered at each location in the sampling apparatus train (Dunbar and Mitchell 2005), as illustrated schematically in Figure 24.19. The type of chemical assay methods that are in use to quantify API mass is outside the scope of this chapter, but such information can be found in monographs for the specific API(s) where published in the pharmacopeial compendia. More often, individual organizations will have developed in-house validated methods for their own APIs.

In 2013, the United States Pharmacopeia deleted detailed instructions on data analysis from normative Chapter <601> that covers the testing of most classes of inhaler except nebulizing systems. Since then, a joint committee comprising members of the Aerosols and Statistics sub-committees of the General Chapters Dosage Forms Committee has been working on the replacement of this missing information in a form that is more suited to current regulatory needs. The present intention is to create a new informative chapter in the <1000> series, in which advice will be provided on the topic, and what follows in this section is largely a distillation of an approach that has been proposed as a stimulus to revision article from this sub-committee that appeared in mid-2017 (Mitchell et al. 2017).

It is important to be aware that the upper bound size of the particles captured on a particular stage must be known for the mass of API collected there to contribute to the APSD (Mitchell et al. 2017). For example, although stage "0" of the ACI in its standard configuration (Table 24.1) has its nominal D_{50} at 9.0 μm aerodynamic diameter, the mass of particles that collect on this stage do not have a defined upper size. This information is absent because the component in the sampling train (induction port or pre-separator) located immediately before this stage does not have a defined D_{50} value. Furthermore, in the case of the induction port, particle size separation may not take place purely in terms of differences in inertia in laminar flow (Zhang et al. 2004). The situation in the case of the first impaction stage of the NGI (stage "1") is different if the NGI pre-separator is used, because the latter was designed to behave in accordance with inertial impactor theory (Marple et al. 2003a) and furthermore has its D_{50} value defined between 30 L/min and 100 L/min by archival calibration.

The APSD is strictly defined as the multivariate mathematical description relating the mass of drug substance collected in the CI and the particle aerodynamic diameter. Its construction from stage deposition profile data is described in detail by Dunbar and Mitchell (2005). Most inhaler-generated aerosols have a single mode (unimodal), but some, particularly from nebulizing systems, may be bi-modal

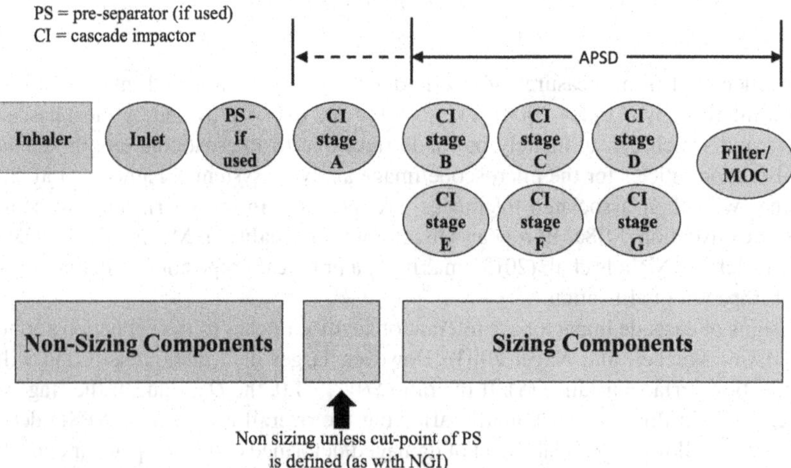

FIGURE 24.19 Schematic representation of non-sizing and sizing components in a complete sampling train from the inhaler via the induction port, pre-separator (if used) to the multi-stage cascade impactor; the upper bound size of the particles captured on a particular stage must be known for the mass of API collected there to contribute to the APSD.

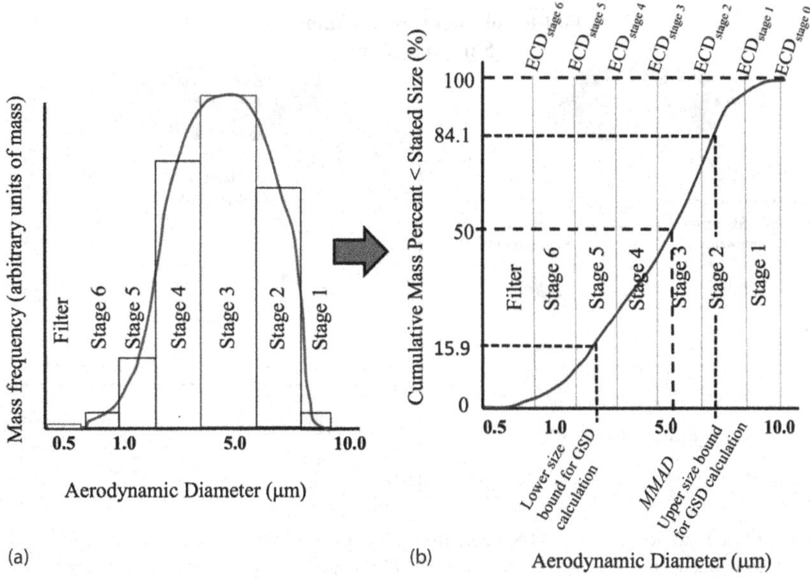

FIGURE 24.20 Unimodal and close to log-normal APSD typical of aerosols from orally inhaled products presented as (a) mass frequency curve showing stage size boundaries and (b) cumulative by mass curve showing how stage ECDs relate and significant sizes concerning determination of MMAD and GSD.

(Carvalho and McConville 2016). For the sake of simplicity, a unimodal APSD is assumed in the following explanation concerning cascade impactor-derived APSDs.

There are many formats in which size distribution data can be presented (International Standards Organization 1998). However, APSDs derived from the testing of orally inhaled products are most often plotted as either mass frequency curves (Figure 24.20a) or in the cumulative mass-weighted form, often normalized to *ISM* (Figure 24.20b). The latter presentation format is the easiest to interpret in terms of the various mass sub-fractions that are relatable to different size ranges. It follows from Figure 24.19, that whichever format for presenting the APSD is chosen, its intrinsic size resolution is limited to the number of impaction stages that contribute, typically no more than seven. This restriction has been seen as a limitation, particularly when time-of-flight measurements (discussed in Section 24.7) offer far greater resolution (Mitchell and Nagel 1999). However, it will become evident later in this section, that high size resolution is unnecessary, given the relatively poor size selectivity of the various regions in the respiratory tract to differences in particle size (ICRP 1994) as well as current regulatory expectations based around stage groupings (United States Food and Drug Administration 2018, Health Canada 2006, European Medicines Agency 2006).

In general, the APSD contains more information that most users require to describe the aerodynamic performance of their inhaler. The task is therefore to extract enough information to provide an adequate description of the particle ensemble, and the various options are illustrated in Figure 24.21. The cumulative mass-weighted APSD has useful properties in terms of simplifying its description (Dunbar and Mitchell 2005). In particular, the size corresponding to the 50% percentile is the MMAD, and, if the APSD is log-normal (or close to log-normal as a first approximation), the GSD is readily calculated from the relationship:

$$\text{GSD} = \sqrt{D_{84.1} / D_{15.9}} \tag{24.16}$$

in which $D_{15.9}$ and $D_{84.1}$ are the sizes corresponding to the 15.9th and 84.1st percentiles, respectively. Alternatively, the ratio D_{90}/D_{10} can be calculated, and as such, is often referred to as the span of the APSD. This approach is more suitable if the size distribution is clearly not log-normal, but still unimodal.

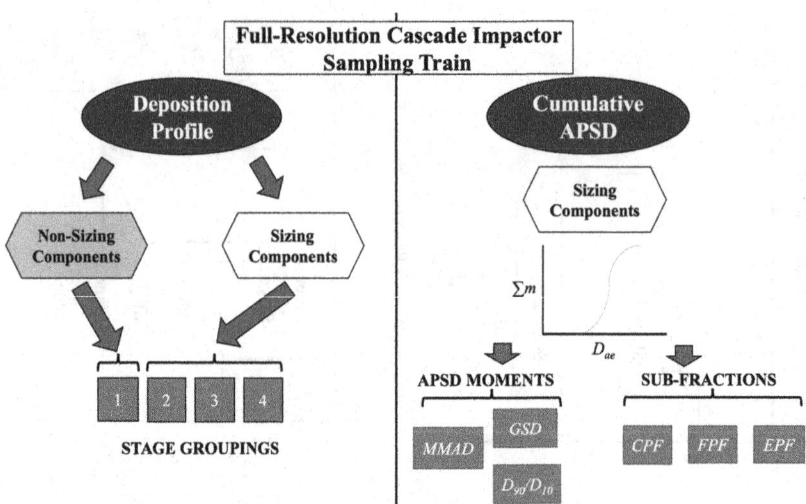

FIGURE 24.21 Derived metrics from the APSD determined by cascade impactor sampling train for an orally inhaled product; the stage grouping approach compares the mass of API grouped in various locations broadly indicative of likely deposition in the respiratory tract. In addition, or alternatively, the APSD may be interpreted in terms of its moments or sub-fractions.

It is often helpful to determine the various sub-fractions comprising the APSD, as these can be qualitatively related to potential deposition locations in the respiratory tract. The commonly encountered sub-fractions are:

1. The coarse particle fraction, representing large particles most likely to deposit in the oropharynx;
2. The fine particle fraction (FPF), indicative of particles likely to penetrate as far as the airways of the lungs; and
3. The extra fine particle fraction, indicative of particles capable of penetrating to the distal airways and the alveolar sacs of the lungs.

These mass fractions may also be expressed in absolute mass terms or as the respective fractions of the inhaled dose. In general, precise size limits for each sub-fraction are undefined with the exception of the boundary size between FPF and coarse particle fraction, which is fixed at 5.0 μm aerodynamic diameter in the European Pharmacopoeia monograph for the evaluation of pMDI and DPI products (European Directorate for Quality in Medicines 2018a). To date, however, there has been no such fixed limit in the United States Pharmacopeia, as there is regulatory guidance to report the APSD data reduced to stage groupings (see next paragraph), rather than expressed as either mass fractions or moments of the distribution. Applicants are currently encouraged by the USFDA to propose acceptance criteria for groupings of consecutive stages rather than proposing an acceptance criterion for each individual stage, and in most cases, three or four groupings should be sufficient to characterize the APSD adequately (United States Food and Drug Administration 2018). The precise size boundaries between each grouping are not defined as the applicant is expected to justify this choice as part of their submission to the USFDA.

The upper bound for extra fine particle fraction is commonly fixed at 1.0 μm aerodynamic diameter, distinguishing such particles as "sub-micron" in size, but there is no pharmacopeial or regulatory definition of this limit at the present time.

Current regulatory practice in the United States, Canada, and the European Union (United States Food and Drug Administration 2018, Health Canada 2006, European Medicines Agency 2006) is to assess the API deposition profile(s) obtained by the cascade impactor methodologies in the pharmacopeias, in groupings of components of the sampling train (in Canada and Europe, termed "stage pooling"). The precise particle sizes for the boundaries between extra fine, fine, and coarse fractions are dependent upon the distribution exhibited by the particular drug product and in both Canada and Europe, these boundaries have to be justified for each product. In the United States, as mentioned above, there is an expectation of a minimum of three to four groupings to ensure future batch-to-batch consistency of the APSD. In a four-group protocol, the following divisions are likely to be chosen:

1. *Group 1*: Mass of API recovered from the nonsizing components;
2. *Group 2*: Mass of API recovered from stages representing relatively the coarse fraction of the dose;
3. *Group 3*: Mass of API recovered from stages representing relatively the fine fraction of the dose; and
4. *Group 4*: Mass of API recovered from stages, representing the extra fine fraction of the dose.

It is probable that selection of stage grouping size ranges used for quality control, once made for a particular product, would not be changed at a later stage in the product lifecycle without the approval of the regulatory agency(ies) concerned.

Both the number of groupings and the number of stages within a specific group for a given drug product normally depend on several factors. These may include masses of deposited particles on critical stages and components of the cascade impactor, as well as minor shifts in APSDs observed during stability studies. Appropriate selection of stages in a group is critical in order to decrease analytical efforts for routine testing while maintaining discriminatory capability of the method for the detection of particle size distribution changes (e.g. in comparative studies for evaluation of changes in the drug product).

24.6 Simplifying the Cascade Impactor and Applying an Alternative, but Highly Effective Procedure for Data Interpretation

The abbreviated impactor measurement (AIM) and effective data analysis (EDA) concepts are two independent, but linked solutions that address the twin issue of impactor complexity and sensitivity of data analysis discrimination of changes to the inhaler-generated APSD in association with product quality control (Tougas et al. 2011) and at the same time provide a simpletoimplement, yet powerful, way to interpret particle size related data (Tougas et al. 2013).

The AIM concept simplifies the measurement of aerodynamic particle size related data into two components, large particle mass (LPM) and small particle mass (SPM), by the reduction of the full-resolution CI from seven or eight impaction stages to two size fractionating stages (Figure 24.22). The first stage is required to define the upper size for LPM, whereas the second stage separates LPM from SPM, and the latter is captured on the back-up filter/MOC. The induction port and preseparator (if needed) are retained (Mitchell et al. 2012a). Various types of abbreviated impactor in current use are illustrated in Figure 24.23. In some cases, the abbreviated apparatus has been constructed from the full-resolution parent impactor, either by removing stages, as can be done with the Andersen viable and non-viable cascade impactors to create the Fast Screening Andersen (FSA) and Fine Particle Dose - Andersen Viable Cascade Impactor (FPD-AVCI) abbreviated apparatuses, respectively. However, other abbreviated impactors, such as the twin impinger and the fast screening impactor (FSI) do not have a parent apparatus. Nevertheless, in many cases, FSI-generated data have been successfully compared with the NGI as the full-resolution apparatus (Tougas et al. 2013).

In Europe, the AIM concept has been simplified further still so that there is only a single impaction stage having its D_{50} fixed at 5 μm aerodynamic diameter, in compliance with the European Pharmacopeia definition for FPM (European Directorate for Quality in Medicines 2018a). Under these circumstances, the fine particle mass fraction ($FPF_{<5\,\mu m}$) is calculated in relation to TEM in accordance with:

$$FPF_{<5\mu m} = FPM_{<5\mu m} / TEM \tag{24.17}$$

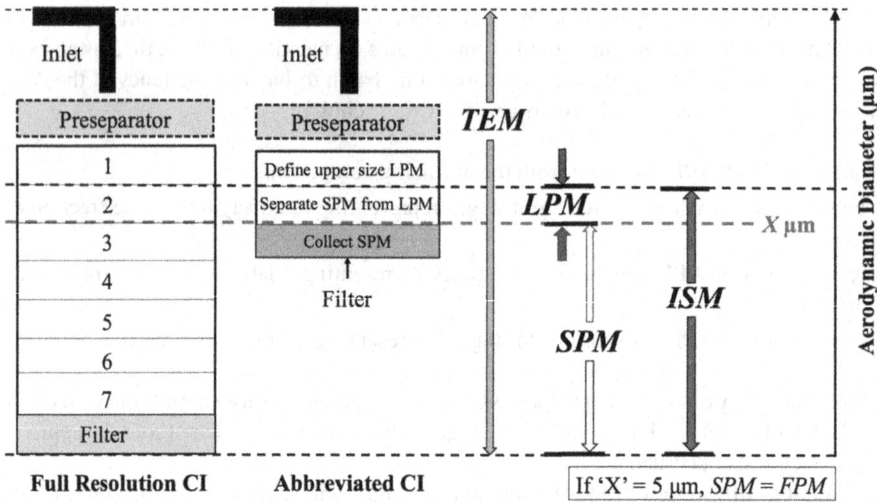

FIGURE 24.22 The principle of the AIM concept. A full resolution cascade impactor is reduced to two impaction stages, the first stage defines the upper size limit for LPM, the second stage collects the LPM, allowing the SPM to pass through to be collected on the back-up filter/MOC.

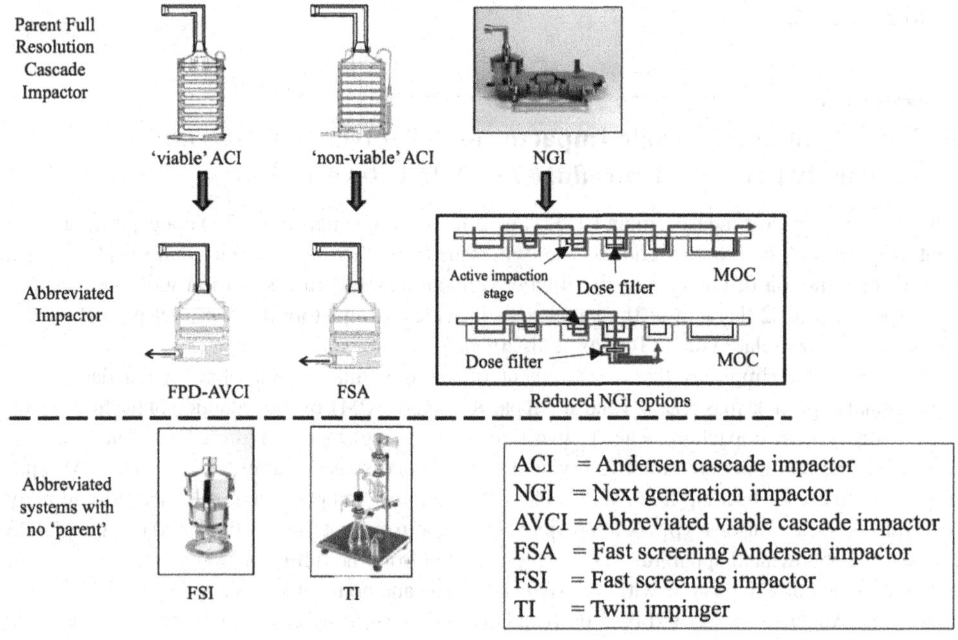

FIGURE 24.23 Various abbreviated impactors showing relation to "Parent" full-resolution cascade impactor where one exists.

It is important to be aware that apparatuses offering this simplified configuration cannot be used in conjunction with EDA, because neither ISM nor LPM are defined.

The twin impinger (apparatus A of the European Pharmacopeia) can be considered as being the earliest AIM-based apparatus of the European type (Hallworth and Westmoreland 1987). However, it is designed to operate only at a flow rate of 60 L/min, where its D_{50} is 6.4 μm aerodynamic diameter. The measurement and data analysis components associated with the acquisition of pertinent orally inhaled product aerodynamic particle size information for both abbreviated and full-resolution cascade impactor

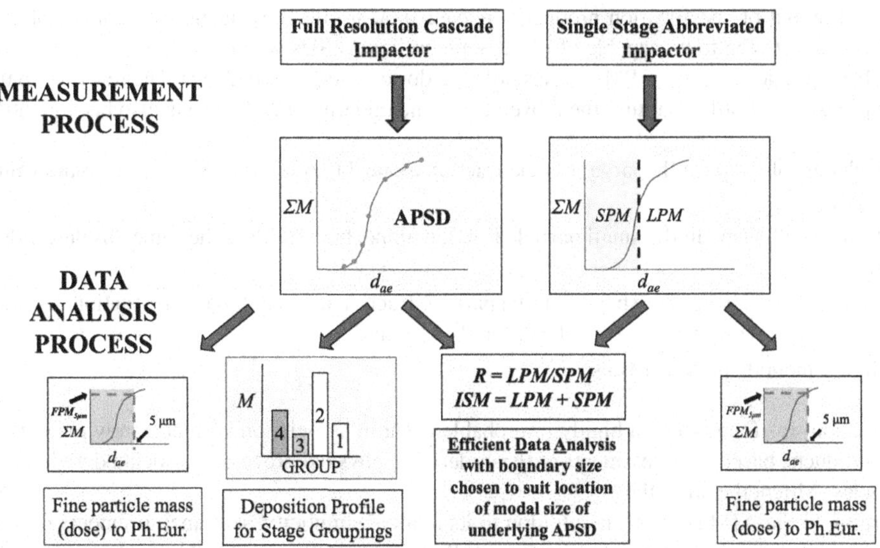

FIGURE 24.24 The measurement and data analysis components associated with the acquisition of OIP aerodynamic particle size information, showing the relationships between the AIM and EDA concepts and current European and United States regulatory requirements based on FPD <5-µm aerodynamic diameter and deposition profile stage groupings, respectively. (Courtesy of Inhalation Magazine, St Paul, MN.)

apparatuses are presented schematically in Figure 24.24. The European approach to abbreviated impactor measurement data analysis is one alternative for data reduction, alongside stage groupings (see Section 24.5) and EDA (see later in this section).

The EDA concept relies on the determination of two quantities, namely ISM, which is the sum of LPM and SPM, and the ratio metric (LPM/SPM) (Figure 24.24). These metrics, taken together, have the capability to detect significant changes in the underlying APSD in both particle size (abscissa scale) and API mass (ordinate scale) (Tougas et al. 2009, 2010). The advantages of the EDA concept, when used with either full-resolution cascade impactor data or in conjunction with AIM-apparatus derived metrics, is summarized in Table 24.7.

Through the assessment of a large database of different commercially available orally inhaled product-generated APSDs, the EDA approach has been demonstrated to have the potential for fewer false positive results (i.e. acceptable product is rejected) compared with a stage grouping-based approach in batch release (Christopher and Dey 2011). At the same time, EDA was shown to preserve patient safety-related considerations, through a similarly low level of false negative outcomes to that associated with stage

TABLE 24.7

Features of Effective Data Analysis Approach Compared with Compendial Full Resolution Cascade Impactor Methodology

Property	EDA with Full Resolution Cascade Impactor	EDA with AIM-Derived Measurements
Measurement Outcome	Complete APSD, which is useful for diagnosis in the event of Out of Specification (OOS)/Out of Tolerance (OOT) scenarios with AIM system	Similar sensitivity to APSD changes compared to current methods
Method Complexity	Same as for EDA with AIM with addition of full resolution APSD, if needed	Only two metrics required to detect APSD shifts in both API mass and aerodynamic diameter
Decision-making Capability	EDA offers fewer falsepositive results in batch release; full resolution APSD is available as backup, but at cost of increased method complexity	Time savings offer potential for more powerful experiment designs improving "coverage" of the batch; EDA offers fewer false positive results in batch release

groupings (i.e. out-of-specification product is released). More recently, using the same database, EDA has been demonstrated to be capable of identifying outlier APSDs where the European Pharmacopeial method based on determining $FPM_{<5\,\mu m}$ has failed to do so (Tougas et al. 2017). The few potential modes in which EDA could fail to capture the movement in the underlying APSD have also been identified:

1. A change of shape in the large particle fraction alone, but retaining the same absolute value of LPM;
2. A change of shape in the small particle fraction alone, but retaining the same absolute value of SPM;
3. Simultaneous changes of shape in large particle fraction and small particle fraction, but resulting in the same absolute values of SPM and LPM; and
4. Highly monodisperse aerosols.

Each situation was found to be a highly improbable event in association with currently marketed orally inhaled products, based on assessments of the underlying physical processes associated with these aerosol particles (Mitchell et al. 2011b).

Returning to the AIM concept, in addition to its relative simplicity, such measurements have numerous advantages compared to procedures using a full-resolution CI (see Table 24.8). These include the use of fewer components and the associated reduced amount of API recovery solvent needed, resulting in a shorter overall assay time per determination. Furthermore, because all of the mass of the API entering the impactor is divided into only two or three portions, depending on which type of abbreviated apparatus configuration is being used, the capability for good precision in association with single actuation measurements is improved in comparison with full-resolution CI determinations, where the incoming API mass typically is fractionated into seven or eight components, depending on the number of stages of the CI.

Although the benefits of the AIM concept have been identified by several independently undertaken studies assessed by Tougas et al. (2013), there are several precautions that potential users should consider before adopting this approach:

1. Stringent care is nearly always necessary to prevent particle bounce in abbreviated impactors. In one study involving measurements of pMDI-delivered aerosols using a modified FSA impactor in which a second impaction stage was used to collect the EPM fraction, it was found that the normal practice of coating the collection plate with a surfactant resulted in displacement of the coating beneath the exit of each of the nozzles (Mitchell et al. 2010). This process created a surface that behaved as if no coating had been applied. It was found necessary to place a surfactant-coated filter on top of the collection surface to provide a surface that was both energy-absorbent, but at the same time resisted re-location by the incoming high velocity air flow.

TABLE 24.8

Features of Abbreviated Impactor Measurement Approach Compared with Compendial Full Resolution Cascade Impactor Methodology

Property	Full Resolution Cascade Impactor Alone	AIM Alone
Measurement Outcome	Provides complete APSD	Provides EDA metrics directly
Method Complexity	Has the most components to assemble and disassemble	Reduced number of components to assemble and disassemble
API Recovery and Assay	Up to 12 separate samples: low sensitivity at stages where mass of API is close to lower limit of detection	Four separate samples to recover if used with EDA with reduced risk of stages collecting low API mass
Time per Determination	Typically up to 2-hr	Typically about 30-min
Decision-making Capability	Offers choice of EDA and/or APSD analysis with increased method complexity	If used with EDA, confers sensitivity benefits to shifts in underlying APSD

2. It is important to match the dead-space upstream of the first impaction stage of the abbreviated impactor to that of the full-resolution system before its initial impaction stage in order to get equivalent results for metrics obtained from full-resolution cascade impactor testing. This precaution is particularly important if the product being tested contains low volatile excipient, such as ethanol (Mitchell et al. 2009b, Keegan and Lewis 2012).
3. Matching the overall dead-space of the abbreviated system and the full-resolution impactor is important to achieve comparable flow rate rise times in DPI testing (Daniels and Hamilton 2011, Pantelides et al. 2011). In this context, it should be noted that the full-resolution results are not inherently "correct," as the flow rate takes some time to reach the final stable value after the vacuum source is applied to the impactor (Section 24.3.2). However, full-resolution impactor measurements remain the stakeholder-recognized benchmark.

The evidence from comparative testing of all classes of orally inhaled product is that AIM-based measurements in general provide realistic, if not exactly equivalent, measurements of key metrics compared with those derived from full-resolution cascade impactor measurements. This finding is illustrated by two cross-industry comparative experiments conducted recently. In the first study (Nichols et al. 2016), undertaken through the EPAG organization, following methodology that was focused on evaluation of $FPM_{<5.0\ \mu m}$, five different participating laboratories were involved with abbreviated apparatuses including a FSI and three slightly different configurations of the FSA. One participant used a reduced NGI created by retaining stage 3 of a full-resolution NGI to size-fractionate coarse from fine particle portions of the incoming aerosol. The NGI was used as the full-resolution reference impactor in measurements comparing the FSI and reduced NGI abbreviated apparatuses, while the non-viable ACI was used otherwise. Even though each participating laboratory used a single full-resolution impactor, they did not use the same impactor (i.e. this was not a "round-robin," study). Similarly, each participant also used their own AIM-based apparatuses. The investigation also involved several different pMDI (two products) and DPI (five products) commercially available formulations. Furthermore, two of the DPI and one of the pMDI products contained two drug products in combination. Nine out of the ten data sets collected fulfilled the main equivalence criterion, that the 90% confidence interval of the ratio ($FPD_{AIM}/FPD_{full\text{-}resolution\ CI}$) was contained within the predefined 85%–118% acceptance interval. However, $FPM_{<5.0\ \mu m}$ determined by AIM-type techniques, based on a survey of the outcomes for all ten products, was found on average to be 5% greater than the equivalent measure made by the full-resolution impactors. Some of the difference could be explained by slightly reduced internal losses associated with the smaller surface area available for such deposition within some designs of abbreviated impactor apparatuses. The EPAG group (Nichols et al. 2016) concluded that these findings provide good support for statistical equivalence across different formulations and delivery device classes for AIM-based and full-resolution impactor-measured $FPD_{<5.0\ \mu m}$. They further showed that an AIM-based approach has the potential of being used as an alternative to full-resolution cascade impactor measurements for determining $FPM_{<5.0\ \mu m}$ as the critical quality attribute with their orally inhaled product aerosols. Finally, they counseled that the validation of an AIM-based technique as an alternative to the full-resolution CI method should (always) be undertaken on a product-by-product basis.

In the second study, a two-centre laboratory study was undertaken under the supervision of the International Pharmaceutical Aerosol Consortium on Regulation and Science, with the goal of expanding the understanding of the performance of FSA-type abbreviated apparatuses capable of use with the EDA concept. In this designed experiment, the focus was on the assessment of pMDI-delivered aerosols containing the same albuterol/salbutamol-based API, compared with data derived from full-resolution ACIs (Christopher et al. 2017). Both centers used representative commercial pMDIs sourced at random points throughout the manufacture of a particular batch. The results demonstrated that the AIM-based measurements undertaken by both participating laboratories in combination with EDA had at least 7.5 levels of discrimination for MMAD shifts (Wheeler 2006) (0.75 μm measurement precision/0.1 μm allowable range of acceptable values = 7.5). For this study at least, the authors concluded that the AIM approach had adequate discrimination to detect changes in the MMAD of the underlying APSD, to be employable for routine product quality control. This group repeated the advice from the EPAG-led group, that transition from an ACI (used in product development) to an appropriate AIM/EDA methodology (used later in product quality control) should be evaluated and supported by data on a product-by-product basis.

24.7 The Tension Between Cascade Impactor Method Simplicity and Clinical Relevance

Until now, the focus of this chapter has been firmly in the camp of determining orally inhaled product APSDs primarily for the purpose of quality control. However, the support of the clinical program is an important part in the product lifecycle (Tougas et al. 2011). There is now an increasing understanding by regulatory agencies and clinicians, from the perspective of patient care, that data derived from quality control testing alone are quite limited in their scope and application, particularly when it comes to informing the prescribing clinician and pharmacist about the way the product is likely to perform in the hands of the patient or caregiver (Mitchell and Suggett 2014). These considerations are especially important in establishing sound IVIVCs and in the assessment of bioequivalence between inhalers (Forbes et al. 2015). A robust IVIVC could permit a laboratory model to be used as a development tool (Delvadia et al. 2012) and potentially replace in-patient tests for product registration.

The development of so-called "clinically appropriate" laboratory test methods has implications for the assessment of APSDs of orally inhaled products in the following ways:

1. There is a driver for simplicity, by reconciling the need to minimize complexity in the realization of the oropharynx as the inlet to the cascade impactor apparatus, but recognizing that critical dimensions of this part of the human anatomy change with patient age, and that there is no single sized oropharynx even with adults and
2. The conflict needs to be resolved between the requirement that the cascade impactor is ideally operated at a constant flow rate throughout the entire sampling period, whereas at the same time the patient interface of the inhaler should experience the continuously varying flow rate associated with an inhalation maneuver specific to the class of orally inhaled product under consideration (pMDIs, soft mist inhalers, and DPIs), or with tidal breathing for nebulizing systems.

Even when these obvious differences between pharmacopeial compendia-based laboratory methods and patient use are considered, there is the further aspect of being able to simulate potential patient misuse/imperfect use, which is widely encountered with inhalers (Crompton et al. 2006, Melani et al. 2011, 2012). The simulation of a delayed inhalation in the testing of valved holding chambers (Section 24.3.4) is a good example in which progress has recently been made to incorporate the patient experience into a compendial methodology (US Pharmacopeial Convention 2018c).

Looking further at the first implication identified above, it has been widely known for many years that the right-angled Ph. Eur./USP induction port is only a rudimentary representation of the complex geometry of the adult oropharynx (Zhou et al. 2011). There have therefore been two separate streams of development towards the design of commercially available more patient-realistic inlets. Early attempts with anatomically accurate oropharyngeal representations were both non-representative of the patient population at large and the process of making use of cadaver-prepared casts or dental impressions resulted in some distortions to the rendered inlets (Swift 1992). Nevertheless, this was the only available approach to the problem until the mid 1990s. The first stream in recent patient-realistic inlet development has been the creation of oropharyngeal airway models that are representative of low, medium, and high particle retention from many magnetic resonance images taken of adult volunteers by the European-based Oropharyngeal Consortium (McRobbie et al. 2003, Burnell et al. 2007); these models are commercially available from Emmace Consulting AB, Lund, Sweden. Chrystyn et al. (2015) have since compared the medium-sized model inlet with the USP/PhEur induction port for the sampling of Spiromax and Turbuhaler® DPI-generated aerosols. They found that measures of FPM and MMAD consistently indicated that the compendial induction port underestimates the deposition of larger particles that takes place in the adult oropharynx.

The second approach towards more representative inlets has been built partly on the work of the Oropharyngeal Consortium, but modeling the fluid flow properties of aerosols passing through age-appropriate airways. These studies were undertaken over a several-year period by Finlay and colleagues at the University of Alberta, Edmonton, Canada (Grgic et al. 2004), in which upper airway modeling was based on anatomic measurements of airways of patients selected initially from adult, then from small child and infant sub-populations. The approach resulted in a series of "idealized" inlets, each having greatly simplified internal geometry compared with anatomic reality, but with comparable aerosol transport properties. Adult (Stapleton et al. 2000), small child (Golshahi and Finlay 2012), and infant (Carrigy et al. 2014) inlets (termed "Alberta" idealized throats) are available from Copley Scientific Ltd., Nottingham, United Kingdom. APSDs measured for both pMDI- and DPI-based products are significantly shifted to finer sizes compared with the situation in which the USP/PhEur inlet is used, again indicative that the compendial inlet underestimates the deposition of larger particles (Copley et al. 2012, Mitchell et al. 2012b).

Early attempts to resolve the conflict between the requirement that the cascade impactor must be operated at a fixed flow rate to maintain stable stage D_{50} values, and the fact that in use, inhalers are always subjected to changing flow rate profile, resulted in several adaptations involving the use of cascade impactors with breathing simulation equipment to operate the inhaler (Finlay 1998, Foss and Keppel 1999). However, none of these apparatuses transported the aerosol released by the inhaler to the impactor without the risk of introducing turbulence where air from the breathing simulator and make-up air for the impactor met the in-flow of aerosol from the inhaler. The Electronic Lung®, developed around the same time by GSK plc, attempted to overcome this difficulty by sampling the aerosol from the inhaler (typically a DPI) into a large vertical cylindrical vessel, mimicking an inhalation maneuver. After shutting off suction from the breathing simulator, the retained aerosol from the chamber can be sampled by applying a vacuum source to a cascade impactor which is located at the tapered based of the chamber (Brindley et al. 1994). Although elegant in terms of aerosol handling, it is possible that gravitational sedimentation, taking place continuously during any delay between operating the inhaler and sampling the aerosol, could be a potential source of APSD bias. An alternative and slightly simpler setup involves the use of the Nephele Mixing Inlet (Miller 2002), available from Copley Scientific Ltd., Nottingham, United Kingdom, or RDD-Online, Richmond, VA, United States. This device, which is operated between the inhaler and a cascade impactor (Figure 24.26) makes use of tapered surfaces of the inner tube containing the aerosol stream from the inhaler at the merge with the make-up air for the impactor. This gradual merging of the two streams mitigates particle losses to internal surfaces of the mixing inlet due to turbulence. At the same time, the impactor measurement takes place almost simultaneously with the aerosol generation process as the inhaler is actuated (Figure 24.25). Olsson et al. have used this

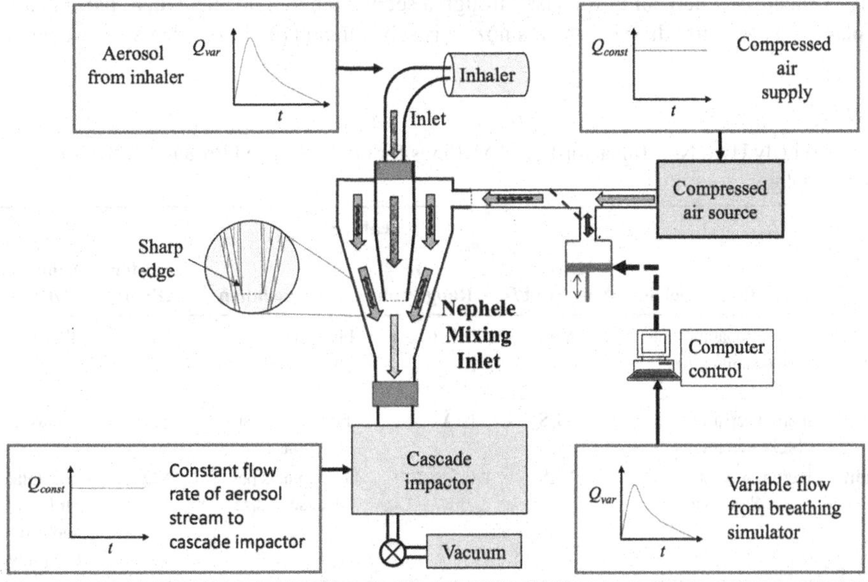

FIGURE 24.25 The Nephele mixing inlet in use between an inhaler subjected to continuously changing airflow from a breathing simulator; aerosol from the inhaler enters the mixing inlet via an anatomic or idealized induction port. Make-up air is supplied to ensure a constant flow rate to the cascade impactor whose entry is aligned with the exit from the mixing inlet. In the mixing zone, aerosol and make-up flow streams converge in laminar conditions. (Courtesy of Inhalation Magazine, St Paul, MN.)

inlet in conjunction with the NGI to achieve remarkably good IVIVCs for budesonide delivered from pMDI, DPI, and nebulizer platforms by mouthpiece to small, medium, and large adult oropharyngeal inlets referred to previously, that were developed from the Oropharyngeal Consortium work, mimicking appropriate patient-derived breathing patterns (Olsson et al. 2013). This approach to more clinically appropriate assessments of inhaler-generated APSDs appears to be gaining in importance (Abdelrahim 2011, Chrystyn 2015, Bagherisadeghi et al. 2017, Svensson et al. 2018).

24.8 Alternatives to the Cascade Impactor for Inhaler APSD Measurement

Although the cascade impactor is the most widely encountered apparatus for the determination of APSD for orally inhaled products, there are two alternative methodologies that are simpler-to-use, permit more rapid determinations, and have better intrinsic size resolution (Table 24.9).

The first of these techniques makes use of measurement of the TOF of individual aerosol particles as they are accelerated in ultra-Stokesian flow regime by passing through a tapered nozzle located immediately above the measurement zone (Baron et al. 1993). The TOF measurement method has been extensively reviewed (Mitchell and Nagel 1999, Mitchell et al. 2011a), so only its highlights are presented here. In essence, the time of flight of the particle between two well-defined locations in the measurement zone is a monotonic function of D_{ae}. Longer flight times are associated with larger-sized particles due to their enhanced drag in the accelerating flow field (Figure 24.26). There have been several TOF-based instruments developed in the past 30 years (Mitchell et al. 2011a), but nowadays, the model 3321 Aerodynamic Particle Sizer (APS®) aerosol spectrometer (TSI Inc., St. Paul, MN, United States), that has undergone several improvements in its 30-year lifetime, is the most likely example to be encountered. The information provided in Table 24.9 is therefore based on the present specification for that instrument.

The aerosol has to be introduced into the APS at a fixed flow rate of 5 L/min. This flow rate is generally too small for direct sampling from most orally inhaled products, except perhaps for the evaluation of certain pediatric products intended for infant use. A flow of clean sheath air is created by removing 80% of the incoming aerosol stream, filtering it, and returning it to the outer nozzle, which is aligned coaxially with the tapered focusing nozzle that carries the remaining aerosol flow to the measurement zone. The combined sheath and aerosol flows pass through a second tapered nozzle, where particle acceleration takes place. The pressure drop below this nozzle is sub-critical (13 kPa) so that sonic velocity is not

TABLE 24.9

Comparison of Widely Used Non-Impactor-Based Methods for Orally Inhaled Product APSD with Cascade Impactor Methodology

		Features				
Technique	**Operating Principle**	**Direct Measure of D_{ae}**	**Size Range (μm)**	**Size Resolution**	**Assay for API(s)**	**Applicability to OIP Classes**
Full Resolution Cascade Impactor	Inertial separation in Stokesian regime	YES	0.1–10	Five stages between 0.5 μm and 5.0 μm	YES	All classes
Abbreviated Impactor	Inertial separation in Stokesian regime	YES	N/A	Two or three size fractions	YES	All classes
Time-of-Flight	Inertial separation in ultra-Stokesian	YES	0.5 to 20	32 channels per decade of size	NO	Less suitable for DPIs without sophisticated sampling
Laser Diffraction	Low-angle laser light scattering	NO	0.1 to several mm	>15 channels per decade of size	NO	Most suitable for aqueous preparations/ products for nebulization

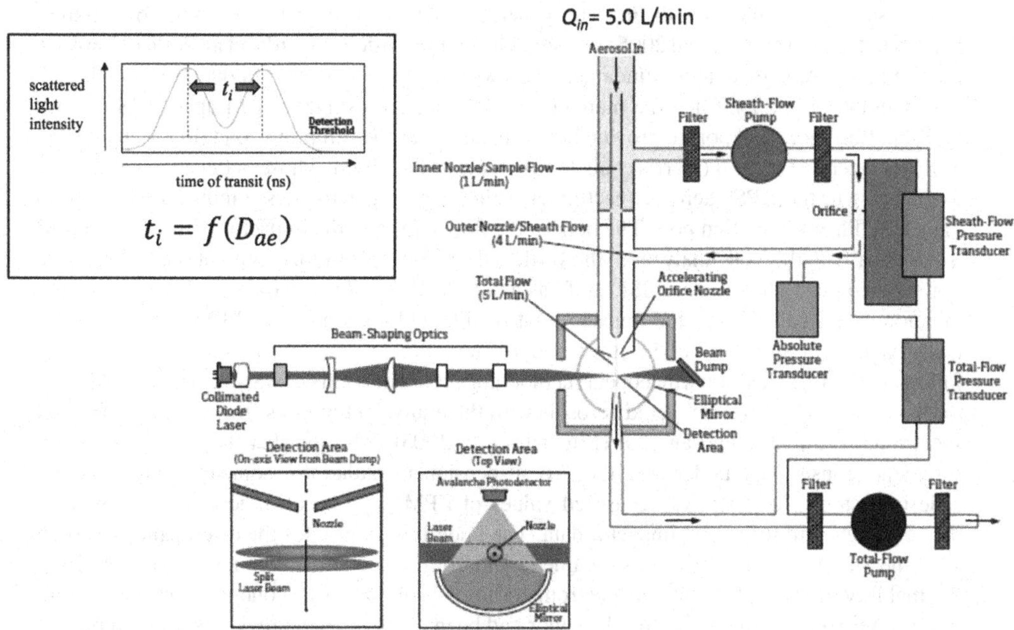

FIGURE 24.26 Schematic diagram of the aerodynamic particle sizer® aerosol spectrometer, showing how the TOF measurement (t_i) per particle traverse across the split laser beam is unambiguously determined using overlapping signals from the particle detection system. (Courtesy of TSI Inc., Shoreview, MN.)

attained (Chen et al. 1985). The flow rates of sheath air and total air are separately controlled by needle valves and monitored with thermal mass flow meters; overall flow control is supervised by a dedicated microprocessor. When the incoming aerosol concentration is sufficiently low, particles leaving the distal end of the acceleration nozzle pass individually through the laser beams, causing two pulses to be detected from which the TOF for the particle is determined (Figure 24.26). Larger particles have longer TOF values, as their inertia has prevented them being accelerated as much as they leave the nozzle. The interpretation of the detector signals in terms of D_{ae} requires fast signal processing and a dedicated microcomputer. The overall particle size range of the currently available instrument (model 3321) is from 0.5 μm to 20 μm aerodynamic diameter, in 52 size channels that equates to 32 channels per decade of size within the range of greatest interest from 0.5 μm–5.0 μm aerodynamic diameter.

Despite the attractiveness of this approach to APSD determination, there are several limitations that have limited its use as a supporting technique to the multi-stage cascade impactor. These are as follows:

1. Since the TOF technique is based on the determination of the transit times of individual particles, the base APSD is number-weighted. Transformation to the more usual mass-weighted form required the multiplication of the particle count in each size channel (j) by the factor ($\pi D_j^3/6$), which assumes the particles are spherical. D_j is the logarithmic average of the upper and lower size bounds for channel "*j*." It follows that the contributions from a few particles that may be present at the large end of the APSD are overemphasized in the mass-weighted presentation. They can therefore have a disproportionate effect on metrics, such as the MMAD and the various size sub-fractions.
2. In comparisons with cascade impactor-based measurements, care needs to be given to the handling of pMDI formulations containing ethanol as a low volatile excipient. Ideally, the co-solvent should be fully evaporated in both apparatuses, however, in reality, some liquid ethanol may be present in the aerosol entering the upper stages of the impactor. The dead space associated with the entry to the APS* aerosol spectrometer is relatively small compared with that which exists with most cascade impactors. Various attempts have been made to achieve comparative

TOF-based measurements with impactor-generated APSDs using extension tubes of different lengths (Mogalian and Myrdal 2005), as well as heated extensions (Myrdal et al. 2006). However, the need to overcome the more fundamental drawback that there is no API quantification by the TOF-method (Table 24.9) led the manufacturer to develop a single-stage impactor (SSI) with USP/Ph. Eur. induction port to provide better matching of the sampling conditions between the TOF analyzer and an ACI (Harris et al. 2006). In the SSI addition, whose outlet attaches directly to the entry to the APS* aerosol spectrometer, the incoming aerosol is sampled at 28.3 L/min via a USP/PhEur induction port. The bulk of the flow passes to the impactor with <1% sampled isokinetically to the TOF analyzer in the vertical direction to minimize gravitational sedimentation-created bias. The standard SSI itself has its D_{50} fixed at 4.7 µm aerodynamic diameter, and therefore acts as an abbreviated impactor that is suitable for determining $FPM_{<4.7\ \mu m}$. A version is available with its D_{50} set at 5.0 µm aerodynamic diameter for comparisons with $FPM_{<5.0\ \mu m}$ following the European Pharmacopeia methodology. Comparisons of SSI-measured $FPM_{<4.7\ \mu m}$ for three different pMDI-delivered aerosols with the equivalent metrics from the APS* aerosol spectrometer, an ACI, and an NGI (Mitchell et al. 2003) indicated that the TOF-based measurements consistently undersized the two suspension formulations, compared with the cascade impactors. However, SSI-measured values of $FPM_{<4.7\ \mu m}$ were in closer agreement with the equivalent full resolution impactor data. The underlying cause for the discrepancy between TOF-measured data and the results obtained by inertial impaction was believed to be related to the inability of the APS* aerosol spectrometer to discriminate API-containing particles from those comprising excipient. Similar behavior had been observed in a previous study sampling a pMDI-delivered product in which surfactant particles had been present, using an earlier type of TOF analyzer (Mitchell et al. 1999). Agreement in $FPM_{<4.7\ \mu m}$ between the TOF-derived measure and the corresponding values from the two full-resolution cascade impactors was better for the solution formulated product, but incomplete evaporation of ethanol co-solvent was believed to have caused the SSI-derived values to be smaller than expected.

3. Differences in particle density as well as shape from their reference values are known to be associated with potential for bias with TOF-based analysis. Particle density values greater than ca. 2.0×10^3 kg.m^{-3} have been associated with detectable shifts in TOF-measured APSDs towards larger sizes than would have been the case had particle density been at its reference value for the aerodynamic diameter scale of 1.0×10^3 kg.m^{-3} (Cheng et al. 1990). In contrast, deformation, observed with liquid droplets larger than about 2 µm diameter causes systematic shifts to smaller sizes (Griffiths et al. 1986, Cheng et al. 1990). Deviations in solid particle shape from spherical (dynamic shape factor, $\chi > 1.00$ (Equation 24.1)), likely to be more important when assessing DPI-derived aerosols, have also been shown to have the same effect on TOF-measured APSD data as droplet deformation (Marshall et al. 1991).

Taken together, these considerations have very likely prevented TOF-based instruments from becoming recognized as an alternative to the cascade impactor for APSD assessments by incorporation into the pharmacopeia compendial methodologies. However, an adaptation of the TOF-based analysis method, termed SPAMS (Morrical et al. 2015, Jetzer et al. 2017) may offer a way around the non-specificity for API that has limited the application of straightforward TOF analysis. SPAMS is a single particle characterization technique, similar to conventional TOF analysis, but determines both D_{ae} and chemical composition of many individual particles in real-time. The instrument is a hybrid of the rapid single particle mass spectrometry technique introduced earlier by Carson et al. (1995) and aerodynamic time-of-flight mass spectrometry. SPAMS allows the determination of the aerodynamic diameter of the particles being analyzed while saturating the detection system at far higher concentrations of particles than the capability of previous Aerodynamic Time-of-Flight Mass Spectrometry (ATOFMS) systems such as that described by Noble and Prather (1998). Aerosol particles are introduced into the SPAMS instrument described by Morrical et al. (2015) via a pre-separator (if necessary) through the port on top of the instrument, passing through a series of aerodynamic focusing lenses (Figure 24.27). The system is maintained under vacuum so that the aerosol interface has a pressure flow reducer pathway with a patented aerodynamic focusing lens stack for the effective sampling of particles (Gard et al. 2008). The lenses focus the particles into a tight beam and also accelerate them to a final velocity

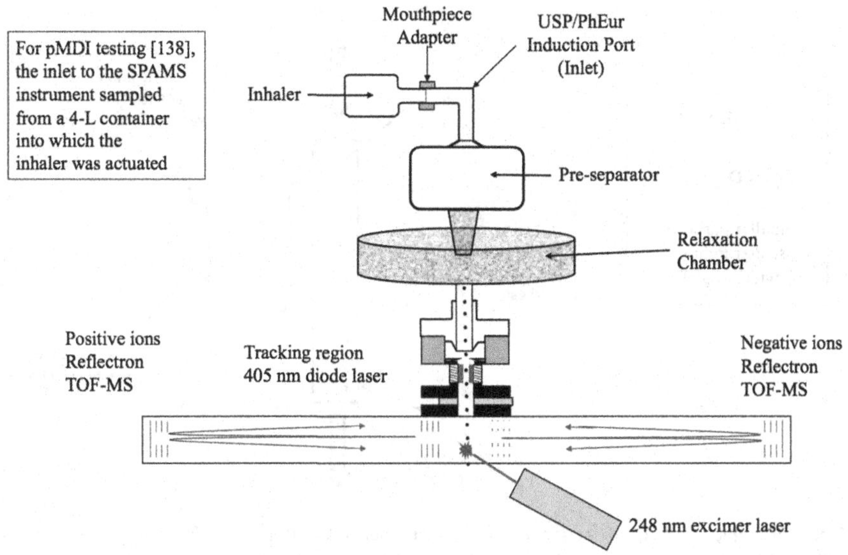

FIGURE 24.27 Schematic diagram showing the operating principle for the TOF-SPAMS instrument which is a hybrid of rapid single particle mass spectrometry and aerodynamic time-of-flight mass spectrometry allowing the determination of the APSD of the particles being analyzed.

as a function of D_{ae} in the range from 0.1 µm–12 µm aerodynamic diameter. Each particle continues across a continuous wave visible light laser. The top and bottom of the laser beam are parallel and its height of the beam is defined. As the particle passes through the beam, it scatters light which is detected by a photomultiplier tube. The duration of the light scattering event provides particle velocity, which is used to compute its aerodynamic diameter. API quantification occurs by collecting a laser mass spectrum of the small molecules (up to 350 Daltons in both positive and negative polarities simultaneously) from individual aerosol particles. Measurements made of various pMDI-delivered aerosols from commercially available products containing both single and two-API components resulted in comparable NGI-measured APSDs (Morrical et al. 2015). The authors of this study claimed that a similar amount of data that would normally require approximately 3 days of experimentation and analysis by conventional multi-stage cascade impactor-based approach was collected in a 5-minute period with automatic API analysis. Although these claims are promising, the equipment is expensive (ca. US$350,000 for the 3rd generation instrument), and its technical limitations have yet to be fully understood when used with all the different classes of Orally Inhaled Product (OIP).

In a further study, the same group has recently used the SPAMS technique to study particle interactions of fluticasone propionate and salmeterol xinafoate associated with both pMDI- and DPI-delivered aerosols (Jetzer et al. 2017). They found that the majority of the aerodynamically size-separated detected salmeterol particles were found to be in co-association with fluticasone from both inhaler types. Another significant finding was that rather coarse fluticasone particles from the DPI and fine salmeterol particles from both the pMDI and DPI were involved in forming these particle co-associations. This study represents an extension of this aerodynamic particle size analysis-based technique towards identifying how different API-containing particles interact in transit from the inhaler to the measurement apparatus and potentially may offer the ability to provide a greater understanding of such behavior when inhaled.

The second widely encountered alternative technique to the multi-stage cascade impactor is LD. LD instruments operate on the basis of the interpretation of the light scattering pattern that is set up by an ensemble of either solid particles or liquid droplets in a collimated beam of coherent light (Figure 24.28) (Swithenbank et al. 1977). The light scattering pattern is converted into a volume-weighted particle size distribution by the application of a model (either Fraunhofer theory, for droplets >> λ, where λ is the wavelength of the light source, or Lorenz-Mie theory, which is applicable for all droplet sizes (International Standards Organization 1999). Either model describes the relationship between scattered light energy and angle of scattering in relation to the axis defined by the light

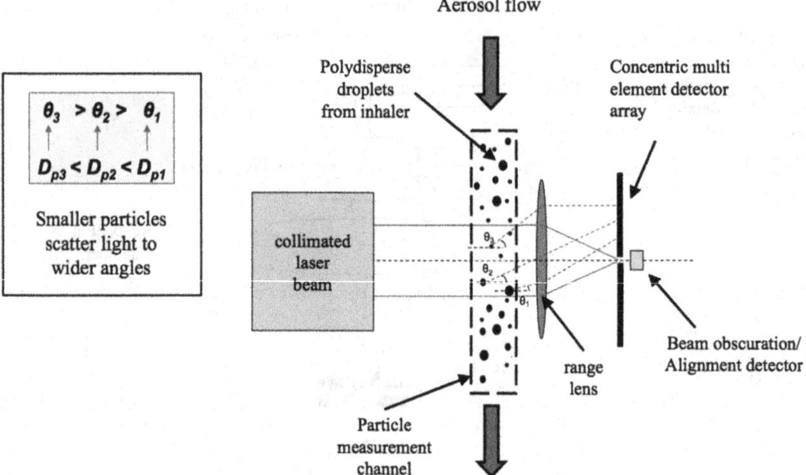

FIGURE 24.28 Principles of laser diffraction: the polydisperse aerosol is illuminated by coherent light typically from a He-Ne laser; the entire population of illuminated particles scatters light simultaneously (ensemble scattering) with the light interacting with the smallest particles scattering to the largest angles. A concentric ring diode collects the scattered light after passing through the range lens that focuses the light onto the detector array.

source, aerosol, and detection optics. The refractive index of the aerosol droplets does not need to be known to apply the Fraunhofer model (International Standards Organization 1999). However, both the light deflection and absorption components comprising the complex refractive index must be known to apply Lorenz-Mie theory (Van de Hulst 1981). The digital signal is deconvoluted into the size distribution, using an iterative process that finds the distribution of equivalent spherical light scattering bodies using the appropriate theory with the best fit of the calculated intensity/angle relationship to the corresponding measured values (Figure 24.29) (Mitchell et al. 2006). LD measurements are rapid; a typical time per determination being of the order of a few seconds (Figure 24.29).

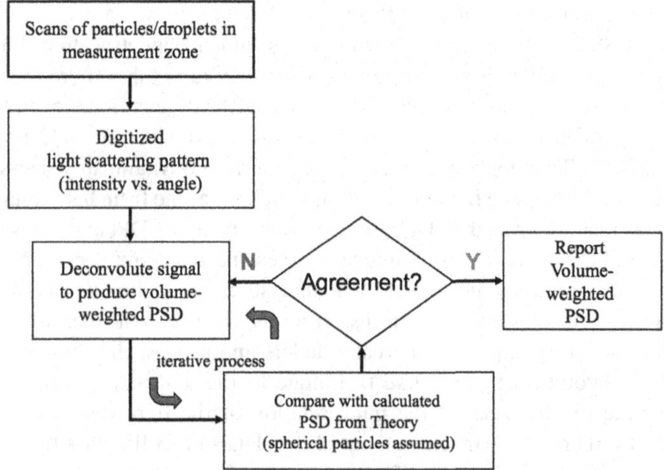

FIGURE 24.29 Conversion of the light scattering pattern recorded by the concentric diode detector array to a volume-weighted particle size distribution (PSD). The digital signal is deconvoluted into the size distribution, using an iterative process that finds the distribution of equivalent spherical light scattering bodies with the best fit of the calculated intensity/angle relationship to the corresponding measured values.

The LD technique as applied to the size characterization of aerosols from orally inhaled products has been reviewed more recently by Mitchell et al. (2011a). It is important to appreciate that LD does not directly measure particle aerodynamic diameter; the size that is measured approximates to the physical diameter (D_p, Equation (24.1), as long as the particle shape is close to spherical). The reason for mentioning LD in the context of the topic covered in this chapter is because for aqueous droplets produced from nebulizing systems, to a first approximation: $D_p = D_{ae}$. LD has therefore become widely adopted for the assessment of droplet distributions from this class of orally inhaled product (Mitchell et al. 2006). Importantly, the measured size distribution data are volume-weighted, making it unnecessary to transform the distribution from a number to mass-weighted basis, as is the case for the equivalent TOF analyzer-measured data. The underlying assumption is made that droplet density is independent of size, which is probably acceptable given the dilute nature of nebulizer-delivered solutions, which are typically administered in physiological normal saline (0.9% w/v NaCl). Nebulizer-generated droplets can be measured non-invasively by the open-bench technique, in which the droplet stream passes through the illuminating zone and is then dispersed into the open surroundings (Mitchell et al. 2006). Alternatively, the droplets can be drawn from the nebulizer through a closed cell by applying a vacuum; windows in the cell allow for droplet illumination and sheath air can be provided to avoid window fouling by deposited droplets. The closed cell procedure enables better control of the local relative humidity surrounding the droplet stream, which can be important with nebulizing systems that do not entrain ambient air as part of their normal operation (Mitchell et al. 2006) (see Section 24.3.3).

Although LD has been used predominantly with nebulizing systems for droplet APSD determinations, a significant number of studies have applied this technique to the characterization of aerosols from other classes of orally inhaled product (de Boer et al. 2002, Smyth and Hickey 2002, Jones et al. 2004, Krarup and Kippax 2004, Simons and Stein 2005). In response to the desire to be able to relate LD-measured data to an APSD from the same inhaler using a cascade impaction-based technique, one manufacturer (Malvern Panalytical Ltd., Great Malvern, UK) has developed an "inhalation cell," into which the aerosol from the inhaler is drawn by a vacuum source. LD measurements are carried out simultaneously with sampling from the inhalation cell to a cascade impactor located orthogonally from the illuminating axis of the LD system (Haynes et al. 2004). In this way, the LD-measured particle size distribution can be directly compared to a reference cascade impactor-determined APSD as a means of qualifying the LD measurement approach.

Despite its simplicity and measurement rapidity, the LD approach to particle sizing has several limitations:

1. There is no assay for the API(s) that are present, so the technique is non-specific if excipients are present or if there is more than one API in the formulation being assessed.
2. The underlying theories for LD treat the light scattering by particles as if they were spherical; while this assumption may be acceptable for compact non-spherical particles, it may result in bias if their geometry deviates significantly from spherical (i.e. for fiber-like particles).
3. Beam steering caused by high local concentrations of propellant from pMDI products may result in the appearance of anomalously large particles in the size distribution data. Some instruments have a "kill channel" feature that disables the detector rings closest to the axis of the incoming beam in order to avoid bias from this source.
4. Multiple scattering may occur with highly concentrated droplets from certain nebulizing systems. Under such circumstances, the assumption that the angle of scattering is related to the droplet size breaks down because the scattered photons interact with at least one other droplet resulting in further scattering before reaching the detector. Manufacturers of LD instruments provide a beam obscuration detection feature so that users can ensure they are working with aerosol concentrations that do not result in significant bias from this cause, and users should therefore err on the cautious side by ensuring that they work within the recommended obscuration range for their LD system.

In summary, LD systems have a significant role to play, especially in the rapid screening of formulations likely to be used with a particular orally inhaled dosage form. However, apart from the measurement of aqueous droplets from nebulizing systems, where it is recommended in the compendial chapters that this technique may be used if validated against a cascade impaction method (US Pharmacopeial Convention

2018b, European Directorate for Quality in Medicines 2018b), it is unlikely to replace traditional multi-stage cascade impaction as the primary measurement technique to determine APSDs of aerosols from orally inhaled products.

24.9 Personal Observations

Development of existing test procedures for orally inhaled products for APSD is currently at a mature stage, with the choice of several well defined, if complex-in-use methods for the different inhaler classes that are based on multi-stage cascade impactors. The GCIP framework that is currently being developed to support the use and maintenance of both abbreviated and full resolution cascade impactors will undoubtedly assist in reducing the incidence of measurements that fail because of a measurement apparatus-related cause. Given the conservative nature of the regulatory environment, it is unlikely that developments moving away from existing pharmacopeial methods in connection with product registration and quality control will take place in the near future. Nevertheless, there continues to be significant interest from industrial stakeholders in the benefits of simplifying the measurement approach utilizing the AIM concept. This is particularly the case in early stage product development where it is often necessary to conduct many determinations of APSD-related metrics as part of formulation screening and prototype delivery device evaluations. Likewise, there is significant continued interest from developers of orally inhaled products in the rapid, high size resolution techniques, such as TOF aerodynamic particle size analysis and laser diffractometry, with the latter already a mainstream technique for nebulizing systems. Developments to make TOF-based analysis traceable in terms of API mass may result in increased uptake by users, provided the cost of these techniques can become more affordable than at present.

Determination of either the full resolution underlying aerosol APSD, or more often a reduced data set based on three or four stage groupings, is likely to remain essential both in support of the clinical program and to provide reference data in the context of quality control. However, EDA offers the opportunity to follow shifts in terms of both API mass concentration and particle size associated with the underlying APSD, with a high degree of sensitivity, utilizing just two metrics describing ISM and the ratio LPM/SPM. In Europe, the use of $FPM_{<5\ \mu m}$ aerodynamic diameter, determined either by full resolution or abbreviated impactor, is likely to continue, given the fact that the European Pharmacopeial chapter in which this metric is defined for pMDI and DPI products has legal force within the European Union.

The goal of achieving meaningful IVIVCs across the different inhaler classes and API products currently available will clearly depend on the adoption of clinically appropriate testing methodologies for APSD determinations. However, at the present time, it is difficult to see when convergence between the test methods associated with product quality control and the more sophisticated measurement procedures associated with supporting the clinical program will take place, or if it even needs to occur. Indeed, there is a strong argument in favor of remaining with the existing compendial methods for quality control, as long as the relationships with more clinically appropriate procedures are well understood by all stakeholders associated with a given orally inhaled product.

REFERENCES

Abdelrahim, M. 2011. Aerodynamic characteristics of nebulized terbutaline sulphate using the Andersen cascade impactor compared to the next generation impactor. *Pharm Dev Technol* 16(2):137–145.

Asking, L., and B. Olsson. 1997. Calibration at different flow rates of a multistage liquid impinger. *Aerosol Sci Technol* 27(1):39–49.

Bagger-Jörgensen, H., D. Sandell, H. Lundbäck, and M. Sundahl. 2005. Effect of inherent variability of inhalation products on impactor mass balance limits. *J Aerosol Med.* 18(4):367–378.

Bagherisadeghi, G., E.H. Larhrib, and H. Chrystyn. 2017. Real life dose emission characterization using COPD patient inhalation profiles when they inhaled using a fixed dose combination (FDC) of the medium strength Symbicort* Turbuhaler*. *Int J Pharm* 522:137–146.

Baron, P.A., M.K. Mazumder, and Y.S. Cheng. 1993. Direct-reading techniques using optical particle detection. *Aerosol measurement: Principles, Techniques and Applications*, Eds. K. Willeke, P.A. Baron. 381–409. New York: Van Nostrand Reinhold.

de Boer, A.H., D. Gjaltema, P. Hagedoorn et al. 2002. Characterization of inhalation aerosols: A critical evaluation of cascade impactor and laser diffraction technique. *Int J Pharm* 249(1–2):219–231.

Bonam, M., D. Christopher, D. Cipolla et al. 2008. Minimizing variability of cascade impaction measurements in inhalers and nebulizers. *AAPS PharmSciTech* 9(2):404–413.

Brindley, A., B.S. Sumby, and I.J. Smith. 1994. The characterization of inhalation devices by an inhalation simulator: The Electronic Lung. *J Aerosol Med* 7(2):197–200.

Burnell, P.K.P., L. Asking, L. Borgström et al. 2007. Studies of the human oropharyngeal airspaces using magnetic resonance imaging IV—The oropharyngeal retention effect for four inhalation delivery systems. *J Aerosol Med* 20(3):269–281.

Canadian Standards Association. 2002 revised 2008 reaffirmed 2016. *Spacers and Holding Chambers for Use with Metered-Dose Inhalers*. Mississauga, ON, Canada. CAN/CSA/Z264.1-02: Available at URL: https://store.csagroup.org/ccrz__Products? .cartID=&operation=quickSearch&searchText=CAN%2FCSA-Z264.1-02%20%28R2016%29&searchFilter=all&isCSRFlow=true&portalUser=&store=&cclcl=en_US Visited June 20, 2018.

Carrigy, N.B., C. O'Reilly, J. Schmitt, M. Noga et al. 2014. Effect of facial material softness and applied force on face mask dead volume, face mask seal, and inhaled corticosteroid delivery through an idealized infant replica. *J Aerosol Med Pulmon Deliv.* 27(4):290–298.

Carson, P.G., K.R. Neubauer, M.V. Johnston et al. 1995. On-line analysis of aerosols by rapid single-particle mass spectrometry. *J Aerosol Sci* 26(4):535–545.

Carvalho, T.C., and J.T. McConville. 2016. The function and performance of aqueous aerosol devices for inhalation therapy. *J Pharm Pharmacol* 68(5):556–578.

Chambers, F., A. Ali, J. Mitchell, C. Shelton, and S. Nichols. 2010. Cascade impactor (CI) mensuration: An assessment of the accuracy and precision of commercially available optical measurement systems. *AAPS PharmSciTech* 11(1):472–484.

Chen, B.T., Y.S. Cheng, and H.C. Yeh. 1985. Performance of a TSI aerodynamic particle sizer. *Aerosol Sci Technol* 4(1):89–97.

Cheng, Y.-S., B.-T. Chen, and H.C. Yeh. 1990. A study of density effect and droplet deformation in the TSI aerodynamic particle sizer. *Aerosol Sci Technol* 12(2):278–285.

Christopher, D., P. Curry, W. Doub et al. 2003. Considerations for the development and practice of cascade impaction testing including a mass balance failure investigation tree. *J Aerosol Med* 16(3):235–247.

Christopher, D., and M. Dey. 2011. Detecting differences in APSD: Efficient data analysis (EDA) vs. stage grouping. *Respiratory Drug Delivery-Europe 2011*, Eds. Dalby, R.N., Byron, P.R., Peart, J., Suman, J.D., and Young, P.M. 215–224. River Grove, IL: Davis Healthcare International Publishing.

Christopher, J.D., R.J. Patel, J.P. Mitchell et al. 2017. Discriminating ability of abbreviated impactor measurement approach (AIM) to detect changes in mass median aerodynamic diameter (MMAD) of an albuterol/salbutamol pMDI aerosol *AAPS PharmSciTech* 18(8):3296–3306.

Chrystyn, H., G. Safioti, J.R. Keegstra et al. 2015. Effect of inhalation profile and throat geometry on predicted lung deposition of budesonide and formoterol (BF) in COPD: An in-vitro comparison of Spiromax with Turbuhaler. *Int J Pharm* 491(1–2):268–276.

Copley, M. 2008. The importance of stage mensuration in cascade impaction. *Pharm Technol Europe* September. 2008. Available at: http://www.copleyscientific.com/files/ww/news/COP%20JOB%20013_The%20importance%20of%20stage%20mensuration%20for%20cascade%20impaction.pdf. (accessed 22 September 2017).

Copley, M., J. Mitchell, and D. Solomon. 2012. Evaluating the Alberta throat: An innovation to support the acquisition of more clinically applicable aerosol aerodynamic particle size distribution (APSD) data in oral inhaled product (OIP) development. *Inhalation* 5(1):12–16.

Copley, M., M. Smurthwaite, D.L. Roberts, and J.P. Mitchell. 2005. Revised internal volumes to those provided by Mitchell JP and Nagel MW in cascade impactors for the size characterization of aerosols from medical inhalers: Their uses and limitations. *J Aerosol Med* 18(3):364–366.

Crompton, G.K. 1982. Problems patients have using pressurized aerosol inhalers. *Eur J Respir Dis* Suppl.119:101–104.

Crompton, G.K., P.J. Barnes, M. Broeders et al. 2006. The need to improve inhalation technique in Europe: A report from the aerosol drug management improvement team. *Respir Med* 2006;100(9):1479–1494.

Dalby, R., M. Spallek, and T. Voshaar. 2004. A review of the development of Respimat® Soft Mist™ inhaler. *Int J.Pharm* 283(1–2):1–9.

Daniels, G.E., and M. Hamilton. 2011. Assessment of early screening methodology using the reduced next generation and fast screening impactor systems. *Respiratory Drug Delivery-Europe 2011*, Eds. Dalby, R.N., Byron, P.R., Peart, J., Suman, J.D., and Young, P.M. 327–330. River Grove, IL: Davis Healthcare International Publishing.

Delvadia, R., L.P. Worth, and P. Byron. 2012. *In vitro* tests for aerosol deposition I: Scaling a physical model of upper airways to predict drug deposition variation in normal humans. *J Aerosol Med Pulmon Drug Deliv* 25(1):32–40.

Dennis, J.H. 2007. Nebulizer efficiency: Modeling versus *in vitro* testing. *Respir Care* 52(8):984–988.

Dennis, J., E. Berg, D. Sandell et al. 2008. Cooling the NGI: An approach to size a nebulised aerosol more accurately. *Pharm Europa Sci Notes* 2008(1):27–30.

Dennis, J.H., C.A. Pieron, and O. Nerbrink. 2000. Standards in assessing in vitro nebulizer performance. *Eur Resp Rev* 10-72:178–182.

Dolovich, M.B., R.C. Ahrens, D.R. Hess et al. 2005. Device selection and outcomes of aerosol therapy: Evidence-based guidelines. *Chest* 127(1):335–371.

Dolovich, M., N.R. MacIntyre, P.J. Anderson et al. 2000. Consensus statement: Aerosols and delivery devices. *Respir Care* 45(6):589–596.

Dolovich, M.B., and J.P. Mitchell. 2004. Canadian standards association standard CAN/CSA/Z264.1-02:2002: A new voluntary standard for spacers and holding chambers used with pressurized metered-dose inhalers. *Can Respir J* 11(7):489–495.

Dunbar, C.A., and A.J. Hickey. 2000. Evaluation of probability density functions to approximate particle size distributions of representative pharmaceutical inhalers. *J Aerosol Sci* 31(7):813–831.

Dunbar, C., and J.P. Mitchell. 2005. Analysis of cascade impactor mass distributions. *J Aerosol Med* 18(4):439–451.

Esmen, N.A., and T.C. Lee. 1980. Distortion of cascade impactor measured size distribution due to bounce and blow-off. *Am Ind Hyg Assoc J* 41(6):410–419.

European Directorate for Quality in Medicines (EDQM). 2018a. *European Pharmacopeia 9.0, monograph 2.9.18. Preparations for inhalations: Aerodynamic assessment of fine particles.* Strasburg, France: EDQM.

European Directorate for Quality in Medicines (EDQM). 2018b. *European Pharmacopeia 9.0, Monograph 2.9.44. Preparations for Nebulization.* Strasburg, France: EDQM. 2017

European Medicines Agency (EMA). 2006. Guideline on the pharmaceutical quality of inhalation and nasal products. EMEA/CHMP/QWP/49313/2005 Corr. 2006. http://www.ema.europa.eu/docs/en_GB/document_library/Scientific_guideline/2009/09/WC500003568.pdf Accessed September 1, 2017.

European Medicines Agency (EMA). 2009. Requirements for clinical documentation for orally inhaled products (OIP) including the requirements for demonstration of therapeutic equivalence between two inhaled products for use in the treatment of asthma and chronic obstructive pulmonary disease (COPD) in adults and for use in the treatment of asthma in children and adolescents. London, UK. CPMP/EWP/4151/00 Rev. 1, 2009. Available at URL: http://www.ema.europa.eu/docs/en_GB/document_library/Scientific_guideline/2009/09/WC500003504.pdf Accessed June 20, 2018.

European Committee for Standardization (CEN). 2009. European Standard CSN-EN. Respiratory therapy equipment - Part 1: Nebulizing systems and their components. BS EN 13544-1:2007+A1:2009. British Standards Institute. London, UK. https://shop.bsigroup.com/ProductDetail/?pid=000000000030189969.

Finlay, W.H. 1998. Inertial sizing of aerosol inhaled during pediatric tidal breathing from an MDI with attached holding chamber. *Int J Pharm* 168(2):147–152.

Forbes, B., P. Bäckman, D. Christopher et al. 2015. *In vitro* testing for orally inhaled products: Developments in science-based regulatory approaches. *AAPS J* 17(4):837–852.

Foss, S.A., and J.W. Keppel. 1999. *In vitro* testing of MDI spacers: A technique for measuring respirable dose output with actuation in-phase or out-of-phase with inhalation. *Respir Care* 44(12):1474–1485.

Galván, C.A., and J.C. Guarderas. 2012. Practical considerations for dysphonia caused by inhaled corticosteroids. *Mayo Clin Proc* 87(9):901–904.

Gard, E.E., V.I. Riot, K.R. Coffee et al. 2008. Pressure flow reducer for aerosol focusing devices. U.S. Patent 7,361,891. Lawrence Livermore National Security, LLC, CA.

Golshahi, L., and W.H. Finlay. 2012. An idealized child throat that mimics average pediatric oropharyngeal deposition. *Aerosol Sci Technol* 46(5):i–iv.

Grgic, B., A.F. Heenan, P.K.P. Burnell et al. 2004. *In vitro* intersubject and intrasubject preposition measurements in realistic mouth-throat geometries. *J Aerosol Sci* 35(8):1025–1040.

Griffiths, W.D., P.J. Iles, and N.P. Vaughan. 1986. The behavior of liquid droplets in an APS3300. *J Aerosol Sci* 17(6):921–930.

Hallworth, G.W., and D.G. Westmoreland. 1987. The twin impinger: A simple device for assessing the delivery of drugs from metered dose pressurized aerosol inhalers. *J Pharm Pharmacol.* 39(12): 966–972.

Harris, J., S.W. Stein, and P.B. Myrdal. 2006. Evaluation of the TSI aerosol impactor 3306/3321 system using a redesigned impactor stage with solution and suspension metered-dose inhalers. *AAPS PharmSciTech* 7(1): Article 20. available at: www.ncbi.nlm.nih.gov/pmc/articles/PMC2750727/pdf/12249_2008_Article_710138.pdf visited September 27, 2017.

Haynes, A., M.S. Shaik, H. Krarup et al. 2004. Evaluation of the malvern spraytec with inhalation cell for the measurement of particle size distribution from metered dose inhalers. *J Pharm Sci* 93(2):349–363.

Health Canada. 2006. Pharmaceutical quality of inhalation and nasal products. https://www.canada.ca/en/health-canada/services/drugs-health-products/drug-products/applications-submissions/guidance-documents/chemical-entity-products-quality/guidance-industry-pharmaceutical-quality-inhalation-nasal-products.html. Accessed September 1, 2017.

Hess, D.R. 2000. Nebulizers: Principles and performance. *Respir Care* 45(6):609–622

Heyder, J., J. Gebhart, G. Rudolf, C.F. Schiller, and W. Stahlhofen. 1986. Deposition of particles in the human respiratory tract in the size range 0.005–15 μm. *J Aerosol Sci.* 17(5):811–825.

Heyder, J., and M.U. Svartengren. 2002. Basic principles of particle behavior in the human respiratory tract. In *Drug Delivery to the Lung*, eds. H. Bisgaard, C. O'Callaghan, and G.C. Smaldone. 21–45. New York: Marcel Dekker.

Hinds, W.C. 1999. *Properties, Behavior, and Measurement of Airborne Particles*, Second Edition, New York: Wiley-Interscience.

(Annals of the) International Commission on Radiological Protection (ICRP). 1994. *Human Respiratory Tract Model for Radiological Protection.* Tarrytown, NY: Pergamon Press (Elsevier Science).

International Standards Organization (ISO). 1998. *Representation of Results of Particle Size Analysis—Part 1: Graphical Representation.* ISO 9276-1. Geneva, Switzerland. https://www.iso.org/standard/25860.html. Visited June 20 2018.

International Standards Organization (ISO). 1999. *Particle Size Analysis—Laser Diffraction Methods: General Principles.* ISO 13320-1: Geneva, Switzerland. https://www.iso.org/standard/21706.html. Visited June 20 2018.

International Standards Organization (ISO). 2013. *Anaesthetic and Respiratory Equipment—Nebulizing Systems and Components.* ISO 24727. Geneva, Switzerland. https://www.iso.org/standard/59482.html. Visited June 20 2018.

Jetzer, M.W., B.D. Morrical, D.P. Fergensen et al. 2017. Particle interactions of fluticasone propionate and salmeterol xinafoate detected with single particle aerosol mass spectrometry (SPAMS). *Int J Pharm* 532(1):218–228.

Jones, S.A., G.P. Martin, and M.B. Brown. 2004. Development of a rapid pre-formulation screen for HFA-suspension metered dose inhalers. *Respiratory Drug Delivery IX.* Eds. Dalby, R.N., Byron, P.R., Peart, J., Suman, J.D., and Farr, S.J. 529–531. River Grove, IL: Davis Healthcare International Publishers.

Keegan, G.M., and D.A. Lewis. 2012. Formulation-dependent effects on aerodynamic particle size measurements using the Fast Screening Andersen (FSA). *Respiratory Drug Delivery 2012*, Eds. Dalby, R.N., Byron, P.R., Peart, J., Suman, J.D., and Young, P.M. 465–468. River Grove, IL: Davis Healthcare International Publishing.

Krarup, H.G., and P.G. Kippax. 2004. Rapid screening of dry powder inhalers by laser diffraction. *Respiratory Drug Delivery IX.* Eds. Dalby, R.N., Byron, P.R., Peart, J., Suman, J.D. and Farr, S.J. 541–544. River Grove, IL: Davis Healthcare International Publishers.

Kwok, P.C.L., and H.-K. Chan. 2005. Electrostatic charge in pharmaceutical systems. *Encyclopedia of Pharmaceutical Technology*, 2nd ed. 1–14. New York: Taylor & Francis.

Kwok, P.C.L., and H.-K. Chan. 2008. Effect of relative humidity on the electrostatic charge properties of dry powder inhaler aerosols. *Pharm Res* 25(2):277–288.

Marple, V.A., and B.Y.H. Liu. 1974. Characteristics of laminar jet impactors. *Environ. Sci. Technol* 8(7): 648–654.

Marple, V.A., D.L. Roberts, F.J. Romay et al. 2003a. Next generation pharmaceutical impactor, part I: Design. *J Aerosol Med* 16 (3):283–299.

Marple, V.A., B.A. Olson, and N.C. Miller. 1995. A low-loss cascade impactor with stage collection cups: Calibration and pharmaceutical inhaler applications. *Aerosol Sci. Technol* 22(1):124–134.

Marple, V.A., B.A. Olson, K. Santhanakrishnan et al. 2003b. Next generation pharmaceutical impactor. Part II: Archival calibration. *J Aerosol Med* 16(3):301–324.

Marple, V.A., B.A. Olson, K. Santhanakrishnan et al. 2004. Next generation pharmaceutical impactor. Part III: Extension of archival calibration to 15 L/min. *J Aerosol Med* 17(4):335–343.

Marple, V.A., and K. Willeke. 1976. Impactor design. *Atmos. Environ* 10:891–896.

Marshall, I.A., J.P. Mitchell, and W.D. Griffiths. 1991. The behavior of regular-shaped, non-spherical particles in a TSI aerodynamic particle sizer. *J Aerosol Sci* 22(1):73–89.

McFarland, A.R., J.B. Wedding, and J.E. Cermak. 1977. Wind tunnel evaluation of a modified Andersen impactor and an all-weather sampler inlet. *Atmos Environ* 11(6):535–539.

McRobbie, D.W., S. Pritchard, and R.A. Quest. 2003. Studies of the human oropharyngeal airspaces using magnetic resonance imaging. I. Validation of a three-dimensional MRI method for producing *ex vivo* virtual and physical casts of the oro-pharyngeal airways during inspiration. *J Aerosol Med* 16(4):401–415.

Melani, A.S., M. Bonavia, V. Cilenti et al. 2011. Inhaler mishandling remains common in real life and is associated with reduced disease control. *Respir Med* 105(6):930–938.

Melani, A.S., P. Canessa, I. Coloretti et al. 2012. Inhaler mishandling is very common in patients with chronic airflow obstruction and long-term home nebulizer use. *Respir Med* 106(5):668–676.

Merkus, H.G. 2009. Particle size, size distributions and shape. In *Particle Size Measurements: Fundamentals, Practice, Quality*, Ed. H.G. Merkus, 13–42. Dordrecht, the Netherlands: Springer.

Miller, N.C. 2002. Apparatus and process for aerosol size measurement at varying gas flow rates. US Patent 6,435,004-B1.

Mitchell, J.P. 2005. Good practices of qualifying cascade impactors (CIs): A survey of members of the European Pharmaceutical Aerosol Group (EPAG). In: *Drug Delivery to the Lungs*, 189–192. Edinburgh, UK: The Aerosol Society.

Mitchell, J.P., and M.W. Nagel. 1999. Time-of-flight aerodynamic particle size analyzers: Their use and limitations for the evaluation of medical aerosols. *J Aerosol Med* 12(4):217–240.

Mitchell, J.P., and M.W. Nagel. 2003. Cascade impactors for the size determination of aerosols from medical inhalers: Their uses and limitations. *J Aerosol Med* 16(3):341–377.

Mitchell, J.P., and M.B. Dolovich. 2012. Clinically relevant test methods to establish *in vitro* equivalence for spacers and valved holding chambers used with pressurized metered dose inhalers (pMDIs). *J Aerosol Med Pulmon Deliv* 25(4):217–242.

Mitchell, J.P., and J.A. Suggett. 2014. Developing ways to evaluate in the laboratory how inhalation devices will be used by patients and care-givers: The need for clinically appropriate testing. *AAPS PharmSciTech* 15(5):1275–1291.

Mitchell, J., R. Bauer, S. Lyapustina et al. 2011a. Non-impactor-based methods for sizing of aerosols emitted from orally inhaled and nasal drug products (OINDPs). *AAPS PharmSciTech* 12(3):965–988.

Mitchell, J.P., M. Copley, Y. Sizer et al. 2012b. Adapting the abbreviated impactor measurement (AIM) concept to make appropriate inhaler aerosol measurements to compare with clinical data: A scoping study with the "Alberta" idealized throat (AIT) inlet. *J Aerosol Med Pulmon Deliv* 25(4):188–197.

Mitchell, J.P., D.P. Coppolo, and M.W. Nagel. 2007 Electrostatics and inhaled medications: Influence on delivery via pressurized metered-dose inhalers and add-on devices. *Respir. Care* 52(3):283–300.

Mitchell, J.P., P.A. Costa, and S. Waters. 1987. An assessment of an Andersen Mark-II cascade impactor. *J Aerosol Sci* 19(2):213–221.

Mitchell, J.P., M.W., Nagel, and A.D. Archer. 1999. Size analysis of a pressurized metered dose inhaler-delivered suspension formulation by an API Aerosizer* time-of-flight aerodynamic particle size analyzer. *J Aerosol Med* 12(4):255–264.

Mitchell, J.P., M.W. Nagel, K.J. Wiersema et al. 2003. Aerodynamic particle size analysis of aerosols from pressurized metered-dose inhalers: Comparison of Andersen 8-stage cascade impactor, Next Generation Pharmaceutical Impactor, and model 3321 aerodynamic particle sizer aerosol spectrometer. *AAPS PharmSciTech* 4:Article 54. available at: www.ncbi.nlm.nih.gov/pmc/articles/PMC2750647/pdf/12249_2008_Article_44425.pdf visited September 27, 2017.

Mitchell, J.P., M.W. Nagel, H. MacKay et al. 2009a. Developing a "universal" valved holding chamber (VHC) platform with added patient benefits whilst maintaining consistent in vitro performance. In *Respiratory Drug Delivery-Europe 2009*, Eds. Dalby, R.N., and Byron, P.R. 383–386. River Grove IL: Davies Healthcare International Publishing.

Mitchell, J.P., M.W. Nagel, V. Avvakoumova et al. 2009b. The abbreviated impactor measurement (AIM) concept: Part 2—influence of evaporation of a volatile component—evaluation with a "droplet producing" pressurized metered dose inhaler (pMDI)-based formulation containing ethanol as co-solvent. *AAPS PharmSciTech* 10(1):252–257.

Mitchell, J.P., M.W. Nagel, S.C. Nichols et al. 2006. Laser diffractometry as a technique for the rapid assessment of aerosol particle size from inhalers. *J Aerosol Med* 19(4):409–433.

Mitchell, J.P., D. Sandell, J Suggett et al. 2017. Proposals for data interpretation in the context of determination of aerodynamic particle size distribution profile for orally inhaled products. *Pharm, Forum.* 43(3): Available on-line at: http://www.usppf.com/pf/pub/index.html visited June 20, 2018.

Mitchell, J.P., J. Suggett, and M. Nagel. 2016. Clinically relevant in vitro testing of orally inhaled products—Bridging the gap between the lab and the patient. *AAPS PharmSciTech* 17(4):787–804.

Mitchell, J., D. Christopher, T. Tougas et al. 2011b. When could efficient data analysis (EDA) fail? Theoretical considerations. *Respiratory Drug Delivery-Europe 2011*, eds. Dalby, R.N., Byron, P.R., Peart, J., Suman, J.D., and Young, P.M. 237–246. River Grove, IL: Davis Healthcare International Publishing.

Mitchell, J.P., T.P. Tougas, J.D. Christopher et al. 2012a. The abbreviated impactor measurement and efficient data analysis concepts: Why use them and when. *Respiratory Drug Delivery 2012. Volume 3.* Eds. Dalby, R.N., Byron, P.R., Peart, J., Farr, S.J., Suman, J.D., and Young, P.M. 731–736. River Grove, IL: Davis Healthcare International Publishing.

Mogalian, E., and P.B. Myrdal. 2005. Application of USP inlet extensions to the TSI impactor system 3306/3320 using HFA 227 based metered dose inhalers. *Drug Dev Ind Pharm* 31(10):977–985.

Mohammed, H., D.L. Roberts, M. Copley et al. 2012. Effect of sampling volume on dry powder inhaler (DPI)-emitted aerosol aerodynamic particle size distributions (APSDs) measured by the Next-Generation pharmaceutical Impactor (NGI) and the Andersen eight-stage Cascade Impactor (ACI). *AAPS Pharm Sci Tech* 13(3):875–882.

Morrical, B.D., M. Balaxi, and D. Fergenson. 2015. The on-line analysis of aerosol-delivered pharmaceuticals via single particle aerosol mass spectrometry. *Int J Pharm* 489(1–2):11–17.

Myrdal, P.B., E. Mogalian, J.P. Mitchell et al. 2006. Application of heated inlet extensions to the TSI 3306/3321 system: Comparison with the Andersen cascade impactor and next generation impactor. *J Aerosol Med* 19(4):543–554.

Nerbrink, O.L., J. Pagels, C.A. Pieron et al. 2003. Effect of humidity on constant output and breath enhanced nebulizer designs when tested in the EN 13544-1 EC standard. *Aerosol Sci Technol* 37(3): 282–292.

Nichols, S.C., D.R. Brown, and M. Smurthwaite. 1998. New concept for the variable flow rate Andersen cascade impactor and calibration data. *J Aerosol Med* 11S1:S133–S138.

Nichols, S.C, J.P. Mitchell, C.M. Shelton et al. 2013. Good Cascade Impactor Practice (GCIP) and considerations for "in-use" specifications. *AAPS PharmSciTechnol* 14(1):375–390.

Nichols, S., D. Sandell, and J. Mitchell. 2016. A multi-laboratory *in vitro* study to compare data from abbreviated and pharmacopeia impactor measurements for orally inhaled products: A report of the European Pharmaceutical Aerosol Group (EPAG). *AAPS PharmSciTech* 17(6):1383–1392.

Noble, C.A., and K.A. Prather. (1998). Single particle characterization of albuterol metered dose inhaler aerosol in near real-time. *Aerosol Sci Technol* 29(4):294–306.

Olson, B.A., V.A. Marple, J.P. Mitchell et al. 1998. Development and calibration of a low-flow version of the Marple-Miller impactor. *Aerosol Sci Technol* 29(4):307–314.

Olsson, B., and L. Asking. 2003. Methods of setting and measuring flow rates in pharmaceutical impactor experiments. *Pharm Forum* 29(3):879–884.

Olsson, B., L. Borgström, H. Lundbäck et al. 2013. Validation of a general *in vitro* approach for prediction of total lung deposition in healthy adults. *J Aerosol Med Pulmon Drug Deliv.* 26(6):355–369.

Pantelides, P.N., H. Bogard, D. Russell-Graham et al. 2011. Investigation into the use of the fast screening impactor as an abbreviated impactor measurement (AIM) tool for dry powder inhalers. *Respiratory Drug Delivery-Europe 2011*, Eds. Dalby, R.N., Byron, P.R., Peart, J., Suman, J.D., and Young, P.M. 391–395. River Grove, IL: Davis Healthcare International Publishing.

Rao, A.K., and K.T. Whitby. 1978a. Non-ideal collection characteristics of inertial impactors—single stage impactors and solid particles. *J Aerosol Sci* 9(1):77–86.

Rao, A.K., and K.T. Whitby. 1978b. Non-ideal collection characteristics of inertial impactors—cascade impactors. *J Aerosol Sci* 9(1):87–100.

Roberts, D.L. 2009. Theory of multi-nozzle impactor stages and the interpretation of stage mensuration data. *Aerosol Sci Technol* 43(11):1119–1129.

Roberts, D.L., and J.P. Mitchell. 2013. The effect of non-ideal cascade impactor stage collection efficiency curves on the interpretation of the size of inhaler-generated aerosols. *AAPS PharmSciTech* 14(2):497–510.

Roberts, D.L., and J.P. Mitchell. 2017. Spatial aerosol flow maldistribution: A design flaw confounding the proper calibration and data interpretation of stages "0" and "1" of the Andersen eight- stage nonviable cascade impactor. *Aerosol Sci Technol* 51(4):409–420.

Rudolph, G., R. Köbrich, and W. Stahlhofen. 1990. Modeling and algebraic formulation of regional aerosol deposition in man. *J Aerosol Sci* 21(S1):S403–S406.

Simons, J.K., and S.W. Stein. 2005. Replacing cascade impactors with labor saving alternatives—making the methods acceptable to the regulators. *Respiratory Drug Delivery Europe-2005*. Eds. Dalby, R.N., Byron, P.R., Peart, J., and Suman, J.D. 19–27. River Grove, IL: Davis Healthcare International Publishers.

Smyth, H.D.C., and A.J. Hickey. 2002. Comparative particle size analysis of solution propellant driven metered dose inhalers using cascade impaction and laser diffraction. *Respiratory Drug Delivery VIII*. Dalby, R.N., Byron, P.R., Peart, J., and Farr, S.J. 731–734. River Grove, IL: Davis Healthcare International Publishers.

Stapleton, K.W., and W.H. Finlay. 1999. Undersizing of droplets from a vented nebulizer caused by aerosol heating during transit through an Andersen impactor. *J Aerosol Sci* 30(1):105–109.

Stapleton, K.W., E. Guentsch, M.K. Hoskinson et al. 2000. On the suitability of K-e turbulence modeling for aerosol deposition in the mouth and throat: A comparison with experiment. *J Aerosol Sci* 31(6):739–749.

Stein, S.W. 2008. Estimating the number of droplets and drug particles emitted from MDIs. *AAPS PharmSciTech* 9(1):112–115.

Svensson, M., E. Berg, J. Mitchell et al. 2018. Laboratory study comparing pharmacopeial testing of nebulizers with evaluation based on Nephele mixing inlet methodology. *AAPS PharmSciTech* 19(2): 565–572.

Swift, D.L. 1992. Apparatus and method for measuring regional distribution of therapeutic aerosols and comparing delivery systems. *J Aerosol Sci* 23(S1):S495–S498.

Swithenbank, J., J.M. Beer, D.S. Taylor et al. 1977. A laser diagnostic technique for the measurement of droplet and particle size distribution. *Prog Astronaut. Aeronaut* 53:421–447.

Tougas, T.P., D. Christopher, J.P. Mitchell et al. 2009. Improved quality control metrics for cascade impaction measurements of orally inhaled drug products (OIPs). *AAPS PharmSciTech* 10(4):1276–1285.

Tougas, T.P., J.D. Christopher, J.P. Mitchell, and S. Lyapustina. 2010. Efficient data analysis and abbreviated impactor measurement concepts. *Respiratory Drug Delivery 2010*, Eds. Dalby, R.N., Byron, P.R., Peart, J., Suman, J.D, Farr, S.J., and Young, P.M. 599–603. River Grove, IL: Davis Healthcare International Publishing.

Tougas, T.P., A.P. Goodey, G. Hardwell, J. Mitchell, and S. Lyapustina. 2017. A comparison of the performance of efficient data analysis versus fine particle dose as metrics for the quality control of aerodynamic particle size distributions of orally inhaled pharmaceuticals. *AAPS PharmSciTech* 18(2):451–461.

Tougas, T.P., D. Christopher, J. Mitchell et al. 2011. Product lifecycle approach to cascade impaction measurements. *AAPS PharmSciTech*. 12(1):312–322.

Tougas, T.P., J.P. Mitchell, and S.A. Lyapustina. 2013. eds. *Good Cascade Impactor Practices, AIM and EDA for Orally Inhaled Products*. New York: Springer.

United States Food and Drug Administration. Center for Drug Evaluation and Research (CDER). 1998. Draft guidance for industry metered dose inhaler (MDI) and dry powder inhaler (DPI) drug products chemistry, manufacturing, and controls documentation. No longer available on-line.

United States Food and Drug Administration. Center for Drug Evaluation and Research (CDER). 2018. Draft guidance for industry metered dose inhaler (MDI) and dry powder inhaler (DPI) drug products chemistry, manufacturing, and controls documentation. Revision 1. https://www.fda.gov/downloads/drugs/guidances/ucm070573.pdf. Accessed December 11, 2018.

US Pharmacopeial Convention. 2018a. United States Pharmacopeia 41/National Formulary 36, Chapter <601> Aerosols, Nasal Sprays, Metered-Dose Inhalers, and Dry Powder Inhalers. Rockville, MD. https://online.uspnf.com/uspnf. Accessed December 11, 2018.

US Pharmacopeial Convention. 2018b. United States Pharmacopeia 41/National Formulary 36, Chapter <1601> Products for Nebulization. Rockville, MD. https://online.uspnf.com/uspnf. Accessed December 11, 2018.

US Pharmacopeial Convention. 2018c. United States Pharmacopeia 39/National Formulary 34, Chapter <1602> Spacers and valved holding chambers used with inhalation aerosols – Characterization tests. Rockville, MD. https://online.uspnf.com/uspnf. Accessed December 11, 2018.

Van de Hulst, H.C. 1981. *Light Scattering by Small Particles*. New York: Dover.

Van Oort, M. 1995. *In vitro* testing of dry powder inhalers. *Aerosol Sci Technol* 22(4):364–373.

Vaughan, N.P. 1989. The Andersen impactor: Calibration, wall losses and numerical simulation. *J Aerosol Sci* 20(1):67–90.

Wheeler, D.J. *EMP III*. 2006. (Evaluating the measurement process): Using imperfect data. Knoxville, TN: SPC Press.

Wilcox, J.D. 1956. Isokinetic sampling. *J Air Pollut Control Assoc* 5(4):226–245.

Wyka, B., T. Tougas, J.P. Mitchell et al. 2007. Comparison of two approaches for treating cascade impaction mass balance measurements. *J. Aerosol Med* 20(3):236–256.

Zhang, Y., W.H. Finlay, and E.A. Matida. 2004. Particle deposition measurements and numerical simulation in a highly-idealized mouth-throat. *J Aerosol Sci* 35(7):789–803.

Zhou, Y., J.J. Sun, and Y.S. Cheng. 2011. Comparison of deposition in the USP and physical mouth-throat models with solid and liquid particles. *J Aerosol Med Pulmon. Drug Deliv* 24(6):277–284.

Section VIII

Regulatory Considerations

25

Scanning the Intricate Regulatory Landscape and Trying to Peek Over the Horizon

Stephen T. Horhota, Stefan Leiner, and Allen Horhota

CONTENTS

25.1 Common Basis, Different Outcomes

A recently published chronology of the history of therapeutic aerosols (Stein and Thiel 2017) examined the major pharmacologic and technology advances related to the delivery of medicinal agents to the lungs. The article only briefly mentions the companion regulatory history which has its own narrative that significantly impacted some of those advances particularly in the discipline of chemistry, manufacturing, and controls (CMC).

Before 1990, there were few governmental regulations or guidances specific to inhalation aerosols, with pharmacopoeial monographs providing most of the direction. The current regulatory landscape for pharmaceutical inhalation products has grown to be frustratingly complex. It is best described as "tribal" with at least a dozen identifiable agencies, standard setting bodies, and scientific groups influencing the present landscape and its future evolution (Horhota and Leiner 2011, Hochhaus et al. 2015). A large measure of this diversity dates to the period 1975–2005 during which United States and European agencies dominated. These regions were the innovative centers for scientific/technological advances in the field and also the economic regions where products were first introduced commercially. Australian and Canadian authorities also had a presence. Since the legal foundation for the regulation of pharmaceutical products in these regions was and remains markedly different (Sifuentes and Giuffrida 2015, Van Norman 2016), each group of regulators adopted separate views on technical requirements to be fulfilled. There were also divergent interpretations of scientific studies leading to dissimilar risk evaluations and judgments about the criticality of various features of product performance and specifications.

This situation was not unique to inhalation products and affected nearly all pharmaceutical products. The excessive financial burden of dealing with so many differing, sometimes conflicting, registration requirements coupled with the general globalization of the pharmaceutical industry prodded cooperation between academics, regulators, and industry to bring about the International Conference on Harmonization (ICH), the synchronization of major pharmacopoeia, international agreement on key quality aspects, and other consolidation initiatives. Strong emphasis was given to orally administered dosage forms, a natural consequence of their preeminence in the pharmaceutical armamentarium.

25.2 Filling the Void

Harmonization for pharmaceutical inhalation aerosols did not attract the same level of attention and thus drew very little research effort, funding, or regulatory collaboration. This unintended prioritization through neglect unfortunately occurred at a critical point in the early 1990s when three significant trends emerged:

- More therapies for asthma, emphysema, chronic obstructive pulmonary disease (COPD), and cystic fibrosis became available
- Patents on the short acting beta-agonist albuterol (salbutamol) expired and generic market opportunities opened up
- Concerns grew about the accelerating morbidity and mortality associated with asthma

In the absence of any coordinated harmonization effort, individual agencies began issuing their own guidances and guidelines as submissions and requests for marketing authorizations began to show up (European Medicines Agency 1993, Food and Drug Administration 1993, 1994). With these guidances came demands for more extensive data on the physical stability of the drug product, uniformity of delivered dose, and aerodynamic particle size distribution (APSD) data using test platforms adapted from environmental monitoring. CMC regulators began to question if impurities and unwanted materials in increasingly utilized inhalation products, especially pressurized metered dose inhalers (pMDIs) might be a contributing factor to the observed morbidity/mortality rise (Schroeder 2005). If so, reducing their levels and generally elevating the quality of inhalation products might have a positive outcome.

Exactly in this timeframe, questions about how to establish bioequivalence for locally acting inhalation aerosol products gained prominence as a consequence of two driving factors. The first was a growing demand for generic substitutes of albuterol chlorofluorocarbon (CFC) pMDI's as already mentioned. The second factor was the need to reformulate equivalents to existing CFC-based products in response to the mandated phase out of CFC propellants according to the 1987 Montreal Protocol. Both fell victim to the lack of valid in vitro and in vivo methods with metrics for assessing bioequivalence (BE) for this class of locally acting drug products.

25.3 The Unanticipated Impact of the Montreal Protocol

Initial investigations into the reformulation of CFC-based pMDIs showed that the problem was more than just a simple substitution of propellants having a lower ozone depleting potential. Compatibility issues meant that all components in the system, i.e. valves, elastomers, canisters, mouthpieces, excipients, and suspending agents needed to be addressed. The 1987 Montreal Protocol called for the elimination of CFC propellants by January 1996 although orally inhaled MDI products were exempt from this ban until medically acceptable alternatives became available. Facing the uncertain timing as to when high purity CFCs would no longer be available, hundreds of scientists, engineers, analysts, and technicians across industry and academia were mobilized to investigate these problems and identify solutions. Many companies which were at this same time developing new compounds for the treatment of respiratory diseases, chose the pathway of dry powder inhalation as the delivery technology hoping to avoid the mounting perils of using the replacement hydrofluoroalkanes (HFA). Into the mix came other innovators who sought to exploit the lung as a systemic delivery portal, with insulin being the forefront candidate.

Additionally, analytical method technologies with dramatically lowered limits of detection and quantitation were applied in the investigation of new in vitro models for pulmonary airways, resulting in novel, sometimes surprising, insights into inhaled particle behavior.

25.4 Devices Bring Their Own Divisiveness

Medical device technologies also began their intrusion into the pharmaceutical world with a whole host of options for generating liquid and powder aerosols, improving lung deposition efficiency, and attempts to address patient compliance or errors due to incorrect device usage. This exacerbated the dual identity problem of orally inhaled products (OIP) because they possess features of both pharmaceutical objects and medical devices. Historically, this regulatory review problem was solved by classifying the device elements as adjuncts to the formulation or an extension of packaging. This framework became increasingly stressed as the device portion and delivery mechanics of inhalation products grew in sophistication. The concomitant growth of the medical device industry spawned its own regulatory structures, again dominated by United States (US) and European Union (EU) agencies, to deal with risks and their management (Van Norman 2016). The conflicting overlap of technical drug and device issues and the matter of jurisdictional priority was partially resolved by defining a separate class known as "combination products" in the US or "borderline products" in EU that would borrow regulatory direction from both domains and identify where approval authority would reside (Food and Drug Administration 1991, European Commission DG Enterprise and Industry 2010). This partially solved some problems while adding new ones to the confusing landscape of regulatory processes.

25.5 Shortcomings of the Pharmacopoeial System, Diverging Risk Assessments, and Consequences

The explosion in new scientific and technical data disrupted the established risk management and quality control paradigms based on pharmacopoeial standards which were slow to respond and did so in an uncoordinated manner. As pharmacopeia focus on quality control questions and are not regulating development or bioequivalence aspects, regulatory agencies continued to find it necessary to proceed independently. US and EU regulators followed different pathways in defining critical test parameters, sample sizes, determination of specification limits, and elaborating the types of information to be included in submissions. Their methods of communicating requirements also differed.

FDA's concerns and ideas were initially conveyed via two routes. Publicly, this was done through presentations at various meetings/symposia that proliferated to meet the onslaught of new research findings. Out of public view, comments were also sent to individual companies as a part of licensing application reviews. As these individual responses principally dealt with proprietary issues, there was not a strong desire by the sponsors to share the information publicly. It wasn't until late 1998 that the FDA formally documented its general recommendations on technical requirements for materials, components, and performance testing in a draft guidance (Food and Drug Administration 1998). As recommendations, these were not official requirements, but became the de facto framework for chemistry, manufacturing, and control modules in US submissions. There were a number of criticisms of the draft guidelines citing a high degree of empiricism in the content, heavy emphasis on end product testing, and lack of flexibility towards alternative testing/control approaches. It is of interest to note that the 1998 FDA guidance, while having significant impact, was never converted to a formal guideline. In early 2018, the FDA issued an update to the draft guidance (Food and Drug Administration 2018). The core content of the new document dealing with required information and data to be submitted in drug applications remains largely unchanged. It does acknowledge that MDI and dry powder inhalation products (DPIs) are combination products, meaning that elements of 21 CFR 820 governing Quality Systems for medical devices, design controls in particular, are now formal requirements. It also states that Good Manufacturing Practices extend to components and constituent parts of the final product.

Simultaneously, EU regulators re-examined the topics of test parameters, sample sizes, and specification limits, but took a less prescriptive approach to risk management and product control. The EU position reflected the stronger legal standing of the pharmacopoeia in that region and the different structure for the regulation of pharmaceutical products and medical devices compared to the US. Additionally, the EU position highlighted differences in risk assessment and the resulting ways to control such risks compared to the FDA. One of the first cooperative efforts to harmonize inhalation aerosol requirements came about with the 2006 joint guideline on "the pharmaceutical quality of inhalation and nasal products" from EMA and Health Canada (European Medicines Agency 2006). This guideline remains substantially unchanged after more than a decade.

The lack of consensus among the major regulatory authorities and the uncertainty this created for the industry prompted a number of companies to join together forming the International Pharmaceutical Aerosol Consortium on Regulation and Science (IPAC-RS) (International Pharmaceutical Aerosol Consortium on Regulation and Science 2018). The goal was to objectively advance the science of orally inhaled and nasal drug products (OINDP) by collecting and analyzing data as well as conducting joint research and development projects. The consortium is managed by a legal firm that allowed companies to share information in a way that protected proprietary content while permitting them to exchange technical data in a manner that avoided violation of anti-trust regulations. This body was modeled after a similar consortium (International Pharmaceutical Aerosol Consortium 1999) formed to support the toxicological qualification of the HFA series of alternate propellants for industry-wide use in inhalation aerosols. In the EU, a similar expert group, the European Pharmaceutical Aerosol Group (Mitchell 2007) formed primarily to offer opinion and input to regulators in that region. Initiatives from these groups helped bring about consensus approaches on the management of leachables and extractables associated with components (Product Quality Research Institute Leachables and Extractables Working Group 2006), recommendations on supply chain management of components (International Pharmaceutical Aerosol Consortium on Regulation and Science 2017), specific requirements and guidance for Good Manufacturing Practice relating to the manufacture of packaging materials for medicinal products (Pharmaceutical Quality Group 2016), and minimizing variability in aerodynamic particle size measurement (Bonam et al. 2008), all of which have become accepted practices in the field. Proposals on uniform requirements/specifications for Uniformity of Delivered Dose (Novick et al. 2009a, 2009b, Larner et al. 2011) have been incorporated into the 2018 FDA MDI/DPI guidance. The situation with aerodynamic particle size distribution lags behind considerably because there are currently seven different apparatus configurations listed in the pharmacopoeia each providing different views onto the size distribution produced by the same inhalation product. In these latter two cases, this lack of consensus among the major regulatory authorities in the identification of specific risks of inhalation products, in the assessment of their criticalities, and in the identification of suitable control metrics means that uncertainty and confusion will continue to exist for some time to come.

25.6 Unequal Views on Bioequivalence

Bioequivalence, or, more broadly, product interchange/substitution re-emerged as a key issue around 2007 and continues to the present time. As mentioned earlier, there was a rise in activity on this topic in the early 1990s associated with the patent expiry of albuterol (salbutamol). There were two main presentations of albuterol at the time, namely, aqueous solution for nebulization and CFC-based pressurized metered dose inhaler. A number of competitors appeared with solutions for nebulization since there was no in vivo BE study required for a solution formulation. There were few entrants for pMDI due to the lack of trustworthy in vitro/in vivo correlations and definitive clinical protocols that could be carried out using 30 or fewer subjects. Furthermore, the uncertainty in the future availability of CFCs put generic developers in a very tenuous business position of risking considerable effort and resources on a product that would face registration difficulties or in the end they would be unable to procure propellant. Adding to the conundrum, originator companies uncovered new patent opportunities through their investigative work on HFA formulations for pMDIs or new powder inhalation formulations/ devices. It wasn't until this second layer of patent protections expired in the mid 2000s that bioequivalence regained regulatory prominence.

The success of the biopharmaceutical classification system (BCS) and correlating in vitro testing to in vivo outcomes lowered the barriers for establishing bioequivalence and qualification of orally and topically administered generic products. This brought hope that the same could be achieved for inhalation aerosols if only proper in vitro metrics and analysis platforms could be identified (Hastedt et al. 2016). Despite an expansion in the number and type of aerodynamic particle size methods, anatomically representative throat/airway models, and physiologically relevant airflow generators, broadly applicable quantitative or qualitative correlations are not at hand although there have been some promising reports (Olsson et al. 2013).

The US FDA is legally required to actively encourage opportunities that increase the presence of generic competitors without compromising patient risk. In the face of yet to be resolved science, the agency has taken what it calls "the weight of evidence" approach for judging bioequivalence of DPI products (Lee et al. 2009). It is a multifactorial view that posits that if a wide range of criteria can be fulfilled, the risks of bio-inequivalence are sufficiently managed. This approach has been augmented by issuance of drug-specific guidances (e.g. [Food and Drug Administration 2017b]) for locally acting inhalation drug products that require: (1) statistically supported comparison of in vitro analyses, (2) blood or plasma bioequivalence, and (3) pharmacodynamic equivalence between test and reference products. Population-based statistical metrics are demanded. There is also a requirement to show that device appearance, operation, and patient handling are similar enough to permit free and indistinguishable substitution between innovator and generic. For inhalation products where the goal is systemic delivery, no guidances have been issued, but would presumably require in vitro equivalence, pharmacokinetic (PK) bioequivalence, and operational/handling equivalence only.

In the EU, the legal and risk management framework does not require simultaneous demonstration of equivalence in all three areas, but directs a sequential approach through in vitro, pharmacokinetic, and pharmacodynamic protocols, respectively (European Medicines Agency 2009). The statistical evaluations are focused on comparison of mean values. Under this system, it is possible to gain regulatory approval based upon comparative in vitro testing only, but this seems to be rarely done for fear of application rejection because of the uncertainty surrounding the in vivo relevance of existing test models.

25.7 New Entrants to the Regulatory Picture

It does not appear that the differences in scientific and technical opinions or requirements between US and EU authorities will be resolved soon. This has created an interesting situation for many countries with expanding economies and unmet health care needs in their populations. The growing incidence of pulmonary disease worldwide (Forum of International Respiratory Societies 2013) is one of the areas where societies struggle to balance accessibility to and affordability of inhalation therapies. Two countries where this is most evident are Brazil and China. Both are in the process of reconfiguring their health agencies to improve product review and approval processes and meet legislative demands for stronger patient safeguards including enhanced quality standards. They are judiciously evaluating the US and EU regulatory positions and selectively adopting the most suitable and supported ones. This is nicely illustrated in a comparison of BE requirements between US, EU, Brazil, and China (Lee et al. 2015).

While it is eminently logical to integrate the most up to date scientific information to formulate their country-specific requirements, it does add another layer of complexity to the already convoluted regulatory landscape. There is less dissention with regard to supply chain control strategy approaches with both the Brazilian Health Regulatory Agency (ANVISA) and the Chinese FDA (CFDA) appearing to have accepted the PQRI consensus positions on leachables and extractables (Product Quality Research Institute Leachables and Extractables Working Group 2006).

25.8 Where Might We Be Headed?

If past becomes prologue, what then are the current forces that are shaping the next 10 years of regulatory evolution for pharmaceutical inhalation products? Many of the trends are the same ones driving the global pharmaceutical industry overall:

- Massively improved data collection, analysis, and connectivity augmented by expanded use of artificial intelligence and self-learning algorithms to accelerate device design, formulation development, and improve clinical outcomes.

There has been some interesting progress in the last few years on the use of computational fluid dynamics (CFD) to understand and optimize device performance coupled with rapid prototyping of design concepts for delivery devices (Ruzycki et al. 2013). Since the same tools can easily be applied to the evaluation and design of test platforms especially APSD (Dechraksa et al. 2014) that incorporate a stronger physiological basis, further advancements that narrow the in vitro/in vivo correlation gap should be expected in this field.

The "Internet of things" continues reaching into aerosol technology with ideas to connect delivery devices through wireless networks or smartphones (Monroe 2017). Such configurations have the potential to monitor patient compliance, assess patient lung function and patient inhalation technique more readily, and adjust dosing amount/frequency/aerosol particle size. The adjustments could be made remotely by a supervising health care provider or arrived at by artificial intelligence (AI) algorithms crunching information on potential triggers of asthma attacks, i.e. local weather, pollen counts, indices of atmospheric pollution, exertion level, etc. All the technology to achieve this is available, but the current costs can be prohibitive, although these should decrease with time and advances in sensing and manufacturing technologies. Insurers and health care payers are also asking for study data that demonstrate a treatment benefit of the technology before agreeing to reimbursement. Expansions in the use of the technologies in clinical investigation phases are occurring now and will be the proving ground leading up to more widespread use in general populations. The regulatory issues to be addressed will mainly be extensions of medical device requirements that we deal with today such as sensor reliability/validation, adjustable dosing control, data integrity, failure mode analysis, human factors engineering, hacking threats, personal data security (Lyapustina and Armstrong 2018), and fail-safe options in case the device does not function properly in an emergency situation. With this, it should be expected that the ongoing discussion as to how combination products can be defined and which regulatory framework (drug or device) predominates will grow even deeper and more confusing.

- Advances from basic research that accelerate the shift towards personalized medicine and individually tailored treatments which improve treatment success rate.

There are at present a number of interpretations of the term "personalized medicine" (Food and Drug Administration 2013). In its most common context, personalized medicine, or precision medicine, encompasses the use of specific genome information from an individual to diagnose then target or alter a disease condition. A lot of effort is currently concentrated on cancer treatment where the problems of non-specific biodistribution, poor water solubility, limited bioavailability, and rapid clearance must be overcome. Nanoparticles, including liposomes/lipid vesicles with tuned size and surface characteristics to passively or actively deliver anti-cancer drugs to tumor cells are the most common approaches being used in the search for solutions. The pulmonary portal remains attractive as a delivery route for local or systemic targets following precedents set by a number of biologic entities (Morales et al. 2017). The regulatory issues surrounding the device and performance requirements are probably not going to be much different than presently encountered. There may be some special designs or technologies that need to be employed to generate aerosols that do not denature or degrade sensitive biologic therapeutics or significantly alter the function and efficacy of the formulation or delivery vehicle. This will be especially critical where intracellular delivery is necessary and complex formulation approaches are applied to overcome biological barriers to inhaled gene therapy as in the case of gene therapy (Kim et al. 2016). The greatest regulatory barrier is likely to be connected with formulation components that have not been evaluated for local pulmonary safety or qualified toxicologically for long-term use in humans. The fact that many of these formulation materials are already being used in injectable preparations suggests that the overall risks will be low, but the appropriate studies still need to be performed at considerable investment. It is conceivable to see specialty companies in the field forming consortia and jointly sponsoring qualification studies on critical components similar to what was done for HFA propellants.

Within the scope of pharmaceutical inhalation, personalized medicine also encompasses concerns about human factors and minimizing patient administration errors that are a large part of the failure mode picture for these products. FDA and EU regulators have been bringing more focus to this area with recent guidelines or guidances (Food and Drug Administration 2016, Medicines and Healthcare Products Regulatory Agency 2017) that make human factor evaluations mandatory. In 2017, the FDA announced that a proposed generic inhalation product must have comparable human factors test results to the innovator in order to be judged bioequivalent (Food and Drug Administration 2017a). This guideline makes direct reference to pharmaceutical inhalation aerosols as combination products as does the 2018 FDA MDI/DPI guidance, a further signal of regulatory complexity.

- The general desire to drive down drug prices, maintain high-quality levels, and improve accessibility through more rapid approvals of generic drugs.

Patents on a number of therapeutically important respiratory drugs have already or are set to expire shortly with the anticipation that competitors will enter the marketplace resulting in lower pricing. However, regional differences on criteria for evaluating bioequivalence and lack of confidence in in vitro comparisons means that clinical assessment is still needed which naturally increases developmental costs. This potentially limits the extent to which final price reductions can be realized. This will put pressure on regulators to come to some resolution towards harmonization. Until the pressure becomes great enough to drive political action, individual countries will pursue independent pathways, further adding to the thick web of global regulatory requirements.

Insuring quality and consistent performance with inhalation products has always been a challenge because of the number of possible chemical and physical failure modes involving both the drug substance and the mechanical features of the delivery device. This generates a large number of critical quality attributes (CQA) and test parameters that must be measured with each batch of manufactured product. There have been some advances in end product test automation, but widespread deployment seems to be limited. Principles of Quality by Design (QbD) and process analytical technology (PAT) offered up initially by the FDA and later incorporated into the framework of ICH Q8, Q9, Q11 as a way to reduce regulatory and testing burden would appear to be well suited for application to inhalation products. However, they remain largely unexploited. Morton (2011) has suggested that for DPIs, QbD implementation in its true sense remains out of reach. This is certainly an opportunity area for inhaled products, but elements of design control taken from the medical device industry or ISO 20072 probably offer a better pathway to improving efficiency than the pharmaceutical QbD models (de Kruijf et al. 2015). The 2018 FDA MDI/DPI Guidance does acknowledge that upstream controls can be substituted for direct end product testing with appropriate justification and validation.

25.9 Conclusion

The advancing scientific and medical environment for inhalation therapy has also transformed the regulatory sphere making the arena for chemistry, manufacturing, and control aspects very convoluted. That regulatory structure for pulmonary delivery systems has been built up from a variety of guidances, official regulations, compendia, and public standards which categorize these systems as drug products rather than medical devices. This structure borrows heavily from older delivery technologies and struggles to keep up with rapidly evolving innovations which blur the domains of pharmaceuticals and medical devices. Bioequivalence issues will dominate discussion and regulatory activity over the next 5–7 years and possibly beyond. Closely behind will be the necessity for specialized guidances and regulations to deal with inhaled administration of vaccines, gene therapies, insulin, cannabinoids, and antibiotics.

ACKNOWLEDGMENTS

The authors wish to thank Dr. Svetlana Lyapustina and Dr. Lee Nagao of the International Pharmaceutical Aerosol Consortium on Regulation and Science for their contributions of background information.

REFERENCES

Bonam, M., D. Christopher, D. Cipolla et al. 2008. "Minimizing variability of cascade impaction measurements in inhalers and nebulizers." *AAPS PharmSciTech* 9: 404. Accessed June 4, 2018. doi:10.1208/s12249-008-9045-9.

de Kruijf, W., M. Wilby, P. Swanbury, and A. Dundon. 2015. "QbD for inhaler devices." *IPAC-RS*. Accessed June 8, 2018. https://ipacrs.org/assets/uploads/outputs/06_-de_Kruijf_Presentation.pdf.

Dechraksa, J., T. Suwandecha, K. Maliwan et al. 2014. "The comparison of fluid dynamics parameters in an Andersen cascade impactor equipped with and without a preseparator." *AAPS PharmSciTech* 15: 792. doi:10.1208/s12249-014-0102-2.

European Commission DG Enterprise and Industry. 2010. "Medical devices guidance document: Borderline products, drug-delivery products and medical devices incorporating, as an integral part, an ancillary medicinal substance or an ancillary human blood derivative." *MEDDEV 2. 1/3 rev 3.* Accessed June 4, 2018. https://ec.europa.eu/docsroom/documents/10328/attachments/1/translations/en/renditions/pdf.

European Medicines Agency. 1993. "Draft guidance on replacement of chlorofluorocarbons (CFC) in metered dose inhalation products." Accessed June 4, 2018. http://www.ema.europa.eu/docs/en_GB/document_library/Scientific_guideline/2009/09/WC500003559.pdf.

European Medicines Agency. 2006. "Guideline on the pharmaceutical quality of inhalation and nasal products." Committee for Medicinal Products for Human Use. Accessed June 4, 2018. http://www.ema.europa.eu/docs/en_GB/document_library/Scientific_guideline/2009/09/WC500003568.pdf.

European Medicines Agency. 2009. "Guideline on the requirements for clinical documentation for orally inhaled products (OIP) including the requirements for demonstration of therapeutic equivalence between two inhaled products for use in the treatment of asthma and chronic obstructive pulm." Accessed June 8, 2018. http://www.ema.europa.eu/docs/en_GB/document_library/Scientific_guideline/2009/09/WC500003504.pdf.

Food and Drug Administration. 1991. *Intercenter Agreement Between the Center for Drug Evaluation and Research and the Center for Devices and Radiological Health.* Accessed June 4, 2018. https://www.fda.gov/CombinationProducts/JurisdictionalInformation/ucm121177.htm.

Food and Drug Administration. 1993. "Reviewer guidance for nebulizers, metered dose inhalers, spacers and actuators." Accessed June 4, 2018. https://www.fda.gov/downloads/MedicalDevices/DeviceRegulationandGuidance/GuidanceDocuments/ucm081293.pdf.

Food and Drug Administration. 1994. "Interim guidance for documentation of in vivo bioequivalence of albuterol aerosols (metered-dose inhalers)." Publication No. 1-27, Division of Bioequivalence, Office of Generic Drugs, Rockville, MD.

Food and Drug Administration. 1998. *Guidance for Industry Metered Dose Inhaler (MDI) and Dry Powder Inhaler (DPI) Drug Products Chemistry, Manufacturing, and Controls Documentation.* Accessed June 4, 2018. https://wayback.archive-it.org/7993/20170405182634/https://www.fda.gov/ohrms/dockets/ac/00/backgrd/3634b1c_sectiond.pdf.

Food and Drug Administration. 2013. "Paving the way for personalized medicine." Accessed June 8, 2018. http://wayback.archive-it.org/7993/20180125110554/https://www.fda.gov/downloads/ScienceResearch/SpecialTopics/PrecisionMedicine/UCM372421.pdf.

Food and Drug Administration. 2016. "Draft guidancessss Human factors studies and related clinical study considerations for combination product design and development." Accessed June 8, 2018. https://www.fda.gov/downloads/regulatoryinformation/guidances/ucm484345.pdf.

Food and Drug Administration. 2017a. "Draft guidance—Comparative analyses and related comparative use human factors studies for a drug-device combination product submitted in an ANDA." Accessed June 8, 2018. https://www.fda.gov/downloads/Drugs/GuidanceComplianceRegulatoryInformation/Guidances/UCM536959.pdf.

Food and Drug Administration. 2017b. "Draft guidance on glycopyrrolate inhalation powder." Accessed June 8, 2018. https://www.fda.gov/downloads/Drugs/GuidanceComplianceRegulatoryInformation/Guidances/UCM566418.pdf.

Food and Drug Administration. 2018. *Guidance for Industry Metered Dose Inhaler (MDI) and Dry Powder Inhaler (DPI) Products—Quality Considerations.* Accessed June 4, 2018. https://www.fda.gov/downloads/drugs/guidancecomplianceregulatoryinformation/guidances/ucm070573.pdf.

Forum of International Respiratory Societies. 2013. *Respiratory diseases in the World Realities of Today—Opportunities for Tomorrow.* Sheffield, UK: European Respiratory Society. Accessed June 8, 2018. https://www.ersnet.org/pdf/publications/firs-world-report.pdf.

Hastedt, J. M., P. Bäckman, A. R. Clark et al. 2016. "Scope and relevance of a pulmonary biopharmaceutical classification system." *AAPS Open* 2: 1. doi:10.1186/s41120-015-0002-x.

Hochhaus, G., M. Davis-Cutting, M. Oliver, S. L. Lee, and S. Lyapustina. 2015. "Regulatory considerations for approval of generic inhalation drug products in the US, EU, Brazil, China, and India." *AAPS Journal* 17: 1285. doi:10.1208/s12248-015-9791-z.

Horhota, S. T., and S. Leiner. 2011. "Developing performance specifications for pulmonary products." In *Controlled Pulmonary Drug Delivery*, edited by H.D.C. Smyth and A. J. Hickey, pp. 529–541. New York: Springer.

International Pharmaceutical Aerosol Consortium. 1999. *United Nations Framework Convention on Climate Change.* Accessed June 4, 2018. https://unfccc.int/files/methods/other_methodological_issues/interactions_with_ozone_layer/application/pdf/ipacat2.pdf.

International Pharmaceutical Aerosol Consortium on Regulation and Science. 2017. "Recommended baseline requirements for materials used in orally inhaled and nasal drug products (OINDP)." *IPAC-RS.* Accessed June 4, 2018. https://ipacrs.org/assets/uploads/outputs/Baseline_Requirements_for_OINDP_%289_Feb_2017%29.pdf.

International Pharmaceutical Aerosol Consortium on Regulation and Science. 2018. *IPAC-RS.* Accessed June 4, 2018. https://ipacrs.org/.

Kim, N., G. A. Duncan, J. Hanes, and J. S. Suk. 2016. "Barriers to inhaled gene therapy of obstructive lung diseases: A review." *Journal of Controlled Release* (Elsevier) 240: 465–488. doi:10.1016/j.jconrel.2016.05.031.

Larner, G., A. Cooper, S. Lyapustina et al. 2011. "Challenges and opportunities in implementing the FDA default parametric tolerance interval two one-sided test for delivered dose uniformity of orally inhaled products." *AAPS PharmSciTech* 12: 1144. doi:10.1208/s12249-011-9683-1.

Lee, S. L., W. P. Adams, B. V. Li, D. P. Connor, B. A. Chowdhury, and L. X. Yu. 2009. "In vitro considerations to support bioequivalence of locally acting drugs in dry powder inhalers for lung diseases." *AAPS Journal* 11: 414–423. doi:10.1208/s12248-009-9121-4.

Lee, S. L., B. Saluja, A. García-Arieta et al. 2015. "Regulatory considerations for approval of generic inhalation drug products in the US, EU, Brazil, China, and India." *AAPS Journal* 17: 1285. doi:10.1208/s12248-015-9787-8.

Lyapustina, S., and K. Armstrong. 2018. "Regulatory considerations for cybersecurity and data privacy in digital health and medical applications and products." *Inhalation* (CSC Publishing) 12 (1): 16–23. Accessed June 8, 2018. https://www.inhalationmag.com/wp-content/uploads/pdf/inh_20180201_0016.pdf.

Medicines and Healthcare Products Regulatory Agency. 2017. "Human factors and usability engineering—Guidance for medical devices including drug-device combination products." Accessed June 8, 2018. https://www.gov.uk/government/uploads/system/uploads/attachment_data/file/645862/HumanFactors_Medical-Devices_v1.0.pdf.

Mitchell, J. 2007. "European Pharmaceutical Aerosol Group (EPAG): Standards and regulatory guidance development." *Drug Delivery to the Lungs-18*, pp. 79–82. Accessed June 4, 2018. https://www.researchgate.net/publication/288989162_European_Pharmaceutical_Aerosol_Group_EPAG_Standards_and_Regulatory_Guidance_Development.

Monroe, N. 2017. "Connected combination products: US analysis with potential implications worldwide." *ONdrugDelivery* (Frederick Furness Publishing Ltd) 76: 28–33. Accessed June 8, 2018. http://www.ondrugdelivery.com/publications/76/Napoleon_Monroe.pdf.

Morales, J. O., K. R. Fathe, A. Brunaugh et al. 2017. "Challenges and future prospects for the delivery of biologics: Oral mucosal, pulmonary, and transdermal routes." *AAPS Journal* (Springer) 19 (3): 652–668. doi:10.1208/s12248-017-0054-z.

Morton, D. 2011. "QbD in dry powder inhaler development." *AIChE*. Accessed June 8, 2018. https://www.aiche.org/academy/videos/conference-presentations/qbd-dry-powder-inhaler-development.

Novick, S., D. Christopher, M. Dey et al. 2009a. "A two one-sided parametric tolerance interval test for control of delivered dose uniformity part 1—Characterization of FDA proposed test." *AAPS PharmSciTech* 10: 820. doi:10.1208/s12249-009-9270-x.

Novick, S., D. Christopher, M. Dey et al. 2009b. "A two one-sided parametric tolerance interval test for control of delivered dose uniformity—part 2—Effect of changing parameters." *AAPS PharmSciTech* 10: 841. doi:10.1208/s12249-009-9269-3.

Olsson, B., L. Borgström, H. Lundbäck, and M. Svensson. 2013. "Validation of a general in vitro approach for prediction of total lung deposition in healthy adults for pharmaceutical inhalation products." *Journal of Aerosol Medicine and Pulmonary Drug Delivery* 26 (6): 355–369. doi:10.1089/jamp.2012.0986.

Pharmaceutical Quality Group. 2016. "PS 9000:2016. Pharmaceutical packaging materials for medicinal products with reference to Good Manufacturing Practice." *Pharmaceutical Quality Group*. Accessed June 4, 2018. https://www.pqg.org/shop/standards/115-ps-90002016-downloadable.html.

Product Quality Research Institute Leachables and Extractables Working Group. 2006. "Safety thresholds and best practices for extractables and leachables in orally inhaled and nasal drug products." *Product Quality Research Institute*. Accessed June 4, 2018. http://pqri.org/wp-content/uploads/2015/08/pdf/LE_Recommendations_to_FDA_09-29-06.pdf.

Ruzycki, C. A., E. Javaheri, and W. H. Finlay. 2013. "The use of computational fluid dynamics in inhaler design." *Expert Opinion on Drug Delivery* 10 (3): 307–332. doi:10.1517/17425247.2013.753053.

Schroeder, A. C. 2005. "Leachables and extractables in OINDP: An FDA perspective." *PQRI L/E Workshop*, Bethesda, MD. Accessed June 4, 2018. http://pqri.org/wp-content/uploads/2015/08/pdf/AlanSchroederDay1.pdf.

Sifuentes, M. M., and A. Giuffrida. 2015. "Drug review differences across the United States and the European Union." *Pharmaceutical Regulatory Affairs* e156. doi:10.4172/2167-7689.1000e156.

Stein, S. W., and C. G. Thiel. 2017. "The history of therapeutic aerosols: A chronological review." *Journal of Aerosol Medicine and Pulmonary Drug Delivery* 30 (1): 20–41. doi:10.1089/jamp.2016.1297.

Van Norman, G. A. 2016. "Drugs and devices: Comparison of European and U.S. approval processes." *Journal American Association Cardiology: Basic to Translational Science* 1 (5): 399–412. doi:10.1016/j.jacbts.2016.06.003.

26

Pharmacopeial and Regulatory Guidances on Product Quality and Performance

Anthony J. Hickey

CONTENTS

26.1 Introduction

Chapters 24 and 25 gave perspectives on global and European regulatory considerations, respectively. Some specifics were identified in Chapters 10 and 20 with respect to "Quality by Control" and "Quality by Design." This chapter will highlight the standards and guidance documents that govern product quality, performance, and regulatory approval in the United States (Singh and Poochikian 2011). The independence of the United States Pharmacopeia (USP) from the US Food and Drug Administration (FDA) represents a unique separation of responsibility not found in other countries where pharmacopeias carry the sole authority of government regulation. However, it should be noted that there are formal lines of communication between the USP and FDA and staff liaisons that facilitate alignment in response to any important new development.

The history of product monographs, standards, and guidance in the United States can be traced to the nineteenth century when the potential for adulteration of products and need to establish quality standards led to the United States Pharmacopeial Convention (USPC). The intent of producing detailed specifications and testing procedures was to establish the quality of the product in commerce and to assure the accuracy and reproducibility of the dose that in turn relates to safety and efficacy. This was occurring at a time when the scale of manufacturing was limited in comparison with current mass production of dosage forms.

The Food, Drug, and Cosmetics Act passed into law in 1938 (FDA 2009, 2012a; USC 1938). The US FDA was formed to implement the law ensuring the safety of products by following their development closely from manufacturing through preclinical to clinical testing prior to gaining regulatory approval and commercialization. The law also presented a mechanism of following products after commercialization through routine inspection and adverse effects reporting. The Hatch-Waxman Act further expanded the FDA activities to include generic drug products (Rumore 2009; USC 1984). The scope of the FDA review and inspection processes reflects developments in science and technology that had occurred when the agency was formed, almost a century after the USP, and it has continued to evolve to the present day. The need for greater interaction and oversight of companies developing products was apparent as manufacturing transitioned to a large scale and with a level of automation that could not have been imagined at the time of the first United States Pharmacopeial Convention.

Inhaled pharmaceutical products entered the market in the mid-1950s by which time the USP and FDA had been guiding the quality of conventional products in commerce and in development for some time. The initial attempts to address the important properties of aerosol products were focused on dose and particle size, but the methods available, notably microscopy, were limited as quantitative measures of critical quality attributes. As the number and variety of dosage forms to generate inhaled aerosols proliferated in the 1970s, serious efforts began to evaluate methods that might be more suitable for establishing product quality specifications. The current approach has been well documented in the literature (Lee et al. 2015) and is discussed in earlier chapters in this book.

The following overview of the relevant standards and guidance documents issued by the USP and the FDA is intended to place them in context and to guide the reader with respect to their significance. The specifics of each document are not reproduced here as they deal with dosage forms and methods that are described thoroughly throughout this book. Consequently, those looking for detailed descriptions of pressurized metered dose inhalers (inhalation aerosols), dry powder inhalers (inhalation powders), soft mist inhalers (inhalation sprays) nebulizers, cascade impactors (for aerodynamic particle size distribution measurement), and delivered dose samplers should refer to earlier chapters where they are described in detail. The dosage forms described in the previous sentence are referred to by the FDA terminology with the USP terminology in parentheses. Wherever possible the correct term will be used for the organization that is promulgating the standard. Finally, to be consistent with the emphasis of the book, the focus of the present overview is on oral inhalation products and reference to nasal products will only occur where this document refers to both products.

26.2 United States Pharmacopeia

The USP taxonomic framework for general chapters, into which all of its documents are embedded, was established in its current form in the early years of the Millennium (USP41-NF35 2018i). The system is composed of three tiers that broadly define the nature of the product being assessed. Tier 1 identifies the route of administration, tier 2 identifies the dosage form, and tier 3 describes the performance test that is of most biological relevance, but serves as a quality measure.

As a guide to the location of the relevant USP sections to the discussion below, the major headings of "General Notices" and "General Chapters" are starting points in its table of contents. The "General Notices" guide the reader at a high level on the purpose and use of other entries describing aspects of drugs and drug products. Two sub-headings in the "General Chapters" section are of importance, "General Tests and Assays" and "General Information." In the "General Tests and Assays" sub-section, two further sub-headings contain important general chapters, "General Requirements for Tests and Assays," the location for general chapter (GC)<5>, and "Physical Tests and Determinations," the location for GC<601>. The "General Information" section contains three important guides on background to dosage forms (GC<1151>) (USP41-NF36 2018i) and testing of nebulizers (GC<1601>) (USP41-NF36 2018j) and spacer and valved holding chambers (GC<1602) (USP41-NF36 2018k).

The general information chapter, GC<1151> describes pharmaceutical dosage forms and includes a description of the tier 1–3 taxonomy. The specific reference documents that define tier 1 and tier 2 are shown in Figure 26.1. In addition to the general notices, the first general chapter that relates to route of administration is general chapter<1151>. This gives a high-level overview of all dosage forms and routes of administration and gives context to the detailed general chapters describing dosage forms employed to administer drug by specific routes of administration. As depicted in Figure 26.1, general chapters

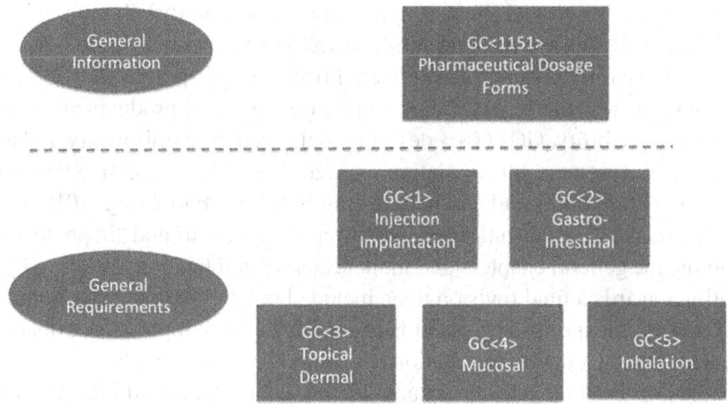

FIGURE 26.1 General chapters describing tier 1, route of administrations and tier 2, dosage forms.

<1> through <5> describe dosage forms employed for injection/implantation GC<1>, gastro-intestinal GC<2>, topical/dermal GC<3>, mucosal GC<4>, and inhalation GC<5> administration. Product descriptions are more detailed in these chapters and general quality tests, focused on the physico-chemical properties of the drug in the dosage form, are listed with references to related chapters on analytical methods where necessary.

Dissolution is the major performance test for products described in general chapters <1> to <4>. It is evident that for these products, the dose is well defined and the relevant quality metric is the bioavailability of the drug, which is in part dictated by immediate, delayed, or extended dissolution. Inhalation aerosols, dry powder inhaler, and nebulizer products frequently generate soluble airborne particles and droplets intended to promote immediate local drug action. GC<5> describes quality tests for inhalation and nasal products (USP41-NF36 2018e). While there is some interest in the role of dissolution in the bioavailability of drugs delivered as aerosols, the current position of the USP is that delivered dose and aerodynamic particle size distribution are the key product performance variables dictating bioavailability.

Figure 26.2 indicates the general chapters describing requirements and test of relevance to inhalation products. The important performance measures for these products are the dose, which is influenced

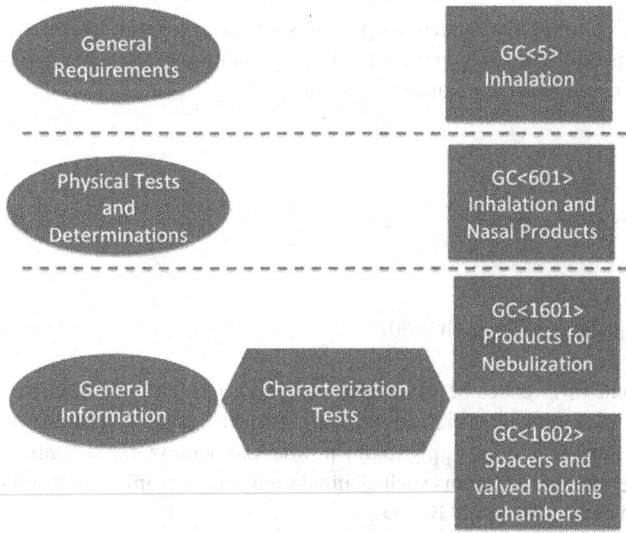

FIGURE 26.2 General chapters describing requirements and tests for inhalation products.

by formulation and device design and the aerodynamic particle size distribution, which influences the deposition in the lungs. Nasal sprays and powders are also dependent on dose-delivered and plume characteristics although it is clear that the aerosol delivered from a nasal spray is unlikely to fully develop in the nasal cavity. Consequently, these performance measures for nasal products are mostly indicators of quality rather than bioavailability. GC<601> describes delivered dose uniformity and aerodynamic particle size distribution measurement for inhalation and nasal products (USP41-NF36 2018f). GC<602> and GC<604> describe propellants and leak rate testing (USP41-NF36 2018g, 2018h).

Pharmaceutical Forum, a USP journal, contains "stimuli to revision" and "in process revision" articles as a means of evolving the general chapters and monographs by publication, followed by a period of public comment iterating towards a final revision to be included in USP-National Formulary (NF) following balloting by the Council of Experts. The intent is to secure as much input as possible before moving to final publication. Recently, "General Information" chapters have been employed as an alternate mechanism to guide readers on broadly relevant issues. In this context, general chapters have appeared on nebulizer output characterization (GC<1601>) and spacers and valved holding chambers (GC<1602>).

26.2.1 General Chapter<5>

The range of inhalation and nasal dosage forms are identified in GC<5> including: inhalation aerosol (pressurized metered dose inhaler); inhalation powder (dry powder inhaler); inhalation spray (soft mist inhaler); inhalation solution (drug solution for nebulizer); inhalation suspension (drug suspension for nebulizer); solution for inhalation (drug solution requiring dilution for nebulizer) and; [drug] for inhalation solution (drug powder that upon addition of a vehicle is delivered by nebulizer) (USP41-NF36 2018e).

Many of the tests described in GC<5> are common to other dosage forms and require very little explanation. Among these are, using "Inhalation Aerosols" (pressurized metered dose inhalers) as an example, the following.

- Identification
- Assay
- Impurities and degradation products
- Water content
- Foreign particulate matter
- Microbial limit

Others are very specific to inhalation aerosol products and emerge from the interaction of the formulation and device that is necessary to generate an effective therapy to the patient. These properties again using "Inhalation Aerosols" as an example are as follows.

- Leachables
- Spray pattern
- Alcohol content (if present)
- Net fill weight
- Leak rate
- Performance quality tests, see GC<601>

GC<5> identifies some differences between each of the dosage forms that may require the addition of other tests and removal of some identified above. For example, "leak rate" is a function of propellant used in inhalation aerosols and would not apply to dry powders or nebulizers. In contrast, pH and osmolality are important to aqueous-based systems such as inhalation sprays or inhalation solutions. Complete lists for each dosage form can be found in GC<5>.

It should be noted that the performance tests for inhalation and nasal products in GC<601> are referenced in GC<5> since they complete the overall evaluation of the quality of the product.

26.2.2 General Chapter<601>

GC<601> is necessarily a complicated chapter for a number of reasons. Firstly, it encompasses a wide range of products as defined by their components and listed above (USP41-NF36 2018f). Secondly, each of the products requires characterization of delivered dose uniformity (nephele tube) and aerodynamic particle size distribution (inertial impaction). Due to the method of generation (active and passive delivery) and the state (solid, liquid) of the aerosol, different configurations of the same equipment are required, and this is itemized in the general chapter in sufficient detail to allow the correct method to be adopted by the user.

The independent supply of drug solutions and suspensions from the nebulizer is a peculiarity of this method of aerosol generation and delivery. Some products, particularly vibrating mesh nebulizers, are now supplied with the drug formulation. However, this is not the most common situation. Consequently, while nebulizer formulations are described in GC<601>, characterization of nebulizer output is not. This is consistent with USP policies, but for many years left a void in information on nebulizer product characterisation. Recently, this was corrected by the publication of an information general chapter describing a nebulizer output method, GC<1601>.

26.2.3 General Chapter<1601>

GC<1601> was an important addition to the USP for those developing nebulizer products (USP41-NF36 2018j). Despite the overall principle of nebulizer testing being known to the scientific community and product developers, no standard guidance was available. Some controls on the method were subject to interpretation in the scientific literature, which would be cause for confusion to those wishing to adopt a standard method. Clear instructions on the instruments to be employed (notably laser diffraction and inertial impaction for particle size determination) and their use in an overall apparatus assembly are available in this general chapter. In addition, a procedure for chilling the impactor overcomes the evaporation that would otherwise occur changing the aerodynamic particle size distribution (APSD) in real-time. This approach circumvents the impact of evaporation on aerodynamic particle size distribution measurement by stipulating an appropriate method.

26.2.4 General Chapter<1602>

Nebulizers are considered devices and are regulated separately from the drug product despite their importance to the desired therapeutic effect. In this regard, they are not the only devices that have impact on product performance that are not supplied or regulated with the drug product. Spacers and valved holding chambers, for which characterization tests are described in GC<1602>, are used for a variety of reasons related to improving therapy (USP41-NF36 2018k). They are also not usually a component of the drug product and are regulated independently. A spacer is simply an open tube into which an inhalation aerosol is administered. A valved holding chamber has a one-way valve that controls the direction of flow to the patient and prevents exhalation into the tube. The purpose of these spacers and holding chambers is to allow for development of the aerosol plume from which a number of advantages occur: (a) the actuation of the device and inhalation by the patient are separate activities which improves adherence; (b) large particles/droplets deposit in the spacer and not in the oropharynx which increases safety, particularly for steroids; (c) the deceleration of the aerosol plume in the stagnant air in the tube lowers the velocity of the droplets; and (d) evaporation occurs in the time the plume develops reducing droplets size. Both (c) and (d) result in reduced deposition in the oropharynx and increased lung deposition compared with an inhalation aerosol product used without these devices.

26.2.5 General Chapter<1603>

As GC<601> has been through revisions, much of the informational material has been removed to conform to the need for only required material to appear in chapters less than <1000> and for clarity to the reader. Recently, a stimuli article has appeared in *Pharmaceutical Forum* describing a proposed general

TABLE 26.1
Recent[a] USP Inhalation and Nasal Product Monographs, USP41-NF36

Active Pharmaceutical Ingredient	Dosage Form	Monograph
Fluticasone Propionate	Inhalation Aerosol	(USP41-NF36 2018d)
Fluticasone Propionate and Salmeterol	Inhalation Aerosol	(USP41-NF36 2018b)
Fluticasone Propionate	Inhalation Powder	(USP41-NF36 2018c)
Fluticasone Propionate and Salmeterol	Inhalation Powder	(USP41-NF36 2018a)

[a] A number of legacy monographs exist for inhalation aerosols in chlorofluorocarbon propellants. Since these are no longer subject to regulatory approval in the United States, they are not shown here.

chapter on good cascade impactor practices which describes issues that are not enumerated in GC<601>, but might arise as questions by those not familiar with this technique. This has yet to appear formally, but it is anticipated that in the near future it will appear as an aid to those interested in this topic.

26.2.6 Monographs

Monographs for inhaled products have appeared infrequently in the last two decades. The phase-out of chlorofluorocarbon propellants and the hiatus that this created in new product development as the industry shifted to alternative propellants and dry powder inhalers is one explanation for this. However, this situation is slowly changing as innovators are beginning to share product specifications. A list of product monographs is shown in Table 26.1.

26.3 United States Food and Drug Administration Guidance for Industry

The FDA is the government agency regulating and enforcing controls on drug products submitted for review and approved for use in the United States. The role of the FDA in reviewing industry data submissions and overseeing the quality of products through on-site inspections gives the agency a high level of scrutiny and the ability to respond quickly to any contingency. In contrast to the USP, the FDA has the opportunity to respond to information on the manufacture and development of the product before it enters commerce. Indeed, it is only after meeting the requirements of the FDA, in part disclosed in guidance documents, that a product will be approved for manufacture, distribution, and sale in the United States. As a consequence, the range of considerations and tests promulgated by the FDA overlaps to some extent with the USP, but often exceeds the USP requirements.

Broadly speaking, the FDA guides parallel the USP general chapters. Figure 26.3 illustrates the way that guides on chemistry manufacturing controls considerations parallel GC<5> and GC<601>, while the guides on specific products are somewhat equivalent (not the same) as drug product monographs in the USP. Importantly, industry submissions contribute to the crafting of these documents directly (USP) or indirectly (FDA).

26.3.1 Guidance on Inhalation Aerosols and Dry Powder Inhalers (2018)

For 20 years, the FDA operated with an initial draft guidance document on the Chemistry, Manufacturing and Controls (CMC) for metered dose inhalers and dry powder inhalers. In 2018, the draft guidance was revised and submitted through the *Federal Register* for comment (FDA 2018). The essence of the revision to the draft guidance, which presumably is near to final guidance, is similar to the previous version and therefore very familiar to the industry. The focus of this document is on the physico-chemical characterization of the product with respect to quality and performance and, in common with GC<5> and GC<601> of the USP, describes innate properties and methods for characterizing delivered dose and aerodynamic particle

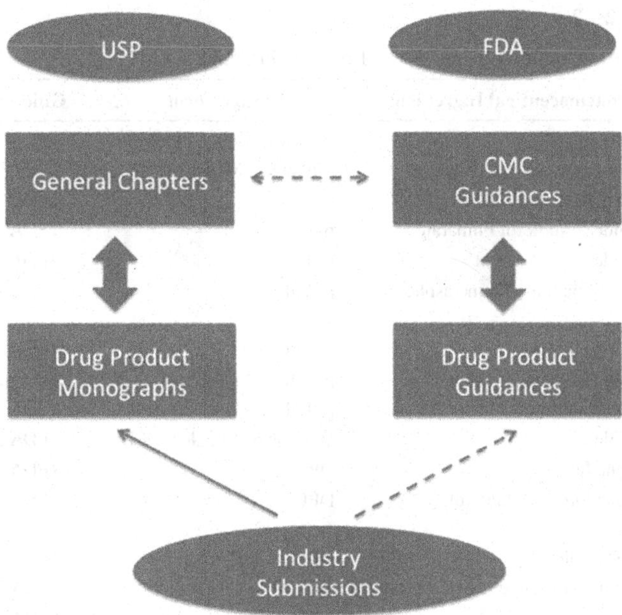

FIGURE 26.3 Parallels USP general chapters and monographs and guidance documents from the FDA.

size distribution. Unlike the USP methods, there are additional requirements in the FDA guidance such as sampling at a range of airflow rates for dry powder inhalers (inhalation powders) that are clearly important tests for a product in development, but would not be as important once the product is in commerce.

26.3.2 Guidance on Drug Products

The FDA also publishes guidance for industry on drug products that define minimally acceptable criteria that would meet the pharmaceutical equivalence and bioequivalence specifications necessary in comparison with currently marketed products. Again, it may be possible that additional information is required, but these documents are intended to form the basis for any interactions between the company and the FDA on the drug product designated (Table 26.2).

26.3.3 Guidance on Quality by Design

It has been an FDA objective for almost two decades to have sufficient control of the product design, manufacture, and characterization to assure the quality of the product (Hickey and Ganderton 2010). This has been described in a number of guidance documents for industry. Since this was discussed in detail in Chapter 20, here we just emphasize in brief that these considerations are prerequisites to subsequent testing and release of products, and underpin any guidance documents on products. At a high level, variables in manufacturing are considered in order to identify critical process variables with respect to defining critical quality attributes that ultimate define product quality and performance with a high probability of meeting defined specifications.

26.3.4 Weight of Evidence Principle

It was noted earlier that only after meeting the requirements of the FDA "in part disclosed in guidance documents" that a product will be approved for market in the US. Since each new product presents different manufacturing and development challenges, it is acknowledged that the guidance documents may not cover every eventuality. Meetings or written questions are part of the industry interaction with

TABLE 26.2
Recent FDA Inhalation and Nasal Product Guidance

Active Pharmaceutical Ingredient	Dosage Form	Guidance [ref]
Albuterol sulfate	Pressurized Metered Dose Inhaler (pMDI)	(FDA 2016j)
Beclomethasone dipropionate	pMDI	(FDA 2016a)
Budesonide/formoterol Fumarate	pMDI	(FDA 2016c)
Ciclesonide	pMDI	(FDA 2016d)
Formoterol Fumarate/mometasone furoate	pMDI	(FDA 2016f)
Mometasone furoate	pMDI	(FDA 2016h)
Ipratropium bromide	pMDI	(FDA 2015d)
Levalbuterol tartrate	pMDI	(FDA 2015c)
Budesonide	Dry powder inhaler (DPI)	(FDA 2016b)
Fluticasone furoate	DPI	(FDA 2016k)
Fluticasone furoate/vilanterol trifenetate	DPI	(FDA 2016e)
Indacaterol maleate	DPI	(FDA 2016g)
Umeclidinium bromide	DPI	(FDA 2016i)
Aclidinium bromide	DPI	(FDA 2015a)
Formoterol fumarate	DPI	(FDA 2015b)
Fluticasone dipropionate and Salmeterol xinafoate	DPI	(FDA 2013)
Budesonide	Nebulizer suspension	(FDA 2012b)

the FDA that help guide the product to meet expectations. In this context, the FDA applies a weight of evidence principle to these discussions to allow for iteration on critical quality and process attributes, product quality, and performance metrics, the latter including preclinical and clinical study design and evaluation (Cormier 2011).

26.4 Conclusion

A brief outline of the USP general chapters and monographs and FDA guidance documents on a variety of inhalation and nasal products has been outlined above. The overarching taxonomic structure employed by the USP considers the pulmonary and nasal routes of administration for which inhalation aerosols and sprays, dry powder inhalers, solutions and suspension for nebulization, and nasal solutions and suspensions have been developed as dosage forms. The performance measures for these dosage forms are delivered dose uniformity and aerodynamic particle size distribution. Special considerations are required for testing nebulizer performance and for inhalation aerosols that use spacers and valved holding chambers. Monographs have appeared infrequently, but are the location of product specifications.

The Food and Drug Administration after 20 years of regulation based on a draft guidance document have recently produced a guidance document on inhalation aerosols and dry powder inhalers. In places, the guidance document is consistent with the USP GC<601>. Deviations are usually based on an understanding of product performance that is required for product approval, but might not be as relevant for commerce, where the USP has an interest. An example of this phenomenon is testing a dry powder product at a variety of flow rates, which is intended to establish its susceptibility to poor performance under certain conditions. Presumably, demonstrating flow rate independence to the FDA to satisfy their requirement for approval would not be a concern in commerce as the device being tested has met its release specifications. Consequently, the USP can focus on a simple assessment as a fixed flow rate.

The United States is unique in its regulatory oversight of drug products in that the pharmacopeia is not an instrument of government as it is in other parts of the world. The Food and Drug Administration is the agency of government tasked with ensuring the safety and quality of drug products, the USP, a non-government document and organization, has a close working relationship with the FDA. The law supports USP standards and monographs. Noting this difference between the two organizations may explain the difficult task of international harmonization. The USP must align with the FDA to be relevant in the United States, but cannot speak for the FDA in its discussions with representatives of other pharmacopeias that are government documents. Despite the slow pace of events, it is a credit to all involved that compendial harmonization is proceeding given the unique situation in the United States.

REFERENCES

Cormier, J. (2011). Advancing FDA's regulatory science through weight of evidence evaluations. *Journal of Contemporary Health Law and Policy, 28*, 1–22.

FDA. (2009). US Food and Drug Administration, The 1938 Food, Drug and Cosmetic Act—FDA. https://www.fda.gov/aboutfda/whatwedo/history/productregulation/ucm132818.htm.

FDA. (2012a). US Food and Drug Administration, 1938 Food, Drug and Cosmetic Act—FDA. https://www.fda.gov/aboutfda/whatwedo/history/origin/ucm054826.htm.

FDA. (2012b). US Food and Drug Administration, budesonide (nebulized) guidance. http://www.fda.gov/downloads/Drugs/GuidanceComplianceRegulatoryInformation/Guidances/UCM319977.pdf.

FDA. (2013). US Food and Drug Administration, fluticasone dipropionate and salmeterol xinafoate guidance. http://www.fda.gov/downloads/Drugs/GuidanceComplianceRegulatoryInformation/Guidances/UCM367643.pdf.

FDA. (2015a). US Food and Drug Administration, aclidinium bromide guidance. http://www.fda.gov/downloads/Drugs/GuidanceComplianceRegulatoryInformation/Guidances/UCM460918.pdf.

FDA. (2015b). US Food and Drug Administration, formoterol fumarate. http://www.fda.gov/downloads/Drugs/GuidanceComplianceRegulatoryInformation/Guidances/UCM461064.pdf.

FDA. (2015c). US Food and Drug Administration, levalbuterol tartrate guidance. http://www.fda.gov/downloads/Drugs/GuidanceComplianceRegulatoryInformation/Guidances/UCM452780.pdf.

FDA. (2015d). US Food and Drug Adminstration, ipratropium bromide guidance. http://www.fda.gov/downloads/Drugs/GuidanceComplianceRegulatoryInformation/Guidances/UCM436831.pdf.

FDA. (2016a). US Food and Drug Administration, belomethasone dipropionate guidance. http://www.fda.gov/downloads/Drugs/GuidanceComplianceRegulatoryInformation/Guidances/UCM481768.pdf.

FDA. (2016b). US Food and Drug Administration, budesonide (DPI) guidance. http://www.fda.gov/downloads/Drugs/GuidanceComplianceRegulatoryInformation/Guidances/UCM533023.pdf.

FDA. (2016c). US Food and Drug Administration, budesonide and formoterol fumarate Guidance. http://www.fda.gov/downloads/Drugs/GuidanceComplianceRegulatoryInformation/Guidances/UCM452690.pdf.

FDA. (2016d). US Food and Drug Administration, ciclesinide guidance. http://www.fda.gov/downloads/Drugs/GuidanceComplianceRegulatoryInformation/Guidances/UCM481787.pdf.

FDA. (2016e). US Food and Drug Administration, fluticasone furoate and vilanterol trifenetate guidance. http://www.fda.gov/downloads/Drugs/GuidanceComplianceRegulatoryInformation/Guidances/UCM495023.pdf.

FDA. (2016f). US Food and Drug Administration, formoterol fumarate and mometasone furoate. http://www.fda.gov/downloads/Drugs/GuidanceComplianceRegulatoryInformation/Guidances/UCM481824.pdf.

FDA. (2016g). US Food and Drug Administration, indacaterol maleate guidance. http://www.fda.gov/downloads/Drugs/GuidanceComplianceRegulatoryInformation/Guidances/UCM495054.pdf.

FDA. (2016h). US Food and Drug Administration, mometasone furoate guidance. http://www.fda.gov/downloads/Drugs/GuidanceComplianceRegulatoryInformation/Guidances/UCM495387.pdf.

FDA. (2016i). US Food and Drug Administration, umeclidinium bromide guidance. http://www.fda.gov/downloads/Drugs/GuidanceComplianceRegulatoryInformation/Guidances/UCM520285.

FDA. (2016j). US Food and Drug Adminstration, albuterol sulfate guidance. http://www.fda.gov/downloads/Drugs/GuidanceComplianceRegulatoryInformation/Guidances/UCM346985.pdf.

FDA. (2016k). US Food and Drug Adminstration, fluticasone furoate (DPI) guidance. http://www.fda.gov/downloads/Drugs/GuidanceComplianceRegulatoryInformation/Guidances/UCM495024.pdf.

FDA. (2018). US Food and Drug Administration, metered dose inhaler (MDI and dry powder inhaler (DPI) quality considerations- Draft guidance for industry—Revision 1. http://www.fda.gov/downloads/Drugs/GuidanceComplianceRegulatoryInformation/Guidances/UCM70573.pdf.

Hickey, A., and Ganderton, D. (2010). Quality by design. In A. Hickey and D. Ganderton (Eds.), *Pharmaceutical Process Engineering* (2nd ed., pp. 193–196). New York: Informa Healthcare.

Lee, S., Saluja, B., Arieta, A. G., Santos, G., Li, Y., Lu, S., and Lyapustina, S. (2015). Regulatory considerations for approval of generic inhalation drug products in the US, EU, Brazil, China and India. *AAPS Journal*, *17*, 1285–1304.

Rumore, M. (2009). The Hatch-Waxman Act—25 years later: Keep the pharmaceutical scales balanced. *Pharmacy Times*. https://www.pharmacytimes.com/publications/supplement/2009/genericsupplement0809/generic-hatchwaxman-0809.

Singh, G., and Poochikian, G. (2011). Development and Approval of inhaled respiratory drugs: A US regulatory perspective. In H. Smyth and A. Hickey (Eds.), *Controlled Pulmonary Drug Delivery* (pp. 489–527). New York: Springer.

USC. (1938). The Food, Drug and Cosmetic Act, Pub. L. No. 75-717, ch. 675, 52 Stat. 1040 (June 25, 1938) (codified as amended at 21 U.S.C. §§ 301–399 (2002) at 21 U.S.C. § 355 (2006).

USC. (1984). The Drug Price Competition and Patent Term Restoration (Hatch-Waxman) Act, Pub. L. No. 98-417, 98 Stat. 1585 (1984) (codified as amended at 21 U.S.C. §355 and 35 U.S.C. §156, 271, and 282.

USP41-NF36. (2018a). Fluticasone dipropionate and salmeterol inhalation powder. https://online.uspnf.com/uspnf/document/GUID-5BD2B30C-5CC9-4003-8ED1-59E4FF6B0CAF_2_en-US.

USP41-NF36. (2018b). Fluticasone propionate and salmeterol inhalation aerosol. *USP-NF Online*. https://online.uspnf.com/uspnf/document/GUID-2E4D271E-08DF-418D-88BC-D15214726312_3_en-US.

USP41-NF36. (2018c). Fluticasone propionate inhalation powder. *USP-NF Online*. https://online.uspnf.com/uspnf/document/GUID-39375AC5-C31B-4C74-AB80-75FD5D95A6A0_1_en-US.

USP41-NF36. (2018d). Fluticasone propionate inhalation aerosol. *USP-NF Online*. https://online.uspnf.com/uspnf/document/GUID-A54661A3-DF23-400A-8763-0213D19A10C6_2_en-US.

USP41-NF36. (2018e). General Chapter<5>. *USP-NF Online*. https://online.uspnf.com/uspnf/document/GUID-63942EFA-FA01-4046-BF63-7C0706FD3924_3_en-US.

USP41-NF36. (2018f). General Chapter<601>. *USP-NF Online*. https://online.uspnf.com/uspnf/document/GUID-FA5F788A-4449-4F16-8435-9B8D5EECB5C9_4_en-US

USP41-NF36. (2018g). General Chapter<602> Propellants. *USP-NF Online*. https://online.uspnf.com/uspnf/document/GUID-93D5843F-E4FC-4D13-B3A5-35D674A9CBC9_1_en-US.

USP41-NF36. (2018h). General Chapter<604> Leak rate. *USP-NF Online*. https://online.uspnf.com/uspnf/document/GUID-99594EDC-4589-4C97-A0A6-4D5884D214B3_1_en-US.

USP41-NF36. (2018i). General Chapter<1151>. *USP-NF Online*. https://online.uspnf.com/uspnf/document/GUID-431F93A9-1FEC-42AE-8556-AA5B604B2E36_2_en-US.

USP41-NF36. (2018j). General Chapter<1601>. *USP-NF Online*. https://online.uspnf.com/uspnf/document/GUID-8C627507-281E-4B5E-923E-796DA0853CD7_2_en-US.

USP41-NF36. (2018k). General Chapter<1602>. *USP-NF Online*. https://online.uspnf.com/uspnf/document/GUID-8C627507-281E-4B5E-923E-796DA0853CD7_2_en-US.

27

The European Union Regulatory Scene

Steven C. Nichols and Dennis Sandell

CONTENTS

27.1 Introduction

The purpose of this chapter is to provide an overview of current European Union (EU) legislation, regulatory process, and guidance. Guidance under review and the proposed work plan will be discussed. We shall only consider those topics that are most current, issues, or where recent changes have or will be made in the near future. How industry interfaces with the regulators to achieve updated and harmonized guidance is critical so the viewpoint of industry is important to achieve an effective product development programme and submissions views of members of the European Pharmaceutical Aerosol Group (EPAG) were canvassed and are reported.

The significant event of the United Kingdom of Great Britain (UK) leaving the EU will be occurring in the short term, and the impact of this on the European regulatory scene and approval process will be discussed. Clearly, this event is expected to influence pharmaceutical company strategies and those of the regulatory authorities. As at the beginning of 2018, little detail is known about this event and what, in the future, the UK regulations and processes will look like.

The European Pharmacopeia (Ph. Eur.) is a significant source of quality standards and methods and is enshrined within the European regulations and guidance. For orally inhaled products (OIPs), the activities of the Inhalanda working party is important in maintaining up to date standards and methodologies. The activities of the Inhalanda working party will be discussed. Also, how Brexit may affect the inhalation sections of the British Pharmacopeia and how this may develop in the future, including its relationship with the Ph. Eur. are worth considering here.

Without doubt, those regulations affecting the development of generic OIPs are challenging and especially regulations governing bioequivalence will be considered in some detail. This whole area is currently a hot topic with recent generic product approvals within the EU illustrating how different regulatory authorities interpret the requirements. This whole area is still evolving so consideration of alternate approaches is relevant at this time.

Within orally inhaled products, there are those products which are "integral," here the drug formulation and device (inhaler) are one product. Further, there are "non-integral" devices that can be acquired and used with a drug formulation purchased separately from a different manufacturer; these devices are often nebulizers, unit-dose dry powder inhalers, and other accessories, e.g. spacers and valved holding chambers (VHCs). These "non-integral" devices are regulated by the Medical Device Directive regulations; this has recently been updated and will be discussed here.

27.2 EU Legislation and Regulations

The EU regulatory procedure applicable to pharmaceuticals is well described, the main source of information being the European Commission and European Medicines Agency (EMA) websites [1,2]. It is not possible here to describe the process and procedures in detail, but be aware that requirements and guidance are updated on a regular basis; therefore it is imperative that users maintain a current awareness by referring to these websites or by utilizing regulatory specialists. A broad outline of the structural backbone will aid understanding before discussing current and future issues affecting the regulatory requirements. Any company working within the OIP field is advised to utilize knowledge and guidance from an experienced person in OIP regulations and development strategies to achieve the most effective development and submission programme.

The EU legislation in the pharmaceutical sector is compiled in ten volumes of the publication *The Rules Governing Medicinal Products in the European Union*, Table 27.1 [1]. Additional to this, medicinal products for pediatric use, orphans, herbal medicinal products, and advanced therapies are governed by other specific rules.

For example, volume 3 contains the scientific guidelines prepared by the Committee for Medicinal Products for Human Use (CHMP) in consultation with the EU member state competent authorities, these help an applicant make a marketing authorization applications (MAA). In Europe, it is from these scientific guidelines that the OIP industry takes its cue for the activities required to develop medicinal products. More detail and discussion of the contents of these volumes can be found on the EMA website [1].

Within the realm of developing orally inhaled products there are two key guidelines, the "Guideline on Pharmaceutical Quality of Inhalation and Nasal Products" [3] and "Guideline on the Requirements for Clinical Documentation for Orally Inhaled Products" [4]. The former is essentially chemistry, manufacturing, and controls (CMC) based requirements and the latter deals with therapeutic equivalence requirements. These were written to complement each other; further information to clarify certain re-occurring points has been dealt with by a "question and answer" document from the EMA [5]. We shall return to discuss some aspects of these important guidelines later.

TABLE 27.1

The Rules Governing Medicinal Products in the European Union

Volume	Title
1	EU pharmaceutical legislation for medicinal products for human use
2	Pharmaceutical legislation on notice to applicants and regulatory guidelines for medicinal products for human use
3	Scientific guidelines for medicinal products for human use
4	Good Manufacturing Practice (GMP) guidelines
5	EU pharmaceutical legislation for medicinal products for veterinary use
6	Notice to applicants and regulatory guidelines for medicinal products for veterinary use
7	Scientific guidelines for medicinal products for veterinary use
8	Maximum residue limits guidelines (MRLs)
9	Pharmacovigilance guidelines
10	Clinical trials guidelines

Marketing Authorization for OIPs within the EU can be applied for by one of three procedures [6]:

- *Centralized procedure*: which is compulsory for products derived from biotechnology, for orphan medicinal products, and for medicinal products for human use which contain an active substance authorized in the community after May 20, 2004 (date of entry into force of Regulation (EC) No 726/2004) and which are intended for the treatment of AIDS, cancer, and neurodegenerative disorders or diabetes.
- *Mutual recognition procedure*: applicable to the majority of conventional medicinal products and based on the principle of recognition of an already existing national marketing authorization by one or more member states.
- *Decentralized procedure*: which was introduced with the legislative review of 2004, is also applicable to the majority of conventional medicinal products. Through this procedure, an application for the marketing authorization of a medicinal product is submitted simultaneously in several member states, one of them being chosen as the "Reference Member State." At the end of the procedure, national marketing authorizations are granted in the reference and in the concerned member states.

It is important to know at the outset of any development program which marketing authorization procedure you are going to use as this will affect the strategy and technical development plans for any given product. Knowledge of the experience that a national authority has of OIPs when selecting which to submit to is a critical component of a development plan for an OIP. The reason is that not all national authorities have the same level of knowledge and experience of assessing OIPs, which can prove problematical in gaining a timely marketing authorization application.

If one is developing a "generic" OIP within the EU, then either a hybrid application or an abridged application [7,8] can be made. The former usually occurs when bioequivalence cannot be demonstrated through bioavailability studies. In the latter case, complete quality data (module 3 of the Common Technical Document [CTD]), appropriate preclinical (module 4), and clinical data (module 5) are required. We shall discuss generic OIPs further later. Guidance on MAAs can be found in "*The Rules Governing Medicinal Products*"—Notice to applicants Volume 2A (Chapter 1).

27.2.1 OIP Guidelines

There are two overarching notes for guidance that impact on OIPs, one dealing with the aspects describing the expected quality [3] and one dealing with clinical documentation that includes establishing therapeutic equivalence of two OIPs [4]. Supplementing this guidance, the EMA has published a "question and answer" document that deals with clarifying some of the guidance requirements [5]. However, experience of these two guidance has raised further issues, questions, and the need to clarify certain aspects, particularly related to therapeutic equivalence, which resulted in the EMA publishing a concept paper [9]. All stakeholders have been able to comment on the topics in the concept paper or raise new topics, the deadline for comments was the end of June 2017. After the EMA drafting team have considered and consulted internally, they will publish a new draft guidance; which will then have a further 3-month consultation period, this may occur during 2018.

Vincenzi [10] noted that the concept paper was well received by industry and all the proposals were supported; over 70 principle comments were received from stakeholders providing further insights for consideration by the drafting group. Vincenzi [10] summarized the common topics that were raised by the stakeholders, Table 27.2, illustrating those areas of concern to the OIP industry.

Outside of this process a number of quality topics have been covered in recent EMA scientific advices and business pipeline meetings [10]. These topics included: "in vitro" bioequivalence for life cycle management, extractable and leachables, add-on devices and e-connective apps, and Conformité Européene (CE)-marking and the new requirements mandated by the new medical device regulation.

So, a considerable number of key guidance activities and extra-guidance activities have occurred and are occurring within the EU regulatory process. The EMA is very responsive to the OIP industry, and the

TABLE 27.2

Stakeholder Common Topics

Topic Area	Number of Comments
Spacer-holding chambers	15
New device technologies	9
ICH Q8/9/10 and life cycle management	8
Consistency over all EMA guidance	7
Flow rate dependency	6
Fine particle dose specification	5
Impactor stage grouping	6
Data in eCTD document	4

working relationship appears to be strong and beneficial to all stakeholders. These activities will make the guidance "fit for purpose" ensuring quality and safe products are produced while industry has clear regulatory guidance as we move forward in the twenty-first century.

In terms of the future, it is imperative that further developments occur and that a holistic multidisciplinary approach is developed further and managed across all the regulatory bodies that issue OIP relevant regulations and guidance. This not only includes intra-EMA groups, but also extra-EMA groups, such as International Standards Organization (ISO) and Ph. Eur., United States Pharmacopeia (USP), International Conference on Harmonization (ICH), World Health Organization (WHO), etc. For industry to work effectively to produce safe OIPs, consistency and clarity in regulations and guidance are critical.

27.3 Brexit

The UK joined the European Economic Community (EEC) in 1973, which then evolved into the EU; the UK subsequently became an influential member especially with respect to OIPs regulations and guidance. The UK has been particularly able to provide much OIP expert regulatory advice through various committees and working groups as it has a well-established industry developing this product type. Generally, within the life science sector it has been estimated [11] that the UK licensing body, the Medicines and Healthcare Products Regulatory Agency, provides 20%–25% of the overall European expertise into the European system. It is further estimated that 65% of the pharmacovigilance qualified persons operate out of the UK. The potential removal of this expertise is of concern to the continued operation of the system within Europe and to European public health.

The UK has an enviable history of developing orally inhaled drugs and their devices from early pMDIs and DPIs through the propellant change issues and beyond. This technical and scientific knowledge would ensure the UK was at the leading edge of product development given that the UK is a significant market for respiratory drugs, particularly asthma and now COPD. A number of major companies have their R & D and/or headquarters in the UK, making the country a skills base. This base helped to build a regulatory agency with significant OIP knowledge which would help: (a) development guidance, (b) advice to industry, and (c) market authorizations through the EU processes.

The UK held a referendum on June 23, 2016 which resulted in the nation voting to leave the EU. The date the UK will leave the EU, following the necessary procedures, will be March 29, 2019. The significance of this first and foremost will be that the UK will be outside the EU product approval process, thereby requiring its own registration process and requirements. While in the EU the UK has a regulatory process, so the question is "will the process change post-Brexit, and, if so, in what way?"

In the first instance, the UK government has proposed a European Union (withdrawal) Bill, which is to transfer all the current EU legislation into UK law in one go. This bill is being debated and taken through the necessary processes to be law within the UK, currently the outcome of this is unknown; however, the UK will have to create its own national regulatory process. Although the current EU requirements may be transferred directly into UK law, it is inevitable that over time differences will develop. What is critical will be the future working relationship between the new UK agency and the EMA. Currently, there is little information available as the whole process is ongoing, however, a number of EU-based and UK-based committees and stakeholders are busily working on this. The Medicines and Healthcare Products Regulatory Agency quickly issued comment on leaving the EU and making a success of Brexit [12] and subsequently provides updates as available.

There will be many significant affects; both for the UK and EU, by the UK leaving the EU, some of the key general issues have already been set-out [11]. Many of these affect processes and requirements and are not specific to OIPs. With respect to the latter, it is the potential loss of the expertise to the EU that may have the largest impact on OIPs and their approval.

Finally, both the EU and Medicines and Healthcare Products Regulatory Agency have issued statements concerning Brexit, these are often updated, therefore readers are advised to check the respective agency websites for the latest information and decisions.

27.4 European Industry Perceptions of the European Regulatory Scene

To understand better the current industry thinking, concerns, and needs with respect to the European regulations and procedures, a number of questions were asked to the European Pharmaceutical Aerosol Group, an industry pressure group; the key responses are summarized here. This information should be of use by both regulators and industry to bring about improvements to regulations where needed.

Overall, industry satisfaction of the procedures and the available guidance is high. There is always the dilemma of guidance not being too prescriptive (particularly as the Quality by Design principles are increasingly being applied to OIPs following ICH guidance), yet sufficiently indicative and clear as to the regulatory authorities requirements. Inevitably, different companies have different views on this, influenced by whether they are developing innovative or generic products, so finding the right level of guidance is challenging. Further, within Europe, the issue of the different interpretation of the guidance by different regulatory authorities (therefore potential inconsistencies) can be challenging at times. It was summed-up by one response which indicated that the decentralized procedure (DCP) can lead to different regulatory authority comments and is slow, but one can choose the reference member state (RMS). The centralized procedure (CP) is quicker and dependent on the experience of the rapporteur/co-rapporteur, but one has no choice of agency then.

The main areas that cause industry concern or where clear/improved guidance and understanding are required were:

- Requirements for similarity and comparability of in vitro data for generic drug products, further clarity and definition is requested.
- Delivered dose uniformity requirements.
- Guidance relating to pediatric product development.
- Guidance on early clinical studies, especially dealing with proof of concept and first in man activities.
- For products in different presentations or with different drug substance suppliers.
- Include "product change management" into the guidance.

When considering areas where cross industry-regulatory authority co-operation would be of benefit the following areas were identified:

- Delivered dose uniformity for inter- and intra-pMDI inhaler variability—Inhalanda monograph.
- Assessment of in vitro data for generic product similarity/comparability. Including how these can be extrapolated to clinical outcomes.

Being able to hold a technical meeting ("scientific advice") with the regulatory authorities was seen as a very useful activity, although it was recognized that it was easier to hold meetings with some European agencies than others. An official end of phase 2 meeting may be a useful requirement to have. Further, sometimes advice can be difficult to interpret and may require clarification. One strategy is to sample a number of key agencies on a topic to gain the range of advice which then allows a technical strategy to be established.

Although some of these points are being addressed as part of the recent concept paper [9] and the revised guidance, it is clear that there are several other areas where industry and regulators need to work together. With regard to the future, the regulatory authority requirement for a greater quantity of data was considered very likely. If this is so, then data analysis and interpretation tools and skills by both the pharmaceutical industry and regulatory assessors will be key areas where training and education is continually enhanced.

Comments on the effect of the UK leaving the EU included the following:

- It would not affect EU submissions or requirements, but may increase the time required for a UK submission.
- Not clear yet, it is anticipated that at least the process should remain similar. There is potential for divergence. The UK will have no influence on EU guidance in the future.
- Different standards in different countries will be difficult to control. An increase in bureaucracy is likely.

In summary, the EU regulatory procedure is mature and is generally accepted by industry as satisfactory. As always, it is only with use that the strengths and weaknesses of regulations are discovered; it is always the latter that have to be resolved. Additionally, the OIP industry is developing new drugs and devices for inhalation which challenge existing guidance or necessitates new guidance. Much of the guidance will come directly or indirectly from industry, and its role in steering regulations is required as much now as ever it was.

27.5 European Pharmacopeia

The Ph. Eur. sets a whole range of quality standards (specifications) for packaging, materials, products, and active pharmaceutical ingredients (APIs).

Most significantly, it provides standard test methods without which like-for-like data comparisons would be very difficult. Within the EU these become official methods which are referred to in EMA guidelines. However, inhalers and nebulizers come in many design and usability variations, and it is inevitable that there will be exceptions which means a standard method cannot always be applied. As now, it is therefore essential that Ph. Eur. does allow other methods to be used where justified and approved. The interpretation of this requirement is often not clear to all users, but a little commonsense usually provides the answer, e.g. documenting why the Ph. Eur. method is not applicable to that particular OIP. Irrespective of the method used (the Ph. Eur., a Ph. Eur. variant, or complete alternative) method validation is still required. Whenever possible this should include comparative data generated with the Ph. Eur. method.

The principle monographs relating to orally inhaled product testing are: (a) preparations for inhalation (0671), (b) preparations for inhalation; aerodynamic assessment of fine particles (2.9.18), and (c) preparations for nebulization: characterization (2.9.44). These monographs can form the basis of product testing through development and when the product receives marketing authorization.

The Ph. Eur. can establish expert groups and working parties (WPs) to review and propose updates to monographs; one such working party is the inhalation WP (Inhalanda), and this has been operative and effective for a considerable number of years. During this time OIPs have not just evolved, but a step change has occurred in their design and capabilities. Some of the step change has been brought about by technology developments, devices and test method advances, and mandated requirements by regulatory authorities, e.g. dose counters, issued within guidance by the EMA. The Inhalanda WP has produced many revisions to the Ph. Eur. monographs to ensure the most up to date monographs possible. As part of this, it has taken the bold step of removing many of the older methods from the monographs so as to ensure that producers also move ahead and don't continue with out-dated methodology that often does not provide the quality of data that is required today.

The Inhalanda WP has worked hard over the years to maintain these monographs; very little external publication [13] of its work occurs outside the official European Pharmacopeia channels, which is a shame as people change in industry and may not be as aware as they should of its activities. The Inhalanda WP usually meets twice a year in Strasbourg, currently it is a good mix of experts from industry, national authorities, and academia. Interestingly, the Ph. Eur. does not have to declare the names or affiliations of the members for any expert group or working party. For an open public sponsored body, this seems overly protective, similarly, the minutes of the meetings are not made public. So, this means that people willing to participate or wanting to communicate need to know how to do so, this may not be clear either, the first stop is to contact one's national authority or respond to requests that are published by the Ph. Eur., usually in its publication *PharmEuropa*.

The Inhalanda WP does have a work plan [14] that is presented to the European Commission and approved along with all the work that the Ph. Eur. proposes. The current (Q3 2017) Inhalanda work plan consists of: (a) revisions on preparations for inhalation and (b) drafting of a new general Section 2.9.53 uniformity of delivered dose of inhalation. Recent proposals on nasal preparations (Nasalia) can be found in the "knowledge data base" [15] which can be reviewed and searched. This knowledge data base may often contain information of interest to those developing OIPs.

One of the many strengths of the Inhalanda working party has been the willingness to agree to collaborative studies either internally or with other stakeholders. One of the earliest industry collaborative studies was the comparison of impingers and impactors given in the Ph. Eur. monograph [16]. This was initiated by the then Inhalanda WP party, in recent times other groups have presented to Inhalanda WP, notably the industry Next Generation Impactor (NGI) Consortium and the European Pharmaceutical Aerosols Group. The former drove the NGI through the Ph. Eur. monograph update process by providing much comparative data [17]. The latter is currently assessing possible Nasalia product methodology for determining the particle fraction less than 10 μm aerodynamic diameter. These types of interactions are vital if the monographs are to have a real value in assessing product quality and usability by the stakeholders.

27.6 British Pharmacopoeia

In recent years, the British Pharmacopoeia (BP) had undertaken a review of the relevant inhalation related monographs and had undertook to update and align with the corresponding Ph. Eur. monographs. Some exceptions were made where an old monograph/test method was kept to ensure that "mature" existing products could be maintained on the UK market. It was considered by some manufacturers that it would be unlikely that these "mature" products would meet today's higher quality criteria when using the modern methods, therefore, the specifications would have to alter, which would present many challenges to marketed "effective" products, especially to prescribers and patients.

It is important that any national pharmacopoeias maintain regular review and a Ph. Eur. harmonization process to ensure marketed product quality uses the latest standards. We should accept that standards and methodology will change (i.e. improve); this is a challenge for industry, but good for the welfare of a nation's people.

Following the UK EU "leave" vote, the BP issued a statement that said that "the BP will continue to play a full and active role with all our international stakeholders including the European Pharmacopoeia, part of the European Directorate for the Quality of Medicines and Healthcare under the Council of Europe. We continue to incorporate the contents of the Ph. Eur., including in-year update" [18].

This is what one would expect to occur, but what of the future, which is being discussed, but not yet decided, will the BP be the only national pharmacopeia allowed in UK marketing authorizations or will the use of the Ph. Eur. (e.g. in specifications, etc.) be permitted in place of the BP?

27.7 Medicinal Devices

There is a need for clear requirements for devices used in OIPs. "Integral" devices are regulated under the Medical Product Directive (2001/83/EC) and "non-integral" devices under the Medical Device Directive (93/42/EEC). It is expected there will be a concept paper on drug-device combinations entitled "Developing a guideline on quality requirements of medicinal products containing a device component for delivery or use of the medicinal product" [10]. Unlike in the United States, there is no legal definition of "drug-device" combination in the EU, which clearly there needs to be.

There will be new medical device regulations (MDR 2017/745) within Europe that come into force in 2020. The regulations were published in the *Official Journal of the European Union* in May 2017 after much debate and compromise among the EU member states and other affiliated countries. The intervening period is to be used as a transition period. Significant changes in the regulations occur in the following areas, it is particularly important that the impact of these are understood and strategies for dealing with them are developed.

- Product scope extension (annex 1);
- Clinical evidence requirements;
- Labeling changes (Annex V, part c);
- European authorization representative;
- Notified body; and
- CE marking.

Several reviews of the new regulations have been published and webinars etc. held by specialists to help industry. Even though usually devices for orally inhaled products fit at the low end of the device risk scale, it will, nevertheless, require changes to the detail and the work required for these devices to be approved. The following quote captures the essence of the new working environment [19].

> It is evident that this regulation is vastly more "legal" in nature than its predecessor, which took more of a "good will" approach in many ways. This will have consequences for staffing at CAs, NBs, and the EOs, manufacturers included. Although the proposed regulation may have many similarities with the MDD, the devil is in the details. The regulation will change the European regulatory environment as more stringent clinical data requirements, extended data management, more complex conformity assessment procedures (particularly for high-risk medical devices), and product liability and penalties will be introduced. NBs are already signaling they will not be able to process all this extra work, which may lead to compliant devices losing access to the European market. It is important to note that EN ISO 13485:2016, which was released in March 2016, also becomes mandatory in early 2019, thus heralding a very busy 2017 and 2018 for all parties involved in QA/RA compliance.

The OIP industry needs to ensure that it has understood and discussed with regulatory authorities the details of what is needed and how to present this during the transition period to avoid delays to market authorizations and appropriate new activities are embedded into the development programs.

27.8 Generic Orally Inhaled Products

In this section, we focus on the in vitro requirements and considerations related to these requisites for generic OIPs.

Currently, approval of a generic/hybrid orally inhaled product in the EU follows a 3-step procedure (Figure 27.1) described in [4] where approval can be granted in step 1 based on in vitro data only. If the

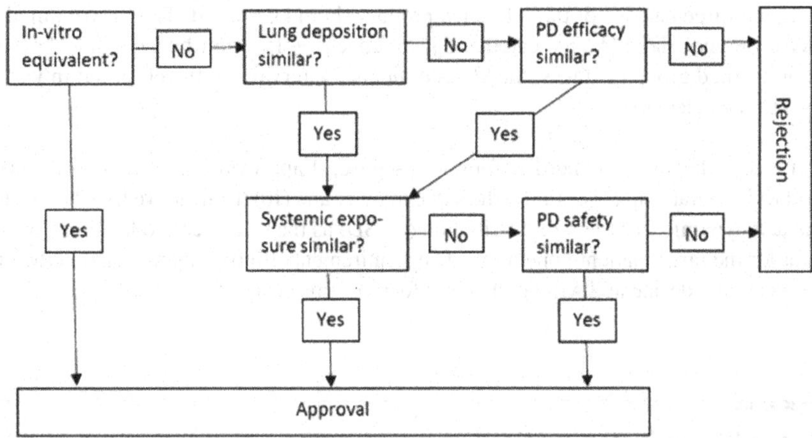

FIGURE 27.1 Decision tree for the development and regulatory assessment of orally inhaled products in the European Union. PD, pharmacodynamics.

conditions for this are not fulfilled, in vivo work is required to show pharmacokinetic (PK; step 2) or pharmacodynamic (PD; step 3) equivalence to the reference product.

The EU Guidance [4] states that therapeutic equivalence to the reference product may be concluded in step 1 (in vitro only) provided the following criteria all are fulfilled:

1. The product contains the same active substance (i.e. same salt, ester, hydrate or solvate, etc.).
2. The pharmaceutical dosage form is identical (e.g. pMDI, non-pressurized MDI, DPI, etc.).
3. The active substance is in the solid state (powder, suspension): any differences in crystalline structure and/or polymorphic form should not influence the dissolution characteristics, the performance of the product, or the aerosol particle behavior.
4. Any qualitative and/or quantitative differences in excipients should not influence the performance of the product (e.g. delivered dose uniformity, etc.), aerosol particle behavior (e.g. hygroscopic effect, plume dynamic and geometry), and/or be likely to affect the inhalation behavior of the patient (e.g. particle size distribution affecting mouth/throat feel or "cold Freon" effect).
5. Any qualitative and/or quantitative differences in excipients should not change the safety profile of the product.
6. The inhaled volume through the device to enable a sufficient amount of active substance into the lungs should be similar (within ± 15%).
7. Handling of the inhalation devices for the test and the reference products in order to release the required amount of the active substance should be similar.
8. The inhalation device has the same resistance to airflow (within ± 15%).
9. The target delivered dose should be similar (within ± 15%).
10. Data from the complete particle size distribution profile of individual stages of a validated multistage impactor/impinger method should be provided. Unless justified otherwise, comparative in vitro data on flow rate dependence should be obtained with a range of flow rates. This range should be justified in relation to the intended patient population. The minimum (e.g. 10th percentile), median, and maximum (e.g. 90th percentile) achievable flow rate in this patient population(s) should be investigated. The comparison should be performed per impactor stage or justified group of stages. At least four groups of stages are expected. Justification should be based on the expected deposition sites in the lungs. At least three consecutive batches of the test

product and three batches of the reference product should be tested. The maximum allowable in vitro difference should be indicated and justified, e.g. ± 15% may be justifiable. Per impactor stage or justified group of stages, the 90% confidence intervals for the observed in vitro differences must be calculated.

In practice, it is seen that the main hurdles for obtaining step 1 approval are the requirements (7) that the alternate product is operated in (essentially) the same manner and (10) (from above list) that the test product has the same aerodynamic particle size distribution (APSD) as the reference product, for flow rates in the range relevant for the target patient population. The requirement (10) (from above list) is the one that has caused most issues and debate and will be the main focus of this chapter.

27.9 In Vitro Bioequivalence (IVBE)

The standard approach to investigate criterion (10) above is to characterize three test (T) and three reference (R) batches for APSD at each of three flow rates (for dry powder inhalers only). These are usually determined in an inhalation flow study showing what peak inspiratory flow rates (PIFR) the relevant patient population generate with the test device. In the IVBE study, typically ten devices are investigated per batch, and both beginning and end APSD are determined using some pharmacopoeial impactor such as the NGI [20]. In total, three flow rates × (3T+3R) batches × 10 devices × 2 life-stages = 360 NGI determinations are required (per strength)—a significant measurement effort. The evaluation of data follows standard practice for statistically equivalence testing: a 90% confidence interval (CI) for the mean T/R ratio is determined based on all data pooled and equivalence is concluded if the CI is completely contained in a pre-specified acceptance interval (C, 1/C), where C = 0.85 unless otherwise justified. Many alternative approaches of how to calculate the CI are available. The most common is the log-transformation approach, possibly combined with estimation of variance components. Alternatively, a Fieller interval may be used. A very efficient approach is to use matched pairs, but then the data collection must be organized to allow this in a unique way.

Very few OIPs have been approved in the EU based on in vitro data only. Apart from some local approvals of marginal products, the only significant "in vitro only" approval is for Circassia fluticasone pMDI in 2015 (50 µg/actuation, 125 µg/actuation, and 250 µg/actuation, generic to GSK's Flixotide).

There are several reasons for the difficulties encountered in gaining approval, these are listed below:

- Although the EU guidance opens for an IVBE comparison based on groups of stages, there is still no consensus of what groupings have most clinical relevance. The trend however appears towards a set including throat (+ pre-separator if used), stage 1, and stage 6 to filter, and with a split of the set stage 2 to stage 5 in two groups of approximately equal size. This approach is, however, suboptimal in that groups are not possible to compare between flow rates (as the impactor stage cut-offs depend on the flow rate) for the purpose of having a consistent approach between flow rates, it is better to use end-points defined by particle size ranges (for example <1 µm, 1–3 µm, 3–6 µm, and >6 µm). Such parameters are also better suited for assessment of flow dependence.
- Due to the debate on groupings, and due to growing evidence that extra fine particles may play an important role for PK outcomes, it is commonly required to show IVBE for all individual stages. As several of the stages typically contain very little drug (<5% of delivered dose), and thus are associated with significant relative variability, this causes a practically impossible task to show that the mean T/R ratio is within ±15% for these. Indeed, it has been shown that many originator products cannot fulfill this requirement when compared to themselves; thus it is unreasonable to require a candidate generic to meet acceptance criteria that the originator itself cannot fulfill. This issue has been noted by regulators and is hopefully considered in the ongoing revision of the EU guidance [4].

- Associated with a request to assess individual stages is the "multiplicity issue": the more tests are performed, the larger is the risk that some fail due to pure chance. As an example, for a combination DPI product available in three strengths, one would need to pass 180 tests to get all strengths approved (3 strengths × 3 flows × 10 stages × 2 active pharmaceutical ingredients). Even if the risk to wrongly fail an individual test is only 1%, the risk to fail at least one of the 180 may be up to 84% ($1-0.99^{180}$)! One way to reduce the issue is to remove the requirement to compare the products at the middle flow rate; this is justified as it seems both theoretically and practically impossible to fail IVBE for the middle flow if data have passed at the low and high flows. Furthermore, a multiplicity correction can be considered; that is, to scale the confidence level according to the number of tests being performed.
- Another issue is related to the sometimes high between batch variability of the reference product. If this is the case, the selection of the three R batches becomes critical as a pool of batches representing the product is required. The easiest way to ensure "representativity" is to increase the number of batches. This need not be associated with any increase in the total amount of testing as one could decrease the amount of testing per batch; for example, one can include six batches and assess five devices per batch instead of three batches and ten devices per batch, and ten batches and three devices per batch would be an even better choice. The approach to increase the number of batches reduces the risk to fail IVBE due to "bad luck" when purchasing batches for the study. The use of more than three batches should not be a regulatory concern; on the contrary, this improves the confidence and relevance of the results. Similarly, increasing the total sample size (possibly different for test and reference products) should be acceptable as this improves the precision of estimates, gives shorter Cis, and might be required to have a chance to show BE for end-points with high variability. It is wise to make a formal power calculation for sizing the IVBE study.
- A related issue (which might partly be the cause of the between batch variability) is the possible aging of the reference product, typically leading to reduction of the amount of finer particles as batches get older. This opens the question whether it is relevant to compare relatively fresh test product to mid-age reference product (which is typically done). Due to this issue, regulators are now sometimes asking generic sponsors to study the stability also for the reference product and possibly perform two IVBE studies—one with as fresh material as possible and one at the end of shelf life.
- As noted above, pMDIs need not as DPIs to be assessed at different flow rates. On the other hand, it is commonly required that IVBE to the reference product is shown both without and with the recommended spacer or VHC. Furthermore, in the study with spacer/VHC, it is sometimes requested to compare test and reference with different breathing patterns (especially tidal breathing) or inhalation profiles in addition to constant flow, as well as using different delay time (0 seconds, 2 seconds, 5 seconds, and 10 seconds) between pMDI firing and onset of aerosol collection. If test and reference products are required to be compared at all combinations of strength, spacer/VHC brands, breathing patterns, and delay time, the amount of testing might exceed that needed for DPI.

The list above explains the main reasons why so few in vitro only approvals have been seen to date. Still, the 3-step approach taken by the EU regulators is a brave step towards a more streamlined process for generic/hybrid OIP approvals. What is needed now is to consider the practical experiences after 9 years of use and to improve the short-comings found. Most important seems to introduce some procedure how IVBE acceptance criteria are determined based on the variability of the reference product, so there is a realistic possibility to comply with these. One proposal on how to scale the acceptance limits was proposed in [21]. Note that this would most likely lead to different acceptance limits for different end-points. Further in the future it is likely that clinically more relevant test methods are preferred for the test to reference comparisons. These methods could include the use of anatomically more correct mouth/throat (M/T) models, such as the Alberta [22], VCU [23], or OPC [24] models, together with different inhalation profiles (IPs) relevant for the intended patient population. The IPs selected for the study could be chosen from profiles recorded for real patients or realistic simulated profiles may be used. An approach on how the desired inhalation profiles could be constructed from representative values of peak inspiratory flow rates, time to peak inspiratory flow rates ("acceleration"), inhalation time, and volume is described in [25].

One feasible alternative to the current standard of comparing the test and reference products at three different flow rates was proposed in [26], suggesting performing only one IVBE study, but comparing the products using nine different IPs spanning the full range of IPs of the patient population. This is expected to provide a clinically more realistic comparison and thus be a better basis for judging equivalence of the products, especially if combined with using some anatomic M/T models. A similar approach has recently been proposed for nasal sprays in [27]; here, factors such as firing pressure, insertion angle, and inhalation/firing relation, as well as nasal geometry are varied to create a set of conditions representing usage by the full patient population.

One significant issue with current prescribed in vitro characterizations is that there are indications that batches with very similar in vitro properties occasionally show substantial differences in PK. This is a sign that there is some critical in vitro parameter that is not measured properly at present. Most focus in the search for this has been on dissolution of OIPs, but still no generally acceptable method for assessing this has been agreed. Despite this, regulators are asking for dissolution comparisons of test and reference products.

As discussed above, approval based on IVBE is still a rare event. Thus, companies typically are entering a PK program. This may also be very challenging, again due to high between batch variability leading to differences between reference product batches. Indeed, in two PK studies [28,29], each including three Advair Diskus 100/50 batches, none of all possible pair-wise R-to-R comparisons resulted in bioequivalence. Different batches of reference product are thus not bioequivalent to each other—so it is not a surprise that companies fail to show PK BE for their test product. These results show that the current regulatory paradigm for showing PK BE (comparing one T batch to one R batch in a two-period cross-over study) is not appropriate for products with high between batch variability. BE in such a study is no sure sign that the products are BE, only that the investigated batches are. Similarly, non-BE results are no reliable proof that the products are in-equivalent. In cases with high between batch variability a single randomly selected batch cannot represent the product and thus the standard two-period cross-over design is not suitable. To solve this issue, it has been proposed that representative batches should be selected for the PK comparison, but this has been shown difficult due to the still limited understanding of what in vitro parameters the selection should be based on. An alternative simple and efficient approach comprising multiple batches to better represent the product has been proposed in [30] as a possible solution to this problem.

Finally, it is noted that the regulatory recommendations for how to assess APSD equivalence between a candidate generic and an originator is (rightly) increasingly used for other types of test-to-reference comparisons. Typical examples include additions of dose counters, material changes, dimensional changes of components, scale up, introduction of breath triggered actuators, comparison of VHC brands, etc. The list is endless and illustrates the wide use of the principles for statistical equivalence testing. The issues associated with all these various types of comparisons are similar as those discussed for the generic/originator IVBE comparison.

27.10 Dose Linearity

In the case the reference product has several strengths and PK BE has been shown in one of these, the EU guidance [4] opens for waiving the requirement for showing therapeutic equivalence in the other strengths, provided in vitro dose linearity has been shown: "If dose linearity is demonstrated in vitro when different dose strengths of a known active substance are sought it may be sufficient to establish therapeutic equivalence clinically with only one strength of the active substance." The guidance further clarifies that a biowaiver in this case is only possible if the reference product also is linear; however, a bio-waiver might still be possible also if the test product is non-linear, provided the reference product shows the same non-linearity. In essence, thus, it does not matter if the test product has linear strengths or not, as long as the reference shows the same behavior. This is a logical consequence from the possibility to obtain approval in step 1 based in in vitro data only.

To investigate linearity, the standard approach is to fit a power model $X = \alpha \cdot \text{strength}^{\beta}$ [or $\ln(X) = \alpha + \beta \cdot \ln(\text{strength})$ after log-transformation to obtain a linear model] to the data and make a confidence interval for the "linearity parameter" β; for perfect linearity $\beta = 1$. Linearity is then concluded if this CI is completely contained in some acceptance interval. However, no linearity acceptance interval has been published by any EU regulator. In the absence of guidance, the interval 0.80–1.20 is suggested.

If the product has only two strengths, an alternative linearity evaluation is suggested in [31]; in the case of two strengths, the term "proportionality" is often used rather than linearity.

The EU guidance [4] is silent on what parameters (the X above) should be investigated for linearity. A common choice is delivered dose and fine particle dose <5 µm (FPD<5). However, for a more detailed assessment the same groupings/end-points as justified for the IVBE evaluation are a natural choice; if these are the best suited for that assessment, they should also be appropriate for investigating dose linearity/proportionality.

Finally, as noted above, the key question for obtaining a biowaiver is whether the two products have the same "linearity factor β." This is simply investigated using the same type of statistical equivalence testing as recommended for IVBE assessment: a 90% confidence interval for the β_T/β_R ratio is constructed, and equivalence is concluded if the CI is included in a pre-specified acceptance interval. As for linearity, there is no agreed acceptance interval; it is suggested that 1 ± 0.20 is used until better recommendations are available.

As for IVBE, the scaling of acceptance intervals with the variability of the reference product should be considered also for dose linearity investigations and the use of different acceptance intervals for different end-points should be acceptable.

There is a regulatory trend for requiring the formal key in vitro studies (bioequivalence, dose linearity, flow dependence, drug product characterization tests, and stability) to be pre-specified in a protocol more detailed than historically has been the case. Although the situation still is far from what is required for clinical studies, the trend is surely in that direction. At a minimum, the protocol should pre-specify the material and test methods, detailed testing design, power considerations, primary and secondary end-points, statistical evaluation approach, significance and confidence levels as appropriate, and acceptance criteria. The protocol should be approved and signed before data collection is initiated.

REFERENCES

1. EudraxLex – EU legislation. https://ec.europa.eu/health/documents/eudralex_en (accessed January 29, 2018).
2. Knowledge Database – EDQM. https://extranet.edqm.eu/publications/recherches_sw.shtml (accessed December 1, 2017).
3. European Medicines Agency. 2005. Guideline on pharmaceutical quality of inhalation and nasal products. EMEA/CHMP/QWP/49313/2005 Corr.
4. European Medicines Agency. 2007. Guideline on the requirements for clinical documentation for orally inhaled products (OIP) including the requirements for demonstration of therapeutic equivalence between two inhaled products for use in the treatment of asthma and chronic obstructive pulmonary disease (COPD). CPMH/EWP/4151/00 Rev. 1.
5. European medicines Agency. Quality of medicines questions and answers – part 2. http://www.ema.europa.eu/ema/index.jsp?curl=pages/regulation/q_and_a/q_and_a_detail_000072.jsp&mid=WC0b01ac058002c2b0#section14 (accessed October 24, 2017).
6. European commission. https://ec.europa.eu/health/human-use/legal-framework_en (accessed October 24, 2017).
7. Gov. UK. Apply for a licence to market a medicine in the UK. https://www.gov.uk/guidance/apply-for-a-licence-to-market-a-medicine-in-the-uk (accessed January 29, 2018).
8. European Medicines Agency. Generic and hybrid applications. www.ema.europa.eu/ema/index.jsp?curl=pages/regulation/general/general_content_000179.jsp&mid=WC0b01ac0580022717 (accessed January 29, 2018).

9. Committee for Medicinal Products for Human use (CHMP). 2017. Concept paper on revision of the guideline on the pharmaceutical quality of inhalation and nasal products. February 16, 2017 EMA/CHMP/QWP/115777/2017.
10. Vencenzi, C. 2017. Update on the guideline on the pharmaceutical quality of inhalation and nasal products. *Drug Deliv Lung.* 2017:30.
11. Jefferys, D. 2017. Licensing medicines: Consequences of the UK "Brexit" vote to leave the European Union. *Resp Drug Deliv Eur* 2017:95–100.
12. www.gov.uk/government/news/medicines-and-healthcare-products-regulatory-agency-statement-on-the-outcome-of-the-eu-referendum. June 27, 2016.
13. Nichols. S C. 2009. European Pharmacopeia Inhalanda: Help or hindrance. *Drug Deliv Lung* 20:14–17.
14. Council of Europe – work programme. http://www.edqm.eu/en/european-pharmacopoeia-work-programme-607.html (accessed October 24, 2017).
15. Council of Europe – databases. https://www.edqm.eu/en/edqm-databases-10.html (accessed October 24, 2017).
16. Aiache, J-M, Bull H, Ganderton D, Haywood P, Olsson B, and Wright P. 1993. Inhalations; Collaborative study on the measurement of the fine particle dose using inertial impactors. *Pharmeuropa* 5:386–389
17. Marple, V A, Roberts, D L, Romay, F J, Miller, N C, Truman, K G, Van Oort, M, Olsson, B, Holroyd, M J, Mitchell, J P, and Hochrainer, D. 2004. Next generation pharmaceutical impactor (a new impactor for pharmaceutical inhaler testing). *Part I: Design J Aerosol Med* 16:283–299. doi:10.1089/089426803769017659.
18. Update statement on the EU referendum from the British Pharmacopoeia. Hppts://www.pharmacopoeia.com/news/208 (accessed October 4, 2017).
19. Lah, E and Boumans, R. White paper "Understanding Europe's new medical device regulation MDR 2017/745." https//www.emergogroup.com/resources/articles/whitepaper-understanding-europes-medical-devices-regulation (accessed November 20, 2017).
20. USP. USP39–NF34. <601> *Inhalation and Nasal Drug Products: Aerosols, Sprays, and Powders-Performance Quality Tests.* Rockville, MD: United States Pharmacopeial Convention. (accessed November 2, 2015).
21. Sandell, D and Mitchell, J. 2015. Considerations for designing in vitro bioequivalency (IVBE) studies for pressurized metered dose inhalers (PMDIS) with spacer or valved holding chamber (S/VHC) Add-on Devices. *J Aerosol Med* 28:156–181.
22. Zhang, Y, Gilbertson, K, and Finlay, WH. 2007. In vivo–in vitro comparison of deposition in three mouth–throat models with QVAR® and Turbuhaler® inhalers. *J Aerosol Med* 20:227–235.
23. Delvadia, R R, Longest, P W, and Byron, P R. 2012. In vitro tests for aerosol deposition. I: Scaling a physical model of the upper airways to predict drug deposition variation in normal humans. *J Aerosol Med* 25:32–40.
24. Burnell, P K, Asking, L, Borgström, L, Nichols, S C, Olsson, B, Prime, D, and Scrubb, I. 2007. Studies of the human oropharyngeal airspaces using magnetic resonance imaging IV–the oropharyngeal retention effect for four inhalation delivery systems. *J Aerosol Med* 20:269–281.
25. Delvadia, R R, Wei, X, Longest, P W, Venitz, J, and Byron, P R. 2015. In vitro tests for aerosol deposition. IV: Simulating variations in human breath profiles for realistic DPI testing. *J Aerosol Med* 28:1–11.
26. Sandell, D. 2016. Assessing in vitro BE using realistic inhalation profiles for regulatory approval of generic inhalers. In *Respiratory Drug Delivery 2016.* Volume 1. Edited by Dalby, R N, Byron, P R, Peart, J, Suman, J D, Farr, S J, Young, P M, and Traini, D. DHI Publishing; River Grove, IL:133–143.
27. Azimi, M, Longest, P W, Shur, J, Price, R, and Hindle, M. 2016. Clinically relevant in vitro tests for the assessment of innovator and generic nasal spray products. *Drug Deliv Lung* 27:12–15.
28. Burmeister Getz, E, Carroll, K J, Mielke, J, Benet, L Z, and Jones, B. 2017. Between-batch pharmacokinetic variability inflates type I error rate in conventional bioequivalence trials: A randomized Advair Diskus clinical trial. *Clin Pharmacol Ther* 101:331–340.
29. Burmeister Getz, E, Carroll, K J, Jones, B, and Benet, L Z. 2016. Batch-to-batch pharmacokinetic variability confounds current bioequivalence regulations: A dry powder inhaler randomized clinical trial. *Clin Pharmacol Ther* 100:223–231.
30. Sandell, D, Olsson, B, and Borgström, L. 2017. PK Bioequivalence testing when the between batch variability is high: A multiple-batch proposal. *Inhalation Magazine* (December 2017).
31. Garcia-Arieta, A. 2014. A European perspective on orally inhaled products: in vitro requirements for a biowaiver. *J Aerosol Med* 27:419–429.

Section IX

Preclinical Testing

28

Reconstituted 2D Cell and Tissue Models

Nicole Schneider-Daum, Patrick Carius, Justus C. Horstmann, and Claus-Michael Lehr

CONTENTS

28.1 Cell and Tissue-Based (Reconstituted) 2D *In Vitro* Models

28.1.1 Pulmonary Drug Delivery—Medical Opportunities and Pharmaceutical Needs

According to data from the World Health Organization (WHO), respiratory and lung diseases are listed within the top five death causing conditions worldwide, following ischemic heart disease and stroke (World Health Organization 2016). The administration of pharmacologically active substances via the lungs has been used to treat pulmonary maladies for ages. Within the lung, the unique morphology provides a vast contact area between pharmacologically active ingredients and the diseased tissue, immediately after inhalation. Through modern pulmonary delivery technologies, a targeted and efficient application of high local doses of aerosol medicines may be achieved with a simultaneous reduction of systemic drug exposure to the rest of the body (Ruge et al. 2013). However, the very thin epithelium of the respiratory mucosa in concert with its extensive surface area make the lung also suitable for systemic drug application since low enzymatic activity circumvents first-pass metabolism and a rapid onset is achieved (Labiris and Dolovich 2003; Patton and Byron 2007). While there has been an improvement in the topical treatment of pulmonary diseases through optimized deposition of inhaled medicines, the development of systemic pulmonary delivery of, e.g. peptides and proteins has been facing setbacks (Newman 2017). This backlog is or a large part based on insufficient knowledge about the mechanisms that take place after particle deposition (Patton et al. 2010). Therefore, contemporary models are needed that take cellular as well as non-cellular barriers like mucus, mucociliary clearance, and surfactant into account to gain insights about the fate of a tested substance and the underlying uptake mechanisms (Hittinger et al. 2015).

In vivo animal models have been utilized to study toxicologically or pharmacodynamic properties, but also systemic uptake (Andes and Craig 2002). However, the translation of results from animal-based *in vivo* studies to humans is difficult and needs to be critically evaluated (Leist and Hartung 2013; Seok et al. 2013).

Ex vivo models, comprising cultured lung slices, cultured essential lung constituents, or perfused lungs are further accepted methods in laboratory research (Sturton et al. 2008; Nelson et al. 2014). They can be applied to challenge isolated complex tissues or organs while maintaining their structural nature. Although such models allow to conduct studies with a higher level of physiological complexity, their usefulness is restricted by a short life-span and rather complex protocols.

Cell and tissue-based 2D *in vitro* models have been beneficial tools to reduce the complexity of the lung and its tissues into more controllable individual constituents. The following sections will describe different *in vitro* models starting from monocultures up to complex co-cultures.

28.1.2 Basics of Lung Anatomy

The path of an aerosol particle through the human airways starts at the nasal region, continues along the trachea, and subsequently passes the conducting airways of the central lung, as shown in Figure 28.1, until it eventually reaches the terminal respiratory airways of the peripheral lung. In order to cross the air-blood barrier, it has to traverse both cellular as well as non-cellular barriers, with different characteristics depending on the site of deposition (central versus peripheral lung). These barriers display significant differences in their structure and morphology, depending on their physiological function.

A partially ciliated pseudostratified epithelium characterizes the trachea as well as the large bronchi of the central lung, where columnar ciliated epithelial cells are adjacent to mucus secreting goblet cells both supported by basal cells (McDowell et al. 1978).

Mucus, which mainly consists of water (~95%), the high molecular glycoprotein mucin (~2%–5%), as well as low concentrations of lipids forms a hydrogel that lines the upper conducting airways (Boegh and Nielsen 2015). Through its mesh-like network, mucus traps particulate matter or microorganisms which are then transported to the pharynx via synchronized cilia movement in a process termed "mucociliary clearance." Along the ramifications of the conducting airways, a columnar ciliated epithelium lines the bronchioles with several club cells and scattered goblet cells. Club cells show a non-ciliated, cuboidal morphology with a dome-shaped apical cell surface, and they secrete high levels of secretoglobins (Reynolds et al. 2002). The bronchioles develop into respiratory bronchioles with repeated ramifying of the bronchial tree, then transform into the pulmonary acinus.

The pulmonary acinus comprises the alveolar ducts that terminate in two or three alveolar sacs each. One alveolar sac consists of many alveoli, whereby one alveolus forms the functional unit of gas exchange. Each alveolus in turn is lined by cells of the alveolar epithelium. The expansion of the respiratory airways makes it possible that the surface area covered by the alveolar epithelium (~100 m^2) amounts to more than 99% of the internal surface area of the lungs (Gehr et al. 1978; Mercer et al. 1994).

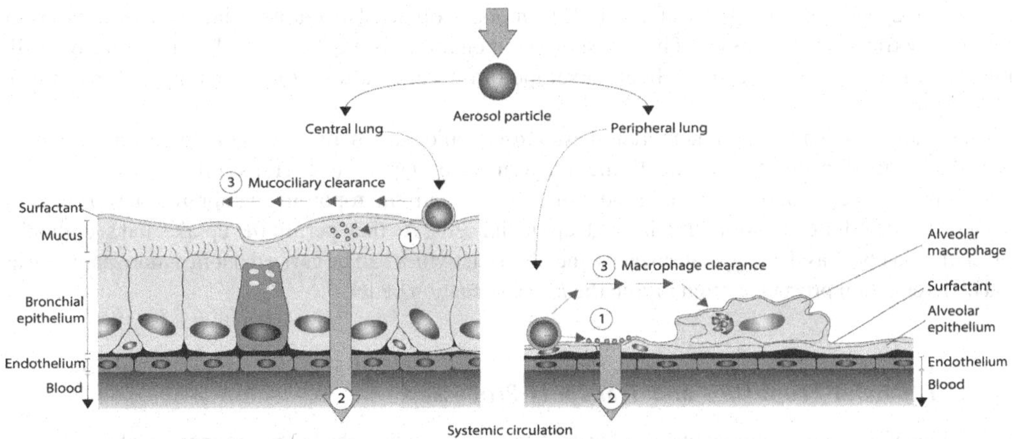

FIGURE 28.1 Cellular and non-cellular barriers of the human lung. A deposited particle, containing the active pharmaceutical ingredient (API) and eventually some excipients, initially interacts with the pulmonary lining fluid. Thereby, it primarily needs to deal with the surfactant layer that covers the central as well as the peripheral lung. After dissolution, a particle must penetrate the non-cellular barriers, as represented by mucus (central lung) and surfactant (central and peripheral lung) (1). To become systemically bioavailable some drugs need to be taken up by the pulmonary epithelium in order to reach the systemic circulation (2). Unless it dissolves very rapidly, a deposited aerosol particle needs to bypass the clearance mechanisms of the lung, that are exhalation, or active clearance by the mucociliary escalator in the conductive airways and phagocytosis by macrophages in the respiratory airways (3) (Modified from Ruge et al. 2013).

The alveolar epithelium is formed by AT I and AT II pneumocytes that separate the air-filled respiratory lumen from the bloodstream, thereby forming the "air-blood barrier." The flat AT I cells have a share of 8% of all lung cells, with one AT I cell covering a vast area of ~5000 µm² on average, comprising 95%–98% of the internal surface area (Crapo et al. 1982).

The cuboidal AT II cells represent 14% of all lung cells, contributing 2%–5% to the surface area (Stone et al. 1992). AT I cells are in their function mainly responsible for gas exchange as well as transport of fluids and solutes, while AT II cells ensure surfactant homeostasis, support immune responses, and serve as progenitors to AT I cells.

The respiratory epithelium and specifically the alveoli are coated with the alveolar lining fluid which is a thin aqueous layer comprising water and pulmonary surfactant. Pulmonary surfactant mainly reduces the surface tension of the alveolar epithelium, thereby preventing each alveolus from collapsing.

A lesser extent of pulmonary surfactant is also secreted by bronchial epithelial cells. Formed to around 90% of lipids, surfactant additionally contains ~10% of proteins including the bioactive surfactant proteins (SP-A, -B, -C, and -D) (Goerke 1998). Besides having an antimicrobial activity, the protein constituents of pulmonary surfactant influence the dissolution as well as the surface composition of nanoparticles.

28.2 How to Put the Lung in a Test Tube?

28.2.1 From Native Tissue to Epithelial Cell Cultures

First attempts to study transport across an epithelium were made by use of the Ussing chamber, developed by Ussing and Zerhan in the early 1950s (Ussing and Zerahn 1999). Starting with the analysis of frog skin, it was further used in combination with excised bullfrog alveolar epithelium

(Kim and Crandall 1983; Wall et al. 1993) amongst other also mammalian epithelia to study pulmonary transport processes. The classic Ussing chamber is nowadays still commercially available, but also newer devices have been developed in order to allow for diffusion or electrophysiological measurements.

These can be combined with membrane-based inserts allowing them to accommodate various tissues as well as cultured primary cells or cell lines on permeable supports (e.g. Transwell®).

Such permeable supports (even as stand-alone device) with microporous membranes have become a standard method for cultivation of polarized, epithelial cells. As they permit the uptake and secretion of molecules on both basal and apical surfaces, metabolic activities can be carried out in a more natural way and differentiation processes often mimic the *in vivo* situation better.

28.2.1.1 Barrier Properties and Transport Processes

Regardless of the *in vitro* model utilized for drug transport studies, the barrier properties of such model are an essential feature and can be evaluated by measuring the transepithelial electrical resistance (TEER). This value (typically: $\Omega*cm^2$) corresponds to the tightness of intercellular junctions in the cell monolayer and is formed as a consequence to the expression of intercellular tight junctions during cellular differentiation. TEER can be measured online using a chopstick electrode connected to a Volt-Ohm-meter (EVOM).

The presence of drug transporters within the lung was neglected for a long time. However, over the past years it has become evident that drug transporters also play an important role in pulmonary drug absorption, distribution, and elimination processes as well as drug-drug interactions. Different tissue and cell populations of the lung have distinct transporter expression patterns (Nickel et al. 2016). Although the lungs express high levels of both efflux and uptake drug transporters, little has been known of the impact on the pharmacokinetics of inhaled drugs (Bosquillon 2010). To close this gap, *in vitro* models of lung epithelium have been extensively used for uptake and transport studies. P-glycoprotein (P-gp) and organic cation transporters are among the most investigated ones, but also multidrug resistance proteins, peptide transporters, and several others have been intensively studied.

In vitro models of the alveolar epithelium (A549 and NCI-H441), for instance, have been used to prove a possible interaction between organic cation transporter 1 and the clinically relevant β_2-adrenergic agonists salbutamol sulfate, formoterol fumarate, and salmeterol xinafoate (Salomon et al. 2015). Thereby, transporters have been found to influence drug absorption processes *in vitro.*

Recent *ex vivo* experiments using isolated, perfused lung models, however, suggest that mainly efflux pumps significantly alter absorption into the pulmonary circulation (Nickel et al. 2016). Obviously, elucidating the role of pulmonary transport processes in the context of drug absorption and delivery via the lung is a timely topic in pharmaceutical research, for which cell and tissue based 2D *in vitro* models are an important tool.

28.2.1.2 Air Liquid Interface versus Submerged Conditions

The number of pulmonary *in vitro* models is dramatically increasing. Thereby, it has been realized that cultivation of cells as thin (mono)layers on plastic surfaces under submerged conditions may not adequately reflect the situation *in vivo*, especially when it comes to the lungs. This has led to the development of more complex models that better mimic cell interactions in their natural environment *in vivo.* Especially when modeling the air-blood barrier of the lungs, it is important to distinguish between so called air-liquid interface (ALI) conditions and liquid-covered culture (LCC) conditions: ALI conditions are not only critical in promoting cellular differentiation (Jong et al. 1994). An important advantage of the ALI models is that they allow the deposition of aerosolized liquids and powders using the air exposure route being representative for pulmonary application (Hiemstra et al. 2017).

28.2.1.3 Stretching/Breathing

Many models display only a specific part of the lung and are static. However, this still does not yet reflect physiological stretching of the lungs during respiration/breathing. Mounting bullfrog lung into a modified permeation system for studying transpulmonary drug permeation kinetics, Yu and Chien (2001) reported that respiratory dynamics dramatically enhanced the pulmonary permeation of progesterone as a model penetrant without causing a damage of the physical barrier of the membrane. In one of the pioneering lung-on-chip devices, breathing motions emulated on chip led to an increased transport of ultrafine silica nanoparticles through a cellular monolayer as well as a simultaneous increase in reactive oxygen species production (Huh et al. 2010). In a technically improved lung-on-chip device it could be shown that transport of Fluorescein isothiocyanate (FITC)-sodium was significantly increased by the cellular *in vivo*-like stretching (Stucki et al. 2015). At the same time, first efforts have been described to implement particle dynamics and deposition in true scale acinar models (Fishler et al. 2015).

Taken together, these findings demonstrate that respiration has an effect on pulmonary drug permeation through possible alterations in the properties of the pulmonary *in vitro* model.

28.2.2 Primary Cells

In oral drug delivery, the human intestinal epithelial cell line Caco-2, which forms relatively tight monolayers (300–400 $\Omega*cm^2$) when grown on Transwells, has dramatically affected pharmaceutical research and meanwhile developed to a worldwide industry and regulatory standard (Hidalgo et al. 1989; Artursson and Karlsson 1991). In pulmonary drug delivery, a suitable cell line which can be conveniently cultivated and displaying relevant barrier properties (>1500 $\Omega*cm^2$) of the alveolar epithelium was for a long time not available and researchers were therefore bound to the use of primary cells.

Cells that have been isolated from animal or human tissue and subsequently cultured *in vitro* are referred to as primary cells. They are usually regarded as the closest approximation of *in vivo* physiology as they directly originate from native tissues or organs and hence resemble a differentiated multiphenotype model with distinct cellular responses after taken into cell culture. Primary epithelial cells can be sub-cultured for a couple of passages after the initial isolation, but then may lose the ability to form high TEER values, lose barrier functions, or the capacity to differentiate (Yoon et al. 2000; Zabner et al. 2003). In addition to their shorter survival period compared to continuous cell line cultures, primary cells show donor-to-donor variations that impede the generation of reproducible results.

Although considered as the gold standard to study barrier-transport *in vitro*, limited access to human lung tissue and performing the costly isolation are accompanied by ethical issues, and financial limitations, which aggravate widespread usage of primary cells for drug transport studies.

28.2.2.1 Primary Bronchial Epithelial Cell Monocultures

Primary cells which originate from the conducting airways can be directly isolated from bronchial brushes or biopsies, resected bronchial tissue, or commercially purchased (Epithelix, Lonza, MaTek) (Devalia et al. 1999; Bucchieri et al. 2002). Isolation protocols are available for a broad range of species covering cow (Sisson et al. 1991), dog (Welsh 1985), ferret (Chung et al. 1991), guinea pig (Robison et al. 1993), hamster (Kaufman 1976), horse (Sime et al. 1997), human (Galietta et al. 1998; Lin et al. 2007), mouse (Oreffo et al. 1990), and rabbit (Mathias et al. 1995; Sporty et al. 2008).

Expanded on collagen 1-coated growth supplies and supplemented with defined growth medium under LCC conditions, primary bronchial epithelial cells do not polarize, thereby forming monolayers that resemble a basal cell-like phenotype (Hackett et al. 2011).

Such epithelial cell monolayers have been, for example, used to study the effect of external noxae, showing that the dysregulation of the basal cell transcriptome at the chronic obstructive pulmonary disease risk locus 19q13.2 could be directly linked to the influence of cigarette smoke (Ryan et al. 2014). Some advanced applications of primary bronchial epithelial cells are described further below in the paragraph 28.2.4.

28.2.2.2 Primary Alveolar Epithelial Cell Culture

Alveolar epithelial cells are mostly collected from lung tissue of patients who underwent lung surgery or from perfused animal lungs. Cell isolation is in principle performed via different methods of proteolytic digestion, followed by purification via positive or passive selection methods, and subsequently followed by culturing cells *in vitro*. Protocols for the isolation of AT II cells had been reported first for rodents (Dobbs 1990; Gonzalez and Dobbs 2013; Sinha and Lowell 2016). The differentiation of AT II into AT I cells and the formation of tight intercellular junctions, however, have not been in the focus of such research.

While AT II cells normally show a restricted proliferation *in vitro*, Bove et al. (2014) could retain AT II cell characteristics by co-culturing primary human AT II cells together with feeder cells from mouse and simultaneously treating the cells with a Rho kinase inhibitor "Y-27632." By this method, some epithelial barrier function with a TEER of ~350–400 Ω*cm^2 could be established (Bove et al. 2014). Methods to primary isolate AT I cells have so far only been described for rat tissue (Borok et al. 2002; Chen et al. 2004; Gonzalez and Dobbs 2013). None of these methods, however, was intended for the generation of electrically tight barriers after *in vitro* cultivation. Interestingly enough, AT II cells can be trans-differentiated into AT I-like cells, forming monolayers with significant barrier properties when cultivated *in vitro* which was reported first for rats (Danto et al. 1995) and later for humans (Elbert et al. 1999; Fuchs et al. 2003). By further improving the protocol, isolated human alveolar epithelial cells (hAEpC) seeded on permeable supports can be trans-differentiated into AT I-like cells, developing tight intercellular junctions and reaching TEER values of ~2000–2500 Ω*cm^2 within 1 week (Daum et al. 2012). Even though such procedures allow for transport and uptake studies, the poor availability of human tissue still limits their wider application.

28.2.3 Cell Lines

Clear advantages of cell lines over primary cells are that cell lines can be conveniently expanded *in vitro* over several passages, and that they can be easier cryo-preserved for long time storage. Over the years, cell lines of several pulmonary epithelia have been established to explore general barrier functionality or to investigate pulmonary absorption and toxicity *in vitro*. Pulmonary epithelial cell lines are typically derived from and therefore representative for either the bronchial or alveolar region of the lung. However, because often originating from tumors, some cell lines do no longer represent the typical phenotype of the original tissue.

This may result in an altered morphology, impaired barrier properties, and incomplete expression of transporters.

28.2.3.1 Cell Lines of Bronchial Epithelial Cells

The Calu-3 and the 16HBE14o- cell lines are most common to evaluate transport mechanisms across the bronchial epithelium. For both cell lines, the permeability of a series of pharmaceutical compounds was evaluated in a study among different laboratories (Forbes and Ehrhardt 2005). Especially the human Calu-3 cell line has turned out to be easy in handling which might have contributed to its frequent usage. The Calu-3 cell line originates from a lung adenocarcinoma and can be purchased from the American Type Culture Collection (ATCC). It has been utilized in several drug transport studies on a regular basis (Foster et al. 2000; Mathia et al. 2002; Grainger et al. 2006).

In a recent study, the permeability of seven substances (imipramine, propranolol, metoprolol, terbutaline, mannitol, dextran, and formoterol) was evaluated for three cell lines (Calu-3, 16HBE14o-, and NHBE) and for an isolated perfused rat lung *ex vivo* model (Bosquillon et al. 2017). These permeability data were then compared to an *in vivo* absorption dataset that was already published. While the permeability measurements were comparable between all three cell lines, the Calu-3 cell line was proposed best suited for standardized permeability screening studies, because of its availableness and convenient handling.

Further, the Calu-3 cell line has been used to study nanoparticle effects on cellular monolayers (Fiegel et al. 2003; Cooney et al. 2004; Amidi et al. 2006).

The 16HBE14o- cell line was established via transformation of human bronchial epithelial cells with the SV40 large-T antigen and can be received from Dieter C. Gruenert at the California Pacific Medical Center (Cozens et al. 1994). The barrier integrity of this cell line strongly depends on the cell culture conditions. Grown under LCC conditions, 16HBE14o- cells show a polarized monolayer with TEER values up to 800 Ω*cm^2, the formation of a formidable barrier for solutes with increasing TEER, and the expression of several drug transporters (Ehrhardt et al. 2002, 2003). However, this effect was reversed under ALI conditions through unknown mechanisms.

Another frequently studied continuous cell line are the BEAS-2B bronchial airway cells that were generated by transfection of NHBE cells with an adenovirus 12-SV40 hybrid virus (Reddel et al. 1988).

BEAS-2B cells do not yield TEER values >100 Ω*cm^2, thus lacking sufficient barrier function as would be needed for transport studies (Noah et al. 1995). Nonetheless, they are commonly used for toxicological studies on the toxicity of exhaust fumes, pathogens, or nanoparticles (Steerenberg et al. 1998; Opitz et al. 2004; Xia et al. 2008).

28.2.3.2 Cell Lines of Alveolar Epithelial Cells

Compared to the bronchial epithelium, where several useful cell lines are easily accessible for transport studies, the situation for the alveolar epithelium is more challenging.

This is made even more evident considering the vast surface area together with the thickness of under 1 µm for the alveolar epithelium, which rises interest particularly in standardized transport studies over the "air-blood barrier" (Low 1953; Gehr et al. 1978).

The NCI-H441 cell line which can be obtained from ATCC was isolated from adenocarcinoma tissue of the human lung and bridges the gap between bronchial and alveolar epithelial cell lines (Brower et al. 1986). Formerly described as having morphological and functional analogies to bronchiolar club cells, the NCI-H441 cell line was further characterized showing surfactant protein secretion and lamellar body formation similar to AT II pneumocytes (Gazdar et al. 1990; Duncan et al. 1997; Rehan et al. 2002).

Cultured under LCC conditions on permeable growth supports, NCI-H441 monolayers, however, showed the formation of an electrically tight barrier and TEER values of ~1000 Ω*cm^2 after 8 days–12 days in culture (Salomon et al. 2014). Furthermore, the function of the drug transporter P-glycoprotein or the expression patterns of tight junction protein ZO-1 resembled the phenotype of AT I cells.

By adding insulin-transferrin-selenium (ITS) and dexamethasone to the cell culture medium of NCI-H441 monolayers, the TEER values measured under ALI conditions before supplementation (<100 Ω*cm^2) could be elevated to ~400 Ω*cm^2 making absorption studies possible (Ren et al. 2016).

A549 cells are an adenocarcinoma cell line which is probably most frequently applied to emulate AT II-like pneumocyte function *in vitro* (Giard et al. 1973). The initially reported formation of lamellar bodies in A549 cells categorized them as AT II-like cells, whereas this functional characteristic is lost during longer culture times (Lieber et al. 1976; Speirs et al. 1991). Even though A549 cells show characteristic features of AT II cells with respect to drug transport and metabolism, their inability to form functional tight junctions disqualifies the A549 cell line from being used for transport studies because the discontinuous barrier shows no selectivity for low molecular weight compounds (Foster et al. 1998; Winton et al. 1998).

Another cell line, transformed type 1 (TT1), demonstrates functional expression of the AT I cell markers caveolin-1 and the receptor for advanced glycation end products (RAGE) as well as a flattened morphology similar to AT I cells (Kemp et al. 2008). This cell line allows an expansion of AT I-like cells over multiple passages through an initial transformation of primary AT II cells with the catalytic subunit of human telomerase (hTERT) and a temperature sensitive mutant of simian virus 40 large antigen (U19tsA58). Unfortunately, low expression of ZO-1 and the leakiness of the permeability barrier with TEER values around ~50 Ω*cm^2 make them non-applicable for transport studies (van den Bogaard et al. 2009).

The recently introduced human alveolar epithelial lentivirus immortalized (hAELVi) cell line shows AT I-like pneumocyte physiology; it preserves electrically tight barrier properties under different culture conditions, and it is as well suitable for continuous expansion (Kuehn et al. 2016). Available from InSCREENeX GmbH, the hAELVi cell line showed the expression of caveolin-1 as an AT I cell marker, as well as the expression of the tight junction proteins ZO-1 and Occludin. Cultured hAELVi cells showed TEER value formation of ~1000 Ω*cm^2 under LCC conditions and >2000 Ω*cm^2 under ALI while simultaneously preserving a permeability barrier for the paracellular transport marker sodium fluorescein. The data support the hAELVi cell line as a promising candidate for the standardization of transport studies over the alveolar epithelium, since they resemble functional barrier properties and AT I cell markers equivalent to primary AT I-like cells *in vitro*.

28.2.4 Co-cultures and Tissue-Like *In Vitro* Models

Reproducing the full complexity of pulmonary epithelia through an *in vitro* model represents a demanding challenge. Aside from the difficulties of culturing different cell types in the same environment, the relation of cell numbers must also be adequate. Moreover, designs get even more intricate, if tissue morphology is also taken into account.

Co-cultures and tissue-like *in vitro* models thereby aim to investigate the interplay among the various differentiated cells within an epithelium or between epithelial cells and other cell types like immune cells or endothelial cells. As mentioned in Section 28.2.2.1, primary bronchial epithelial cells can be differentiated into complex epithelia *in vitro*.

When grown on collagen-coated membrane supports under ALI conditions with supplementation of retinoic acid, primary bronchial epithelial cells form a columnar pseudostratified epithelium with ciliated epithelial cells and goblet cells supported by basal cells, that resemble *in vivo* morphology after 2 weeks in culture (Karp et al. 2002).

With this in mind, primary NHBE cells (Lonza) have been differentiated under ALI conditions and were characterized according to their barrier functionality and transport of lipophilic compounds (Lin et al. 2007; Bosquillon et al. 2017). Two additional commercially available primary bronchial cells are MucilAir™ (Epithelix) and EpiAirway™ (MatTek). Both comprise initially de-differentiated cells which are gradually differentiated under ALI conditions over time, forming multicellular polarized epithelia. Ciliated epithelia with TEER values of ~400 Ω*cm^2 are formed after 14 days–21 days in the case of MucilAir or after 20 days–45 days with regard to EpiAirway (Gordon et al. 2015). Characterization of drug absorption and transport studies was performed for MucilAir as well as for EpiAirway (Leonard et al. 2005, 2007; Agu et al. 2006; Reus et al. 2014). Although bronchial differentiated epithelia *in vitro* may possess a high biorelevance, they seem to have the same predictivity in relation to transport or permeability studies than continuous cell lines (Bosquillon et al. 2017). By contrast, based on a co-culture model of Rothen-Rutishauser et al. (2005) where three different cell types (A549 cells, macrophages, and dendritic cells) have been cultured in parallel, Müller et al. (2010) could show that co-cultures were more suitable to investigate the toxicological effects of nanoparticle exposure than monocultures. The authors proposed a synergistic effect between lung epithelial cells and the cells of the immune system in case of cytokine secretion and total antioxidant capacity. This model was recently used, after further characterization and enhancement, as a predictivity model for the immunogenicity of gold nanoparticles (Fytianos et al. 2017). By adding a dendritic cell-specific intracellular adhesion molecule 3-grabbing non-integrin (DCSIGN) antibody to gold nanoparticles, the authors could show an enhanced targeting of monocyte derived dendritic cells, whereas unmodified nanoparticles mainly targeted monocyte derived macrophages.

It is, however, interesting to note that barrier integrity is also affected by the culture of epithelial cells together with other cell types. A co-culture of the cell line 16HBE41o- together with human umbilical vein endothelial cells (HUVECs) led to a significant increase in TEER value compared to a monolayer of 16HBE41o- cells only (Chowdhury et al. 2010). In another study by Hittinger et al. (2016a), TEER values decreased in two out of three isolations, when a growing number of autologous alveolar macrophages was added to confluent hAEpC. In a further example, co-culturing the AT I-like hAELVi cell line together with differentiated THP-1 cells did not have an impact on the tightness of the barrier (Kletting et al. 2017).

28.3 Hardware Considerations

In vitro testing of aerosols remains as a major challenge, both for efficiency testing of APIs as well as for safety testing of accidentally inhaled other substances. Evaluation of aerosols in Transwell-based 2D *in vitro* models are ethically preferable to inhalation testing in animals and, once validated, could be more cost- and time-efficient (Hein et al. 2010). In any event, such models will definitely improve our scientific understanding of the interactions between inhaled particles and the lung in general. Safety testing of formulations must include both acute and chronic toxicity, as described by the respective Guidelines (OECD 2009, 2017). Whereas for efficiency testing, inhalable pharmaceutic compounds must comply with quality standards of EMA (EMA 2006) or FDA (FDA/CDER 2002). Generally, in comparison to other epithelial barriers, such as, e.g. the intestinal mucosa or the blood-brain barrier, the air-blood barrier of the lung requires to address ALI conditions and eventually also the presence of mucus and alveolar lining fluid.

As the depth of the alveolar lining fluid is only 0.2 μm (Bastacky et al. 1995), 1/10 smaller than an average inhalable particle, dissolution behavior, and drug release are likely to be much different compared to LCC conditions (Fiegel et al. 2003). The same is true for *in vitro* transport studies (Bur et al. 2010) and cellular uptake (Lenz et al. 2014) that has been reported to be higher after aerosol deposition under ALI conditions.

28.3.1 Aerosol Deposition Without Particle Size Differentiation

Simple, but effective deposition devices are the Dry Powder Insufflator™ for solid aerosols or the MicroSprayer® Aerosolizer for liquid aerosols. Initially developed for *in vivo* research, these devices are also able to apply small clouds of aerosols on cell cultures (Blank et al. 2006; Bur et al. 2010). However, differentiation between particle size distributions is lacking and possible cell damage as well as decreasing TEER values after such non-physiological impaction have been reported (Meindl et al. 2015).

28.3.2 Modified Impactors

In order to classify aerosols in respect to their aerodynamic behavior, impactors as described in United States Pharmacopeia (USP) and European Pharmacopoeia (Ph. Eur.) are widely used (Mitchell and Nagel; Hickey 2014). Instead of measuring the amount of particles in each stage of an impactor, some authors modified these impactors and placed cell culture inserts inside the stages, as done for the Twin Stage Impinger (Grainger et al. 2009; Haghi et al. 2012), for the Anderson Cascade Impactor (Cooney et al. 2004; Ong et al. 2015), and for the Multistage Liquid Impinger (Fiegel et al. 2003; Bur et al. 2009). Even though particles were deposited successfully in ALI condition, impactor models have the disadvantage that particles are hitting the cells rather bluntly. Therefore, new approaches are needed which better reflect physiological processes of aerosol deposition in the lung.

28.3.3 Electrostatic Deposition

In addition to conventional deposition of aerosols, electrostatic deposition has emerged in the last decade. Basically, particles are charged and consecutively precipitated on cell culture inserts in order to increase deposition efficiency. Figure 28.2b illustrates the operating mode of the Nano aerosol chamber for in vitro toxicity (NACIVT) device, where aerosols are charged unipolar, heated up to body temperature, and are humidified to be guided short-distanced on cell culture inserts.

Particles are size-selected previously, a deposition efficiency of 15% was reported (Jeannet et al. 2015). In contrast to depositing particles vertically, the NAVETTA device uses a laminar horizontal flow approach (Frijns et al. 2017). The authors claim that this approach is more physiologic which, indeed, could hold true in the case of bronchial airway cells, but not necessarily for alveolar epithelial cells. With the help of an electric field, a deposition efficiency of 95% is reached.

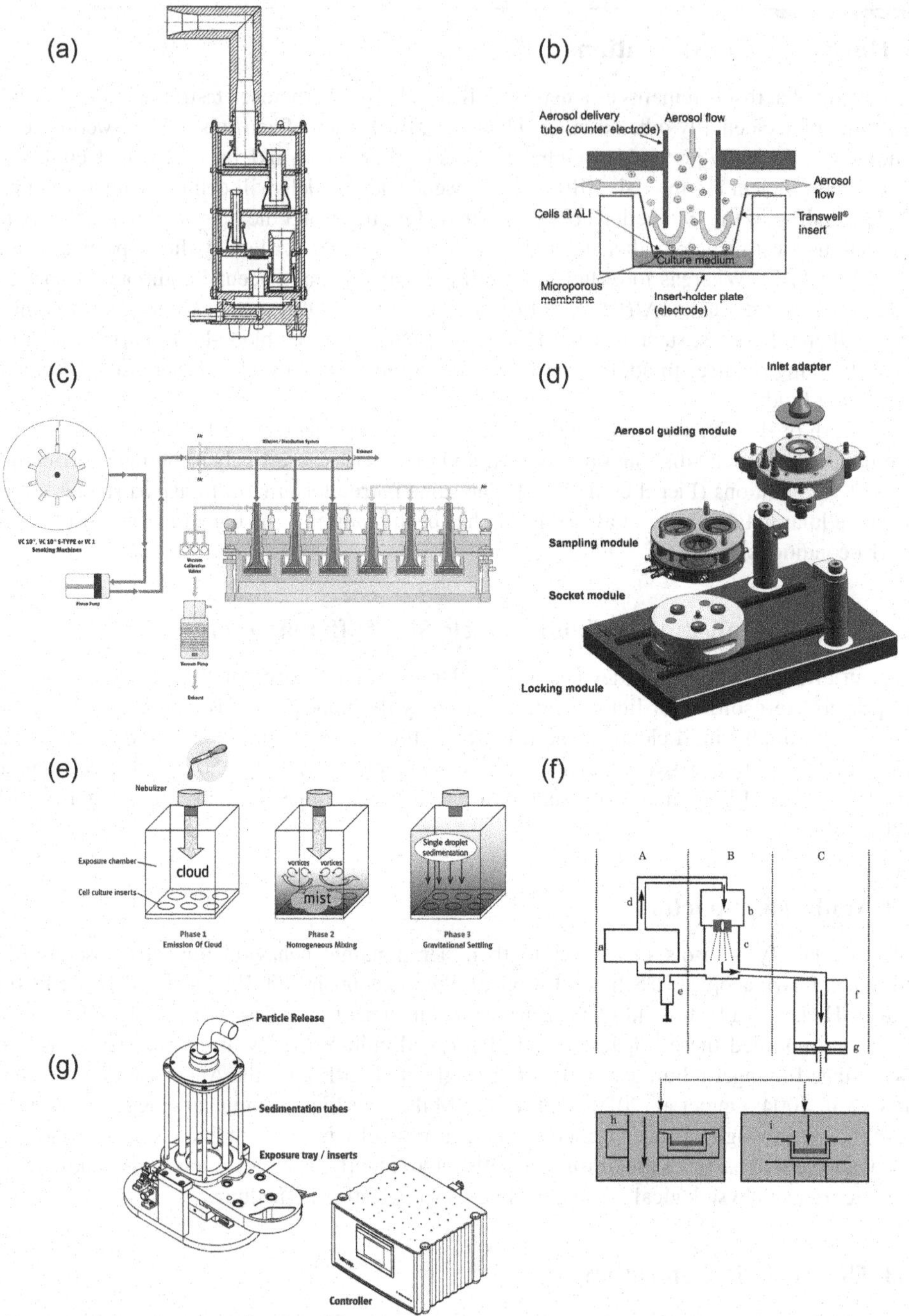

FIGURE 28.2 Pictures of different devices for testing safety and efficacy of inhalable substances. (a) Modified Multi Stage Liquid Impinger, cell culture insert upside down surrounded by lining fluid on stage three. (From Bur, M. et al., *Eur. J. Pharm. Biopharm.*, 72, 350–357, 2009.) (b) NACIVT: unipolar charged particles deposit electrostatically on Transwell insert. (From Jeannet, N. et al., *Nanotoxicology*, 9, 34–42, 2015.) (c) Vitrocell® Smoking Robot linked to exposure system, "trumpet" shaped air exposure outlet. (d) Cultex® RFS (Second Generation): Aerosol is divided equally on cell culture inserts. (From Aufderheide, M. et al., *Exp. Toxicol. Pathol.*, 69, 359–365, 2017.) (e) Vitrocell Cloud: nebulized aerosol is floating on the ground in vortices, ending in sedimentation of the droplets. (f) PADDOCC with air-flow control unit, aerosolization, and deposition unit. (From Hein, S. et al., *Altern. Lab, Anim.*, 38, 285–295, 2010.) (g) Vitrocell Powder Chamber: Dry powder inhaler connected to L-shaped inlet directing aerosol in four different channels, allowing sedimentation type of deposition. (Figure 28.2c, 28.2e, 28.2g: Courtesy of Tobias Krebs, Vitrocell, Germany.)

Following the principle of electrostatic deposition, not only experimentally developed devices are available. The Cultex® Electrical Deposition Device is commercially available and follows a similar principle. Experiments have been performed on organic derived aerosols (Yu et al. 2017).

28.3.4 Innovative Developments in Aerosol Deposition on Cell Cultures

First described some 20 years ago, Cultex Systems have meanwhile developed to a commercially available system for controlled aerosol deposition in ALI conditions. Originally described as an innovative device for cell culture on Transwell inserts at ALI conditions (Aufderheide and Mohr 1999, 2000), the application of gaseous compounds (Ritter et al. 2001), diesel exhaust (Knebel et al. 2002), and cigarette smoke (Aufderheide et al. 2001) were evaluated thereafter. This first generation is made of glass, containing three individual housings for Transwell inserts. Continuous temperature control via water and medium supply are controlled individually. The air flows on cell cultures through a cylindrical structure and exits at the sides to flow back. A second generation device called Cultex Radial Flow System (RFS) generates more consistent particle distribution, as the air flows equally on the cell culture inserts, not in a row like in the first generation (Aufderheide et al. 2017). Experiments have mainly been conducted with different inorganic material, cigarette or e-cigarette aerosol (Aufderheide and Emura 2017). A modified Cultex system presented an enhanced module with hyperboloid-shaped air exposition inlets, improving air flow, and preventing swirls (Aufderheide and Mohr 2004). Later, Vitrocell® developed a range of exposure systems for small to higher throughput. Typical applications are exposure to nanoparticles, gases, and complex mixtures, like in a comparison between cigarette and e-cigarette aerosol (Neilson et al. 2015).

28.3.4.1 Alice-Cloud

To improve the simulation of depositing aerosols in the deep lung, the Alice-Cloud System (Air-Liquid Interface Cell Exposure System) provides a nebulizer-based *in vitro* approach. The first developed apparatus uses aerosolization of suspensions via piezoelectrically driven vibrating membrane to produce fine droplets of the size of around 5 μM. The process of depositing these on cell cultures is divided in three phases: First, a dense cloud of droplets is produced and sinks in the exposure chamber. Then, the cloud falling down on the bottom of the chamber spreads out to all sides forming swirls. In a third phase, particles start to fall down on the bottom via sedimentation forces. The authors used this system to evaluate cytotoxicity (Lenz et al. 2009). Later, the system was improved and equipped with a vibrating mesh cloud generator, that allows deposition of the cloud without external air flow (Alice-Cloud). The authors tested the effect of aerosolized Bortezomib on cells, proving reliability for drug screening in ALI conditions (Lenz et al. 2014). As it is the only system representing sedimentation-like properties of liquid aerosols, the system has been used frequently for testing safety and efficacy of drugs and airborne particles (Chortarea et al. 2017; Röhm et al. 2017).

28.3.4.2 Dry Powder Deposition

Only few innovations happened in the field of dry powder deposition mimicking sedimentation-like processes, instead, most systems were optimized on testing aerosol toxicity. In order to optimize controlled deposition of dry powder inhalers (DPIs)/pressurized metered dose inhalers (pMDIs), one of the few devices developed is the PADDOCCs (Pharmaceutical Aerosol Deposition Device On Cell Cultures). DPIs can be connected to the PADDOCCs and the powder is aerosolized within the PADDOCCs. Via controlled air-flow, particles are able to enter the deposition unit containing three Snapwell™ inserts.

The authors could prove that drugs and lactose carriers were separated via impaction and remaining drug particles (<10 μm) deposited on cell culture inserts via sedimentation (Hein et al. 2010, 2011), which reflects the situation in the deep lung. The PADDOCC has been used since, e.g. for delivery of IL-10 containing microparticles (Hittinger et al. 2016a, 2016b) and clarithromycin microparticles (Dimer et al. 2015).

Continuing the concept of depositing aerosols, the Vitrocell Powder Chamber has been developed recently. Based mainly on the same principles of deposition, i.e. sedimentation and diffusion, lactose carriers and adherent drug particles can be separated size-dependent by the time they are floating through the device. Further experiments on alveolar epithelial cells are planned (Hittinger et al. 2017).

28.3.5 General Difference Between Metered and Non-metered Aerosol Deposition

It is crucial to fundamentally distinguish between metered aerosol deposition, i.e. the application of a defined dose of APIs in order to most efficiently deposit the drugs on each insert and non-metered deposition, where the mass of aerosol itself is not relevant, but safety questions are best being answered with. The development of testing devices that allows to deposit a finite amount of drug as generated by commercially available DPI on pulmonary cell cultures under physiologically relevant conditions represents a certain milestone in this research. Chronologically, several intermediate steps were made before, like the combination of impactors as aerosol classification devices that assure physiological particle size distribution and finite amounts of drugs in DPIs with the disadvantage of drug impaction on cells. In return, the Alice-Cloud system displays sedimentation of particles instead of impaction, but the nebulizer theoretically produces infinite drug amounts, that are measured as deposited on the cells.

However, the PADDOCC and the new invented Vitrocell Powder Chamber work with DPIs, display separation of lactose carriers from adherent drugs by impaction, and afterwards sedimentation properties on cells. A single puff as inhaled by a patient is investigated.

Regardless how the aerosol under investigation is being generated, ALI conditions are relevant with respect to drug deposition and transcellular drug transport as well as possible effects of the formulation on pulmonary barrier integrity. Deposition by impaction might negatively affect cell viability and therefore should be avoided. Instead, deposition by sedimentation and/or diffusion is preferred, especially regarding the alveolar epithelium of the deep lung. In API testing, finite amounts of drugs (i.e. dry powder reservoirs in DPIs) are administered and particle properties should realistically simulate the inhalation procedure. As an example, lactose carrier particles, which do not normally enter the lung after inhalation *in vivo*, must be separated from the smaller, respirable drugs before deposition on cells. Table 28.1 provides an overview of selected examples of different deposition methods for particles on cell culture inserts.

28.4 Future Directions

28.4.1 Non-cellular Barriers: Mucus and Surfactant

The previous sections mainly covered cell- and tissue-based *in vitro* models as well as possible aerosol deposition devices. However, the respiratory tract comprises also non-cellular barriers, such as mucus and surfactant, to protect from external noxae. During the last years, the role of the constituents and the functionality of mucus and surfactant have been extensively studied—biochemically and biophysically. In the case of mucus, this knowledge has led to drug delivery approaches like mucoadhesion or mucopenetration, exploiting the molecular architecture of mucus in order to sustain drug release or to enhance drug permeability in case of the latter (Murgia et al. 2017). Nevertheless, the role and importance of non-cellular barriers is still a matter of current research and, due to its complexity, cannot be further elucidated within this chapter.

28.4.2 Disease-Relevant Models

There is a huge gap in understanding and treating human lung diseases. It has been recognized in the last decade that animal models suffer from severe limitations: lung anatomy, cellular morphology, and crosstalk significantly differ between humans and animals, such as rodents. In addition, several animal-based *in vivo* models are naturally not permissive to some zoonotic infections or do not reflect the clinical course of the disease in humans (Zscheppang et al. 2018). Furthermore, species-specific variations in drug efficacy are a major drawback.

Taken together, there is a high necessity for the development and evaluation of human-based pulmonary disease models. The capability of mimicking pathophysiological conditions could thereby contribute to our understanding of lung disease mechanisms and could help to identify improved or even novel diagnostics and therapies.

TABLE 28.1

Selected Examples of Different Deposition Methods for Particles on Cell Culture Inserts

General Classification	Device	Aerosol Generation	Manufacturer/ Source	Mechanism of Deposition	Specification	Deposition Efficiency	Cell Type	Substance/ Formulation Tested	Reference
Aerosol deposition without particle size differentiation	DP-4 Dry Powder Insufflator™	(DPI)	Penn-Century, Inc., Wyndmoor, USA	Impaction	Spray deposition of aerosols on cell culture inserts in set distance	–	Calu-3	Micronized Salbutamol sulfate and Budenoside microparticles	(Bur et al. 2010)
						3%–28%	Calu-3	Budesonide, Formoterol fumarate, sodium Fluorescein, Rhodamine 123 microparticles	(Meindl et al. 2015)
	MicroSprayer® Aerosolizer IA-1C	Atomizer		Impaction		39% (inside cells)	A549	Polystyrene microparticles	(Blank et al. 2006)
						24%–30%	Calu-3	Budesonide, Formoterol fumarate, sodium Fluorescein, Rhodamine 123 solution	(Meindl et al. 2015)

(Continued)

TABLE 28.1 (*Continued*)

Selected Examples of Different Deposition Methods for Particles on Cell Culture Inserts

General Classification	Device	Aerosol Generation	Manufacturer/ Source	Mechanism of Deposition	Specification	Deposition Efficiency	Cell Type	Substance/ Formulation Tested	Reference
Modified impactors	Twin Stage Impinger (TSI)	(DPI)	Ph. Eur.	Impaction	Single Transwell insert located directly under second stage inlet	–	Calu-3	FITC-Dextran microparticles	(Grainger et al. 2009)
						–	Calu-3	Salbutamol, Salbutamol sulfate microparticles	(Haghi et al. 2012)
	Andersen Cascade Impactor (ACI)	Nebulizer, DPI	USP/Ph. Eur.	Impaction	Three Transwell inserts inserted under stage 4 of an ACI	–	SAEC, Calu-3	FITC-Dextran suspension, Disodium fluorescein lactose microparticles	(Cooney et al. 2004)
		Nebulizer, DPI, pMDI			Eight Snapwell™ inserts on 3D printed, wetted stage that replace stage 4 or 5 of the ACI	–	Calu-3	Salbutamol sulfate solution and microparticles	(Ong et al. 2015)
	Multistage Liquid Impinger (MSLI)	DPI		Impaction	Single Transwell® insert located directly under second stage inlet	–	Calu-3	PLGA microparticles	(Fiegel et al. 2003)
					Two Transwell inserts located shifted under inlet and upside down in stage 2 or 3	–	Calu-3	Salbutamol sulfate and Budenoside microparticles	(Bur et al. 2009)

(*Continued*)

TABLE 28.1 (*Continued*)

Selected Examples of Different Deposition Methods for Particles on Cell Culture Inserts

General Classification	Device	Aerosol Generation	Manufacturer/ Source	Mechanism of Deposition	Specification	Deposition Efficiency	Cell Type	Substance/ Formulation Tested	Reference
Electrostatic deposition	NACIVT	Nebulizer, spark generator	Institute of Anatomy, U Bern, CH	Electrostatic deposition	Positive charged particles, humidified air-flow directed short-distanced on 24 Transwell inserts	15% (Poly-styrene particles)	BEAS-2B, p. HBE cells, p. porcine lung macrophages	Polystyrene latex submicron particles suspension, silver nanoparticles	(Jeannet et al. 2015)
	NAVETTA	Atomizer	Vito NV, Mol, Belgium	Electrostatic deposition	Unipolar charged nanoparticles deposited via sideward air stream on 12 well plate	95%	A549 reporter cells	CuO nanoparticle suspension	(Frijns et al. 2017)
	Cultex RFS Compact+EDD	Aerosol generator	Cultex Laboratories GmbH, Hannover, D	Electrostatic deposition	Electrical Deposition Device produces positive charged particles to be deposited in Cultex Radial Flow System	–	BEAS-2B	Secondary organic aerosol from α-Pinene or D-Limonene	(Yu et al. 2017)
Deposition of non-metered (infinite) aerosol doses	Original Cultex Device Cultex RFS	Smoke machine		Impaction	Smoking machine coupled to exposure chamber, ALI cond. under medium supply	–	HFBE-21	Cigarette smoke	(Aufderheide et al. 2001)
					See above, radial composition of exposure chamber, more consistent deposition	–	NHBE	Cigarette smoke, e-cigarette aerosol	(Aufderheide and Emura 2017)
	P.R.I.T. ExpoCube	Gas generator	Fraunhofer ITEM Hannover, D	Impaction	Compact aerosol deposition device, stagnation flow setup on multiwell plates	–	A549	Air, Formaldehyde, Ozone	(Ritter and Knebel 2014)

(*Continued*)

TABLE 28.1 (*Continued*)

Selected Examples of Different Deposition Methods for Particles on Cell Culture Inserts

General Classification	Device	Aerosol Generation	Manufacturer/ Source	Mechanism of Deposition	Specification	Deposition Efficiency	Cell Type	Substance/ Formulation Tested	Reference
	Alice, Alice-Cloud Vitrocell Cloud 12	Nebulizer	Helmholtz Zentrum München, Neuherberg, D	Cloud-settling, Sedimentation	Droplet cloud entering exposure chamber, then distribution and settling on inserts	7%	A549	ZnO suspension	(Lenz et al. 2009)
					See above, slightly changed nebulizer	17%	A549 reporter cells	Fluoresceine, Mannitol, Bortezomib solution	(Lenz et al. 2014)
			Vitrocell® Systems GmbH, Waldkirch, D			–	RPMI 2650	IgG Fab, IgG solution	(Röhm et al. 2017)
	Vitrocell 12/6 CF	Smoking robot		Impaction	Smoking robot VC1 attached to exposure module at ALI condition	–	EpiAirway	Cigarette smoke, e-cigarette aerosol	(Neilson et al. 2015)
	Vitrocell 6 PT-CF	Nebulizer			PARI LC Sprint® nebulizer attached to exposure model, cells at ALI cond.	<7%	A549	Polystyrene submicron particles, carbon nanotubes	(Fröhlich et al. 2013)
Deposition of metered (finite) aerosols doses	Vitrocell Powder Chamber	DPI		Sedimentation	DPI connected at inlet to chamber and distribution of aerosol in four channels	–	–	Salbutamol sulfate microparticles	(Hittinger et al. 2017)
	PADDOCC	DPI	Biopharmaceutics and Pharmaceutical Technology, UdS, Saarbrücken, D	Sedimentation	Separated air-flow control unit, aerosolization and deposition unit, 3 Snapwell® Inserts	–	Calu-3	Salbutamol sulfate, Budenoside microparticles	(Hein et al. 2010)
						–	AT2 cells, pr. alveolar macrophages	IL-10 microparticles	(Hittinger et al. 2016a, 2016b)

REFERENCES

Agu, Remigius U., Satyanarayana Valiveti, Kalpana S. Paudel, Mitch Klausner, Patrick J. Hayden, and Audra L. Stinchcomb. 2006. "Permeation of WIN 55,212-2, a potent cannabinoid receptor agonist, across human tracheo-bronchial tissue in vitro and rat nasal epithelium in vivo." *The Journal of Pharmacy and Pharmacology* 58 (11): 1459–1465. doi:10.1211/jpp.58.11.0006.

Amidi, Maryam, Stefan G. Romeijn, Gerrit Borchard, Hans E. Junginger, Wim E. Hennink, and Wim Jiskoot. 2006. "Preparation and characterization of protein-loaded N-trimethyl chitosan nanoparticles as nasal delivery system." *Journal of Controlled Release* 111 (1–2): 107–116. doi:10.1016/j.jconrel.2005.11.014.

Andes, David R., and William A. Craig. 2002. "Animal model pharmacokinetics and pharmacodynamics: A critical review." *International Journal of Antimicrobial Agents* 19 (4): 261–268.

Artursson, Per, and Johan E. Karlsson. 1991. "Correlation between oral drug absorption in humans and apparent drug permeability coefficients in human intestinal epithelial (Caco-2) cells." *Biochemical and Biophysical Research Communications* 175 (3): 880–885. doi:10.1016/0006-291X(91)91647-U.

Aufderheide, Michaela, and Makito Emura. 2017. "Phenotypical changes in a differentiating immortalized bronchial epithelial cell line after exposure to mainstream cigarette smoke and e-cigarette vapor." *Experimental and Toxicologic Pathology* 69 (6): 393–401. doi:10.1016/j.etp.2017.03.004.

Aufderheide, Michaela, Wolf-Dieter Heller, Olaf Krischenowski, Niklas Möhle, and Dieter Hochrainer. 2017. "Improvement of the CULTEX® exposure technology by radial distribution of the test aerosol." *Experimental and Toxicologic Pathology* 69 (6): 359–365. doi:10.1016/j.etp.2017.02.004.

Aufderheide, Michaela, and Ulrich Mohr. 1999. "CULTEX—a new system and technique for the cultivation and exposure of cells at the air/liquid interface." *Experimental and Toxicologic Pathology* 51 (6): 489–490. doi:10.1016/S0940-2993(99)80121-3.

Aufderheide, Michaela, and Ulrich Mohr. 2000. "CULTEX—an alternative technique for cultivation and exposure of cells of the respiratory tract to airborne pollutants at the air/liquid interface." *Experimental and Toxicologic Pathology* 52 (3): 265–270. doi:10.1016/S0940-2993(00)80044-5.

Aufderheide, Michaela, and Ulrich Mohr. 2004. "A modified CULTEX system for the direct exposure of bacteria to inhalable substances." *Experimental and Toxicologic Pathology* 55 (6): 451–454. doi:10.1078/0940-2993-00348.

Aufderheide, Michaela, Detlef Ritter, Jan W. Knebel, and Gerhard Scherer. 2001. "A method for in vitro analysis of the biological activity of complex mixtures such as sidestream cigarette smoke." *Experimental and Toxicologic Pathology* 53 (2–3): 141–152. doi:10.1078/0940-2993-00187.

Bastacky, Jacob, Candice Y. Lee, Jon Goerke, Homayoon Koushafar, Dorne Yager, Leah Kenaga, Terence P. Speed, Ya Chen, and John A. Clements. 1995. "Alveolar lining layer is thin and continuous: Low-temperature scanning electron microscopy of rat lung." *Journal of Applied Physiology (Bethesda, Md.: 1985)* 79 (5): 1615–1628.

Blank, Fabian, Barbara M. Rothen-Rutishauser, Samuel Schurch, and Peter Gehr. 2006. "An optimized in vitro model of the respiratory tract wall to study particle cell interactions." *Journal of Aerosol Medicine* 19 (3): 392–405. doi:10.1089/jam.2006.19.392.

Boegh, Marie, and Hanne M. Nielsen. 2015. "Mucus as a barrier to drug delivery – Understanding and mimicking the barrier properties." *Basic & Clinical Pharmacology & Toxicology* 116 (3): 179–186. doi:10.1111/bcpt.12342.

Borok, Zea, Janice M. Liebler, Richard L. Lubman, Martha J. Foster, Beiyun Zhou, Xian Li, Stephanie M. Zabski, Kwang-Jin Kim, and Edward D. Crandall. 2002. "Na transport proteins are expressed by rat alveolar epithelial type I cells." *American Journal of Physiology. Lung Cellular and Molecular Physiology* 282 (4): L599-L608. doi:10.1152/ajplung.00130.2000.

Bosquillon, Cynthia. 2010. "Drug transporters in the lung--Do they play a role in the biopharmaceutics of inhaled drugs?" *Journal of Pharmaceutical Sciences* 99 (5): 2240–2255. doi:10.1002/jps.21995.

Bosquillon, Cynthia, Michaela Madlova, Nilesh Patel, Nicola Clear, and Ben Forbes. 2017. "A comparison of drug transport in pulmonary absorption models: Isolated perfused rat lungs, respiratory epithelial cell lines and primary cell culture." *Pharmaceutical Research* 34 (12): 2532–2540. doi:10.1007/s11095-017-2251-y.

Bove, Peter F., Hong Dang, Chaitra Cheluvaraju, Lisa C. Jones, Xuefeng Liu, Wanda K. O'Neal, Scott H. Randell, Richard Schlegel, and Richard C. Boucher. 2014. "Breaking the in vitro alveolar type II cell proliferation barrier while retaining ion transport properties." *American Journal of Respiratory Cell and Molecular Biology* 50 (4): 767–776. doi:10.1165/rcmb.2013-0071OC.

Brower, Michael, Desmond N. Carney, Herbert K. Oie, Adi F. Gazdar, and John D. Minna. 1986. "Growth of cell lines and clinical specimens of human non-small cell lung cancer in a serum-free defined medium." *Cancer Research* 46 (2): 798–806.

Bucchieri, Fabio, Sarah M. Puddicombe, James L. Lordan, Audrey Richter, Diane Buchanan, Susan J. Wilson, Jon Ward et al. 2002. "Asthmatic bronchial epithelium is more susceptible to oxidant-induced apoptosis." *American Journal of Respiratory Cell and Molecular Biology* 27 (2): 179–185. doi:10.1165/ajrcmb.27.2.4699.

Bur, Michael, Hanno Huwer, Leon Muys, and Claus-Michael Lehr. 2010. "Drug transport across pulmonary epithelial cell monolayers: Effects of particle size, apical liquid volume, and deposition technique." *Journal of Aerosol Medicine and Pulmonary Drug Delivery* 23 (3): 119–127. doi:10.1089/jamp.2009.0757.

Bur, Michael, Barbara Rothen-Rutishauser, Hanno Huwer, and Claus-Michael Lehr. 2009. "A novel cell compatible impingement system to study in vitro drug absorption from dry powder aerosol formulations." *European Journal of Pharmaceutics and Biopharmaceutics* 72 (2): 350–357. doi:10.1016/j.ejpb.2008.07.019.

Chen, Jiwang, Zhongming Chen, Telugu Narasaraju, Nili Jin, and Lin Liu. 2004. "Isolation of highly pure alveolar epithelial type I and type II cells from rat lungs." *Laboratory Investigation* 84 (6): 727–735. doi:10.1038/labinvest.3700095.

Chortarea, Savvina, Hana Barosova, Martin J. D. Clift, Peter Wick, Alke Petri-Fink, and Barbara Rothen-Rutishauser. 2017. "Human asthmatic bronchial cells are more susceptible to subchronic repeated exposures of aerosolized carbon nanotubes at occupationally relevant doses than healthy cells." *ACS nano* 11 (8): 7615–7625. doi:10.1021/acsnano.7b01992.

Chowdhury, Ferdousi, William J. Howat, Gary J. Phillips, and Peter M. Lackie. 2010. "Interactions between endothelial cells and epithelial cells in a combined cell model of airway mucosa: Effects on tight junction permeability." *Experimental Lung Research* 36 (1): 1–11. doi:10.3109/01902140903026582.

Chung, Yiu, Carolyn M. Kercsmar, and Pamela B. Davis. 1991. "Ferret tracheal epithelial cells grown in vitro are resistant to lethal injury by activated neutrophils." *American Journal of Respiratory Cell and Molecular Biology* 5 (2): 125–132. doi:10.1165/ajrcmb/5.2.125.

Cooney, Daniel, Masha Kazantseva, and Anthony J. Hickey. 2004. "Development of a size-dependent aerosol deposition model utilising human airway epithelial cells for evaluating aerosol drug delivery." *Alternatives to Laboratory Animals: ATLA* 32 (6): 581–590.

Cozens, Alison L., M. J. Yezzi, Karl Kunzelmann, Takashi Ohrui, Lynda Chin, Kurt Eng, Walter E. Finkbeiner, Jonathan H. Widdicombe, and Dieter C. Gruenert. 1994. "CFTR expression and chloride secretion in polarized immortal human bronchial epithelial cells." *American Journal of Respiratory Cell and Molecular Biology* 10 (1): 38–47. doi:10.1165/ajrcmb.10.1.7507342.

Crapo, James D., Brenda E. Barry, Peter Gehr, Marianne Bachofen, and Ewald Rudolf Weibel. 1982. "Cell number and cell characteristics of the normal human lung." *The American Review of Respiratory Disease* 126 (2): 332–337. doi:10.1164/arrd.1982.126.2.332.

Danto, Spencer I., John M. Shannon, Zea Borok, Stephanie M. Zabski, and Edward D. Crandall. 1995. "Reversible transdifferentiation of alveolar epithelial cells." *American Journal of Respiratory Cell and Molecular Biology* 12 (5): 497–502. doi:10.1165/ajrcmb.12.5.7742013.

Daum, Nicole, Anna Kuehn, Stephanie Hein, Ulrich F. Schaefer, Hanno Huwer, and Claus-Michael Lehr. 2012. "Isolation, cultivation, and application of human alveolar epithelial cells." *Methods in Molecular Biology (Clifton, N.J.)* 806: 31–42.

Devalia, Jagdish L., Hasan Bayram, Muntasir M. Abdelaziz, Raymond J. Sapsford, and Robert J. Davies. 1999. "Differences between cytokine release from bronchial epithelial cells of asthmatic patients and non-asthmatic subjects: Effect of exposure to diesel exhaust particles." *International Archives of Allergy and Immunology* 118 (2–4): 437–439. doi:10.1159/000024157.

Dimer, Frantiescoli, Cristiane de Souza Carvalho-Wodarz, Jörg Haupenthal, Rolf Hartmann, and Claus-Michael Lehr. 2015. "Inhalable clarithromycin microparticles for treatment of respiratory infections." *Pharmaceutical Research* 32 (12): 3850–3861. doi:10.1007/s11095-015-1745-8.

Dobbs, Leland G. 1990. "Isolation and culture of alveolar type II cells." *The American Journal of Physiology* 258 (4 Pt 1): L134–L147. doi:10.1152/ajplung.1990.258.4.L134.

Duncan, James E., Jeffrey A. Whitsett, and Ann D. Horowitz. 1997. "Pulmonary surfactant inhibits cationic liposome-mediated gene delivery to respiratory epithelial cells in vitro." *Human Gene Therapy* 8 (4): 431–438. doi:10.1089/hum.1997.8.4-431.

Ehrhardt, Carsten, Carsten Kneuer, Jennifer Fiegel, Justin Hanes, Ulrich Schaefer, Kwang-Jin Kim, and Claus-Michael Lehr. 2002. "Influence of apical fluid volume on the development of functional intercellular junctions in the human epithelial cell line 16HBE14o-: Implications for the use of this cell line as an in vitro model for bronchial drug absorption studies." *Cell and Tissue Research* 308 (3): 391–400. doi:10.1007/s00441-002-0548-5.

Ehrhardt, Carsten, Carsten Kneuer, Michael Laue, Ulrich F. Schaefer, Kwang-Jin Kim, and Claus-Michael Lehr. 2003. "16HBE14o- human bronchial epithelial cell layers express P-glycoprotein, lung resistance-related protein, and caveolin-1." *Pharmaceutical Research* 20 (4): 545–551. doi:10.1023/A:1023230328687.

Elbert, Katharina J., Ulrich F. Schäfer, Hans-Joachim Schäfers, Kwang-Jin Kim, Vincent H. Lee, and Claus-Michael Lehr. 1999. "Monolayers of human alveolar epithelial cells in primary culture for pulmonary absorption and transport studies." *Pharmaceutical Research* 16 (5): 601–608. doi:10.1023/A:1018887501927.

EMA. 2006. *Guideline on the Pharmaceutical Quality of Inhalation and Nasal Products.* London, UK. Report No.: EMEA/CHMP/QWP/49313/2005 Corr.

FDA/CDER. 2002. *Guidance for Industry - Nasal Spray and Inhalation Solution, Suspension, and Spray Drug Products - Chemistry, Manufacturing, and Controls Documentation.* Rockville, MD. https://www.fda.gov/downloads/drugs/guidancecomplianceregulatoryinformation/guidances/ucm070575.pdf.

Fiegel, Jennifer, Carsten Ehrhardt, Ulrich F. Schaefer, Claus-Michael Lehr, and Justin Hanes. 2003. "Large porous particle impingement on lung epithelial cell monolayers--Toward improved particle characterization in the lung." *Pharmaceutical Research* 20 (5): 788–796. doi:10.1023/A:1023441804464.

Fishler, Rami, Philipp Hofemeier, Yael Etzion, Yael Dubowski, and Josué Sznitman. 2015. "Particle dynamics and deposition in true-scale pulmonary acinar models." *Scientific Reports* 5: 14071.

Forbes, Ben, and Carsten Ehrhardt. 2005. "Human respiratory epithelial cell culture for drug delivery applications." *European Journal of Pharmaceutics and Biopharmaceutics* 60 (2): 193–205. doi:10.1016/j.ejpb.2005.02.010.

Foster, Kimberly A., Michael L. Avery, Mehran Yazdanian, and Kenneth L. Audus. 2000. "Characterization of the Calu-3 cell line as a tool to screen pulmonary drug delivery." *International Journal of Pharmaceutics* 208 (1–2): 1–11.

Foster, Kimberly A., Christine G. Oster, Mary M. Mayer, Michael L. Avery, and Kenneth L. Audus. 1998. "Characterization of the A549 cell line as a type II pulmonary epithelial cell model for drug metabolism." *Experimental Cell Research* 243 (2): 359–366. doi:10.1006/excr.1998.4172.

Frijns, Evelien, Sandra Verstraelen, Linda C. Stoehr, Jo van Laer, An Jacobs, Jan Peters, Kristof Tirez et al. 2017. "A novel exposure system termed NAVETTA for in vitro laminar flow electrodeposition of nanoaerosol and evaluation of immune effects in human lung reporter cells." *Environmental Science & Technology* 51 (9): 5259–5269. doi:10.1021/acs.est.7b00493.

Fröhlich, Eleonore, Gudrun Bonstingl, Anita Höfler, Claudia Meindl, Gerd Leitinger, Thomas R. Pieber, and Eva Roblegg. 2013. "Comparison of two in vitro systems to assess cellular effects of nanoparticles-containing aerosols." *Toxicology in Vitro* 27 (1): 409–417. doi:10.1016/j.tiv.2012.08.008.

Fuchs, Sabine, Andrew J. Hollins, Michael Laue, Ulrich F. Schaefer, Klaus Roemer, Mark Gumbleton, and Claus-Michael Lehr. 2003. "Differentiation of human alveolar epithelial cells in primary culture: Morphological characterization and synthesis of caveolin-1 and surfactant protein-C." *Cell and tissue research* 311 (1): 31–45. doi:10.1007/s00441-002-0653-5.

Fytianos, Kleanthis, Savvina Chortarea, Laura Rodriguez-Lorenzo, Fabian Blank, Christophe von Garnier, Alke Petri-Fink, and Barbara Rothen-Rutishauser. 2017. "Aerosol delivery of functionalized gold nanoparticles target and activate dendritic cells in a 3D lung cellular model." *ACS Nano* 11 (1): 375–383. doi:10.1021/acsnano.6b06061.

Galietta, Luis J. V., Sabina Lantero, Andrea Gazzolo, Oliviero Sacco, Luca Romano, Giovanni A. Rossi, and Olga Zegarra-Moran. 1998. "An improved method to obtain highly differentiated monolayers of human bronchial epithelial cells." *In Vitro Cellular & Developmental Biology-Animal* 34 (6): 478–481. doi:10.1007/s11626-998-0081-2.

Gazdar, Adi F., R. Ilona Linnoila, Yukio Kurita, Herbert K. Oie, James L. Mulshine, Jean C. Clark, and Jeffrey A. Whitsett. 1990. "Peripheral airway cell differentiation in human lung cancer cell lines." *Cancer Research* 50 (17): 5481–5487.

Gehr, Peter, Marianne Bachofen, and Ewald R. Weibel. 1978. "The normal human lung: Ultrastructure and morphometric estimation of diffusion capacity." *Respiration Physiology* 32 (2): 121–140. doi:10.1016/0034-5687(78)90104-4.

Giard, Donald J., Stuart A. Aaronson, George J. Todaro, Paul Arnstein, John H. Kersey, Harvey Dosik, and Wade P. Parks. 1973. "In vitro cultivation of human tumors: Establishment of cell lines derived from a series of solid tumors." *Journal of the National Cancer Institute* 51 (5): 1417–1423.

Goerke, Jon. 1998. "Pulmonary surfactant: Functions and molecular composition." *Biochimica et Biophysica Acta (BBA) - Molecular Basis of Disease* 1408 (2–3): 79–89. doi:10.1016/S0925-4439(98)00060-X.

Gonzalez, Robert F., and Leland G. Dobbs. 2013. "Isolation and culture of alveolar epithelial Type I and Type II cells from rat lungs." *Methods in Molecular Biology (Clifton, N.J.)* 945: 145–159.

Gordon, Sarah, Mardas Daneshian, Joke Bouwstra, Francesca Caloni, Samuel Constant, Donna E. Davies, Gudrun Dandekar et al. 2015. "Non-animal models of epithelial barriers (skin, intestine and lung) in research, industrial applications and regulatory toxicology." *ALTEX* 32 (4): 327–378. doi:10.14573/altex.1510051.

Grainger, Christopher I., Leona L. Greenwell, David J. Lockley, Gary P. Martin, and Ben Forbes. 2006. "Culture of Calu-3 cells at the air interface provides a representative model of the airway epithelial barrier." *Pharmaceutical Research* 23 (7): 1482–1490. doi:10.1007/s11095-006-0255-0.

Grainger, Christopher I., Leona L. Greenwell, Gary P. Martin, and Ben Forbes. 2009. "The permeability of large molecular weight solutes following particle delivery to air-interfaced cells that model the respiratory mucosa." *European Journal of Pharmaceutics and Biopharmaceutics* 71 (2): 318–324. doi:10.1016/j.ejpb.2008.09.006.

Hackett, Neil R., Renat Shaykhiev, Matthew S. Walters, Rui Wang, Rachel K. Zwick, Barbara Ferris, Bradley Witover, Jacqueline Salit, and Ronald G. Crystal. 2011. "The human airway epithelial basal cell transcriptome." *PLoS One* 6 (5): e18378. doi:10.1371/journal.pone.0018378.

Haghi, Mehra, Daniela Traini, Mary Bebawy, and Paul M. Young. 2012. "Deposition, diffusion and transport mechanism of dry powder microparticulate salbutamol, at the respiratory epithelia." *Molecular Pharmaceutics* 9 (6): 1717–1726. doi:10.1021/mp200620m.

Hein, Stephanie, Michael Bur, Tobias Kolb, Bernhard Muellinger, Ulrich F. Schaefer, and Claus-Michael Lehr. 2010. "The pharmaceutical aerosol deposition device on cell cultures (PADDOCC) in vitro system: Design and experimental protocol." *Alternatives to Laboratory Animals: ATLA* 38 (4): 285–295.

Hein, Stephanie, Michael Bur, Ulrich F. Schaefer, and Claus-Michael Lehr. 2011. "A new Pharmaceutical Aerosol Deposition Device on Cell Cultures (PADDOCC) to evaluate pulmonary drug absorption for metered dose dry powder formulations." *European Journal of Pharmaceutics and Biopharmaceutics* 77 (1): 132–138. doi:10.1016/j.ejpb.2010.10.003.

Hickey, Anthony J. 2014. "Controlled delivery of inhaled therapeutic agents." *Journal of Controlled Release* 190: 182–188.

Hidalgo, Ismael J., Thomas J. Raub, and Ronald T. Borchardt. 1989. "Characterization of the human colon carcinoma cell line (Caco-2) as a model system for intestinal epithelial permeability." *Gastroenterology* 96 (3): 736–749. doi:10.1016/0016-5085(89)90897-4.

Hiemstra, Pieter S., Gwendolynn Grootaers, Anne M. van der Does, Cyrille A. M. Krul, and Ingeborg M. Kooter. 2017. "Human lung epithelial cell cultures for analysis of inhaled toxicants: Lessons learned and future directions." *Toxicology In Vitro* 47: 137–146.

Hittinger, Marius, Sarah Barthold, Lorenz Siebenbürger, Kilian Zäh, Alexander Gress, Sabrina Guenther, Birgit Wiegand et al. 2017. "Proof of concept of the VITROCELL® dry powder chamber: A new in vitro test system for the controlled deposition of aerosol formulations." In *RDD Europe 2017*, Vol. 2, edited by Richard N. Dalby, Joanne Peart, Julie D. Suman, Paul M. Young, and Daniela Traini, pp. 283–288.

Hittinger, Marius, Julia Janke, Hanno Huwer, Regina Scherliess, Nicole Schneider-Daum, and Claus-Michael Lehr. 2016a. "Autologous co-culture of primary human alveolar macrophages and epithelial cells for investigating aerosol medicines. Part I: Model characterisation." *Alternatives to Laboratory Animals: ATLA* 44 (4): 337–347.

Hittinger, Marius, Jenny Juntke, Stephanie Kletting, Nicole Schneider-Daum, Cristiane de Souza Carvalho, and Claus-Michael Lehr. 2015. "Preclinical safety and efficacy models for pulmonary drug delivery of antimicrobials with focus on in vitro models." *Advanced Drug Delivery Reviews* 85: 44–56.

Hittinger, Marius, Nico A. Mell, Hanno Huwer, Brigitta Loretz, Nicole Schneider-Daum, and Claus-Michael Lehr. 2016b. "Autologous co-culture of primary human alveolar macrophages and epithelial cells for investigating aerosol medicines. Part II: Evaluation of IL-10-loaded microparticles for the treatment of lung inflammation." *Alternatives to Laboratory Animals: ATLA* 44 (4): 349–360.

Huh, Dongeun, Benjamin D. Matthews, Akiko Mammoto, Martín Montoya-Zavala, Hong Y. Hsin, and Donald E. Ingber. 2010. "Reconstituting organ-level lung functions on a chip." *Science (New York, N.Y.)* 328 (5986): 1662–1668. doi:10.1126/science.1188302.

Jeannet, Natalie, Martin Fierz, Markus Kalberer, Heinz Burtscher, and Marianne Geiser. 2015. "Nano aerosol chamber for in-vitro toxicity (NACIVT) studies." *Nanotoxicology* 9 (1): 34–42. doi:10.3109/17435390.2014.886739.

Jong, Peter M. de, Marian A. van Sterkenburg, S. C. Hesseling, Johanna A. Kempenaar, Adriaan A. Mulder, A. Mieke Mommaas, Joop H. Dijkman, and Maria Ponec. 1994. "Ciliogenesis in human bronchial epithelial cells cultured at the air-liquid interface." *American Journal of Respiratory Cell and Molecular Biology* 10 (3): 271–277. doi:10.1165/ajrcmb.10.3.8117445.

Karp, Philip H., Thomas O. Moninger, S. P. Weber, Tamara S. Nesselhauf, Janice L. Launspach, Joseph Zabner, and Michael J. Welsh. 2002. "An in vitro model of differentiated human airway epithelia. Methods for establishing primary cultures." *Methods in Molecular Biology (Clifton, N.J.)* 188: 115–137.

Kaufman, David G. 1976. "Biochemical studies of isolated hamster tracheal epithelium." *Environmental Health Perspectives* 16: 99–110.

Kemp, Sarah J., Andrew J. Thorley, Julia Gorelik, Michael J. Seckl, Michael J. O'Hare, Alexandre Arcaro, Yuri Korchev, Peter Goldstraw, and Teresa D. Tetley. 2008. "Immortalization of human alveolar epithelial cells to investigate nanoparticle uptake." *American Journal of Respiratory Cell and Molecular Biology* 39 (5): 591–597. doi:10.1165/rcmb.2007-0334OC.

Kim, Kwang-Jin, and Edward D. Crandall. 1983. "Heteropore populations of bullfrog alveolar epithelium." *Journal of Applied Physiology: Respiratory, Environmental and Exercise Physiology* 54 (1): 140–146. doi:10.1152/jappl.1983.54.1.140.

Kletting, Stephanie, Sarah Barthold, Urska Repnik, Gareth Griffiths, Brigitta Loretz, Nicole Schneider-Daum, Cristiane de Souza Carvalho-Wodarz, and Claus-Michael Lehr. 2018. "Co-culture of human alveolar epithelial (hAELVi) and macrophage (THP-1) cell lines." *ALTEX* 35 (2): 211–222. doi:10.14573/altex.1607191.

Knebel, Jan W., Detlef Ritter, and Michaela Aufderheide. 2002. "Exposure of human lung cells to native diesel motor exhaust—Development of an optimized in vitro test strategy." *Toxicology In Vitro* 16 (2): 185–192. doi:10.1016/S0887-2333(01)00110-2.

Kuehn, Anna, Stephanie Kletting, Cristiane de Souza Carvalho-Wodarz, Urska Repnik, Gareth Griffiths, Ulrike Fischer, Eckart Meese et al. 2016. "Human alveolar epithelial cells expressing tight junctions to model the air-blood barrier." *ALTEX* 33 (3): 251–260. doi:10.14573/altex.1511131.

Labiris, Nancy Renee, and Myrna B. Dolovich. 2003. "Pulmonary drug delivery. Part I: Physiological factors affecting therapeutic effectiveness of aerosolized medications." *British Journal of Clinical Pharmacology* 56 (6): 588–599. doi:10.1046/j.1365-2125.2003.01892.x.

Leist, Marcel, and Thomas Hartung. 2013. "Inflammatory findings on species extrapolations: Humans are definitely no 70-kg mice." *Archives of Toxicology* 87 (4): 563–567. doi:10.1007/s00204-013-1038-0.

Lenz, Anke, Erwin Karg, Bernd Lentner, Vlad Dittrich, Christina Brandenberger, Barbara Rothen-Rutishauser, Holger Schulz, George A. Ferron, and Otmar Schmid. 2009. "A dose-controlled system for air-liquid interface cell exposure and application to zinc oxide nanoparticles." *Particle and Fibre Toxicology* 6 (1): 32. doi:10.1186/1743-8977-6-32.

Lenz, Anke-Gabriele, Tobias Stoeger, Daniele Cei, Martina Schmidmeir, Nora Semren, Gerald Burgstaller, Bernd Lentner, Oliver Eickelberg, Silke Meiners, and Otmar Schmid. 2014. "Efficient bioactive delivery of aerosolized drugs to human pulmonary epithelial cells cultured in air-liquid interface conditions." *American Journal of Respiratory Cell and Molecular Biology* 51 (4): 526–535. doi:10.1165/rcmb.2013-0479OC.

Leonard, Alexis K., Anthony P. Sileno, Gordon C. Brandt, Charles A. Foerder, Steven C. Quay, and Henry R. Costantino. 2007. "In vitro formulation optimization of intranasal galantamine leading to enhanced bioavailability and reduced emetic response in vivo." *International Journal of Pharmaceutics* 335 (1–2): 138–146. doi:10.1016/j.ijpharm.2006.11.013.

Leonard, Alexis K., Anthony P. Sileno, Conor MacEvilly, Charles A. Foerder, Steven C. Quay, and Henry R. Costantino. 2005. "Development of a novel high-concentration galantamine formulation suitable for intranasal delivery." *Journal of Pharmaceutical Sciences* 94 (8): 1736–1746. doi:10.1002/jps.20389.

Lieber, Michael, George Todaro, Barry Smith, Andras Szakal, and Walter Nelson-Rees. 1976. "A continuous tumor-cell line from a human lung carcinoma with properties of type II alveolar epithelial cells." *International Journal of Cancer* 17 (1): 62–70. doi:10.1002/ijc.2910170110.

Lin, Hongxia, Hong Li, Hyun-Jong Cho, Shengjie Bian, Hwan-Jung Roh, Min-Ki Lee, Jung S. Kim, Suk-Jae Chung, Chang-Koo Shim, and Dae-Duk Kim. 2007. "Air-liquid interface (ALI) culture of human bronchial epithelial cell monolayers as an in vitro model for airway drug transport studies." *Journal of Pharmaceutical Sciences* 96 (2): 341–350. doi:10.1002/jps.20803.

Low, Frank N. 1953. "The pulmonary alveolar epithelium of laboratory mammals and man." *Anatomical Record* 117 (2): 241–263. doi:10.1002/ar.1091170208.

Mathia, Neil R., Julita Timoszyk, Paul I. Stetsko, John R. Megill, Ronald L. Smith, and Doris A. Wall. 2002. "Permeability characteristics of calu-3 human bronchial epithelial cells: In vitro-in vivo correlation to predict lung absorption in rats." *Journal of Drug Targeting* 10 (1): 31–40. doi:10.1080/10611860290007504.

Mathias, Neil R., Kwang-Jin Kim, Timothy W. Robison, and Vincent H. Lee. 1995. "Development and characterization of rabbit tracheal epithelial cell monolayer models for drug transport studies." *Pharmaceutical Research* 12 (10): 1499–1505.

McDowell, Elizabeth M., Lucy A. Barrett, Fred Glavin, Curtis C. Harris, and Benjamin F. Trump. 1978. "The respiratory epithelium. I. Human bronchus." *Journal of the National Cancer Institute* 61 (2): 539–549.

Meindl, Claudia, Sandra Stranzinger, Neira Dzidic, Sharareh Salar-Behzadi, Stefan Mohr, Andreas Zimmer, Eleonore Fröhlich, and Shama Ahmad. 2015. "Permeation of therapeutic drugs in different formulations across the airway epithelium in vitro." *PLoS One* 10 (8): e0135690. doi:10.1371/journal.pone.0135690.

Mercer, Robert R., Michael L. Russell, Victor L. Roggli, and James D. Crapo. 1994. "Cell number and distribution in human and rat airways." *American Journal of Respiratory Cell and Molecular Biology* 10 (6): 613–624. doi:10.1165/ajrcmb.10.6.8003339.

Mitchell, Jolyon P., and Mark W. Nagel. "Cascade impactors for the size characterization of aerosols from medical inhalers: Their uses and limitations." *Journal of Aerosol Medicine* 16: 341–377.

Müller, Loretta, Michael Riediker, Peter Wick, Martin Mohr, Peter Gehr, and Barbara Rothen-Rutishauser. 2010. "Oxidative stress and inflammation response after nanoparticle exposure: Differences between human lung cell monocultures and an advanced three-dimensional model of the human epithelial airways." *Journal of the Royal Society, Interface* 7 Suppl 1: S27–S40.

Murgia, Xabier, Brigitta Loretz, Olga Hartwig, Marius Hittinger, and Claus-Michael Lehr. 2017. "The role of mucus on drug transport and its potential to affect therapeutic outcomes." *Advanced Drug Delivery Reviews* 124: 82–97. doi:10.1016/j.addr.2017.10.009.

Neilson, Louise, Courtney Mankus, David Thorne, George Jackson, Jason DeBay, and Clive Meredith. 2015. "Development of an in vitro cytotoxicity model for aerosol exposure using 3D reconstructed human airway tissue; Application for assessment of e-cigarette aerosol." *Toxicology in Vitro* 29 (7): 1952–1962. doi:10.1016/j.tiv.2015.05.018.

Nelson, Kevin, Christopher Bobba, Samir Ghadiali, Don Hayes, Sylvester M. Black, and Bryan A. Whitson. 2014. "Animal models of ex vivo lung perfusion as a platform for transplantation research." *World Journal of Experimental Medicine* 4 (2): 7–15. doi:10.5493/wjem.v4.i2.7.

Newman, Stephen P. 2017. "Drug delivery to the lungs: Challenges and opportunities." *Therapeutic Delivery* 8 (8): 647–661. doi:10.4155/tde-2017-0037.

Nickel, Sabrina, Caoimhe G. Clerkin, Mohammed A. Selo, and Carsten Ehrhardt. 2016. "Transport mechanisms at the pulmonary mucosa: Implications for drug delivery." *Expert Opinion on Drug Delivery* 13 (5): 667–690. doi:10.1517/17425247.2016.1140144.

Noah, Terry L., James R. Yankaskas, Johnny L. Carson, Todd M. Gambling, Lisa H. Cazares, Karen P. McKinnon, and Robert B. Devlin. 1995. "Tight junctions and mucin mRNA in BEAS-2B cells." *In Vitro Cellular & Developmental Biology-Animal* 31 (10): 738–740. doi:10.1007/BF02634112.

OECD. 2009. *Guidance Document on Acute Inhalation Toxicity Testing - OECD Environment, Health and Safety Publications Series on Testing and Asessment No. 39.* Organisation for Economic Co-operation and Development (OECD), Paris, France.

OECD. 2017. *Guideline for the Testing of Chemicals - 90-Day (Subchronic) Inhalation Toxicity Study, Test Guideline 413.* Organisation for Economic Co-operation and Development (OECD), Paris, France.

Ong, Hui X., Daniela Traini, Ching-Yee Loo, Lala Sarkissian, Gianluca Lauretani, Santo Scalia, and Paul M. Young. 2015. "Is the cellular uptake of respiratory aerosols delivered from different devices equivalent?" *European Journal of Pharmaceutics and Biopharmaceutics* 93: 320–327.

Opitz, Bastian, Anja Püschel, Bernd Schmeck, Andreas C. Hocke, Simone Rosseau, Sven Hammerschmidt, Ralf R. Schumann, Norbert Suttorp, and Stefan Hippenstiel. 2004. "Nucleotide-binding oligomerization domain proteins are innate immune receptors for internalized Streptococcus pneumoniae." *The Journal of Biological Chemistry* 279 (35): 36426–36432. doi:10.1074/jbc. M403861200.

Oreffo, Victor I. C., Arthur Morgan, and Roy J. Richards. 1990. "Isolation of Clara cells from the mouse lung." *Environmental Health Perspectives* 85: 51.

Patton, John S., Joseph D. Brain, Lee A. Davies, Jennifer Fiegel, Mark Gumbleton, Kwang-Jin Kim, Masahiro Sakagami, Rita Vanbever, and Carsten Ehrhardt. 2010. "The particle has landed—Characterizing the fate of inhaled pharmaceuticals." *Journal of Aerosol Medicine and Pulmonary Drug Delivery* 23 Suppl 2: S71–S87.

Patton, John S., and Peter R. Byron. 2007. "Inhaling medicines: Delivering drugs to the body through the lungs." *Nature Reviews. Drug Discovery* 6 (1): 67–74. doi:10.1038/nrd2153.

Reddel, Roger R., Yang Ke, Brenda I. Gerwin, Mary G. McMenamin, John F. Lechner, Robert T. Su, Douglas E. Brash, Joo-Bae Park, Johng S. Rhim, and Curtis C. Harris. 1988. "Transformation of human bronchial epithelial cells by infection with SV40 or adenovirus-12 SV40 hybrid virus, or transfection via strontium phosphate coprecipitation with a plasmid containing SV40 early region genes." *Cancer Research* 48 (7): 1904–1909.

Rehan, Virender K., John S. Torday, Sara Peleg, Lynn Gennaro, Paul Vouros, James Padbury, D. S. Rao, and G. S. Reddy. 2002. "1Alpha,25-dihydroxy-3-epi-vitamin D3, a natural metabolite of 1alpha,25-dihydroxy vitamin D3: Production and biological activity studies in pulmonary alveolar type II cells." *Molecular Genetics and Metabolism* 76 (1): 46–56.

Ren, Hui, Nigel P. Birch, and Vinod Suresh. 2016. "An optimised human cell culture model for alveolar epithelial transport." *PLoS One* 11 (10): e0165225. doi:10.1371/journal.pone.0165225.

Reus, Astrid A., Wilfred J. M. Maas, Harm T. Jansen, Samuel Constant, Yvonne C. M. Staal, Jos J. van Triel, and C. F. Kuper. 2014. "Feasibility of a 3D human airway epithelial model to study respiratory absorption." *Toxicology In Vitro* 28 (2): 258–264. doi:10.1016/j.tiv.2013.10.025.

Reynolds, Susan D., Paul R. Reynolds, Gloria S. Pryhuber, Jonathan D. Finder, and Barry R. Stripp. 2002. "Secretoglobins SCGB3A1 and SCGB3A2 define secretory cell subsets in mouse and human airways." *American Journal of Respiratory and Critical Care Medicine* 166 (11): 1498–1509. doi:10.1164/rccm.200204-285OC.

Ritter, Detlef, Jan W. Knebel, and Michaela Aufderheide. 2001. "In vitro exposure of isolated cells to native gaseous compounds—Development and validation of an optimized system for human lung cells." *Experimental and Toxicologic Pathology* 53 (5): 373–386. doi:10.1078/0940-2993-00204.

Ritter, Detlef, and Jan Knebel. 2014. "Investigations of the biological effects of airborne and inhalable substances by cell-based in vitro methods: Fundamental improvements to the ALI concept." *Advances in Toxicology* 2014 (1): 1–11. doi:10.1155/2014/185201.

Robison, Timothy W., Raymond J. Dorio, and Kwang-Jin Kim. 1993. "Formation of tight monolayers of guinea pig airway epithelial cells cultured in an air-interface: Bioelectric properties." *BioTechniques* 15 (3): 468–473.

Röhm, Martina, Stefan Carle, Frank Maigler, Johannes Flamm, Viktoria Kramer, Chrystelle Mavoungou, Otmar Schmid, and Katharina Schindowski. 2017. "A comprehensive screening platform for aerosolizable protein formulations for intranasal and pulmonary drug delivery." *International Journal of Pharmaceutics* 532 (1): 537–546. doi:10.1016/j.ijpharm.2017.09.027.

Rothen-Rutishauser, Barbara M., Stephen G. Kiama, and Peter Gehr. 2005. "A three-dimensional cellular model of the human respiratory tract to study the interaction with particles." *American Journal of Respiratory Cell and Molecular Biology* 32 (4): 281–289. doi:10.1165/rcmb.2004-0187OC.

Ruge, Christian C., Julian Kirch, and Claus M. Lehr. 2013. "Pulmonary drug delivery: From generating aerosols to overcoming biological barriers-therapeutic possibilities and technological challenges." *The Lancet Respiratory Medicine* 1 (5): 402–413. doi:10.1016/S2213-2600(13)70072-9.

Ryan, Dorothy M., Thomas L. Vincent, Jacqueline Salit, Matthew S. Walters, Francisco Agosto-Perez, Renat Shaykhiev, Yael Strulovici-Barel et al. 2014. "Smoking dysregulates the human airway basal cell transcriptome at COPD risk locus 19q13.2." *PLoS One* 9 (2): e88051. doi:10.1371/journal.pone.0088051.

Salomon, Johanna J., Yohannes Hagos, Sören Petzke, Annett Kühne, Julia C. Gausterer, Ken-ichi Hosoya, and Carsten Ehrhardt. 2015. "Beta-2 adrenergic agonists are substrates and inhibitors of human organic cation transporter 1." *Molecular Pharmaceutics* 12 (8): 2633–2641. doi:10.1021/mp500854e.

Salomon, Johanna J., Viktoria E. Muchitsch, Julia C. Gausterer, Elena Schwagerus, Hanno Huwer, Nicole Daum, Claus-Michael Lehr, and Carsten Ehrhardt. 2014. "The cell line NCl-H441 is a useful in vitro model for transport studies of human distal lung epithelial barrier." *Molecular Pharmaceutics* 11 (3): 995–1006. doi:10.1021/mp4006535.

Seok, Junhee, H. S. Warren, Alex G. Cuenca, Michael N. Mindrinos, Henry V. Baker, Weihong Xu, Daniel R. Richards et al. 2013. "Genomic responses in mouse models poorly mimic human inflammatory diseases." *Proceedings of the National Academy of Sciences of the United States of America* 110 (9): 3507–3512. doi:10.1073/pnas.1222878110.

Sime, A., Quintin Mckellar, and Andrea Mary Nolan. 1997. "Method for the growth of equine airway epithelial cells in culture." *Research in Veterinary Science* 62 (1): 30–33. doi:10.1016/S0034-5288(97)90176-4.

Sinha, Meenal, and Clifford A. Lowell. 2016. "Immune defense protein expression in highly purified mouse lung epithelial cells." *American Journal of Respiratory Cell and Molecular Biology* 54 (6): 802–813. doi:10.1165/rcmb.2015-0171OC.

Sisson, Joseph H., Dean J. Tuma, and Stephen I. Rennard. 1991. "Acetaldehyde-mediated cilia dysfunction in bovine bronchial epithelial cells." *The American Journal of Physiology* 260 (2 Pt 1): L29–L36. doi:10.1152/ajplung.1991.260.2.L29.

Speirs, Valerie, K. P. Ray, and Robert Ian Freshney. 1991. "Paracrine control of differentiation in the alveolar carcinoma, A549, by human foetal lung fibroblasts." *British Journal of Cancer* 64 (4): 693–699. doi:10.1038/bjc.1991.383.

Sporty, Jennifer L., Lenka Horálková, and Carsten Ehrhardt. 2008. "In vitro cell culture models for the assessment of pulmonary drug disposition." *Expert Opinion on Drug Metabolism & Toxicology* 4 (4): 333–345. doi:10.1517/17425255.4.4.333.

Steerenberg, Peter A., J. A. Zonnenberg, Jan A. Dormans, P. N. Joon, Inge M. Wouters, Leendert van Bree, Paul T. Scheepers, and Henk van Loveren. 1998. "Diesel exhaust particles induced release of interleukin 6 and 8 by (primed) human bronchial epithelial cells (BEAS 2B) in vitro." *Experimental Lung Research* 24 (1): 85–100. doi:10.3109/01902149809046056.

Stone, Kimberly C., Robert R. Mercer, Peter Gehr, Barbara Stockstill, and James D. Crapo. 1992. "Allometric relationships of cell numbers and size in the mammalian lung." *American Journal of Respiratory Cell and Molecular Biology* 6 (2): 235–243. doi:10.1165/ajrcmb/6.2.235.

Stucki, Andreas O., Janick D. Stucki, Sean R. R. Hall, Marcel Felder, Yves Mermoud, Ralph A. Schmid, Thomas Geiser, and Olivier T. Guenat. 2015. "A lung-on-a-chip array with an integrated bio-inspired respiration mechanism." *Lab on a Chip* 15 (5): 1302–1310. doi:10.1039/c4lc01252f.

Sturton, Richard G., Alexandre Trifilieff, Andrew G. Nicholson, and Peter J. Barnes. 2008. "Pharmacological characterization of indacaterol, a novel once daily inhaled 2 adrenoceptor agonist, on small airways in human and rat precision-cut lung slices." *The Journal of Pharmacology and Experimental Therapeutics* 324 (1): 270–275. doi:10.1124/jpet.107.129296.

Ussing, Hans H., and K. Zerahn. 1999. "Active transport of sodium as the source of electric current in the short-circuited isolated frog skin. Reprinted from Acta. Physiol. Scand. 23: 110-127, 1951." *Journal of the American Society of Nephrology: JASN* 10 (9): 2056–2065. doi:10.1111/j.1748-1716.1951.tb00800.x.

van den Bogaard, Ellen H. J., Lea A. Dailey, Andrew J. Thorley, Teresa D. Tetley, and Ben Forbes. 2009. "Inflammatory response and barrier properties of a new alveolar type 1-like cell line (TT1)." *Pharmaceutical Research* 26 (5): 1172–1180. doi:10.1007/s11095-009-9838-x.

Wall, Doris A., Doreen Pierdomenico, and Glynn Wilson. 1993. "An in vitro pulmonary epithelial system for evaluating peptide transport." *Journal of Controlled Release* 24 (1–3): 227–235. doi:10.1016/0168-3659(93)90181-4.

Welsh, Michael J. 1985. "Ion transport by primary cultures of canine tracheal epithelium: Methodology, morphology, and electrophysiology." *The Journal of Membrane Biology* 88 (2): 149–163.

Winton, H.L., H. Wan, M. B. Cannell, D. C. Gruenert, P. J. Thompson, D. R. Garrod, G. A. Stewart, and C. Robinson. 1998. "Cell lines of pulmonary and non-pulmonary origin as tools to study the effects of house dust mite proteinases on the regulation of epithelial permeability." *Clinical & Experimental Allergy* 28 (10): 1273–1285. doi:10.1046/j.1365-2222.1998.00354.x.

World Health Organization. 2016. "Global Health Estimates 2015: Deaths by cause, age and sex, by country and by region, 2000–2015." Geneva, Switzerland. News release, 2016. Accessed February 6, 2018. http://www.who.int/healthinfo/global_burden_disease/estimates/en/index1.html.

Xia, Tian, Michael Kovochich, Monty Liong, Lutz Mädler, Benjamin Gilbert, Haibin Shi, Joanne I. Yeh, Jeffrey I. Zink, and Andre E. Nel. 2008. "Comparison of the mechanism of toxicity of zinc oxide and cerium oxide nanoparticles based on dissolution and oxidative stress properties." *ACS Nano* 2 (10): 2121–2134. doi:10.1021/nn800511k.

Yoon, Joo-Heon, Kyung-Su Kim, Jeung-Gweon Lee, Sung-Shik Kim, and In Yong Park. 2000. "Secretory differentiation of serially passaged normal human nasal epithelial cells by retinoic acid: Expression of mucin and lysozyme." *The Annals of Otology, Rhinology, and Laryngology* 109 (6): 594–601. doi:10.1177/000348940010900612.

Yu, Jianwei, and Yie W. Chien. 2001. "An in vitro pulmonary permeation system with simulation of respiratory dynamics." *Pharmaceutical Development and Technology* 6 (3): 363–371. doi:10.1081/PDT-100002618.

Yu, Zechen, Myoseon Jang, Tara Sabo-Attwood, Sarah E. Robinson, and Huanhuan Jiang. 2017. "Prediction of delivery of organic aerosols onto air-liquid interface cells in vitro using an electrostatic precipitator." *Toxicology In Vitro* 42: 319–328.

Zabner, Joseph, Phil Karp, Michael Seiler, Stacia L. Phillips, Calista J. Mitchell, Mimi Saavedra, Michael Welsh, and Aloysius J. Klingelhutz. 2003. "Development of cystic fibrosis and noncystic fibrosis airway cell lines." *American Journal of Physiology. Lung Cellular and Molecular Physiology* 284 (5): L844–L854. doi:10.1152/ajplung.00355.2002.

Zscheppang, Katja, Johanna Berg, Sarah Hedtrich, Leonie Verheyen, Darcy E. Wagner, Norbert Suttorp, Stefan Hippenstiel, and Andreas C. Hocke. 2018. "Human pulmonary 3D models for translational research." *Biotechnology Journal* 13 (1). doi:10.1002/biot.201700341.

[illegible] Hallal [illegible] [illegible] Comparison [illegible] zinc oxide and [illegible]

[illegible] 2000. [illegible]

[illegible] 2002. 302–128.

[illegible]

29

3D In Vitro/Ex Vivo *Systems*

Bethany M. Young, Alexandria Ritchie, Laleh Golshahi, and Rebecca L. Heise

CONTENTS

29.1 Introduction

The systems discussed in this chapter provide an intermediate between two dimensional (2D) systems and whole animal studies for the discovery, deposition, and cellular response of inhaled pharmaceuticals. This chapter will review the state-of-the-art in many bioengineering and additive manufacturing techniques that are being utilized to develop 3D models of the lung. This chapter discusses hydrogel co-culture systems, lung on a chip devices, 3D printed airways, *ex vivo* perfused lungs, precision cut lung slices, decellularized lung matrices, and bioprinting. The advantages of these systems are that they can typically include multiple human cell types, take into account mechanical and geometrical influences for drug delivery, and are higher throughput than conventional animal studies. These systems retain some disadvantages for pharmaceutical aerosol testing; however, if they are utilized in concert with other methods described in this textbook, they can be a valuable part of the design and analysis of new inhaled pharmaceuticals. The overall use of each system and the advantages and limitations are detailed in this chapter.

29.2 3D Hydrogel Co-culture Systems

It is difficult to predict the human body's response to different drugs, stimulation, and disease. Currently, the most common way to do so is via *in vitro* culture assays and *in vivo* animal experiments which are generally very expensive. However, recent advancements in the field of biomaterials have contributed to the creation of three-dimensional hydrogels that are encapsulated by cells. As a result, researchers are now able to model the response of tissue *in vitro* to certain drugs. Through this advancement, *in vitro* studies have the potential to be revolutionized in order to provide a flexible and unique platform for *in vitro* modeling (Ahmed 2015).

Hydrogels have evolved from being constructed of natural materials to synthetic polymers. This transition allowed the researcher to have greater control over different components of the hydrogel system such as absorbency and flexibility to increase the accuracy of their models (Ahmed 2015). Hydrogels are widely utilized in the field of regenerative medicine because they possess many properties of tissue. Recently, three-dimensional hydrogels have been created from an advanced network of polymer chains and water filling the open spaces between the macromolecules. These systems are multi-component in comparison to the original natural and synthetic hydrogels. They are hydrophilic and have been made to accurately resemble living tissue because they can absorb large amounts of water. They are also porous and possess an overall soft consistency. As a result, these three-dimensional hydrogel models can successfully represent the tissue macro and microenvironment. Thus, researchers can gain a more accurate and comprehensive understanding of the cells being studied (Caló and Khutoryanskiy 2015).

Also, the creation of these three-dimensional hydrogels has given rise to an increase in co-culture modeling. Two-dimensional hydrogel culture has been the conventional method for *in vitro* modeling of cellular environments. However, many groups have demonstrated that cells respond in a manner that more closely resembles their natural behavior when cultured in a three-dimensional environment. The hydrogel environment plays a very active role in the function of the cells within the culture. The simulated microenvironment influences cell signaling and ultimately the cellular phenotype. As a result, it is critical to understand the utilization of hydrogel culture systems. Microporous scaffolds provide cells with an environment capable of encapsulating them. However, since the average size of their pores is larger than the average cell, they are only providing a two-dimensional environment with a limited degree of curvature (Tibbitt and Anseth 2009). On the other hand, nanofibrous scaffolds effectively provide the cells with a three-dimensional topology which can more accurately resemble the environment formed by extracellular matrix proteins. The problem with these scaffolds is that they are not adequately handling the stress due to mechanotransduction of forces. As a result, they are limited in their ability to completely mimic a realistic cellular environment. Hydrogel co-culture systems do not possess these limitations. They can effectively demonstrate the interaction and impact that different cell types have on each other. The hydrogel material allows for a greater amount of flexibility than most other materials. Also, their cross-linked, chain-like structure contains a high water content and with free diffusion. Three-dimensional hydrogels can also be modified to possess different viscoelastic and degradative properties which allow for researchers to create models that closely resemble the environment they are trying to simulate. Overall, three dimensional hydrogels can successfully promote and allow for cellular function.

Three-dimensional hydrogel systems have emerged as a model for drug delivery and treatment of diseases related to the lung. More specifically, these systems are utilizing organoids which are 3D developing tissues that provide researchers with an accurate representation of microanatomy (Fang and Eglen 2017). Figure 29.1 shows the overall scheme for developing organoid tissues. Organoids are essentially a collection of cell types that are specific to the organ of interest. Organoids are typically formed from stem cells and organize into the cell type in a manner similar to this process *in vivo*. Also, tissue organoids are cultured as being mesenchyme-free. These cells are most commonly studied in the lung because they directly apply to epithelial cells due to their capabilities to organize into structures resembling this tissue.

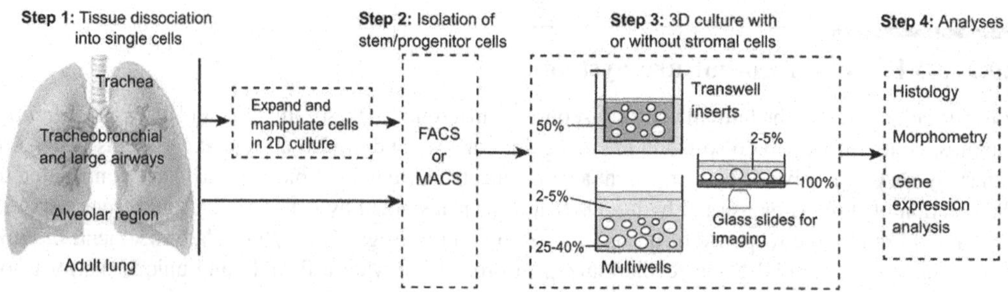

FIGURE 29.1 Process for isolating and culturing 3D organoids for pharmaceutical testing. (Reproduced from Barkauskas, C.E. et al., *Development*, 144, 986–997, 2017. With permission.)

Current researchers are using these *in vivo* organoid models to resemble the lung tissue microanatomy and environment. As a result, these models accurately demonstrate the impact of certain drugs on lung tissue. Furthermore, all of these qualities and characteristics of multi-dimensional hydrogels provide researchers with the ability to culture different cell types in the same environment to gain a complete understanding of their interactions.

29.3 Lung on a Chip

Organs on a chip have been a hot topic over the past two decades. The promise of these systems is that they provide high-throughput drug screening with multiple human cell types, along with physiologic spatial relationships. The general workflow for developing these "on a chip" systems is to first perform photolithography to create microchannels typically made from polydimethylsiloxane (PDMS). Following the microchannel formation, hydrogels (as described in Section 29.2) or extracellular matrix coatings may be used to fill or coat the channels. Next, cell types are sequentially added. For mimicking the airways, these cell types may be smooth muscle cells and bronchial epithelial cells. For mimicking the alveoli, these cell types may be endothelial cells and alveolar epithelial cells. Once cells are then lining the microchannels, air or media may flow through the channels. These devices are designed to fit on a microscope stage for real-time imaging. These "on a chip" devices have been used to screen drugs for applications in cancer, the immune system, skin, bone, kidney, cardiovascular, liver, gut, muscle, brain, and lung (Ahadian et al. 2018).

For the lung on a chip, the Ingber group pioneered the "breathing lung" (Huh et al. 2010), which includes a two-layer channel structure made from polydimethylsiloxane. The upper chamber contains alveolar epithelial cells, and the lower surface contains vascular endothelial cells. The flow of media and the internal pressure in the chambers are controlled, mimicking the mechanical conditions in the breathing lung. The same group has also developed a "small airway on a chip," which involves co-culture of bronchial epithelium and microvascular endothelium (Figure 29.2) (Benam et al. 2016b). This general setup can be used for lung disease and injury modeling and pharmaceutical screening. However, the use of these microfluidic lung on a chip devices for examining aerosolized therapeutics has not yet been reported. This lack of aerosol testing is likely due to the size limitation of the physiologically relevant microfluidic channels.

In recent years, there has been a push to combine multiple "on a chip" setups to mimic the interaction between multiple organs. These setups are termed "body on a chip," and they may prove to be an important technology for assessing the systemic effects of inhaled pharmaceuticals in the future.

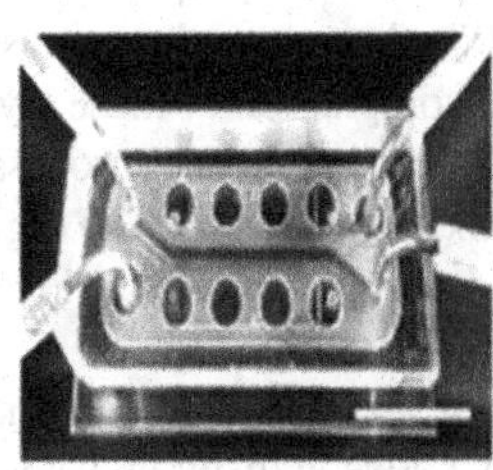

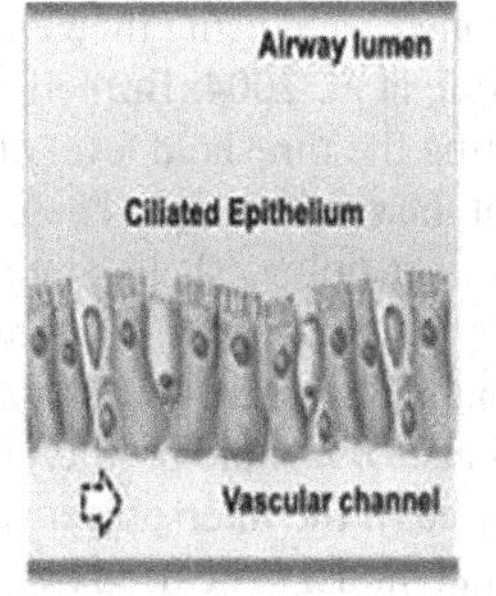

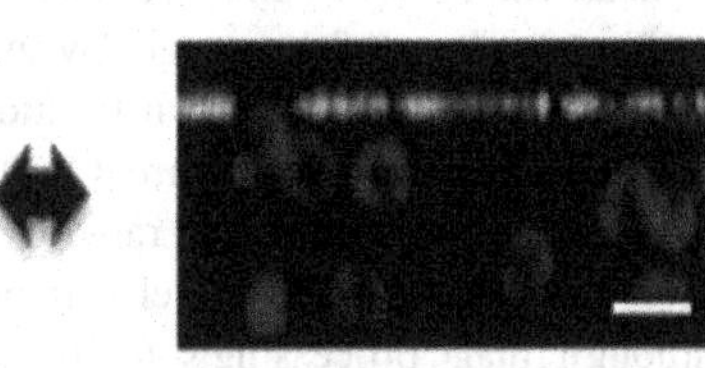

FIGURE 29.2 Lung-on-a-chip set up. From left to right: a photograph of a small airway-on-a-chip microdevice (bar, 1 cm), a schematic diagram showing differentiated human mucociliated airway epithelium cultured in the top channel of the device, and a confocal fluorescence orthogonal micrograph showing cross-section of pseudostratified bronchiolar epithelium cultured on-chip for 4 weeks lined by apical cilia (green/top white line, β-tubulin IV; blue/bottom gray disks, DAPI-stained nuclei; bar, 10 μm). (Reproduced from Benam, K.H. et al., *Cell Syst.*, 3, 456–466.e4, 2016. With permission.)

29.4 3D Printed Airways

The 3D printed anatomical airway models combined with physiological breathing profiles have been found useful for reliably predicting respiratory deposition of inhaled aerosol and suggesting the optimal combination of device and formulation for pulmonary drug delivery (Golshahi et al. 2015). High-resolution images of the airways are required for the development of 3D printed anatomical airway models. However, the radiation dose associated with computed tomography (CT) imaging of the lower respiratory tract has mostly been found too high to be justified. Although radiation is not a concern with magnetic resonance imaging (MRI), the drawback of this imaging method is the cost, time, and the need for minimum movements of airway walls to prevent motion artifacts during imaging. Thus, due to the difficulties with the acquisition of high-resolution images of the lower airways, the majority of anatomical airway models have been limited to the upper airways. A common approach is to estimate total lung dose (TLD) by fabricating anatomical extrathoracic airway models, mainly mouth-throat region for adult subjects, and infer the total lung dose by subtracting the amount deposited in the mouth-throat region from the dose delivered to the models.

Despite the usefulness of TLD in discriminating between devices, the efficacy of local-acting pulmonary drugs naturally depends on the regional deposition of inhaled pharmaceutical aerosols in the intrathoracic airways. In the absence of intrathoracic airway models, impactors such as Anderson cascade impactors (ACI) or next generation impactors (NGI) have commonly been used to estimate the dose reaching different regions in the intrathoracic airways. However, multiple studies have shown a significant amount of intersubject variability in the respiratory deposition of inhaled aerosol, which is difficult to be captured by impactors (Grgic et al. 2004; Golshahi et al. 2012, 2013a, 2013b). The main source of this variability has been suggested to be the difference in the anatomy of extrathoracic airways (Borgstrom et al. 2006). Thus, to avoid variability between the tests routinely performed to evaluate inhalers and/or drug formulations in liquid or dry powder forms, standardized inlets to impactors have long been used to represent the 90° bend, which is observed in the mouth-throat region of human subjects.

A 90° elbow pipe bend was suggested as a standardized mouth-throat region by British Pharmacopeia in 1988 and later was adopted by the United States Pharmacopeia as well as the European Pharmacopeia ("USP. General Chapter <601> Aerosols, Nasal Sprays, Metered Dose Inhalers, and Dry Powder Inhalers" 2009; Olsson et al. 2013). This simplified inlet to impactors was used for many years as a common representation of the upper oral airways. However, further research emphasized the importance of the anatomy of the oral airways in accurately predicting the amount of drug "lost" in the mouth-throat region (Olsson Borgstrom et al. 1996; Stapleton et al. 2000; Grgic et al. 2004; Ehtezazi et al. 2005; McRobbie and Pritchard 2005; Burnell et al. 2007; Xi and Longest 2007). Initially, cadaver-based casts were used as the anatomical oral airway models, but there was a concern with the change in the dimensions of the airways due to postmortem shrinking (Swift 1992). Later with the improvements in medical imaging and 3D printing technology, anatomical geometries are constructed using images (e.g. computed tomography or MRI) of the head and neck of human subjects (Grgic et al. 2004; Burnell et al. 2007). The air regions are segmented in each layer of the images by selecting the threshold level of air, and compilation of these layers eventually forms a 3D solid reconstruction of the oral airways. These solid airways can be post-processed in computer-aided design software (CAD) to form hollow shells representing the airway walls. The digital shells can then be printed using rapid prototyping machines. A more detailed review and illustrations of the most recent anatomical models can be found elsewhere (Golshahi et al. 2015).

Although image processing software packages and rapid prototyping technology have made the generation of anatomical airway models relatively easy, the intersubject variability between different subjects calls for consensus on a standard mouth-throat model to be used by the industry and regulatory agencies. This need for standardization led to the development of idealized, simplified geometries, which include the critical dimensions of the airways. However, to capture large variability in clinical trials, the *in vitro* test results with anatomical models should capture the mean, minimum, and maximum extremes in a human population, which are expected to be represented by the lower and upper 95% confidence interval limits (International Commission on Radiological Protection 1994).

Different approaches have been taken by different researchers for the production of an oral airway model that can represent the average deposition. A widely used anatomical mouth-throat model, representing the oral airways of an average adult is the Alberta Idealized Throat (AIT), which was developed beginning with the work of Stapleton et al. (2000). This is a geometry that was developed based on CT and MRI scans, airway dimensions given in the literature, and direct observation of healthy subjects. Experiments with anatomical oral airway models showed the square root of volume over the length of airways is a characteristic dimension that predominantly controls the intersubject variability in mouth-throat deposition (Grgic et al. 2004). Thus, AIT was developed in a way to represent the average value of square root of volume over length in a human population (Grgic et al. 2004). Good agreement has been found between *in vitro* data taken with the AIT model and *in vivo* data (Grgic et al. 2004; Zhang et al. 2007; Zhou et al. 2011). The AIT model has been found a good model to represent the average mouth-throat deposition of pharmaceutical aerosols in adults during both steady and spontaneous breathing (Grgic et al. 2004; Golshahi et al. 2013a). Later, Golshahi and Finlay developed an Alberta Idealized Child Mouth-Throat model as a model representing average mouth-throat deposition in children 6 years–14 years old (Golshahi and Finlay 2012).

To represent the range of variability in pulmonary drug delivery in human subjects, three anatomical oral airway models including average, small, and large versions that can capture 95% of the normal adult human population have been developed at VCU (Delvadia et al. 2012). The three models incorporate mouth-throat region including the larynx, trachea, and upper bronchi including trachea and extend to the upper bronchi (generation 3). The large and small models were developed by scaling the average model in a way to capture mean ±2 standard deviations of the volume of airways reported for a human population by Burnell et al. (2007). An existing model of an adult mouth-throat was selected as the average mouth-throat model based on preliminary data (Delvadia et al. 2012). Similarly, the medium tracheobronchial model was an existing model (Yeh and Schum 1980), which was scaled using the same scale factors that were used for the attached small and large mouth-throat models (Delvadia et al. 2012). These three anatomical models have been used in a series of studies performed to improve the accuracy of *in vitro-in vivo* correlations for pulmonary drug delivery (IVIVC) (Delvadia et al. 2013a, 2013b).

In addition to the preceding anatomical oral airway models, anatomical nasal airway replicas including face have been used to study pediatric aerosol therapy. Mainly facemasks are used to administer pharmaceutical aerosols to this age group, who typically struggle to hold onto a mouthpiece for pulmonary drug delivery through the mouth. A widely used pediatric infant airway replica is known as the Sophia Anatomical Nose-Throat model, which is an anatomical nasal airway model of a 9-month-old girl and is described by Janssens et al. (2001). Later, a nasal airway model of a premature male infant of 32-week gestational age, known as premature infant nose throat model was developed using MRI scans (Minocchieri et al. 2008). This model, similar to the Sophia Anatomical Nose-Throat model, included the face of the infant in addition to the entire nasal airway from the nostrils to 4 mm below glottis (Minocchieri et al. 2008). Similar to oral airways, significant intersubject variability exists in the nasal deposition of inhaled pharmaceutical aerosols. To capture pediatric intersubject variability in a nasal deposition, a series of studies have recently been performed in Aerosol Research Laboratory of Alberta with multiple neonates (5 days–79 days) (Tavernini et al. 2017), infants (3 months–18 months old) (Storey-Bishoff et al. 2008), and children and adolescents (4 years–14 years old) (Golshahi et al. 2011). Idealized nasal models have also been developed for neonates and infants (Javaheri et al. 2013; Tavernini et al. 2018).

In conclusion, while by using anatomical airway models useful information has been obtained regarding the comparison of different pulmonary drug delivery devices and formulations regarding drug dose reaching tracheobronchial region, several limitations of these airway models must be borne in mind. First, a single anatomical model cannot capture the effect of anatomical differences between different individuals. Idealized geometries developed based on multiple subjects can partly resolve this issue. Second, most anatomical airway replicas are made from polymers, which may leach when solvents are used to extract the deposited drug from their surfaces. This leached material can make the analytical methods needed to quantify the deposited drug complicated. Use of metal materials or certain resins without added color have been found useful to address this potential incompatibility of materials used for the production of anatomical airway models with common solvents (e.g. methyl alcohol, etc.).

Finally, patient's interaction with pharmaceutical drug delivery devices is difficult to be captured with rigid anatomical airway models, since the motion of tongue, teeth, lips and oropharynx, or nasopharynx is difficult to be captured with rigid models. *In vivo* studies present a realism that may not be fully captured by *in vitro* anatomical airway models.

29.5 *Ex Vivo* Perfused Lungs

As described in the previous section, it is critical to evaluate pharmaceutical aerosols and their dispersal behaviors in an anatomically and physiologically correct model. Complexities of the human lung geometry and removal mechanisms, such as the mucociliary escalator and immune phagocytosis, can drastically alter the pharmacokinetics of aerosols. The behavior of an aerosol particle *in vivo* can only be predicted in a similarly complex environment and is vital for drug and drug delivery design. While *in vivo* testing of inhaled drugs is optimal for combining systemic and local effects, it can be an experimentally challenging task and has ethical restrictions that limit testability. Conversely, the *ex vivo* perfused lung (EVPL) is a highly translatable analysis platform for aerosol behavior such as airway dispersal, mucosal interaction, and transport across the air-liquid interface that can show cellular response and simplify the experimental results by eliminating systemic complications.

Sources of healthy or diseased lungs are commonly acquired from recently deceased non-transplant candidate human donors or xenographic sources such as pigs or rodents, which require some understanding of the physiological differences from humans. Lung isolation for EVPL includes surgical removal of the lung and transfer to a negative pressure artificial chest cavity. There are several standard EVLP protocols, including the Lund, Toronto, and portable EVLP protocols, that all vary in the amount of time before connection to the chamber and assessment strategies (Sakagami 2006, Makdisi et al. 2007). All of the protocols require a biomimetic artificial environment for preservation and testing. There are four commercially available EVLP devices including Organ Care System™, XPS™, Lung Assist®, and Vivoline® LS1 that all vary in the portability and availability (Makdisi et al. 2007). All artificial chambers consist of two main circuits. The first is the vascular circulation circuit that deoxygenates and filters media leaving the pulmonary vein (PV) canula and then returns it to the pulmonary artery (Figure 29.1). The other circuit contains the ventilator that is connected to the trachea cannula and delivers oxygenated air to the lungs. Perfusion flow rate, pulmonary vascular resistance, lung compliance, glucose levels, lactate levels, and arterial blood gas levels must be monitored and maintained within a physiological range for accurate testing.

EVPLs have advantages and disadvantages over *in vivo* or *in vitro* models. EVPLs are seen as a highly translatable testing system that can be continuously monitored in a way that would be considered invasive *in vivo*. Compared to *in vitro* methods, they can analyze the behavior of multiple tissues and cell types that perform normal physiological functions such as bronchoconstriction and vasoconstriction (Ewing et al. 2010). While this is a very promising tool for aerosol testing, there are aspects of the system that may be problematic. Inflammatory mediators within the lung during removal can cause substantial inflammation and cause damage to the tissue. There can also be an injury caused by the chosen protocol as well, including, but not limited to, compromised blood supply (Tanaka et al. 2015; Tane et al. 2017) and complications caused by ventilator-induced lung injury that is seen with any lung placed on a ventilator for a prolonged amount of time. EVPL is recommended for only deposition and initial lung function assessments because of the decrease in lung viability after only several hours. Even with these substantial limitations for the EVPL, this is a suitable predictive model that closely correlates to *in vivo* results when concerning kinetics and deposition (Sakagami 2006; Selg et al. 2012).

Ex vivo lung perfusion was used as early as the 1980s (Mehendale et al. 1981; Hardesty and Griffith 1987), but this procedure was mostly attempted to extend transplant travel times. Over decades, the EVPL has improved with the capability of functioning for days and can offer vital data on absorption and deposition of inhaled pharmaceuticals. EVPL methods have been used with humans, rats, guinea pigs, rabbits, dogs, and monkeys. To most effectively test pharmaceutical aerosols, the EVPL can be used in conjunction with meter dose propellant-based intratracheal dosing cartridge, nebulizers, inhalable dry powder exposures, or dust gun aerosol technology with healthy or diseased lungs (Figure 29.3). This technology has been utilized with both therapeutic aerosols (Beck-Broichsitter et al. 2010; Morris et al. 2011;

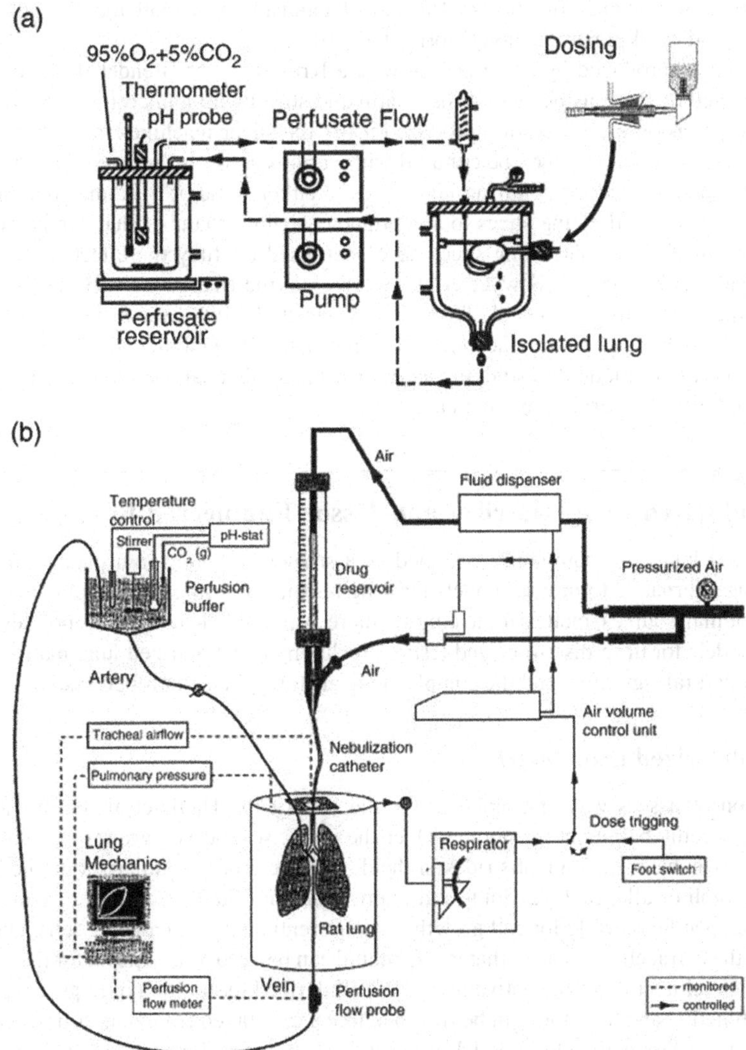

FIGURE 29.3 (a,b) *Ex vivo* perfused lung nebulizer aerosol dosing apparatus. (Reproduced from Sakagami, M., *Adv. Drug Deliv. Rev.*, 58, 1030–1060, 2006. With permission.)

Ong et al. 2014) and particulate air pollution (Nemmar et al. 2005). More recently, *ex vivo* lungs have been used in conjunction with a plastinated head to give a model of the full respiratory tract for accurate deposition kinetics (Perinel et al. 2017). EVLP is expected to play a large role in pharmaceutical aerosol drug discovery and testing as an effective alternative to *in vivo* models.

29.6 Precision Cut Lung Slices

Precision cut lung slices are a beneficial alternative to *in vivo* animal models for pharmacotoxicology experimentation. While liver and kidney slices are more frequently used in the field of pharmacology, the use of lung slices for aerosols is also useful for assessing cytotoxicity and metabolism. The main advantage of these systems is that the cell-cell and cell-Extracellular Matrix (ECM) interactions are maintained with the controllability of a culture system. These slices can maximize the output of *ex vivo* lungs by giving multiple replicates and less expensive culturing conditions. Lung slices, if maintained correctly, preserve physiological function such as vascular and airway smooth muscle contraction, mucociliary function, and cytokine production (Morin et al. 2013).

Lung slices can be produced by either slicing with a Krumdieck or Brendel slicer to keep the lung cells alive or embed the lung using agarose or gelatin and sliced with a microtome (Morin et al. 2013). Currently, most precision lung slices are produced using the slicer machines to allow for the uniform thickness of live tissues that can then be cultured with various aerosols. Submerged culture systems or multi-well plates can be used for culturing lung slices in either static or dynamic conditions. Aerosols can be tested by exposing the lung slices to a continuous airflow chamber that can be added to many different culture systems. To date, lung slices have been used to study the effects of several aerosols such as chemical warfare agents (Sawyer et al. 1995), cytokine treatments such as IL-6 (Kida et al. 2005), environmental hazards (Fall et al. 2007; Henjakovic et al. 2008), and drug discovery and testing (Nassimi et al. 2010). Lung slices produced from bleomycin-challenged rodents (Bosnar et al. 2017) are an example of an *in vitro* method to studying an *ex vivo* model that can lead to therapies for idiopathic fibrosis (IPF) and testing of drugs already in use.

29.7 Decellularized Lung Matrices and Tissue Engineered Lungs

Tissue-engineered lungs are commonly designed as a strategy for lung transplantation, but they are also a promising alternative to *in vivo* models for drug testing. By using tissue from an animal or non-transplantable human sources, models for testing are more available. There are currently several naturally derived lung models for drug discovery and testing, including decellularized lung matrices, bioprinted lungs that offer natural signaling, and the complex lung anatomy, in a controlled system.

29.7.1 Decellularized Lung Matrix

Decellularization of tissues was first pioneered in the late 1970s (Hjelle et al. 1979) with the aim of isolating tissue-specific basement membrane. Over the years, several key groups, such as the Badylak and Ott laboratories, have made great strides in the development of decellularization methods that can extend to xenograph or allograph scaffolds and many different organs. The goal of this research is to develop a tissue-specific scaffold for cell growth and differentiation of a patient's cells. Once cells have been removed, the extracellular matrix that is left behind can be used as a scaffold for tissue engineering by providing the architecture of the native organ. Decellularized tissues do not require the preservation of the cellular function and therefore can be frozen before use or taken from donors unsuitable for transplant. This creates a less demanding model, in terms of sterility and controlled environmental conditions, compared to an *ex vivo* perfused model. It is important to note that this technology can be costly and usually requires further methods, such as recellularization, to make this a useful experimental tool.

Removal of cellular material to produce a decellularized tissue is done with chemical reagents, mechanical abrasion, or freeze-thaw procedures. The most common method of lung decellularization includes perfusion of chemical reagents such as acids and bases, hypertonic or hypotonic solutions, non-ionic detergents such as Triton X-100, ionic detergents such as sodium dodecyl sulfate or sodium deoxycholate, zwitterionic detergents such as 3-[(3-cholamidopropyl)dimethylammonio]-1-propanesulfonate (CHAPS), or enzymatic solutions such as nucleases, trypsin, or dispase through both the trachea and vasculature. Some of the physical methods include pressure, electroporation, or agitation. Most protocols use a combination of various chemicals and mechanical methods to ensure removal of all cellular remanence within the tissue (Ott et al. 2008; Petersen et al. 2010; Price et al. 2010). A gold standard for this procedure has not definitively been established because there are disadvantages to some reagents over others. Some reagents are more effective at removing cellular material such as sodium dodecyl sulfate and sodium deoxycholate, but they can also cause damage to the ECM. Less harsh chemicals such as Triton X-100, trypsin, or CHAPS do not disrupt the ECM composition, but are inefficient at cellular removal. All tissues are different and require tailoring of the decellularization protocol based on the tissue's density or lipid content (Crapo et al. 2012). For the lung specifically, there is low lipid content, and the airways and vasculature arrangement allows for efficient distributing of the reagents to all parts of the tissue, making it a great candidate for decellularization research. Quality control for removal of DNA, proteins, or α-galactosidase in cases of xenogeneic tissues, is important to eliminate immunological reactions or other adverse effects. To be considered a fully decellularized scaffold, the lung must pass the standard of less than 50 ng dsDNA per mg ECM dry weight and less than 200 base pair DNA fragment length, with lack of visible nuclear staining (Crapo et al. 2011). Quality control is done by histological nuclei staining with DAPI or hematoxylin and eosin and dsDNA quantification methods such as PicoGreen assay, propidium iodide, or gel electrophoresis (Crapo et al. 2011).

In cases of aerosol testing, a more appropriate and complete model can be produced from recellularization of the scaffold with human cell lines. Lungs engineered in this way will give many of the benefits of decellularized lungs that have already been discussed, but this will also allow the researcher to gain information on lung mechanics and cellular response. There are currently two main unanswered questions in the field of lung recellularization. (1) What are the best cell lines for recellularisation that will differentiate into all cell types of the adult lung? (2) What are the best cell delivery and culturing methods to produce viable, long-lasting tissues? Both sides of the gas exchange barrier, epithelial and endothelial, need to be recellularized fully to produce functional tissue. Heterogeneous populations of primary lung cells from a human donor can offer multiple cell types with the least amount of effort, but this will not always result in the full cellular profile. Another promising option for epithelial recellularization are lung stem cells such as basal progenitor cells (Trp63+, Krt5+) (Gilpin et al. 2017), alveolar type 2 cells (sftpc+, sftpb+) (Price et al. 2010), club cells (scgb1a1+, Cyp2f2–), induced pluripotent stem cells (IPSCs) (Shafa et al. 2018), or resident mesenchymal stem cells (MSCs) from either a bone marrow or adipose lineage (Schilders et al. 2016). As for revascularization, similar cell options are available, such as heterogeneous mixture of vascular cells (Le et al. 2017), human umbilical vein endothelial cells (HUVECs) (Ott et al. 2010), induced pluripotent stem cells, endothelial stem cells (Chavakis et al. 2008; Heise et al. 2016), or mesenchymal stem cells. The ideal recellularization protocol has not been determined, but will ultimately include multiple cell types at a perfect concentration, providing a physiological niche similar to the native lung.

Recellularization of decellularized lung scaffolds is improved by culturing in a dynamic bioreactor system to simulate the physiological environment and innovative protocols that allow for the most effective seeding of cells (Ren et al. 2015; Gilpin et al. 2017; Le et al. 2017). Bioreactor designs began with hollow fiber bioreactors that allow for basic perfusion of media around the tube and air within the tube for lung cell differentiation (Guyot and Hanrahan 2002) to more complex and regulated whole lung perfusion systems. Bioreactors have been developed for both decellularization and recellularization procedures to ensure reproducibility. The most common system performs cell seeding and culture with pulsatile or continuous vascular perfusion and negative pressure breathing (Ott et al. 2010; Bonvillain et al. 2013). This system can be outfitted with various aerosol delivery systems such as pressure metered-dose inhaler, dry powder inhalers, nebulizers, solution mist inhalers, or nasal sprays (Cheng 2014) at the inlet of the tracheal canula to test pharmacokinetics and toxicity.

29.7.2 3D Bioprinted Lungs

Bioprinting of tissues and organs is another resource that allows for customization to the anatomy and complexity of a living 3D lung model. Bioprinting includes both cells and bioactive, cross-linkable materials that are printed using extrusion, inkjet methods, or laser assistance (Figure 29.4) (Murphy and Atala 2014). Another challenge for this technology is to produce a bio-ink that will give the organ structure and resolution, contain culture medium, have biodegradability, and maintain bioactive and non-cytotoxic characteristics. Bioinks are commonly hydrogels composed of synthetic polymers such as polyethylene glycol (PEG) or pluronic to give rigidity and/or natural polymers, such as collagen (Michael et al. 2013), chitosan (Geng et al. 2005), fibrin (Gruene et al. 2011), gelatin (Wang et al. 2006), Matrigel (Schiele et al. 2009), or alginate (Jia et al. 2014) to offer biocompatibility and signaling components. Embedding cells into a cross-linkable hydrogel is often a challenge from the standpoint of cytotoxicity. Choosing a cross-linker that will not damage cells or change cellular processes is crucial. There can be temperature dependent cross-linking, chemically cross-linked, enzymatic cross-linking, or photopolymerization using ultraviolet light, but some of these methods have cytotoxic effects and should be taken into consideration

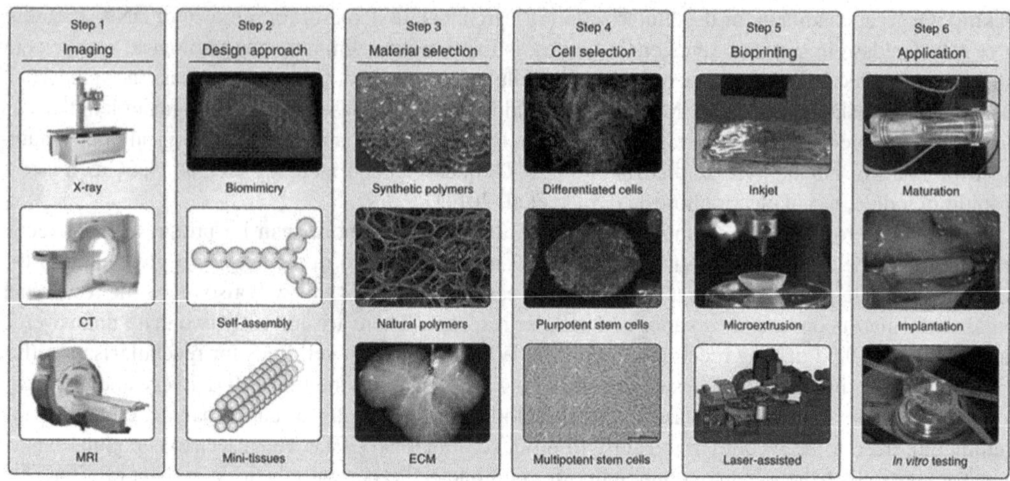

FIGURE 29.4 Various process for bioprinting tissues. (Reproduced from Murphy, S.V., and Atala, A., *Nat. Biotechnol.*, 32, 773, 2014. With permission.)

(Hospodiuk et al. 2017). The main limiting factor with lung bioprinting is that it is difficult to produce the level of resolution needed to create distal lung structures, while making this technology affordable. However, as bioprinting and additive manufacturing techniques improve, the bioprinted alveoli and airway may be utilized for future aerosol technology testing.

29.8 Conclusions

The technology in these areas is rapidly developing. As the push towards more sophisticated 3D cultures, 3D printing, and tissue-engineered lungs continues, the possibility for highly biologically accurate *in vitro* systems for inhaled aerosol development becomes more of a reality. These 3D systems can provide valuable pre-clinical data for drug development.

REFERENCES

Ahadian, Samad, Robert Civitarese, Dawn Bannerman, Mohammad Hossein Mohammadi, Rick Lu, Erika Wang, Locke Davenport-Huyer et al. 2018. "Organ-on-a-chip platforms: A convergence of advanced materials, cells, and microscale technologies." *Advanced Healthcare Materials* 7 (2). doi:10.1002/adhm.201700506.

Ahmed, Enas M. 2015. "Hydrogel: Preparation, characterization, and applications: A review." *Journal of Advanced Research* 6 (2): 105–121. doi:10.1016/j.jare.2013.07.006.

Barkauskas, Christina E., Mei-I. Chung, Bryan Fioret, Xia Gao, Hiroaki Katsura, and Brigid L. M. Hogan. 2017. "Lung organoids: Current uses and future promise." *Development* 144 (6): 986–997. doi:10.1242/dev.140103.

Beck-Broichsitter, Moritz, Julia Gauss, Tobias Gessler, Werner Seeger, Thomas Kissel, and Thomas Schmehl. 2010. "Pulmonary targeting with biodegradable salbutamol-loaded nanoparticles." *Journal of Aerosol Medicine and Pulmonary Drug Delivery* 23 (1): 47–57.

Benam, Kambez H., Richard Novak, Janna Nawroth, Mariko Hirano-Kobayashi, Thomas C. Ferrante, Youngjae Choe, Rachelle Prantil-Baun et al. 2016a. "Matched-comparative modeling of normal and diseased human airway responses using a microengineered breathing lung chip." *Cell Systems* 3 (5): 456–466.e4. doi:10.1016/j.cels.2016.10.003.

Benam, Kambez H., Remi Villenave, Carolina Lucchesi, Antonio Varone, Cedric Hubeau, Hyun-Hee Lee, Stephen E. Alves et al. 2016b. "Small Airway-on-a-chip enables analysis of human lung inflammation and drug responses in vitro." *Nature Methods* 13 (2): 151–157. doi:10.1038/nmeth.3697.

Bonvillain, Ryan W., Michelle E. Scarritt, Nicholas C. Pashos, Jacques P. Mayeux, Christopher L. Meshberger, Aline M. Betancourt, Deborah E. Sullivan, and Bruce A. Bunnell. 2013. "Nonhuman primate lung decellularization and recellularization using a specialized large-organ bioreactor." *JoVE (Journal of Visualized Experiments)*, 82 (December): e50825. doi:10.3791/50825.

Borgstrom, Lars, Bo Olsson, and Lars Thorsson. 2006. "Degree of throat deposition can explain the variability in lung deposition of inhaled drugs." *Journal of Aerosol Medicine* 19 (4): 473–483. doi:10.1089/jam.2006.19.473.

Bosnar, Martina, Daniela Belamaric, Matea Cedilak, Andrea Paravic Radicevic, Ivan Faraho, Krunoslav Ilic, Mihailo Banjanac, Ines Glojnaric, and Vesna Erakovic Haber. 2017. "Lung tissue explants and precision-cut lung slices from bleomycin treated animals as a model for testing potential therapies for idiopathic pulmonary Fibrosis." *American Journal of Respiratory and Critical Care Medicine* 195: A2386.

Burnell, Patricia K., Lars Asking, Lars Borgstrom, Steve C. Nichols, Bo Olsson, David Prime, and Ian Shrubb. 2007. "Studies of the human oropharyngeal airspaces using magnetic resonance imaging iv—The oropharyngeal retention effect for four inhalation delivery systems." *Journal of Aerosol Medicine* 20 (3): 269–281. doi:10.1089/jam.2007.0566.

Caló, Enrica, and Vitaliy V. Khutoryanskiy. 2015. "Biomedical applications of hydrogels: A review of patents and commercial products." *European Polymer Journal*, 50 Years of European Polymer Journal, 65 (April): 252–267. doi:10.1016/j.eurpolymj.2014.11.024.

Chavakis, Emmanouil, Carmen Urbich, and Stefanie Dimmeler. 2008. "Homing and engraftment of progenitor cells: A prerequisite for cell therapy." *Journal of Molecular and Cellular Cardiology*, Special Issue: Stem Cells and Regenerative Medicine, 45 (4): 514–522. doi:10.1016/j.yjmcc.2008.01.004.

Cheng, Yung Sung. 2014. "Mechanisms of pharmaceutical aerosol deposition in the respiratory tract." *AAPS PharmSciTech* 15 (3): 630–640. doi:10.1208/s12249-014-0092-0.

Crapo, Peter M., Thomas W. Gilbert, and Stephen F. Badylak. 2011. "An overview of tissue and whole organ decellularization processes." *Biomaterials* 32 (12): 3233–3243. doi:10.1016/j.biomaterials.2011.01.057.

Crapo, Peter M., Christopher J. Medberry, Janet E. Reing, Stephen Tottey, Yolandi van der Merwe, Kristen E. Jones, and Stephen F. Badylak. 2012. "Biologic scaffolds composed of central nervous system extracellular matrix." *Biomaterials* 33 (13): 3539–3547. doi:10.1016/j.biomaterials.2012.01.044.

Delvadia, Renishkumar, Michael Hindle, P. Worth Longest, and Peter R. Byron. 2013a. "In vitro tests for aerosol deposition II: Ivivcs for different dry powder inhalers in normal adults." *Journal of Aerosol Medicine and Pulmonary Drug Delivery* 26 (3): 138–144. doi:10.1089/jamp.2012.0975.

Delvadia, Renishkumar R., P. Worth Longest, and Peter R. Byron. 2012. "In vitro tests for aerosol deposition. I: Scaling a physical model of the upper airways to predict drug deposition variation in normal humans." *Journal of Aerosol Medicine and Pulmonary Drug Delivery* 25 (1): 32–40. doi:10.1089/jamp.2011.0905.

Delvadia, Renishkumar R., P. Worth Longest, Michael Hindle, and Peter R. Byron. 2013b. "In vitro tests for aerosol deposition. III: Effect of inhaler insertion angle on aerosol deposition." *Journal of Aerosol Medicine and Pulmonary Drug Delivery* 26 (3): 145–156. doi:10.1089/jamp.2012.0989.

Ehtezazi, Touraj, Kevin W. Southern, David R. Allanson, I. Jenkinson, and Christopher O'Callaghan. 2005. "Suitability of the upper airway models obtained from mri studies in simulating drug lung deposition from inhalers." *Pharmaceutical Research* 22 (1): 166–170.

Ewing, Pär, Åke Ryrfeldt, Carl-Olof Sjöberg, Paul Andersson, Staffan Edsbäcker, and Per Gerde. 2010. "Vasoconstriction after inhalation of budesonide: A study in the isolated and perfused rat lung." *Pulmonary Pharmacology & Therapeutics* 23 (1): 9–14. doi:10.1016/j.pupt.2009.09.004.

Fall, Mamadou, Michel Guerbet, Barry Park, Frantz Gouriou, Frédéric Dionnet, and Jean-Paul Morin. 2007. "Evaluation of cerium oxide and cerium oxide based fuel additive safety on organotypic cultures of lung slices." *Nanotoxicology* 1 (3): 227–234. doi:10.1080/17435390701763090.

Fang, Ye, and Richard M. Eglen. 2017. "Three-dimensional cell cultures in drug discovery and development." *Slas Discovery* 22 (5): 456–472. doi:10.1177/1087057117696795.

Geng, Li, Wei Feng, Dietmar W. Hutmacher, Yoke San Wong, Han Tong Loh, and Jerry Y. H. Fuh. 2005. "Direct writing of chitosan scaffolds using a robotic system." *Rapid Prototyping Journal* 11 (2): 90–97. doi:10.1108/13552540510589458.

Gilpin, Sarah E., Qiyao Li, Daniele Evangelista-Leite, Xi Ren, Dieter P. Reinhardt, Brian L. Frey, and Harald C. Ott. 2017. "Fibrillin-2 and tenascin-C bridge the age gap in lung epithelial regeneration." *Biomaterials* 140 (September): 212–219. doi:10.1016/j.biomaterials.2017.06.027.

Golshahi, Laleh, and Warren H. Finlay. 2012. "An idealized child throat that mimics average pediatric oropharyngeal deposition." *Aerosol Science and Technology* 46 (5): i–iv.

Golshahi, Laleh, Warren H. Finlay, and Herbert Wachtel. 2015. "Use of airway replicas in lung delivery applications." In *The ISAM Textbook of Aerosol Medicine*, edited by R. Dhand, pp. 221–252. International Society for Aerosols in Medicine.

Golshahi, Laleh, Michelle L. Noga, and Warren H. Finlay. 2012. "Deposition of inhaled micrometer-sized particles in oropharyngeal airway replicas of children at constant flow rates." *Journal of Aerosol Science* 49: 21–31. doi:10.1016/j.jaerosci.2012.03.001.

Golshahi, Laleh, Michelle L. Noga, Richard B. Thompson, and Warren H. Finlay. 2011. "In vitro deposition measurement of inhaled micrometer-sized particles in extrathoracic airways of children and adolescents during nose breathing." *Journal of Aerosol Science* 42 (7): 474–488.

Golshahi, Laleh, Michelle L. Noga, Reinhard Vehring, and Warren H. Finlay. 2013a. "An in vitro study on the deposition of micrometer-sized particles in the extrathoracic airways of adults during tidal oral breathing." *Annals of Biomedical Engineering* 41 (5): 979–989.

Golshahi, Laleh, Reinhard Vehring, Michelle L. Noga, and Warren H. Finlay. 2013b. "In vitro deposition of micrometer-sized particles in the extrathoracic airways of children during tidal oral breathing." *Journal of Aerosol Science* 57: 14–21. doi:10.1016/j.jaerosci.2012.10.006.

Grgic, Biljana, Warren H. Finlay, P. K. P. Burnell, and A. F. Heenan. 2004. "In vitro intersubject and intrasubject deposition measurements in realistic mouth–throat geometries." *Journal of Aerosol Science* 35 (8): 1025–1040. doi:10.1016/j.jaerosci.2004.03.003.

Gruene, Martin, Michael Pflaum, Christian Hess, Stefanos Diamantouros, Sabrina Schlie, Andrea Deiwick, Lothar Koch et al. 2011. "Laser printing of three-dimensional multicellular arrays for studies of cell–cell and cell–environment interactions." *Tissue Engineering Part C: Methods* 17 (10): 973–982. doi:10.1089/ten.tec.2011.0185.

Guyot, Annick, and John W. Hanrahan. 2002. "ATP release from human airway epithelial cells studied using a capillary cell culture system." *The Journal of Physiology* 545 (Pt 1): 199–206. doi:10.1113/jphysiol.2002.030148.

Hardesty, R. L., and B. P. Griffith. 1987. "Autoperfusion of the heart and lungs for preservation during distant procurement." *The Journal of Thoracic and Cardiovascular Surgery* 93 (1): 11–18.

Heise, Rebecca L., Patrick A. Link, and Laszlo Farkas. 2016. "From here to there, progenitor cells and stem cells are everywhere in lung vascular remodeling." *Frontiers in Pediatrics* 4 (August). doi:10.3389/fped.2016.00080.

Henjakovic, Maja, Christian Martin, Heinz-Gerd Hoymann, Katherina Sewald, Anne R. Ressmeyer, Constanze Dassow, Gerhard Pohlmann, Norbert Krug, Stefan Uhlig, and Armin Braun. 2008. "Ex vivo lung function measurements in precision-cut lung slices (pcls) from chemical allergen–sensitized mice represent a suitable alternative to in vivo studies." *Toxicological Sciences* 106 (2): 444–453. doi:10.1093/toxsci/kfn178.

Hjelle, J. Thomas, Edward C. Carlson, Klaus Brendel, and Elias Meezan. 1979. "Biosynthesis of basement membrane matrix by isolated rat renal glomeruli." *Kidney International* 15 (1): 20–32. doi:10.1038/ki.1979.3.

Hospodiuk, Monika, Madhuri Dey, Donna Sosnoski, and Ibrahim T. Ozbolat. 2017. "The bioink: A comprehensive review on bioprintable materials." *Biotechnology Advances* 35 (2): 217–239. doi:10.1016/j.biotechadv.2016.12.006.

Huh, Dongeun, Benjamin D. Matthews, Akiko Mammoto, Martín Montoya-Zavala, Hong Yuan Hsin, and Donald E. Ingber. 2010. "Reconstituting organ-level lung functions on a chip." *Science* 328 (5986): 1662–1668. doi:10.1126/science.1188302.

International Commission on Radiological Protection, ICRP. 1994. "Human respiratory tract model for radiological protection." *Annals of the ICRP* 24 (1–3): 1–482.

Janssens, Hattie M., Johan C. de Jongste, Wytske J. Fokkens, Simon G. Robben, Kris Wouters, and Harm A. Tiddens. 2001. "The Sophia Anatomical Infant Nose-Throat (Saint) Model: A valuable tool to study aerosol deposition in infants." *Journal of Aerosol Medicine* 14 (4): 433–441. doi:10.1089/08942680152744640.

Javaheri, Emadeddin, Laleh Golshahi, and Warren H. Finlay. 2013. "An idealized geometry that mimics average infant nasal airway deposition." *Journal of Aerosol Science* 55: 137–148. doi:10.1016/j.jaerosci.2012.07.013.

Jia, Jia, Dylan J. Richards, Samuel Pollard, Yu Tan, Joshua Rodriguez, Richard P. Visconti, Thomas C. Trusk et al. 2014. "Engineering Alginate as Bioink for Bioprinting." *Acta Biomaterialia* 10 (10): 4323–4331. doi:10.1016/j.actbio.2014.06.034.

Kida, Hiroshi, Mitsuhiro Yoshida, Shigenori Hoshino, Koji Inoue, Yukihiro Yano, Masahiko Yanagita, Toru Kumagai et al. 2005. "Protective effect of IL-6 on alveolar epithelial cell death induced by hydrogen peroxide." *American Journal of Physiology-Lung Cellular and Molecular Physiology.* doi:10.1152/ajplung.00016.2004.

Le, Andrew V., Go Hatachi, Arkadi Beloiartsev, Mahboobe Ghaedi, Alexander J. Engler, Pavlina Baevova, Laura E. Niklason, and Elizabeth A. Calle. 2017. "Efficient and functional endothelial repopulation of whole lung organ scaffolds." *ACS Biomaterials Science & Engineering* 3 (9): 2000–2010. doi:10.1021/acsbiomaterials.6b00784.

Makdisi, George, Tony Makdisi, Tambi Jarmi, and Christiano C. Caldeira. 2017. "Ex vivo lung perfusion review of a revolutionary technology." *Annals of Translational Medicine* 5 (17). doi:10.21037/atm.2017.07.17.

McRobbie, Donald W., and Susan E. Pritchard. 2005. "Studies of the human oropharyngeal airspaces using magnetic resonance imaging. III. The effects of device resistance with forced maneuver and tidal breathing on upper airway geometry." *Journal of Aerosol Medicine* 18 (3): 325–336. doi:10.1089/jam.2005.18.325.

Mehendale, Harihara M., Linda S. Angevine, and Yoshio Ohmiya. 1981. "The isolated perfused lung—A critical evaluation." *Toxicology* 21 (1): 1–36. doi:10.1016/0300-483X(81)90013-5.

Michael, Stefanie, Heiko Sorg, Claas-Tido Peck, Lothar Koch, Andrea Deiwick, Boris Chichkov, Peter M. Vogt, and Kerstin Reimers. 2013. "Tissue engineered skin substitutes created by laser-assisted bioprinting form skin-like structures in the dorsal skin fold chamber in mice." *PLoS One* 8 (3): e57741. doi:10.1371/journal.pone.0057741.

Minocchieri, Stefan, Juerg Martin Burren, Marc Aurel Bachmann, Georgette L. Stern, Johannes H. Wildhaber, Stefan Buob, Ralf Schindel, Richard Kraemer, Urs P. Frey, and Mathias Nelle. 2008. "Development of the Premature Infant Nose Throat-Model (PrINT-Model): An upper airway replica of a premature neonate for the study of aerosol delivery." *Pediatric Research* 64 (2): 141–146. doi:10.1203/PDR.0b013e318175dcfa.

Morin, Jean-Paul, Jean-Marc Baste, Arnaud Gay, Clément Crochemore, Cécile Corbière, and Christelle Monteil. 2013. "Precision cut lung slices as an efficient tool for in vitro lung physio-pharmacotoxicology studies." *Xenobiotica* 43 (1): 63–72. doi:10.3109/00498254.2012.727043.

Morris, Christopher J., Mathew W. Smith, Peter C. Griffiths, Neil B. McKeown, and Mark Gumbleton. 2011. "Enhanced pulmonary absorption of a macromolecule through coupling to a sequence-specific phage display-derived peptide." *Journal of Controlled Release* 151 (1): 83–94. doi:10.1016/j.jconrel.2010.12.003.

Murphy, Sean V., and Anthony Atala. 2014. "3D bioprinting of tissues and organs." *Nature Biotechnology* 32 (8): 773. doi:10.1038/nbt.2958.

Nassimi, Matthias, Carsten Schleh, Hans D. Lauenstein, Razan Hussein, Heinz-Gerd Hoymann, Wolfgang Koch, Gerhard Pohlmann et al. 2010. "A toxicological evaluation of inhaled solid lipid nanoparticles used as a potential drug delivery system for the lung." *European Journal of Pharmaceutics and Biopharmaceutics* 75 (2): 107–116. doi:10.1016/j.ejpb.2010.02.014.

Nemmar, Abderrahim, Julien Hamoir, Benoit Nemery, and Pascal Gustin. 2005. "Evaluation of particle translocation across the alveolo-capillary barrier in isolated perfused rabbit lung model." *Toxicology* 208 (1): 105–113. doi:10.1016/j.tox.2004.11.012.

Olsson, Bo, Lars Borgstrom, Lars Asking, and Eva B. Bondesson. 1996. "Effect of inlet throat on the correlation between measured fine particle dose and lung deposition." In *Respiratory Drug Delivery V*, edited by P. R. Byron, R. N. Dalby and S. J. Farr, pp. 273–281. Buffalo Grove, AZ: Interpharm Press Inc.

Olsson, Bo, Lars Borgstrom, Hans Lundback, and Marten Svensson. 2013. "Validation of a general in vitro approach for prediction of total lung deposition in healthy adults for pharmaceutical inhalation products." *Journal of Aerosol Medicine and Pulmonary Drug Delivery* 26 (6): 355–369. doi:10.1089/jamp.2012.0986.

Ong, Hui Xin, Faiza Benaouda, Daniela Traini, David Cipolla, Igor Gonda, Mary Bebawy, Ben Forbes, and Paul M. Young. 2014. "In vitro and ex vivo methods predict the enhanced lung residence time of liposomal ciprofloxacin formulations for nebulisation." *European Journal of Pharmaceutics and Biopharmaceutics* 86 (1): 83–89. doi:10.1016/j.ejpb.2013.06.024.

Ott, Harald C., Ben Clippinger, Claudius Conrad, Christian Schuetz, Irina Pomerantseva, Laertis Ikonomou, Darrell Kotton, and Joseph P. Vacanti. 2010. "Regeneration and orthotopic transplantation of a bioartificial lung." *Nature Medicine* 16 (8): 927. doi:10.1038/nm.2193.

Ott, Harald C., Thomas S. Matthiesen, Saik-Kia Goh, Lauren D. Black, Stefan M. Kren, Theoden I. Netoff, and Doris A. Taylor. 2008. "Perfusion-decellularized matrix: Using nature's platform to engineer a bioartificial heart." *Nature Medicine* 14 (2): 213. doi:10.1038/nm1684.

Perinel, Sophie, Jérémie Pourchez, Lara Leclerc, John Avet, Marc Durand, Nathalie Prévôt, Michèle Cottier, and Jean M. Vergnon. 2017. "Development of an ex vivo human-porcine respiratory model for preclinical studies." *Scientific Reports* 7: 43121. doi:10.1038/srep43121.

Petersen, Thomas H., Elizabeth A. Calle, Liping Zhao, Eun Jung Lee, Liqiong Gui, MichaSam B. Raredon, Kseniya Gavrilov et al. 2010. "Tissue-engineered lungs for in vivo implantation." *Science (New York, N.Y.)* 329 (5991): 538–541. doi:10.1126/science.1189345.

Price, Andrew P., Kristen A. England, Amy M. Matson, Bruce R. Blazar, and Angela Panoskaltsis-Mortari. 2010. "Development of a decellularized lung bioreactor system for bioengineering the lung: The matrix reloaded." *Tissue Engineering. Part A* 16 (8): 2581–2591. doi:10.1089/ten.tea.2009.0659.

Ren, Xi, Philipp T. Moser, Sarah E. Gilpin, Tatsuya Okamoto, Tong Wu, Luis F. Tapias, Francois E. Mercier et al. 2015. "Engineering pulmonary vasculature in decellularized rat and human lungs." *Nature Biotechnology* 33 (10): 1097–1102. doi:10.1038/nbt.3354.

Sakagami, Masahiro. 2006. "In vivo, in vitro and ex vivo models to assess pulmonary absorption and disposition of inhaled therapeutics for systemic delivery." *Advanced Drug Delivery Reviews*, Challenges and innovations in effective pulmonary systemic and macromolecular drug delivery, 58 (9): 1030–1060. doi:10.1016/j.addr.2006.07.012.

Sawyer, Thomas W., Paul E. Wilde, Paul Rice, and M. Tracy Weiss. 1995. "Toxicity of sulphur mustard in adult rat lung organ culture." *Toxicology* 100 (1): 39–49. doi:10.1016/0300-483X(95)03055-K.

Schiele, Nathan R., Ryan A. Koppes, David T. Corr, Karen S. Ellison, Deanna M. Thompson, Lee A. Ligon, Thomas K. M. Lippert, and Douglas B. Chrisey. 2009. "Laser direct writing of combinatorial libraries of idealized cellular constructs: biomedical applications." *Applied Surface Science*, Laser and Plasma in Micro- and Nano-Scale Materials Processing and Diagnostics, 255 (10): 5444–5447. doi:10.1016/j.apsusc.2008.10.054.

Schilders, Kim A. A., Evelien Eenjes, Sander van Riet, André A. Poot, Dimitrios Stamatialis, Roman Truckenmüller, Pieter S. Hiemstra, and Robbert J. Rottier. 2016. "Regeneration of the lung: Lung stem cells and the development of lung mimicking devices." *Respiratory Research* 17 (April): 44. doi:10.1186/s12931-016-0358-z.

Selg, Ewa, Pär Ewing, Fernando Acevedo, Carl-Olof Sjöberg, Åke Ryrfeldt, and Per Gerde. 2012. "Dry powder inhalation exposures of the endotracheally intubated rat lung, ex vivo and in vivo: The pulmonary pharmacokinetics of fluticasone furoate." *Journal of Aerosol Medicine and Pulmonary Drug Delivery* 26 (4): 181–189. doi:10.1089/jamp.2012.0971.

Shafa, Mehdi, Lavinia Iuliana Ionescu, Arul Vadivel, Jennifer J. P. Collins, Liqun Xu, Shumei Zhong, Martin Kang et al. 2018. "Human induced pluripotent stem cell–Derived lung progenitor and alveolar epithelial cells attenuate hyperoxia-induced lung injury." *Cytotherapy* 20 (1): 108–125. doi:10.1016/j.jcyt.2017.09.003.

Stapleton, Kevin W., E. Guentsch, M. K. Hoskinson, and Warren H. Finlay. 2000. "On the suitability of k–ε turbulence modeling for aerosol deposition in the mouth and throat: A comparison with experiment." *Journal of Aerosol Science* 31 (6): 739–749. doi:10.1016/S0021-8502(99)00547-9.

Storey-Bishoff, John, Michelle Noga, and W. H. Finlay. 2008. "Deposition of micrometer-sized aerosol particles in infant nasal airway replicas." *Journal of Aerosol Science* 39 (12): 1055–1065. doi:10.1016/j.jaerosci.2008.07.011.

Swift, David L. 1992. "Apparatus and method for measuring regional distribution of therapeutic aerosols and comparing delivery systems." *Journal of Aerosol Science* 23 (Suppl): 495–498. doi:10.1016/0021-8502(92)90457-7.

Tanaka, Yuya, Kentaro Noda, Kumiko Isse, Kimimasa Tobita, Yoshimasa Maniwa, Jay Kumar Bhama, Jonathan D'Cunha, Christian A. Bermudez, James D. Luketich, and Norihisa Shigemura. 2015. "A novel dual ex vivo lung perfusion technique improves immediate outcomes in an experimental model of lung transplantation." *American Journal of Transplantation* 15 (5): 1219–1230. doi:10.1111/ajt.13109.

Tane, Shinya, Kentaro Noda, and Norihisa Shigemura. 2017. "Ex vivo lung perfusion: A key tool for translational science in the lungs." *Chest* 151 (6): 1220–1228. doi:10.1016/j.chest.2017.02.018.

Tavernini, Scott, Tanya K. Church, David A. Lewis, Andrew R. Martin, and Warren H. Finlay. 2018. "Scaling an idealized infant nasal airway geometry to mimic inertial filtration of neonatal nasal airways." *Journal of Aerosol Science* 118: 14–21. doi:10.1016/j.jaerosci.2017.12.004.

Tavernini, Scott, Tanya K. Church, David A. Lewis, Michelle L. Noga, Andrew R. Martin, and Warren H. Finlay. 2017. "Deposition of micrometer-sized aerosol particles in neonatal nasal airway replicas." *Aerosol Science and Technology*, December. doi:10.1080/02786826.2017.1413489.

Tibbitt, Mark W., and Kristi S. Anseth. 2009. "Hydrogels as extracellular matrix mimics for 3d cell culture." *Biotechnology and Bioengineering* 103 (4): 655–663. doi:10.1002/bit.22361.

"USP. 2009. General Chapter <601> Aerosols, nasal sprays, metered dose inhalers, and dry powder inhalers." *United States Pharmacopeia—National Formulary.*

Wang, Xiaohong, Yongnian Yan, Yuqiong Pan, Zhuo Xiong, Haixia Liu, Jie Cheng, Feng Liu et al. 2006. "Generation of three-dimensional hepatocyte/gelatin structures with rapid prototyping system." *Tissue Engineering* 12 (1): 83–90. doi:10.1089/ten.2006.12.83.

Xi, Jinxiang, and Philip Worth Longest. 2007. "Transport and deposition of micro-aerosols in realistic and simplified models of the oral airway." *Annals of Biomedical Engineering* 35 (4): 560–581. doi:10.1007/s10439-006-9245-y.

Yeh, Hsu-Chi, and G. M. Schum. 1980. "Models of human lung airways and their application to inhaled particle deposition." *Bulletin of Mathematical Biology* 42 (3): 461–480. doi:10.1007/BF02460796.

Zhang, Yu, Kyle Gilbertson, and Warren H. Finlay. 2007. "In vivo-in vitro comparison of deposition in three mouth-throat models with Qvar and Turbuhaler inhalers." *Journal of Aerosol Medicine* 20 (3): 227–235. doi:10.1089/jam.2007.0584.

Zhou, Yue, Jaijie Sun, and Yung-Sung Cheng. 2011. "Comparison of deposition in the USP and physical mouth–throat models with solid and liquid particles." *Journal of Aerosol Medicine and Pulmonary Drug Delivery* 24 (6): 277–284.

30

Preclinical Models for Pulmonary Drug Delivery

Jibriil P. Ibrahim, Robert J. Bischof, and Michelle P. McIntosh

CONTENTS

30.1 Introduction

While not as common in the public conscious as other drug delivery routes, inhalable medicines have been in use since at least 1554 BC. Today, pulmonary drug delivery is an expanding field, with new therapeutics either approved or in development for a range of diseases (Price 2018, Sanders 2011, Stein and Theil 2017). The use of suitable animal models for preclinical studies (small animals such as rodents, guinea pigs and rabbits as well as the larger dog, sheep and non-human primate models), presents an unrivalled opportunity to advance our understanding of pulmonary drug development and delivery at a preclinical stage, and to maximize the likelihood of successful clinical translation of drug development and preclinical testing outcomes (Sakagami 2006).

The central value of preclinical animal models is derived from the ability to evaluate drug efficacy, safety, and dosages before investing in more comprehensive, decisive, and expensive human trials (Fernandez and Vanbever 2009). Animal models are therefore important not simply to measure drug efficacy, but also to investigate drug administration, absorption, clearance, tolerance, and toxicity (Price 2018). From these studies, important data can be generated around drug formulation characteristics, particle dispersion dynamics, and pharmacokinetic and pharmacodynamic variables. Consequently, the process of selecting an appropriate animal model requires careful consideration of both physiological specificity and suitability of animal models for proposed studies, as well as the availability of resources and expertise to maximize the utility of selected animal models (Figure 30.1).

This chapter discusses some of the important factors that researchers should consider when developing preclinical models for pulmonary drug delivery studies, and also reviews the current use of animal models in a research and preclinical setting, while reflecting on animal models currently in use or development.

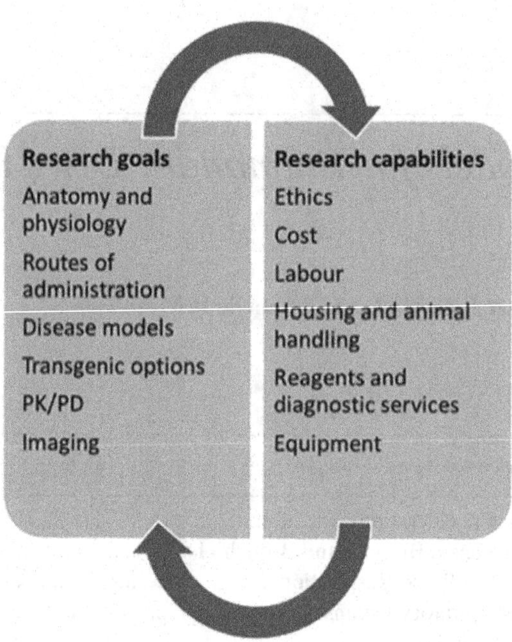

FIGURE 30.1 Researchers proceeding with preclinical studies must consider their research goals and research capabilities when selecting animal models. A superior physiologically relevant animal model is of little value if a laboratory does not have the adequate experience or resources necessary for their study to be conducted.

30.2 Research Capabilities

Before considering the physiological suitability of preclinical animal models, research groups must evaluate their research capabilities and objectives in order to develop a realistic list of animals that they can utilize. A preliminary review of ethical, analytical, and financial constraints can often help in the selection process.

The financial costs associated with the use of animals in preclinical studies are significant. Some estimates suggest that up to 95% of all financial and logistical resources in preclinical trials are attributed to studies which use animals, compared to those that utilize *in vitro* or *ex vivo* methods (Dickson and Gagnon 2004, Kuman and Longstreth 2011). There is also variance in these attributed costs based on species, and often species size, with one study (from 1983) calculating that chimpanzee, dog, and mice studies were 3.59%, 1.33%, and .02% the cost of a human equivalent, respectively, though these figures have certainly changed (Fitzgerald 1983). The relationship between species size and financial cost is important to consider. Larger animals require larger housing facilities, have greater feeding and waste management needs, and require specialized transport and more laborious management. While rodents can be managed by a single researcher, procedures involving larger animals may often require utilization of a number of research staff.

Larger animal models are also limited by the number of reagents and diagnostic services that are available, due to the dominance of smaller animal models in preclinical studies. For instance, a review performed by the authors found over 1.1 million commercial antibodies were available for mice compared to 31,000 for sheep on a public online antibody catalogue. Further expenses can accrue if custom reagents need to be manufactured or acquired. Similarly, the equipment required to conduct experiments with larger animals can often be more expensive due to increases in material requirements and a reduced demand generally in the market, though occasionally this can be circumvented by using equipment designed for human use.

Finally, and most importantly, the selection and use of animals for preclinical studies must be based on sound ethical considerations. Many articles have discussed the ethical use of animals in medical research.

We direct the reader to recent articles that investigate the validation and suitability of animal models for preclinical studies (Varga et al. 2010) and the ethical and regulatory considerations in animal studies (Carbone 2011). Importantly, the ethical use of animals extends beyond individual animal welfare and includes the number of animals used for trials. This can be evaluated during the study design and in collaboration with biostatisticians to evaluate proposed statistical methods and determine the number of animals required for the proposed study (Aban and George 2015).

30.3 Research Goals

One of the more significant challenges that arise when selecting an animal model for preclinical pulmonary studies is evaluating the considerable differences in respiratory anatomy and physiology across species. While the respiratory system across mammals may appear generally comparable from a gross perspective, these similarities often give way to noticeable differences under closer scrutiny. Researchers must therefore consider how species variances may affect the outcome of preclinical pulmonary drug delivery studies and whether a selected species is an appropriate model for their research interests.

30.3.1 Anatomical Considerations

Despite gross similarities in respiratory anatomy across species, the differences in size, geometry, and position of these anatomical structures can have a significant impact on the outcome of respiratory drug studies. The respiratory system has two fundamental purposes: (1) to regulate respiration, oxygen transfer, and carbon dioxide removal and (2) to protect the lungs from foreign or noxious particle inhalation so that respiration remains uninterrupted. These two goals are supported by the basic anatomical structure of the airways, comprising the trachea, bronchi and bronchioles, and the terminal alveoli. The airways are lined by the mucosal respiratory epithelium, beneath which there is a complex cellular tissue makeup that varies in its composition along the respiratory tree, but which includes the underlying loose connective tissue of the submucosa that may comprise cartilage, neuronal and capillary networks, and interstitial cells such as airway smooth muscle, myofibroblasts, fibroblasts, and immune cells.

In mammals, the respiratory tree is defined by branching of the airways, the extent of which varies to some degree between species. The anatomical architecture of the respiratory tract consists of the upper and lower airways. The upper airways include the nasal cavity, pharynx, and larynx, while the lower airways are made up of the trachea and bronchial branchings of the lung (Figure 30.2). The structures within these regions can be further grouped into conducting and respiratory zones, based on structural features and their role in the process and regulation of respiration. The conducting zone is the first stage, which includes the nose, pharynx, larynx, trachea, bronchi, bronchioles, and terminal bronchioles. The respiratory zone includes the deeper, more distal structures such as the respiratory bronchioles, the alveolar ducts, and alveoli.

Evolution has led to species differences in anatomy, structure, and function of the airways (Table 30.1), which may have a defining influence on the suitability of a particular animal model for pulmonary drug delivery and human respiratory function. The tracheobronchial branching of the airways begins at the distal point of the trachea, with the first bifurcation (carina) leading to the bronchi of the left and right lungs (Patra 1986). From the trachea, the two main bronchi enter the two lungs and, depending on the species, divide into a number of branches that serve the one, two, three, or more lobes of the left and right lung. The branching pattern of the airways is complicated, and depending on the species, can be classified as monopodial (branching point where a small daughter segment branches from the parent stem), dichotomous (parent stem branches into two smaller, but equal daughter segments), or polychotomous (parent stem branches into many daughter segments).

30.3.1.1 Trachea, Bronchi and Bronchioles

The trachea, the conducting unit of the airways that links the upper and lower regions of the respiratory tract, is critical for respiration and is one of the few organs that shows a degree of uniformity across all mammals in terms of shape and size, particularly with relation to body size (Pinkerton et al. 2015).

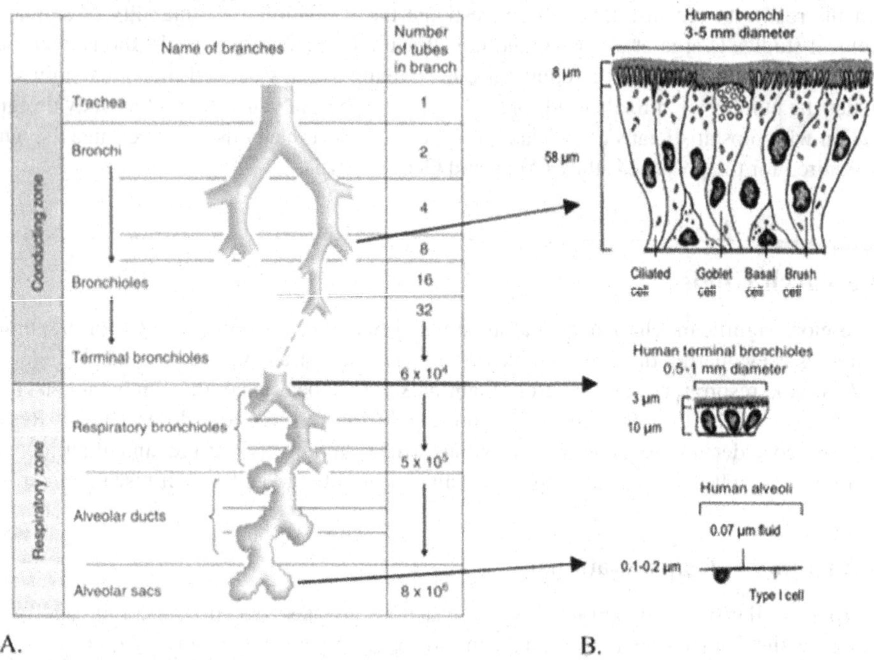

FIGURE 30.2 (A) Structures of the airways (Reprinted from Human Physiology, 8th Edition, 2001. McGraw Hill© with permission from the publisher); (B) Changes in epithelial cell morphology and size within the lung, and of epithelial lung fluid. (Modified from Patton, J.S., *Nat. Rev. Drug Discov.*, 6, 67–74, 2007. With permission.)

At the histological level, the trachea is made up of the mucosal epithelium (comprising ciliated and secretory epithelial cells, goblet cells, and clara or club cells), the submucosa (blood vessels, neurons and secretory glands throughout loose connective tissue), and a cartilaginous layer, trachealis muscle and outer adventitia. Variations between species at this level may impact on model suitability for pulmonary drug delivery studies (Table 30.2). Epithelial thickness, for example, ranges from <25 µm (in rodents) to 50 µm–100 µm (in larger models including human) (Reynolds 2015).

Further changes can be seen as the trachea branches into bronchi and deeper bronchioles. Branching symmetry of these conducting airways is highly variable between species and also within lobes and between branching generations (Pinkerton et al. 2015). While humans have the least symmetrical branching pattern compared to other species, the angle of branching between generations is greater in rodents, particularly past the 2nd and 3rd generation (Schlesinger and McFadden 1981). Furthermore, the total number of terminal bronchioles in the deeper lung is far greater in the "larger" lungs of the human (~26,000) compared to smaller animal models such as mice (<3000) (Pinkerton et al. 2015).

While considering species variation, researchers should also reflect on the age of their preclinical model, as studies have shown absorption rates across the respiratory epithelium vary depending on age in the rat, with larger molecular weight compounds absorbed faster across the airway epithelium of younger rats (Schanker and Hemberger 1983). Similarly, age can be a factor when investigating the mechanics of premature lung function and development, and lambs have become a well validated model for premature lung studies due to their comparative developmental lung physiology (and structural similarities) to human newborn infants (Inocencio et al. 2017, Niemarkt et al. 2014).

30.3.1.2 Alveoli and Respiration

Past the bronchioles lie the alveolar ducts which enter alveolar sacs at the most distal position of the respiratory tree (Figure 30.2). In all species, the alveoli play a critical role in gas exchange between the lung air spaces and the capillaries lining the alveoli. Histologically, the alveolar epithelium is very thin (0.1 µm –0.2 µm)

TABLE 30.1
Comparative Anatomy and Physiology of the Mammalian Lung

Characteristics	Human	Sheep	Non-human Primate	Dog	Rabbit	Guinea Pig	Rat	Mouse
Body weight (kg)	70	30–80	6–38	10–15	2.5–3.5	0.4	0.25–0.35	0.02–0.04
Nose and/or mouth breather	nose and mouth	nose and mouth	nose and mouth	nose and mouth	obligate nose breather	obligate nose breather	obligate nose breather	obligate nose breather
Turbinate complexity	simple scroll	double scroll	simple scroll	complex scroll	complex scroll	complex scroll	complex scroll	complex scroll
Lung weight (g)	1000	507	–	100	18	3.2	1.5	0.012
Lung symmetry	dichotomous	dichotomous	dichotomous	monopodial	monopodial	monopodial	monopodial	monopodial
Trachea length/diameter (cm)	12/2	–	3/0.3	17/1.6	6/.5	5.7/.4	2.3/.26	.7/.12
Number of alveoli (x10⁶)	950	–	81.8	1040	135	69	43	18
Diameter of alveoli (μm)	219	74	–	126	88	65	70	47
minute volume (l/min)	7.98	4.5–10	1.67	–	1.5	0.8	0.12	1.02
Respiratory rate (breaths/min)	12	16–34	38	23	51	90	85	163
Tidal volume (ml)	400–616	197–491	20–21.2	11.4–16.6	15.8	1.72–1.75	0.87–2.08	0.15–0.18
Mucus clearance rate (mm/min)	3.6–21.5	10.5–17.3	–	7.5–21.6	3.2	2.7	1.9–5.9	–
Particle size for deep lung delivery (μm)	1–5	–	1–3	1–3	–	–	3.5	3

Source: Ball, L. et al., *Ann. Transl. Med.*, 5, 2017; Cross, K.W. et al., *J. Physiol.*, 146, 316–343, 1959; Hales, J.R.S. and Webster, M.E.D., *J. Physiol.*, 190, 241–260, 1967; Price, D.N. et al., *KONA Powder Part. J.*, 2019008, 2018; Soane, R.J. et al., *Int. J. Pharm.*, 217, 183–191, 2001.

TABLE 30.2

Species Variations in Cellular Composition of the Trachea

	Tracheal Epithelium		Tracheal Submucosal glands	
Species	**Cell Type**	**Density**	**Cell Type**	**Density**
Hamster	Clara	+ + +	Mucous	+/−
	Mucous	+		
Rat	Serous	+ + +	Serous	+
	Mucous	+	Mucous	+
Mouse	Mucous	+	Serous	+/−
			Mucous	+/−
Rabbit	Mucous	+	Mucous	+/−
	Clara	+ + +		
Canine	Mucous	+ +	Serous	++
			Mucous	++
Cat	Mucous	+ +	Serous	++++
	Serous	+	Mucous	++++
Pig	Mucous	+	Serous	++
			Mucous	++
Sheep	Mucous	+ +	Serous	++
	Clara	++	Mucous	++
Non-human primate	Mucous	+ +	Serous	++
			Mucous	++
Human	Mucous	+ + +	Serous	+++
			Mucous	+++

Source: Plopper, C.G. et al., *Exp. Lung Res.*, 1, 155–169, 1980; Reynolds, S.D. et al., Epithelial cells of trachea and bronchi, in *Comparative Biology of the Normal Lung* (2nd ed.), pp. 61–81, Elsevier, Amsterdam, the Netherlands, 2015; St George, J.A., Secretory glycoconjugates of the trachea and bronchi, in *Comparative Biology of the Normal Lung* (2nd ed.), pp. 53–60, Elsevier, Amsterdam, the Netherlands, 2015.

and comprises type I and type II alveolar epithelial cells responsible for gas exchange, epithelial repair, and immune responses (Chuquimia et al. 2013, Guillot et al. 2013, Whitsett and Alenghat 2015).

Species differences exist in the respiratory zone at the level of the terminal bronchioles. For example, in contrast to humans and other animals, respiratory bronchioles are either absent (mice) or significantly underdeveloped (rats) in the small rodent species (Mercer and Crapo 2015, Yeh et al. 1979). Differences are also observed in the alveolar sacs which are made up of the alveoli and alveolar ducts. For instance, humans have a 50-fold larger number of alveolar sacs compared to mice and a 170-fold greater internal volume of these alveolar sacs (Mercer and Crapo 2015). These alveolar sacs can also vary in size by more than 15-fold along the same bronchi, depending on depth, which may have important ramifications on particle deposition due to dead space (Mercer and Crapo 2015, Mercer et al. 1991). The ratio of alveolar ducts to alveolar sacs also varies from smaller rodent models to larger species and humans across different bronchial generations (Mercer and Crapo 2015, Mercer et al. 1991). Similarly, as seen in the trachea and bronchi, the cellular composition in the deeper lung is diverse across species, with humans having a greater epithelial cell density in the bronchiolar and alveolar regions compared to smaller species such as mice (Mercer and Crapo 2015).

Furthermore, the airway smooth muscle (ASM) found throughout the airways in all species is noticeably absent in the alveolar ducts of mice and rats (Allen et al. 2009, Mercer and Crapo 2015), while changes in ASM dynamics between species has also been reported previously (Allen et al. 2009, Lecarpentier et al. 2002).

The regional absence of ASM in smaller animals, coupled with the uniform thinning of the epithelial layer deeper in the airways of all species, should also be considered with respect to drug deposition, as changes in the cellular composition of deeper lung regions may affect drug absorption.

30.3.1.3 Respiratory Defenses

The role of the respiratory system to maintain respiration and life is clear, but to ensure this process remains unobstructed, evolutionary changes in respiratory physiology have led to important pulmonary defense mechanisms (Nicod 1999). Innate defense mechanisms include anatomical structures such as the oropharynx, the action of beating cilia on epithelial cells, and production and clearance of mucus at the surface of the respiratory mucosa, as well as the resident "front-line" leukocyte host defense system (Wilkinson et al. 2012). The physical action of coughing also serves in mucus clearance and to protect the airways from unwanted entry of foreign particles (Nicod 1999). The success of these pulmonary defense mechanisms is vital for ensuring unobstructed respiratory function, however, their actions can also be responsible for impaired pulmonary drug delivery and require due consideration in the context of preclinical studies.

The impact that these pulmonary defense mechanisms have on drug delivery to the airways is often not straightforward. The oropharynx, for instance is the first structure that foreign particles must avoid, is easier to traverse in rodents than humans due to the reduced angle of entry. This can make rodents a poor model for investigating the rate of drug loss due to deposition in the oropharynx and clearance via swallowing. Understanding the early loss of drug bioavailability due to deposition in the oropharynx is important as previous studies have shown significant portions of emitted doses from metered dose inhalers and dry powder inhalers are frequently lost in the oropharynx of patients during administration, with some studies reporting less than 20% of inhaled drug successfully clearing the oropharynx (Cheng 2014, Gonda 2016).

Drug that does pass the oropharynx region must still traverse multiple generations of branching airways that are lined with mucosa and cilia before reaching deeper lung regions where absorption can more readily take place. Drug compounds deposited early in the branching bronchi regions may become trapped within the mucus and lost due to mucociliary clearance. This involves the trapping of foreign particles in mucus and subsequent movement, via the beating action of cilia, back to the throat to be swallowed (a processed termed the mucociliary escalator) (Bustamante-Marin et al. 2017). A range of animal models have been used to study the secretion and clearance of mucus, although there are some notable species differences (King 1988). Humans have a faster rate of mucociliary clearance compared to rats, though the overall time it takes for drugs to reach the throat and be cleared may be slower due to the deeper generational branching and length of the trachea (Fröhlich and Salar-Behzzadi 2014, Kreyling 1990). Species size can also impact the research capabilities in mucociliary studies due to the use of radiolabels and resolution limits associated with scintigraphy imaging (Foster et al. 2001), and while there are methods available for use with smaller rodent models (Hua et al. 2009, Koelsch et al. 2017), larger animals such as dogs and sheep are good candidates for mucociliary studies (King 1998). These larger animal models have the advantage of allowing long-term serial measurements to be taken and to make integrated measurements of the clearance of mucus, ciliary function, epithelial ion transport, and the rheology of mucus in the same preparation.

When drugs succeed in avoiding early clearance and reach the deeper lung there are still barriers that can inhibit their absorption. Leukocytes, and airway or alveolar macrophages in particular, are integral to lung defense, and these cells are significantly regulated by the local lung environment and involved in the phagocytosis and clearance of foreign particles (Hussell and Bell 2014). For compounds and drugs that are foreign to the body (Folkesson et al. 1996), this can mean phagocytosis and clearance via lymphatic drainage or mucociliary clearance and digestion, which under the influence of local tissue factors or conditions may take place over an extended period of time (Martonen 1993). Again, however, understanding these barriers to pulmonary drug delivery is likely compounded by species differences in airway macrophage distribution and function.

For instance, alveolar macrophages in smaller rodents show greater sensitivity to changes in local acidity levels while displaying less lethality and slower phagocytic activity compared to humans (Nguyen 1982, Schlesinger et al. 1992). The size and morphology of alveolar macrophages are also larger in humans compared to other species, though the total number of alveolar macrophages is proportional based on species weight and lung fluid volume (Haley et al. 1991, Warheit et al. 1988). A number of species differences in leukocyte-derived nitric oxide pathways as well as chemokine and cytokine functions have also been reported, while further differences have been reported in matrix metalloproteinase activity and in nerve-mediated bronchoconstriction (Borzone et al. 2014, Garcia-Delgado 2012, Matute-Bello et al. 2008, Schlepütz et al. 2012). While there is no clear link between these observations, presented together they demonstrate the importance of reviewing and understanding the animal model system being used and the challenges that can arise with the translation of preclinical findings to humans.

30.4 Experimental Considerations

30.4.1 Methods of Administration

In humans, pulmonary drug delivery is performed via direct drug administration orally into the lungs during normal respiratory inhalation. Replicating this mechanism is not straightforward in animal models. Breathing behavior differs between species, with rabbits, guinea pigs, rats, and mice all obligate nasal breathers, compared to larger animals and humans, who breathe via the mouth or nose and mouth (Allen et al. 2009). This can create challenges during pulmonary drug delivery studies. The current methods that are available for administering pulmonary drug formulations into the lungs of animals are limited in their representation of human delivery systems and can be classified based on their passive or active route of administration (Table 30.3).

The passive delivery methods, which are exclusively used in smaller animal models, include whole body chamber or nasal and head chamber delivery systems. Whole body chambers allow for conscious, unassisted inhalation of administered drug, though this comes at the expense of drug administration specificity, as drug may be absorbed through the skin, mucus membranes and gastrointestinal tract (Fernandes and Vanbever 2009).

TABLE 30.3

Comparison of Methods Available for *in vivo* Pulmonary Drug Delivery. Modified from

	Whole Body	Head/Nose Only	Small Animal Intratracheal Delivery	Large Animal Intratracheal Delivery	Tracheostomy
Conscious	Yes	Yes	No	Yes[1]	No
Free breathing	Yes	Yes	Yes	Yes	No
Restrained	No	Yes	Yes	Yes	Yes
Direct dosing	No	No	Yes	Yes	Yes
Suitable for long term or repeat dose studies	Yes	Yes	No	Yes	No
Efficient use of material	No	Yes	Yes	Yes	Yes
Efficient for large numbers of animals	Yes	Yes	No	No	No
Associated stress	Low	High	Low	Low	Low
Routes of exposure	Respiratory/ GI tract, Skin/Fur	Respiratory/ GI tract	Trachea, Respiratory tract	Trachea, Respiratory tract	Trachea, Respiratory tract
Does air mixing need to be monitored	Yes	Yes	No	No	No
Can excreta interact with pollutants	Yes	No	No	No	No
Monitor thermoregulation	No	Yes	No	No	No
Labor intensive	No	Yes	Yes	Yes	Yes
Bypass respiratory defenses	No	No	Yes	Yes	Yes
Technically difficult	No	No	Yes	Yes	Yes
Surgery required	No	No	No	No	Yes
Terminal procedure	No	No	No	No	Yes

Source: Cheng, Y.S., *AAPS PharmSciTech*, 15, 630–640, 2014; Guillon, A. et al., *Int. J. Pharm.*, 434, 481–487, 2012; Meeusen, E.N. et al., *Drug Discov. Today Dis. Models*, 6, 101–106, 2009; Prankerd, R.J. et al., *PLoS One*, 8, e82965, 2013; Price, D.N. et al., *KONA Powder Part. J.*, 2019008, 2018; Wolff, R.K., *Mol. Pharm.*, 12, 2688–2696, 2015; Wylie, J.L. et al., *Ther. Deliv.*, 9, 387–404, 2018.

[1] Depending on regional animal welfare guidelines some research facilities can perform intratracheal delivery on large animals with topical analgesic/anesthesia alone.

This in turn can affect pharmacokinetic and pharmacodynamic profiles. Furthermore, determining the quantity of drug administered to animals is difficult. Some of these obstacles can be overcome by using nose-only drug administration devices, however, these delivery systems come with other challenges such as the need to ensure animals are positioned comfortably and under minimal stress (Wong 2007).

Alternatively, researchers can avoid some of these obstacles by administering drug formulations directly into the trachea of research animals using commercially available drug delivery devices.

Intratracheal delivery is a more invasive, but precise alternative for pulmonary drug delivery, as the drug can be administered directly into the lung, bypassing other drug absorption routes and avoiding deposition in the oropharynx (Fernandes and Vanbever 2009). However, this can be technically challenging in smaller animals: not only do smaller animals require anesthesia and surgical preparation, but the small airway size can make the insertion of tubing or instruments into the trachea difficult, and increase the risk of respiratory damage or inflammation (Massara et al. 2004, McCluskie et al. 2000). Furthermore, due to their size and independent respiratory control, drugs must be actively administered directly into the lungs of smaller animals. The active delivery of drug, or even control bolus air, may cause significant lung damage that can impact on drug absorption and pharmacokinetics (Guillon et al. 2012) or even lead to fatalities (Morello et al. 2009) if not performed by a skilled technician.

Subtle changes in delivery methods or technique may also lead to significant differences in delivery outcomes due to the size of respiratory organs in smaller animals, as has been shown previously in the rat (Codrons et al. 2004). Similarly, the volume of administered drugs must be considered with respect to lung size, and in particular, the volume of extracellular lung fluid in smaller animal models. The volume of lung fluid in the rat and mouse, for instance, is sufficiently small enough that minor changes to dosing methods can induce high variability during data collection.

While the advantages and disadvantages seen with these delivery methods are clear, there is one major exception. Direct drug administration in large animals, unlike their smaller counterparts, can be performed without the limitations that are common in smaller animal models.

Furthermore, the larger size of some animals, combined with the ability to maintain conscious respiratory function means drug formulations can, in effect, be administered passively if timed carefully to release the formulation in coordination with inhalation. In sheep, for example, intratracheal and intranasal drug administration has been performed using dry powder, and liquid formulations without sedation.

Intranasal delivery for pulmonary drug administration is also possible, though drug may be delivered (Prankerd et al. 2013) to the nasal region rather than the lungs, which may in turn be absorbed or transported via mucociliary action to the throat and swallowed, affecting pharmacokinetic dynamics and safety/tolerability (Wolff 2015).

30.4.2 Pharmacokinetic and Pharmacodynamic Sample Collection

Pharmacokinetic (PK) and pharmacodynamic (PD) modeling are essential components during preclinical drug development. Understanding the rates and mechanisms of drug absorption, distribution, metabolization, excretion (ADME), and action can give early indications regarding the likelihood of a drug progressing or succeeding in later developmental stages.

In PK studies, this is performed by collecting and analyzing physiological samples including plasma, saliva, bronchoalveolar lavage, or excreta for drug or metabolite concentrations. In addition to collection and analysis, however, researchers must consider the influence animal models can have on PK measurements and whether the preclinical observations can be extrapolated to humans.

For instance, despite physiological parameters across species being comparable when scaled to body size, drug clearance is often more rapid in smaller animals that have a pharmacokinetically distinct space-time continua (Mordenti 1986). Animal size can also determine sampling capability.

Physiological realities restrict the amount and frequency of blood that can be taken from small animals (Diehl et al. 2001, Parasuraman et al. 2010). Some blood sampling sites require general anesthesia and when repeated bleeds are necessary, new injection sites should be used which can be difficult to achieve in smaller animals (Diehl et al. 2001). In contrast, larger animal models have a greater tolerance to repeated bleeds and collections. Similarly, bronchoalveolar lavage (BAL) sample collections from airways in smaller animals can require lengthy or terminal surgical procedures, whereas in large animals, multiple samples can be collected from targeted lobes (Meeusen et al. 2009, Qamar 2015). While the time it takes to urinate is surprisingly consistent across all species, urine volume is variable and reflective of species size (Yang 2013). This is also true for defecation times, although volume of excrement varies (Yang 2017). These factors should be considered, particularly for studies that are investigating drug metabolization, clearance, and excretion.

30.4.3 Measurements of Respiratory Mechanics

An important step in preclinical drug development generally, and pulmonary drug delivery specifically, is ensuring drugs are safe and tolerable for human administration. While understanding the potential toxicological effects of drugs is vital, in pulmonary drug delivery studies the fundamental requirement to maintain respiratory function for survival means it is critical to have a detailed understanding of how drugs affect respiratory function. However, investigating the effects of pulmonary drug administration on respiration has historically been difficult, and the phenotyping uncertainty principle first published in 2003, which states that more precise measures of respiratory animals require more invasive procedures (in smaller animals) still holds true today, despite continual improvements in our technological and scientific capabilities (Bates et al. 2003).

Methods for studying respiratory dynamics have often been divided into invasive and non-invasive categories, with the sensitivity and range of quantifiable respiratory parameters (the rate of respiration, tidal flow, airway resistance, and hyperresponsiveness) increasing with invasiveness, at the expense of normal, or unaltered, respiratory function. While this is still accurate for smaller animal models, large animals present a unique opportunity to collect sensitive data for a range of parameters while under normal respiratory conditions. Many good reviews have been published that discuss individual methods used to study respiratory dynamics in animal models in greater detail (Glaab et al. 2007, Irvin and Bates 2003), and a summary of these methods is presented in Table 30.4.

Due to their size, studies involving small animal models are able to utilize plethysmography to investigate basic changes in respiratory function and detect early signs of respiratory impairment. As the least

TABLE 30.4

Methods for *in vivo* Lung Function Testing

	Non Invasive		*Invasive*	
	Plethysmography	**Large Animal Measurements**	**Forced Oscillation**	**Small Animal Measurements**
Surgery required	No	No	Yes	Yes
Technically difficult	No	Yes	Yes	Yes
Conscious	Yes	Yes	No	No
Labor intensive	No	Yes	Yes	Yes
Restrained	No	Yes	Yes	Yes
Free breathing	Yes	Yes	No	No
Terminal procedure	No	No	Yes	Yes
Respiratory rate	Yes	Yes	Controlled	Controlled
Respiratory volume	Yes	Yes	Controlled	Controlled
Respiratory force	Yes	Yes	Controlled	Controlled
Tidal volume	Yes	Yes	Controlled	Controlled
Lung resistance	No	Yes	Yes	Yes
Lung compliance	No	Yes	Yes	Yes
Diffusion capacity	No	Yes	Yes	Yes

Source: Brashier, B. and Salvi, S., Breathe, 11, 57, 2015; Dellacà, R.L. et al., *Intensive Care Med.*, 37, 1021, 2011; Irvin, C.G. and Bates, J.H.T., *Respir. Res.*, 4, 1, 2003; Glaab, T. et al., Respir. Res., 8, 63, 2007; Meeusen, E.N. et al., *Drug Discov. Today Dis. Models*, 6, 101–106, 2009; Nakano, S. et al., *BMC Anesthesiol.*, 16, 32, 2015; Prankerd, R.J. et al., *PLoS One*, 8, e82965, 2013; Tepper, J.S. and Costa, D.L., Methods, measurements, and interpretation of animal lung function in health and disease, in *Comparative Biology of the Normal Lung* (2nd ed.), pp. 305–351, Elsevier, Amsterdam, the Netherlands, 2015.

invasive procedure, it also allows researchers to conduct studies without the need for surgery. Unfortunately, the range of parameters that can be measured are limited and less sensitive than other techniques, though improvements have been made with new developments such as barometric, whole body, or double chamber plethysmography, enriching the scientific output from these studies (Tepper and Costa 2015).

On the other hand, while more invasive techniques which require anesthesia and forced ventilation may not reflect normal respiratory conditions, they do give researchers the ability to study lung resistance and compliance and generate more comprehensive and sensitive data (Tepper and Costa 2015). However, performing respiratory function studies in smaller animal models can be challenging due to additional demands on technical and surgical skills (Hoymann 2012, Irvin and Bates 2003, Zosky and Sly 2007). This approach has recently been enhanced by the development of the forced oscillation technique, which allows researchers to measure changes in airway resistance and hyperresponsiveness, as well as changes in tissue resistance in humans and small and large animal models such as rabbits, pigs and sheep (Brashier and Salvi 2015, Dellacà et al. 2011, Nakano et al. 2015, Oostveen et al. 2003, Porra et al. 2018).

Unlike smaller animal models, however, large animals are not rigidly bound to the phenotyping uncertainty principle and can be used to measure sensitive changes in lung resistance and compliance without undergoing the invasive procedures that are necessary in smaller animals. Whereas rodents must be anesthetized and often tracheotomized, large animals can be studied while conscious and breathing freely. Sheep for instance have been used to measure changes in airway resistance and hyperresponsiveness without the need for sedation or surgical intervention: their large size means individual lobes within the sheep lung can be studied to create a more detailed and comprehensive reflection of respiratory mechanics (Meeusen et al. 2009).

As a final note, enhanced pause (Penh) has also been used as a measure of respiratory function in animal models and humans, though significant controversy surrounds its acceptance and the wider scientific community generally rejects its suitability as a marker for respiration function (Bates et al. 2004, Sly et al. 2005).

30.5 Genes

Historically, one of the key advantages with smaller animal models, and particularly mice, has been the ability to efficiently and economically edit their genome, allowing for the development of knock-out, knock-in, and disease models (Barrangou and Horvath 2012, Maeder et al. 2016, Wang et al. 2017). Recently, however, the development of tools such as Crispr/Cas9 have greatly expanded our approach to studying and altering the genome of small and larger animal species alike, establishing an era where editing the genome of larger animal models can be realistically considered. Recently, for instance, a sheep knock-out model was developed using Crispr/Cas9 technology (Crispo et al. 2015). Certain realities are unavoidable, however, with both the length of time required for larger animals to reach sexual maturity and the gestational period presenting (time) barriers for the use of large animals as models for genome editing (Tu et al. 2015).

On the other hand, these gene editing technologies could lead to future treatments and new medicines rather than the development of disease models. The pulmonary delivery of a gene therapy using Crispr/Cas9 for the treatment of cystic fibrosis, for instance, has recently been suggested and demonstrates the possibilities that arise when combining pulmonary drug delivery with genome editing (Marangi 2018). Recent studies in sheep have shown the potential of aerosolized gene therapy (McLachlan and Baker 2007), and pulmonary DNA vaccination and induction of gene expression changes in the lung (McLachlan et al. 2011). Rats have also been used to show antibody generation after nebulization of a DNA vaccine, while mouse models have demonstrated the potential use of viral vectors to treat lung cancer via pulmonary delivery (Hong et al. 2015, Rajapaksa et al. 2014). A bleomycin-induced model of pulmonary fibrosis in the rat also showed significant improvements in survival after pulmonary delivery of a small interfering RNA (Sung 2013).

30.6 Imaging

Some of the most valuable tools available for preclinical studies are those that allow researchers the capability to image the lungs and deposition of drug into the lungs. These include X-ray, ultrasound, electrical impendence tomography, gamma scintigraphy, positron emission tomography (pet), single photon emission computer tomography (SPECT), and magnetic resonance imaging (Ball et al. 2017, Fouras and Dubsky 2015). Of these different technologies, the radionuclide labeling methods (gamma scintigraphy, PET, and SPECT) are frequently used for pulmonary drug delivery studies as they provide a range of techniques for investigating the deposition and absorption of drugs as well as changes in respiratory function (Newman 2014). While these technologies have been used broadly in small animal studies, their increasing availability to researchers means that such studies are becoming more feasible for use in larger animal models. In the mouse, SPECT has been used to conduct pharmacokinetic studies and investigate the rate of clearance post administration of albumin into the lungs while scintigraphy has been used to measure drug biodistribution in the rat (Hureaux et al. 2017, Woods et al. 2015). PET has also been used to investigate particle deposition in the lungs of rhesus monkeys (Dabisch et al. 2017). Similarly, MRI is a viable radionuclide-free alternative that is capable of imaging deposition of particles in the lungs, as demonstrated in the mouse (Thompson and Finlay 2012). However, unlike methods that use radionuclides, MRI is complicated by the need to use helium or other gases to enhance the resolution from contrasting agents (Guillon et al. 2018). Many good reviews on imaging technologies have been produced, and we direct the reader to some recent publications for greater detail (Ball et al. 2017, Fouras and Dubsky 2015).

30.7 Summary

Preclinical research is vital to improve the long-term outcome for drug discovery and commercialization. The successful preclinical development and testing of candidate pulmonary therapeutics requires careful consideration of drug design and delivery, the desired treatment outcomes, and selection and use of an appropriate animal model system. For researchers, success during the early preclinical stage can facilitate translation of this work into the clinic and improve the prospect and pathway for new respiratory drugs becoming available to patients in need.

REFERENCES

Aban, IB, and B George. "Statistical considerations for preclinical studies." *Experimental Neurology* 270 (2015): 82–87.

Allen, JE, RJ Bischof, HYS Chang, JA Hirota, SJ Hirst, MD Inman, W Mitzner, and TE Sutherland. "Animal models of airway inflammation and airway smooth muscle remodelling in asthma." *Pulmonary Pharmacology & Therapeutics* 22, no. 5 (2009): 455–465.

Ball, L, V Vercesi, F Costantino, K Chandrapatham, and P Pelosi. "Lung imaging: How to get better look inside the lung." *Annals of Translational Medicine* 5, no. 14 (2017).

Barrangou, R, and P Horvath. "A decade of discovery: crispr functions and applications." *Nature Microbiology* 2, no. 7 (2017): 17092.

Bates, JHT, and CG Irvin. "Measuring lung function in mice: The phenotyping uncertainty principle." *Journal of Applied Physiology* 94, no. 4 (2003): 1297–1306.

Bates, J, C Irvin, V Brusasco, J Drazen, J Fredberg, S Loring, D Eidelman et al. "The use and misuse of penh in animal models of lung disease." *American Journal of Respiratory Cell and Molecular Biology* 31, no. 3 (2004): 373–374.

Borzone, G, P Ayala, J Araos, R Contreras, A Cutiño, and M Meneses. "Orotracheal instillation of gastric juice: Species variations in acute lung injury relate to differences in matrix metalloproteinase activity." *European Respiratory Journal* 44, no. Suppl 58 (2014): P3922.

Brashier, B, and S Salvi. "Measuring lung function using sound waves: Role of the forced oscillation technique and impulse oscillometry system." *Breathe* 11, no. 1 (2015): 57.

Bustamante-Marin, XM, and LE Ostrowski. "Cilia and mucociliary clearance." *Cold Spring Harbor Perspectives in Biology* 9, no. 4 (2017): a028241.

Carbone, L. "Pain in laboratory animals: The ethical and regulatory imperatives." *PLoS One* 6, no. 9 (2011): e21578.

Cheng, YS. "Mechanisms of pharmaceutical aerosol deposition in the respiratory tract." *AAPS PharmSciTech* 15, no. 3 (2014): 630–640.

Chuquimia, OD, DH Petursdottir, N Periolo, and C Fernández. "Alveolar epithelial cells are critical in protection of the respiratory tract by secretion of factors able to modulate the activity of pulmonary macrophages and directly control bacterial growth." *Infection and Immunity* 81, no. 1 (2013): 381–389.

Codrons, V, F Vanderbist, B Ucakar, V Préat, and R Vanbever. "Impact of formulation and methods of pulmonary delivery on absorption of parathyroid hormone (1–34) from rat lungs." *Journal of Pharmaceutical Sciences* 93, no. 5 (2004): 1241–1252.

Crispo, M, AP Mulet, L Tesson, N Barrera, F Cuadro, PC dos Santos-Neto, TH Nguyen et al. "Efficient generation of myostatin knock-out sheep using Crispr/Cas9 technology and microinjection into zygotes." *PLoS One* 10, no. 8 (2015): e0136690.

Cross, KW, GS Dawes, and JC Mott. "Anoxia, oxygen consumption and cardiac output in new-born lambs and adult sheep." *The Journal of Physiology* 146, no. 2 (1959): 316–343.

Dabisch, PA, Z Xu, JA Boydston, J Solomon, JK Bohannon, JJ Yeager, JR Taylor et al. "Quantification of regional aerosol deposition patterns as a function of aerodynamic particle size in rhesus macaques using PET/CT imaging." *Inhalation Toxicology* (2017): 1–10.

Dellacà, RL, E Zannin, P Kostic, MA Olerud, PP Pompilio, G Hedenstierna, A Pedotti, and P Frykholm. "Optimisation of positive end-expiratory pressure by forced oscillation technique in a lavage model of acute lung injury." *Intensive Care Medicine* 37, no. 6 (2011): 1021.

Dickson, M, and JP Gagnon. "Key factors in the rising cost of new drug discovery and development." *Nature Reviews Drug discovery* 3, no. 5 (2004): 417.

Diehl, KH, R Hull, D Morton, R Pfister, Y Rabemampianina, D Smith, JM Vidal, and CVD Vorstenbosch. "A good practice guide to the administration of substances and removal of blood, including routes and volumes." *Journal of Applied Toxicology* 21, no. 1 (2001): 15–23.

Fernandes, CA, and R Vanbever. "Preclinical models for pulmonary drug delivery." *Expert Opinion on Drug Delivery* 6, no. 11 (2009): 1231–1245.

Fitzgerald, TA. "Comparison of research cost: Man—Primate Animal—Other animal models." *Journal of Medical Primatology* 12, no. 3 (1983): 138–145.

Folkesson, HG, MA Matthay, BR Westrom, KJ Kim, BW Karlsson, and RH Hastings. "Alveolar epithelial clearance of protein." *Journal of Applied Physiology* 80, no. 5 (1996): 1431–1445.

Foster, WM, DM Walters, M Longphre, K Macri, and LM Miller. "Methodology for the measurement of mucociliary function in the mouse by scintigraphy." *Journal of Applied Physiology* 90, no. 3 (2001): 1111–1118.

Fouras, A, and S Dubsky. "The role of functional lung imaging in the improvement of pulmonary drug delivery." *Pulmonary Drug Delivery: Advances and Challenges* (2015): 19–34.

Fröhlich, E, and S Salar-Behzadi. "Toxicological assessment of inhaled nanoparticles: Role of in vivo, ex vivo, in vitro, and in silico studies." *International Journal of Molecular Sciences* 15, no. 3 (2014): 4795–4822.

García-Delgado, M, I Navarrete-Sánchez, V Chamorro-Marín, JC Díaz-Monrové, J Esquivias, and E Fernández-Mondéjar. "Alveolar overdistension as a cause of lung injury: Differences among three animal species." *The Scientific World Journal* 2012 (2012).

Glaab, T, C Taube, A Braun, and W Mitzner. "Invasive and noninvasive methods for studying pulmonary function in mice." *Respiratory Research* 8, no. 1 (2007): 63.

Gonda, I. "Targeting by deposition." In *Pharmaceutical Inhalation Aerosol Technology, Second Edition*, 84–104: CRC Press, 2016.

Guillon, A, J Montharu, L Vecellio, V Schubnel, G Roseau, J Guillemain, P Diot, and M De Monte. "Pulmonary delivery of dry powders to rats: tolerability limits of an intra-tracheal administration model." *International Journal of Pharmaceutics* 434, no. 1–2 (2012): 481–487.

Guillon, A, T Sécher, LA Dailey, L Vecellio, M de Monte, M Si-Tahar, P Diot, CP Page, and N Heuzé-Vourc'h. "Insights on animal models to investigate inhalation therapy: Relevance for biotherapeutics." *International Journal of Pharmaceutics* 536, no. 1 (2018/01/30/ 2018): 116–126.

Guillot, L, N Nathan, O Tabary, G Thouvenin, PL Rouzic, H Corvol, S Amselem, and A Clement. "Alveolar epithelial cells: Master regulators of lung homeostasis." *The International Journal of Biochemistry & Cell Biology* 45, no. 11 (2013): 2568–2573.

Hales, JRS, and MED Webster. "Respiratory function during thermal tachypnoea in sheep." *The Journal of Physiology* 190, no. 2 (1967): 241–260.

Haley, PJ, BA Muggenburg, DN Weissman, and DE Bice. "Comparative morphology and morphometry of alveolar macrophages from six species." *Developmental Dynamics* 191, no. 4 (1991): 401–407.

Hong, SH, SJ Park, S Lee, CS Cho, and MH Cho. "Aerosol gene delivery using viral vectors and cationic carriers for in vivo lung cancer therapy." *Expert Opinion on Drug Delivery* 12, no. 6 (2015): 977–991.

Hoymann, H. "Lung function measurements in rodents in safety pharmacology studies." [In English]. *Frontiers in Pharmacology* 3, no. 156 (2012-August-28 2012).

Hua, X, KL Zeman, B Zhou, Q Hua, BA Senior, SL Tilley, and WD Bennett. "Noninvasive real-time measurement of nasal mucociliary clearance in mice by pinhole gamma scintigraphy." *Journal of Applied Physiology* 108, no. 1 (2009): 189–196.

Hureaux, J, F Lacoeuille, F Lagarce, MC Rousselet, A Contini, P Saulnier, JP Benoit, and T Urban. "Absence of lung fibrosis after a single pulmonary delivery of lipid nanocapsules in rats." *International Journal of Nanomedicine* 12 (2017): 8159.

Hussell, T, and TJ Bell. "Alveolar macrophages: Plasticity in a tissue-specific context." *Nature Reviews Immunology* 14, no. 2 (2014): 81.

Inocencio, IM, RJ Bischof, SD Xiang, VA Zahra, VY Nguyen, T Lim, D LaRosa et al. "Exacerbation of ventilation-induced lung injury and inflammation in preterm lambs by high-dose nanoparticles." *Scientific Reports* 7, no. 1 (2017): 14704.

Irvin, CG, and JHT Bates. "Measuring the lung function in the mouse: the challenge of size." *Respiratory Research* 4, no. 1 (2003): 1.

King, M. "Experimental models for studying mucociliary clearance." *European Respiratory Journal* 11, no. 1 (1998): 222–228.

Koelsch, S, U Sent, P Nickolaus, and W Abraham. "Effect of ambroxol on whole lung mucociliary clearance in sheep." *European Respiratory Society* (2017): PA1054.

Kreyling, WG. "Interspecies comparison of lung clearance of 'insoluble' particles." *Journal of Aerosol Medicine* 3, no. s1 (1990): S-93–S-110.

Kumar, M, and J Longstreth. "Risks and benefits of conducting preclinical studies in the global setting." (2011).

Lecarpentier, Y, FX Blanc, S Salmeron, JC Pourny, D Chemla, and C Coirault. "Myosin cross-bridge kinetics in airway smooth muscle: A comparative study of humans, rats, and rabbits." *American Journal of Physiology-Lung Cellular and Molecular Physiology* 282, no. 1 (2002): L83–L90.

Maeder, ML, and CA Gersbach. "Genome-editing technologies for gene and cell therapy." *Molecular Therapy* 24, no. 3 (2016): 430–446.

Marangi, M, and G Pistritto. "Innovative therapeutic strategies for cystic fibrosis: Moving forward to Crispr technique." *Frontiers in Pharmacology* 9 (2018).

Martonen, TB. "Mathematical model for the selective deposition of inhaled pharmaceuticals." *Journal of Pharmaceutical Sciences* 82, no. 12 (1993): 1191–1199.

Massaro, D, GD Massaro, and LB Clerch. "Noninvasive delivery of small inhibitory RNA and other reagents to pulmonary alveoli in mice." *American Journal of Physiology-Lung Cellular and Molecular Physiology* 287, no. 5 (2004): L1066–L1070.

Matute-Bello, G, CW Frevert, and TR Martin. "Animal models of acute lung injury." *American Journal of Physiology-Lung Cellular and Molecular Physiology* 295, no. 3 (2008): L379–L399.

McCluskie, MJ, RD Weeratna, and HL Davis. "Intranasal immunization of mice with cpg DNA induces strong systemic and mucosal responses that are influenced by other mucosal adjuvants and antigen distribution." *Molecular Medicine* 6, no. 10 (2000): 867.

McLachlan, G, H Davidson, E Holder, LA Davies, IA Pringle, SG Sumner-Jones, A Baker et al. "Pre-clinical evaluation of three non-viral gene transfer agents for cystic fibrosis after aerosol delivery to the ovine lung." *Gene Therapy* 18, no. 10 (2011): 996.

McLachlan, G, A Baker, P Tennant, C Gordon, C Vrettou, L Renwick, R Blundell et al. "Optimizing aerosol gene delivery and expression in the ovine lung." *Molecular Therapy* 15, no. 2 (2007): 348–354.

Meeusen, EN, KJ Snibson, SJ Hirst, and RJ Bischof. "Sheep as a model species for the study and treatment of human asthma and other respiratory diseases." *Drug Discovery Today: Disease Models* 6, no. 4 (2009): 101–106.

Mercer, RR, S Anjilvel, FJ Miller, and JD Crapo. "Inhomogeneity of ventilatory unit volume and its effects on reactive gas uptake." *Journal of Applied Physiology* 70, no. 5 (1991): 2193–2205.

Mercer, RR, and JD Crapo. "Architecture of the gas exchange region of the lungs." In *Comparative Biology of the Normal Lung (Second Edition)*, 93–104. Amsterdam, the Netherland: Elsevier, 2015.

Mordenti, J. "Man versus beast: Pharmacokinetic scaling in mammals." *Journal of Pharmaceutical Sciences* 75, no. 11 (1986): 1028–1040.

Morello, M, CL Krone, S Dickerson, E Howerth, WA Germishuizen, YL Wong, D Edwards, BR Bloom, and MK Hondalus. "Dry-powder pulmonary insufflation in the mouse for application to vaccine or drug studies." *Tuberculosis* 89, no. 5 (2009): 371–377.

Nakano, S, J Nakahira, T Sawai, Y Kuzukawa, J Ishio, and T Minami. "Perioperative evaluation of respiratory impedance using the forced oscillation technique: A prospective observational study." *BMC Anesthesiology* 16, no. 1 (2015): 32.

Newman, SP. "Imaging pulmonary drug delivery." *Drug Delivery Applications of Noninvasive Imaging: Validation from Biodistribution to Sites of Action* (2014): 333–366.

Nguyen, BY, PK Peterson, HA Verbrugh, PG Quie, and JR Hoidal. "Differences in phagocytosis and killing by alveolar macrophages from humans, rabbits, rats, and hamsters." *Infection and Immunity* 36, no. 2 (1982): 504–509.

Nicod, LP. "Pulmonary defence mechanisms." *Respiration* 66, no. 1 (1999): 2–11.

Niemarkt, HJ, E Kuypers, R Jellema, D Ophelders, M Hütten, M Nikiforou, A Kribs, and BW Kramer. "Effects of less-invasive surfactant administration on oxygenation, pulmonary surfactant distribution, and lung compliance in spontaneously breathing preterm lambs." *Pediatric Research* 76, no. 2 (2014): 166.

Oostveen, E, D MacLeod, H Lorino, R Farre, Z Hantos, K Desager, and F Marchal. "The forced oscillation technique in clinical practice: Methodology, recommendations and future developments." *European Respiratory Journal* 22, no. 6 (2003): 1026–1041.

Parasuraman, S, R Raveendran, and R Kesavan. "Blood sample collection in small laboratory animals." *Journal of Pharmacology & Pharmacotherapeutics* 1, no. 2 (2010): 87.

Patra, AL. "Comparative anatomy of mammalian respiratory tracts: The nasopharyngeal region and the tracheobronchial region." *Journal of Toxicology and Environmental Health, Part A Current Issues* 17, no. 2–3 (1986): 163–174.

Patton, JS. "Inhaling medicines: Delivering drugs to the body through the lungs." *Nature Reviews Drug Discovery* 6, no. 1 (2007): 67–74.

Pinkerton, KE., LSV Winkle, CG. Plopper, S Smiley-Jewell, EC Covarrubias, and JT McBride. "Chapter 4—Architecture of the tracheobronchial tree A2—Parent, Richard A." In *Comparative Biology of the Normal Lung (Second Edition)*, 33–51. San Diego, CA: Academic Press, 2015.

Plopper, CG, AT Mariassy, and LH Hill. "Ultrastructure of the nonciliated bronchiolar epithelial (clara) cell of mammalian lung: II. A comparison of horse, steer, sheep, dog, and cat." *Experimental Lung Research* 1, no. 2 (1980): 155–169.

Porra, L, L Dégrugilliers, L Broche, G Albu, S Strengell, H Suhonen, GH Fodor et al. "Quantitative imaging of regional aerosol deposition, lung ventilation and morphology by synchrotron radiation Ct." *Scientific Reports* 8, no. 1 (2018): 3519.

Prankerd, RJ, TH Nguyen, JP Ibrahim, RJ Bischof, GC Nassta, LD Olerile, AS Russell et al. "Pulmonary delivery of an ultra-fine oxytocin dry powder formulation: potential for treatment of postpartum haemorrhage in developing countries." *PLoS One* 8, no. 12 (2013): e82965.

Price, DN, NK Kunda, and P Muttil. "Challenges associated with the pulmonary delivery of therapeutic dry powders for preclinical testing." *KONA Powder and Particle Journal* (2018): 2019008.

Qamar, W. "Technical considerations and precautions in situ bronchoalveolar lavage and alveolar infiltrating cells isolation in rats." *Toxicology Mechanisms and Methods* 25, no. 7 (2015): 547–551.

Rajapaksa, AE, JJ Ho, A Qi, R Bischof, TH Nguyen, M Tate, D Piedrafita et al. "Effective pulmonary delivery of an aerosolized plasmid DNA vaccine via surface acoustic wave nebulization." *Respiratory Research* 15, no. 1 (2014): 60.

Reynolds, SD, KE Pinkerton, and AT Mariassy. "Epithelial cells of trachea and bronchi." In *Comparative Biology of the Normal Lung (Second Edition)*, 61–81. Amsterdam, the Netherlands: Elsevier, 2015.

Sakagami, M. "In vivo, in vitro and ex vivo models to assess pulmonary absorption and disposition of inhaled therapeutics for systemic delivery." *Advanced Drug Delivery Reviews* 58, no. 9–10 (2006): 1030–1060.

Sanders, M. "Pulmonary drug delivery: An historical overview." In *Controlled Pulmonary Drug Delivery*, 51–73: Springer, 2011.

Schanker, LS., and JA Hemberger. "Relation between molecular weight and pulmonary absorption rate of lipid-insoluble compounds in neonatal and adult rats." [In eng]. *Biochemical Pharmacology* 32, no. 17 (Sep 1 1983): 2599–2601.

Schlepütz, M, AD Rieg, S Seehase, J Spillner, A Perez-Bouza, T Braunschweig, T Schroeder et al. "Neurally mediated airway constriction in human and other species: A comparative study using precision-cut lung slices (Pcls)." *PLoS One* 7, no. 10 (2012): e47344.

Schlesinger, RB, JM Fine, and LC Chen. "Interspecies differences in the phagocytic activity of pulmonary macrophages subjected to acidic challenge." *Fundamental and Applied Toxicology* 19, no. 4 (1992): 584–589.

Schlesinger, RB, and LA McFadden. "Comparative morphometry of the upper bronchial tree in six mammalian species." *The Anatomical Record* 199, no. 1 (1981): 99–108.

Sly, PD., DJ Turner, RA Collins, and Z Hantos. "Penh is not a validated technique for measuring airway function in mice." *American Journal of Respiratory and Critical Care Medicine* 172, no. 2 (2005): 256–256.

Soane, RJ, M Hinchcliffe, SS Davis, and L Illum. "clearance characteristics of chitosan based formulations in the sheep nasal cavity." *International Journal of Pharmaceutics* 217, no. 1–2 (2001): 183–191.

St George, JA. "Secretory glycoconjugates of the trachea and bronchi." In *Comparative Biology of the Normal Lung (Second Edition)*, 53–60. Amsterdam, the Netherlands: Elsevier, 2015.

Stein, SW, and CG Thiel. "The history of therapeutic aerosols: A chronological review." *Journal of Aerosol Medicine and Pulmonary Drug Delivery* 30, no. 1 (2017): 20–41.

Sung, DK, WH Kong, K Park, JH Kim, MY Kim, H Kim, and SK Hahn. "Noncovalenly pegylated ctgf sirna/ pdmaema complex for pulmonary treatment of bleomycin-induced lung fibrosis." *Biomaterials* 34, no. 4 (2013): 1261–1269.

Tepper, JS, and DL Costa. "Methods, measurements, and interpretation of animal lung function in health and disease." In *Comparative Biology of the Normal Lung (Second Edition)*, 305–351: Amsterdam, the Netherlands: Elsevier, 2015.

Thompson, RB, and WH Finlay. "Using Mri to measure aerosol deposition." *Journal of Aerosol Medicine and Pulmonary Drug Delivery* 25, no. 2 (2012): 55–62.

Tu, Z, W Yang, S Yan, X Guo, and XJ Li. "Crispr/Cas9: A powerful genetic engineering tool for establishing large animal models of neurodegenerative diseases." *Molecular Neurodegeneration* 10, no. 1 (2015): 35.

Varga, OE, AK Hansen, P Sandøe, and IAS Olsson. "Validating animal models for preclinical research: a scientific and ethical discussion." *Alternatives to Laboratory Animals: ATLA*, 38, no. 3 (2010): 245–248.

Wang, HX, M Li, CM Lee, S Chakraborty, HW Kim, G Bao, and KW Leong. "Crispr/Cas9-based genome editing for disease modeling and therapy: Challenges and opportunities for nonviral delivery." *Chemical Reviews* 117, no. 15 (2017): 9874–9906.

Warheit, DB, MA Hartsky, and MS Stefaniak. "Comparative physiology of rodent pulmonary macrophages: In vitro functional responses." *Journal of Applied Physiology* 64, no. 5 (1988): 1953–1959.

Whitsett, JA, and T Alenghat. "Respiratory epithelial cells orchestrate pulmonary innate immunity." *Nature Immunology* 16, no. 1 (2015): 27.

Wilkinson, ST, JM Sallenave, and J Simpson. "Pulmonary defence mechanisms." *Current Respiratory Medicine Reviews* 8, no. 3 (2012): 149–162.

Wolff, RK. "Toxicology studies for inhaled and nasal delivery." *Molecular Pharmaceutics* 12, no. 8 (2015): 2688–2696.

Wong, BA. "Inhalation exposure systems: Design, methods and operation." *Toxicologic Pathology* 35, no. 1 (2007): 3–14.

Woods, A, A Patel, D Spina, Y Riffo-Vasquez, A Babin-Morgan, RTM de Rosales, K Sunassee et al. "In vivo biocompatibility, clearance, and biodistribution of albumin vehicles for pulmonary drug delivery." *Journal of Controlled Release* 210 (2015): 1–9.

Wylie, JL, A House, PJ Mauser, S Sellers, J Terebetski, Z Wang, and JD Ehrick. "Inhaled formulation and device selection: Bridging the gap between preclinical species and first-in-human studies." *Therapeutic Delivery* 9, no. 5 (2018): 387–404.

Yang, PJ, M LaMarca, C Kaminski, DI Chu, and DL Hu. "Hydrodynamics of defecation." *Soft Matter* 13, no. 29 (2017): 4960–4970.

Yang, PJ, JC Pham, J Choo, and DL Hu. "Law of urination: All mammals empty their bladders over the same duration." *Arxiv Preprint Arxiv:1310.3737* (2013).

Yeh, HC, GM Schum, and MT Duggan. "Anatomic models of the tracheobronchial and pulmonary regions of the rat." *The Anatomical Record* 195, no. 3 (1979): 483–492.

Zosky, GR, and PD Sly. "Animal models of asthma." *Clinical & Experimental Allergy* 37, no. 7 (2007): 973–988.

Section X

Clinical Testing

31

Bioequivalence of Orally Inhaled Drug Products: Challenges and Opportunities

Jayne E. Hastedt and Elise Burmeister Getz

CONTENTS

31.1 Introduction

Most clinicians and pharmaceutical scientists today are familiar with the bioequivalence concept, even if not with the details and variations of its implementation; bioequivalence testing plays a central role in today's pharmaceutical industry. Bioequivalence allows innovator products to bridge across changes in manufacturing process, scale, or location, and to link batches of product used in safety and efficacy testing to those manufactured for commercial use. Importantly, bioequivalence provides a means by which copies of approved drugs, referred to as generics, can be offered to the patient as a lower-cost alternative to the innovator drug. Without doubt, the advent of the bioequivalence concept has not only improved the quality of pharmaceutical products, but has also saved the industry (and therefore the patient) considerable cost by eliminating unnecessary and redundant clinical testing. In the United States (U.S.), nine out of every ten prescriptions are filled by a generic.[1] But this cost efficiency has not reached the locally acting, orally inhaled drug product sector. Currently, there is only one orally inhaled, locally acting generic drug product on the U.S. market. In this chapter, we illustrate the challenges and opportunities for the bioequivalence concept when applied to locally acting, orally inhaled drug products (OIDPs). The challenges associated with the current approaches utilized to establish clinical bioequivalence emphasize the need to establish a bridge between the OIDP technologies discussed in the earlier chapters of this text and the biology. To this end, we close out this chapter by exploring ways to utilize the principles of biopharmaceutics as a means to establish a linkage between pulmonary drug delivery products and the biology of the lung.

31.1.1 Origin and Definition of the Bioequivalence Standard

The need for, and concept of, bioequivalence arose from evidence that clinical substitutability is not always guaranteed by chemical equivalence or even by pharmaceutical equivalence. Pharmaceutical equivalence is defined as an identical dosage form and route of administration with quantitatively similar amounts of the same active ingredients. Pharmaceutically equivalent products can, however, differ in shape and size, shelf life, drug release mechanisms, and excipients; these differences may affect the *in vivo* performance of the product. For example, variability between topical glucocorticoid products containing the same active ingredient led scientists and regulators to conclude "that incorporating identical concentrations of the same drug into two different topical vehicles (chemical equivalency) does not necessarily produce dosage forms that will deliver the active drug to the biosystem at the same rate or to the same extent."[2] The requirement for evidence of bioequivalence was introduced into FDA regulation in 1977 and formalized in the 1984 Drug Price Competition and Patent Term Restoration Act (the "Hatch-Waxman Act"). When bioequivalence and pharmaceutical equivalence are both demonstrated, the products are concluded to be therapeutically equivalent. In the years since the Hatch-Waxman Act, the field of bioequivalence has endeavored to define testing conditions and criteria that ensure clinical substitutability. In this chapter, we present considerations for the continued development of "an appropriate bioequivalence standard," as required by the Hatch-Waxman Act, as it pertains to locally acting inhaled medicinal products.

Bioequivalence is defined as "the absence of a significant difference in the rate and extent to which the active ingredient or active moiety in pharmaceutical equivalents or pharmaceutical alternatives becomes available at the site of drug action when administered at the same molar dose under similar conditions in an appropriately designed study."[3] That is, when the chemical entity that exerts a biological effect appears at its site of action in a similar amount, and with similar kinetics, in two formulations or products, these two formulations or products will be assumed to "have the same clinical effect and no greater chance of adverse effect."[4]

For the majority of drug products intended for systemic absorption, "an appropriately designed study" is a pharmacokinetic study in healthy volunteers, chosen because of its sensitivity to product differences and relevance to the means by which the active pharmaceutical ingredient is delivered to its pharmacologic target (namely, via the systemic circulation). The "absence of a significant difference" is defined as a 90% confidence interval around the geometric mean product ratio on pharmacokinetic metrics that is fully contained within 80.00%–125.00%. For drugs that reach their pharmacological target via the blood, this bioequivalence definition has ensured good agreement in the rate and extent of drug appearance at the site of action; amongst products that have passed this bioequivalence test, the difference between innovator and copy is, on average, within approximately 5%.[5] The definition of a "significant difference" has evolved in recent years to include accommodation for highly variable drug products,[6] narrow therapeutic index drug products,[7] and drug products with dichotomous endpoints.[8]A comprehensive presentation of the history, fundamentals, and current methodology of bioequivalence testing in the United States can be found in the comprehensive text authored by FDA scientists.[9]

31.1.2 Challenges in the Application of Bioequivalence to Orally Inhaled Drug Products

For OIDPs, heterogeneity of the site of application (the airways and lungs) and widespread distribution of local biological targets suggest that the rate and extent of drug appearance at more than one biological location may be important. Further, the orally inhaled drug product itself is complex,[10] involving not only a drug product formulation, but also a delivery device; both formulation and device, as well as interactions of these constituent parts with each other and with the user, influence *in vivo* performance. Perhaps the most substantial bioequivalence challenge for OIDPs is that there is no direct or surrogate measure of drug concentration at the site of action; blood plasma concentration may not reflect the therapeutic effect, and concentration at the local pulmonary site of action is not easily measured. Today, it is commonly appreciated that locally acting, orally inhaled drug products will require a multifaceted bioequivalence approach. The challenge for application of the bioequivalence concept to locally acting OIDPs, therefore, is to identify a suite of assessments that collectively ensures that an alternative formulation or alternative product (aka, the "Test" product) will produce a similar desired clinical effect and no greater chance of adverse effect under the various conditions present in commercial use as the approved formulation or product (aka, the "Reference" product).

Interpretation of bioequivalence studies, when partnered with pharmaceutical equivalence, as evidence of therapeutic equivalence relies on a clear understanding of the means by which a drug product achieves its clinical safety and efficacy profile. For locally acting, orally inhaled products, this understanding is typically not adequately complete. For example, while the molecular mechanism(s) of action may be well understood, the exact location(s) of the pharmacological targets in the airways is rarely known. That is, it's not typically known how the drug deposition pattern within the respiratory tract, the physicochemical properties of the drug and formulation, the interaction of drug and device, etc., ultimately contribute to the overall safety and efficacy profile of the drug product. The FDA, therefore, has taken an approach to bioequivalence that relies not on one test, but instead on a panel of tests that collectively attempt to characterize the performance of the Test and Reference products with sufficient completeness that, despite the gaps in understanding, a claim of therapeutic equivalence has a low risk of error if all the tests in the panel are passed. This aggregate testing is termed the "weight-of-evidence" approach.[11]

Currently, the components of the bioequivalence assessment for OIDPs are: (i) qualitative and quantitative formulation sameness, (ii) *in vitro* bioequivalence of drug delivery metrics, (iii) pharmacokinetic bioequivalence, and (iv) pharmacodynamic or clinical endpoint bioequivalence. Since 2013, 39 product-specific draft guidance for orally inhaled and nasal drug products have been issued by FDA to define, on a by-product basis, the details of these four categories of testing.[12] Most orally inhaled drug-specific guidances currently require all four weight-of-evidence bioequivalence tests. These regulatory recommendations are a necessary step towards successful bioequivalence testing for OIDPs; the sufficiency, necessity, and biorelevance of the current recommendations, however, remain an active area of research and investigation. In this chapter, we discuss these weight-of-evidence bioequivalence components, including the value each adds to the overall bioequivalence assessment, opportunities to refine comparative testing, and challenges still facing the field of bioequivalence as applied to OIDPs. Our focus is on approaches appropriate for the U.S. market, where pharmacy-level generic substitution is allowed, noting that in some instances the U.S. approach diverges from that applied in other regulatory domains (e.g. Europe).

31.2 Pulmonary Physiology and the Fate of Inhaled Drugs

Regulatory standards underpinning bioequivalence testing are grounded in pharmaceutical science. While the earlier chapters of this book have addressed the influence of formulation, delivery device, and human factors on the OIDP dose, in this chapter we begin with the pulmonary dose and consider the downstream events during and following inhalation, e.g. regional deposition, local clearance, dissolution, diffusion, permeation, and tissue interaction (Figure 31.1). In this context, the biorelevant attributes of the OIDP dose can be identified and form the basis for the necessary and sufficient components of a bioequivalence assessment. We note that biorelevant characterization of the OIDP dose is important not only for bioequivalence testing, but also for the establishment of clinically relevant drug product specifications.

When we breathe, our lungs perform a gas exchange that transfers oxygen into the blood, and removes carbon dioxide, a waste gas, from the blood. Anatomically, the lungs, though quite complex, are often

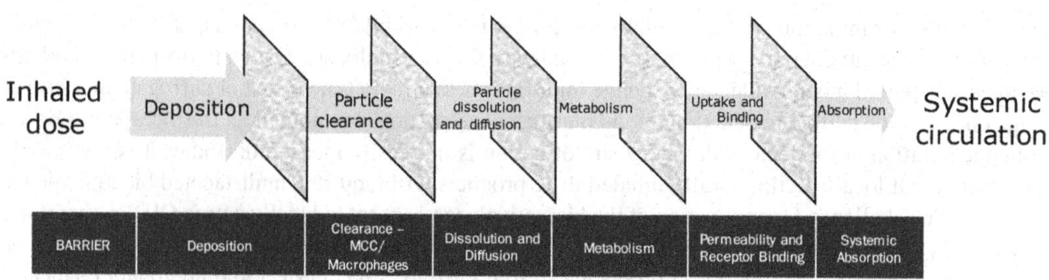

FIGURE 31.1 Pulmonary drug delivery barriers.

Zone	Generation		d (cm)	l (cm)	number	cross-section area (cm^2)	cartilage	epithelial cell type
conducting zone	trachea	0	1.8	12.0	1	2.54	open rings	columnar ciliated
	bronchi	1	1.22	4.8	2	2.33		
		2	0.83	1.9	4	2.13	plates	
		3	0.56	0.8	8	2.00		
	bronchioles	4	0.45	1.3	16	2.48		
	terminal bronchioles	5	0.35	1.07	32	3.11		
		↓	↓	↓	↓	↓		
		16	0.06	0.17	6×10^4	180.0		cuboidal
respiratory zone	respiratory bronchioles	17	↓	↓	↓	↓	absent	cuboidal to alveolar
		18						
		19	0.05	0.10	5×10^5	10^3		
	alveolar ducts	20	↓	↓	↓	↓		alveolar
		21						
		22						
	alveolar sacs	23	0.03	0.03	8×10^6	10^4		

FIGURE 31.2 Description of the regions of the human lung. (Adapted from Hastedt, J.E. et al., *AAPS Open*, 2, 2016.)

described as consisting of two general regions: the conducting and the non-conducting zones. The conducting zone, as the name implies, conducts the inhaled air from the mouth and nose to the areas of gas exchange; the conducting (central) airways include the trachea, bronchi, bronchioles, and the terminal bronchioles. The non-conducting zone (the respiratory or peripheral airways) consists of respiratory bronchioles, alveolar ducts, and alveoli. It is within the alveoli that the gas exchange occurs. Anatomical and physiological differences between the zones are substantial, as described below.

The airway zones reduce in size from the trachea to the alveoli or aleveolar sacs (Figure 31.2). The surface area of the central airways is approximately 1 m^2–2.5 m^2, whereas that of the peripheral airways is on the order of 100 m^2–140 m^2 in adults.[14]

The airway surface liquid (ASL) or lung "fluid" composition and volume vary by location within the lung and play an important role in the fate of inhaled drugs.[15,16] The composition of the ASL by region is provided in Table 31.1. The values provided are for healthy subjects and therefore do not reflect changes to the composition, pH, and volume that can be impacted by a disease state. The ASL is not a free-flowing liquid, but a film lining the walls of the airways. At the air/ASL interface, both the upper and lower airways are covered with a thin layer of lung surfactant. Underneath this layer, the upper airways are lined with a non-Newtonian layer of hydrophilic mucin-rich mucus, the thickness of which varies by location. The airways (except for the alveolar regions) are also ciliated to allow for mucociliary clearance (MCC) of undissolved particles. The alveolar regions are covered with a thin layer of Newtonian surfactant-rich fluid.

TABLE 31.1
Airway Surface Liquid Composition by Zone

	Conducting Airways	**Peripheral Alveolar Airways**
Description	Non-Newtonian hydrophilic viscous mucus; ciliated	Newtonian hydrophobic lipid; non-ciliated
Composition[17]	1% inorganic salts 1% proteins 2% glycoproteins (mucins) 1% lipids 95% water	85% phospholipids 5% cholesterol 10% proteins
Estimated Volume of ASL	10 mL–20 mL	10 mL
Surface area	1 m^2–2.5 m^2	100 m^2–140 m^2
pH	6.69 ± 0.07[18]	

Source: Eixarch, H. et al., *J. Epithelial Biol. Pharmacol.*, 3, 1–14, 2010.
Note: Volumes are estimated by multiplying average film thickness by the average surface area provided in Eixarch et al.

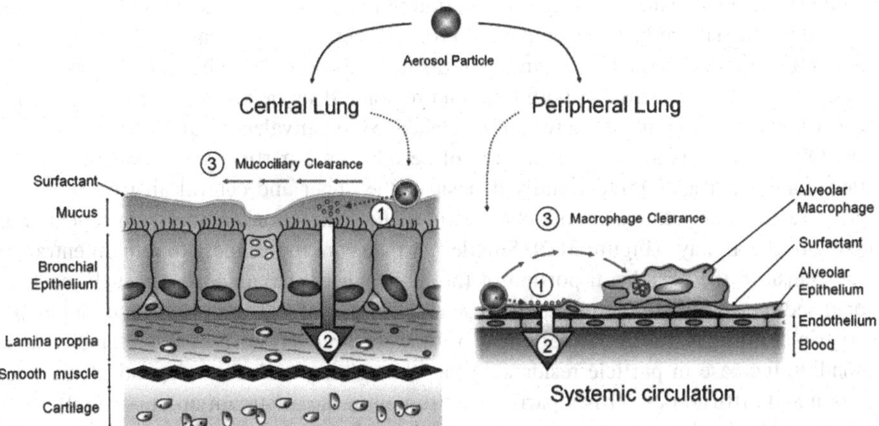

FIGURE 31.3 The fate of inhaled drugs. (With kind permission from Taylor & Francis: *AAPS Open*, Scope and relevance of a pulmonary biopharmaceutical classification system AAPS/FDA/USP workshop March 16–17th, 2015 in Baltimore, MD, 2, 2016, Hastedt, J.E. et al.)

Thus, the environment of the central conducting airways is very different from that of the peripheral airways. The fate of an inhaled drug therefore depends on the location within the lung where the drug particle deposits.[20,21]

Following deposition, the fate of the inhaled drug particle is determined by the physical and chemical properties of the drug substance(s), the formulation, and the deposition environment as illustrated in Figure 31.3. Particles deposited in the conducting airways land in the hydrophilic mucin-rich viscous environment of the lung. Clearance from the central conducting airways can occur through binding to the negatively charged mucin or clearance of undissolved drug, both facilitated by mucociliary clearance. The thickness of the ASL in the upper airways, as well as its viscosity, can hinder diffusion and reduce the rate of transport to the epithelium. In the alveolar space, the ASL layer is thin and the composition is lipophilic, therefore favoring dissolution and rapid transport of lipophilic compounds into the blood. Undissolved compounds in the alveolar space can undergo clearance by the interaction with macrophages whose role is to scour the inside of these air sacs. Regardless of the airway location, the thicker the diffusion barrier, the slower the rate of transport to the epithelial surface and *vice versa*. The greater the concentration gradient across the barrier, the faster the transport.

After dissolution and diffusion, transport across the epithelium can occur via passive transcellular or paracellular transport, active transport, or a combination of these mechanisms. Lipophilic drugs tend to undergo transcellular transport, whereas hydrophilic compounds transport paracellularly through the hydrophilic space between the cells (e.g. tight junctions). The molecular weight of a compound also contributes to the efficiency of transport.

The relative importance of the barriers to transport are expected to be drug- and formulation-specific. For example, absorption relies on the ability of the dissolved drug to partition into and transport through biological membranes. Because of the composition of biological membranes, drugs that are highly permeable are typically more lipophilic, have a higher potential to partition, and therefore have a higher passive absorption potential. Hydrophilic or charged drugs are less permeable, but more soluble in an aqueous environment. Therefore, the ionization potential (pKa) and the local pH can impact the transport properties of a drug.

31.3 The Weight-of-Evidence Approach to OIDP Bioequivalence

31.3.1 *In Vitro* Bioequivalence of Drug Delivery Metrics

If bioequivalence testing for oral medicinal products can be considered a two-dimensional problem (i.e. matching the rate and extent of drug presentation to the systemic circulation), bioequivalence testing for inhaled medicinal products encompasses a third dimension: the location of drug presentation in the airways and lungs, due to the heterogeneity of the lungs as described above. Current FDA guidance relies heavily on *in vitro* measures of both total and regional drug deposition, for a range of flow rates and container life stages, as part of the weight-of-evidence bioequivalence paradigm.

For most OIDPs, there is a wide distribution of aerodynamic particle sizes, sometimes of varying composition. Larger particles preferentially deposit in the upper and central airways because, due to inertia, they are less likely to follow the changes in airflow direction arising from repeated anatomical branching of the airways (Figure 31.2). Smaller particles are more likely to remain entrained in the airflow and transit to the peripheral portion of the lungs where they deposit via such mechanisms as gravitational sedimentation and Brownian diffusion. The vast increase in cross-sectional area towards the later (peripheral) generations of the lungs[22] results in a reduction in airflow velocity *in vivo* and a corresponding increase in particle residence time, thus giving such time-dependent mechanisms as sedimentation and diffusion of aerosol particles entrained in the airstream an opportunity to influence deposition. Thus, the *in vivo* lung deposition pattern depends on inhalation flow rate, airway geometry, aerodynamic particle size, and the interaction of the patient with the drug delivery device.

In vitro bioequivalence methods of aerosol sizing do not mimic the *in vivo* anatomy or airflow velocity profile; the results are not necessarily correctly interpreted as indicating *in vivo* deposition pattern. Rather, the bioequivalence objective is to use measures of (flow rate dependent) emitted dose and aerodynamic particle size as assays to characterize product differences (e.g. as a quality control test), on the basis that these metrics are primary determinants of regional deposition pattern. The cascade impactor is the most commonly used instrument for aerodynamic particle size measurement in bioequivalence testing. An induction port, typically designed to mimic the right angle turn of the throat, is attached to a series of stages, each comprising: (i) one or more nozzles through which the airstream flows and (ii) collection plates onto which particles with sufficient inertia as to be unable to follow bends in the airstream impact. The cascade impactor operates entirely via the inertial impaction mechanism, stepwise separating the aerosol into size "bins" according to the aerodynamic diameter which itself is a composite parameter that collectively represents the effects of such features as particle density and particle shape. Test and Reference products that are qualitatively and quantitatively similar in composition, have similar emitted dose, aerodynamic particle size distribution, pharmacokinetics, and local response, are deemed unlikely to have detectable differences in the rate and extent to which they present drug to the site(s) of action (both pharmacologic and toxicologic), i.e. are considered to be bioequivalent. Issues that potentially confound the use of inertial impaction as an assay of aerosol particle size distribution (APSD) sameness include product differences in particle composition (important when there are multiple solid-phase ingredients in a formulation) and dry powder inhaler (DPI) emptying rate (which affects the flow rate experienced by the formulation *in vivo* and the extent to which the inspiratory air in which the drug particle is entrained will penetrate the lungs).

Dose measurements, both total (emitted dose) and regional (via APSD), are compared between products using population bioequivalence (PBE) methods. The PBE test as applied to aerosol characteristics is described in detail.[23] This test differs from average bioequivalence in that it compares not only the means, but also the variances of the product sample distributions. The proximity of product means required for a bioequivalence conclusion is determined in the context of product variability; to be considered bioequivalent, the Test mean must sit closer to the mean of a Reference product with consistent performance than to the mean of a widely varying Reference product. A minimum of three manufacturing batches of both Test and Reference products must be included in the bioequivalence assessment, presumably to ensure that the bioequivalence conclusion will be generalizable despite naturally occurring batch-to-batch differences. Recent characterization of emitted dose measurements from 856 individual batches across 20 pressurized metered dose inhaler (pMDI) products by PBE Working Group of the International Pharmaceutical Aerosol Consortium on Regulation and Science (IPAC-RS) identified substantial between-batch variability in most products, accounting for 0%–90% of total variability with the 10th percentile, 50th percentile, and 90th percentile at 0%, 14%, and 48% of total variability, respectively.[24] The FDA's current specification of the PBE method does not account for between-batch differences directly and instead assumes that all data come from a single "superbatch," i.e. ignores batch identification in the statistical model. The consequence is an inflated false equivalence (type I) error rate due to overestimated confidence in both mean and variance estimates. As will be seen also in the following section on *in vivo* bioequivalence assessments, differences between manufacturing batches may require modification to OIDP bioequivalence methods.

31.3.2 Systemic *In Vivo* Bioequivalence

In vivo bioequivalence testing is used only when *in vitro* bioequivalence approaches are considered to be, on their own, insufficient evidence that the active ingredient(s) will reach the site(s) of action with the same rate and to the same extent in two different formulations, two different products, or following changes in manufacturing process, scale, or location between clinical trial batches and the to-be-marketed product. Currently, OIDP *in vitro* characterization is not considered adequate to waive the *in vivo* components of the bioequivalence assessment. A pharmacokinetic study is typically used as the bioassay of product differences in systemically available drug. Theory and implementation of the pharmacokinetic bioequivalence bioassay are discussed here, with a subsequent section devoted to the pharmacodynamic or clinical endpoint study used to assess product differences in the rate and extent of drug appearance at local targets.

31.3.2.1 Basic Design Principles of the Pharmacokinetic Bioassay

The pharmacokinetic bioequivalence study for OIDPs is conducted using the same design principles used for a solid oral pharmacokinetic bioequivalence study, on the basis that these design features increase sensitivity to product or formulation differences in rate and extent to which the active ingredient(s) is released from the drug product. The study is typically run as a randomized, open-label, single-dose crossover in healthy adult male and (non-pregnant) female volunteers, with samples of the blood compartment collected frequently during the absorption phase and extending until 80%–90% of total systemic exposure has been observed.[25,26] The pharmacokinetic bioequivalence study is typically not blinded, i.e. study participants and clinic staff are aware of whether it is the Test or the Reference treatment that has been administered, because the pharmacokinetic endpoints are not readily influenced by the actions, behaviors, or decisions of clinical trial participants or clinic staff. Use of a single dose, even for products intended for chronic use, improves the sensitivity of the maximum observed plasma concentration (Cmax) to absorption rate differences by avoiding a contribution from prior doses (for which absorption rate differences are no longer relevant due to completion of absorption).[27]

Use of healthy subjects (if it is ethically acceptable to do so) instead of the target patient population allows each subject to better serve as their own control in the crossover design, by avoiding variability arising from the underlying disease. This design feature is particularly relevant to OIDPs, for which the dose is administered, in patients, directly to the diseased organ; both natural fluctuations in disease severity and the effect of treatment on disease status are expected to complicate a crossover design in the patient population. An adequately long washout between treatments could address the latter, but not the former, concern. Further, some OIDPs yield lower blood concentrations in asthmatic patients relative to healthy subjects. For example, both total blood exposure and peak blood concentration of inhaled fluticasone propionate in asthmatic patients are observed to be less than half of healthy subject values.[28,29] Thus, less of the inhaled dose is observable. For these reasons, healthy adults are the preferred OIDP pharmacokinetic bioequivalence study population. The essential point is that the pharmacokinetic bioequivalence study is a comparative bioassay, not a clinical pharmacology trial; the objective is to assess similarity in release of the active ingredient(s) from the drug product, not to assess basic pharmacokinetic properties (e.g. clearance, volume of distribution, absolute bioavailability, etc.) in the target patient population.

Most FDA OIDP guidance documents recommend a two-way crossover design, in which each subject receives one administration of the Test product and one administration of the Reference product across two treatment occasions according to a randomly assigned sequence (TR or RT) with an adequate washout (approximately five elimination half-lives) between the treatments. The crossover design substantially improves the ability of the study to separate a formulation or product difference from measurement variability, because the product or formulation comparison is always *within* a subject, not between subjects. Differences between subjects are typically large, due, for example, to different inhalation techniques, different airway geometries, and/or different body sizes. The difference in pharmacokinetic profile magnitude or shape *between* subjects is irrelevant in the crossover design; it is only the Test-versus-Reference product comparison *within* each subject that is of interest. The two-way crossover, however, assumes that all variation in the within-subject Test/Reference ratio is attributable to measurement error, i.e. assumes that the true Test/Reference value is the same for all subjects. True variation in the Test/Reference ratio from subject to subject is termed a subject-by-formulation interaction,[30,31] several examples are provided in Chapter 2 of the FDA's textbook on bioequivalence standards.[32] This subject-by-formulation variability, if it exists, is combined with within-subject measurement error for construction of the Test/Reference ratio confidence interval in the standard two-way crossover design. Treatment replication is required to separately estimate these components of total variance. Statistical pharmacokinetic bioequivalence approaches that separately consider the subject-by-formulation interaction from within-subject residual error, i.e. individual bioequivalence, are no longer commonly used by FDA, in accord with the two-way crossover design recommendation in draft product-specific guidance. These and other design and analysis considerations are detailed in several FDA guidances,[29,30,33] as well as in the FDA-authored text on bioequivalence testing, see, for example, Chapters 2 and 3.[36]

Even with a crossover design, clinical study participants must be trained thoroughly and repeatedly to ensure that their inhalation technique is consistent among the treatment periods, thereby avoiding confounding treatment differences with variability in inhalation technique. Recent FDA guidance documents for OIDPs specifically include a recommendation regarding subject training. This may reflect an attempt to prevent OIDPs from appearing to be highly variable drug products when high variability is only an artifacts of a variable inhalation maneuver caused by inadequate training and practice. Although the Reference-scaled average bioequivalence method (RSABE) detailed in the draft Progesterone guidance[6] is considered broadly applicable, it is not the intent to allow bioequivalence goalpost expansion in instances of avoidable variability.

31.3.2.2 Pharmacokinetic Bioequivalence Metrics

The primary endpoints in a pharmacokinetic bioequivalence study are Cmax (the maximum observed plasma concentration) and AUC (the area under the plasma concentration-versus-time curve). AUC is expressed in terms of the dose and primary physiology-derived pharmacokinetic parameters:

$$\mathrm{AUC} = \frac{F \cdot D}{\mathrm{CL}} \tag{31.1}$$

where F, or bioavailability, is the fraction of the dose that is absorbed into the blood, D is the total administered dose, and CL, or clearance, is the rate at which the body eliminates the drug. An increase in total dose or the bioavailable fraction of the dose will increase the body's exposure to drug (AUC), as will a decrease in the clearance rate. A comparison of bioavailability between Test (T) and Reference (R) products can then be expressed from Equation 31.1 as:

$$\frac{F_T}{F_R} = \frac{\text{AUC}_T \cdot \text{CL}_T \cdot D_R}{\text{AUC}_R \cdot \text{CL}_R \cdot D_T} \tag{31.2}$$

In a bioequivalence study, the Test and Reference products are administered at the same dose, $D_T = D_R$. Further, it is assumed that the drug clearance rate is unaffected by the formulation or delivery device, $\text{CL}_T = \text{CL}_R$. Thus, Equation 31.2 becomes:

$$\frac{F_T}{F_R} = \frac{\text{AUC}_T}{\text{AUC}_R} \tag{31.3}$$

demonstrating that the AUC product ratio represents relative bioavailability, i.e. the extent to which drug in the Test product is available to the circulation relative to the extent the same drug in the Reference product is available to the circulation. An AUC product ratio of 1.0 indicates that equal amounts of the drug are absorbed into the circulation from the Test and Reference products. For systemically acting products; this implies that the extent to which drug is presented to the site of action is the same across the products; this implication has clear relevance in bioequivalence testing. For locally acting OIDPs, an AUC product ratio of 1.0 implies equality of the systemically available dose, but not necessarily equality of the "bioavailable" dose (the dose available to pharmacological targets), since some (perhaps, most) targets are local to the lungs. Thus, for OIDPs, the AUC product ratio reflects the relative amounts of drug presented to systemic targets. These systemic targets are often associated with undesirable effects, and so the AUC comparison is considered to be an assessment of the relative safety of the Test and Reference products. Clearly, however, the appearance of inhaled drug in the blood is not entirely independent of the dose deposited in the lungs. The question of the extent to which plasma AUC is informative regarding the pharmacological dose is a topic of ongoing discussions. Some inhaled drugs (e.g. fluticasone propionate, fluticasone furoate) are almost fully metabolizsed to inactive metabolites on first pass through the liver, and so the plasma AUC entirely reflects drug absorbed from the lungs. For others, the plasma AUC is the sum of drug absorbed from the lungs and drug absorbed from the gut after swallowing (following deposition in the mouth or throat, or resulting from mucociliary clearance from the central airways).

The innovator's pharmacokinetic characterization of a drug will typically involve a compartmental analysis in which the plasma concentration-versus-time profile is expressed as a linear combination of exponential functions. The analysis is termed "compartmental" because it considers theoretical body "compartments" through and between which the drug moves as it is absorbed, distributed, metabolized, and eliminated. Movement of drug between the "compartments" is determined by physiological parameters such as clearance, volume of distribution, bioavailability (or systemic availability), and absorption rate. These physiological parameters uniquely determine the drug's concentration-versus-time profile. Integration of plasma concentration over time, then, yields the AUC. In the bioequivalence context, however, AUC is computed empirically, by adding up each trapezoidal contribution to the total area under the concentration-versus-time curve. This is referred to as a non-compartmental analysis (to distinguish it from compartmental analysis). For example, if linear interpolation between two concentration data points is used, the AUC contribution between the time points is given by:

$$\text{AUC}_{t_1 \to t_2} = \frac{1}{2}(C_1 + C_2)(t_2 - t_1) \tag{31.4}$$

where $\frac{1}{2}(C_1 + C_2)$ is the average concentration in the time window, and $(t_2 - t_1)$ is the duration over which this average concentration appears in the plasma. When this calculation is applied to all the data points, the sum is the AUC from the time of drug administration to the time of the last quantifiable drug concentration (t_{last}); this metric is commonly notated as AUC(0–t) or, more simply, AUC_t. AUC_t represents the total observed systemic exposure to drug. Although different assumptions about the shape of the concentration profile can be made (e.g. logarithmic, instead of linear, decline), the linear trapezoidal method is commonly used for bioequivalence analyses.

OIDPs are specifically designed to minimize systemic exposure to drug; the inhalation route delivers drug directly to the site of action. Accordingly, plasma concentrations are typically low. The later samples in a pharmacokinetic profile will often contain drug concentrations below the bioanalytical lower limit of quantitation (LOQ). These concentrations are excluded from the non-compartmental AUC analysis because no concentration value is estimated for them. Each pharmacokinetic profile will therefore have an AUCt value that is calculated to the time of the last quantifiable concentration *for that particular profile.* In a crossover study, the consequence is that AUCt may be calculated over a different time window for Test than for Reference (Figure 31.4). The resulting bias in AUCt can be easily corrected by using a common t_{last} value across all profiles (i.e. both Test and Reference) for a given subject.[34,35] Use of a subject-specific common t_{last} ensures that the reported AUCt product ratio does not exaggerate the difference in exposure between the products in a bioequivalence assessment.

As previously described, AUC_t represents the *observed* systemic exposure to drug. For bioequivalence testing, AUC_t is considered alongside an estimate of the *total* systemic exposure. Total exposure is the area under the entire concentration-versus-time profile and is obtained by extrapolating the concentration profile from t_{last} to infinite time, i.e. extrapolating to zero plasma concentration. Total systemic exposure is commonly indicated as AUC(0–inf) or AUC_∞. Concentration extrapolation is based on an assumption of single-exponential concentration decline, with the half-life of this exponential decline estimated from the last few (three or more) plasma concentrations. AUC_∞ is then computed according to:

$$AUC_\infty = AUC_t + \frac{C_{tf}}{\lambda_z} \tag{31.5}$$

where C_{tf} is the final plasma concentration ≥ LOQ, and λ_z, the elimination rate constant, is ln(2) divided by the estimated half-life (i.e. derived directly from the single-exponential decay assumption).

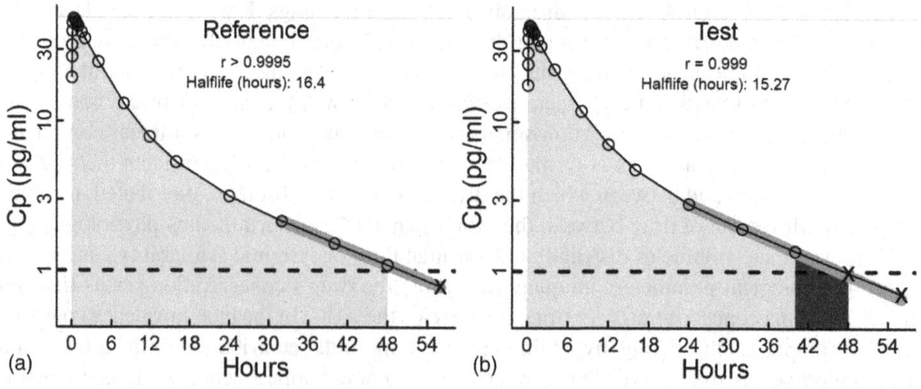

FIGURE 31.4 Plasma concentration vs. time profiles for Reference and Test products illustrating that the use of profile-specific tlast biases the AUCt comparison. Hypothetical plasma concentration (Cp) profiles from a single subject in a two-way bioequivalence crossover study are displayed on semi-log coordinates for Reference (left) and Test (right) products. Values for Test are exactly 90% of the values for Reference. A thin horizontal line appears in both panels at Cmax of Reference. With an LOQ of 1.00 pg/mL (dashed line), circles represent "observed" samples and X indicates samples reported as <LOQ. The AUC0-t calculation for Reference includes the area through 48 hours, whereas AUC0-t for Test is truncated at 40 hours. As a result, the dark gray shaded region (hours 40–48) is included in the calculation of AUC0-t for Reference but not Test. Half-life (calculated from linear regression of the log of the final 3 samples >LOQ) is slightly longer for Reference than Test (*r* for the linear regression is displayed). The fit of the linear regression (extrapolated through hour 56) is shown as a thick gray line.

Although AUC is a direct measure of the extent to which drug is available to the systemic circulation, Cmax is not a direct measure of the rate of availability. Firstly, Cmax is influenced by not only the rate, but also the extent, of absorption (and also the kinetics of the processes of distribution and elimination that remove drug from the circulation, although these are assumed to be characteristics of the drug, not the product, and therefore constant across Test and Reference). After dosing, all plasma drug concentrations will increase in proportion to the extent of absorption, Cmax included. While this issue can be solved by considering the Cmax/AUC ratio,[36–38] the second issue is that Cmax (and Cmax/ AUC) is relatively insensitive to absorption rate. Differences in absorption rate of two- to three-fold were shown to result in a bioequivalence conclusion based on Cmax or Cmax/AUC,[39] because Cmax reflects a balance of absorption and distribution/elimination rates. Thus, Cmax is not correctly interpreted as providing evidence that the rate of drug availability is within the standard –20% to +25%. The time after dosing at which Cmax occurs, Tmax, is relatively more sensitive to absorption rate, but as a categorical metric, Tmax is more difficult to handle in the statistical bioequivalence analysis (nonetheless, Tmax values are a mandatory reported metric in all pharmacokinetic bioequivalence studies). After considerable discussion, the FDA determined that the conventional view of pharmacokinetic bioequivalence as based on measures of the rate and extent of systemic availability should be replaced by a view that the objective of pharmacokinetic bioequivalence is to demonstrate a similar shape of the plasma concentration-versus-time curve. This became known as the "exposure" concept.[43] The maximum concentration (Cmax) and total exposure (AUC) can be directly linked to efficacy and tolerability outcomes for most systemically acting drugs.[40] The "exposure" view of Cmax and AUC applies equally well to the systemic safety assessment of OIDPs, although it remains to be seen how pharmacokinetics will be used to comment on similarity of local drug presentation.

Both Cmax and AUC are assumed to be log-normally distributed, based on both observational and theoretical grounds; values are log-transformed prior to statistical analysis. Consequently, the bioequivalence goalposts, 80.00%–125.00%, are asymmetric on the original scale.

31.3.2.3 Dose Selection

Historically, characterization of the *in vivo* absorption, distribution, metabolism, and elimination of OIDPs often required doses exceeding the labeled dose level and/or measurements in urine instead of plasma. For example, the NDA-enabling single-dose pharmacokinetic studies of low-strength Advair Diskus DPI (fluticasone propionate/salmeterol xinafoate) and low-strength Symbicort pMDI (budesonide/formoterol fumarate) relied on multiple consecutive inhalations to achieve doses five- and six-fold higher, respectively, than the marketed therapeutic doses.[41] Improvements in bioanalytical technology now allow most studies of *in vivo* drug movement to use the marketed dose and to track plasma concentrations instead of urine amounts. These improvements allow improved kinetic resolution of dissolution and subsequent absorption phenomena, which are not readily observable in urine data, and avoid potential loss of product discrimination arising from absorption saturation at supra-marketed dose levels, thereby ensuring that bioequivalence conclusions are directly applicable to the commercial setting. When fronted by liquid-chromatography (LC), advances in tandem mass spectroscopy (MS/MS), in which two stages of mass analysis are used to discriminate chemical signal from chemical noise (for example, from the plasma matrix), allow LC-MS/MS methods to reach sub-pg/mL sensitivity with acceptably small sample volume (≤500 μL). However, most OIDP FDA draft guidance documents continue to recognize the difficulty to pharmacokinetics of the low (by design) plasma concentrations and allow the pharmacokinetic bioequivalence study to be run with the "[m]inimum number of inhalations that is sufficient to characterize a PK profile by using a sensitive analytical method" (e.g.[42–46]).

31.3.2.4 Sensitivity

As a bioassay of product differences, pharmacokinetics is both sensitive and, in some cases, orthogonal to *in vitro* tests. In one example, comparison of Advair Diskus® to a reservoir powder inhalation device (RPID), both containing 250 μg fluticasone propionate with 50 μg salmeterol in a powder formulation,

TABLE 31.2

Dose-Normalized Aerodynamic Particle Size of Fluticasone Propionate from Advair Diskus®

	Dose-normalized emitted mass (μg/μg)	Dose-normalized impactor sized mass (μg/μg)	Dose-normalized <5 μm mass (μg/μg)	Dose-normalized <2 μm mass (μg/μg)
Advair Diskus® 100/50	0.888 ± 0.013	0.297 ± 0.012	0.201 ± 0.014	0.062 ± 0.008
Advair Diskus® 250/50	0.885 ± 0.017	0.278 ± 0.009	0.202 ± 0.005	0.062 ± 0.003
Advair Diskus® 500/50	0.894 ± 0.029	0.279 ± 0.018	0.211 ± 0.019	0.064 ± 0.009

All measurements were collected on a Next Generation Impactor using 4 L of air at a flow rate of 60 L/min. The mass of particles with aerodynamic diameter <5 μm and <2 μm was calculated by Copley Inhaler Testing Data Analysis Software (CITDAS). All inertial impaction data were collected during the dosing period of the corresponding clinical study, whose data are shown in Figure 31.5, below. Thirty (30) individual devices were measured per batch, across a total of 13 batches, 8 batches, and 10 batches of low-, mid-, and high-strength Advair Diskus®. Values represent mean ± standard deviation (SD) of the batch means. All values are normalized by the nominal dose (100 μg, 250 μg, or 500 μg fluticasone propionate). Data courtesy of Oriel Therapeutics, an indirect wholly-owned subsidiary of Novartis Pharma AG.

showed nearly indistinguishable inertial impaction profiles, but approximately two-fold differences in both fluticasone propionate and salmeterol pharmacokinetics.[47] Separately, comparison of fluticasone propionate absorption rate across the Advair Diskus® product strengths demonstrates a formulation effect not apparent in inertial impaction data. Despite dose-proportional aerodynamic particle size distributions (Table 31.2), fluticasone propionate Cmax is proportionally higher for the 100 μg product (median: 48 pg/mL) compared to the 250 μg and 500 μg products (median: 68 pg/mL and 125 pg/mL, respectively) (Figure 31.5).[48] The relatively higher Cmax of the low-strength product is a consequence of faster transfer of drug from the formulation into the blood; median time to peak plasma concentration (T_{max}) is 8 minutes, 30 minutes, and 45 minutes for the 100 μg, 250 μg, and 500 μg strength products, respectively. The Cmax results are not influenced by variation in total systemic dose; AUC is dose proportional. Nor is a direct influence of dose level likely; the pharmacokinetics of fluticasone propionate formulated as an aerosol suspension (specifically, a hydrofluoroalkane metered dose inhaler) are strictly dose-proportional.[49] Thus, fluticasone propionate pharmacokinetics appear to contain information about formulation differences that is not detected by inertial impaction. Current mechanistic models do not describe the dependence of fluticasone propionate dry powder inhaler absorption rate on product strength;[50] pharmacokinetic data were needed to reveal this phenomenon. A number of possibilities exist to explain product differences observable *in vivo*, but not by inertial impaction, including differences in particle composition and microstructure and/or differences in aerosol delivery rate.[51]

The sensitivity of the pharmacokinetic bioassay allows detection even of differences between manufacturing batches of a single product. Lähelmä et al. reported that both budesonide and formoterol Cmax and AUC ratios ranged from ≤0.80 to approximately 0.90 when two batches of Symbicort® Turbuhaler® were compared to each other in a crossover design.[52] Burmeister Getz and colleagues demonstrated differences between manufacturing batches of Advair Diskus® 100/50, also a dry powder inhaler, large enough to meet the FDA's definition of bio-*in*equivalence[53] in two independent studies (Figure 31.6).[54,55] Thus, the sensitivity of the pharmacokinetic assay allowed identification of substantial differences between commercial batches that had passed all *in vitro* release tests.

31.3.2.5 Biorelevance

The goal of bioequivalence testing of pharmaceutically equivalent products is to assess the impact of product and formulation on *in vivo* performance. Once the drug is separated from the formulation, the assumption is that subsequent *in vivo* movement will be independent of whether Test or Reference was administered. The question, then, is: to what extent are circulating blood levels informative of the safety and efficacy consequences of inhaler and formulation differences? The relevance of pharmacokinetic differences to the safety of OIDPs is clear; the adverse effect profile is typically driven by drug exposure at sites accessible by the blood. Additionally, however, pharmacokinetics are influenced by the same factors (inhaler and formulation) that influence dose to the local targets in the lungs (Figure 31.7).

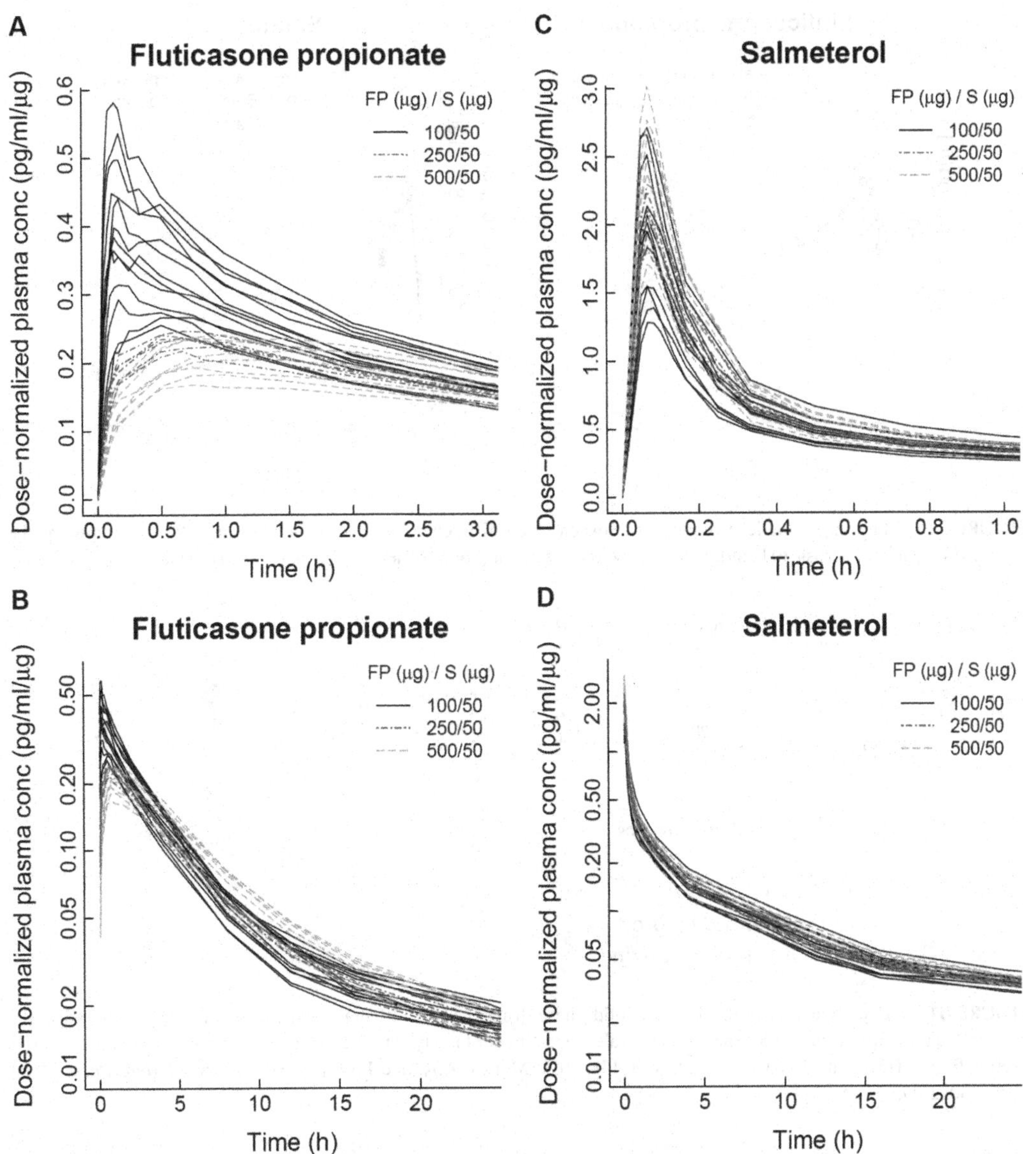

FIGURE 31.5 Pharmacokinetic detection of strength-dependent differences in the rate of drug transfer from formulation to blood for Advair Diskus®. Each profile represents the geometric mean plasma concentration vs nominal time following a single inhalation from a single Advair Diskus® manufacturing batch (A and C: linear scale; B and D: semi-log scale). Fluticasone propionate dose levels are distinguished by shading and line type (100 µg: solid black; 250 µg: dot-dash dark gray; 500 µg: dashed light gray). Concentration values (y-axis) are normalized by the nominal dose (100 µg, 250 µg or 500 µg for FP; 50 µg for salmeterol) to more easily assess the dependence of profile shape on dose level.

As stated by the Pharmaceutical Science Advisory Committee,[56] "it is clear that the connection of PK to product quality is the same whether the site of action is downstream or upstream." For both systemically and locally acting products, pharmacokinetic differences between a Test and a Reference product arise from differences that are upstream of target engagement, regardless of whether or not these targets are accessed via the circulation. However, for locally acting products, the connection between pharmacokinetics and efficacy is not as direct as for drugs that reach their targets via the circulation. For OIDPs, the biorelevance of pharmacokinetics in the bioequivalence assessment, beyond safety, relies on the extent to which pharmacokinetics reflect the portion of the dose giving rise to the therapeutic effect.

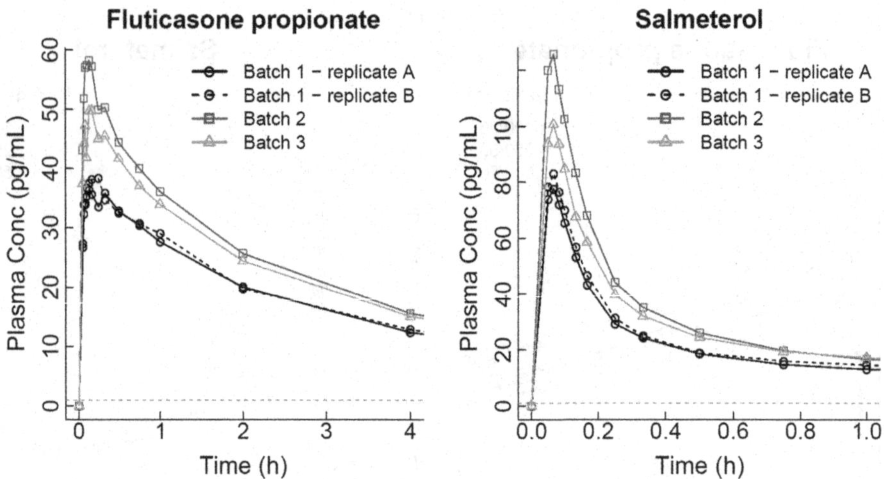

FIGURE 31.6 Pharmacokinetic detection of between-batch differences within Advair Diskus®. Results represent the average by treatment across 30 healthy adults in a four-treatment, four-sequence, four-period crossover design.

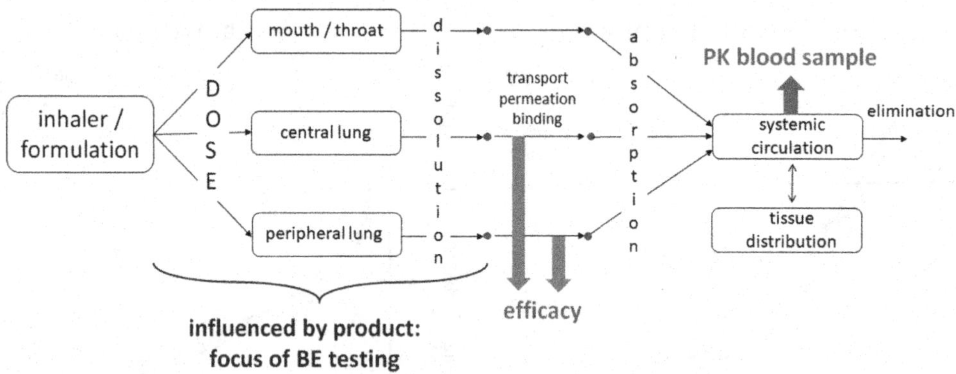

FIGURE 31.7 Locally acting orally inhaled solid phase drugs. (Adapted from Background Information for Advisory Committee for Pharmaceutical Science: Bioequivalence testing for locally acting gastrointestinal drugs, October 20, 2004; Weber, B. and Hochhaus, G., *AAPS J.*, 15, 159–171, 2013; Martin, A.R. and Finlay, W.H., *J. Aerosol Med. Pulm. Drug Deliv.*, 30, 2017.)

31.3.3 Local *In Vivo* Bioequivalence

Notwithstanding the potential for future development, systemic exposure (pharmacokinetics) is currently not considered by the FDA to be a surrogate for local efficacy. There are two primary reasons for this. First, pharmacokinetics can be influenced by absorption of swallowed drug from the gut. Second, pharmacokinetics may reflect drug absorbed from a different part of the lungs than that giving rise to the therapeutic effect. While the first consideration is irrelevant for drugs that experience complete hepatic first-pass metabolism (e.g. fluticasone propionate), some orally inhaled drug substances have >20% oral bioavailability (e.g. beclomethasone, flunisolide). To separate pulmonary and gastrointestinal contributions to total systemic exposure, the European Medicines Agency favors an approach involving two companion pharmacokinetic studies: one with charcoal block, to eliminate the contribution of swallowed drug, thus providing a pharmacokinetic profile that reflects only the lung dose (taken to be a surrogate for efficacy) and one without charcoal block, to measure total systemic exposure (taken to be a surrogate for safety) following product use per the labeled instructions. The FDA, on the other hand, does not recommend charcoal block pharmacokinetic studies on the basis that systemic pharmacokinetics may reflect drug absorbed from a different part of the lungs than that giving rise to the therapeutic effect.

The charcoal block does not address this second issue and so does not allow interpretation of pharmacokinetic bioequivalence as evidence of bioequivalence at the local site of action.

In the U.S., bioequivalence of the local dose is assessed via either a pharmacodynamic (PD) study, using a biomarker that reflects the drug's local pharmacological action or a clinical endpoint (CE) study, using a measure of clinical efficacy. Often, the maximum volume of air that can be forcibly exhaled in one second (FEV_1) is used to measure the drug's effect on lung function. Short-acting β-adrenergic agonists (e.g. albuterol) are commonly assessed using either a bronchoprovocation (dose of an agent, such as methacholine, required to provoke bronchoconstriction, determined as a 20% reduction in FEV_1) or bronchodilatation (area under the FEV_1-versus-time curve for approximately 6 hours post-dose) endpoint following a single dose. Long-acting β-adrenergic agonists (e.g. salmeterol, vilanterol, formoterol) are also assessed using single-dose bronchodilatation (area under the FEV_1-versus-time curve), but for a longer time post-dose, typically to 12 hours or 24 hours. Considerable effort has been invested in evaluating fractional exhaled nitric oxide as a biomarker of the local anti-inflammatory action of inhaled corticosteroids, but to date this assay has not demonstrated satisfactory dose-discriminating ability.[59–65] Instead, bioequivalence of the local corticosteroid dose relies on a measure of pre-dose (trough) FEV_1 following 4 weeks of treatment.

To maximize sensitivity to differences in dose, the PD/CE bioassay is performed at the lowest marketed dose of the Reference product. PD endpoints may be evaluated in a crossover design using the dose-scale method described in the FDA's Draft Guidance on Orlistat,[66] in which bioequivalence is assessed on the product dose ratio (relative bioavailability) corresponding to equal PD effects. The non-linear (saturating) feature of the dose-response curve may be accommodated by widening the bioequivalence goalposts to 67%–150%. Clinical endpoints can be evaluated in either a parallel group or crossover design; while the crossover design requires fewer patients than the parallel design, some drugs (e.g. corticosteroids) may have a washout period that leads to more favorable timelines (and patient retention rates) with a parallel design. Both PD and CE studies involve a placebo treatment arm, which serves to anchor the dose-response curve (for the dose-scale analysis of PD endpoints) or to confirm that the CE product comparison comes from a study with enough dose sensitivity to distinguish active from placebo treatment.

The relative insensitivity to dose is a substantial limitation for the assessment of local OIDP bioequivalence. Not only does this preclude PD/CE evaluation of the higher product strengths, but the low signal:noise ratio, especially for CE studies, leads to very large study sizes (1,000 patients or more). Often, the CE bioequivalence study requires more subjects than were used in the innovator's original confirmatory (phase III) safety and efficacy assessments; this presents a substantial barrier to product development. CE testing is acknowledged, even by regulators, as "an expensive and time-consuming way to attempt to infer the bioequivalence of drug products" and "is the least accurate and reproducible" of the available *in vivo* bioequivalence methodologies.[30] Current regulations require use of "the most accurate, sensitive, and reproducible approach available,"[67] yet despite the shortcomings, to date, no surrogate for the local PD/CE study has been accepted. Clinical endpoint testing is a currently necessary, but unsatisfying, bioequivalence requirement for most locally acting, orally inhaled products. This suggests unrealized potential in our collective understanding of aerosol products and their methods of characterization.

31.3.4 Patient Interface and Product Robustness

Bioequivalence determinations based on the components of the FDA's weight-of-evidence assessment model (qualitative and quantitative formulation sameness, and sameness of emitted dose, aerodynamic particle size distribution, pharmacokinetics, and local effect) can be invalidated if the patient uses the Test product differently than the Reference product. In the extreme, if the Test product is more difficult or less convenient to use, the patient may simply miss more doses with the Test product as compared to the Reference; bioequivalent generics can't match an innovator's safety and efficacy profile if there are differences in compliance with the treatment regimen. Errors in product use, such as incorrect inhalation technique, incorrect priming, or incorrect dose actuation, can also lead to different safety and efficacy profiles of otherwise bioequivalent products. Familiarity with the innovator product is not always adequate to ensure substitutability on the market; sometimes the second-entry product will be the first prescription filled for a new patient. Thus, Test and Reference products should be similar with regard to the ways in which patients interpret instructions for use (including, for example, cleaning), manipulate the device, and make decisions based on feedback from the device (including, for example, information from a dose counter). As stated in the January 2017 draft guidance on drug-device combination product human factors,[68] "FDA expects that end-users of generic [drug-device combination] products ... can use the generic combination product when it is substituted for the RLD without the intervention of the health care provider and/or without additional training prior to use of the generic combination product."

Due to the added complexity inherent in a drug-device combination product, the bioequivalence of a Test product to its Reference listed drug is also potentially affected by differences in product robustness under conditions of patient use. The FDA's 1998 guidance[69] predicted that maintaining critical attributes of DPIs such as dose and particle size distribution under patient-use conditions would "probably present the most formidable challenge" to ensuring the proper functionality of the product over its lifetime. While the intervening 20 years have exposed even greater challenges to development of bioequivalent OIDPs, demonstration of equivalent product robustness remains an important component of the overall assessment of product comparability.

31.4 Future Directions: Clinically Relevant Product Characterization

For systemically acting drug products, the bioequivalence assessment is directly linked to clinical action: the pharmacokinetic bioequivalence assay directly comments on delivery of drug to both therapeutic and toxicological targets. Further, *in vitro* test methods, such as dissolution rate, intestinal permeability, and solubility tests have been developed, standardized, and demonstrated to be indicative of *in vivo* performance for many systemically acting drug products. Standardized procedures to measure solid oral drug product dissolution characteristics and confirm dissolution profile similarity (e.g. using the f_2-test) provide an opportunity for streamlined development, meaningful product specifications, and reduced *in vivo* bioequivalence burden.[70,71] Can a similar approach be identified for OIDPs? Clinically relevant analytical tools could, at least, decrease the need for repetitious and exploratory *in vivo* testing during OIDP development. Importantly, as stated by industry and regulators in the summary report of the March 2009 Product Quality Research Institute (PQRI) workshop on OIDP bioequivalence, "[a] predictive link between the *in vitro* and *in vivo* performance would be highly desirable, and is central to the concept of [bioequivalence],"[72] Efforts to develop clinically relevant *in vitro* testing methods for OIDPs will benefit from synergies amongst related focus areas, including development of physiologically based pharmacokinetic models,[73] understanding the impact of device performance and drug delivery rates,[74] and classification of drug products according to biopharmaceutical properties.[75]

31.4.1 Biopharmaceutics Classification Approaches and Biowaivers

Biopharmaceutics is the relationship between the physical and chemical properties of the drug substance and its dosage form (the drug product) and the rate and extent of drug delivery to the site of action. For systemically acting orally ingested drugs, the rate and extent of systemic absorption are primarily determined by drug dissolution and gastrointestinal permeability. On this basis, the Biopharmaceutical Classification System (BCS) for orally administered drugs divides drug products into four categories: high solubility/high permeability (BCS I), low solubility/high permeability (BCS II), high solubility/low permeability (BCS III), and low solubility/low permeability (BCS IV).[75]

For oral immediate release dosage forms, biowaivers are the regulatory mechanism by which the FDA waives the requirement for *in vivo* bioequivalence testing. For these drug products, current FDA policy allows biowaivers in four general instances: (i) pharmaceutically equivalent solution formulations with no excipient that could significantly affect absorption, (ii) proportionally similar strengths of a drug product that has already demonstrated *in vivo* bioequivalence, (iii) high solubility (BCS Class 1 and 3) drug substances, assuming they meet certain other requirements such as rapid dissolution (Class 1) and very rapid dissolution and the same excipients as the reference product (Class 3) and a therapeutic index that is not narrow, and (iv) demonstration of a validated *in vitro / in vivo* correlation (IVIVC), for instances of manufacturing scale-up or post-approval changes.[76]

Most OIDPs do not conform to any of the scenarios described above for reduced *in vivo* bioequivalence burden. The majority of OIDPs are formulated as a suspension or powder, not a solution. Most do not have active and excipient proportionality across the product strengths. Many, notably the corticosteroids, are poorly soluble. None have a validated IVIVC (at least not one that has been published). *In vitro* tests are not easily validated as assays of biorelevant product comparison. Biorelevant *in vitro* tests have limitations; particle size determination is blind to the chemical composition or physicochemical properties of the particle, and dissolution test methods have yet to be harmonized and validated and therefore no similarity tests can be conducted. Differences in drug product device design between an innovator device and that of a generics product can impact the dose, deposition pattern, and the rate of the drug delivery to the lungs. As a consequence, the bioequivalence assessment of most OIDPs involves *in vivo* testing. Can *in vitro* test methods be developed to assess the relevant physicochemical properties and thus help to reduce the regulatory burden of OIDP bioequivalence as has been done for solid oral immediate release dosage forms?

31.4.1.1 Physicochemical Properties of Orally Inhaled Drugs and the BCS

The physiology of the delivery site for orally administered drugs differs substantially from that of inhaled drugs (Table 31.3). Therefore, the equations and relationships derived for the oral BCS approach cannot be directly applied to orally inhaled drugs without making the appropriate adjustment to the transport models to take into account parameters associated with lung physiology.

Also, as a "drugability" guide, the oral BCS is not directly applicable to locally acting inhaled products. While oral drugs rely on efficient systemic absorption for their therapeutic effect, locally acting inhaled drugs are designed specifically to minimize systemic exposure. The desired product profile for an oral therapeutic is therefore significantly different from a locally acting pulmonary therapeutic (Table 31.4).

Since the desired product profile is different for inhaled drugs, the physicochemical properties of inhaled therapeutics with local activity are expected to differ from their oral counterparts. A comparison of the physicochemical properties of oral versus inhaled therapeutics was published in 2011 by Selby et al.[76] Selby and colleagues at Pfizer evaluated 28 compounds spanning five classes of inhalation compounds from the patent literature and concluded that inhaled drugs have more hydrogen bonding, a higher polar surface area, and a larger number of rotatable bonds when compared to oral therapeutics (Table 31.5). These findings are further supported by Ritchie et al.,[77] who concluded that the locally acting compounds delivered via the inhaled route, and marketed at the time of the evaluation, have a higher

TABLE 31.3
Physiological Comparison Between the gastrointestinal (GI) and the Lung in Healthy Humans

Property	Gastrointestinal Tract	Lung
Typical Site of Action	Systemic	Local
Transit Time/Residence Time	199 minutes (mean intestinal transit time)	1 hour–24 hours
"Fluid" Volume	50 mL–1100 mL average: 500 mL	10 mL–70 mL[15,78,79]
"Fluid" Properties	Bulk liquid Location specific pH	Surface fluid layers. Location-specific viscosity, composition, and thickness.
pH Range **(fasted state)**	Range: 1.4–7.4 Stomach: 1.4–2.1 Duodenum: 4.4–6.6 Ileum: 6.5–7.4	6.69 ± 0.07[18]
Surface area	Mucosal surface area:[80] 30 m²–40 m²	Central: 1 m²–2.5 m² Peripheral: 100 m²–140 m²

Source: Hastedt, J.E., The lung as a dissolution vessel? *Inhalation Magazine*, December, 18–22, 2014.

TABLE 31.4

Desired Properties of Oral versus Inhaled Therapeutics

Properties	Oral Drugs	Inhaled Drugs with Local Target
Distribution	Systemic	Local to Lung
Systemic Absorption	Rapid	Low to None
Systemic Clearance	Slow	Rapid
Protein Binding or Retention Time	Low	High
Oral Bioavailability	High	Low

Source: Yeadon, M., *Future Med. Chem.*, 3, 1581–1583, 2011.

TABLE 31.5

Physicochemical Properties of Oral versus Inhaled Therapeutics by Class

Class	Avg. Mol. Weight (SD)	Avg. H-bond Count (SD)	Avg. Polar Surface Area (Å²) (SD)	Avg. Rotatable Bond Count (SD)
LABA	498 (80.29)	11.00 (2.12)	116.63 (28.53)	13.00 (4.30)
LAMA	385 (63.39)	3.50 (1.50)	43.15 (11.80)	6.00 (2.35)
MABA	717 (58.22)	12.82 (1.80)	148.5 (23.97)	16.73 (2.83)
PDE4 Muscarinic duals	691 (32.29)	11.25 (1.30)	122.50 (9.66)	12.25 (1.30)
Phosphate prodrugs	969 (102.88)	13.20 (2.48)	173.00 (31.72)	26.2 (2.32)
Oral	305 (91.00)	6.04 (2.92)	60.37 (32.27)	4.70 (2.69)
Inhaled	370 (103.00)	8.31 (3.25)	89.20 (38.65)	5.10 (2.76)

Source: Selby, M.D. et al., *Future Med. Chem.*, 3, 1679–1701.

Abbreviations: LABA, long-acting beta-2 agonist; LAMA, long-acting muscarinic antagonist; MABA, muscarinic antagonist-beta 2 agonist; PDE4, phosphodiesterase type 4 inhibitors; and SD, standard deviation.

polar surface area, a higher molecular weight, and trend towards lower lipophilicity relative to oral therapeutics. Edwards et al. defined a quantitative structure-activity relationship (QSAR) model that linked physicochemical properties to pulmonary absorption.[82] The authors generated data from an isolated perfused respiring rat lung model for 82 drug discovery compounds and 17 marketed drugs and built a quantitative structure-activity relationship based on physicochemical properties of permeability, hydrophobicity, ionization, and molecular size. Both increased permeability and hydrophobicity enhanced pulmonary absorption (and therefore systemic exposure), while the increasing charge and molecule size negatively impacted absorption from the lung (decreased systemic exposure). All of these identified trends for OIDPs deviate from the Lipinski Rule of five which describes physicochemical guideposts for drugs delivered systemically by the oral route of administration.[83]

31.4.1.2 Critical Product Attributes of Orally Inhaled Drugs

For all drug products, the establishment of a clinically relevant specification requires the understanding of key molecular properties of the drug that influence performance (e.g. solubility, dissolution, and membrane permeability), the development of *in vitro* product performance test methods capable of measuring these attributes using biorelevant conditions, and an understanding of how the *in vivo* environment influences drug disposition. For OIDPs, in addition to the basic physiochemical properties of the drug, the physiology of the lung coupled with the patient, device, and formulation influence aerosol deposition and disposition and therefore impact *in vivo* product performance.

Qualitative and quantitative formulation sameness and sameness of the delivered dose and APSD are required attributes for the Test and Reference products in an OIDP BE assessment. Therefore, given the same dose, deposition pattern, and formulation sameness, an assumption can be made that product-specific attributes such as differences in the release of the drug from the formulation (e.g. dissolution rate) will be more impactful on the overall BE than the molecule-specific properties (e.g. absorption, diffusion, and solubility). However, even though an OIDP BE assessment may require only a subset of drug and drug product properties, all of the attributes are important to the development of an inhalation BCS. Streamlined product development and scientifically justified regulatory relief pathways based on *in vitro* assessment for OIDP products will require OIDP classification in a manner similar to the oral BCS. Therefore, in the following sections, the mechanistic and molecular principles that impact overall pulmonary product performance, such as pulmonary deposition and regional dose, regional dissolution, regional permeability, and tissue retention will be discussed.

31.4.1.2.1 Pulmonary Deposition: Total and Regional Dose

The mass of drug deposited in a lung region can be considered in the context of the solubility of the drug and the volume of fluid available for dissolution; this dimensionless value is referred to as the dose number and derived in the oral BCS model. It has been demonstrated that distribution of the lung dose can be estimated for various pulmonary compartments (e.g. central and peripheral airways) by using mathematical modeling and aerosol deposition patterns obtained by gamma scintigraphy as a function of time[84,85] as well as mathematically derived *in vitro* regional deposition patterns using various anatomical throat models.[86,87] If the central and peripheral pulmonary deposited doses can be measured, then the regional dose numbers can be calculated using a modified version of the gastrointestinal BCS relationship shown in Equation 31.6 for centrally deposited drug (Do_c) and Equation 31.7 for peripherally deposited drug (Do_p).

$$\mathrm{Do}_c = \frac{M_c / V_c}{C_{\mathrm{sc}}} \tag{31.6}$$

$$\mathrm{Do}_p = \frac{M_p / V_p}{C_{\mathrm{sp}}} \tag{31.7}$$

where M is the amount of drug deposited in the central or peripheral compartment, V is the effective volume of ASL available for dissolution in the central or peripheral compartment, and C_s is the solubility in the biorelevant media associated with the compartment at neutral pH. If the dose number is less than 1, the delivered dose is assumed to be fully dissolved and therefore once the drug is released from the formulation, it will be in solution. Calculating regional dose numbers means that the volume and accessibility of the ASL per region as well as the media compositions to be used to measure solubility need to be determined, which is not trivial. Numerous researchers are making advances in this research area in an effort to identify standardized biorelevant media.[88–93]

As an illustrative example, assuming an aqueous ASL volume of 10 mL in the central airways and an estimated centrally deposited dose (M_c), the centrally deposited dose number (Do_c) can be calculated using Equation 31.6 (Table 31.6).[94] Drugs with dose numbers greater than 1 may be dissolution limited in the central airways and therefore susceptible to mucociliary clearance, which impacts the effective regional dose to the central lung. The ICS drugs are a class of potent compounds that have low aqueous solubility values in the range of 0.1 mcg/mL. These compounds, especially fluticasone propionate, have been extensively studied and besides being of low solubility, are known to have high receptor affinity and long receptor half-lives, which are thought to contribute to a long residence time in lung tissue.[95–98]

TABLE 31.6
Central Deposition Dose Number Estimates

Drug	Class	Dose Number (Do)
Amphotericin B	AB	150
Fluticasone propionate	ICS	27
Beclomethasone dipropionate	ICS	15
Ciprofloxacin betaine	AB	12
Mometasone furoate	ICS	3
Tobramycin sulfate	AB	0.1
Salmeterol xinafoate	LABA	0.005
Albuterol sulfate	SABA	0.0001
Ipratropium bromide	SAMA	0.00002
Formoterol fumarate	LABA	0.00001
Tiotropium bromide	LAMA	0.00001

Abbreviations: AB, antibiotic, ICS, inhaled corticosteroid, LABA, long-acting beta-2 agonist; LAMA, long-acting muscarinic antagonist; MABA, muscarinic antagonist-beta 2 agonist; PDE4, phosphodiesterase type 4 inhibitors; and SD, standard deviation.

31.4.1.2.2 Regional Dissolution and Diffusion of the Deposited Dose

Dissolution is defined as the rate of solution of solid in a liquid. The rate of dissolution is described by equations such as the Noyes Whitney[99] equation as shown below in Equations 31.8 and 31.9; and the dissolution rate constant, *k*, as provided in Equation 31.10.

$$\frac{dM}{dt}=\frac{\mathrm{DS}}{h}(C_s-C) \tag{31.8}$$

$$\frac{dC}{dt}=k(C_s-C) \tag{31.9}$$

$$k=\frac{D\times S}{h\times V} \tag{31.10}$$

The relationship demonstrates that the dissolution of a solid (expressed as mass of drug (*M*) in Equation 31.8 or concentration of drug (*C*) in Equation 31.9) as a function of time (*t*) in a liquid is dependent upon the diffusion coefficient of the drug (*D*), the surface area available for dissolution (*S*), the thickness of the diffusion layer (*h*), the volume of liquid available for dissolution (*V*), and the concentration gradient between the solid surface and in the surrounding solution ($C_s - C$) or (ΔC), where C_s is the solubility of the drug in the media and *C* is the concentration of the drug in the bulk solution. Under sink conditions, $C = 0$, and for this specific condition, the driving force for dissolution is the solubility of the compound in the dissolution media.

In addition to the dose number, the BCS model defines a dimensionless value to describe the relative rate of dissolution as the ratio between the residence time and the time for dissolution. For the lung, if the time for complete dissolution is greater than the residence time, then the undissolved drug could be cleared by mucociliary clearance (central deposition) or macrophages (alveolar deposition). If the dissolution time is less than the residence time, then it is expected that complete dissolution will occur.

Using a biorelevant dissolution test method (appropriate regional media, volume, dose, particle size, and distribution), a dissolution rate constant could be measured. However, since there are non-dissolution-related mechanisms that impact transport as well as clearance in both the central and peripheral regions of the lung, dissolution testing alone cannot predict observed *in vivo* differences. For instance, the relationship that describes both dissolution and diffusion needs to be utilized (Equation 31.11) in situations where dissolution and diffusion contribute to transport to the epithelium. This relationship includes both Fick's second law and the Noyes Whitney equation.

$$\frac{\partial C}{\partial t} = D\frac{\partial^2 C}{\partial x^2} + k(C_s - C) \tag{31.11}$$

When dissolution is the rate limiting component, Equation 31.11 becomes the Noyes Whitney equation. When diffusion is the rate limiting component, the relationship becomes Fick's second law, which describes the change in concentration over time of a diffusing species. Solving this relationship in these two extremes results in the following[100]:

$$\frac{M_t}{M_\infty} = 2\frac{C_s}{C_0}\sqrt{\frac{Dk}{h^2}}\left(\frac{1}{2k} + t\right) \tag{31.12}$$

$$\frac{M_t}{M_\infty} = 4\frac{C_s}{C_0}\left(\frac{Dt}{\pi h^2}\right)^{\frac{1}{2}} \tag{31.13}$$

Where Equation 31.12 describes the dissolution dominated transport, and Equation 31.13 describes the diffusion dominated transport, and M_∞ is the total mass of drug deposited per unit area. Based on these relationships, we can conclude that diffusion dominated transport will be square root time based and dissolution dominated transport will be linear with time. It is anticipated that transport to the epithelium in the ciliated, mucus-lined, upper airways will be diffusion controlled, whereas transport to the epithelium layer in the alveoli will be dissolution controlled due to the thin layer of lipid lining the alveoli.

31.4.1.2.3 Regional Absorption and Permeability of the Deposited Dose

Once the dissolved drug reaches the epithelium, in order to reach the bloodstream, it must have the ability to partition into and diffuse across the epithelium. This is a molecule-specific transport process and therefore, once the drug is dissolved, absorption will be dictated by the physicochemical properties of the chemical species. Also, for OIDPs, which are locally acting, the appearance of the drug in the systemic circulation does not necessarily reflect its therapeutic effect since the site of action is in the lung. Since measuring blood levels is easier than measuring the concentration at the local pulmonary site of action, and it plays an important role in establishing the safety of the inhaled drug product, an understanding of absorption is important for inhaled drug product development. Absorption is also an attribute that will be used in the inhalation BCS, but it may not be relevant for bioequivalence assessment for generic drugs.

According to Fick's first law, the amount of material flowing through a unit cross section of a barrier in unit time (*t*), the flux (*J*) is proportional to the concentration gradient across the barrier, *dC/dx* (Equation 31.14). The proportionality term in this equation is the diffusion coefficient of the drug in the media, *D*. For biological systems, this relationship can be modified to include the partition coefficient (*K*) and the membrane thickness (*h*) to describe membrane permeability (*P*) (Equation 31.15). Replacing the diffusion coefficient with permeability results in Equation 31.16, which states that the flux across a membrane is driven by the concentration gradient across the membrane where the proportionality term is the membrane permeability.

$$J = \frac{dM}{S \cdot dt} = -D\frac{dC}{dx} \tag{31.14}$$

$$P = \frac{DK}{h} \tag{31.15}$$

$$J = P\Delta C \tag{31.16}$$

Like dissolution, absorption rates are expected to differ across the lung regions, and, therefore, the deposition pattern is critical to understanding the time course of the appearance of the drug in the blood.

The absorptive flux across biological membranes is driven by the permeability and the concentration gradient as described by Equation 31.16. The absorption number (An) from the BCS is the ratio of the residence time to the absorption time and is inversely related to the absorption rate constant. In order to determine the absorption number, data from pharmacokinetic studies and/or permeability using well-characterized/standardized cell cultures are needed. It is anticipated that absorption rates from the central airways will be different than from the peripheral airways. Therefore, more than one cell culture model may be needed to describe permeability.

The oral BCS absorption number (An) is calculated using the derived equations provided below (Equations 31.17 and 31.18).

$$\text{An} = \frac{P_{\text{eff}}}{R} \cdot t_{\text{res}} = \frac{t_{\text{res}}}{t_{\text{abs}}} \tag{31.17}$$

and

$$\frac{1}{t_{\text{abs}}} = k_{\text{abs}} = \left(\frac{S}{V}\right) \cdot P_{\text{eff}} = 2 \cdot \frac{P_{\text{eff}}}{R} \tag{31.18}$$

where $1/t_{abs}$ is the effective absorption rate constant, P_{eff} is the effective permeability through the membrane, S is the surface area available for absorption, R is the radius of the tubular space, and V is the volume. Again, since the residence time in the lung for a pulmonary therapeutic is molecule dependent, the absorption number cannot be calculated *a priori.* However, assuming that absorption can be modeled by a first-order reaction, the apparent first-order absorption rate constant, k_{abs}, can be used to determine the absorption time and the absorption half-life can be calculated using Equation 31.19.

$$k_{\text{abs}} = \frac{\ln 2}{t_{1/2}} \tag{31.19}$$

Numerous cell cultures have been used to measure permeability of drugs. For GI transport, the Caco-2 cell monolayers have been extensively used. Correlations have been attempted to link *in vivo* transport across lung epithelium to *in vitro* Caco-2 permeability values using physicochemical properties.[101] These authors found a strong correlation between absorption and permeability for the ten small molecules investigated.

The various cellular models for pulmonary absorption are provided in Table 31.7. Much needed efforts aimed at the understanding of the limitations and impact of cellular models and the role of drug transporters in the lung are underway.[102]

31.4.1.2.4 Pulmonary Retention Time

It is important to note that the residence time in the lung is not a parameter that can be estimated using the simple fluid flow in a tube approach used for the oral BCS. Instead, the residence time in the lung is dictated by the clearance mechanisms of "the bucket" (e.g. mucociliary clearance and macrophages), regional solubility, receptor binding at the local site of action, and transport mechanisms.

Retention time in an inhalation BCS model may not be possible to calculate if receptor binding is the rate limiting factor to systemic bioavailability for locally acting drugs. Instead, factors such as deposition pattern, regional dissolution, and diffusional transport to the receptor location may be more important attributes that impact efficacy. Bioequivalence will be complicated by receptor affinity and retention.

TABLE 31.7
Cellular Models for Inhalation

Name	Species	Origin	Region	Characteristics
Caco-2	Human	Colorectal adenocarcinoma	Small intestine	Enterocytes Tight junctions Microvilli Enzymes and transporters
NHBE	Human	Primary cells	Bronchi	Mucus production Functional tight junctions Confluent layers
Calu-3		Bronchial adenocarcinoma		Expression of tight junctions Metabolic capacity Mucus production under AIC
16HBE14o-		Transformed bronchial epithelial cells		Basal cell morphology Tight junctions, microvilli, cilia
Alveolar epithelial cells	Rat Human Pig	Primary cells	Alveoli	Type II type I trans-differentiation Tight epithelial barrier

Source: Ehrhardt, C. et al., *J. Pharm. Sci.*, 106, 2234–2244, 2017; Exiarch, H. et al., *J. Epithel. Biol. Pharmacol.*, 3, 1–14, 2010.

31.4.2 Trends in Understanding Regional Drug Deposition and Disposition

The use of computational fluid dynamics (CFD) and physiologically based pharmacokinetic models (PBPK) has increased in the field of pulmonary drug delivery. When mechanistic computer-based models are coupled with techniques such as gamma scintigraphy, they can aid in our understand of dose, deposition, and disposition of OIDPs. The sections that follow review a few references that are relevant to this effort.

31.4.2.1 Total and Regional Drug Deposition

In vitro testing conditions that mimic clinical use are valuable for predicting clinical outcome, optimizing patient use instructions and providing guidance to health care providers.[103] While cascade (i.e. inertial) impaction testing has a long history of use in routine quality control testing, its ability to deliver biopredictive sizing within the respirable particle population (typically considered to be particles with aerodynamic diameter less than approximately 5 μm) is still an area of active development. Use of anatomically realistic models of the human respiratory tract, especially models of the human mouth and throat used in place of the standard induction port, as well as use of physiological inspiratory flow rates, have been investigated as a means to improve the *in vivo* predictive ability of APSD information coming from the cascade impactor. In some instances, the use of realistic head/throat models and physiological air flows have resulted in *in vitro* predictions of total lung deposition and systemic availability that show agreement with *in vivo* pharmacokinetic measures.[97] Computational fluid dynamics techniques, using complex mathematical models of lung morphology and airflow, have been also investigated with the goal of describing the probability of regional deposition for a given OIDP under a specific set of use conditions. Excellent reviews of *in vitro* approaches to estimate or predict the extent and pattern of deposition are available in the review of the 2015 Congress of the International Society for Aerosols in Medicine[104] and from a 2010 session on pharmaceutical aerosol deposition modeling.[105] Importantly, for pulmonary drug products that are neither highly soluble nor rapidly absorbed, the clinical relevance of *in vitro* dissolution and permeability test methods is predicated on the accurate estimation of deposition pattern because of the expected differences in dissolution and permeation across lung regions, as described above.

31.4.2.2 *Physiologically Based Models and Drug Disposition*

Physiologically based mechanistic and pharmacokinetic models for OIDPs are composite models incorporating information about not only regional deposition pattern, but also regional airway surface liquid volumes and clearance mechanisms, drug dissolution characteristics, and drug disposition processes to collectively describe the *in vivo* fate of an OIDP actuation.[58,73,106] The underlying hypothesis is that, although the complete path of an inhaled medicinal drug particle (involving initial entrainment in the inspiratory airflow, formulation dispersion, respiratory tract deposition, dissolution, absorption, tissue distribution, and ultimately elimination from the body), is complex, it is predictable. Recent advances in computational modeling are being used to predict exposure based on an understanding of the fundamental mechanisms that control the rate and extent of delivery in the lungs. However, to be beneficial, these models need to include values for dose deposition patterns, and location-based solubility, dissolution, permeability, and non-absorptive clearance. Standardized and validated approaches to measure these quantities are currently unavailable; however, several publications have appeared within the last few years that provide insight into the role these parameters can play on bioequivalence, especially for poorly soluble OIDPs, as described below.

To understand the impact of physicochemical properties on absorption and drug retention in the lungs, a cell-based computational model was developed.[107] Using cells and tissues of excised rat lungs, the authors were able to demonstrate that both the physicochemical properties of monobasic molecules and the regional lung location directly impacted the absorption half-life and distribution in the lung. Absorption rate constants calculated based on the pKa, logP, and the molecular radius of nine monocharged molecules compared fairly well to experimental findings. This research supports the concept that an understanding of the physicochemical properties and lung location are important to understand drug disposition in the lung.

For a poorly soluble drug, a series of deposition models for dose were shown to correlate poorly with AUC clinical data.[108] Using the physicochemical properties of the drug, dose deposition patterns, and systemic PK parameters, the authors were able to successfully simulate systemic plasma exposure using GastroPlus™ software for the same series of various formulations of the insoluble drug. The authors concluded that the predicted dominating regional bioavailability from the alveolar region (100%) relative to the low percent predicted from the central airways does not lead to a good understanding of regional deposition when assessing PK data. This research suggests that for poorly soluble drugs, the rate and extent of absorption is impacted by the regional distribution of the deposited drug.

In a retrospective analysis, two semi-mechanistic simulation models were used to predict the systemic pharmacokinetics of inhaled corticosteroids delivered with dry powder inhalers.[54] This research utilized *in vitro* data as model input parameters to predict plasma concentration-time profiles. For the poorly soluble lipophilic drugs, the authors assumed that dissolution was the rate-limiting step to absorption. One approach used solubility in a "biorelevant" media to predict the *in vivo* solubility while the other used *in vitro* dissolution to determine the mean dissolution time (MDT) to predict the pulmonary absorption rate. Both approaches were used to compare the *in vitro* data to the *in vivo* data with some success, but the MDT approach was less labor intensive. This research demonstrates the need for generating standardized biorelevant media and dissolution test methods to better characterize poorly soluble drugs.

31.4.3 Biorelevant Critical Attributes for OIDPs

Based on the mechanistic and molecular properties and the research efforts discussed in the previous sections, assuming the same delivery device, the most critical biorelevant attributes of an OIDP formulation are *regional deposition patterns and dose and physicochemical properties*. The amount of drug deposited regionally (regional dose), the physicochemical properties of the drug, and where it lands will determine the time it takes to dissolve, diffuse, and appear both at the local pharmacological target and in the blood. Based on the biopharmaceutical principles discussed, the appearance of drug in systemic circulation for drugs with high solubility in all regions of the lung will be dependent upon the rate of drug diffusion to the epithelium and permeability through the epithelium. Drugs of low solubility in lung fluids may be dissolution limited. The regional dose and deposition patterns of low solubility drugs will impact the rate and extent of absorption of the deposited drug. Therefore, *in vitro* test methods will need to focus on biopredictive tools to determine the *pulmonary dose as a function of deposition location* as well as the media and volumes available for solubility and dissolution measurements. The permeability of a compound is driven by biology and molecular properties of the drug, and, given the same dose deposition rate, pattern, and dissolution rate, shouldn't play a major role in bioequivalence, but will remain an important attribute for pulmonary drug classification. In addition, the *in vitro* data generated using methods based on an understanding of local pulmonary physiology, pulmonary drug deposition patterns, regional dose, and dissolution using biorelevant media and conditions will inform the mechanistic computer modeling approaches and lead to a better understanding of the properties needed to develop successful pulmonary drug products.

31.5 Conclusions

The regulatory pathway for bioequivalence testing in the U.S., including generic substitution, is well defined for OIDPs by the FDA's weight-of-evidence paradigm. This panel of tests acknowledges administration site heterogeneity and local drug action, as well as the dependence of product performance on characteristics of patient use. *In vitro* tests provide sensitive product discrimination in emitted dose and aerodynamic particle size for a wide range of test conditions (e.g. inspiratory flow rate, device life stage, orientation), but do not capture patient use interactions or particle composition. The pharmacokinetic bioassay provides sensitive *in vivo* product discrimination based on well-established systemic exposure metrics, but is not directly linked to the local effect. Pharmacodynamic or clinical endpoint comparisons are directly relevant to the local therapeutic effect, but often lack dose-discriminating sensitivity and can, therefore, require large clinical studies. Consistent with the bioequivalence objective to avoid unnecessary repetition in clinical testing, improvements in product understanding and characterization may eventually allow the field of inhalation medicine to meet the challenges of complex OIDPs without substantial clinical burden.

Approaches based on molecular and mechanistic properties of the drug and drug product, like an iBCS coupled with CFD approaches and mechanistic computational models, have the potential to streamline both the development and regulatory review of inhalation drug products. Development of a classification system for inhaled drugs could lead to a better understanding of the key *in vitro* attributes impacting product *in vivo* performance by "class" of drug (or drug product) and when combined with computational approaches may lead to similar streamlined development and regulatory benefits as achieved for immediate release oral drug products. Identifying biopharmaceutical attributes of a drug substance and/or drug product that impact *in vitro* product performance provide not only the ability to control product quality, but can lead to a better understanding of product performance *in vivo*. With this "enlightened" understanding, test methods become more than quality control tools; they become clinically relevant test methods, and therefore bio-predictive.

For locally acting OIDPs, the physiologically important mechanisms that determine drug delivery to the site of action include dissolution of the inhaled dose and uptake by pulmonary tissue (analogous to oral drugs), but also regional airway deposition pattern and perhaps additional post-deposition events, e.g. particle clearance rates and diffusion from the deposition site to the epithelial surface and protein binding. Events occurring after dissolution are not directly influenced by formulation or delivery device; after dissolution, the body does not distinguish a "Test product" drug molecule from a "Reference product" drug molecule. However, the relevance of a dissolution test may be predicated on whether dissolution is rate-limiting relative to the other physiological processes.

The inhalation BCS is more complex than its gastrointestinal counterpart because of the interactions between the formulation, the delivery device, and the human user confound the interpretation of any one test, and therefore the dose delivered to the site of action, and the rate at which that delivery is achieved, are not entirely controlled by the formulation. If the interactions can be understood by combining the classification system approach with computational fluid dynamics modeling and mechanistic computer models, or at least captured by a relevant span of testing conditions, an adequate repertoire of validated *in vitro* tests methods, combined with *in vivo* pharmacokinetics, may eventually be able to replace the high-resource clinical endpoint/pharmacodynamic *in vivo* studies in the weight-of-evidence paradigm.

REFERENCES

1. https://www.fda.gov/Drugs/ResourcesForYou/Consumers/BuyingUsingMedicineSafely/GenericDrugs/default.htm
2. Smith, E. W., Meyer, E., Haigh, J. M., Maibach, H. I. 1991. "The human skin blanching assay for comparing topical corticosteroid availability." *Journal of Dermatological Treatment* 2 (2): 69–72.
3. Code of Federal Regulations—Title 21 [21 CFR], Part 314.3
4. Peters, J. R., Hixon, D. R., Conner, D. P., Davit, B. M., Catterson, D. M., Parise, C. M. 2009. "Generic drugs—Safe, effective, and affordable." *Dermatologic Therapy 22*: 229–240.
5. Davit, B. M., Nwakama, P. E., Buehler, G. J., Conner, D., Haidar, S. H., Patel, D.T. et al. 2009. "Comparing generic and innovator drugs: A review of 12 years of bioequivalence data from the United States Food and Drug Administration." *Annals of Pharmacotherapy* 43(10): 1583–1597.
6. Draft Guidance on Progesterone. *U.S. Department of Health and Human Services, Food and Drug Administration Center for Drug Evaluation and Research*, February 2011.
7. Draft Guidance on Warfarin Sodium. *U.S. Department of Health and Human Services, Food and Drug Administration Center for Drug Evaluation and Research*, December 2012.
8. Draft Guidance on Permethrin. *U.S. Department of Health and Human Services, Food and Drug Administration*, October 2017.
9. Yu, L. X. and Li, B. V., eds. *FDA Bioequivalence Standards*. Springer. New York. 2014.
10. Hickey, A. J. 2017. "Complexity in pharmaceutical powders for inhalation: A perspective." *KONA Powder and Particle Journal* 1–11.
11. Adams, W. P., Ahrens, R. C., Chen, M. L., Christopher, D., Chowdhury, B. A., Conner, D. P., Dalby, R. et al. 2010. "Demonstrating bioequivalence of locally acting orally inhaled drug products (OIPs): Workshop summary report." *Journal of Aerosol Medicine and Pulmonary Drug Delivery* 23(1): 1–29.
12. https://www.fda.gov/Drugs/ResourcesForYou/Consumers/BuyingUsingMedicineSafely/GenericDrugs/ucm592245.htm, accessed 25 March 2018).
13. Newman, S. 2009. Chapter 1: The background to pulmonary drug delivery in man, In *Respiratory Drug Delivery Essential Theory & Practice* (p. 30). RDD Online: Richmond, VA.
14. Hastedt, J. E. 2014. "The lung as a dissolution vessel?" *Inhalation Magazine*. December, 18–22.
15. Widdicombe, J. G. 1997. "Airway liquid: A barrier to drug diffusion?" *European Respiratory Journal* 10 (October): 2194–2197. doi:10.1183/09031936.97.10102194.
16. Patton, J. S. 1996. "Mechanisms of macromolecule absorption by the lungs." *Advanced Drug Delivery Reviews* 19: 3–36.
17. Eixarch, H., Haltner-Ukomadu, E., Beisswenger, C., Bock, U. 2010. "Drug delivery to the lung: Permeability and physicochemical characteristics of drugs as the basis for a pulmonary biopharmaceutical classification system (pBCS)." *Journal of Epithelial Biology & Pharmacology* 3: 1–14.
18. Effros, R. M., and Chinard, F. P. 1969. "The in vivo pH of the extravascular space of the lung." *Journal of Clinical Investigation* 48: 1983–1996. doi:10.1172/JCI106164.
19. Hastedt, J. E., Bäckman, P., Clark, A. R., Doub, W., Hickey, A., Hochhaus, G., Kuehl, P. J. et al. 2016. "Scope and relevance of a pulmonary biopharmaceutical classification system AAPS/FDA/USP workshop March 16–17th, 2015 in Baltimore, MD." *AAPS Open* 2 (1). AAPS Open: 1. doi:10.1186/s41120-015-0002-x.
20. Patton, J. S., Brain, J. D., Davies, L. A., Fiegel, J., Gumbleton, M., Kim, K. J., Sakagami, M., Vanbever, R. and Ehrhardt, C. 2010. "The particle has landed—Characterizing the fate of inhaled pharmaceuticals." *Journal of Aerosol Medicine and Pulmonary Drug Delivery* 23 (Suppl 2): S71–S87. doi:10.1089/jamp.2010.0836.
21. Ehrhardt, C. 2017. "Inhalation biopharmaceutics: Progress towards comprehending the fate of inhaled medicines." *Pharmaceutical Research*., 1–3. doi:10.1007/s11095-017-2304-2.
22. Weibel E. R. (1963) "Geometry and dimensions of airways of the respiratory zone." In: *Morphometry of the Human Lung*. Springer-Verlag, Berlin, Heidelberg.
23. Draft Guidance on Budesonide. *U.S. Department of Health and Human Services, Food and Drug Administration*, September 2012.

24. Morgan, B., Chen, S., Christopher, D., Långström, G., Wiggenhorn, C., Burmeister Getz, E. et al. 2018. "Performance of the population bioequivalence (PBE) statistical test using an IPAC-RS database of delivered dose from metered dose inhalers." *AAPS PharmSciTech*, 19 (3): 1410–1425. doi: 10.1208/s12249-017-0941-8. [Epub ahead of print]).
25. Bioequivalence: Blood level bioequivalence study. VICH GL52. VICH Steering Committee, September 2014.
26. Guidance for Industry: *Bioavailability and Bioequivalence Studies Submitted in NDAs or INDs—General Considerations*. U.S. Department of Health and Human Services, Food and Drug Administration Center for Drug Evaluation and Research, March 2014.
27. El-Tahtawy, A. A., Jackson, A. J., Ludden, T. M. 1994. "Comparison of single and multiple dose pharmacokinetics using clinical bioequivalence data and monte carlo simulations." *Pharmaceutical Research 11* (9): 1330–1336.
28. Daley-Yates, P. T., Tournant, J., Kunka R. L. 2000. "Comparison of the systemic availability of fluticasone propionate in healthy volunteers and patients with asthma." *Clinical Pharmacokinetics. 39* (1): 39–45.
29. Brutsche, M. H., Brutsche, I. C., Munavvar, M., Langley, S. J., Masterson, C. M., Daley-Yates, P. T., Brown, R., Custovic, A., Woodcock, A. 2000. "Comparison of pharmacokinetics and systemic effects of inhaled fluticasone propionate in patients with asthma and healthy volunteers: A randomised crossover study." *Lancet 356*: 556–561.
30. Schall, R., Luus, H. G. 1993. "On population and individual bioequivalence." *Stat. Med. 12*: 1109–1124.
31. Hauck, W. W., Hyslop T., Chen, M. L., Patnaik, R., Williams, R. L. 2000. "Subject-by-formulation interaction in bioequivalence: Conceptual and statistical issues." *FDA Population/Individual Bioequivalence Working Group. Food and Drug Administration. Pharmaceutical Research 17* (4): 375–380.
32. Yu, L. X. and Li, B. V. Eds. *FDA Bioequivalence Standards*. Springer. New York. 2014.
33. Guidance for Industry: *Statistical Approaches to Establishing Bioequivalence*. U.S. Department of Health and Human Services, Food and Drug Administration, Center for Drug Evaluation and Research, Silver Spring, MD, January 2001.
34. Allen, A, Bal, J., Moore, A., Stone, S., Tombs, L. 2014. "Bioequivalence and dose proportionality of inhaled fluticasone furoate." *Journal of Bioequivalence & Bioavailability 6* (1): 24–32.
35. Fisher, D., Kramer, W., Burmeister Getz, E. 2016. "Evaluation of a scenario in which estimates of bioequivalence are biased and a proposed solution: Tlast (Common)." *The Journal of Clinical Pharmacology 56* (7): 794–800.
36. Endrenyi, L., Fritsch, S., Yan, W. 1991. "Cmax/AUC is a clearer measure than Cmax for absorption rates in investigations of bioequivalence." *International journal of clinical pharmacology, therapy, and toxicology 29* (10): 394–399.
37. Endrenyi, L., Yan, W. 1993. "Variation of Cmax and Cmax/AUC in investigations of bioequivalence." *International journal of clinical pharmacology, therapy, and toxicology 31* (4): 184–189.
38. Tothfalusi, L., Endrenyi, L. 1995. "Without extrapolation, Cmax/AUC is an effective metric in investigations of bioequivalence." *Pharmaceutical Research 12* (6): 937–942.
39. Tozer, T. N., Bois, F. Y., Hauck, W. W., Chen, M. L., Williams, R. L. 1996. "Absorption rate Vs. exposure: Which is more useful for bioequivalence testing?" *Pharmaceutical Research 13* (3): 453–456.
40. Chen, M. L., Lesko, L., Williams, R. L. 2001. "Measures of exposure versus measures of rate and extent of absorption." *Clinical Pharmacokinetics 40* (8): 565–572.
41. NDA 21-077, submitted Mar 24, 1999, GlaxoSmithKline, https://www.accessdata.fda.gov/drugsatfda_docs/nda/2000/21077_AdvairDiskus.cfm, NDA 021929, submitted September 23, 2005, AstraZeneca, https://www.accessdata.fda.gov/drugsatfda_docs/nda/2006/021929_symbicort_toc.cfm.
42. Draft Guidance on Mometasone Furoate. *U.S. Department of Health and Human Services, Food and Drug Administration*, October 2017.
43. Draft Guidance on Tiotropium Bromide. *U.S. Department of Health and Human Services, Food and Drug Administration*, October 2017.
44. Draft Guidance on Fluticasone Propionate. *U.S. Department of Health and Human Services, Food and Drug Administration*, October 2017.

45. Draft Guidance on Indacaterol Maleate. *U.S. Department of Health and Human Services, Food and Drug Administration*, April 2016.
46. Draft Guidance on Budesonide, *Formoterol fumarate dihydrate. U.S. Department of Health and Human Services, Food and Drug Administration*, June 2015.
47. Daley-Yates, P. T., Parkins, D. A., Thomas, M. J., Gillett, B., House, K. W., Ortega, H. G. 2009. "Pharmacokinetic, pharmacodynamic, efficacy, and safety data from two randomized, double-blind studies in patients with asthma and an in vitro study comparing two dry-powder inhalers delivering a combination of salmeterol 50 μg and fluticasone propionate 250 μg: Implications for establishing bioequivalence of inhaled products." *Clinical Therapeutics 31* (2): 370–385.
48. Maffia, A. 2016. *Sandoz Citizen Petition*. Docket ID FDA–P: 1–20.
49. Kunka, R., Andrews, S., Pimazzoni, M., Callejas, S., Ziviani, L., Squassante, L., Daley-Yates, P. T. 2000. "Dose proportionality of fluticasone propionate from hydrofluoroalkane pressurized metered dose inhalers (pMDIs) and comparability with chlorofluorocarbon pMDIs." *Respiratory Medicine 94* (Suppl B): S10–S16.
50. Bhagwat, S., Schilling, U., Chen, M. J., Wei, X., Delvadia, R., Absar, M., Saluja, B., Hochhaus, G. 2017. "Predicting pulmonary pharmacokinetics from In vitro properties of dry powder inhalers." *Pharmaceutical Research., 34* (12): 2541–2556. doi:10.1007/s11095-017-2235-y.
51. Ziffels, S., Bemelmans, N. L., Durham, P. G., Hickey, A. J. 2015 "In vitro dry powder inhaler formulation performance considerations." *Journal Controlled Release* 199: 45–52.
52. Lähelmä, S., Sairanen, U., Haikarainen, J., Korhonen, J., Vahteristo, M., Fuhr, R., Kirjavainen, M. 2015. "Equivalent lung dose and systemic exposure of budesonide/formoterol combination via easyhaler and turbuhaler." *Journal of Aerosol Medicine and Pulmonary Drug Delivery 28*(6): 462–473.
53. Background Information for Advisory Committee for Pharmaceutical Science: Concept and Criteria of BioINequivalence. October 20, 2004, https://www.fda.gov/ohrms/dockets/ac/04/briefing/2004-4078B1_06_BioINequivalence.pdf, accessed 25 Mar 2018.
54. Burmeister Getz, E., Carroll, K. J., Jones, B., Benet, L. Z. 2016. "Batch-to-batch pharmacokinetic variability confounds current bioequivalence regulations: A dry powder inhaler randomized clinical trial." *Clinical Pharmacology & Therapeutics 100* (3): 223–231.
55. Burmeister Getz, E., Carroll, K. J., Mielke, J., Benet, L. Z., Jones, B. 2017. "Between-batch pharmacokinetic variability inflates type I error rate in conventional bioequivalence trials: A randomized Advair Diskus clinical trial." *Clinical Pharmacology & Therapeutics 101* (3): 331–340.
56. Background Information for the Pharmaceutical Science Advisory Committee meeting on locally-acting gastrointestinal drugs in October 2004.
57. Weber, B., and Hochhaus, G. 2013. "A pharmacokinetic simulation tool for inhaled corticosteroids." *The AAPS Journal* 15 (1): 159–171. doi:10.1208/s12248-012-9420-z.
58. Martin, A. R., and Finlay, W. H. 2017. "Model calculations of regional deposition and disposition for single doses of inhaled liposomal and dry powder ciprofloxacin." *Journal of Aerosol Medicine and Pulmonary Drug Delivery* 30. doi:10.1089/jamp.2017.1377.
59. Lanz, M. J., Eisenlohr, C., Llabre, M. M., Toledo, Y., Lanz, M. A. 2001. "The effect of low-dose inhaled fluticasone propionate on exhaled nitric oxide in asthmatic patients and comparison with oral zafirlukast." *Ann Allergy Asthma Immunol. 87* (4): 283–288.
60. Silkoff, P. E., Wakita, S., Chatkin, J., Ansarin, K., Gutierrez, C., Caramori, M., McClean, P., Slutsky, A. S., Zamel, N., Chapman, K. R. 1999. "Exhaled nitric oxide after beta2-Agonist inhalation and spirometry in asthma." *American Journal of Respiratory and Critical Care Medicine 159* (3): 940–944.
61. Silkoff, P. E., McClean, P., Spino, M., Erlich, L., Slutsky, A. S., Zamel, N. 2001. "Dose-response relationship and reproducibility of the fall in exhaled nitric oxide after inhaled beclomethasone dipropionate therapy in asthma patients." *Chest 119* (5): 1322–1328.
62. Anderson, W. J., Short, P. M., Williamson, P. A., Lipworth, B. J. 2012. "Inhaled corticosteroid dose response using domiciliary exhaled nitric oxide in persistent asthma—The fenotype trial." *Chest 142*: 1553–1561.
63. Weiler, J. M., Sorkness, C. A., Hendeles, L., Nichols, S., Zhu, Y. 2017. "Randomized, double-blind, crossover, clinical-end-point pilot study to examine the use of exhaled nitric oxide as a bioassay for dose separation of inhaled fluticasone propionate." *The Journal of Clinical Pharmacology*. doi:10.1002/jcph.1043.

64. Jatakanon, A., Kharitonov, S., Lim, S., Barnes, P. J. 1999. "Effect of differing doses of inhaled budesonide on markers of airway inflammations in patients with mild asthma. *Thorax* 54: 108–114.
65. Jones, S. L., Herbison, P., Cowan, J. O., Flannery, E. M., Hancox, R. J., McLachlan, C. R., Taylor, D. R. 2002. "Exhaled NO and assessment of anti-inflammatory effects of inhaled steroid: Dose-response relationship" *European Respiratory Journal* 20: 601–608.
66. Draft Guidance on Orlistat. U.S. Department of Health and Human Services, Food and Drug Administration, August 2010.
67. CFR Title 21 Part 320.24.
68. Comparative Analyses and Related Comparative Use Human Factors Studies for a Drug-Device Combination Product Submitted in an *ANDA: Draft Guidance for Industry*. U.S. Department of Health and Human Services, Food and Drug Administration, Center for Drug Evaluation and Research, Silver Spring, MD, January 2017.
69. Guidance for Industry: *Metered Dose Inhaler (MDI) and Dry Powder Inhaler (DPI) Drug Products*. U.S. Department of Health and Human Services, Food and Drug Administration, Center for Drug Evaluation and Research, Silver Spring, MD, October 1998.
70. CDER/FDA. 2015. "Guidance for industry, waiver of in vivo bioavailability and bioequivalence studies for immediate release solid oral dosage forms based on a biopharmaceutics classification system." *Center for Drug Evaluation and Research*, May: 1–2.
71. EMEA Guideline on the Investigation of Bioequivalence, 2010.
72. Adams, W. P., Ahrens, R. C., Chen, M. L., Christopher, D., Chowdhury, B. A., Conner, D. P., Dalby, R. et al. 2010. "Demonstrating bioequivalence of locally acting orally inhaled drug products (OIPs): Workshop summary report." *Journal of Aerosol Medicine and Pulmonary Drug Delivery* 23 (1): 1–29.
73. Bäckman, P., Arora, S., Couet, W., Forbes, B., de Kruijf, W., Paudel, A. 2017. "Advances in experimental and mechanistic computational models to understand pulmonary exposure to inhaled drugs." *European Journal of Pharmaceutical Sciences 113*: 41–52. doi:10.1016/j.ejps.2017.10.030.
74. Dunbar, C. A., Hickey, A. J., Holzner, P. 1998. "Dispersion and characterization of pharmaceutical dry powder aerosols." *Kona Powder and Particle Journal* 16 (16): 7–45. doi:10.14356/kona.1998007.
75. Amidon, G. L., Lennernäs, H., Shah, V. P., Crison, J. P. 1995. "A theoretical basis for a biopharmaceutical drug classification: The correlation of in vitro drug product dissolution and in vivo bioavailability." *Pharmaceutical Research* 12 (3): 413–420.
76. Selby, M. D., de Koning, P. D., Roberts, D. F. 2011. "A perspective on synthetic and solid-form enablement of inhalation candidates." *Future Medicinal Chemistry* 3 (13): 1679–1701. doi:10.4155/fmc.11.125.
77. Ritchie, T. J., Luscombe, C. N. and Macdonald, S. J. 2009. "Analysis of the calculated physicochemical properties of respiratory drugs: Can we design for inhaled drugs yet?" *Journal of Chemical Information and Modeling* 49 (4): 1025–1032. doi:10.1021/ci800429e.
78. Rennard, S. I., Basset, G., Lecossier, D., O'Donnell, K. M., Pinkston, P., Martin, P. G. and Crystal, R. G. 1986. "Estimation of volume of epithelial lining fluid recovered by lavage using urea as marker of dilution." *Journal of Applied Physiology* 60 (2): 532–538.
79. Das, S. C., and Stewart, P. J. 2016. "The influence of lung surfactant liquid crystalline nanostructures on respiratory drug delivery." *International Journal of Pharmaceutics* 514 (2): 465–474. doi:10.1016/j.ijpharm.2016.06.029.
80. Helander, H. F., and Fändriks, L. 2014. "Surface area of the digestive tract—Revisited." *Scandinavian Journal of Gastroenterology* 49 (6): 681–689. doi:10.3109/00365521.2014.898326.
81. Yeadon, M. 2011. "The paradox of respiratory R&D, and why 'inhaled-by-design' heralds a new dawn in asthma and chronic obstructive pulmonary disease treatments." *Future Medicinal Chemistry* 3 (13): 1581–1583. doi:10.4155/fmc.11.97.
82. Edwards, C. D., Luscombe, C., Eddershaw, P., Hessel, E. M. 2016. "Development of a novel quantitative structure-activity relationship model to accurately predict pulmonary absorption and replace routine use of the isolated perfused respiring rat lung model." *Pharmaceutical Research* 33 (11) 2604–2616. doi:10.1007/s11095-016-1983-4.
83. Lipinski, C. A., Lombardo, F., Dominy, B. W., Feeney, P. J. 1997. "Experimental and computational approaches to estimate solubility and permeability in drug discovery and development settings." *Advanced Drug Delivery Reviews* 23 (March): 3–25. http://www.ncbi.nlm.nih.gov/pubmed/11259830.

84. Clark, A. R. 2012. "Understanding penetration index measurements and regional lung targeting." *Journal of Aerosol Medicine and Pulmonary Drug Delivery.* 25 (4): 179–187. doi:10.1089/jamp.2011.0899.
85. Newman, S. P., Wilding, I. R., Hirst, P. H. 2000. "Human lung deposition data: The bridge between in vitro and clinical evaluations for inhaled drug products?" *International Journal of Pharmaceutics* 208 (1–2): 49–60. http://www.ncbi.nlm.nih.gov/pubmed/11064211.
86. Finlay, W. H., Lange, C. F., King, M., Speert, D. P. 2000. "Lung delivery of aerosolized dextran." *American Journal of Respiratory and Critical Care Medicine* 161 (1): 91–97. doi:10.1164/ajrccm.161.1.9812094.
87. Olsson, B., Borgström, L., Lundbäck, H., Svensson. M. 2013. "Validation of a general in vitro approach for prediction of total lung deposition in healthy adults for pharmaceutical inhalation products." *Journal of Aerosol Medicine and Pulmonary Drug Delivery* 26 (6): 355–369. doi:10.1089/jamp.2012.0986.
88. Son, Y. J., Horng, M., Copley, M., Mcconville, J. T. 2010. "Optimization of an in vitro dissolution test method for inhalation formulations." *Dissolution Technologies* 17 (2): 6–13.
89. Rohrschneider, M., Bhagwat, S., Krampe, R., Michler, V., Breitkreutz, J., Hochhaus, G. 2015. "Evaluation of the transwell system for characterization of dissolution behavior of inhalation drugs: Effects of membrane and surfactant." *Molecular Pharmaceutics* 12 (8): 2618–2624. doi:10.1021/acs.molpharmaceut.5b00221.
90. Arora, D., Shah, K. A., Halquist, M. S., Sakagami, M. 2010. "In vitro aqueous fluid-capacity-limited dissolution testing of respirable aerosol drug particles generated from inhaler products." *Pharmaceutical Research* 27 (5): 786–795. doi:10.1007/s11095-010-0070-5.
91. Son, Y. J. and Mcconville, J. T. 2012. "A prospective dissolution test design: Controlling the important variables." *Respiratory Drug Delivery* 177–184.
92. Bicer, E. M., Kumar, A., Somers, G., Hassall, D., Blomberg, A., Behndig, A., Mudway, I., Forbes, B. 2014. "Towards biorelevant dissolution media to model human respiratory tract lining fluid," 465–468.
93. Kumar, A., Terakosolphan, W., Hassoun, M., Vandera, K. K., Novicky, A., Harvey, R., Royall, P. G. et al. 2017. "A biocompatible synthetic lung fluid based on human respiratory tract lining fluid composition." *Pharmaceutical Research.* 34 (12): 2454–2465. doi:10.1007/s11095-017-2169-4.
94. Weers, J. G. 2015. From particle dissolution in the lung slides presented during scope and relevance of a pulmonary biopharmaceutical classification system AAPS/FDA/USP Workshop March 16–17, Baltimore, MD.
95. Edsbäcker, S., Wollmer, P., Selroos, O., Borgström, L., Olsson, B., Ingelf, J. 2008. "Do airway clearance mechanisms influence the local and systemic effects of inhaled corticosteroids?" *Pulmonary Pharmacology & Therapeutics* 21: 247–258. doi:10.1016/j.pupt.2007.08.005.
96. Georgitis, J. W. 1999. "The 1997 asthma management guidelines and therapeutic issues relating to the treatment of asthma. National heart, lung, and blood institute." *Chest* 115 (2): 210–217.
97. Högger, P. 2014. "Optimizing ICS suspensions for nasal use: The influence of solubility, stability, spray volume, dose, Log P, and receptor binding." *RDD 2014:* 75–88.
98. Esmailpour, N., Högger, P., Rabe, K. F., Heitmann, U., Nakashima, M., Rohdewald, P. 1997. "Distribution of inhaled fluticasone propionate between human lung tissue and serum in vivo." *The European Respiratory Journal: Official Journal of the European Society for Clinical Respiratory Physiology* 10: 1496–1499. doi:10.1183/09031936.97.10071496.
99. Noyes, A. S. and Whitney, W. R. 1897. "The rate of solution of solid substances in their own solutions." *Journal of the American Chemical Society* 19: 930–934.
100. Chandrasekaran, S. K. and Paul, D. R. 1982. "Dissolution-controlled transport from dispersed matrixes." *Journal of Pharmaceutical Sciences* 71 (12): 1399–1402. doi:10.1002/jps.2600711222.
101. Tronde, A., Nordén, B. O., Jeppsson, A. B., Brunmark, P., Nilsson, E., Lennernäs, H. and Bengtsson, U. H. 2003. "Drug absorption from the isolated perfused rat lung—Correlations with drug physicochemical properties and epithelial permeability." *Journal of Drug Targeting* 11 (1): 61–74. doi:10.1080/1061186031000086117.
102. Ehrhardt, C., Bäckman, P., Couet, W., Edwards, C., Forbes, B., Fridén, M., Gumbleton, M. et al. 2017. "Current progress toward a better understanding of drug disposition within the lungs: Summary proceedings of the 1st workshop on drug transporters in the lungs." *Journal of Pharmaceutical Sciences* 106 (9): 2234–2244. doi:10.1016/j.xphs.2017.04.011.
103. Dolovich, *IPAC/UF Inhalation Conference, March 2014 "Best Practices Bioequivalence Testing for pMDIs with Spacer/VHC"*) https://ipacrs.org/assets/uploads/outputs/14-Day_2_OIC_2014_Dolovich.pdf.

104. Darquenne, C., Fleming, J. S., Katz, I., Martin, A. R., Schroeter, J., Usmani, O. S. et al. 2016. "Bridging the gap between science and clinical efficacy: Physiology, imaging, and modeling of aerosols in the lung. *Journal of Aerosol Medicine and Pulmonary Drug Delivery* 29(2): 107–126.
105. Byron, P. R., Hindle, M., Lange, C. F., Longest, P. W., McRobbie, D., Oldham, M. J. et al. 2010 "In vivo-in vitro correlations: Predicting pulmonary drug deposition from pharmaceutical aerosols. *Journal of Aerosol Medicine and Pulmonary Drug Delivery* 23(2): S59–S69.
106. Eriksson, J., Sjögren, E., Thörn, H., Rubin, K., Bäckman, P. and Lennernäs, H. 2018. "Pulmonary absorption—Estimation of effective pulmonary permeability and tissue retention of ten drugs using an ex vivo rat model and computational analysis." *European Journal of Pharmaceutics and Biopharmaceutics* 124: 1–12. doi:10.1016/j.ejpb.2017.11.013.
107. Yu, J. Yu, and Rosania, G. R. 2010. "Cell-based multiscale computational modeling of small molecule absorption and retention in the lungs." *Pharmaceutical Research* 27 (3): 457–467. doi:10.1007/s11095-009-0034-9.
108. Bäckman, P., and Olsson, B. O. 2017. "Predicting exposure after oral inhalation of the selective glucocorticoid receptor modulator AZD5423 based on dose, deposition pattern and mechanistic modeling of pulmonary disposition." *Journal of Aerosol Medicine and Pulmonary Drug Delivery* 29 (0): 1–10. doi:10.1089/jamp.2016.1306.

32

General Conclusions

Anthony J. Hickey and Sandro R.P. da Rocha

The demand for thoroughly documented, accurate, and reproducible performance of inhaled aerosols has driven a revolution in inhalation drug product design. The overall principle of maintaining high quality products that can be used by well-trained patients or in clinical settings with the support of auxiliary systems to enhance adherence is intended to assure the desired therapeutic outcome while minimizing adverse events.

Control begins with the manufacture of the active pharmaceutical ingredient and formulation where critical physico-chemical properties are monitored and controlled. The formulation is then evaluated for metering system and device compatibility and performance in generating a therapeutic aerosol. Each category of device requires different considerations because of the nature of the drug, the medium in which it is dispersed, and the aerosol generation mechanism.

Therapeutic aerosols are unique in that with one exception, nebulizers, they do not exist in kinetic equilibrium. The aerodynamic properties of the aerosol and their lung deposition are dictated by the temporal and spacial sampling method/inhalation.

Pressurized metered dose disperse aerosols under the propulsive force of a propellant that is rapidly evaporating and expanding, result in the production of high velocity droplets whose size decreases with the developing plume. There is not enough time for the aerosol droplets to reach their equilibrium state before they are inhaled, and the nature of the aerosol depends on direct inhalation, possibly the use of spacers, all coordinated with the inspiratory flow cycle.

Dry powder inhalers most frequently use the inspiratory flow of the patient to disperse the aerosol. The extent of dispersion may depend on the formulation, pressure-drop, and flow rate generated by the patient in response to the resistance of the device.

In contrast, nebulizers generate an aerosol under controlled conditions for a defined period and the patient passively inhales the aerosol. In this case, the co-ordination and inspiratory flow rate have less impact on the efficiency of aerosol delivery, but the condition of the aerosol between inspiratory cycles may result in loss of aerosol and overall inefficiency of the approach. This does vary depending on the device and control systems employed.

Soft mist inhalers are aqueous-based metered dose systems that combine the facility of formulation associated with nebulizers with the capacity to accurately meter small doses of liquid aerosols in appropriate sizes as usually associated with pressurized metered dose inhalers. These devices have the obvious advantages of efficient delivery of therapeutic doses from a hand-held, discreet, and convenient device without the environmental impact associated with propellant based systems.

It is important to remember the patient-related factors involved in effective inhaled drug delivery as these are overlaid on the product performance. It is essential to control the components, manufacturing processes, and analytical methods sufficiently to ensure the quality of the product since the sources of biological variability will be amplified by deviation in the accuracy and reproducibility of drug delivery.

Throughout this volume, monitoring and control of quality has been emphasized. It is only through adequate measures to define the product that its performance can be assured. The importance of this strategy cannot be understated in the context of bioequivalence considerations comparing generic and innovator products.

Assuring the performance of any product will facilitate its integration with emerging personalized medicine tools that aid in patient use. It is likely that as electronic and mechanical feedback devices are developed with the capacity to link to data storage systems that patients and their physicians will enjoy a level of control over symptoms and underlying causes of disease that will significantly reduce the impact of disease and the cost of care.

A revolution in inhaled drug therapy can be envisaged as pharmaceutical inhalation science and technology converges with electronic monitoring and the information age. We are on the brink of a disruptive shift in product development, government regulation, and personalized medicine including gene therapy and nanomedicine that will bring greater symptom relief and improved treatment platforms for pulmonary and systemic diseases through the delivery of pharmaceutical aerosols.

Index

Note: Page numbers in italic and bold refer to figures and tables, respectively.

Printed in the United States
by Baker & Taylor Publisher Services